Rickham's Neonatal Surgery

Paul D. Losty • Alan W. Flake
Risto J. Rintala • John M. Hutson
Naomi Iwai
Editors

Rickham's Neonatal Surgery

Volume II

Springer

Editors
Paul D. Losty
Division of Child Health
Alder Hey Children's NHS
Foundation Trust
Liverpool
United Kingdom

Risto J. Rintala
Childrens Hospital
University of Helsinki
Helsinki
Finland

Naomi Iwai
Department of Surgery
Meiji University of Integrative Medicine
Kyoto
Japan

Alan W. Flake
University of Pennsylvania
Philadelphia
Pennsylvania
USA

John M. Hutson
Royal Children's Hospital
University of Melbourne
Parkville
Victoria
Australia

ISBN 978-1-4471-4720-6 ISBN 978-1-4471-4721-3 (eBook)
https://doi.org/10.1007/978-1-4471-4721-3

Library of Congress Control Number: 2017964011

Printed on acid-free paper

This Springer imprint is published by the registered company Springer-Verlag London Ltd. part of Springer Nature
The registered company address is: The Campus, 4 Crinan Street, London, N1 9XW, United Kingdom

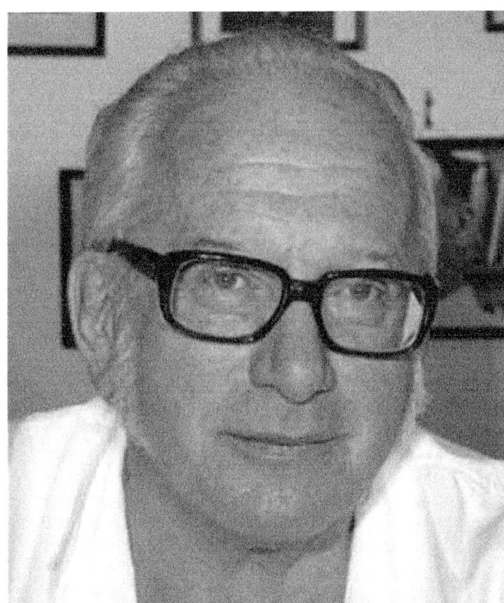

Peter Paul Rickham (1917–2003)

This textbook is dedicated to Peter Paul Rickham, pioneering surgeon, who co-founded the world's First neonatal surgical unit at Alder Hey Children's Hospital Liverpool, United Kingdom.

Foreword

Peter Paul Rickham graduated in medicine from Queens' College, Cambridge, and St Bartholomew's Hospital, London, in 1941. He trained in paediatric surgery at the Hospital for Sick Children, Great Ormond Street, London, under Sir Denis Browne and under Isabella Forshall at Alder Hey Children's Hospital, Liverpool, where he was appointed consultant paediatric surgeon in 1953.

At Alder Hey, Rickham established the hospital as a regional centre for neonatal surgery, he instituted a neonatal transport system for the safe transfer of surgical neonates from a wide area around Liverpool to Alder Hey and he inaugurated the world's first neonatal surgical intensive care unit which was the prototype emulated at centres throughout the world. As a result of the developments, neonatal surgical mortality decreased from 78% to 26% over a period of only 3 years. The subject of his MD thesis was "The Metabolic Response of the Newborn to Surgery".

Rickham remained in Liverpool until 1971 when he was then appointed Professor of Paediatric Surgery at the University Children's Hospital, Zurich, Switzerland, where he remained until retirement in 1983. At Alder Hey he trained numerous surgeons throughout the world particularly from the United States, Japan, Europe, Asia and South Africa.

He was the recipient of many awards and distinctions including the Denis Browne Gold Medal of the British Association of Paediatric Surgeons of which he was founder member and later President, the Legion d'Honneur, France, the Commander Cross, Germany, Ladd Medal Surgical Section of the American Academy of Pediatrics and two Hunterian Professorships from the Royal College of Surgeons of England.

The first edition of *Neonatal Surgery* co-edited with J. Herbert Johnston was published in 1969. It was the first textbook devoted entirely to neonatal surgery based on the accumulating experience of newborn surgery carried out at Alder Hey Children's Hospital from 1953 to 1968. It was, in its time, the "bible" of neonatal surgery and I read it from cover to cover before, during and after my time as a Smith and Nephew Fellow studying under Peter Paul Rickham in 1970. Two subsequent editions of *Neonatal Surgery* were later published in 1978 and 1990. The scope of these publications was expanded, and new contributions from a range of experts of international repute were included.

It is pleasing now to witness a major new international textbook launched from Alder Hey titled *Rickham's Neonatal Surgery* edited by Paul Losty

(Liverpool, UK), Alan Flake (Philadelphia, USA), Risto Rintala (Helsinki, Finland), Naomi Iwai (Kyoto, Japan) and John Hutson (Melbourne, Australia). This new textbook has a truly international list of distinguished contributors covering the full range of neonatal surgical conditions and related topics. Among many key themes comprehensively included in the new book attention also focuses on advances in fetal surgery, minimal invasive surgery, long-term outcomes and evidence-based surgery.

The textbook is a fitting tribute to the life and work of Peter Paul Rickham who was my mentor and good friend.

London, UK Lewis Spitz

Editors' Preface: Rickham's Neonatal Surgery

In 1969, Peter Paul Rickham and Herbert Johnston published the first edition of Neonatal Surgery from Alder Hey Children's Hospital Liverpool which for many paediatric surgeons was considered to be one of the leading textbooks in the world dedicated to newborn surgery. The huge success of the first edition was followed with further editions of this landmark textbook published in 1978 and 1990. Peter Paul Rickham is credited with establishment of the world's first neonatal surgical unit at Alder Hey in 1953 co-founded together with Isabella Forshall. Indeed, it is perhaps then no great surprise that several generations of young paediatric surgeons travelled to Liverpool to work with Rickham and the team of surgical staff based at Alder Hey. Peter Rickham was fortunate to also have Jackson Rees a pioneer in neonatal anaesthesia as a consultant colleague during that era. The "impossible became possible". Many young surgeons who visited Alder Hey later advanced to become world leaders in paediatric surgery across four continents.

This new textbook "Rickham's Neonatal Surgery" is dedicated to Peter Paul Rickham including past and present staff at Alder Hey. The team of editors have assembled leading experts with co-authors to provide state-of-the-art chapters covering the speciality field of neonatal surgery and its related disciplines including fetal medicine, fetal surgery, radiology, newborn anaesthesia, intensive care, neonatal medicine, medical genetics, pathology, cardiac surgery and urology. Contributions from the basic sciences and laboratory research are highlighted in the textbook reflecting steady progress in our current working knowledge and understanding of many neonatal surgical disorders. Evidence-based studies and "best practice" provide the reader wide-ranging information including the latest developments in many chapters. As huge advances have been made in neonatal surgery with improved survival particularly in the past decade(s), ethical issues, long-term outcomes and quality of life are also emphasised by the individual contributors. We hope the textbook will be an authoritative reference for surgical residents in training, consultant surgeons, general surgeons with an interest in paediatric surgery, neonatologists, paediatricians, intensive care specialists and nursing staff. The editors are greatly indebted to the many authors from across the world for their excellent contributions and for some their lifelong professional associations having trained or worked as surgeons at Alder Hey.

Special thanks must go to Barbara Lopez Lucio who worked tirelessly with all authors, editor-in-chief and editorial team to make the project possible. We greatly value and appreciate the skills of the artist(s) and illustrators for their high-quality work. Finally, enormous gratitude is owed to Julia Megginson, Wyndham Hacket Pain and Melissa Morton at Springer, London, UK, for the final production of the textbook.

Liverpool, UK	Paul D. Losty
Philadelphia, PA, USA	Alan W. Flake
Helsinki, Finland	Risto J. Rintala
Melbourne, VIC, Australia	John M. Hutson
Kyoto, Japan	Naomi Iwai

Contents

Volume I

Part I General

Volume II

Part IV Gastrointestinal System

Part V Liver, Biliary Tract, Pancreas

Part VI Abdominal Wall Defects

Part VII Nervous System

Part VIII Oncology

Part IX Urology

Part X Outcomes in Newborn Surgery

Contributors

Laurence Abernethy, MD, FRCR Department of Radiology, Alder Hey Children's Hospital, Liverpool, UK

N. Scott Adzick, MD, FACS Department of Pediatric Surgery, University of Pennsylvania Perelman School of Medicine, Children's Hospital of Philadelphia, Philadelphia, PA, USA

Michael Ashworth, MB, BCh, FRC(Path) Camelia Botnar Laboratories, Great Ormond Street Hospital for Children NHS Foundation Trust, London, UK

Pietro Bagolan, MD Department of Medical and Surgical Neonatology, Bambino Gesù Children's Hospital, Rome, Italy

Colin T. Baillie, MB, ChB, DCH, MCh, FRCS(Paed) Department of Paediatric Surgery, Alder Hey Children's Hospital NHS Foundation Trust, Liverpool, UK

Chris Barton, MB, ChB, BSc(Hons), MRCPCH Department of Oncology, Alder Hey Children's Hospital, Liverpool, Merseyside, UK

Spencer W. Beasley, MB, ChB(Otago), MS(Melbourne) Department of Paediatric Surgery, Christchurch School of Medicine, University of Otago, Christchurch, New Zealand

Leanne Bricker, MB, BCh, MRCOG Corniche Hospital, Abu Dhabi, United Arab Emirates

James Bruce, MB, ChB, FRCS(Ed), FRACS Department of Paediatric Surgery, Central Manchester Children's Hospital, Manchester, UK

Steven W. Bruch, MD, MSc Department of Surgery, Section of Pediatric Surgery, C.S. Mott Children's Hospital, University of Michigan, Ann Arbor, MI, USA

Shijie Cai, MD, PhD, MPhil Radcliffe Department of Medicine, University of Oxford, Oxford, UK

Carmen Capito, MD Department of Pediatric Surgery, AP-HP, Université Paris Descartes, Hôpital Necker Enfants-Malades, Paris, France

Robert Carachi, MBE, MD, PhD, FRCS(Gla) Department of Surgical Paediatrics, University of Glasgow, School of Medicine, Glasgow, UK

Luc De Catte, MD, PhD Department of Obstetrics and Gynecology, University Hospitals Leuven—Campus Gasthuisberg, Leuven, Belgium

Joel Cazares, MD Department of Pediatric General and Urogenital Surgery, Juntendo University School of Medicine, Tokyo, Japan

Emily R. Christison-Lagay, MD Department of Surgery, Yale School of Medicine, New Haven, CT, USA

Andrea Conforti, MD Department of Medical and Surgical Neonatology, Bambino Gesù Children's Hospital, Rome, Italy

Arnold G. Coran, MD Department of Surgery, Section of Pediatric Surgery, C.S. Mott Children's Hospital, University of Michigan, Ann Arbor, MI, USA

Paolo De Coppi, MD, PhD Surgery Unit, Institute of Child Health, London, UK

Martin T. Corbally, MB, BCh, BAO, MCh, FRCS(Ed) Department of Surgery, RCSI Medical University, King Hamad University Hospital, Al Sayh, Bahrain

Harriet J. Corbett, MD, FRCS(Paed) Regional Department of Paediatric Urology, Alder Hey Children's Hospital NHS Foundation Trust, Liverpool, UK

David C.G. Crabbe, MD, FRCS Department of Paediatric Surgery, Leeds General Infirmary, Leeds, UK

Paul Cullis, BSc(Hons), MB, ChB(Hons), MRCS University of Glasgow, Glasgow, Scotland, UK

Royal Hospital for Children, Glasgow, Scotland, UK

Mark Davenport, ChM, FRCS(Eng), FRCPS(Glas) Department of Paediatric Surgery, Kings College Hospital, London, UK

Jan Deprest, MD, PhD, FRCOG University Hospital Leuven, Leuven, Belgium

Roland Devlieger, MD, PhD Department of Obstetrics and Gynecology, University Hospitals Leuven—Campus Gasthuisberg, Leuven, Belgium

Stephen C. Donnell, MB, ChB, FRCS(Paed) Department of Paediatric Surgery, University Hospital of the North Midlands and Alder Hey Children's Hospital, Liverpool, UK

Harikrishna Doshi, MBBS, MS, FRCS(CTh) Department of Heart and Lung Transplantation, Papworth Hospital, Papworth, UK

Christopher P. Driver, MB, ChB, FRCS(Paed) Department of Surgical Paediatrics, Royal Aberdeen Children's Hospital, Aberdeen, UK

Simon Eaton, PhD Department of Paediatric Surgery, UCL Institute of Child Health and Great Ormond Street Children's Hospital, London, UK

Ian Ellis, BSc, MBBS, FRCP Department of Clinical Genetics, Liverpool Women's Hospital, Liverpool, UK

Dario O. Fauza, MD, PhD Department of Surgery, Boston Children's Hospital and Harvard Medical School, Boston, MA, USA

R. Dawn Fevurly, MD Department of Surgery, Children's Hospital Boston, Boston, MA, USA

Steven J. Fishman, MD Department of Surgery, Vascular Anomalies Center, Children's Hospital Boston, Boston, MA, USA

Florian Friedmacher, MD, MSc National Children's Research Centre, Our Lady's Children's Hospital, Dublin, Ireland

Jörg Fuchs, MD Department of Pediatric Surgery and Urology, University of Tuebingen, Tuebingen, Germany

John P. Gearhart, MD, FACS, FRCS(Hon) (Ed) Pediatric Urology, Johns Hopkins Hospital, James Brady Urological Institute, Baltimore, MD, USA

Anju Goyal, MCh, FRCS(Paed) Royal Manchester Children's Hospital, Manchester, UK

Graham Haddock, MBChB, MD, FRCS(Paed) Royal Hospital for Children, Glasgow, Scotland, UK

Nigel J. Hall, PhD, MRCPCH, FRCS(Paed) Faculty of Medicine, University of Southampton, Southampton, UK

Andrew Healey, BSc, MB, ChB, FRCR Department of Radiology, Alder Hey Children's Hospital, Liverpool, UK

Holly L. Hedrick, MD Perelman School of Medicine at the University of Pennsylvania, Philadelphia, PA, USA

Department of Pediatric General, Thoracic, and Fetal Surgery, Children's Hospital of Philadelphia, Philadelphia, PA, USA

Ryuichiro Hirose, MD, PhD Department of Pediatric Surgery, Graduate School of Medical Sciences, Kyushu University, Fukuoka, Fukuoka, Japan

Ryan Hodges, MD Department of Obstetrics and Gynecology—Maternal Fetal Medicine, Monash Medical Centre, Clayton, VIC, Australia

Joshua N. Honeyman, MD Pediatric Surgery, Department of Surgery, Memorial Sloan-Kettering Cancer Center, New York, NY, USA

Mark A. Hughes, MBChB, BSc(Hons), MRCS, MSc, PhD Department of Clinical Neurosciences, Western General Hospital, Edinburgh, UK

Caroline Ann Jones, MBChB, FRCPCH, MD Department of Paediatric Nephrology, Alder Hey Children's NHS Foundation Trust, Liverpool, UK

Colin Jones, MBBS, FRACP, PhD Department of Nephrology, Royal Children's Hospital, Melbourne, VIC, Australia

Jothy Kandasamy, FRCS(Neuro Surg) Department of Neurosurgery, Royal Hospital for Sick Children, Edinburgh, Lothian, UK

Joshua Kausman, MBBS, FRACP, PhD Department of Nephrology, Royal Children's Hospital, University of Melbourne, Murdoch Children's Research Institute, Melbourne, VIC, Australia

Basem A. Khalil, MPH, PhD, FRCS(Paed) Department of Pediatric Surgery, SIDRA, Doha, Qatar

Edward Kiely, FRCSI, FRCS(Eng), FRCPCH(Hons) Department of Paediatric Surgery, Great Ormond Street Hospital for Children NHS Foundation Trust, London, UK

Peter C. Kim, MD, PhD Department of General and Thoracic Surgery, Sheikh Zayed Institute for Pediatric Surgical Innovation, Children's National Hospital, Washington, DC, USA

Yoshiaki Kinoshita, MD, PhD Department of Pediatric Surgery, Graduate School of Medical Sciences, Kyushu University, Fukuoka, Japan

Dietrich Kluth, MD, PhD Research Laboratories of the Department of Pediatric Surgery, University Hospital, University Leipzig, Leipzig, Saxony, Germany

Antti I. Koivusalo, MD, PhD Department of Pediatric Surgery, Children's Hospital, University of Helsinki, Helsinki, Finland

Pablo Laje, MD Department of Surgery, The Children's Hospital of Philadelphia, Philadelphia, PA, USA

Graham L. Lamont, MBChB, DM, FRCS, FRCS(Paed) Department of Paediatric Surgery, Alder Hey Children's NHS Trust, Liverpool, UK

Michael P. La Quaglia, MD Pediatric Surgery, Department of Surgery, Memorial Sloan-Kettering Cancer Center, New York, NY, USA

Michael W.Y. Leung, MBChB, FRCS(Ed, Paed), FCSHK Division of Paediatric Surgery, Department of Surgery, Queen Elizabeth Hospital, Kowloon, Hong Kong

Marc A. Levitt, MD Center for Colorectal and Pelvic Reconstruction, Nationwide Children's Hospital, The Ohio State University, Columbus, OH, USA

Liesbeth Lewi, MD, PhD Department of Obstetrics and Gynecology, University Hospitals Leuven—Campus Gasthuisberg, Leuven, Belgium

Kelvin K.W. Liu, MBBCh, FRCS(Glas), FRACS, FRCS(Ed) Department of Surgery, United Christian Hospital, Hong Kong, Kowloon, China

Stavros P. Loukogeorgakis, MBBS, BSc, PhD, MRCS Department of Stem Cells and Regenerative Medicine, UCL Great Ormond Street Institute of Child Health, London, UK

Gordon Alexander MacKinlay, OBE, MB, BS, LRCP, FRCS (Ed) Paediatric Surgery, University of Edinburgh, The Royal Hospital for Sick Children, Edinburgh, UK

Conor L. Mallucci, MBBS, FRCS(Surgical Neurology) Department of Neurosurgery, Alder Hey Children's NHS Foundation Trust, Liverpool, UK

Toshiharu Matsuura, MD, PhD Department of Pediatric Surgery, Graduate School of Medical Sciences, Kyushu University, Fukuoka, Japan

Helen Fiona McAndrew, MD, FRCS(Paed) Regional Department of Paediatric Urology, Alder Hey Children's Hospital NHS Foundation Trust, Liverpool, UK

Alastair J.W. Millar, FRCS, FRACS(Paed Surg) Paediatric Surgery, University of Cape Town, Red Cross War Memorial Children's Hospital, Cape Town, South Africa

Roman Metzger, MD, PhD Department of Paediatric and Adolescent Surgery, Uniklinikum Salzburg, Salzburg, Austria

Antonino Morabito, MD, FRCS(Ed), FRCS(Eng), FICS Department of Pediatric Surgery, University of Florence, Florence, Italy

Henry Morgan, MB, ChB, MRCPCH Department of Paediatric Nephrology, Aldery Hey Children's NHS Foundation Trust, Liverpool, UK

Dhanya Mullassery, PhD, FRCS(Paed) Institute of Translational Medicine, Alder Hey Children's Hospital NHS Foundation Trust, University of Liverpool, Liverpool, UK

Alp Numanoglu, MBChB(Turkey), FCS(SA) Department of Paediatric Surgery, Red Cross War Memorial Children's Hospital, University of Cape Town, Cape Town, South Africa

Mike O'Brien, PhD, FRCSI, FRCSI(Paed) Department of Paediatric Urology, Royal Children's Hospital, Melbourne, VIC, Australia

Bruce Okoye, MBBS, MD, FRCS(Paeds) Department of Paediatric Surgery, St. Georges Hospital, London, UK

Shigeru Ono, MD, PhD Department of Pediatric Surgery, Kyoto Prefectural University of Medicine, Kyoto, Japan

Daniel Orbach, MD Department of Pediatric, Adolescent, Young Adult, Institut Curie, Paris, France

Mikko P. Pakarinen, MD, PhD Section of Pediatric and Pediatric Transplantation Surgery, Children's Hospital, University Central Hospital, University of Helsinki, Helsinki, Finland

Stephano R. Parlato, MD Alder Hey Children's NHS Foundation Trust, Liverpool, UK

Emily Partridge, MD, PhD Center for Fetal Research, Children's Hospital of Philadelphia, Philadelphia, PA, USA

Andy Petros, MD, MSc, MA, FRCP Paediatric Intensive Care Unit, London, UK

Benedetta Pettorini, MD Department of Neurosurgery, Alder Hey Children's Hospital, Liverpool, Merseyside, UK

Agostino Pierro, MD, FRCS(Eng), OBE Division of Pediatric Surgery, The Hospital for Sick Children, Toronto, ON, Canada

Barry Pizer, MB, ChB, MRCP, FRCPCH, PhD Department of Oncology, Alder Hey Children's Hospital, Liverpool, Merseyside, UK

Francis A. Potter, MBChB, FRCA, FFICM Jackson Rees Department of Paediatric Anaesthesia, NHS Foundation Trust, Alder Hey Children's Hospital, Liverpool, UK

Prem Puri, MS, FRCS, FRCS(ED), FACS National Children's Research Centre and Consultant Paediatric Surgeon, National Children's Research Centre, Our Lady's Children's Hospital, Dublin, Ireland

Helen L. Rees, FRCPCH Medical Oncology, Bristol Royal Hospital for Children, Bristol, UK

Nicola Reilly, BSc Pharmacy Department of Pharmacy, Alder Hey Children's NHS Foundation Trust, Liverpool, UK

Devender Roberts, MB, ChB, MRCOG Obstetrics and Fetal Medicine, Liverpool Women's Hospital, Liverpool, UK

Timothy N. Rogers, MBBCh, FCS(SA), FRCS(Paed) Department of Paediatric Surgery, Bristol Royal Hospital for Children, Bristol, UK

Richard E. Sarginson, BSc, MB, ChB, FRCA Jackson Rees Department of Paediatric Anaesthesia, Alder Hey Children's NHS Foundation Trust, Liverpool, Merseyside, UK

Sabine Sarnacki, MD, PhD Department of Pediatric Surgery, Hôpital Necker Enfants-Malades, AP-HP, Université Paris Descartes, Paris, France

Emma L. Sidebotham, BSc, MB, ChB, MD, FRCS Department of Paediatric Surgery, Leeds General Infirmary, Leeds, UK

Rona Slator, DPhil, FRCS, FRCS(Plast) Birmingham Children's Hospital, Birmingham, UK

Lewis Spitz, PhD, FRCS(Eng), FRCS(Ed), FRCSI Department of Paediatric Surgery, Great Ormond Street Hospital, London, UK

Andrew A. Stec, MD Department of Urology, The Medical University of South Carolina, Charleston, SC, USA

Charles Stiller, MSc Lead on Childhood Cancer, Public Health England, National Cancer Registration and Analysis Service, Oxford, UK

Charles J.H. Stolar, MD Rudolph N. Schullinger Professor Emeritus of Surgery and Pediatrics, College of Physicians and Surgeons, Columbia University, New York City, NY, USA

California Pediatric Surgical Group, Santa Barbara, CA, USA

Peter P. Stuhldreher, MD Johns Hopkins Hospital, James Buchanan Brady Urological Institute, Baltimore, MD, USA

Nada Sudhakaran, MBBS, MRCS, FRCS(Paeds) Department of Paediatric Surgery, Gold Coast University Hospital, Gold Coast, QLD, Australia

Sanaulla K. Syed, MBBS, DA, FRCA Jackson Rees Department of Paediatric Anaesthesia, Alder Hey Children's NHS Foundation Trust, Liverpool, Merseyside, UK

Tomoaki Taguchi, MD, PhD Department of Pediatric Surgery, Graduate School of Medical Sciences, Kyushu University, Fukuoka, Japan

Mark Tattersall, MA, BM, BCh, MRCOG Obstetrics and Gynaecology, Department of Women's and Children's Health, Liverpool Women's Hospital, University of Liverpool, Liverpool, UK

Nia Taylor, MPhil Institute of Ageing and Chronic Disease, University of Liverpool, Liverpool, UK

Arul S. Thirumoorthi, MD Department of Pediatric Surgery, Columbia University Medical Center, New York, NY, USA

Dick Tibboel, MD, PhD Department of Intensive Care, Erasmus Medical Center, Sophia Children's Hospital, Rotterdam, The Netherlands

Juan A. Tovar, MD, PhD, FEBPS, FAAP(Hon) Department of Pediatric Surgery, Hospital Universitario La Paz, Madrid, Spain

Alexander M. Turner, BSc, MB, ChB, FRCS(Paeds), PhD Department of Paediatric Urology, Leeds Children's Hopsital, Leeds, UK

Christopher G. Turner, MD, MPH Department of Surgery, Boston Children's Hospital, Boston, MA, USA

John N. van den Anker, MD, PhD Erasmus Medical Center, Sophia Children's Hospital, Rotterdam, The Netherlands

Tim Van Mieghem, MD, PhD Department of Obstetrics and Gynecology—Maternal Fetal Medicine, Mount Sinai Hospital, Toronto, ON, Canada

Hendrik K.F. van Saene, MD, PhD, FRCPath Institute of Ageing and Chronic Disease, University of Liverpool, Liverpool, UK

Prem Sundar Venugopal, MS, FRCS(CTh) Lady Cilento Children's Hospital, Queensland Paediatric Cardiac Service, Brisbane, QLD, Australia

Steven W. Warmann, MD Deparment of Pediatric Surgery and Urology, University of Tuebingen, Tuebingen, Germany

Robert Wheeler, FRCS MS LLB(Hons) LLM Department of Clinical Law, Wessex Regional Centre for Paediatric Surgery, University Hospital of Southampton, Southampton, UK

Alexandra L. Williams, MBChB, MRCS(Ed), FRCR Department of Radiology, Alder Hey Children's NHS Foundation Trust, Liverpool, UK

Richard J. Wood, MD Associate Director, Center for Colorectal and Pelvic Reconstruction, Nationwide Children's Hospital, Columbus, OH, USA

Assistant Professor of Surgery, The Ohio State University, Columbus, OH, USA

Atsuyuki Yamataka, MD, PhD FAAP(Hon) Department of Pediatric General & Urogenital Surgery, Juntendo University School of Medicine, Tokyo, Japan

Jawad Yousaf, MBBS, MRCS Department of Neurosurgery, Alder Hey Children's NHS Foundation Trust, Liverpool, UK

Editors

Alan W. Flake, MD, FACS Surgery and Obstetrics & Gynecology, University of Pennsylvania School of Medicine, Philadelphia, PA, USA

Children's Center for Fetal Research, Children's Hospital of Philadelphia, Philadelphia, PA, USA

John M. Hutson, BS, MD(Monash), MD, DSc(Melb) Department of Paediatrics, University of Melbourne, Parkville, VIC, Australia

Department of Urology, Royal Children's Hospital, Parkville, VIC, Australia

Naomi Iwai, MD, PhD Department of Surgery, Meiji University of Integrative Medicine, Kyoto, Japan

Paul D. Losty, MD, FRCS(Paed), FEBPS Department of Paediatric Surgery, Alder Hey Children's Hospital NHS Foundation Trust, Institute of Translational Medicine, University of Liverpool, Liverpool, UK

Risto J. Rintala, MD, PhD Section of Paediatric Surgery, Children´s Hospital, University Central Hospital, University of Helsinki, Helsinki, Finland

Part IV

Gastrointestinal System

Inguinal Hernia

29

Antti I. Koivusalo

Abstract

Inguinal hernia is one of the most common surgical conditions in infancy. Practically all infant hernias are of congenital indirect type. Medical conditions causing increased intra-abdominal pressure and connective tissue weakness predispose to inguinal hernias. Close to 5% of infants undergo hernia repair before the age of 6 months and in every fourth of those infants an emergent repair for incarceration, strangulation or repeated difficult reduction is performed. Thus hernia repair is indicated whenever a diagnosis has been made. Incarcerated or strangulated hernia is a paediatric surgical emergency and requires either manual reduction and subsequent repair or immediate surgery if reduction is not achieved. Elective repair of uncomplicated neonatal inguinal hernia is scheduled not later than 2–4 weeks following the diagnosis. In premature infants complicated hernias are repaired before discharge from NICU. In small infants the risk of apnoea requires appropriate facilities for postoperative monitoring after hernia repair.

Neonatal inguinal hernia is repaired in the standard fashion of division and high ligation of the sac, but for a pediatric surgeon mastery of alternative incisions and laparoscopy is very useful. In a unilateral repair routine exploration of the asymptomatic contralateral groin is not recommended in any infant. Complication rate in the repair neonatal inguinal hernia is 1–5% including recurrence, testicular ascent, testicular atrophy, injury to vas deferens and injury to intestine, ovary, bladder and uterus. Neonatal hernia repair should have 0% mortality rate.

Keywords

Inguinal hernia • Newborn • Newborn surgery • Outcomes

A.I. Koivusalo, MD, PhD
Department of Pediatric Surgery, Children's Hospital, University of Helsinki, Helsinki, Finland
e-mail: antti.koivusal@hus.fi

P.D. Losty et al. (eds.), *Rickham's Neonatal Surgery*, https://doi.org/10.1007/978-1-4471-4721-3_29

29.1 Introduction

Inguinal hernia is one of the most common surgical conditions in infancy and consequently repair of the hernia is a common surgical procedure in neonates. The peak incidence of inguinal hernia is during the first months of life and approximately one third of children are aged less than 6 months at the time of the repair. The recent developments in paediatric anaesthesia and intensive care have enabled safe hernia repair in premature babies. The basic operation for an indirect inguinal hernia, high ligation and division of the hernia sac at the internal inguinal orifice, remains the mainstay of the surgical technique, but the introduction of laparoscopy in children has provided a new surgical approach also for neonatal hernia repair. Hernia repair in infants must take in consideration anaesthetic risks, appropriate postoperative care and the risk of inguinal hernia related complications. Proper timing, awareness of risks, mastery of proper techniques and the ability to treat complications are basic skills of a paediatric surgeon for safe and efficient neonatal hernia repair. These issues are discussed in this chapter.

29.2 Etiology

At the neonatal period practically all inguinal hernias are of congenital indirect type, whereas direct inguinal or femoral hernias are rare [1–3]. Indirect inguinal hernias are the result of failure of the processus vaginalis to close. Processus vaginalis is an outpouching of the peritoneum through inguinal canal identifiable from the third month of the gestation. Processus vaginalis elongates as it accompanies gubernaculum and testes during their descent, and it reaches the scrotum by the seventh month of gestation. Processus vaginalis obliterates after the descent of the testes, but the process of obliteration continues after birth. In the female, processus vaginalis accompanies the round ligament and reaches the labia major as the canal of Nuck. The rate of patency of processus vaginalis has been reported to sink from 89–94% in the newborn period to 57% in the 4–12 month age group and 20% in adulthood [4]. Patent processus vaginalis is a potential hernia but not an equivalent to an inguinal hernia. It has been estimated that although at the age of 2 years processus vaginalis may be bilaterally open in 40% of children, only 6–12% of those who have undergone unilateral hernia repair by the age of 2 years, develop a metachronous contralateral inguinal hernia [5–7].

29.3 Epidemiology

The incidence of indirect inguinal hernia in full-term neonates ranges from 3.5–5% [8]. The incidence in preterm infants commensurates with the patency of the processus vaginalis and highest incidence rates ranging from 16% to 30% are reported in premature infants [8–10]. During the birth hospitalization, the incidence of inguinal hernia for premature infants is reported to range from 3% to 9% and for infants weighing less than 1500 and 1000 g, 11% and 17%, respectively [10, 11]. Males are much more likely to develop hernias with a reported male-female ratio of 3:1 to 10:1 [8]. In both sexes, approximately 60% of the hernias are right-sided, 25–30% left-sided and 10% are bilateral [12, 13]. In premature infants the incidence of bilateral hernias may reach 50% [11].

Approximately 11.5% of patients have family history of inguinal hernia [8, 13]. The incidence of hernia is increased in twins as well [14, 15].

29.4 Associated Conditions with an Increased Incidence of Inguinal Hernia

There is an increased incidence of inguinal hernia in patients with the following conditions:

- Urogenital
  - Undescended testis
  - Bladder exstrophy
  - Cloacal exstrophy
- Increased peritoneal fluid
  - Ascites
  - Ventriculoperitoneal shunt
  - Peritoneal dialysis

- Increased intraabdominal pressure
  - Repair of omphalocele/gastroschisis
  - Meconium peritonitis
  - Necrotizing enterocolitis
  - Chylous ascites
- Chronic respiratory disease
  - Cystic Fibrosis
- Disorders of the connective tissue [16]
  - Marfan syndrome [17]
  - Loeys-Dietz syndrome [18]
  - Williams syndrome [19, 20]
  - Cutis laxa [16]
  - Costello syndrome [16]
  - Menkes disease and OHS [16]
  - Ehlers-Danlos syndrome [21]
- Mucopolysaccharidoses [16]
  - Osteogenesis imperfecta
  - Hurler syndrome, Hunter syndrome
- Disorders of sexual differentiation
  - Complete androgen insensitivity syndrome [22]
  - Persistent Mullerian duct syndrome [16]
  - Chromosomal disorders and gene defects such as XXYY males, Opitz syndrome Aarskog syndrome, Fragile X [16]
  - Etiology unknown: Velocardiofacial–syndrome
  - DiGeorge syndrome [16]

29.5 Clinical Presentation

Inguinoscrotal hernia may be diagnosed prenatally by ultrasonographic screening [23]. In the newborn the presenting feature is a firm bulge in the groin lateral to the pubic tubercle which increases size and extends toward or into the scrotum or in the female the ipsilateral labia major with crying and straining. In the female the bulge is less obvious and may contain often a nonreducible ovoid-shaped mass corresponding with the herniated ovary. The bulge may disappear spontaneously when the patient is relaxed or sometimes remain visible and palpable causing crying, discomfort and vomiting. The bulge can be reduced with gentle pressure. After reduction 'silk glove sign', thickening or silkiness of the spermatic cord as it crosses the pubic tubercle or, in the female on palpating the processus vaginalis over the pubic tubercle, may be felt on palpation. Silk glove sign has been reported to detect indirect inguinal hernia or patent processus vaginalis with as high as 93% sensitivity and 97% and specificity [24], but the accuracy of silk glove sign in the female is lower and probably varies between examiners. A positive silk glove sign together with a reliable clinical history is, however, highly suggestive of inguinal hernia. Stretching a supine infant on the bed with legs extended and arms held straight above the head may cause the infant to struggle and push out the hernia. When the physical examination with clinical history is not diagnostic a new evaluation should be arranged. Digital photographs of the hernia taken by the parents may confirm the diagnosis accurately and prevent repeated visits to the attending surgeon [25]. The diagnosis of neonatal inguinal hernia can be made by clinical history and physical examination and radiologic investigations are generally not needed. Groin ultrasound scan may disclose patent processus vaginalis, presence of mass in the inguinal canal or movement of an intestinal loop through the internal ring. In older children ultrasonographic diameter of the inguinal canal may be used to differentiate between patent processus vaginalis and a true inguinal hernia [26, 27]. Ultrasound scan may be also used in differential diagnostics to detect disorders of testis, abnormal inguinal lymph node, abscess or hydrocele.

29.6 Management

An inguinal hernia does not resolve spontaneously and because of the incarceration risk which is particularly high during the first months of life repair is always indicated. An irreducible incarcerated or strangulated hernia requires immediate surgery. A reduced incarcerated hernia should be repaired as soon as the patient is stable and the swelling in the sac has subsided usually by the second day after the reduction. Delaying the surgery 5 days or more after reduction carries a significant risk of reincarceration [28].

Most paediatric surgeons recommend that an uncomplicated inguinal hernia in full-term neonates and in infants under 3 months of age is repaired as soon as convenient not later than four but preferably within 2 weeks following the diagnosis. Undue delay of elective repair increases the risk of incarceration [29] and should an incarceration occur the parents must be informed where to take the infant for immediate paediatric surgical care. From a daily clinical point of view it is rational to plan a semi-emergent repair within a couple of days if an otherwise uncomplicated hernia has been difficult to reduce, or, if an infant is brought day after day to the emergency ward for the reduction of the hernia.

In premature infants timing of repair for hernias should follow same guidelines as in full-term infants. A complicated inguinal hernia or a hernia requiring repeated difficult reductions during birth hospitalization should be repaired before discharge from neonatal intensive care unit (NICU). Premature infants with uncomplicated inguinal hernias may be discharged and scheduled for a repair at an age when postoperative observation at NICU is not required. If, however, the hernia causes complications or repeated reductions, the need for overnight observation at NICU should not delay a semi-emergent repair.

29.7 Anaesthesia

General anaesthesia with endotracheal intubation, laryngeal mask or face mask is the method of choice. The use of regional techniques such as spinal, epidural or caudal anaesthesia, local anaesthetic instilled in the operative field reduce the need for postoperative analgesics. Neonates carry at least a 5% risk of postoperative apnoea and consequently they usually undergo a 24 h period of postoperative respiratory and circulatory monitoring. The risk of postoperative apnoea has been reported particularly high among preterm neonates but it is also associated with low postmenstrual age, anaemia, and a history of recurrent apnoea [30–32]. Use of regional or local anaesthetics may reduce but does not eliminate the risk of apnoea within the 24 h following the surgery [32, 33]. It has been estimated that the risk of postoperative apnoea does not drop below 1% until 56 weeks for a 32-week premature infant and 54 weeks for 34-week premature infant [30].

In the authors institution day surgery is performed to healthy infants with a minimum corrected age of 3 months (i.e. the estimated day of birth after full-term pregnancy plus 3 months), whereas infants with the corrected age less than 3 months stay overnight at paediatric surgical ward. Infants with gestation age a minimum of 37 weeks and aged less than 4 weeks and infants with gestation age of less than 37 weeks and postmenstrual age under 45 weeks are observed overnight in neonatal intensive care unit.

29.8 Operative Technique

29.8.1 Males

The operative technique aims for ligation of the hernia at the internal inguinal ring. The patient lies supine with the genitals included in the sterile operative field. The use of magnifying surgical telescope glasses is recommended. A short incision is placed with the medial end just superior and lateral to the pubic tubercle. Thus placed the incision lays a little superior to the external ring. The incision is carried through the subcutaneous fat and Scarpa's fascia until the level of aponeurosis of the external oblique muscle. Division of the epigastric vein above Scarpa's fascia should be avoided but if inadvertently divided careful haemostasis is required in order to prevent bleeding and postoperative haematoma. In small children the inguinal canal is short and external and internal rings overlap and the entire operation can be performed through the external ring without splitting the external aponeurosis unless more exposition is needed. The cremasteric muscle and fascia are grasped and raised with blunt forceps the hernia sac is exposed spreading and opening the cremasteric fibers. The hernia sac is grasped with forceps and elevated with the structures of the spermatic cord. The testicular vessels and vas deferens are identified and dissected from the hernia sac without touching them by gently separating the thin tissue adhering them to the wall of the hernia sac. The dissection of the cord structures is carried to the level at or just above of the internal ring. The proximal hernia sac is freed of all adherent connective tissue and at this stage the hernia sac may be opened for checking its contents, and then divided between small clamps when at the same time the separated cord structures are gently kept out of harms way. No attempt is made to dissect further the distal sac because of the risk of ischemic orchitis or haematoma. If the dissection of the sac is complete, gentle traction on the scrotal skin should now take the testis into the scrotum without any traction felt in the proximal sac. The proximal sac is twisted on itself and suture-ligated at the internal ring with absorbable monofilament thread while again the cord structures are protected from twisting with the sac or from being inadvertently included in the ligature. Scarpa's fascia and the subcuticular layer are closed with absorbable monofilament thread and the cutis is closed with adhesive tape. Finally the position of the testis is controlled once more (Fig. 29.1).

29.8.2 Females

The surgical approach to the inguinal canal is same as in males. The hernia sac is identified and always opened for inspecting the contents or a sliding component. The wall of the hernia sac may contain the fallopian tube which can be found by following the round ligament. If the hernia sac is empty it is divided together with the round ligament between clamps, twisted on itself and suture-ligated with absorbable monofilament thread, and the distal end of the transected round ligament is cauterized with diathermy (Fig. 29.2).

If a sliding component such as fallopian duct, ovary, uterus or bladder is identified in the wall of within the hernia sac, the sac may be closed with purse string above the structure, inverted at the internal ring and then the internal ring is closed with interrupted sutures [34]. Alternatively a peritoneal flap procedure [35, 36] or laparoscopic approach [37] may be used.

29.8.3 Laparoscopic Repair

Laparoscopic repair of paediatric inguinal hernias have gained popularity especially in children past the neonatal age. The relative advantages of laparoscopic repair include the possibility to synchronous inspection and repair of the contralateral side or a bilateral hernia, easy diagnosis of a direct inguinal hernia, repair of a recurred hernia without renewed dissection of the cord structures and the possibility to identify sliding components of the hernia. In terms of pain, cosmetic appearance of the scar, length of hospitalization and the length of the required theatre time, paediatric laparoscopic repair has no significant advantages compared with the open procedure which in children is considerably less invasive than in adults.

In small infants weighing from one and a half to five kilograms laparoscopic hernia repair is reported feasible and technically simple when performed by expert laparoscopic surgeons [38, 39]. Adequate studies comparing open and laparoscopic hernia repair in neonates do not exist and presently no guidelines for the choice of operative technique, except surgeons' expertise and preference, can be given [40]. Laparoscopic hernia repair in children has carried a 2–3% recurrence rate but recently recurrence rates below 2% has been reported [41]. Although cord structures are not dissected in laparoscopic repair there is a reported rate of 4% of postoperative testicular ascent requiring subsequent orchidopexy [39]. For many surgeons the risk of injury to the cord structures and testicular perfusion have been of concern. In the hands of experienced laparoscopic surgeons, the risk of impaired testicular perfusion or testicular atrophy is, however, low [39, 41]. Some centres perform routinely all or most paediatric hernia repairs laparoscopically. In other centres, the authors centre included, laparoscopic hernia repair is performed in selected indications including incarceration, sliding hernia and recurrence. In premature low-weight infants open approach is preferable to laparoscopy because the small abdominal domain provides limited working space to handle friable tissues, and there is a risk for respiratory problems because of CO_2 pneumoperitoneum.

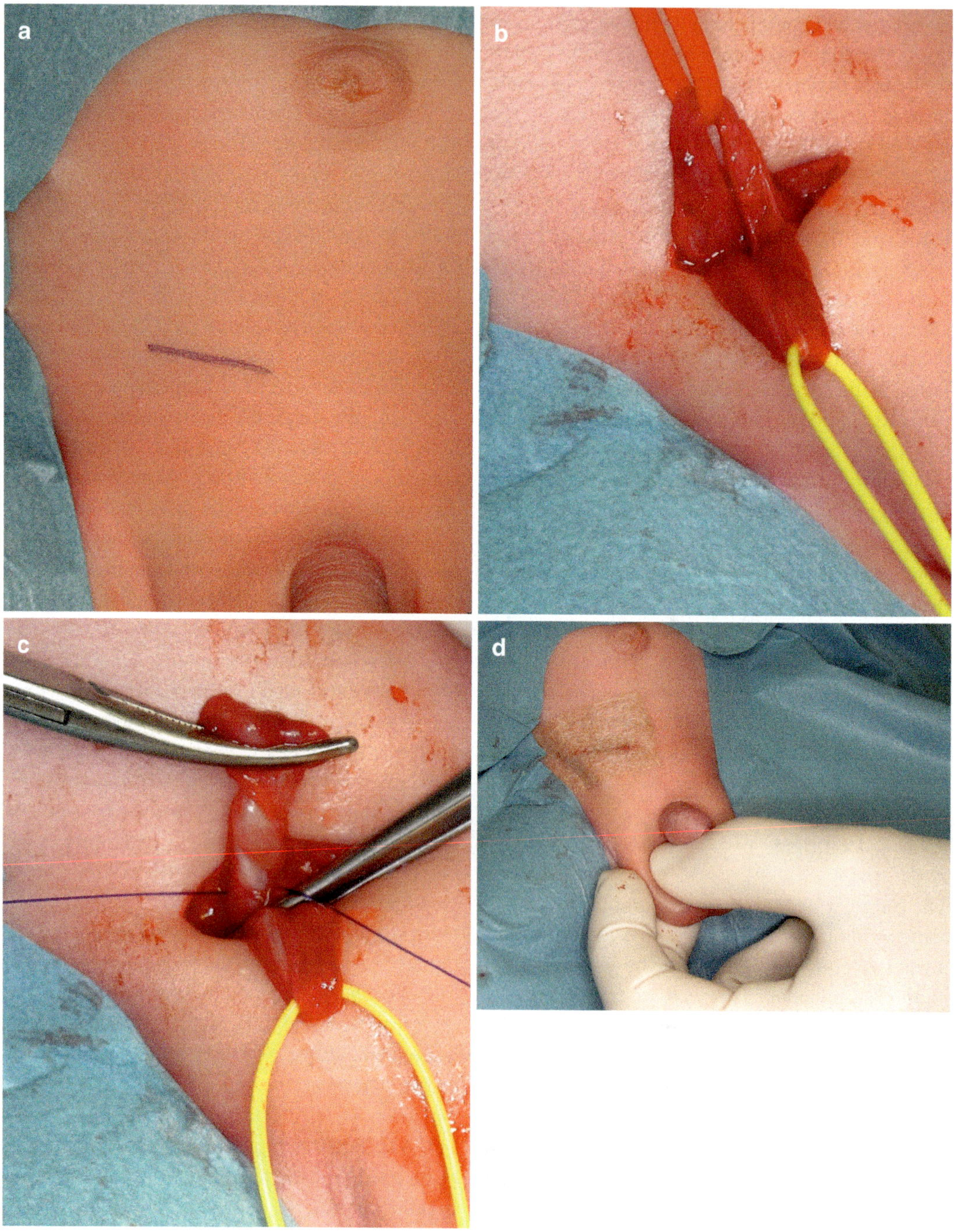

Fig. 29.1 Open repair in male. (**a**) Placement of the incision; (**b**) vas and spermatic vessels (surrounded by *yellow loop*) are dissected free from the sac (*red loop*); (**c**) sac has been diveded, proximal sac is twisted and ligated, distal part is allowed to retract; (**d**) after closure, location of the testicle is checked once more

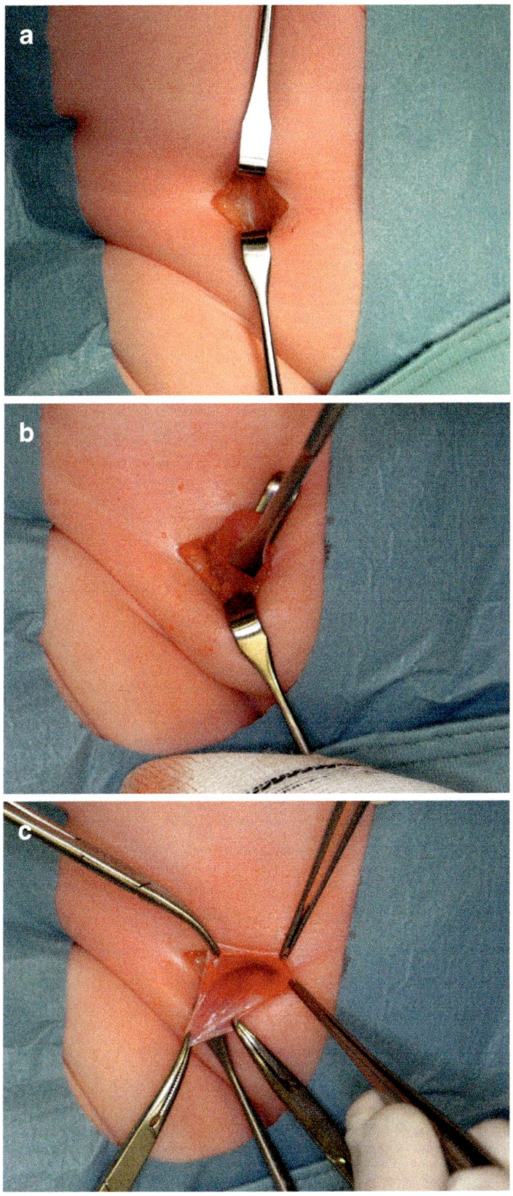

Fig. 29.2 Open repair in female. (**a**) Incision, Scarpa's fascia seen at the bottom of the incision; (**b**) a small retractor is passed below the sac and round ligament; (**c**) hernia sac is opened for examination of its contents

Laparoscopic techniques include closure of the peritoneum at the inguinal ring by a running suture or a purse string suture [41], use of peritoneal flap [42], or division of the periorificial peritoneum from inside, collapse of the sac and subsequent closure of the peritoneal margins [43]. Hernia repair may also be achieved with laparoscopically guided extraperitoneal suture closure surrounding the internal ring [44].

Authors preferred technique of laparoscopic repair in male infants and neonates is performed with the patient supine under general anaesthesia. Urinary bladder is emptied by compression method (Crede's manouver) or, alternatively, urinary catheter may be inserted. The patient must be securely attached to the operating table in order to allow Trendelenburg's position and turning to both sides. Five or three millimeter trocars and instruments are used. Alternatively, laparoscopic instruments can be inserted through stab incisions without trocars. A small incision is made in the infraumbilical fold for open placement of a trocar for videocamera and insufflation. After insufflation two small stab wounds in the left and right abdomen are made for two needle holders. A thread of appropriate length is then placed into abdominal cavity either through abdominal wall or through a trocar. The internal ring is closed with a suture taking general bites of the peritoneum including the medial aspect of the internal ring but excluding the cord structures. Absorbable or unabsorbable thread may be used. The thread is then tightened and tied intracorporeally. A second suture may be added if the course of the cord structures is clear. Trocar incisions are closed in layers and injected with local anaesthetic (Fig. 29.3).

In the female the procedure is similar except that round ligament may be included in the suture that closes the internal ring.

29.9 Incarcerated Inguinal Hernia

Incarceration occurs when the contents of the hernia sac cannot easily be reduced into the abdominal cavity. If there is delay in the reduction of the hernia, incarceration progresses rapidly to strangulation. Strangulation is characterized by irreducible mass, constant pain, vomiting, and in later stages signs of hypovolemic chock. The contents of the hernia sac, small bowel, appendix, omentum, ovary and the fallopian tube or even parts of uterus and urinary bladder become tightly constricted and swollen in the

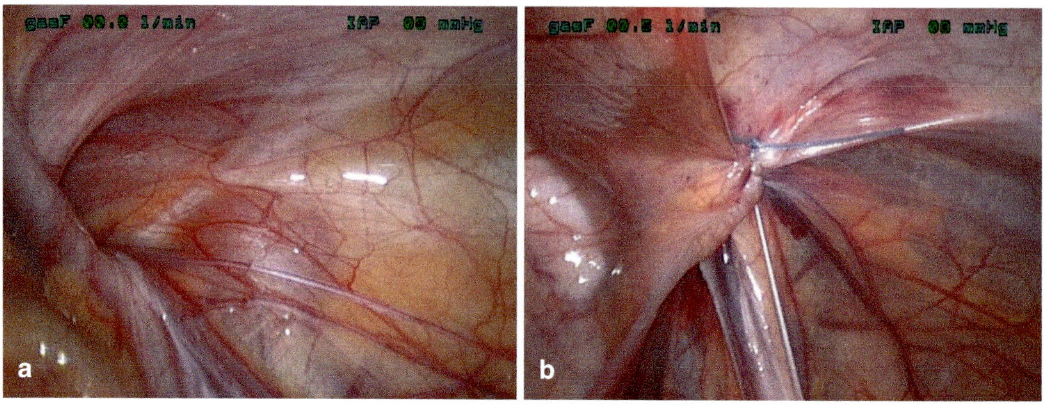

Fig. 29.3 Laparoscopic repair. (**a**) Open internal inguinal ring; (**b**) peritoneum at the internal ring has been closed with a purse string suture

inguinal canal rendering the hernia irreducible. After constriction occludes venous and arterial blood circulation the contents of the hernia sac become gangrenous and intestinal necrosis end even a faecal fistula may result [45, 46].

An incarcerated or strangulated hernia may occlude the testicular vessels located in the spermatic cord and in infants younger than 3 months testicular infarction or cyanotic testis has been reported in 30%. The rate of testicular atrophy after operation for an incarcerated hernia is however estimated to be lower from 9% to 17%. Neither operative or early postoperative testicular assessment correlates with testicular survival, and the pathology may become evident only after puberty. Unless a testis is frankly necrotic it should not be removed [47].

The incidence of incarceration in neonatal infants is relatively high, but due to different practices in reporting the numbers are variable and sometimes unreliable [48]. In infancy incarceration rates as high as 30% has been reported [45, 49], and among infants undergoing their hernia repair during the first year an incarceration rate of 28% has been reported [10]. During their birth hospitalization up to 16% of premature infants need surgery for the incarceration, and later on the incarceration risk approaches that of full term infants [10, 11, 48],

Approximately 5% of the infant female inguinal hernias contain a herniated irreducible ovary without signs of strangulation [50]. Of the irreducible ovaries a torsion rate of 19% has been reported [51] and a semi-emergent hernia repair within days is indicated.

29.10 Management of an Incarcerated Inguinal Hernia

An incarcerated or strangulated inguinal hernia is always a paediatric surgical emergency and treated without delay. In a clinically stable infant an incarcerated irreducible inguinal hernia should initially be managed nonoperatively. Firm compression with fingers on all sides of the mass concentrated to the external inguinal ring along the axis of the inguinal canal may reduce the incarcerated mass. Several minutes of patient compression may be required. The procedure causes discomfort and pain to the infant, and analgesia or sedation may be required. If sedative agents are used the infants must stay under appropriate observation because of the risk of respiratory depression.

After the reduction of a hernia the palpable mass should disappear. In the male with the ipsilateral testis normally descended, the testis should after reduction return downwards into the scrotum by gentle traction. If there is any doubt of successful reduction the manual compression should be continued to complete reduction, and the reduction ascertained by ultrasound examination.

After the reduction the infant is observed until clinically stable. Preferably the hernia repair should be performed during the same hospitalization. Open repair is usually performed 48 h after reduction when the swelling of the hernia sac and the spermatic cord has subsided. Laparoscopic repair may be performed soon after the reduction because there is less or no peritoneal swelling at the internal ring interfering with the closure.

If there are clear signs of strangulated hernia or an incarcerated mass cannot be reduced immediate operative treatment is indicated. Reduction under general anaesthesia without exploration is not recommended, because unrecognized gangrenous contents of the hernia sac may be returned into abdominal cavity. Antibiotic prophylaxis covering the microbes of both upper and lower gastrointestinal tract is given at the induction of the anaesthesia.

The standard surgical approach used in elective open hernia repair can be used, but the incision must allow ample exposure The first step is to free the herniated sac by opening the external oblique aponeurosis through and upwards the external ring or, if the constriction still exist, the internal ring must be freed. The hernia sac is opened and the contents inspected. If the small intestine looks cyanotic, enough length of viable intestine is drawn out to determine the length and condition of the ischemic segment. The ischemic segment is covered with warm saline moistened cloth and inspected after 5 min for colour, arterial pulsation and peristalsis and if deemed viable, returned into abdominal cavity and the hernia is repaired in the standard fashion. Nonviable intestine is resected and anastomosed end-to-end. If the resection cannot be performed through the hernia incision or if the suspectedly gangrenous contents of the sac are spontaneously reduced before the sac is opened a separate abdominal incision may be needed. Transperitoneal Pfannenstiel approach gives excellent exposure to deal with ischemic intestine, visualisation of contralateral inner ring and a cosmetically acceptable scar [52]. Alternatively, preperitoneal approach [53] may be used.

Repair of an incarcerated hernia can demanding because of the friable but thickened sac is difficult to separate from the cord structures. Laparoscopic approach enables inspection of the reduced contents and closure of the internal ring without dissection of the cord structures and the operation may be performed as soon as reduction is accomplished [54, 55]. In irreducible incarcerated strangulated hernias it is advisable to combine laparoscopy with open approach to free the sac [56] because pulling the constricted contents of the sac with laparoscopic instruments from inside may not be possible even with the help of synchronized manual compression of the mass from outside and tearing of the herniated tissue may result.

29.11 Sliding Hernia and Atypical Herniated Organs

Except the fallopian tube and ovary, the sliding component of the hernia may consist of large intestine, appendix, uterus, or the urinary bladder. If a sliding component is at risk of injury, the hernia sac must be opened and a purse string ligature placed at an appropriate level after which the sac is inverted and the internal ring closed. An inguinal hernia may contain appendix (Amyand's hernia), Meckel's diverticulum (Littre's hernia) or a wall of a viscera (Richter's hernia).

29.12 Direct Hernia and Femoral Hernia

Although rare in infants a direct inguinal or femoral hernias may be encountered and should be suspected if in an exploration for a clinically evident hernia the indirect sac cannot be found [1, 2]. In direct hernia a fascial defect medial to epigastric vessels may be palpated and in femoral hernia the bulge and hernia opening lie below the inguinal ligament. A direct hernia may occur together with an indirect hernia in a pantaloon fashion. A direct inguinal hernia and femoral hernia can be diagnosed reliably in laparoscopy [2,

57]. Although laparoscopic repair of direct hernia has been described, in open repair the anatomic landmarks are easier to recognize. Open repair is performed by suturing the internal oblique and transversalis fascia to Cooper's ligament.

29.13 Contralateral Exploration and Metachronous Hernia

Contralateral inguinal exploration and closure of the eventual patent processus vaginalis has been widely practised routinely in premature infants because the high incidence of bilateral hernia among them. Justification for this practise has been the supposed elimination of the renewed risks associated with repair of a metachronous contralateral hernia. More recently there have been a move away from this practice because the risk of a patent processus vaginalis to develop a metachronous clinical hernia is less than 15% [57–59]. In addition an open exploration may be harmful to the structures of the spermatic cord. At laparoscopic hernia repair exploration and closure of the contralateral inguinal orifice are safe and easy.

Alternatively, open hernia repair may be combined with exploration of the contralateral inguinal orifice with a videolaparoscope introduced through the opened ipsilateral hernia sac [60]. The hernia sac in small children may, however, be too narrow to allow this procedure. In addition, routine use of laparoscopy for the sake of contralateral exploration requires resources and increases the theatre time.

It is reported that the overall incidence of metachronous hernias up to the age of 19 years is 7.2% and incidence is below 11% from infants aged less than 6 months to children at 7 years of age, and thus 9–14 contralateral explorations are required to prevent one metachronous inguinal hernia [61, 62]. Without a medical condition that significantly increases the risk of inguinal hernia or high risk of complications of anaesthesia, routine contralateral exploration by any technique in an infant with unilateral inguinal hernia and a normal asymptomatic contralateral groin is not indicated.

29.14 Differential Diagnostics

29.14.1 Hydrocele

Hydocele develops when patent processus vaginalis allows accumulation of peritoneal fluid in the space surrounding the testicle between the layers of tunica vaginalis. Hydrocele presents as a nontender swelling which may vary in size because its draining is dependent of the position of the infant. Usually it is possible to get above the swelling and palpate the cord structures. If hernia is doubted, ultrasound scan is preferable to transillumination to detect herniated intestine in infants. Hydrocele may contain a strip of herniated omentum. Repair is delayed to the age of 2–3 years.

29.14.2 Testicular Torsion

Testicular torsion presents as a tender mass in the scrotum. The testicle is located higher up than in the contralateral scrotum. In intravaginal torsion it is possible to palpate above the mass.

29.14.3 Inguinal Lymphadenitis

Vaccination site, infected wound or insect bite in the draining area of the inguinal lymph nodes may be found. Cord and testes are found to be normal.

29.15 Complications

Mortality rate in neonatal inguinal hernia repair should be 0%.The overall rate of major complications is 5.2% but after elective repair should be less than 1% [63, 64]. Complication rate increases in association with incarceration to [54] and prematurity [64].

Haematoma in the operative field or in the scrotum can be avoided with meticulous haemostasis. Only rarely is evacuation of the haematoma needed.

Wound infection occurs in 1% of patients and can be treated in most cases by irrigation and minimal drainage of the wound.

Recurrence rate in an uncomplicated hernia repair in children is usually 1% [65, 66]. In neonates or premature infants recurrence rate is 3–8% [67, 68]. Recurrence rate is increased in medical conditions which predispose to the development of inguinal hernia. Large hernia sacs and ruptured sacs with technically difficult closure [65] and incarceration [69] are associated with increased risk of recurrence. In rare instances the supposed recurrence turns out to be an undiagnosed direct inguinal hernia. By laparoscopy the nature of the recurrence is easily clarified and laparoscopic repair of the indirect recurrence is recommended [70].

29.15.1 Iatrogenic Ascent of the Testis

Iatrogenic ascent of the testis occurs in 1–4% of patients [39, 63, 67]. It is probably due to entrapment of the testis in the scar tissue, failure to pull the testis down into the scrotum at the end of the operation, or technical difficulties resulting in incomplete mobilisation and division of the hernia sac. Funiculolysis and orchidopexy should be done according to the same principles as in congenital undescended testis.

29.15.2 Injury to Reproductive Organs

Injury to vas deferens during hernia repair is estimated at 0.1–2% [63, 66, 71, 72] but injuries because of overzealous dissection may remain unrecognized. Injury to vas may result in obstructive azoospermia or formation of spermatic antibodies and cause male infertility. Apposition of the ends of a transected vas under magnification with 8-0 sutures should be attempted, but also secondary microsurgical repair even in adulthood may be successful [72]. Vascular compromise of the testicle or ovary are associated with irreducible or incarcerated hernias [67, 68]. Testicular manipulation in an elective repair should not compromise circulation [73].

Injury to urinary bladder is a rare but potentially severe complication. In infants the bladder lies in a relative superficial position and the lateral angles of the bladder may herniate into the inguinal canal and become injured during the division and closure of the sac. A recognized injury should immediately be repaired and an urinary catheter inserted. An unrecognized injury may lead to urinary peritonitis and subsequent scarring and dysfunction of the bladder and the ipsilateral ureter [74].

References

1. Wright JE. Direct inguinal hernia in infancy and childhood. Pediatr Surg Int. 1994;9:161–3.
2. Schier F, Klizaite J. Rare inguinal hernia forms in children. Pediatr Surg Int. 2004;20:748–52.
3. Gorsler CM, Schier F. Laparoscopic herniorrhaphy in children. Surg Endosc. 2003;17:571–3. Epub 2003 Feb 17
4. Nakayama DK, Rowe MI. Inguinal hernia and the acute scrotum in infants and children. Pediatr Rev. 1989;11:87–93.
5. Tackett LD, Breuer CK, Luks FI, Caldamone AA, Breuer JG, DeLuca FG, et al. Incidence of contralateral inguinal hernia: aprospective analysis. J Pediatr Surg. 1999;34:684–8.
6. Kiesewetter WB, Parenzan L. When should hernia in the infant be treated bilaterally? JAMA. 1959;171:287–90.
7. Chin T, Liu C, Wei C. The morphology of the contralateral internal inguinal ring is age-dependent in children with unilateral inguinal hernia. J Pediatr Surg. 1995;30:1663–5.
8. Bronsther B, Abrams MW, Elboim C. Inguinal hernias in children—a study of 1,000 cases and a review of the literature. J Am Med Womens Assoc. 1972;27:522–5.
9. Rajput A, Gauderer MW, Hack M. Inguinal hernias in very low birth weight infants: incidence and timing of repair. J Pediatr Surg. 1992;27:1322–4.
10. Lautz TB, Raval MV, Reynolds M. Does timing matter? A national perspective on the risk of incarceration in premature neonates with inguinal hernia. J Pediatr. 2011;158:573–7. Epub 2010 Oct 30
11. Kumar VH, Clive J, Rosenkrantz TS, Bourque MD, Hussain N. Inguinal hernia in preterm infants (< or = 32-week gestation). Pediatr Surg Int. 2002;18:147–52.
12. Rowe MI, Clatworthy HW. Incarcerated and strangulated hernias in children. A statistical study of high-risk factors. Arch Surg. 1970;101:136–9.
13. Czeizel A. Epidemiologic characteristics of congenital inguinal hernia. Helv Paediatr Acta. 1980;35:57–67.
14. Czeizel A, Gárdonyi J. A family study of congenital inguinal hernia. Am J Med Genet. 1979;4:247–54.
15. Bakwin H. Indirect inguinal hernia in twins. J Pediatr Surg. 1971;6:165–8.

16. Barnett C, Langer JC, Hinek A, Bradley TJ, Chitayat D. Looking past the lump: genetic aspects of inguinal hernia in children. J Pediatr Surg. 2009;4:1423–31.
17. Finkbohner R, Johnston D, Crawford ES, Coselli J, Milewicz DM. Marfan syndrome. Long-term survival and complications after aortic aneurysm repair. Circulation. 1995;91:728–33.
18. Loeys BL, Schwartze U, Holm T, et al. Aneuruysm syndromes caused by mutations in the TGF-beta receptor. N Engl J Med. 2008;358:2787–95.
19. Williams JC, Barrat-Boyes BG, Lowe JB. Supravalvular aortic stenosis. Circulation. 1961;24:1311–8.
20. Amenta S, Sofocleous C, Kolialexi A, Thomaidis L, Giouroukos S, Karavitakis E, Mavrou A, Kitsiou S, Kanavakis E, Fryssira H. Clinical manifestations and molecular investigation of 50 patients with Williams syndrome in the Greek population. Pediatr Res. 2005;57:789–95. Epub 2005 Mar 17
21. Liem MS, van der Graaf Y, Beemer FA, van Vroonhoven TJ. Increased risk for inguinal hernia in patients with Ehlers-Danlos syndrome. Surgery. 1997;122:114–5.
22. Viner RM, Teoh Y, Williams DM, Patterson MN, Hughes IA. Androgen insensitivity syndrome: a survey of diagnostic procedures and management in the UK. Arch Dis Child. 1997;77:305–9.
23. Sharma S, Perni SC, Predanic M, Kalish RB, Zervoudakis IA, Chasen ST. Atypical sonographic presentation of fetal unilateral inguinoscrotal hernia in a multiple gestation. J Perinat Med. 2004;32: 378–80.
24. Luo CC, Chao HC. Prevention of unnecessary contralateral exploration using the silk glove sign (SGS) in pediatric patients with unilateral inguinal hernia. Eur J Pediatr. 2007;166:667–9. Epub 2006 Dec 30
25. Kawaguchi AL, Shaul DB. Inguinal hernias can be accurately diagnosed using the parent's digital photographs when the physical examination is nondiagnostic. J Pediatr Surg. 2009;44:2327–9.
26. Erez I, Rathause V, Vacian I, Zohar E, Hoppenstein D, Werner M, Lazar L, Freud E. Preoperative ultrasound and intraoperative findings of inguinal hernias in children: a prospective study of 642 children. J Pediatr Surg. 2002;37:865–8.
27. Hata S, Takahashi Y, Nakamura T, Suzuki R, Kitada M, Shimano T. Preoperative sonographic evaluation is a useful method of detecting contralateral patent processus vaginalis in pediatric patients with unilateral inguinal hernia. J Pediatr Surg. 2004;39:1396–9.
28. Gahukamble DB, Khamage AS. Early versus delayed repair of reduced incarcerated inguinal hernias in the pediatric population. J Pediatr Surg. 1996;31:1218–20.
29. Chen LE, Zamakhshary M, Foglia RP, Coplen DE, Langer JC. Impact of wait time on outcome for inguinal hernia repair in infants. Pediatr Surg Int. 2009;25:223–7. Epub 2008 Dec 16
30. Coté CJ, Zaslavsky A, Downes JJ, Kurth CD, Welborn LG, Warner LO, Malviya SV. Postoperative apnea in former preterm infants after inguinal herniorrhaphy. A combined analysis. Anesthesiology. 1995;82:809–22.
31. Murphy JJ, Swanson T, Ansermino M, Milner R. The frequency of apneas in premature infants after inguinal hernia repair: do they need overnight monitoring in the intensive care unit? J Pediatr Surg. 2008;43:865–8.
32. Davidson A, Frawley GP, Sheppard S, Hunt R, Hardy P. Risk factors for apnea after infant inguinal hernia repair. Paediatr Anaesth. 2009;19:402–3.
33. Kim J, Thornton J, Eipe N. Spinal anesthesia for the premature infant: is this really the answer to avoiding postoperative apnea? Paediatr Anaesth. 2009;19:56–8.
34. Bevan A. Sliding hernias of the ascending colon and caecum, the descending colon, sigmoid, and the bladder. Ann Surg. 1930;92:754.
35. Shaw A, Santulli TV. Management of sliding hernias of the urinary bladder in infants. Surg Gynecol Obstet. 1967;124:1314–6.
36. Goldstein IR, Potts WJ. Inguinal hernia in female infants and children. Ann Surg. 1958;148:819–22.
37. Patle NM, Tantia O, Prasad P, Khanna S, Sen B. Sliding inguinal hernias: scope of laparoscopic repair. J Laparoendosc Adv Surg Tech A. 2011;21:227–31.
38. Turial S, Enders J, Krause K, Schier F. Laparoscopic inguinal herniorrhaphy in premature infants. Eur J Pediatr Surg. 2010;20:371–4.
39. Turial S, Enders J, Krause K, Schier F. Laparoscopic inguinal herniorrhaphy in babies weighing 5 kg or less. Surg Endosc. 2011;25:72–8. Epub 2010 Jun 8
40. Chan KL, Chan HY, Tam PK. Towards a near-zero recurrence rate in laparoscopic inguinal hernia repair for pediatric patients of all ages. J Pediatr Surg. 2007;42:1993–7.
41. International Pediatric Endosurgery Group. IPEG guidelines for inguinal hernia and hydrocele. J Laparoendosc Adv Surg Tech. 2010;20:xii–vi.
42. Yip KF, Tam PK, Li MK. Laparoscopic flip-flap hernioplasty: an innovative technique for pediatric hernia surgery. Surg Endosc. 2004;18:1126–9.
43. Montupet P, Esposito C. Fifteen years experience in laparoscopic inguinal hernia repair in pediatric patients. Results and considerations on a debated procedure. Surg Endosc. 2011;25:450–3.
44. Endo M, Watanabe T, Nakano M, Yoshida F, Ukiyama E. Laparoscopic completely extraperitoneal repair of inguinal hernia in children: a single-institute experience with 1,257 repairs compared with cut-down herniorrhaphy. Surg Endosc. 2009;23:1706–12.
45. Stylianos S, Jacir NN, Harris BH. Incarceration of inguinal hernia in infants prior to elective repair. J Pediatr Surg. 1993;28:582–3.
46. Roshan Khan T, Maletha M, Tandon R. Neonatal incarcerated inguinal hernia with spontaneous scrotofecal fistula. J Pediatr Surg. 2009;44:1846–7.
47. Walc L, Bass J, Rubin S, Walton M. Testicular fate after incarcerated hernia repair and/or orchiopexy performed in patients under 6 months of age. J Pediatr Surg. 1995;30:1195–7.

48. Gholoum S, Baird R, Laberge JM, Puligandla PS. Incarceration rates in pediatric inguinal hernia: do not trust the coding. J Pediatr Surg. 2010;45:1007–11.
49. Lee SL, Gleason JM, Sydorak RM. A critical review of premature infants with inguinal hernias: optimal timing of repair, incarceration risk, and postoperative apnoea. J Pediatr Surg. 2011;46:217–20.
50. Huang CS, Luo CC, Chao HC, Chu SM, Yu YJ, Yen JB. The presentation of asymptomatic palpable movable mass in female inguinal hernia. Eur J Pediatr. 2003;162:493–5. Epub 2003 Apr 26
51. Merriman TE, Auldist AW. Ovarian torsion in inguinal hernias. Pediatr Surg Int. 2000;16:383–5.
52. Koga H, Yamataka A, Ohshiro K, Okada Y, Lane GJ, Miyano T. Pfannenstiel incision for incarcerated inguinal hernia in neonates. J Pediatr Surg. 2003;38:E16–8.
53. Kamaledeen SA, Shanbhogue LK. Preperitoneal approach for incarcerated inguinal hernia in children. J Pediatr Surg. 1997;32:1715–6.
54. Nah SA, Giacomello L, Eaton S, de Coppi P, Curry JI, Drake DP, Kiely EM, Pierro A. Surgical repair of incarcerated inguinal hernia in children: laparoscopic or open? Eur J Pediatr Surg. 2011;21:8–11. Epub 2010 Oct 11
55. Koivusalo A, Pakarinen MP, Rintala RJ. Laparoscopic herniorrhaphy after manual reduction of incarcerated inguinal hernia. Surg Endosc. 2007;21:2147–9. Epub 2007 May 19
56. Takehara H, Hanaoka J, Arakawa Y. Laparoscopic strategy for inguinal ovarian hernias in children: when to operate for irreducible ovary. J Laparoendosc Adv Surg Tech A. 2009;19(Suppl 1):S129–31.
57. Schier F. Direct inguinal hernias in children: laparoscopic aspects. Pediatr Surg Int. 2000;16:562–4.
58. Levitt MA, Ferraraccio D, Arbesman MC, Brisseau GF, Caty MG, Glick PL. Variability of inguinal hernia surgical technique: a survey of North American pediatric surgeons. J Pediatr Surg. 2002;37:745–51.
59. Nassiri SJ. Contralateral exploration is not mandatory in unilateral inguinal hernia in children: a prospective 6-year study. Pediatr Surg Int. 2002;18:470–1. Epub 2002 Jul 20
60. Steven M, Greene O, Nelson A, Brindley N. Contralateral inguinal exploration in premature neonates: is it necessary? Pediatr Surg Int. 2010;21:703–6. Epub 2010 May 8
61. Klin B, Efrati Y, Abu-Kishk I, Stolero S, Lotan G. The contribution of intraoperative transinguinal-laparoscopic examination of the contralateral side to the repair of inguinal hernias in children. World J Pediatr. 2010;6:119–24.
62. Ron O, Eaton S, Pierro A. Systematic review of the risk of developing metachronous contralateral inguinal hernia children. Br J Surg. 2007;94:804–11.
63. Vogels HD, Bruijnen CJ, Beasley SW. Establishing benchmarks for the outcome of herniotomy in children. Br J Surg. 2010;97:1135–9.
64. Baird R, Gholoum S, Laberge JM, Puligandla P. Prematurity, not age at operation or incarceration, impacts complication rates of inguinal hernia repair. J Pediatr Surg. 2011;46:908–11.
65. Vogels HD, Bruijnen CJ, Beasley SW. Predictors of recurrence after inguinal herniotomy in boys. Pediatr Surg Int. 2009;25:235–8. Epub 2009 Jan 16
66. Ein SH, Njere I, Ein A. Six thousand three hundred sixty-one pediatric inguinal hernias: a 35-year review. J Pediatr Surg. 2006;41:980–6.
67. Phelps S, Agrawal M. Morbidity after neonatal inguinal herniotomy. J Pediatr Surg. 1997;32:445–7.
68. Nagraj S, Sinha S, Grant H, Lakhoo K, Hitchcock R, Johnson P. The incidence of complications following primary inguinal herniotomy in babies weighing 5 kg or less. Pediatr Surg Int. 2006;22:500–2. Epub 2006 May 16
69. Steinau G, Treutner KH, Feeken G, Schumpelick V. Recurrent inguinal hernias in infants and children. World J Surg. 1995;19:303–6.
70. Chan KL. Laparoscopic repair of recurrent childhood inguinal hernias after open herniotomy. Hernia. 2007;11:37–40. Epub 2006 Sep 28
71. Steigman CK, Sotelo-Avila C, Weber TR. The incidence of spermatic cord structures in inguinal hernia sacs from male children. Am J Surg Pathol. 1999;23:880–5.
72. Sheynkin YR, Hendin BN, Schlegel PN, Goldstein M. Microsurgical repair of iatrogenic injury to the vas deferens. J Urol. 1998;159:139–41.
73. Palabiyik FB, Cimilli T, Kayhan A, Toksoy N. Do the manipulations in pediatric inguinal hernia operations affect the vascularization of testes? J Pediatr Surg. 2009;44:788–90.
74. Aloi IP, Lais A, Caione P. Bladder injuries following inguinal canal surgery in infants. Pediatr Surg Int. 2010;26:1207–10.

Gastric Outlet Obstruction

30

Graham Lawrence Lamont

Abstract

Primary intrinsic obstruction to the outlet of the stomach in the neonate is a rare phenomenon, and in the previous edition of this book only five cases had been identified in the preceding 20 year period at the regional neonatal centre in Liverpool. The numbers are of course far outweighed by those children presenting with what is the most common surgically correctable cause of vomiting in the first few weeks of life—infantile hypertrophic pyloric stenosis (IHPS). The justification for including it in a textbook on neonatal surgery is two-fold. Not only do a percentage of the cases present within the true neonatal period, but given the numbers that present to regional neonatal units for management it is often the fledgling Paediatric Surgical trainee's first exposure to the skills required to successfully manage neonatal cases, both in diagnostic and in operative management terms. This chapter will mainly focus on the current state of knowledge around IHPS; its aetiology, diagnosis and management, before concluding with comments around the pathologies leading to intrinsic obstruction.

Keywords

Pyloric stenosis • Pyloromyotomy • Gastric outlet obstruction • Surgery Outcomes

30.1 Introduction

Primary intrinsic obstruction to the outlet of the stomach in the neonate is a rare phenomenon, and in the previous edition of this book only five cases had been identified in the preceding 20 year period at the regional neonatal centre in Liverpool [1]. The numbers are of course far outweighed by those children presenting with what is the most common surgically correctable cause of vomiting in the first few weeks of life—infantile hypertrophic pyloric stenosis (IHPS). The justification for including it in a textbook on neonatal surgery is two-fold. Not only do a percentage of the cases present within the true neonatal period, but given the numbers that present to regional neonatal

G.L. Lamont, MBChB, DM, FRCS, FRCS(Paed)
Department of Paediatric Surgery, Alder Hey Children's NHS Trust, Liverpool, UK
e-mail: graham.lamont@alderhey.nhs.uk

P.D. Losty et al. (eds.), *Rickham's Neonatal Surgery*, https://doi.org/10.1007/978-1-4471-4721-3_30

units for management it is often the fledgling Paediatric Surgical trainee's first exposure to the skills required to successfully manage neonatal cases, both in diagnostic and in operative management terms. This chapter will mainly focus on the current state of knowledge around IHPS; its aetiology, diagnosis and management, before concluding with comments around the pathologies leading to intrinsic obstruction.

30.2 Infantile Hypertrophic Pyloric Stenosis (IHPS)

The first recorded description of pyloric stenosis is thought to be from Hildanus who described a child with spastic vomiting in 1646 [1] but there were only further sporadic reports of the condition in the literature until Hirschsprung presented what is recognised as the first accurate depiction of the clinical features and pathological anatomy [2]. Though the condition initially was treated medically, the operation of pyloromyotomy was first introduced by Dufour and Fredet in [3] and further developed and popularised by Ramstedt [4] resulting in the procedure now commonly bearing this eponymous title.

30.3 Incidence

The incidence of pyloric stenosis has shown considerable variation over time, and quoted incidences have varied from as low as 1.5 per 1000 [5] to as high as 3 per 1000 [6]. Reported incidences are higher in Western countries than in Asian and African countries [7–10]. This trend towards a differing incidence in different racial groups is also seen within Western countries where a lower incidence is often found in non-Caucasian groups compared to Caucasian populations in the same geographic area [11].

It has also been well documented that there is a variable incidence of the disease in different areas over different time periods. There has however been little evidence of a consistent pattern of change. While some studies have shown increases in parts of the UK, [5, 6, 12, 13] other papers have identified a decrease over later time periods [14]. In the 1960s the rate in Belfast was identified as 3 per 1000 live births [6] but the later work from Scotland [14] had shown a decrease from 4.4 per 1000 live births to 1.4 per 100 live births between 1981 and 2004. A European wide study also identified variable patterns of increase and decrease over similar time patterns between different European regions with no consistency [15]. In searching for explanations of this change a number of risk factors have been studied. A paper from Scandinavia [16] reported a potential link between a decrease in the incidence of Sudden Infant Death Syndrome (SIDS) and a fall in the incidence of pyloric stenosis, suggesting this may be in some way linked to the success of campaigns to change sleeping posture. This area was further explored in a paper by Sommerfield [14] which showed similar decreases in the two conditions in Scotland yet identified that the fall in pyloric stenosis incidence preceded that of SIDS by at least 2 years. Further environmental influences will be discussed in the subsequent sections.

What has clearly come through on every review and paper is the influence of genetics on the disease. There is a marked male preponderance with a generally accepted ratio of four affected males to every female [17]. Of interest is one paper showing that a rise seen in incidence in a specific area of the USA was largely due to a widening of the gender ratio with a male to female ratio of over 6 to 1 in that series [18].

More recently we have been analysing Health Episode Statistic (HES) data at Alder Hey. The exercise has shown that the incidence in England over the latest 10 year period for which data was available (2000—2009) has been remarkably consistent, with a mean incidence over this time of 1.6 per 1000 live births. The male to female ratio over this time period was 5.4 to 1.

30.4 Aetiology

30.4.1 General Considerations

The variability in incidence described above and the well recognised risk of recurrence in family members have pointed strongly to a multifactorial aetiology and led to numerous attempts to identify candidate causative factors over the years.

The aetiology of pyloric stenosis has received much attention over the years. As understanding of disease processes has progressed from the investigation of overall physiological and anatomical phenomena to investigation at the molecular level, so the search for the 'cause' for pyloric stenosis has become more focussed on abnormalities at the ultra-structural level. Clinical observational studies have given way to more sophisticated laboratory based techniques, and yet a single unifying theory for the aetiology of pyloric stenosis remains elusive.

It is recognised that the stenosis of the pyloric canal is secondary to hypertrophy of the smooth muscle of the pyloric sphincter [19], first postulated as the primary causative factor by Hirschsprung [2]. This has been supported by observational studies showing this occurring in both foetuses [20] and premature infants [21]. However given the more common occurrence of the condition at the end of the neonatal period and into early infancy, it is generally accepted that the hypertrophy is itself a secondary phenomenon as originally proposed by Thomson [22] as far back as the late nineteenth century. The more difficult question to answer relates to what are the triggers and, indeed, what are the underlying mechanisms that lead ultimately to the hypertrophy.

The pyloric region is recognised as the sphincter that controls the rate of gastric emptying and thus delivery of the stomach contents to the duodenum for further digestion and onward passage. The sphincter consists of thickened circular muscle that is tonically active giving a high pressure zone separating the stomach from duodenum. It exerts its' effect on the regulation of gastric emptying by the transient relaxation of the muscle in a co-ordinated fashion allowing stomach contents to pass in to the duodenum [23, 24]. This interplay involving muscle contraction and relaxation, and the associated neural signalling mechanisms has proven to be a fruitful area for investigation as our understanding of the complexity of these processes has increased.

30.4.2 Genetic Factors

From the earliest descriptions of series of pyloric stenosis occurring in families, [25] it has been clear that heritable factors play a part in the aetiology, and with the increased sophistication of analytical techniques it is now becoming possible to determine specific gene loci that seem to have a role in the causation [26]. It is well recognised that males are more likely to be affected than females in a ratio generally quoted as 4:1 [17, 27–30]. In addition, the risk to subsequent siblings is higher than in those children without a family history, a risk described as being as great as 15 times [31]. Indeed, as many as seven affected children were described in one family [32]. An increased risk is also passed down to the next generation, with sons of affected mothers being most at risk with as many as 5% developing the condition [28].

The possibility of a single gene being responsible for the condition was first proposed by Cockaigne and Penrose in their paper from 1934 [32], and though it is associated with other known genetic syndromes such as Smith-Lemli-Optiz [33] and Cornelia de Lange [34], there has been no convincing evidence of a single candidate gene. Though there have been described a small number of cases on whom the inheritance seems to follow a monogenic pattern [35, 36], the majority of cases follow a model of inheritance that is described as a multifactorial sex-modified threshold model [37]. In this model the risk of developing the disease is determined by the additive effects of various genetic and environmental factors.

In recent years the techniques used to study specific loci in different genes have identified areas that seem to be associated with the development of pyloric stenosis and include regions on chromosomes 16 (16p12-p13; 16q24) and on chromosome 11 (11q14-q22) as well as the X-chromosome [27, 38]. In addition, work on chromosome 12q has suggested that the gene encoding neuronal nitric oxide synthetase is a susceptibility locus for pyloric stenosis [39, 40].

30.4.3 Environmental Factors

The role of environmental factors has been felt to be of importance and would help to explain the variability of incidence reported over time. As noted above, various candidate factors have been sought but none have been clearly identified. For example, a possible role for maternal smoking was highlighted in the Scandinavian literature [41] though it was unclear whether this would have been a pre- or post-natal influence. A further link sought to relate the fall in pyloric stenosis to the changing incidence of SIDS [16]. However, research on a Scottish population [14] identified that the decrease in incidence seen occurred prior to the change in incidence of SIDS.

Other potential environmental factors have been investigated but no consistent pattern has been found. While, in at least one study [42], breast feeding has been identified as a potential risk factor, this potential link has been challenged by work from Italy identifying that in a series in Naples it was more common among bottle fed babies [43]. Neither paper however made any claim for a direct causal link though both explored the potential physiological basis for their results. In other papers the influence of feeding has been explored with particular reference to the potential for transpyloric feeding tubes to be associated with an increase in the incidence of the disease [44, 45]. Again the exact mechanism is unclear though it is postulated that mechanical interference or at least an effect to disrupt the normal co-ordination of emptying may be responsible. No recent reports have looked at this issue, and it may be that the use of transpyloric tubes for feeding is not as widely used a technique as it once was.

An interesting insight into a possible aetiology was the recognition of the potential for erythromycin to lead to an increase in the incidence of pyloric stenosis [46]. This would appear to be specifically related to postnatal exposure and is presumed to work via a motilinomimetic effect [47]. While it has been identified in a number of studies the overall effect has been difficult to determine due to different methodologies used in the different studies especially around different dosage regimens that were used [48].

30.4.4 Hormonal Factors

A key feature in the proper functioning of the pylorus as a sphincter region is the interplay between the regulatory hormones that allow for the co-ordination of gastric emptying. The identified mediators are gastrin, cholecystokinin and secretin [49], and their various effects have been studied in pyloric stenosis. The main focus for research has been the role of gastrin, and the experiments of Dodge [50] in which he identified a key role of pentagastrin in an animal model for pyloric stenosis suggested that gastrin was a causative factor. It was postulated that this worked through driving pyloric contractility and thus led to a work hypertrophy of the muscle [49]. However investigations on the animal model could not be replicated [51] and in human studies of pyloric stenosis, results have been confusing with some authors showing an increase in preoperative gastrin levels [52, 53], whereas others found no differences [54, 55] in pre-operative levels. Further theories advanced have sought to define a role for secretin and cholecystokinin through a response to higher gastric acid secretion [56]. Work reported in 1979 by the same group failed to show any increase in cholecystokinin activity [57]. More recently however [58] the central role for hyperacidity has been reframed postulating that a loss of the controlling role of gastrin has a part to play in the pathogenesis.

Another group of compounds that have been investigated for a role in pyloric stenosis are prostaglandins (PG). Both PGE2 and PGF2α have been shown to have an effect on gastrointestinal muscle contraction [59] and La Ferla [60] found elevated levels of these compounds in the gastric juice of infants with IHPS, suggesting a role for the compounds in the causation of the hypertrophy. Other studies however, [61, 62] have shown that PGE2 can also mediate relaxation of muscle, throwing doubt on the place if any, of these compounds on the causation of pyloric stenosis.

30.4.5 Histological Anomalies

As noted earlier, the pyloric sphincter has an inbuilt contractility maintained by myogenic mechanisms [23]. Thus in the search for the cause or effects of the stenosis, the smooth muscle cells (SMC) themselves have been the subject of study to try to elucidate any causative mechanisms. Again any evidence of abnormality has proven contradictory. Dieler on reviewing pathological findings on 37 specimens [63] identified degenerative changes in both the SMC and associated neural network that led him to postulate the existence of two distinctive types of pyloric stenosis: myogenic and neurogenic subsets of the condition. Langer however failed to find such a distinction in the SMC describing them as morphologically normal [64]. This group did identify that there were significant differences in the neurological control of the sphincter in their study population, and also pointed to anomalies in cell-to cell adhesion. Other groups focussing on the structure of the cell and the arrangement of the junctions between them have sought anomalies in the different proteins involved. Again, results have been contradictory, with one group showing clear differences in the expression of desmin, a protein important in the organisation and function of muscle fibres between pyloric stenosis samples and normal controls [65], and others showing no difference [66]. This group did however find anomalies in the proteins talin and dystrophin, which are involved in the interaction between smooth muscle cells and the extracellular matrix. That anomalies have existed within the extra-cellular environment has been recognised from early light-microscopy studies showing increases in the 'connective tissue' elements from hypertrophied pyloric muscle [67, 68]. As the ability to investigate more fully the underlying structure of connective tissue proteins has increased, so the capability to more specifically define the anomalies seen in pyloric stenosis has also improved. Again a number of candidate proteins have been identified with studies showing increases in chondroitin sulphate, fibronectin, laminin and elastin [66, 69, 70]. In addition the described increase in collagen fibres is thought to be a direct result of enhanced synthesis by the abnormal muscle itself [71].

Though the exact changes seen at the cellular level in both the cells and supporting matrix of the pyloric sphincter remain a subject of debate, there is clear recognition that the hypertrophy is genuine and a significant feature of the condition. The mechanisms by which this hypertrophy is brought about have themselves been the focus for research at the cellular level. Growth factors have been shown to be important in the regulation of the growth of SMC in various tissues [72], and so similar relationships with the SMC of the pyloric sphincter again have been sought. An initial candidate peptide investigated was Insulin-like growth factor-I (IGF-I), which had previously been shown to be a mediator for many cellular activities including growth, replication and differentiation [73, 74]. Studies reported in 1998 [28, 75] identified increases in both IGF-I and IGF-I mRNA expression suggesting increased local synthesis of this growth factor plays a significant role in the causation of the muscle hypertrophy. Since then, other mitogenic growth factors have also been shown to be increased. Studies have reported increases in platelet-derived growth factor-BB [76], platelet-derived endothelial cell growth factor [77], transforming growth factor-α [78] and epidermal growth factor [79]. The finding of an increase in a wide range of growth factors suggests that no single factor acts directly but may be part of a cascade process that ultimately leads to the anomalies seen.

30.4.6 Pyloric Innervation

In keeping with the plethora of anomalies identified when looking at both hormonal control and intrinsic structural changes, the study of the neural control pathways has also turned up abnormal findings in many different aspects. Indeed more or less every component of the neural pathways studied has shown some degree of anomaly, making it difficult to determine the relative strength of each effect and to determine which may be a primary causative effect or a secondary phenomenon.

Among the earliest parts of the neural pathway to be studied were the ganglion cells. The recognition that the absence of ganglion cells in Hirschsprung's disease was responsible for the motility disturbances led to the further investigation of their role in the causation of pyloric stenosis [80, 81]. However, while some studies have reported fewer number [64, 67] or a failure of maturation [82] of ganglion cells in biopsies, these findings have not been confirmed by other groups [83]. Further structural anomalies have been found both within individual nerve cells and the supporting cells that maintain the integrity of the neural cells. In addition to identifying potential anomalies in the ganglion cells, Langer's [64] group also identified a decrease in the number of nerve cells, while further degenerative changes in the axons of these nerves have also been identified [84]. The entire neural network depends on a class of supporting cells that help both in the spatial orientation of the cells and in the physiologic functions [85]. In pyloric stenosis a number of studies have shown both quantitative and qualitative abnormalities in the morphology and function of this supporting network [65, 86, 87] suggesting that this in turn can have a deleterious effect on the innervation of the pylorus.

Another major part of this neural network that has a marked bearing on the proper functioning of the enteric nervous system is the interstitial cells of Cajal. This class of cell is recognised as providing an important role in both the mediation of neurotransmission and acting as electrical pacemakers [88, 89]. Results of studies looking at the role of these cells have shown some concordance. Using electron microscopy Langer [64] has shown a reduction in the presence of these cells compared to control specimens, a finding confirmed by other groups using immunoreactive staining [90, 91]. Given the central role of this class of cell in the regulation of GI motility it has been postulated that these may be crucial to the motility disturbance seen in pyloric stenosis [29]. However, it has been argued more recently that while this network of cells is an important facet of the control of GI motility it is too simplistic to see one system as the key factor [89].

As well as structural anomalies within the GI tract neural network, further anomalies at the synaptic junctions between the nerve cells and muscle cells and disorders of the synthesis and release of neurotransmitters at these junctions have been identified. Such anomalies vary from a decrease in the total number of synapses [92], to an indicator of a decreased expression of neural cell adhesion molecule at the muscular level [93] possibly leading to impaired functioning of the synapse.

Finally, studies have demonstrated anomalies in the cholinergic, [86] adrenergic [76] and peptidergic innervation of the pyloric muscle. In particular, compounds that help in the regulation of other neurotransmitters have found to be deficient including enkephalin [94], substance P [95] and vasoactive intestinal polypeptide [96].

The role of nitric oxide (NO) has been well documented. This is the neurotransmitter particularly related to non-adrenergic, non-cholinergic neural transmission (NANC) that has a recognised role in the mediation of pyloric relaxation [97]. The synthesis of this transmitter has been shown to be reduced in pyloric stenosis [90, 93]). In a specific mouse knockout model [98] those lacking the ability to synthesise NO were shown to have marked enlargement of the stomach with hypertrophy of the pyloric sphincter. Further studies on the role of NO immunoreactivity have shown it be decreased or absent in most though not all cases of pyloric stenosis [67, 99–101], and have also linked lack of NO synthesis to anomalies in ICC distribution, identifying a possible interdependency [29].

In short, the aetiology of the condition remains elusive yet the wide identification of potential causative factors at a pathological, physiological and molecular level points ever more firmly to the interplay between genetic and environmental factors in the causation of this condition.

30.5 Clinical Features

The clinical presentation follows a well recognised pattern, with a previously well child being noted to suffer from increasingly frequent and forceful vomiting. The majority of children will present between 4 and 6 weeks of age, though as many as 3% have been noted to occur within the neonatal period [1], with even isolated cases in the first few days of life. The frequency of presentation peters out at the older age range, and the condition is rare after 12 weeks of age [102]. The incidence in children who are born prematurely is similar to those born at term [103] and at least one study suggested that premature infants may present at a later stage than those born at term [104]. One case report of premature twins however showed that the condition can present while the children are still in the premature age range [105].

The vomiting, while intermittent at first, is noted to increase in frequency until it is occurring after every feed. In a similar fashion, the intensity is described as becoming more forceful, until truly being recognised as projectile. It is this gradual onset and worsening of symptoms that can lead to several days delay in diagnosis of the child. It is the author's opinion though that if there is a family history of the condition, then the child should be reviewed earlier in the course of the condition.

The vomit consists of milk, which may appear relatively fresh if the vomiting occurs soon after feeding, or curdled, if the vomit occurs at a later time from the feeding episode. As the condition progresses and vomiting worsens the contents may contain more mucous than milk. Though occasionally being discoloured by altered blood especially if there is any occurrence of gastritis, the vomit never includes any bile.

The child feeds readily especially in the earlier stages. Delay in the recognition of condition can lead to an overall deterioration in the child's clinical condition, at which point they may become disinclined to feed as part of the spectrum of developing dehydration. While the majority of children present with only mild signs of dehydration, there will be those that present more severely affected, with noticeable decrease in skin turgor, sunken fontanelle and sunken eyes.

While weight loss is also seen in some cases, it is perhaps more recognised as a gradual falling off of the expected weight gain. Given this corrects quite quickly after successful treatment then this may be more related to the degree of dehydration rather than true loss of subcutaneous fat.

30.6 Diagnosis

30.6.1 Clinical Examination

The diagnosis is largely suggested by the occurrence of the history described above, and is supported by the findings on clinical examination.

The abdominal examination remains the keystone to the diagnosis of IHPS. If performed appropriately, the palpation of the pyloric tumor has been reported as having a highly positive predictive value [106, 107].

The description given in the previous edition of this book [1] succinctly describes the conditions required to achieve maximum diagnostic yield. The child should have the abdomen exposed so that the examiner can view the area from the lower chest to upper thighs (Fig. 30.1) and should be nursed comfortably, preferably on the mother's lap. There needs to be a good (and if

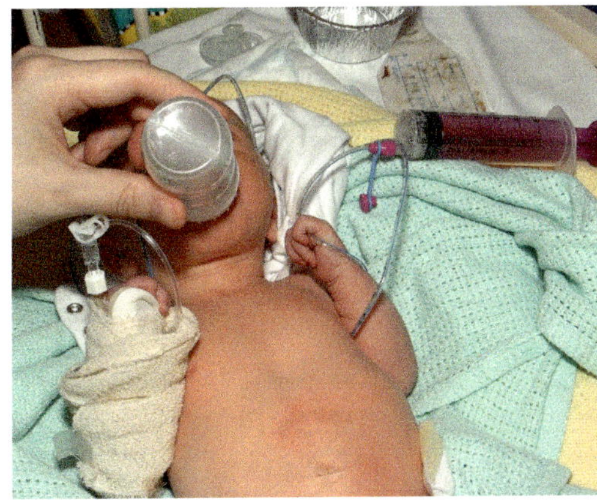

Fig. 30.1 Demonstration of required exposure of infant

possible) natural light shining tangentially on the abdomen. The feed would normally consist of clear fluid, though the actual contents may vary from dextrose to electrolyte solutions. Observation of how the infant feeds can provide the clinician with useful ancillary information, such as inappropriate feeding techniques or whether the infant is apathetic or feeds hungrily, possibly with the swallowing of excess air.

The clinician should inspect the abdomen from the left side looking for a developing fullness in the epigastrium, consistent with the filling stomach. As the stomach continues to distend, visible peristalsis will be seen to develop with the wave spreading from upper left toward the lower right side of the abdomen, before disappearing.

The pyloric tumor is described as having the size and shape as to be consistent with an olive and should be palpable to the right side of the rectus muscle. An initial palpation should start at the transpyloric plane (lying between the tips of the ninth costal cartilages). At this point, one is likely to feel the edge of the liver or possibly even the fullness of the caudate lobe. Working gently below the liver at this point will take the careful examiner to the area where the pyloric tumor can most easily be felt (Fig. 30.2).

It should be noted that this technique can take some time to complete, and indeed may even need to be repeated to confirm the diagnosis. Yet careful and persistent clinical examination will reward the clinician with a positive diagnosis. While it has been recommended that continuous nasogastric suction be employed to aid the diagnosis [108], the author has never found this to be necessary in his own practice.

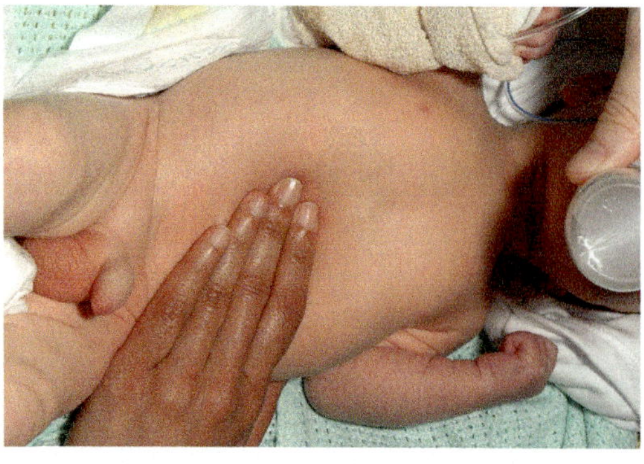

Fig. 30.2 Palpation for the pyloric olive

The pyloric 'olive' is reported to be palpable in approximately 80% of cases [109] and the finding of a palpable tumor has a positive predictive value as high as 99% [106, 107, 110]. There is growing evidence, however, that a rise in the routine use of ultrasound examination is diminishing the confidence with which clinicians will make the diagnosis on clinical grounds alone. In one study [111] the cases diagnosed by clinical means alone fell from 87 to 49% between two study periods separated by 11 years. Indeed in a review of cases from Alder Hey [110] as many as 39% did not have a test feed, the diagnosis being made solely on a positive ultrasound and clinical symptoms. This reported reliance on investigative modalities over clinical examination is not new however. Scharli, in reviewing a large single institution series [109], lamented the fact that of the 254 children undergoing contrast radiological examination, 154 did not require it as the clinical diagnosis was not in doubt. Indeed Cook [1] felt that the triad of visible peristalsis, a palpable pyloric tumor and projectile vomiting was proof positive of the diagnosis.

30.6.2 Biochemistry

A further mainstay in making the diagnosis is the search for specific biochemical abnormalities. As noted, these children present with a variable length of history of vomiting and poor feeding, both of which contribute to a deranged biochemical picture. The losses from the stomach will contain sodium, potassium and hydrochloric acid, leading to the typical picture of hypokalaemic, hypochloraemic metabolic alkalosis, though the individual values quoted may vary from centre to centre due to different reference ranges [7]. In the more severe cases paradoxical aciduria may also be observed as there is an attempt to conserve sodium at the expense of losing hydrogen ions despite metabolic alkalosis [1]. Though described as classic picture it is by no means universal and indeed in the series from this institution reported in 2008 [110] only 55% of cases had evidence of metabolic alkalosis. It may be that a trend to earlier presentation and diagnosis is limiting the degree of biochemical derangement that occurs.

30.6.3 Radiology

In those cases where clinical examination leaves diagnostic doubt then the radiological investigation of choice is now an abdominal ultrasound examination. The routine use in the investigation of pyloric stenosis was first described by Teele and Smith [112], and, as has been alluded to above, it has become the first line investigation of choice for many clinicians. It is a safe, non-invasive technique that, with appropriately trained and experienced operators, can give figures for sensitivity and specificity approaching 100% [113–115]. Over the years different groups have tried to refine the diagnostic criteria moving from initial simple measurements of canal length [116], to the creation of a muscle index [117], but there is no one accepted method. In Alder Hey we use a combination of canal length ≥14 mm and a muscle thickness of ≥4 mm to consider the diagnosis to be positive and with this have demonstrated a positive predictive value of 99.1% for length and 98.7% for muscle thickness [110] (Fig. 30.3).

The place of contrast radiology has, by and large, been consigned to history, though as an investigatory modality it can still find a place in cases of diagnostic doubt to rule out other pathologies (Gastro-oesophageal reflux; other causes of outlet obstruction). Various features have been described as diagnostic including finding a large gastric residue, vigorous peristalsis and a 'string sign' [118]. Again the technique has been felt to be operator dependent but in experienced hands could give sensitivity as high as 95% [119]. This modality is now only used sparingly due to the large dose of radiation that is required and the fact that the results may be either unhelpful or frankly misleading [119, 120].

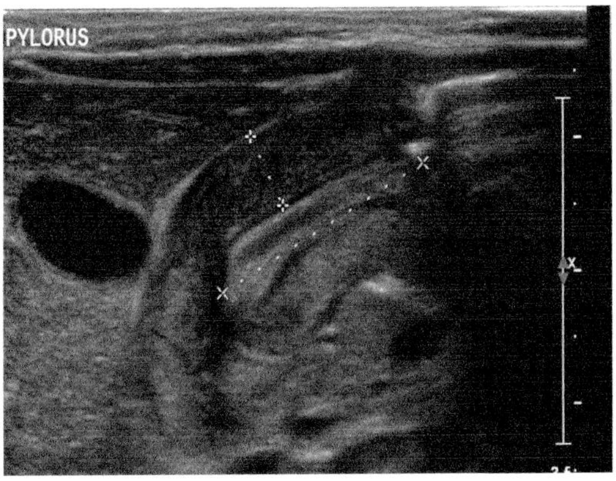

Fig. 30.3 Ultrasound of pyloric tumor

30.6.4 Other Diagnostic Testing

Despite the utility and accuracy of ultrasonographic diagnosis there are still cases when the diagnosis is in doubt and if repeated examination is still not diagnostic it has been the authors practice to undertake an upper GI endoscopy with a view to proceeding to pyloromyotomy if obstruction is confirmed. On two occasions, this has prevented a laparotomy by identifying marked antral gastritis. In both cases the symptoms resolved on medical management. Endoscopy is recognised in other series as a useful adjunct to making the diagnosis [121, 122].

Other modalities to look at the emptying of the stomach have been tried and a technique of measuring electrical resistance to derive an index of stomach emptying 'Applied Potential Tomography' (APT) was shown to provide comparable results to scintigraphy [123]. In one study [124] on a group of infants with pyloric stenosis it was able to demonstrate a significant delay in gastric emptying from a control group. However given the more widespread availability of ultrasound and the improvements over the years in scanning equipment this was never likely to find a widespread application.

30.7 Management

The mainstay of management of this condition remains operative correction following appropriate and adequate pre-operative preparation of the child.

30.7.1 Pre-operative

The condition of pyloric stenosis does not need emergency surgery and time spent adequately resuscitating the child will reduce the likelihood of anaesthetic complications, such as delayed recovery from anaesthesia or even post-operative apnoea [103, 125]. The purpose of resuscitation is to restore the extracellular fluid volume (ECFV) and restore the proper balance of Na^+ and Cl^- to allow for renal correction of the metabolic alkalosis [104]. The preferred fluid therapy in this institution is 0.45% saline with 5% dextrose for maintenance fluid. The actual rate is based on the estimated maintenance of 120 mls/kg/day with an upward adjustment made to correct for the estimated dehydration deficit. Potassium is added to the maintenance fluid, once it has been established that the baby is passing urine, at a maximum value of 3 mmol/kg/day. We would use normal saline to replace any further nasogastric loss, and, in the small number of cases in which dehydration is so severe as to require the use of fluid boluses.

Ongoing monitoring of the child includes an assessment of the state of hydration, evidence of urine output and 12 hourly measurement of blood gases until the alkalosis is corrected. When surgeon and anaesthetist are happy with the clinical state of the baby then arrangements are made for operative correction. Though it is recognised that many babies are now presenting with only minimal signs of dehydration and lesser degrees of biochemical derangement [110, 126], it may yet take 24—48 hrs of fluid therapy before the child is ready for theatre, and in some cases even longer. If there appears to be delayed correction of the abnormality despite adequate fluid therapy consideration should be given to whether there is underlying renal pathology contributing to the clinical picture.

30.7.2 Operative Considerations

The operative management of IHPS was described in 1892 by Cordua [127] who carried out a jejunostomy on a child, who unfortunately did not survive the procedure. The first successful operation described was a gastroenterosotmy carried out by Loebker in 1898, and the first description of a pyloroplasty followed closely in 1903 [128]. Pyloromyotomy was proposed by Dufour and Fredet in [3], but subsequently developed and implemented by Ramstedt in 1912 [4]. This approach of splitting the muscle layer, down to but not through the mucosa of the pyloric canal without suturing, is now the standard technique for operative intervention.

Historically, the initial approaches were either through high midline or pararectal incisions due to a fear of wound dehiscence in malnourished babies, but as pre-operative resuscitation improved the general condition of the children and improvements in anaesthetic techniques were introduced, so these concerns receded. The standard approach in many centres was the use of a transverse incision in the right upper quadrant directly overlying the pylorus [1]. In 1986 Tan and Bianchi [129] published their results of using a circumbilical incision to approach the pylorus, showing this to be an acceptable method of accessing the pylorus and producing a superior cosmetic result. Though in the original paper, the abdomen was originally opened in the midline through the linea alba, [130, 131] many surgeons (including the senior author on that original paper) utilise a transverse muscle cutting approach to enter the abdomen. This is currently the preferred approach at Alder Hey (Fig. 30.4).

Though the cosmetic results are acknowledged as superior, there have been concerns

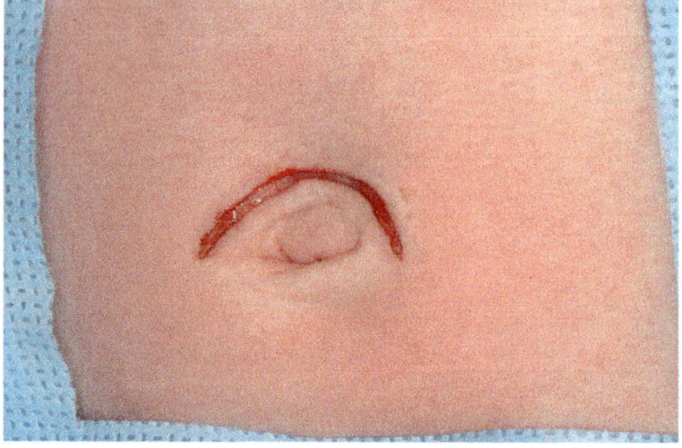

Fig. 30.4 Site of 'circumbilical incision'

raised about the possibility of increased rates of complications including wound infections, incisional hernias or mucosal perforations [132]. This concern has not been replicated in other studies [133–135].

Whatever the approach to the abdominal cavity, the basic tenets of the pyloromyotomy remain the same. The greater curve of the stomach is often the first aspect encountered and is carefully delivered in to the wound. This can then be traced distally to allow identification and extrusion of the pyloric tumor. Care must be taken in this delivery as over enthusiastic traction on the stomach can lead to damage to the antrum. A common cause of difficulty is trying to perform the operation through too small an incision, and enlargement of both skin and muscle incisions may be necessary to facilitate easy delivery of the tumor. It is straightforward to recognise the extent of the pathological thickening at the distal end as there is a sharp demarcation between the abnormal thickened pylorus and the duodenum, though at the proximal margin there may be a more gradual change from antrum to pylorus (Fig. 30.5).

A longitudinal incision is then made in the anterior border of the pylorus avoiding the blood vessels identified there. Distally this should stop at the sharp demarcation with the duodenum but proximally should be carried on to the antrum to ensure that the full extent of the pylorus has been identified. The incision is then deepened using blunt dissection to reach the level of the mucosa at the midpoint. There are various ways that this incision can be deepened and each surgeon has their own preference; use of blunt dissectors, arterial clips or even specially constructed pyloric spreaders. The ultimate aim however is to achieve disruption of the full extent of the pyloric muscle without causing a breach of the mucosa (Fig. 30.6).

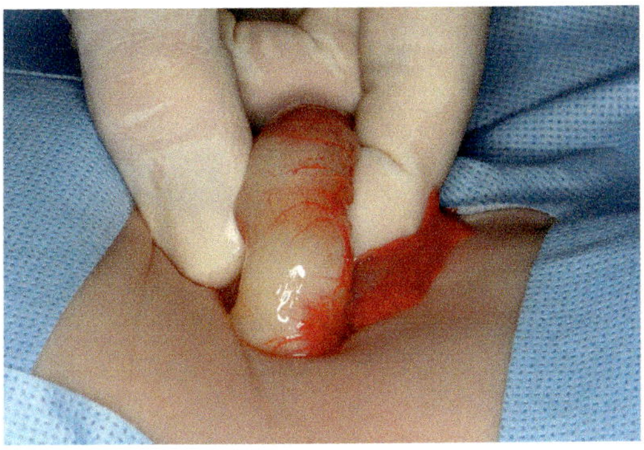

Fig. 30.5 Delivery of 'olive'

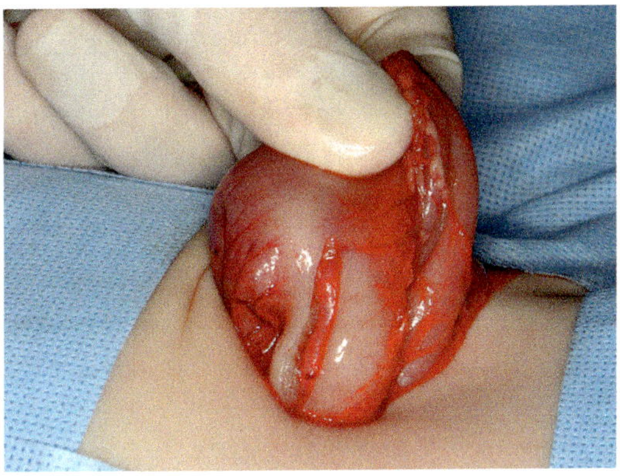

Fig. 30.6 Muscle split to demonstrate mucosa bulging

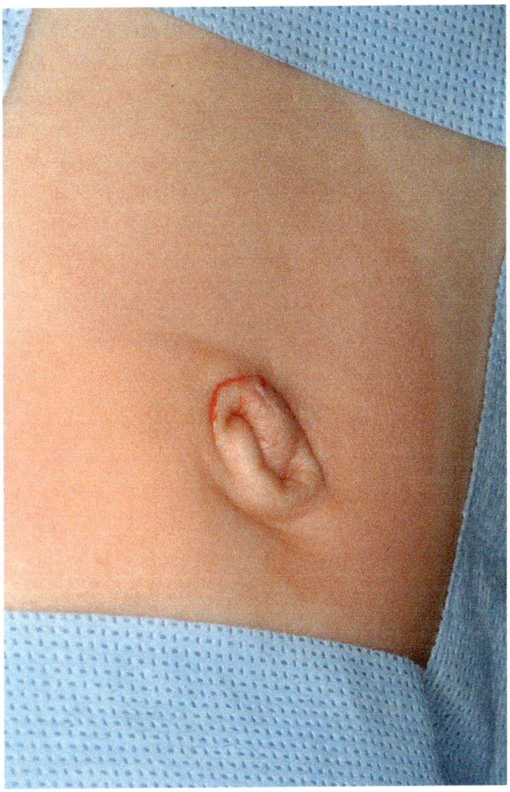

Fig. 30.7 Post-operative appearance

To ensure completeness of the procedure and confirm the integrity of the mucosa, a 'leak-test' can be performed. In this, the anaesthetist is asked to insufflate air into the stomach via the nasogastric tube, and the surgeon then causes the air to be passed form the antrum into the duodenum. The mucosa is inspected to watch for it bulging as the air passes and palpation of the duodenum confirms passage into the duodenum. Breaches in the mucosa can be spotted with this technique, though some surgeons will augment this by instilling saline to the cut surface of the pylorus and looking for bubbles being released during the passage of air.

After aspiration of any remaining air in the stomach, the stomach and pylorus are returned to the abdomen. Though there is occasionally oozing from the cut surface of the pyloric muscle this is usually minimal and will cease once the pylorus is returned to the abdomen.

Closure is carried out in a standard fashion, with my own practice being to close the muscle in two layers using continuous absorbable sutures, followed by a subcuticular absorbable suture for the skin (Fig. 30.7).

While open operation remains the standard practice in many centres, the growing use of laparoscopy has seen this become the standard approach for many. The first reported cases treated via a laparoscopic approach were published in 1991 [136], and subsequent larger series have shown both the efficacy and safety of this approach to pyloromyotomy [133, 134].

30.7.3 Postoperative Management

A further area where there is a divergence of opinion is around the use of a post-operative feeding regime. In many centres and going back some time, there was strict adherence to a specific feeding regime [1] and many units still have their own versions that people abide by. This may commence anywhere from a few hours to even a full day after surgery, and in these regimens there is a gradual increase in volume at every feed and a switch from clear fluid to milk over time. The rationale for this has previously been related to a concern over prolonged gastric stasis [137], with the belief that this graduated approach to feeding decreases the incidence of post-operative vomiting. However, one randomised controlled trial [138] identified that the risk of post-operative emesis was independent of the type of feeding. Observational studies [139, 140] have shown no or only little effect when an accelerated feeding regime is used. Overall there is little evidence to support the use of a specific restriction in post-operative feeding. Once full oral feeding is established the child is ready for discharge.

30.7.4 Outcomes and Complications

The outcomes for pyloromyotomy are generally good with most series reporting zero or minimal mortality and low morbidity for the procedure. This is in contrast to an historical series where, even as recent as the late 1930s, mortality rates as high as 25% were being reported [141]. In the series tracing a single institution's results over a prolonged time period [109], the mortality showed a steady decrease from 13.2% in the period between 1912 and 1930, to 0.5% in the period between 1961 and 1967. Many of the deaths in that series were attributed to infections not directly related to the children's underlying pathology, but in the earlier time period, 7 of 27 deaths were attributed to dehydration and shock. In the latter time period, this cause of death had been eradicated. A review of studies reported from both paediatric and general surgical centres [142] confirmed that this trend had continued, with only one death reported in almost 3500 cases.

This low rate of mortality has meant that most papers focus almost exclusively on the morbidity of various procedures, with quite wide variations in reported outcomes. How much of this variation is due to differences in definition of the evaluation measures used in the various studies is not clear, as it can be difficult to ascertain the parameters used in sufficient detail to allow a comparison between studies.

The complications most reported on in the short term can be divided into those occurring intra-operatively and those in the post operative period.

30.7.5 Intra-operative Complications

The most significant intra-operative complication is that of duodenal perforation. This usually occurs at the junction between the thickened pylorus and the duodenal fornix where there is often a sharp demarcation between abnormal pylorus and normal duodenum. These are usually identified as a result of the 'leak-test' described above, but a number can be missed. The reported rates vary widely with Crabbe [142] calculating an average of 3.2% across specialist paediatric centres versus a rate of 15% in which the operations were performed by non-specialist surgeons. This variation has been highlighted in various studies [143, 144] and it has been postulated this is the effect of specific sub-specialty training. However at least one other study would suggest that it is more related to a case-volume effect [145]. In a review of 11,003 cases, this group identified a better outcome with both higher institutional case volume and higher individual surgeon case volume. This has re-inforced the notion that having protocols for management and ongoing review of surgical outcomes could provide equivalent results to transfer to a specific specialist centre for management. Furthermore, there are other studies showing that, provided the care is provided by appropriately trained staff, then services in district general hospitals can provide equivalent results to specialist centres [106]. This may be of particular importance where the provision of specialist service is limited or the distances for transfer are large [7].

There are only a few reported instances of perforation not being recognised at the time of the procedure [146, 147] that have led to adverse outcomes. It is accepted however, that while the approach to using a leak-test is widespread the test may provide false re-assurance [148]. It behoves the surgeon therefore to have a high index of suspicion for this complication in those cases that do not follow the expected post-operative course.

On recognition of a perforation there is general agreement that primary closure is the treatment of choice, though there is debate about the best way to approach this. The majority of studies, where an approach is identified, describe a primary suture of the perforation plus or minus the addition of an omental patch. An alternative is practised by some surgeons where the perforation is repaired by closure of the primary pyloromyotomy, and the operation completed by rotation of the pylorus and the performance of a secondary pyloromyotomy [149]. Both approaches were compared and contrasted in a series reported in 1995 [150]. No significant differences were found in the efficacy or safety of either procedure. It is the authors practice to opt for a simple primary closure with use of omentum if this is easily manipulated to the area.

There is a small but recognised risk of an incomplete pyloromyotomy being performed. Attention to the detail of the procedure described above should reduce this complication to a minimum, and ensuring free passage of air to the duodenum with observation of both distension of the mucosa of the pylorus and of the distal duodenum should help ensure an adequate pyloromyotomy. However in different reported series the rate varies from less than 1% [106] to as much as 5.6% [151]. In a survey undertaken in the UK in 1995 the overall incidence of incomplete pyloromyotomy was reported as 1% [152]. Though no specific studies of this complication have been undertaken, there are a number of factors that could lead to this, including failure to carry the incision sufficiently proximal onto the gastric antrum, concern over the risk of perforation at the distal extent of the thickened pylorus, or sufficient exposure of the full extent of the tumor either through an open or a laparoscopic approach.

A final intra-operative problem to consider is that of a negative laparotomy. Many studies have not specifically looked at this as an issue but a recent review of practice from our own institution [110] identified that four cases out of a total of 343 underwent a negative exploration. Three of the cases had a positive ultrasound diagnosis (albeit performed at different institutions prior to transfer), and one a positive contrast study.

Prompted by this review, our institutional policy has been revised to ensure that if there is not clear evidence of a positive test-feed and an in-house ultrasound examination identifying specific diagnostic criteria, then operation is not undertaken.

30.7.6 Post-operative

The most commonly reported post-operative complication is that of wound infection. The risk of post-operative infection varies markedly between series [142], with some reporting no post operative infections [153], to other series reporting rates as high as 15% [154, 155]. In the studies reviewed by Crabbe [142] there appears to be a lower rate of infection across all the series reported from paediatric surgical centres compared to series coming from non-specialist centres, with an average difference of 2.2 vs. 9.8%. Though this could be related to differences in the definition of wound infection and the reporting policies, this in itself is unlikely to account for such a marked difference. Of particular interest is those series from paediatric centres that have reported their institutional results comparing the traditional RUQ approach to a circumbilical approach [130, 132, 156]. Each demonstrated a rise in the infection rate when the circumbilical approach has been used. Overall, the collected series quoted [142] have identified a rise from 2.2% with the ‘conventional ‘approach to 9.2% with the circumbilical approach. It has been suggested that this rate can be reduced by the use of prophylactic antibiotics but one study [157] identified that there was no difference in rate of infection related to the use of prophylactic antibiotics. Moreover this study also showed that majority of infants had umbilical colonisation with gut and skin flora and thus contamination at skin level was not necessarily the source of the wound infections identified. The policy in our own institution is to use a single dose of prophylactic antibiotic at the time of induction, and in a postal survey of UK centres [158] 70% of surgeons who used the circumbilical route advocated the use of prophylactic antibiotics. It has been postulated that the higher rate of infection may be related to the difficulty that can be faced in delivering the pylorus through a wound that has not been made sufficiently large, [142] and indeed at least one published study has advocated taking an approach to manage the pyloromyotomy without delivery through the wound and shown a minimal infection rate [159]. In a review of results from our own institution [160] where the circumbilical route has been used since the mid-90s, the overall infection rate was 3.2%, though no infection led to an increase in hospital stay or delay to discharge.

In general, studies on the use of a laparoscopic approach have shown the same or slightly lower incidence of wound infection, but in the majority of reviews this has not shown a significant difference [161–163]. One review did show a reduction in wound infection that was felt to be significant [164], though a subsequent commentary on the methodology used [165] counselled caution in the interpretation of the results citing concerns over sample size and the quality of the overall process of analysis. A further study looked to analyse the impact of using prophylactic antibiotics in laparoscopic pyloromyotomy [166] but this showed no significant difference in the groups with an overall rate of infection of 3%.

As laparoscopy has become more widely available, much of the recent literature has focussed on looking for potential benefits to this technique over open approaches. Different studies have been carried out varying from reporting practice in single centres [162] to reviews of studies and even meta-analysis [161]. Early papers looking at the technique tended to show an increase in length of operation and the risk of incomplete pyloromyotomy, but more recent papers have shown no difference in these parameters. This suggests that once the learning-curve effect has been overcome the technique is both safe and effective. The overall evidence of benefit is lacking in that while some studies will show benefits in some of the parameters, others will not show any benefit from this approach. Though the evidence has so far failed to identify a convincing case for one approach over the other, the use of laparoscopy is both safe and effective and in centres that have both the appropriate experience and available equipment, this will likely be the operative method of choice.

Vomiting is a common finding in the immediate post-operative period and, as previously noted, the risk of vomiting has been used as the rationale for instituting specific feeding regimes. A study on motility [137] had identified disordered gastric peristalsis that may last up to 5 days and proposed this as the reason for vomiting, while at the same time identifying that specific feeding regimes had no influence on the incidence of vomiting. A further risk factor may be a prolonged pre-operative phase of vomiting [140] though it is felt that with earlier presentation most infants should tolerate early and accelerated feedings [7].

The long term sequelae are an area less studied over the years but the most comprehensive recent review occurs in Crabbe [142]. The pylorus heals by the normal processes of wound healing and ultimately there may be little evidence of an operative procedure [167]. There are anecdotal reports of persistence of the hypertrophied muscle in those cases treated by alternatives to surgical approaches [1]. Both radiological [168] and ultrasonographic [169, 170] techniques have been used to study the pyloric muscle in the post-operative period and have shown a gradual resolution of the muscle thickness back towards normal, with most achieving this by 12 weeks. The increase in length of the pyloric canal can persist beyond this time.

A number of studies in adults have reported on the incidence of dyspeptic symptoms in groups who had undergone pyloromyotomy [171–173], though both methodological problems and a reliance on contrast studies to seek out peptic ulcer disease have mitigated against being able to give a true figure for the incidence of ulcers in this group. Indeed in the one study that systematically looked to compare those patients who had had medical treatment for the condition, and a control group there were no significant differences in the occurrence of symptoms [174].

It has been postulated that the occurrence of dyspeptic symptoms may be related to effects on gastric emptying, and indeed in those studies that have used contrast radiology [172, 173]) they have indeed found delay in some of their subjects. However the use of contrast radiology has been shown to give inaccurate results, and in studies using both scintigraphy and ultrasonographic methods, [175–177] no differences have been found as a result of pyloromyotomy.

There have however been case reports relating to prolonged retention of swallowed foreign bodies, particularly coins in children who have had pyloromyotomy [178]. Indeed the author has had a similar case himself and would concur with the advice to remove these coins endoscopically.

30.8 Other Treatment Options

The mainstay of management for almost 100 years now has been the successful use of an operative approach whether by an open or laparoscopic method. An alternative interventional approach has been reported on in studies from Japan [179, 180]. Here, balloon dilatation of the pylorus can be undertaken via an endoscopic technique, analogous to that with oesophageal strictures. However this may be associated with a higher perforation rate and non-resolution of symptoms, and so is unlikely to displace the use of traditional interventions.

Prior to the establishment of the Ramstedt procedure however, medical management was the main approach and is still reported on in some studies from more recent times. In the early twentieth century the treatment was based on trying to maintain feeding regimes until the eventual resolution of the condition [181, 182, 183] though the success was not great. The introduction of an oral form of atropine was reported to give improved success [183] though it was recognised that intensive and prolonged nursing care was required [184].

A number of studies from Japan have identified that the use of atropine as a primary treatment along with both fluid and nutritional support have been effective in managing the condition [186, 187, 188]. The studies have shown success with the use of a regime of intravenous followed by oral atropine. Here though, the in-patient stay was significantly longer than a comparable group undergoing surgery [185] and the total course of treatment was on average 3 months after initial diagnosis. This alone would call into question the economic benefit of the procedure. Yet, given it can be successful and with no reported side-effects, it is a strategy that could be used in children who for varied reasons may not be appropriate for surgical intervention.

30.9 Other Causes of Outlet Obstruction

In contrast to the relatively common occurrence of pyloric stenosis, other causes of gastric outlet obstruction are rare and constitute a diverse and varied range of pathologies.

The most readily recognised pathology would be related to atresia of the pyloric canal. Like other forms of intestinal atresia three distinct types are recognised [188, 189]. Type 1 where there is continuity of the wall but a membrane or web obstructs the lumen, Type 2 in which the pyloric canal is replaced by a thickened cord or type 3 where there is complete separation of the ends.

The incidence is reported as 1:100,000 live births [190]. While many are sporadic cases, there is an association with epidermolysis bullosa (EB), [191] though it is difficult to be clear from the literature just what percentage of cases have the two conditions. Moore [192] published a review which identified 125 cases of gastric outlet obstruction, of which only 18 were also reported to have EB. Both these conditions are inherited with an autosomal recessive pattern [193–195]. Yet other isolated cases have been found to have other intestinal atresias, and congenital cardiac lesions [196, 197].

The exact aetiology remains unclear but the prevailing theories of recanalization of solid organs [197, 198] or neonatal vascular accident [199] have been proposed as being the basic aetiology. However further arguments that there is no evidence of the stomach having ever been occluded [200] or that re-canalisation commences within the duodenum rather than the stomach [20] would mitigate against the re-canalisation theory. A further theory has been postulated that slippage of the epithelial layer may be responsible for the initiation of a diaphragm [201], but again further evidence is felt to be lacking. Work on the association with EB has provided some indirect evidence for this as a possible aetiology [195]. In essence abnormalities of the mucosal layer of the developing intestinal tract lead to the initiation of fibrosis and thus obstruction in narrow areas of the gut such as the pyloric canal. Whether this is the whole story is unclear. However, while there are studies that have shown an inflammatory component to the atretic segment [202] others have not [203].

The presentation tends to be within the neonatal period unless the web is incomplete or perforated. The clinical picture can resemble pyloric stenosis though the onset of vomiting is often earlier in the post gestational period and more progressive. The condition is often diagnosed by a straight abdominal X-Ray with the finding of a 'single bubble', but although this could be viewed as diagnostic, confirmatory evidence can be sought with an upper GI contrast. Treatment consists of managing the pre-operative condition of the child by correcting any electrolyte anomalies as would be required in the management of pyloric stenosis. The type of surgery is dependent on the anatomic variation encountered, and may include a simple pyloroplasty with excision of web, to a formal antroduodenectomy with anastomosis of stomach to duodenum (Bilroth Type I). The use of bypass operative procedures such as gastrojejunostomy is reported to have high failure rates and should be avoided if possible [188]. Overall results for isolated pyloric atresia are good with prompt recognition and treatment of the condition [193]. Mortality seems to be related to associated conditions or a delay in the operative treatment. While the addition of EB as a co-morbidity seemed to herald an almost universally poor prognosis in early published work [192, 203] the recognition that EB itself can have a variable prognosis does not preclude the early recognition and aggressive surgical management of this condition.

A further sub-type related to atresia is the occurrence of a pre-pyloric membrane. Though this often presents in later life [204] previous studies have identified that it is a true congenital anomaly. Family studies have identified this as having a pattern of autosomal recessive inheritance [205]. The condition is amenable to surgical treatment with good results in the cases reported. Any deaths, as in the family series from Libya [205] seem to be related to other co-morbid conditions rather than as a result of the congenital anomaly.

Duplications of the stomach or pyloroduodenal canal are a rare cause of gastric outlet obstruction, which may present in the neonatal period or depending on site and size may present later in childhood [206, 207]. In a series from Philadelphia [208] they represented 8% of all intestinal duplication seen in that institution, though the majority presented beyond the neonatal period. The symptoms can be analogous to hypertrophic pyloric stenosis, but the condition can be distinguished on ultrasonographic and radiological examination by the lack of muscle hypertrophy and the finding of an obstructing lesion, often cystic in nature. In those children (and adults) who present beyond the neonatal period the symptoms more often relate to pain and vomiting or even hematemesis. In the series reported by Clement [206] six of the cases also had ectopic pancreatic tissue as part of the duplication cyst, and three of the cases in the Philadelphia series had a similar pathological finding [208]. The recommended treatment is surgical excision or resection depending on the precise anatomical arrangement of the cyst and the overall results of surgery are reported to be good.

An increasingly recognised cause of obstruction in neonates is related to bezoars. A review of the literature [209] noted that the majority were classed as lactobezoars and some 70% of the published cases occurred in the neonatal period. The aetiology was felt to be multifactorial but factors involved included prematurity and high medium chain triglyceride or casein concentrations in the milk formulae used. Prompt recognition was found to be helpful as it allowed conservative management to be successful, though in some cases, surgery was required secondary to gastric perforation, or non-resolution of symptoms. It should also be noted however that while the majority of reported cases are related to inappropriate milk formulation the use of apparently innocuous therapies can also lead to problems. Gaviscon is widely used for the treatment of reflux, even in neonates and there are reported cases of this also leading to symptoms of gastric outlet obstruction [210]. As with lacto bezoars, if this is promptly recognised then conservative management can be successful.

References

1. Cook RCM. Gastric Outlet Obstruction. In: Lister J, Irving IM, editors. Neonatal Surgery. 3rd ed. London: Butterworth; 1990. p. 403–20.
2. Hirschsprung H. Falle van angeborenen Pylorusstenose, beobachtet bei Saenlingen. Jb kinderheilk. 1888;28:61.
3. Dufour H, Fredet P. La sclerose hypertrophique du pylore chez le nourisson et son traitment chirugical. Rev Chir. 1908;27:208–53.
4. Ramstedt C. Zur operation de angeborenen pylorus stenose. Medsch Klin. 1912;8:1702.
5. Lawson D. The incidence of pyloric stenosis in Dundee. Arch Dis Child. 1951;26:616–7.
6. Dodge JA. Changing incidence of congenital pyloric stenosis. Br Med J. 1974;1:640.
7. Aspelund G, Langer JC. The current management of hypertrophic pyloric stenosis. Semin Pediatr Surg. 2007;16:27–33.
8. Laron Z, Horne LM. The incidence of infantile pyloric stenosis. Am J Dis Child. 1957;94:151–4.
9. Cremin BJ, Klein A. Infantile pyloric stenosis: a 10 year survey. S Afr Med J. 1968;42:1056–60.
10. Swan TT. Congenital pyloric stenosis in the African infant. Br Med J. 1961;1:545–7.
11. McMahon B. The continuing enigma of pyloric stenosis of infancy: a review. Epidemiology. 2006;17:195–201.
12. Kerr AM. Unprecedented rise in incidence of infantile hypertrophic pyloric stenosis. Br Med J. 1980;281:714–5.
13. Knox EG, Armstrong E, Haynes R. Changing incidence of infantile hypertrophic pyloric stenosis. Arch Dis Child. 1983;58:582–5.
14. Sommerfield T, Chalmers J, Youngson G, et al. the changing epidemiology of infantile hypertrophic pyloric stenosis. Arch. Dis. Child. 2008;93:1007–11.
15. Pedersen RN, Garne E, Loane M, et al. Infantile hypertrophic pyloric stenosis: a comparative study of incidence and other epidemiological characteristics in seven European regions. J Matern Fetal Neonatal Med. 2008;21:599–604.

16. Persson S, Ekbom A, Granath F, Nordenskjöld A. Parallel incidences of sudden infant death syndrome and infantile hypertrophic pyloric stenosis; a common cause? Pediatrics. 2001;108:379–81.
17. Stringer MA, Brereton RJ. Current management of infantile hypertrophic pyloric stenosis. Br J Hosp Med. 1990;43:266–72.
18. Jedd MB, Melton JL, Griffin MR, et al. Trends in infantile pyloric stenosis in Olmsted County, Minnesota. Pediatr Perinatol Epidemiol. 1988;2:148–57.
19. Puri P, Lakschmanadass G. Hypertrophic pyloric stenosis. In: Puri P, editor. Newborn Surgery. Oxford: Butterworth-Heinemann; 1996. p. 266–71.
20. Gray S, Skandalakis J. Anomalies of the stomach. In: Gray S, Skandalakis J, editors. Embryology for surgeons. Philadelphia: Saunders; 1972. p. 105–6.
21. Evans NJ. Pyloric stenosis in preterm infants after transpyloric feeding. Lancet. 1982;ii:665.
22. Thomson J. On congenital gastric spasm. Scot Med Surg. 1897;1:511.
23. Gabella G. Structure of muscle and nerves in the gastrointestinal tract. In: Johnson LR, editor. Physiology of the gastrointestinal tract. New York: Raven Press; 1994. p. 751–93.
24. Daniel EE, Tomita T, et al. Sphincters: normal function—changes in diseases. Boca Raton: CRC Press; 1992.
25. Armstrong G. An account of the diseases most incident to children from their birth to the age of puberty etc. London. 1777;
26. Everett KV, Capon F, et al. Linkage of monogenic infantile hypertrophic pyloric stenosis to chromosome 16q24. Eur J Hum Genet. 2008;16(9):1151–4.
27. Carter CO, Evans KA. Inheritance of congenital pyloric stenosis. J Med Genet. 1969;6:233–54.
28. Ohshiro K, Puri P. Pathogenesis of infantile hypertrophic pyloric stenosis: recent progress. Pediatr Surg Int. 1998;13:243–52.
29. Pantelli C. New insights into the pathogenesis of infantile pyloric stenosis. Pediatr Surg Int. 2009;25:1043–52.
30. Finsen VR. Infantile hypertrophic pyloric stenosis- unusual familial incidence. Arch Dis Child. 1979;54:720–1.
31. Garrow E, Hertzler J. Hypertrophic pyloric stenosis with jaundice: a case report of one family. J Pediat Surg. 1966;1:284–7.
32. Cockaigne EA, Penrose LS. Congenital pyloric stenosis in first cousins. Lancet. 1934;2:898.
33. Danzer E, Schier F, et al. Smith-Lemli-Opitz syndrome: case report and literature review. J Pediatr Surg. 2006;35:1840–2.
34. Jackson L, Kline AD, et al. de Lange syndrome: a clinical review of 310 individuals. Am J Med Genet. 1993;47:940–6.
35. Mitchell LE, Risch N. The genetics of infantile hypertrophic pyloric stenosis. A reanalysis. Am J Dis Child. 1991;147:1203–11.
36. Carter CO. Inheritance of congenital pyloric stenosis. Br Med Bull. 1961;17:251–4.
37. Capon F, Reece A, et al. Linkage of monogenic infantile hypertrophic pyloric stenosis to chromosome 16p12-p13 and evidence for genetic heterogeneity. Am J Hum Genet. 2006;79:378–82.
38. Everett KV, Chioza BA, et al. Genome-wide high density SNP-based linkage analysis of infantile hypertrophic pyloric stenosis identifies loci on chromosomes 11q14-q22 and Xq23. Am J Hum Genet. 2008;82:756–62.
39. Chung E, Curtis D, et al. Genetic evidence for the neuronal nitric oxidase synthase gene (NOS1) as a susceptibility locus for infantile pyloric stenosis. Am J Hum Genet. 1996;58:363–70.
40. Saur D, Vanderwinden JM, et al. Single nucleotide promoter polymorphism alters transcription of neuronal nitric oxide synthase exon 1c in infantile hypertrophic pyloric stenosis. Proc Natl Acad Sci U S A. 2004;101:1662–7.
41. Sorensen HT, Skriver MV, Pedersen L, et al. Risk of infantile hypertrophic pyloric stenosis after maternal postnatal use of macrolides. Scand J Infect Dis. 2003;35:104–6.
42. Webb AR, Lari J, Dodge JA. Infantile hypertrophic pyloric stenosis in South Glamorgan 1970-9. Effects of changes in feeding practice. Arch Dis Child. 1983;58:586–90.
43. Pisacane A, de Luca U, et al. Breast feeding and hypertrophic pyloric stenosis: population based case-control study. Br Med J. 1996;312:745–6.
44. Latchaw LA, Jacir NN, et al. The development of pyloric stenosis during transpyloric feeding. J Pediatr Surg. 1989;24:823–4.
45. Muyaed R, Zaber K, Young DG, et al. Pyloric stenosis in sick premature infants. Lancet. 1984;ii:344–5.
46. Mahon BE, Rosenman MB, Kleiman MB. Maternal and infant use of erythromycin and other macrolide antibiotics as risk factors for infantile hypertrophic pyloric stenosis. J Pediatr. 2000;139:380–4.
47. Hauben M, Amsden GW. The association of erythromycin and infantile hypertrophic pyloric stenosis: causal or coincidental? Drug Saf. 2002;25:929–42.
48. Patole S, Rao S, Doherty D. Erythromycin as a prokinetic agent in preterm neonates: a systematic review. Arch Dis Child Fetal Neonatal Ed. 2005;90:F301–6.
49. Fisher R, Lipshutz W, Cohen S. The hormonal regulation of pyloric sphincter function. J Clin Invest. 1973;52:1289–96.
50. Dodge JA. Production of duodenal ulcers and hypertrophic pyloric stenosis by the administration of pentagastrin to pregnant and newborn dogs. Nature. 1970;225:284–5.
51. Janik JS, Akbar AM, Burrington JD. The role of gastrin in congenital hypertrophic pyloric stenosis. J Pediatr Surg. 1978;13:151–4.
52. Spitz L, Zail S. Serum gastrin level congenital hypertrophic pyloric stenosis. J Pediatr Surg. 1976;11:33–5.

53. Wesley JR, Fiddian-Green R, Roi LD. The effects of pyloromyotomy on serum and luminal gastrin in infants with hypertrophic pyloric stenosis. J Surg Res. 1980;20:533–8.
54. Hambourg MA, Mignon M, Ricour C. Serum gastrin levels in hypertrophic pyloric stenosis in infancy. Am J Dis Child. 1979;54:208–12.
55. Grockowski J, Szafran H, Sztetkok K, et al. Blood serum immunoreactive gastrin level in infants with hypertrophic pyloric stenosis. J Pediatr Surg. 1980;15:279–82.
56. Rogers IM, Drainer IK, et al. Plasma gastrin in congenital hypertrophic pyloric stenosis. A hypothesis disproved. Arch Dis Child. 1975;50:467–71.
57. Rogers IM, Drainer IK, et al. Serum cholecystokinin, basal acid secretion and infantile pyloric stenosis. Arch Dis Child. 1979;54:774–5.
58. Rogers IM. The true cause of pyloric stenosis is hyperacidity. Acta Paediatr. 2006;95:132–6.
59. Wada T, Ishizawa M. Effects of prostaglandins on the function of the gastric secretion. Jpn J Clin Med. 1970;28:2465–8.
60. La Ferla G, Watson J, et al. The role of prostaglandins E2 and F2 alpha in infantile hypertrophic pyloric stenosis. J Pediatr Surg. 1986;21:410–312.
61. Goyal RK, Mukhopadhyay A, Rattan S. Effect if prostaglandin E2 on the lower esophageal sphincter in normal subjects and patients with achalasia. Clin Res. 1974;22:358A.
62. Shinohara K, Shimizu T, et al. Correlation of prostaglandin E2 production and gastric acid secretion in infants with hypertrophic pyloric stenosis. J Pediatr Surg. 1998;33:1483–5.
63. Dieler R, Schroder GM, et al. Infantile hypertrophic pyloric stenosis : myopathic type. Acta Neuropathol. 1990;80:295–306.
64. Langer JC, Berezin I, et al. Hypertrophic pyloric stenosis: ultrastructural abnormalities of enteric nerves and the interstitial cells of Cajal. J Pediatr Surg. 1995;30:1535–43.
65. Guarino N, Shima H, et al. Structural immaturity of the pylorus muscle in infantile hypertrophic pyloric stenosis. Pediatr Surg Int. 2000;16:282–4.
66. Gentile C, Romeo C, et al. A possible role of the plasmalemnal cytoskeleton, nitric oxide synthetase, and innervation in infantile hypertrophic pyloric stenosis. A confocal laser scanning microscope study. Pediatr Surg Int. 1998;14:45–50.
67. Belding HH, Kernohan JW. A morphological study of the myenteric plexus with special reference to changes in hypertrophic pyloric stenosis. Surg Gynecol Obstet. 1953;97:323–34.
68. Alarotu H. The histopathologic changes in the myenteric plexus of the pylorus in hypertrophic pyloric stenosis of infants (pylorospasm). Act Paediatr Scan. 1956;45(Suppl 107):1–131.
69. Cass DT, Zhang AL. Extracellular matrix changes in congenital hypertrophic pyloric stenosis. Pediatr Surg Int. 1991;6:190–4.
70. Oue T, Puri P. Abnormalities of elastin and elastic fibres in infantile hypertrophic pyloric stenosis. Pediatr Surg Int. 1999;15:540–2.
71. Miyazaki E, Yamataka T, et al. Active collagen synthesis in infantile hypertrophic pyloric stenosis. Pediatr Surg Int. 1998;13:237–9.
72. Weinstein R, Stemmerma MB, Maciag T. Hormoanl requirements for growth of arterial smooth muscle cells in vitro: an endocrine approach to atherosclerosis. Science. 1981;212:818.
73. Han VKM, D'Ercole AJ, Lund PK. Cellular localization of somatomedin (insulin-like growth factor) messenger RNA in the human fetus. Science. 1987;236:193–7.
74. Czech M. Structural and functional homologies in the receptors for insulin and the insulin-like growth factors. Cell. 1982;31:8–10.
75. Ohshiro K, Puri P. Increased insulin-like growth factor –I mRNA expression in pyloric muscle in infantile hypertrophic pyloric stenosis. Pediatr Surg Int. 1998;13:253–5.
76. Ohshiro K, Puri P. Increased insulin-like growth factor and platelet-derived growth factor system in the pyloric muscle in infantile hypertrophic pyloric stenosis. J Pediatr Surg. 1998;33:378–81.
77. Jablonski J, Gawronska R, et al. Study of insulin-like growth factor-1 (IGF-1) and platelet-derived endothelial cell growth factor(PDEGF) expression on children with infantile hypertrophic pyloric stenosis. Med Sci Monit. 2006;12:CR27–30.
78. Shima H, Puri P. Increased expression of transforming growth factor-alpha in infantile hypertrophic pyloric stenosis. Pediatr Surg Int. 1999;15:198–200.
79. Shima H, Oshiro K, et al. Increased local synthesis of epidermal growth factors in infantile hypertrophic pyloric stenosis. Pediatr Res. 2000;47:201–7.
80. Meeker CS, de Nicola RR. Hypertrophic pyloric stenosis in a newborn infant. J Pediatr. 1948;33:94–7.
81. Friesen SR, Boley JO, Miller DR. The myenteric plexus of the pylorus. Surgery. 1956;39:21–9.
82. Rintoul JR, Jirkham NF. The myenteric plexus in infantile pyloric stenosis. Arch Dis Child. 1961;36:474–80.
83. Tam PKH. Observations and perspectives on the possible aetiology of infantile pyloric stenosis: a histological, biochemical, histochemical and immunochemical study. Ann Acad Med Singap. 1985;14:523–9.
84. Jona JZ. Electron microscopic observations in infantile hypertrophic pyloric stenosis. J Pediatr Surg. 1978;13:17–20.
85. Sugimura K, Haimoto H, Nagura H, et al. Immunohistochemical differential distribution of S-100a and S-100β in the peripheral nervous system of the rat. Muscle Nerve. 1989;12:919–35.
86. Kobyashi H, O'Briain DS, et al. Selective reduction in intramuscular nerve supporting cells in infantile hypertrophic pyloric stenosis. J Pediatr Surg. 1994;29:651–4.

87. Guarino N, Yoneda A, et al. Selective neurotrophin deficiency in infantile hypertrophic pyloric stenosis. Pediatr Surg Int. 2001;36:1280–4.
88. Thuneberg L. Interstitial cells of Cajal: intestinal pacemaker cells. Adv Anat Embryol Cell Biol. 1982;71:1–130.
89. Huizinga JD, Lammers WJ. Gut peristalsis is governed by a multitude of co-operating mechanisms. Am J Physiol Gastrointest Liver Physiol. 2009;296(1):G1–8.
90. Vanderwinden JM, Liu H, et al. Study of the interstitial cells of Cajal in infantile hypertrophic pyloric stenosis. Gastroenterology. 1996;111:279–88.
91. Yamataka A, Fujiwara T, et al. Lack of intestinal pacemaker (C-KIT-positive) cells in infantile hypertrophic pyloric stenosis. J Pediatr Surg. 1996;31:96–8.
92. Okazaki T, Yamataka A, et al. Abnormal distribution of synaptic vesicle proteins in infantile hypertrophic pyloric stenosis. J Pediatr Gastroenterol Nutr. 1994;18:254–5.
93. Kobyashi H, O'Briain DS, et al. Immunochemical characterisation of neural cell adhesion molecule (NCAM), nitric oxide synthase, and neurofilament protein expression in pyloric muscle of patients with pyloric stenosis. J Pediatr Gastroenterol Nutr. 1995;20:319–25.
94. Malmfors G, Sundler F. Peptidergic innervation in infantile hypertrophic pyloric stenosis. J Pediatr Surg. 1986;21:303–6.
95. Wattchow DA, Cass DT, et al. Abnormalities of peptide containing nerve fibers in infantile hypertrophic pyloric stenosis. Gastroenterology. 1987;92: 443–8.
96. Shen Z, She Y, et al. Immunohistochemical study of peptidergic nerves in infantile hypertrophic pyloric stenosis. Pediatr Surg Int. 1990;5:110–3.
97. Blut H, Boeckxstaens GE, Pelckmans PA, et al. Nitric oxide as an inhibitory non-adrenergic noncholinergice neurotransmitter. Nature. 1990;345: 346–7.
98. Vanderwinden JM, Mailleux P, et al. Nitric oxide synthetase activity in infantile hypertrophic pyloric stenosis. N Engl J Med. 1992;327:511–5.
99. Huang PL, Dawson TM, et al. Targeted disruption of the neuronal nitric oxide synthase gene. Cell. 1993;75:1273–86.
100. Huang LT, Tiao MM, et al. Low plasma nitrite in infantile pyloric stenosis patients. Dig Dis Sci. 2006;51:869–72.
101. Subramanian R, Doig CM, et al. Nitric oxide synthase is absent only on a subset of cases of pyloric stenosis. J Pediatr Surg. 2001;36:616–9.
102. Rendle-Short J, Zachary RB. Congenital pyloric stenosis in older babies. Arch Dis Child. 1955;30:70–1.
103. Spicer RD. Infantile pyloric stenosis: a review. Br J Surg. 1982;69:128–35.
104. Bissonette B, Sullivan PJ. Pyloric stenosis. Can J Anaesth. 1991;38(5):668–76.
105. Read HS, Wyatt JP, Lamont GL, et al. Pyloric stenosis in preterm twins. J R Coll Surg Edinb. 1994;39:187–8.
106. White JS, Clements WDB, Heggarty P, et al. Treatment of infantile hypertrophic pyloric stenosis in a district general hospital: a review of 160 cases. J Pediatr Surg. 2003;38:1333–6.
107. Irish MS, Pearl RH, Caty MG, et al. The approach to common abdominal diagnoses in infants and children. Pediatr Clin N Am. 1998;45:729–72.
108. Toyama WM. Infantile hypertrophic pyloric stenosis (an improved technique for diagnosis). Am J Surg. 1969;117:650–2.
109. Scharli AF, Sieber WK, Kiesewetter WB. Hypertrophic pyloric stenosis at the Children's Hospital of Pittsburg from 1912 to 1967. A critical review of current problems and complications. J Pediatr Surg. 1969;4:108–14.
110. Mullassery D, Mallappa S, Shariff S, et al. Negative exploration for pyloric stenosis – is it preventable? BMC Pediatr. 2008;8:37.
111. Macdessi J, Oates RK. Clinical diagnosis if pyloric stenosis: a declining art. Br Med J. 1993;306:553–5.
112. Teele RL, Smith EH. Ultrasound in the diagnosis of idiopathic hypertrophic pyloric stenosis. N Engl J Med. 1977;296:1149–50.
113. Strunden RJ, Le Quesne GW, Little KET. The improved ultrasound diagnosis of hypertrophic pyloric stenosis. Pediat Radiol. 1986;16:200–5.
114. Neilson D, Hollman AS. The ultrasonic diagnosis of infantile hypertrophic pyloric stenosis: technique and accuracy. Clin Radiol. 1994;49:246–7.
115. Godbole P, Sprigg A, Dickson JAS, et al. Ultrasound compared with clinical examination in infantile hypertrophic pyloric stenosis. Arch Dis Child. 1996;75:335–7.
116. Tunnell WP, Wilson DA. Pyloric stenosis: diagnosis by real time ultrasonography, the pyloric muscle length method. J Pediatr Surg. 1984;19:795–9.
117. Carver RA, Okorie M, Steiner GM, et al. Infantile hypertrophic pyloric stenosis- diagnosis from the pyloric muscle index. Clin Radiol. 1988;38:625–7.
118. Meuwissen T, Shoff J. Roentgen examination of the pyloric canal of infants with hypertrophic pyloric stenosis. Am J Dis Child. 1934;48:1304–15.
119. Hernanz-Schulman M, Sells LL, Ambrosino MM, et al. Hypertrophic pyloric stenosis in an infant without a palpable olive: accuracy of sonographic diagnosis. Radiology. 1994;193:771–6.
120. Larsen GL. Limitations of roentgenographic examination in the diagnosis of infantile hypertrophic pyloric stenosis. Surgery. 1966;60:768–72.
121. De Backer A, Bové T, Vandenplas Y, Peeters S, Deconinck P. Contribution of endoscopy to early diagnosis of hypertrophic pyloric stenosis. J Pediatr Gastroenterol Nutr. 1994;18:78–81.
122. Ward E, Easley D, Pohl J. Previously unsuspected infantile hypertrophic pyloric stenosis diagnosed by endoscopy. Dig Dis Sci. 2008;53:946–8.

123. Magnall YF, Baxter AJ, Avill R, et al. Applied potential tomography: a new non-invasive technique for assessing gastric function. Clin Phys Physiol Meas. 1987;8(Suppl A):63–70.
124. Lamont GL, Wright JW, Evans DF, et al. An evaluation of applied potential tomography in the diagnosis of infantile hypertrophic pyloric stenosis. Clin Phys Physiol Meas. 1988;9(Suppl A):65–9.
125. Todres DI, Firestone S. Neonatal emergencies. In: Ryan JF, Cot CJ, Todres DI, Goudsouzian N, editors. A practice of anesthesia for infants and children. Boston: Grune and Stratton Inc.; 1986. p. 152.
126. Benson CD, Lloyd JR. Infantile pyloric stenosis: a review of 1,120 cases. Am J Surg. 1964;107: 429–33.
127. Cordua E. Ein Fall von einem monstrosen Blindsac des Dickdarms. Goettingen: Dieterich; 1892.
128. Cantley E, Dent CT. Congenital hypertrophic pyloric stenosis and its treatment by pyloroplasty. Med Chir Trans. 1903;86:471.
129. Tan KC, Bianchi A. Circumbilical incision for pyloromyotomy. Br J Surg. 1986;73:399.
130. Fitzgerald PG, Lau GY, Langer JC, et al. Umbilical fold incision for pyloromyotomy. J Pediatr Surg. 1990;25:1117–8.
131. Khan AR, Al-Bassam AR. Circumbilical pyloromyotomy: larger pyloric tumours need an extended incision. Pediatr Surg Int. 2000;16:338–41.
132. Leinwand MJ, Shaul DB, Anderson KD. The umbilical fold approach to pyloromyotomy: is it a safe alternative to the right upper quadrant approach? J Am Coll Surg. 1999;189:362–7.
133. Kim SS, Lau ST, Lee SL, et al. Pyloromyotomy: a comparison of laparoscopic, circumbilical, and right upper quadrant operative techniques. J Am Coll Surg. 2005;201:66–70.
134. Blumer RM, Hessel NS, van Baren R, et al. Comparison between umbilical and transverse right upper abdominal incision for pyloromyotomy. J Pediatr Surg. 2004;39:1091–3.
135. Shankar KR, Losty PD, Jones MO, et al. Umbilical pyloromyotomy: an alternative to laparoscopy? Eur J Pediatr Surg. 2001;11:8–11.
136. Alain JL, Grousseau D, Terrier T. Extramucosal pyloromyotomy by laparoscopy. Surg Endosc. 1991;5:174–5.
137. Scharli AF, Leditschke JF. Gastric motility after pyloromyotomy in infants: a reappraisal of postoperative feeding. Surgery. 1968;64:1113–7.
138. Wheeler RA, Najmaldin AS, Stoodley N, et al. Feeding regimens after pyloromyotomy. Br J Surg. 1990;77:1018–9.
139. Georgeson KE, Corbin TJ, Griffen JW, et al. An analysis of feeding regimens after pyloromyotomy for hypertrophic pyloric stenosis. J Pediatr Surg. 1993;28:1478–80.
140. Gollin G, Doslouglu H, Flummerfeldt P, et al. Rapid advancement of feedings after pyloromyotomy for pyloric stenosis. Clin Pediatr. 2000;39:187–90.
141. Robertson DE. Congenital pyloric stenosis. Ann Surg. 1940;112:687–99.
142. Crabbe DCG. Infantile hypertrophic pyloric stenosis. In: Stringer MD, Oldham KT, PDE M, editors. Pediatric surgery and urology. Long-term outcomes. 2nd ed: Cambridge University Press; 2006. p. 296–304.
143. Pranikoff T, Campbell B, Travis J, Hirschl R. Differences in outcome with subspecialty care: pyloromyotomy in North Carolina. J Pediatr Surg. 2002;37:352–6.
144. Langer JC, To T. Does pediatric surgical specialty training affect outcome after Ramstedt pyloromyotomy? A population-based study. Pediatrics. 2004;113(5):1342–7.
145. Safford SD, Pietrobon R, Safford KM, et al. A study of 11,003patients with hypertrophic pyloric stenosis and the associations between surgeon and hospital volume and outcomes. J Pediatr Surg. 2005;40:967–97.
146. Beynon J, Brown R, James C, et al. Pyloromyotomy: can the morbidity be improved? J R Coll Surg Edinb. 1987;32:291–2.
147. Hight DW, Benson CD, Philippart AI, et al. Management of mucosal perforation during pyloromyotomy for infantile pyloric stenosis. Surgery. 1981;90:85–6.
148. Lee SL, Sydorak RM, Lau ST. Air insufflation of the stomach following laparoscopic pyloromyotomy may not detect perforation. JSLS. 2010;14: 60–1.
149. Koop CE. Pyloromyotomy for pyloric stenosis. In: Cooper P, editor. The craft of surgery. Boston, MA: Little Brown; 1964. p. 1450–7.
150. Royal RE, Linz DN, Gruppo DL, et al. Repair of mucosal perforation during pyloromyotomy: surgeon's choice. J Pediatr Surg. 1995;30:1430–2.
151. Sitsen E, Bax NMA, van der Zee DC. Is laparoscopic pyloromyotomy superior to open surgery? Surg Endosc. 1998;12:813–5.
152. British Association of Paediatric Surgeons. Comparative audit service – paediatric surgery. London, UK: Surgical Epidemiology Unit, Royal College of Surgeons of England; 1996.
153. Ford WD, Crameri JA, Holland AJ. The learning curve for laparoscopic pyloromyotomy. J Pediatr Surg. 1997;32:552–4.
154. Eriksen CA, Anders CJ. Audit of results of operations for infantile hypertrophic pyloric stenosis in a district general hospital. Arch Dis Child. 1991;66:130–3.
155. Harvey MH, Humphrey G, Fieldman N, et al. Abdominal wall dehiscence following Ramstedt's operation; a review of 170 cases of infantile hypertrophic pyloric stenosis. Br J Surg. 1991;78: 81–2.
156. Huddart SN, Bianchi A, Kumar V, et al. Ramstedt's pyloromyotomy: circumbilical versus transverse approach. Pediatr Surg Int. 1993;8:395–6.

157. Nour S, MacKinnon AE, Dickson JAS, et al. Antibiotic prophylaxis for infantile pyloromyotomy. J Roy Coll Surg Ed. 1996;41:178–80.
158. Mullassery D, Perry D, Goyal A, et al. Surgical practice for infantile hypertrophic pyloric stenosis in the United Kingdom and Ireland – a survey of members of the British Association of Paediatric Surgeons. J Pediatr Surg. 2008;43:1227–9.
159. Gauderer MW. Experience with a nonlaparoscopic, transumbilical, intracavitary pyloromyotomy. J Pediatr Surg. 2008;43:884–8.
160. Mullassery D, Shariff R, Craigie RJ, et al. Umbilical pyloromyotomy: comparison of vertical linea alba and transverse muscle cutting incisions. J Pediatr Surg. 2007;42:525–7.
161. Hall NJ, Van der Zee J, Tan HL, et al. Meta analysis of laparoscopic versus open pyloromyotomy. Ann Surg. 2004;240:774–8.
162. Siddiqui S, Heidel RE, Angel CA, Kennedy AP Jr. Pyloromyotomy: randomized control trial of laparoscopic vs open technique. J Pediatr Surg. 2012;47:93–8.
163. Jia WQ, Tian JH, Yang KH, Ma B, Liu YL, Zhang P, Li RJ, Jia RH. Open versus laparoscopic pyloromyotomy for pyloric stenosis: a meta-analysis of randomized controlled trials. Eur J Pediatr Surg. 2011;21:77–81.
164. Sola JE, Neville HL. Laparoscopic vs open pyloromyotomy: a systematic review and meta-analysis. J Pediatr Surg. 2009;44:1631–7.
165. Centre for Review and Dissemination. Laparoscopic vs open pyloromyotomy: a systematic review and meta-analysis (structured Abstract) Database of Abstracts of Review of Effects, vol. 3. New York: Wiley\University of York; 2011.
166. Katz MS, Schwartz MZ, Moront ML, et al. Prophylactic antibiotics do no decrease the incidence of wound infections after laparoscopic pyloromyotomy. J Pediatr Surg. 2011;46:1086–8.
167. Wollstein M. Healing of hypertrophic pyloric stenosis after the Fredet-Rammstedt operation. Am J Dis Child. 1922;23:511–7.
168. Steinicke O, Roelsgaard M. Radiographic follow-up in hypertrophic pyloric stenosis. Acta Paediatr. 1960;49:4–16.
169. Okorie NM, Dickson JAS, Carver RA, et al. What happens to the pylorus after pyloromyotomy? Arch Dis Child. 1988;63:1339–40.
170. Tander B, Akalin A, Abbasoglu L, et al. Ultrasonographic follow up of infantile hypertrophic pyloric stenosis after pyloromyotomy: a controlled prospective study. Eur J Ped Surg. 2002;12:379–82.
171. Steinicke Nielson O, Roelsgaard M. Roentgenologically demonstrable gastric abnormalities in cases of previous congenital pyloric stenosis. Acta Radiol. 1956;45:273–82.
172. Solowiejczyk M, Holtzman M, Michowitz M. Congenital hypertrophic pyloric stenosis: a long term follow up of 41 cases. Am Surg. 1980;10:567–71.
173. Wanscher B, Jensen H. Late follow-up studies after operation for congenital pyloric stenosis. Scand J Gastroenterol. 1971;6:597–9.
174. Ludtke FE, Bertus M, Voth E, et al. Gastric emptying 16 to 26 years after treatment of infantile hypertrophic pyloric stenosis. J Pediatr Surg. 1994;29:523–6.
175. Rasmussen L, Oster-Jorgensen E, Hansen LP, et al. Gastric emptying in adults treated for infantile hypertrophic pyloric stenosis. Acta Chir Scand. 1989;155:471–3.
176. Asai A, Takehara H, Harada M, et al. Ultrasonographic evaluation of gastric emptying in normal children and children after pyloromyotomy. Pediatr Surg Int. 1997;12:344–7.
177. Sun WM, Doran SM, Jones KL, et al. Long term effects of pyloromyotomy on pyloric motility and gastric emptying in humans. Am J Gastroenterol. 2000;95:92–100.
178. Stringer MD, Kiely E, Drake DP. Gastric retention of swallowed coins after pyloromyotomy. Br J Clin Pract. 1991;45:66–7.
179. Hayashi A, Giacomantonio JM, Lau HYC, et al. Balloon catheter dilatation for hypertrophic pyloric stenosis. J Pediatr Surg. 1990;25:1119–21.
180. Ogawa Y, Higashimoto Y, Nishijima E, et al. Successful endoscopic balloon dilatation for hypertrophic pyloric stenosis. J Pediatr Surg. 1996;31:1712–4.
181. Tobler L. Ueber Magen verdauung der Milch. Munch Med Wschr. 1907;54:812.
182. Ibrahim J. Die angeborenen Pylorusstenose in Senglingsalter. Berlin: S Karger; 1905.
183. Swensgaard E. Medical treatment of congenital pyloric stenosis. Hospitalstudende. 1935;78:833.
184. Tallerman KH. Discussion on treatment of congenital hypertrophic pyloric stenosis. Proc Roy Soc Med. 1951;44:1055–7.
185. Yamataka A, Tsukada K, Yokoyama-Laws Y, et al. Pyloromyotomy versus atropine sulfate for infantile hypertrophic pyloric stenosis. Surg. 2000;35:338–42.
186. Kawahara H, Imura K, Nishikawa M, Yagi M, Kubota A. Intravenous atropine treatment in infantile hypertrophic pyloric stenosis. Arch Dis Child. 2002;87:71–4.
187. Kawahara H, Takama Y, Yoshida H, et al. Medical treatment of hypertrophic pyloric stenosis: should we always slice the "olive"? J Pediatr Surg. 2005;40:1848–51.
188. Aguayo P, Ostlie DJ. Duodenal and Intestinal Atresia and Stenosis. In: Holcomb III GW, Murphy JP, editors. Ashcraft's Paediatric Surgery. 5th ed. Philadelphia: Saunders Elsevier; 2010. p. 400.
189. Ilce BZ, Erdogan E, Kara C, Celayir S, Sarimurat N, Snyuz OF, Yeker D. Pyloric atresia: 15-year review from a single institution. J Pediatr Surg. 2003;38:1581–4.
190. Koontz SC, Wulkan M. Lesions of the stomach. In: Holcomb III GW, Murphy JP, editors. Ashcraft's paediatric surgery. 5th ed. Philadelphia: Saunders Elsevier; 2010. p. 395–6.

191. Muller M, Morger R, Engert J. Pyloric atresia: report of two cases and review of literature. Pediatr Surg Int. 1990;5:276–9.
192. Moore CCM. Congenital gastric outlet obstruction. J Pediatr Surg. 1989;24:1241–6.
193. Egan N, Ward R, Olmstead M, Marks JG. Junctional epidermolysis bullosa and pyloric atresia in two siblings. Arch Dermatol. 1985;121:1186–8.
194. Bar-Maor JA, Nissan S, Nevo S. Pyloric atresia: a hereditary congenital anomaly with autosomal recessive transmission. J Med Genet. 1972;9:70–2.
195. Chung HJ, Uitto J. Epidermolysis bullosa with pyloric atresia. Dermatol Clin. 2010;28:43–54.
196. Al-Salem AH. Congenital pyloric atresia and associated anomalies. Pediatr Surg Int. 2007;23(6):559–63.
197. Sencan A, Mir E, Karace I, Günşar C, Sencan A, Topçu K. Pyloric atresia associated with multiple intestinal atresias and pylorocholedochal fistula. J Pediatr Surg. 2002;37:1223–4.
198. Tandler J. Zur Emtwicklungsgeschichte des menschlichen Doudenum im fruhen embryonen Stadien. Gegenbaur Morph Jahrbuch. 1900;29:187–216.
199. Louw JH, Barnard CN. Congenital intestinal atresia; observations on its origin. Lancet. 1955;269:1065–7.
200. Tunnel WP, Smith EI. Antral web in infancy. J Pediatr Surg. 1980;15:152–5.
201. Boyden EA, Cope JG, Bill AH. Anatomy and embryology of congenital intrinsic obstruction of the duodenum. Am J Surg. 1967;114:190–2.
202. Maman E, Maor E, Kachko L, et al. Epidermolysis bullosa, pyloric atresia, aplasia cutis congenita: histopathological delineation of an autosomal recessive disease. Am J Med Genet. 1998;78:127–33.
203. Nazzaro V, Nicolini U, De Luca L, et al. Prenatal diagnosis of junctional epidermolysis bullosa associated with pyloric atresia. J Med Genet. 1990;27:244–8.
204. Sloop RD, Montague AC. Gastric outlet obstruction due to congenital pyloric mucosal membrane. Ann Surg. 1967;165:598–604.
205. Gahukamble DB. Familial occurrence of congenital incomplete prepyloric mucosal diaphragm. J Med Genet. 1998;35(12):1040–2.
206. Clement KW, Escamilla HA. Duplication of the stomach. J Nat Med Assoc. 1974;66:292–304.
207. Upadhyaya VD, Srivastava PK, Jaiman R, et al. Duplication cyst of pyloroduodenal canal: a rare cause of neonatal gastric outlet obstruction. Cases J. 2009;2:42.
208. Holcomb GW 3rd, Gheissari A, O'Neill JA Jr, et al. Surgical management of alimentary tract duplications. Ann Surg. 1989;209(2):167–71.
209. Sorbie AL, Symon DN, Sotockdale EJ. Gaviscon bezoars. Arch Dis Child. 1984;59:905–6.
210. Heinz-Erian P, Gassner I, Klein-Franke A, et al. Gastric lactobezoar—a rare disorder? Orphanet J Rare Dis. 2012;7:3.

Duodenal Atresia and Stenosis

31

Emily Partridge and Holly L. Hedrick

Abstract

Congenital duodenal atresia and stenosis is a common cause of intestinal obstruction in the neonate, with an incidence of 1 in 5000 to 10,000 live births and an increased prevalence in males. More than 50% of affected patients have associated congenital anomalies, including annular pancreas, intestinal malrotation, esophageal atresia, Meckel's diverticulum, imperforate anus, renal anomalies, lesions of the central nervous system, and biliary tract malformations. The most common anomalies associated with duodenal atresia include Trisomy 21, diagnosed in one third of patients, and isolated cardiac defects, which occur in approximately 30%. The presence of trisomy carries an increased risk for congenital heart defects requiring operative repair. Approximately 45% of patients are born prematurely, with one-third exhibiting failure to thrive and persistent growth retardation. Presently, laparoscopic or open duodenoduodenostomy has become the standard of care, with survival rates of greater than 95% and mortality primarily attributed to associated anomalies of other organ systems.

Keywords

Congenital duodenal obstruction • Prenatal diagnosis • Associated anomalies • Embryology • Surgery • Outcomes

E. Partridge, MD, PhD
Center for Fetal Research, Children's Hospital of Philadelphia, Philadelphia, PA, USA

Department of Pediatric General, Thoracic, and Fetal Surgery, Children's Hospital of Philadelphia, 34th Street and Civic Center Boulevard, Wood, 5117 Philadelphia, PA, USA

H.L. Hedrick, MD (✉)
Perelman School of Medicine at the University of Pennsylvania, Philadelphia, PA, USA

Department of Pediatric General, Thoracic, and Fetal Surgery, Children's Hospital of Philadelphia, 34th Street and Civic Center Boulevard, Wood, 5117 Philadelphia, PA, USA
e-mail: Hedrick@email.chop.edu

P.D. Losty et al. (eds.), *Rickham's Neonatal Surgery*, https://doi.org/10.1007/978-1-4471-4721-3_31

31.1 Duodenal Atresia and Stenosis

Congenital duodenal atresia and stenosis is a common cause of intestinal obstruction in the neonate, with an incidence of 1 in 5000 to 10,000 live births and an increased prevalence in males [1]. More than 50% of affected patients have associated congenital anomalies, including annular pancreas, intestinal malrotation, esophageal atresia, Meckel's diverticulum, imperforate anus, renal anomalies, lesions of the central nervous system, and biliary tract malformations [2]. The most common anomalies associated with duodenal atresia include Trisomy 21, diagnosed in one third of patients [3], and isolated cardiac defects, which occur in approximately 30% [4]. The presence of trisomy carries an increased risk for congenital heart defects requiring operative repair [5]. Approximately 45% of patients are born prematurely, with one-third exhibiting failure to thrive and persistent growth retardation [6]. Presently, laparoscopic or open duodenoduodenostomy has become the standard of care, with survival rates of greater than 95% and mortality primarily attributed to associated anomalies of other organ systems [7].

31.2 Etiology

Duodenal atresia occurs due to a failure of recanalization of the fetal duodenum, resulting in complete obstruction. Early in the fourth week of gestation, the duodenum develops from the distal foregut and proximal midgut. During the fifth and sixth weeks of gestation, the duodenal lumen is temporarily obliterated due to proliferation of the epithelium. Subsequently, degeneration of the epithelial cells leads to recanalization of the duodenum by the eleventh week of gestation. Embryonic insult during this developmental window may result in an intrinsic web, atresia or stenosis. Unlike atresias distal to the Ligament of Treitz, vascular insult is not thought to play a role in the etiology of duodenal stenosis. Although no specific genetic mutation has been shown to correlate with duodenal atresia, the coincidence of the condition within sibling cohorts supports the likelihood of an underlying genetic predisposition [8].

31.3 Classification

Anatomically, congenital duodenal obstruction is classified as either an atresia or stenosis. Incomplete obstruction due to a fenestrated web or diaphragm is considered a stenosis, while atresias, or complete obstructions, are classified into three morphologic types [9]. Type I atresias account for more than 90% of all congenital duodenal obstructions, and contain a luminal diaphragm including mucosal and submucosal layers with an intact mesentery. A variant of type I duodenal atresia, the 'windsock' deformity, presents with distal dilation of the luminal diaphragm, and may pose particular challenges to surgical repair as a segment of dilated duodenum may persist distally to the point of true obstruction. Type II atresias account for less than 1% of all cases and are characterized by a segment of proximal dilation and distal decompression connected by a fibrous cord with an intact mesentery. Type III atresias account for approximately 7% of all cases, and are distinguished by a V-shaped mesenteric defect. There is no connection between the blind proximal and distal duodenal segments.

31.4 Postnatal Presentation

The postnatal presentation of congenital duodenal obstruction depends greatly on the grade of obstruction and its location in relation to the ampulla of Vater. Neonates classically present with bilious vomiting in the first hours of life, although in approximately 15% of cases the obstruction occurs proximal to the ampulla, resulting in non-bilious emesis [10]. The abdomen is generally scaphoid, and abdominal distension is rarely apparent [11]. Patients with incomplete obstruction, or stenosis, may have a delayed presentation dependent on the initiation of enteral feeds. Delayed diagnosis can result in aspiration, dehydration and the development of acid-base disorders.

Suspected cases of duodenal obstruction may be confirmed by a plain upright X-ray of the abdomen, with the classical finding of the "double bubble" sign generated by the proximal left-sided air- and fluid-filled stomach tapering at the pylorus and the distal dilated proximal duodenum to the right of the midline (Fig. 31.1). Generally the distal bowel is gasless, however in cases of anomalous bifurcated bile duct with termination of one duct distal to the point of obstruction, distal gas may be visualized [12]. In the setting of neonates who have undergone placement of a nasogastric tube, 30–60 mLs of instilled air may reproduce the "double bubble" sign, or a limited upper gastrointestinal contrast study may be performed to confirm the diagnosis and exclude malrotation or volvulus.

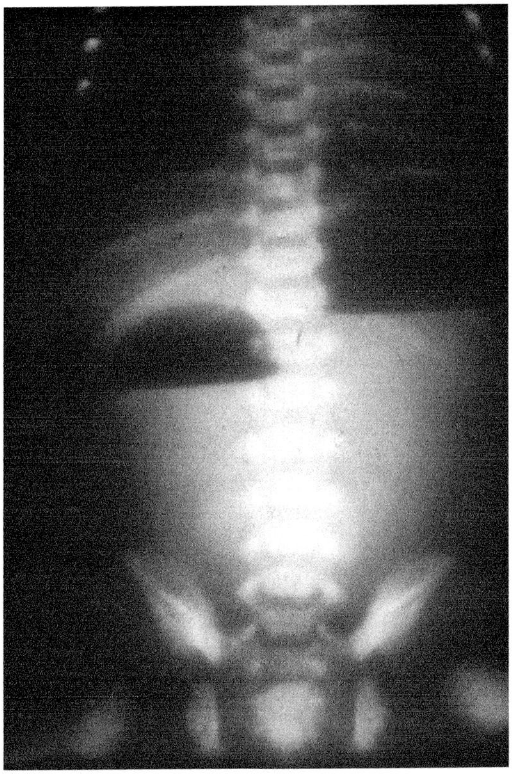

Fig. 31.1 Duodenal atresia showing classic 'double bubble 'sign features indicating proximal foregut obstruction

31.5 Prenatal Diagnosis

Advances in prenatal imaging have led to increased diagnosis of a number of anomalies of the gastrointestinal tract, including stenosis and atresias of the small and large bowel [13]. Prenatal diagnosis may be made in as many as 50% of cases of congenital duodenal obstruction [14]. Prenatal diagnosis is more common in the presence of other congenital anomalies, and is therefore associated with higher overall mortality rates [15]. Polyhydramnios is a frequent complication in the setting of congenital duodenal obstruction [16], and may prompt increased imaging surveillance leading to definitive diagnosis. Prenatal ultrasonography may detect two fluid-filled structures consistent with a double bubble sign (Fig. 31.2a). With the advent of fetal MRI, detailed delineation of soft tissue anomalies has become possible across a wide range of gestational ages, and may be useful in confirming the diagnosis and ruling out other anomalies (Fig. 31.2b). Low fetal and birth weight is also commonly observed, and may be attributed in part to reduced swallowing and transit of amniotic fluid through the fetal bowel [17].

Duodenal atresia is most commonly prenatally diagnosed in the second half of pregnancy [18], although cases of accurate diagnosis in the first of early second trimester have been reported [19, 20]. It has been hypothesized that the relatively late appearance of significant duodenal distension may be attributed to immature fetal swallowing and gastric emptying. Peristaltic movement of the small intestine may be appreci-

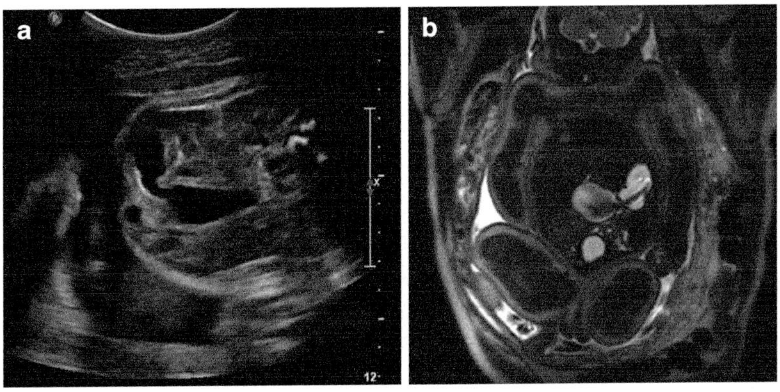

Fig. 31.2 Prenatal radiographic imaging of duodenal stenosis. (**a**) Duodenal stenosis imaged by ultrasonography of the fetus, with a "double-bubble" sign. (**b**) Appearance of duodenal stenosis by fetal magnetic resonance imaging

ated by ultrasonography as early as 6–7 weeks gestational age and may transiently mimic the appearance of dilated intestinal segments, leading to the possibility of a false diagnosis [19]. Importantly, in cases of true obstruction the dilation of the affected segment is observed constantly, therefore scans of several minutes duration are required to minimize the likelihood of false positive diagnoses.

31.6 Postnatal Management

In suspected cases of duodenal stenosis or atresia, placement of a nasogastric tube is an appropriate initial maneuver to achieve gastric decompression and reduce the risk of aspiration. After confirmation of the diagnosis by plain radiograph with or without contrast, a complete metabolic profile is obtained including complete blood cell count, electrolyte panel, blood gas, and coagulation studies. Appropriate resuscitation is required to correct any underlying fluid imbalance or electrolyte disorder. Due to the high risk of congenital heart disease in this patient population, cardiac investigations including an electrocardiogram and echocardiogram should be performed prior to surgical intervention. Generally it is only in the setting of an inability to exclude the possibility of malrotation or volvulus that emergent surgical intervention is undertaken.

Prior to the mid-1970s, duodenojejunostomy was the preferred approach for correction of duodenal atresia [21]. Rarely, gastrojejunostomy was performed as an alternative to duodenojejunostomy [22], but was found to result in a high incidence of marginal ulceration and bleeding [23]. Duodenojejunostomy was found to result in delayed anastomotic function often requiring use of parenteral nutrition or trans-anastomotic feeding tubes [24]. Blind-loop syndrome and megaduodenum also appear to result more commonly in patients treated with duodenojejunostomy, and may require reoperation and conversion to a duodenoduodenostomy to achieve satisfactory functional outcomes [25]. Weitzman and Brennan first reported the results of a direct side-to-side duodenoduodenostomy approach in 1974, with no anastomotic complications in their cohort of 14 patients [26]. The approach was widely adopted, although continued reports of complications including blind loop syndrome and duodenal dilation requiring tapering [27] or duodenoplasty [28] prompted continued technical modifications. In 1977, Kimura and colleagues reported an anastomotic technique with a side-to-side duodenoduodenostomy closed in two layers with the bowel incisions arranged to form a diamond-shaped anastomosis to achieve a larger stoma [29]. The technique was widely adopted with a favorable functional profile, and was further refined by Kimura to incorporate a transverse incision on the distal end of the proximal duodenum and a longitudinal incision in the distal duodenum (Figs. 31.3 and 31.4). By this technique, bowel function is recovered in a significantly shorter time period with a low incidence of complications and good long-term results [30]. The procedure of choice for duodenal atresia, irregardless of type, is presently duodenoduodenostomy with a proximal

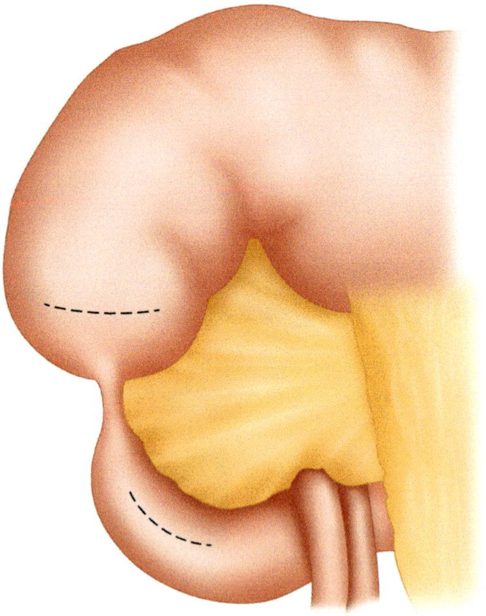

Fig. 31.3 Kimura technique operative duodenal atresia repair. A transverse incision is made in the distal portion of the proximal obstructed duodenum segment. A longitudinal incision is then created in the nearby portion of duodenum distal to the site of the atretic obstruction

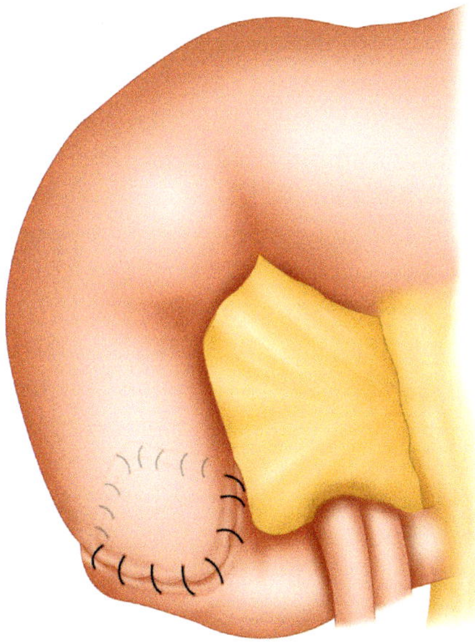

Fig. 31.4 A wide diamond shaped anastomosis is formed by joining the two duodenal segments

transverse to distal longitudinal, or diamond-shaped, anastomosis.

In the open approach, a right upper quadrant supraumbilical incision is made, and the ascending and transverse colon is mobilized medially to expose the duodenum. The position of the bowel should be assessed at this time, as malrotation may occur in up to 30% of cases of congenital duodenal obstruction [31]. Eviscerating and positioning the small bowel and colon cephalad and to the left of the incision achieves ideal exposure of the third and fourth duodenum. The decompressed duodenum is mobilized distal to the point of obstruction to permit a tension-free anastomosis. With the aid of tacking sutures, a transverse duodenotomy is made in the anterior wall of the distal portion of the distended proximal duodenum, and a vertical duodenotomy is made on the anti-mesenteric border of the distal duodenum. To rule out an additional web or windsock deformity, a catheter should be passed proximally into the stomach and distally into the jejunum and pulled back. The ends of the distal vertical duodenotomy incision are then approximated to the mid-portion of the proximal transverse duodenotomy incision with stay-sutures, and the posterior wall of the anastomosis is constructed by placing interrupted sutures using a repeating bisecting technique. The anterior row of the anastomosis is then completed in a similar fashion (Figs. 31.3 and 31.4). In the setting of gross dilation of the proximal segment, an anti-mesenteric tapering duodenoplasty may be performed as to expedite postoperative recovery of bowel function [32]. This may be performed by resection using a gastrointestinal anastomosis (GIA) stapler over a large red rubber catheter. Tapering is performed on the anterior or anterolateral portion of the proximal duodenum to avoid damage to the common bile duct and ampulla of Vater. Finally, the anastomosis is examined for patency, and the intestine is returned to the abdomen. In cases of malrotation, a formal Ladd's procedure is performed. Prior to closure of the abdomen, proper positioning of the nasogastric tube is confirmed. Placement of a transanastomotic feeding tube may hasten the time to tolerance of full oral feeding [33], although the literature on this approach is limited.

The laparoscopic approach to repair of congenital duodenal obstruction was first reported by Rothenberg in [34], with no complications and rapid initiation of oral feeds in the three patients described. The laparoscopic approach begins with insufflation of the abdomen through an umbilical port, with two additional ports placed in the right lower quadrant and the left mid-quadrant. A liver retractor may be placed via a fourth port in the right or left upper quadrant as indicated, or the liver may be retracted by placement of a stay-suture around the falciform ligament secured to the abdominal wall. The duodenum is exposed and mobilized, and rotational position of the bowel inspected. The proximal and distal duodenotomies are performed in a manner similar to that utilized in the open approach, with either running or single interrupted sutures used to anastomose the anterior and posterior walls. Alternatively, U-clips may be used to perform the anastomosis, with favorable outcomes reported in one series to date [35]. Results of an additional series of seventeen neonates undergoing laparoscopic repair following Rothenberg's initial report noted no intraoperative complications, no conversions to open procedures, and no anastomotic leaks [36]. Due to the relatively recent advent of laparoscopic repair of duodenal stenosis, long-term outcomes are not yet reported in the literature. Reports of long-term complications and functional outcomes will facilitate a critical comparison of open versus laparoscopic repair of congenital duodenal obstructions.

Postoperatively, total parenteral nutrition is continued with monitoring of nasogastric tube outputs, and feedings are initiated when the volume of nasogastric output is diminished and non-bilious.

31.7 Outcomes

Early postoperative mortality for duodenal atresia is low. The most common complication encountered in the postoperative course is prolonged feeding intolerance. Prokinetic agents may have some benefit in this population, with one randomized controlled trial reporting shorter duration of TPN requirements, earlier achievement of full enteral feeding, and reduced length of hospitalization in a cohort of 30 neonates undergoing primary anastomosis for congenital small bowel atresias [37]. While some variability in return of bowel function is expected, feeding intolerance beyond the second week postoperatively should prompt concern for residual obstruction, anastomotic stricture, or a complicating motility disorder. An upper gastrointestinal series is helpful to rule out anastomotic stricture, although it should be noted that residual dilation of the proximal duodenum may be apparent for several months in the setting of a fully functional anastomosis.

Long-term complications reported after repair of duodenal obstruction include chronic severe gastrointestinal reflux, bleeding peptic ulcer, megaduodenum, gastritis, blind-loop syndrome, and adhesive bowel obstructions [38]. Patients with additional foregut anomalies, including esophageal atresia and gastroduodenal motility disorders, are the most likely to have gastroesophageal reflux disease [39]. Dysmotility in duodenal atresia may be attributed to smooth muscle cell injury secondary to ischemia or hypoplasia of the enteric nerves [40], while the dilated proximal segment may be associated with impaired transit and low contraction amplitude [41]. Megaduodenum may be diagnosed up to eighteen years postoperatively, and is associated with poor weight gain, frequent emesis, abdominal pain, and blind-loop syndrome [38]. An anti-mesenteric tapering duodenoplasty may be performed to manage cases of megaduodenum manifesting in the postoperative period [42]. Overall survival rates have improved over the past half-century from 45 to 95%, with the majority of deaths attributed to complications arising from associated congenital anomalies [43]. Long-term follow-up is essential for infants treated for congenital duodenal obstruction, with early diagnosis and management of late complications to achieve optimal outcomes.

References

1. Fonkalsrud EW, DeLorimier AA, Hays DM. Congenital atresia and stenosis of the duodenum: a review compiled from members of the Surgical Section of the American Academy of Pediatrics. Pediatrics. 1969;43:79–83.
2. Litwin A, Avidor I, Schujman E, et al. Neonatal intestina perforation caused by congenital defects of the intestinal musculature. Am J Clin Pathol. 1984;81:77–80.
3. Stauffer UG, Irving I. Duodenal atresia and stenosis—long-term results. Prog Pediatr Surg. 1977;10:49–60.
4. Buchin PJ, Levy JS, Schullinger JN. Down's syndrome and the gastrointestinal tract. J Clin Gastroenterol. 1986;8(2):111–4.
5. Keckler SJ, St Peter SD, Spilde TL, Ostlie DJ, Snyder CL. The influence of trisomy 21 on the incidence and severity of congenital heart defects in patients with duodenal atresia. Pediatr Surg Int. 2008;24(8):921–3.
6. Grosfeld JL, Rescorla FJ. Duodenal atresia and stenosis: reassessment of treatment and outcome based on antenatal diagnosis, pathologic variance, and long-term follow-up. World J Surg. 1993;17:301–9.
7. Murshed R, Nicholls G, Spitz L. Intestinal duodenal obstruction: trends in management and outcome over 45 years (1951–1995) with relevance to prenatal counseling. Br J Obstet Gynecol. 1999;106:1197–9.
8. Gahukamble DB, Khamage AS, Shaheen AQ. Duodenal atresia: its occurrence in siblings. J Pediatr Surg. 1994;29(12):1599–600.

9. Gray SW, Skandalakis JE. Embryology for surgeons. Philadelphia, PA: Saunders Elsevier; 1975. p. 147–8.
10. Aguayo P, Ostlie DJ. Duodenal and intestinal atresia and stenosis. In: Holcomb GW, Murphy JP, editors. Ashcraft's pediatric surgery. Philadelphia, PA: Saunders Elsevier; 2005. p. 400–5.
11. Kullendorff CM. Atresia of the small bowel. Annales Chirurgiae et Gyneacologiae. 1983;72(4):192–5.
12. Komuro H, Ono K, Hoshino N, Urita Y, Gotoh C, Fujishiro J, Shinkai T, Ikebukuro K. Bile duct duplication as a cause of distal bowel gas in neonatal duodenal obstruction. J Pediatr Surg. 2011;46(12):2301–4.
13. Benacerraf BB. The Sherlock Holmes approach to diagnosing fetal syndromes by ultrasound. Clin Obstet Gynecol. 2012;55(1):226–48.
14. Hemming V, Rankin J. Small intestinal atresia in a defined population: occurrence, prenatal diagnosis and survival. Prenat Diagn. 2007;27:1205–11.
15. Choudry MS, Rahman N, Boyd P, Lakhoo K. Duodenal atresia: associated anomalies, prenatal diagnosis and outcome. Pediatr Surg Int. 2009;25:727–30.
16. Dalla Vecchia LK, Grosfeld JL, West KW, Rescorla FJ, Scherer LR, Engum SA. Intestinal atresia and stenosis: a 25-year experience with 277 cases. Arch Surg. 1998;133(5):490–6.
17. Francannet C, Robert E. Epidemiological study of intestinal atresias: central-eastern France Registry 1976–1992. Journal de Gynecologie, Obstetrique et Biologie de la Reproduction. 1996;25(5):485–94.
18. Hertzbery BS. Sonography of the fetal gastrointestinal tract: anatomic variants, diagnostic pitfalls and abnormalities. Am J Roentgenol. 1994;162:1175–82.
19. Zimmer EZ, Bronshtein M. Early diagnosis of duodenal atresia and possible sonographic pitfalls. Prenat Diagn. 1996;16:564–6.
20. Tsukerman GL, Krapiva GA, Kirillova IA. First trimester diagnosis of duodenal stenosis associated with oesophageal atresia. Prenat Diagn. 1993;13:371–6.
21. Weber TR, Lewis JE, Mooney D, Connors R. Duodenal atresia: a comparison of techniques of repair. J Pediatr Surg. 1986;21:1133–6.
22. Puri P, Sweed Y. Duodenal obstructions. In: Puri P, editor. Newborn surgery. Oxford: Botterworth-Heinemann; 1996. p. 290–7.
23. Buck P, Sacrez R, Juif JG, Beauvais P. Long delayed compliations of gastrojejunostomy for duodenal stenosis in the newborn. Ann Chir Infant. 1962;3:130–5.
24. Becker JM, Schneider KM. Tube jejunostomy in the treatment of upper intestinal obstruction in the neonate. Surg Gynecol Obstet. 1963;116:123–5.
25. Rescorla FJ, Grosfeld JL. Duodenal atresia in infancy and childhood: improved surgical survival and long-term follow-up. Contemp Surg. 1988;33:22–7.
26. Weitzman JJ, Brennan LP. An improved technique for the correction of congenital duodenal obstruction in the neonate. J Pediatr Surg. 1974;9(3):385–8.
27. Weisgerber G, Boureau M. Resultats immediats et secondaires des duodeno-duodenostomies avec modelage dans le traitement des obstructions duodenales congenitales complete du nouveau-ne. Chirurgie Pediatrique. 1982;23(6):369–72.
28. Dewan PA, Guiney EJ. Duodenoplasty in the management of duodenal atresia. Pediatr Surg Int. 1990;5(4):253–4.
29. Kimura K, Tsugawa C, Oqawa K, Matsumoto Y, Yamamoto T, Asada S. Diamond-shaped anastomosis for congenital duodenal obstruction. Arch Surg. 1977;112(10):1262–3.
30. Kimura K, Mukohara N, Nishijima E, Muraji T, Tsugawa C, Matsumoto Y. Diamond-shaped anastomosis for duodenal atresia: an experience with 44 patients over 15 years. J Pediatr Surg. 1990;25(9):977–9.
31. Bailey PV, Tracy TF Jr, Connors RH, Mooney DP, Lewis JE, Weber TR. Congenital duodenal obstruction: a 32-year review. J Pediatr Surg. 1993;28(1):92–5.
32. Adzick NS, Harrison MR, de Lorimier AA. Tapering duodenoplasty for megaduodenum associated with duodenal atresia. J Pediatr Surg. 1989;21(4):311–2.
33. Arnbjörnsson E, Larsson M, Finkel Y, Karpe B. Transanastomotic feeding tube after an operation for duodenal atresia. Eur J Pediatr Surg. 2002;12(3):159–62.
34. Rothenberg SS. Laparoscopic duodenoduodenostomy for duodenal obstruction in infants and children. J Pediatr Surg. 2002;37(7):1088–9.
35. Spilde TL, St Peter SD, Keckler SJ, Holcomb GW, Snyder CL, Ostlie DJ. Open vs laparoscopic repair of congenital duodenal obstructions: a concurrent series. J Pediatr Surg. 2008;43(6):1002–5.
36. Kay S, Yoder S, Rothenberg S. Laparoscopic duodenoduodenostomy in the neonate. J Pediatr Surg. 2009;44(5):906–8.
37. Razzaq A, Safdar CA, Ali S. Erythromycin establishes early oral feeding in neonates operated for congenital intestinal atresias. Pediatr Surg Int. 2009;25(4):361–4.
38. Spigland N, Yazbeck S. Complications associated with surgical treatment of congenital intrinsic duodenal obstruction. J Pediatr Surg. 1990;25:1127–30.
39. Hassall E. Wrap session: Is the Nissen slipping? Can medical treatment replace surgery for severe gastroesophageal reflux disease in children? Am J Gastroenterol. 1995;90:1212–20.
40. Molenaar JC, Tibboel D, van der Kamp AW, Meijers JH. Diagnosis of innervation-related motility disorders of the gut and basic aspects of enteric nervous system development. Prog Pediatr Surg. 1989;24:173–85.
41. Takahashi A, Tomomasa T, Suzuki N, Kuroiwa M, Ikeda H, Morikawa A, Matsuyama S, Tsuchida Y. The relationship between disturbed transit and dilated bowel, and manometric findings of dilated bowel in patients with duodenal atresia and stenosis. J Pediatr Surg. 1997;32(8):1157–60.
42. Ein SH, Shandling B. The late nonfunctioning duodenal atresia repair. J Pediatr Surg. 1986;21(9):798–801.
43. Escobar MA, Ladd AP, Grosfeld JL, West KW, Rescorla FJ, Scherer LR, Engum SA, Rouse TM, Billmire DF. Duodenal atresia and stenosis: long-term follow-up over 30 years. J Pediatr Surg. 2004;39(6):867–71.

32 Malrotation and Volvulus

Spencer W. Beasley

Abstract

The term malrotation is used to denote the situation where the embryonic bowel, during the period when it herniates into the coelom of the body stalk between the 4th and 10th week of gestation, fails to rotate correctly. This means that when it returns to the abdominal cavity it is not correctly oriented, preventing the normal process of fixation of the midgut and its mesentery to the posterior abdominal wall. This results in a narrowed "universal" mesentery, which predisposes to volvulus. Volvulus is the term given to abnormal twisting of bowel (which, in the case of malrotation, involves most of the midgut) on its mesentery, and may have the consequence of cutting off its blood supply leading to ischaemia or infarction of the bowel.

Keywords

Malrotation • Gut rotation • Human embryology • Volvulus • Ladd's operation

32.1 Introduction

32.1.1 Definition

The term malrotation is used to denote the situation where the embryonic bowel, during the period when it herniates into the coelom of the body stalk between the 4th and 10th week of gestation, fails to rotate correctly. This means that when it returns to the abdominal cavity it is not correctly oriented, preventing the normal process of fixation of the midgut and its mesentery to the posterior abdominal wall. This results in a narrowed "universal" mesentery, which predisposes to volvulus. Volvulus is the term given to abnormal twisting of bowel (which, in the case of malrotation, involves most of the midgut) on its mesentery, and may have the consequence of cutting off its blood supply leading to ischaemia or infarction of the bowel.

32.1.2 Significance

The significance of malrotation relates to the potential for volvulus to supervene. Malrotation alone is usually asymptomatic, and may remain so

S.W. Beasley, MB, ChB(Otago), MS(Melbourne)
Clinical Director, Department of Paediatric Surgery, Christchurch Hospital, Riccarton Avenue, Private Bag 4710, Christchurch 8011, New Zealand
e-mail: spencer.beasley@cdhb.health.nz

P.D. Losty et al. (eds.), *Rickham's Neonatal Surgery*, https://doi.org/10.1007/978-1-4471-4721-3_32

throughout life. Even when asymptomatic, malrotation is dangerous because of its predisposition to midgut volvulus. When volvulus causes ischemia and necrosis of small bowel, the consequences are dire and include death or short gut syndrome.

32.2 Embryology and Pathology

32.2.1 Normal Rotation and Fixation of the Midgut

In simple terms, the normal configuration of the small bowel is acquired in a five stage process (Table 32.1), although there is considerable overlap with some of the stages. For example, rotation commences at the time of herniation.

32.2.1.1 Development of Dorsal Mesentery

The prerequisite for rotation of the midgut is development of the dorsal mesentery at 3–4 weeks gestation [1]. This forms after division of the lateral plate mesoderm into its somatic and splanchnic components to create the coelom, a process facilitated by *Foxf1* [2], with activation of the homeobox gene *Irx3* restricted to the somatic mesoderm.

Table 32.1 Stages leading to the final configuration of the normal midgut

1.	Development of dorsal mesentery
2.	Herniation
3.	Rotation
4.	Return to the abdominal cavity with completion of rotation
5.	Fixation

Intestinal rotation itself is mediated by changes in the dorsal mesentery [3] where mesenchymal cells on the right side of the mesentery become more sparse and cuboidal, and on the left dense and columnar. This is controlled by the transcription factors, *Pitx2* and *Isl1*, which themselves are under the control of *Nodal*. Their effect is that the mesentery is tilted to the left (Fig. 32.1).

32.2.1.2 Herniation

In the fourth week of embryonic life, the midgut (which is primarily supplied by a single vessel, the superior mesenteric artery) starts to protrude ventrally to herniate into the coelom of the body stalk (Fig. 32.2a). This occurs because of the combined effects of the rapid elongation of the intestine and growth of the liver [4]. For convenience, the bowel of the midgut proximal to this vessel is called the "pre-arterial" or "duodenojejunal" segment; and the part distal to the main stem of the superior mesenteric vessel is called the caudal ("post-arterial" or "caeco-colic") segment [5]. Initially, the pre-arterial segment grows more quickly than the post-arterial segment (Fig. 32.2b).

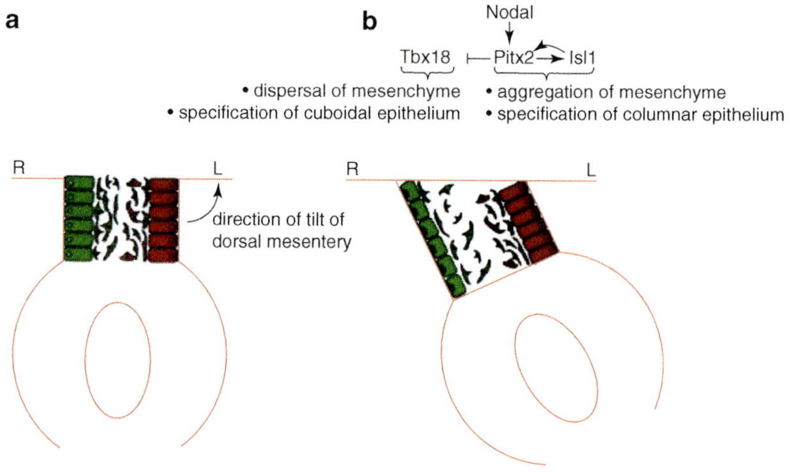

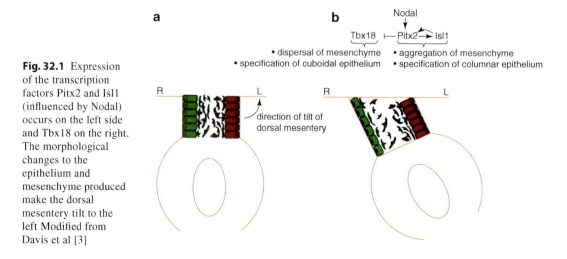

Fig. 32.1 Expression of the transcription factors Pitx2 and Isl1 (influenced by Nodal) occurs on the left side and Tbx18 on the right. The morphological changes to the epithelium and mesenchyme produced make the dorsal mesentery tilt to the left Modified from Davis et al [3]

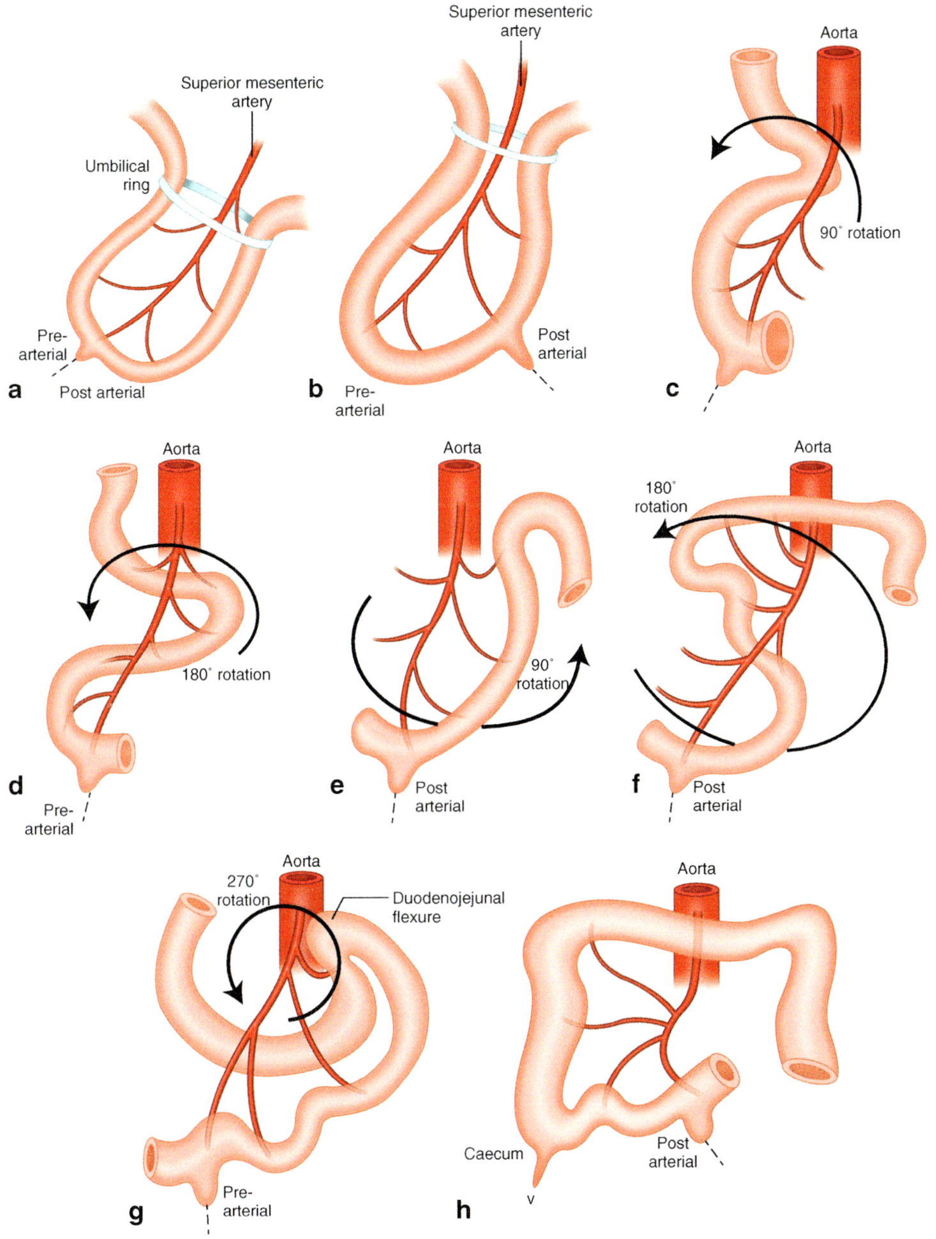

Fig. 32.2 In the fourth week of embryonic life the midgut grows rapidly and soon becomes too big for the space available to it in the abdominal cavity. It herniates through the umbilical ring into the coelom of the body stalk (**a**). The pre-arterial (duodeno-jejunal) segment initially grows more quickly than the post-arterial (ileo-colic) segment (**b**). The pre-arterial segment first rotates 90° counter-clockwise which places it to the right of the SMA (**c**) and then a second 90° (**d**) and in doing so the duodeno-jejunal junction comes to lie posterior to the SMA. Rotation of the post-arterial segment is in the same direction (counter-clockwise) as that of the pre-arterial segment (**e**), initially through 90° (a), followed by a second 90° (b). The 180 degree counter-clockwise twist of the SMA around its axis effectively drags the attached midgut with it. The final configuration of the pre-arterial segment of the midgut after completion of 270° of rotation means that the duodeno-jejunal flexure has altogether rotated 270° counter-clockwise from its original position to now lie to the left of the root of the superior mesenteric artery (**f**). Similarly, the 270° of counter-clockwise rotation brings the caecum down into the right lower quadrant after return of the midgut into the peritoneal cavity

32.2.1.3 Rotation

As the pre-arterial segment protrudes into the coelom, it rotates 90° counter clockwise so that it lies to the right of the SMA (Fig. 32.2c). And as it continues to lengthen it undergoes a further 90° rotation which pulls the duodenojejunal junction posterior to the SMA (Fig. 32.2d), a position it maintains throughout life and is a key feature on imaging by ultrasonography and CT.

Rotation of the post-arterial segment follows that of the pre-arterial segment, such that by the time it returns to the abdominal cavity it is lying ventral to the SMA, effectively having undergone a 180° counter clockwise rotation. The easiest way to understand the process is to imagine the SMA twisting 180° counter clockwise on its axis, drawing the attached midgut with it (Fig. 32.2e).

32.2.1.4 Return to the Abdominal Cavity

By the time the human embryo is about 40 mm in length (10th week) the midgut begins to return into the peritoneal cavity [5]. In doing so, the pre-arterial (duodenojejunal limb) segment completes an additional and final 90° rotation around the SMA, still rotating in a counter clockwise direction (Fig. 32.2f). Similarly, the post-arterial limb, is obliged to undergo a final 90° rotation which brings the caecum down into the right lower quadrant (Fig. 32.2g).

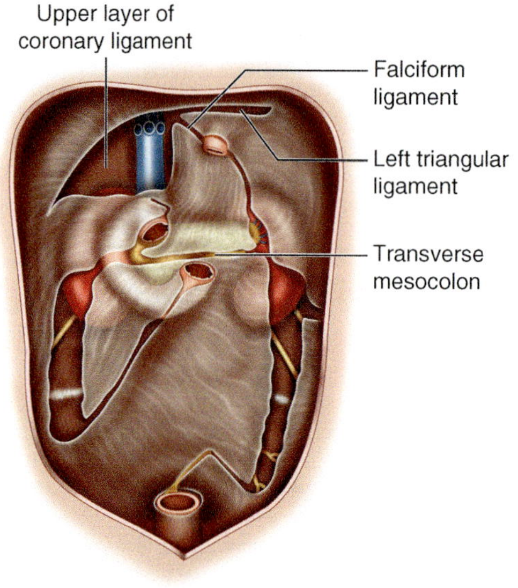

Fig. 32.3 The normal attachment of the root of the small bowel mesentery extends from the ligament of Trietz obliquely downwards and to the right as far as the caecum.

32.2.1.5 Fixation

Within a week or two of its return, the colon, particularly its ascending and descending parts, become adherent to the posterior abdominal wall, within the paracolic gutters. By now the duodenum is well attached to the posterior abdominal wall, with peritoneum running across its anterior surface. The SMA runs downwards ventral to the duodenum's third part. The attachment of the root of the small bowel mesentery extends from the ligament of Trietz obliquely downwards and to the right as far as the caecum (Fig. 32.3). All these events are normally complete by 13 weeks gestation [6]. It is the length and broadness of this attachment that largely prevents the small bowel from undergoing volvulus.

32.2.2 Abnormal Embryology

Incomplete rotation of the duodenum and colon interferes with the process of attachment to the posterior abdominal wall. If the caecum and ascending colon do not rotate a full 270° they cannot become anchored in the right paracolic gutter, and peritoneal condensations run anterior to the duodenum: these tend to tighten and cause obstruction of the duodenum if volvulus occurs.

Where rotation has not occurred, the width of attachment of the small bowel mesentery is much shorter, being largely confined to the region around the SMA (Fig. 32.4). This is sometimes referred to as a "universal mesentery" and is the pedicle around which the midgut can twist. Thus, the predisposition for volvulus is a combination of failure of rotation and failure of adequate fixation, leaving only a narrow attachment of the mesentery of the small bowel (Fig. 32.5). Abnormalities of midgut rotation fall into four broad categories (Table 32.2) of which non-rotation is by far the most common.

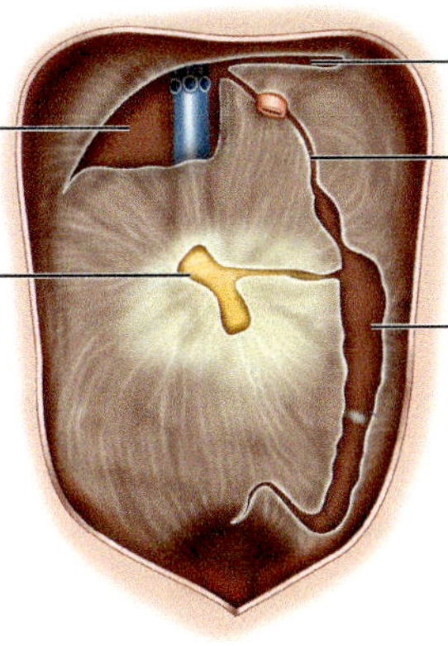

Fig. 32.4 In malrotation, the small bowel mesentery is attached only narrowly to the posterior abdominal wall, and only in the region of the superior mesenteric vessels. It is this lack of breadth of attachment that predisposes to volvulus

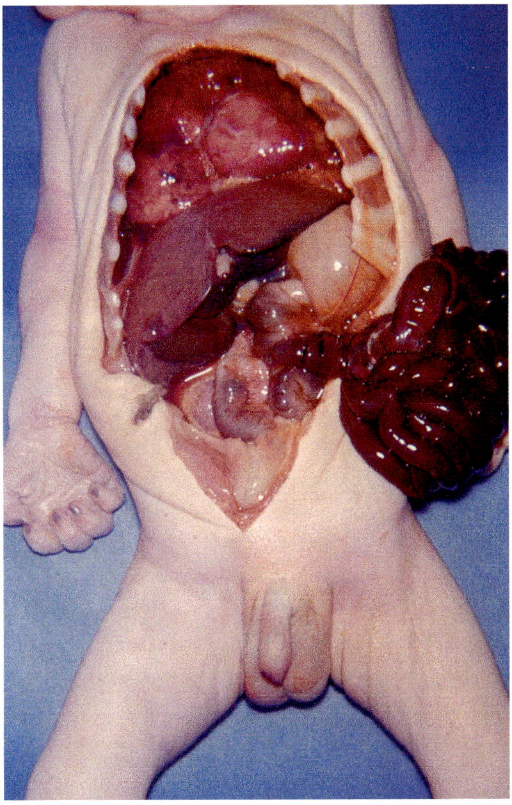

Fig. 32.5 Postmortem appearance of volvulus of the midgut complicating non-rotation where the extremely narrow base to the small bowel mesentery ("universal mesentery") has clearly contributed to the twisting of the small bowel on its mesentery

Table 32.2 Classification of rotational abnormalities of the midgut

Type	Embryology and Pathology
1. Non rotation (most common)	Failure of anticlockwise rotation of both pre and post-arterial segments of midgut Failure of fixation (especially of caecum and ascending colon) Narrow small bowel mesentery (figure)
2. Failure of rotation of pre-arterial segment	Non rotation of duodenojejunal (pre-arterial) segment Normal rotation and fixation of post-arterial segment Broad mesenteric attachment
3. Reverse rotation of midgut	Reverse rotation of pre-arterial segment causes duodenum to lie anterior to SMA May occur in isolation, leading to paraduodenal hernia (which appears as a mesenteric pouch opening to the right) May occur in conjunction with reverse rotation of post-arterial segment, leading to transverse colon lying behind SMA
4. Failure of rotation of post-arterial segment	Failure of the caecum and colon (post-arterial limb) to rotate interferes with its ability to fix to the posterior abdominal wall Leads to narrow small bowel mesentery Peritoneal bands to colon may cause duodenal obstruction Caecal volvulus may occur

32.2.3 Non Rotation

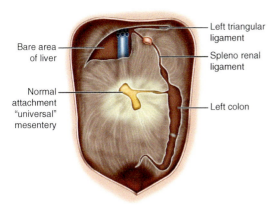

Complete failure of rotation of the midgut is the most frequent abnormality in this spectrum of conditions. Neither the pre-arterial nor post-arterial segments of midgut have rotated. As a consequence, the duodenum remains anterior, and is located mainly to the right of the midline. The ascending colon and caecum are only loosely attached, and can be variable in position, often lying anteriorly in the mid abdomen (Fig. 32.6). It is this variant that is at greatest risk of volvulus. Volvulus occurs around the superior mesenteric artery and tends to tighten the fascial condensations of peritoneum that run across the anterior part of the duodenum (so-called Ladd bands) which causes duodenal

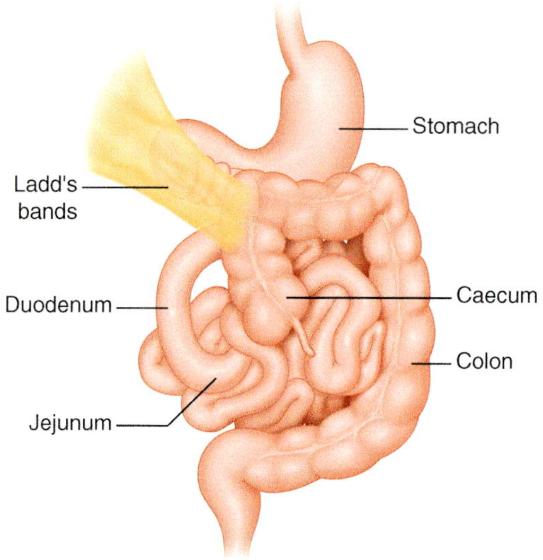

Fig. 32.6 Complete failure of rotation of the midgut (non-rotation with a "universal mesentery"). This is the most common variant, and predisposes to volvulus

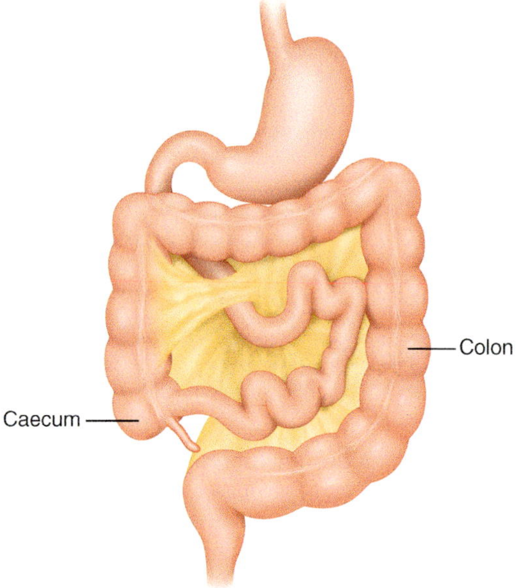

Fig. 32.7 Non-rotation of the pre-arterial (duodeno-jejunal) segment usually presents as duodenal obstruction because of tightening of the Ladd bands which run across the front of the duodenum, but because the caecum has rotated and is lying in the correct position, volvulus is uncommon

obstruction. But of much greater concern is that the twisting may cut off flow through the superior mesenteric artery (and obstruct the superior mesenteric vein) causing the bowel to become ischaemic.

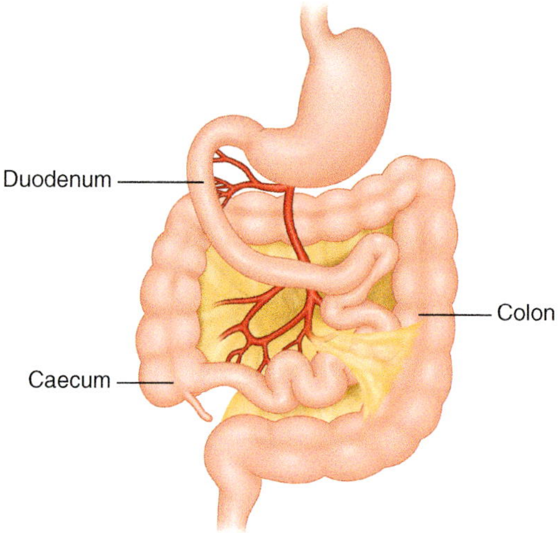

Fig. 32.8 Reverse rotation of the pre-arterial (duodeno-jejunal) segment in such a way that it passes in front of (ventral to) the vascular pedicle, with reverse rotation of the colon behind the superior mesenteric vessels, usually presents with distal bowel obstruction because the vessels compress the transverse colon

32.2.4 Failure of Rotation of Pre-arterial Segment of Midgut

This less common abnormality results from non-rotation of the pre-arterial segment of midgut (duodenojejunal limb), in the presence of normal rotation and fixation of the post-arterial segment (caeco-colic limb) (Fig. 32.7). This abnormality may cause obstruction of the duodenum because mesenteric bands to the ascending colon and caecum still run across the front of the duodenum. However, the risk of midgut volvulus itself is relatively low because of the broad attachment of the base of the mesentery to the posterior abdominal wall.

32.2.5 Reverse Rotation

Extremely rarely, reverse rotation can occur (Fig. 32.8). This brings the duodenum anterior to the SMA (rather than posterior) and causes the

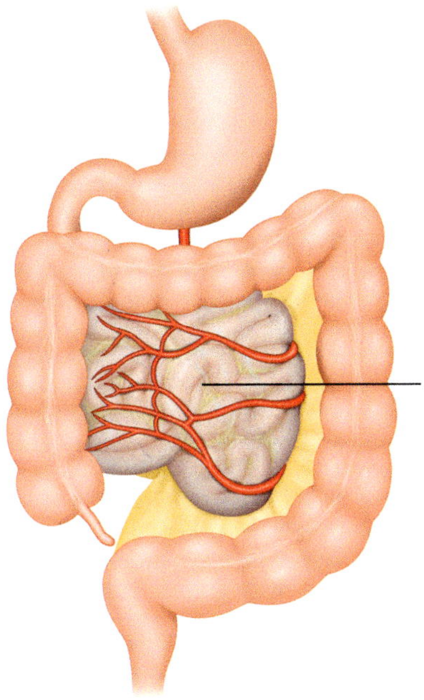

Fig. 32.9 When reverse rotation of the pre-arterial (duodeno-jejunal) segment occurs in conjunction with normal rotation of the post-arterial segment, a paraduodenal hernia is produced. The anterior part of the sac wall is actually the mesentery of the caecum and colon. This may cause some initial confusion on entering the peritoneal cavity because there appears to be a paucity of visible small bowel

transverse colon to lie behind the SMA. This may lead to colonic obstruction. Variants of this, where there are greater or lesser° of reverse rotation of the pre or post-arterial limbs may produce the appearance of paraduodenal hernias (Fig. 32.9), and these also may cause obstruction. (They may also create a challenge for the surgeon who initially may find the appearance confusing, but has to clarify exactly what has occurred in order to rectify it).

32.2.6 Failure of Rotation of the Post-arterial Segment of Midgut

This abnormality prevents adequate fixation of the colon, and produces a narrow mesentery, predisposing to volvulus [5]. It may also predispose to caecal volvulus where there is incomplete fixation of the caecum, and this may happen at any time in life.

32.3 Associated Abnormalities

A wide range of conditions have a recognised association with malrotation (see Table 32.3). Difficulty in making a distinction between true malrotation from incomplete or loose fixation of the midgut to the posterior abdominal wall (in the absence of malrotation) may be responsible for some of the apparent associations listed in Table 32.3. For example, the defects of exomphalos, gastroschisis and congenital diaphragmatic hernia all involve incorrect placement of bowel within the abdominal cavity and this may adversely affect fixation. Malrotation is reported to occur in up to a third of patients with duodenal atresia or stenosis [7]. From a clinical perspective, the co-existence of malrotation with other major congenital gastrointestinal abnormalities may create significant challenges in establishing the correct diagnosis of both conditions [8].

Lack of rotation and excessive mobility of the caecum may predispose to intussusception in some patients [9]: concurrence of intussusception and malrotation is a well-recognised phenomenon [10], accounting for 1.6% of 225 intussusceptions in one series [11]. There is some evidence the intussusceptions may precede the volvulus [12].

In recent years, geneticists have identified malrotation due to mutations in known genes. They fall into two main groups:

1. Mutations in the forkhead box transcription factor FoxF1. Other features include congenital short bowel, alveolar capillary dysplasia, misalignment of the pulmonary veins, and urinary tract malformations. Many have features in common with the heterotaxy syndromes [1].
2. Mutations in genes controlling L-R patterning. It is normal for organs of the torso to be asymmetric in their placement (e.g. heart, stomach, liver, biliary tract, spleen, and bowel) but when mutations occur in genes that specify L-R asymmetry, a number of clinical syndromes result (Table 32.3).

In addition, there are several conditions in which malrotation is likely to have a genetic cause, but for which the chromosomal locus and

Table 32.3 Abnormalities with an apparent association with malrotation

Nature of association	Example
Incorrect placement of bowel within abdominal cavity, or inadequate fixation	Congenital posterolateral (Bochdalek) diaphragmatic hernia Exomphalos Gastroschisis Intussusception
Possible early intrauterine volvulus	Duodenal atresia (including duodenal web or stenosis) Jejunal or ileal atresia
Mutation of known gene	FOXF1 at 16q24.1: alveolar capillary dysplasia, abnormal pulmonary venous drainage, micrognathia, congenital short bowel, annular pancreas, features of heterotaxy syndromes (autosomal dominant) FLNA at xq28: chronic idiopathic intestinal pseudo-obstruction, pyloric stenosis, undescended testes, hydronephrosis, thrombocytopenia (X-linked recessive) Abnormalities of L-R patterning: CFC1, ZIC3, NKX2.5, ACVR2B, LEFTY A (most have congenital heart disease, asplenia/polysplenia, and midline liver)
Non-syndromal malrotation	Familial malrotation
Syndromal malrotation	Martin-Frias syndrome (multiple bowel atresias, foregut appendage abnormalities e.g. biliary atresia, absent gallbladder) Multiple gastrointestinal atresias "apple peel" atresia of jejunum Microgastria, limb reduction defects, oesophageal atresia, ASD, VSD
Chromosomal imbalance	Duplication of long arm of chromosome 16: short bowel syndrome, anorectal malformation, gall bladder agensis Deletion long arm of chromosome 13: Hirschsprung disease, jejunal or ileal atresia
Miscellaneous (unclassified, or part of other syndromes or associations)	Meckel's diverticulum, Trisomy 13, 18, 21, Craniofacial, Prune belly syndrome, Mesenteric cyst, Marfan syndrome, Cornelia de Lange syndrome, Cat eye syndrome, Cantrell's syndrome, Pfeiffer Syndrome Type 2

gene mutations have yet to be identified. They are either non-syndromic (where malrotation occurs in isolation) or syndromic, in which other malformations also occur. The first published example of familial non-syndromic malrotation with volvulus with clear evidence for autosomal dominant inheritance involved eight individuals over three generations [13]. The syndromic conditions usually involve malrotation and other gastrointestinal malformations, and have an autosomal recessive inheritance pattern. They include Martin-Frias syndrome (multiple bowel atresias, biliary atresia and pancreatic abnormalities) [14] and multiple gastro-intestinal atresias (mostly of French-Canadian ethnicity, and include intraluminal calcification [15]. The combination of malrotation with short bowel [16], with MMIH (megacystis, microcolon and intestinal hypoperistalsis) [17], and with "apple peel" atresia [18] is also described.

Sometimes malrotation can be due to chromosomal imbalance [1]. The two situations of most relevance to paediatric surgeons are duplication of the long arm of chromosome 16 [19] (which also includes congenital short bowel, anorectal malformations and agenesis of the gall bladder), and deletions of the long arm of chromosome 13 which occurs with Hirschsprung disease or jejunal and ileal atresia [20].

The clinical geneticist has a role in providing genetic counselling and information about recurrence risk, and for that reason should be consulted whenever malrotation occurs with other abnormalities.

32.4 Incidence

The exact incidence of malrotation has been difficult to establish, mainly because it is so often asymptomatic throughout life. It has been identified in 0.5% of autopsies [21] as an incidental finding, and on upper gastrointestinal contrast studies as an asymptomatic and incidental finding in 0.2% [22], which would be consistent with an incidence of about 1/500 live births [23]. There is a male predominance of 2:1 in neonates who become symptomatic, but the gender difference disappears in older age-groups [24]. A strong concordance between identical twins raises the possibility of genetic factors in its patho-aetiology [25].

32.5 Age At Presentation

In paediatric institutions, more than half the cases of malrotation with volvulus are seen in the first week of life, and about 80% in the first month. If all age groups are taken into account, about half are seen in the first month, 75% by one year, and the remaining 25% occur later in life [26]. In one series 25 of 45 (56%) underwent surgery in the first month of life [27]. At the Royal Children's Hospital, Melbourne, 14 of 32 patients received surgery within a month of birth [28], and a subsequent larger review revealed an age distribution at presentation as shown in Fig. 32.10.

It must be remembered that very occasionally older children, and even adults may present with volvulus or other obstructive symptoms that are secondary to malrotation (see Fig. 32.7). In older children and in adults, the variability in symptomatology and the low index of suspicion for the diagnosis means that delay in making the correct diagnosis is common, with a mean period of delay ranging from 1.7 years [27] to up to 5 years [28–30]. About 70% adults experience symptoms for more than 6 months before diagnosis [31].

The median age at surgery was 9 days in a series of 161 patients from two tertiary centres [32]. Age at presentation is not a good predictor of the likelihood of bowel infarction when volvulus occurs: infarction can be the consequence of volvulus at any age [33], although most cases of volvulus occur in the first few months of life.

32.6 Presentation (Table 32.4)

32.6.1 Antenatal Diagnosis

Malrotation is difficult to diagnose on antenatal ultrasonography in the absence of volvulus. The main clue to malrotation is a horizontally and medially positioned stomach [34], a finding that warrants an early post-natal upper GI contrast study to confirm the diagnosis. There is a higher index of suspicion when abnormalities known to be associated with malrotation (such as congenital diaphragmatic hernia, congenital heart disease and duodenal atresia) are diagnosed.

Volulus is one explanation for unexpected cessation of fetal movement and fetal distress, and may prompt ultrasonographic review of the fetus. It may also precipitate spontaneous rupture of the membranes [35]. It has been conjectured that fetal stress and fetal pain may activate both fetal-placental adrenal and hypothalamic stress hormones leading to premature uterine activity [36]. In these situations, malrotation is more likely to be deduced on antenatal ultrasonography because of features which represent the consequences of volvulus. These include a distended stomach and small bowel dilatation [35], heterogeneous echogenicity within the dilated bowel, the disappearance of peristalsis [37], fetal ascites, dilated loops of bowel [38], and features of meconium peritonitis. A convoluted mass in the mid-abdomen may be seen, and this has a whirlpool or snail configuration and has no peristaltic movement [37, 39]. While none of these alone is pathognomonic, their combination is strongly suggestive of volvulus. Later, peritoneal calcification and pseudocyst

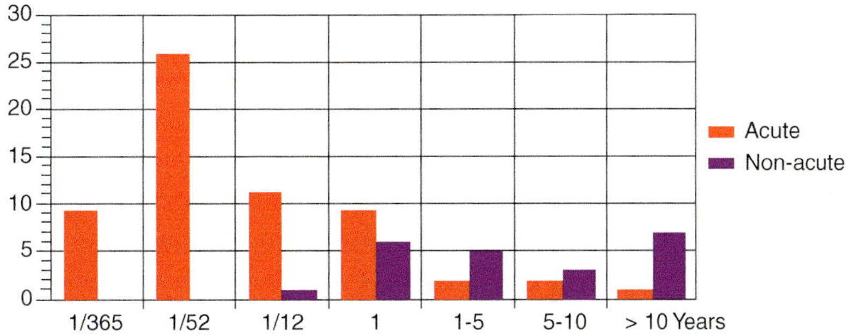

Fig. 32.10 Age at presentation of all cases of malrotation according to acuity. Volvulus can occur at any age, but is more likely in the neonate

Table 32.4 Presentation of malrotation

Antenatal diagnosis	Ultrasound evidence of consequences of volvulus
Postnatal diagnosis	
Malrotation alone	Asymptomatic[a]
	As an incidental finding on imaging (e.g. during upper GI contrast study, ultrasonography)
Malrotation with volvulus	Bile stained vomiting (especially in the neonate)
	Recurrent episodes of acute abdominal pain
	Other nonspecific symptoms (weight loss, early satiety, failure to thrive, intermittent diarrhoea, malabsorption, jaundice)

[a]Sometimes in the absence of volvulus, compression caused by peritoneal bands (Ladd's bands) may cause obstructive symptoms

formation can result from necrosis and perforation [40]. Midgut volvulus may precipitate premature delivery [36, 37].

In "secondary malrotation" [41] a large intra-abdominal cyst that develops early in gestation may prevent the midgut from undergoing normal rotation and fixation. This phenomenon has been described where there has been a large cystic mesenchymal hamartoma of the liver even where it has spontaneously involuted before birth. Teele et al. [41] conjecture that the dilated proximal duodenum seen in duodenal stenosis or atresia may also prevent normal rotation and fixation, which may account for the higher than expected incidence of malrotation in duodenal atresia [7].

Malrotation without volvulus has also been diagnosed antenatally by MRI scan at 35 weeks gestation by the observation of a midline stomach and all loops of small bowel to the right of the midline and all large bowel to the left [42]. However, both false positives and false negative results have been reported for the MRI diagnosis of malrotation [43], and at present it does not have a well defined role antenatally. Malrotation with volvulus can also be diagnosed on MRI antenatally [44].

32.6.2 Presentation in the Neonatal Period

"Volvulus neonatorum" is the term used to describe malrotation with volvulus that is evident at birth. The volvulus is likely to have occurred shortly before birth, and may even precipitate birth [36]. The newborn infant has a markedly tender and distended abdomen, consistent with established peritonitis. Surgical intervention is urgent, but often much of the small bowel is already dead. The mortality rate is high [45]

A more common presentation in the neonatal period is of an infant who appeared well at birth who then has sudden onset of bile stained vomiting. Subsequently, abdominal distension and tenderness may develop, and the infant may show evidence of respiratory distress (in part from elevation and splinting of the diaphragm) and sepsis. If not recognised early, progressive infarction of the midgut leads to signs of peritonitis, shock and eventually death.

32.6.3 Presentation in Older Children

Older children also present with bile stained vomiting, but are more likely to have other symptoms as well. The most common of these is intermittent or chronic abdominal pain which may occur with or without vomiting. Features more clearly indicative of intermittent obstruction may occur, with the addition of episodes of severe colicky pain and abdominal distension. Less usual presentations are often fairly non-specific, and include malabsorption, hypoproteinaemia, solid food intolerance, feeding difficulties, jaundice from common bile duct obstruction [27, 46], aspiration, failure to thrive, abdominal mass and diarrhoea [27]. A poor nutritional state is seen in many, with almost half on or below the third centile [47]. In advanced cases, where the blood supply to the small bowel has been acutely and severely compromised by volvulus, the presentation is of peritonitis and shock. Older children are more likely to have the rarer anatomic variants of malrotation than neonates who become symptomatic [27].

Sometimes malrotation is noted as an incidental finding at abdominal surgery or during abdominal imaging for other conditions. For example, it is sometimes noted for the first time at appendicectomy when the appendix is difficult to locate and cannot be found in the right iliac fossa.

32.6.4 Approach to Clinical Assessment

Malrotation *per se* is asymptomatic. Symptoms develop when volvulus supervenes. In general, acute volvulus produces symptoms related to:

- proximal bowel obstruction
- midgut ischaemia

This means that these patients present with bile-stained vomiting, abdominal pain and distension, and where the blood supply to the gut is compromised, signs of peritonitis (Fig. 32.11). Therefore, the key to clinical assessment is to establish whether there is any evidence of compromised small bowel—as this represents an emergency and demands urgent surgical intervention to untwist the volvulus.

Specific signs at presentation which indicate that the bowel is ischaemic or infarcted include:

- shock
- abdominal tenderness
- guarding
- rectal bleeding

These signs confirm that extreme urgency exists: aggressive resuscitation and urgent laparotomy are indicated, even in the absence of specific imaging beforehand to confirm the diagnosis.

32.7 Investigation/Imaging

32.7.1 Plain Radiology

32.7.1.1 Diagnostic Features

There are few diagnostic features specific to malrotation on plain radiology of the abdomen in the infant in the absence of volvulus.

When volvulus has supervened the plain x-ray typically shows a relatively "gasless" abdomen with air in the stomach and duodenum, but little beyond the first part of the duodenum. Dilatation of the stomach and proximal duodenum (seen as an air bubble) with paucity of gas more distally is indicative of the duodenal obstruction caused by Ladd bands. The radiological appearance may not be dissimilar to that of duodenal atresia or duodenal stenosis with its typical "double bubble", although there is usually more gas distally in malrotation than is evident in duodenal atresia. Also, the small bowel is often distended. On other occasions, the plain radiological appearance can be fairly nonspecific, particularly if the stomach is not distended as might occur after vomiting has emptied it.

In some instances the appearances may be of a complete small bowel obstruction with multiple air fluid levels and dilated loops of small bowel. This is particularly likely to be seen when there is compromised blood flow to the midgut. There

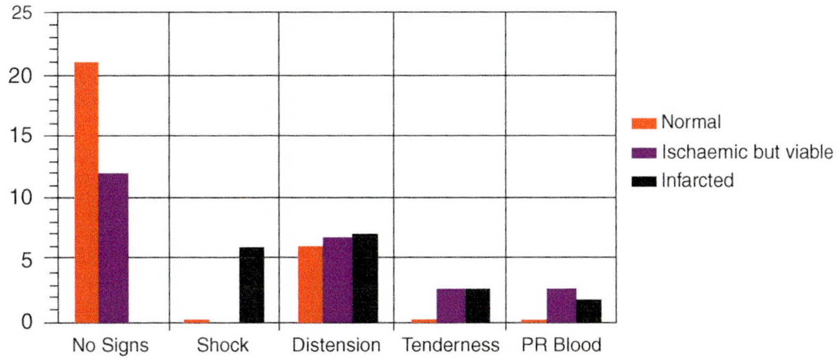

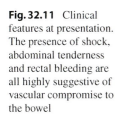

Fig. 32.11 Clinical features at presentation. The presence of shock, abdominal tenderness and rectal bleeding are all highly suggestive of vascular compromise to the bowel

may be evidence of free peritoneal fluid and thickened bowel loops. This radiological appearance will usually be associated with significant abdominal distension and tenderness, and justifies immediate surgical intervention.

32.7.1.2 Limitations

It is important to recognise that a normal abdominal radiograph in an infant with bilious emesis and suspected malrotation does not reliably exclude the diagnosis of malrotation. Even in the presence of volvulus the appearance on plain radiographs can be normal or "nonspecifically abnormal". For this reason, if malrotation and volvulus are suspected, further investigation is required.

32.7.1.3 Role

In the neonate with bile-stained vomiting or abdominal distension, plain radiology of the abdomen is mainly employed to identify or exclude other conditions such as duodenal atresia (no gas or distension distal to the duodenum) or necrotizing enterocolitis (intramural gas, portal venous gas).

32.7.2 Upper Gastrointestinal Contrast Study

32.7.2.1 Diagnostic Features

The upper gastrointestinal contrast study (which can be performed with either barium or a water soluble agent) is the most commonly performed investigation used to confirm the diagnosis of malrotation. Ideally, the examination should be performed by a paediatric radiologist under fluoroscopic control.

It is generally accepted that the key to diagnosis is establishing the exact location of the duodenojejunal junction: in the normal patient the duodenojejunal junction is anchored to the posterior abdominal wall by the ligament of Treitz, so will be to the left of the midline and at the level of the pylorus [28]. But where there is malrotation, the duodenojejunal junction tends to be located more inferiorly and to the right (Fig. 32.12). This gives an appearance of contrast running down through the duodenum in a corkscrew or spiral pattern as it connects with the jejunum, also on the right side (Fig. 32.13). Identification of the exact location of the duodenojejunal junction

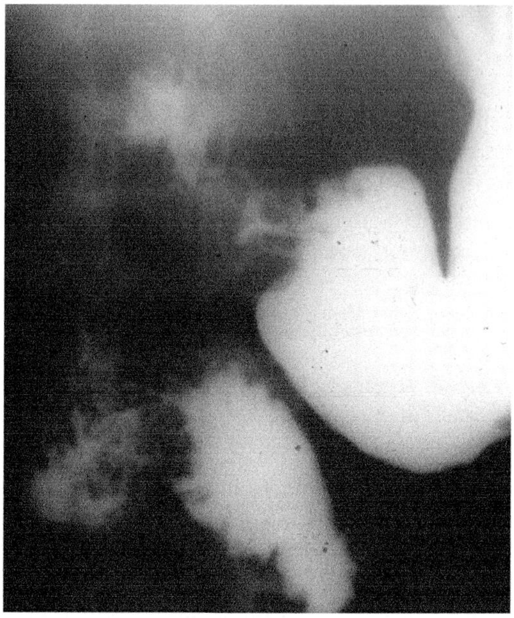

Fig. 32.12 The key to diagnosis of malrotation is demonstration of the duodeno-jejunal junction being inferior and to the right of its normal position and an upper GI contrast study

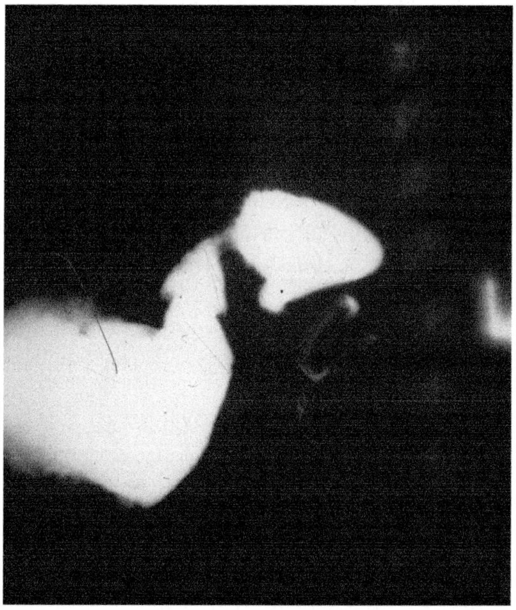

Fig. 32.13 The classical "corkscrew" or "spiral" appearance of the distal duodenum and proximal jejunum to the right of the midline

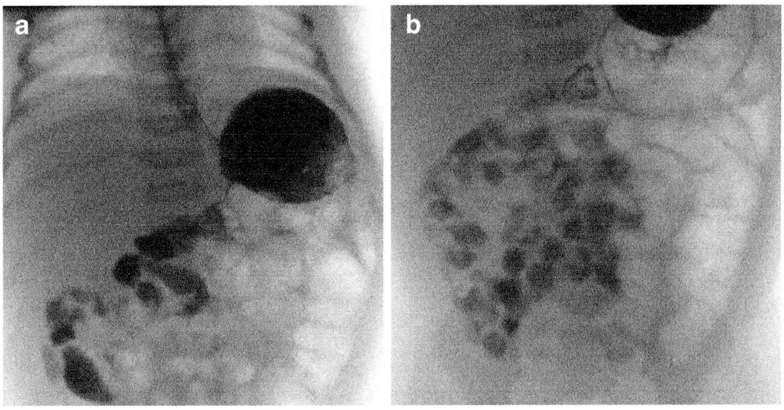

Fig. 32.14 This 4 day old infant presented with bilious vomiting. The upper GI contrast study showed (**a**) the duodenojejunal flexure displaced inferiorly and to the right, and the small bowel filling to the right of the midline; and (**b**) delayed films confirmed the small bowel opacified predominantly in the right side of the abdomen, and the colon (unopacified) to the left

necessitates continuous fluoroscopy to view carefully the flow of contrast as it exits the stomach and passes rapidly through the duodenum into the jejunum. As the contrast continues to pass through the small bowel it is noted to be predominantly on the right side of the abdomen (Fig. 32.14a,b), and later on once colonic filling occurs, the colon can be seen to the left. The caecum is abnormally positioned in 80% patients with malrotation [48].

In the presence of volvulus, obstruction of the mid duodenum is evident (Fig. 32.15)

32.7.2.2 Limitations

Its limitations are that the DJ flexure may be difficult to identify when contrast passes out of the stomach quickly (which is why continuous fluoroscopic control and a paediatric radiologist familiar with the radiological diagnostic criteria and potential pitfalls is required) (Table 32.5). Views are compromised if the stomach is too full of Barium [48]. It should be remembered that the position of the DJ flexure itself is only a consequence of malrotation—that the relationship between the third part of the duodenum and the superior mesenteric vessels is more critical [49], something that can only be inferred from the upper GI meal. Interpretation is complicated further by the normal variations that are seen in the position of the pylorus (given that it is used as the axial landmark in the lateral view for establishing the normal position of the DJ flexure).

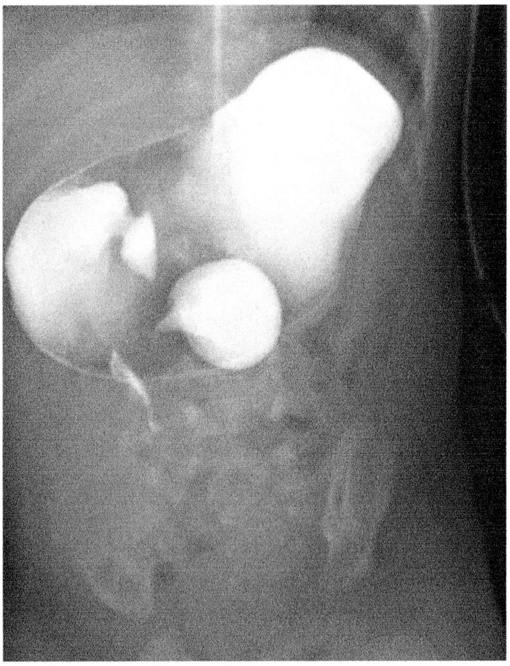

Fig. 32.15 The upper GI contrast study of a one month old infant presenting with sudden onset of bile stained vomiting showing mid-duodenal obstruction and a distended stomach. Notice the relative paucity of distal gas

Immediate follow-through of the contrast shows that the small bowel is predominantly on the right side of the abdomen, and delayed films (usually the next day) show that the colon is predominantly on the left. However, the caecal site and mobility cannot be reliably shown by a barium follow-through examination, and as such, delayed follow-through imaging has no place *per se* in the investigation of malrotation [28]. Nevertheless, the delayed films sometimes provide useful additional information on the location of the caecum and disposition of the colon. Where an upper GI study has proved equivocal in diagnosing malrotation it can be repeated a day or two later. Alternatively, ultrasonography, a distal contrast enema or diagnostic laparoscopy can be performed, depending on the facilities and expertise available, condition of the child, and the degree of uncertainty about the diagnosis.

32.7.2.3 Role

The upper GI contrast study has long been considered the "gold standard" for the diagnosis of malrotation, particularly in the absence of volvulus, although many paediatric institutions increasingly are using ultrasonography as a complementary investigation. A barium meal can also be used to confirm duodenal obstruction in volvulus. It is considered a more reliable investigation than the barium enema to diagnose malrotation, particularly in the neonate [28].

32.7.3 Distal Gastrointestinal Contrast Study

32.7.3.1 Diagnostic Features

For many years the barium enema was considered the procedure of choice, but its shortcomings mean that it is now used less commonly.

The key diagnostic feature on a contrast enema relates to identifying the position of the caecum, which should be in the right iliac fossa but in malrotation tends to be higher than normal, and even on the left side of the abdomen. Often the entire colon will be seen in the left side of the abdomen, and the ascending colon appears relatively short.

32.7.3.2 Limitations

The caecum may be difficult to identify in infants because it is less bulbous than later in life, and redundancy of the colon might obscure it (Table 32.5). The finding of a high and mobile caecum is indicative of malrotation, but this finding may also occur in about 15% of normal infants in the absence of malrotation.

Table 32.5 Summary of short-comings of gastrointestinal contrast studies in diagnosing malrotation

Investigation	Problems	Comment
Barium meal	Failure to correctly identify duodenojejunal (DJ) flexure Normal variation in position of neonatal DJ flexure Variability in position of pylorus	causes include: Inappropriate view Failure to see barium pass rapidly through the flexure, with sudden massive filling of proximal small bowel (that obscures further viewing) Especially if stomach full
Follow-through	site of caecum not reliably seen Mobility of caecum cannot be established	
Barium enema	Difficulty identifying position of caecum Wide normal variation in position of neonatal caecum Failure to demonstrate mobility of caecum Normally-located caecum may still be consistent with malrotation	Especially in neonate (caecum not bulbous) often high-lying

Consequently, the main limitations of a barium enema relate to interpretation of the mobility of the caecum [50], which may produce a false positive result. The degree of attachment of the caecum to the posterior abdominal wall in the right iliac fossa is quite variable, and where this is loose, the caecum will also be quite variable in its position, including being situated higher and more medially than normal. This may give a false impression of post-arterial malrotation, where in fact, it simply represents a degree of non-fixation [28]. Moreover, duodenal obstruction may be caused by pre-arterial malrotation in the presence of a caecum in the normal position. A second limitation in the distal contrast study relates to the fact that the neonatal caecum is not particularly bulbous and may be quite difficult to identify accurately. It is most easily seen with oblique, compression, and left-side down decubitus films.

32.7.3.3 Role

The barium enema is now mainly used to provide further information when an upper GI contrast study has been equivocal, but malrotation is still suspected. In a study of the correlation in 11 patients where both studies were performed, there were no cases where both the upper and lower GI series were negative in the presence of malrotation [28].

32.7.4 Ultrasonography

32.7.4.1 Diagnostic Features

Ultrasound has the advantage that it is non-invasive but is vitally dependent on the expertise of the ultrasonographer: without a well-trained paediatric ultrasonographer it is probably of very limited value.

The key diagnostic feature is the relationship of the superior mesenteric artery to the superior mesenteric vein: if the SMV lies anterior or to the left of the SMA (rather than to its right) it indicates malrotation. Other diagnostic features include: dilatation of the proximal duodenum, a distended (obstructed) superior mesenteric vein (SMV), bowel loops fixed to the midline, the "whirlpool sign" (Fig. 32.16), and location of the third part of the duodenum [51, 52]. The "whirlpool sign" on colour Doppler ultrasonography indicates flow within the SMV as it spirals around the SMA in a clockwise direction [39, 53]. The third part of the duodenum should be retromesenteric if malrotation is to be excluded [49]. In the presence of volvulus, Doppler ultrasonography can provide further information on blood flow through the superior mesenteric vessels, as an indicator of perfusion of the midgut.

32.7.4.2 Limitations

It has a significant false negative rate, perhaps as high as 30% [54] (Table 32.6). In one study [55] identification of the SMV to the left of the SMA proved a more reliable indicator of malrotation than when the SMV was anterior to the SMA. Confirmation of the relationship of the third part of the duodenum to the mesenteric vessels may improve its reliability [49]

32.7.4.3 Role/Indications

Its main use is in the investigation of the infant with vomiting, where malrotation is one of a number of diagnostic possibilities. Particularly when it is used to diagnose pyloric stenosis, it may provide information on the rotation of the gut. Where a high level of paediatric ultrasonographic expertise is available, it is used more routinely as a primary diagnostic tool, and will often be used in conjunction with a upper GI contrast study if there is clinical suspicion of malrotation.

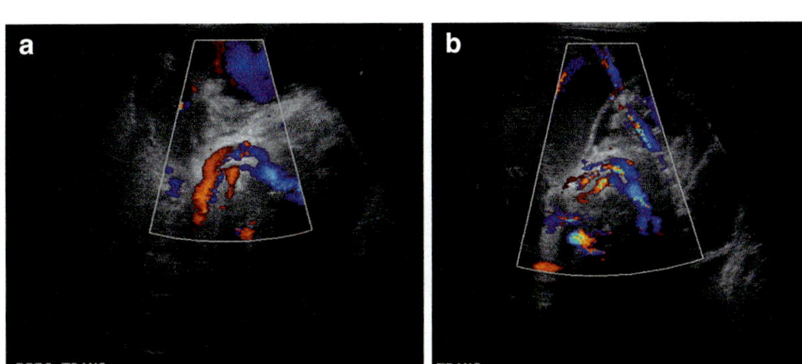

Fig. 32.16 Transverse upper abdominal transverse ultrasound images showing the "whirlpool" configuration of the superior mesenteric vessels at the root of the small bowel mesentery, with aligning dilated loops of small bowel

Table 32.6 Accuracy of imaging in diagnosing malrotation

Investigation	Accuracy	Percentage
Ba meal (Beasley “” “ “)	False negative rate	8
Follow-through study (“ “ “)	Unhelpful or misleading	67
Ba enema (Beasley and de Campo 1987)	False negative rate	17
Ultrasound (Applegate 2009) (Orzech et al. 2006) http://emedicine.medscape etc. Reid	Sensitivity	67–100
	Specificity	75–100
	False negative rate	2
	False positive rate	21
	False negative rate	30
	False positive rate	20
CT scan (Taylor 2011)	False negative rate	28.9
	False positive rate	10

32.7.5 CT Scan

32.7.5.1 Diagnostic Features

Features suggestive of malrotation include the small bowel being predominantly right-sided with the colon located on the left. It can also demonstrate an abnormal relationship between the superior mesenteric vessels (Fig. 32.17), and aplasia of the uncinate process [56]. An abnormal location of the third part of the duodenum has been identified in over 80% of patients with malrotation compared with 0% of controls [57], particularly in relation to the mesenteric vessels [49]. In adults, it is most often seen as an incidental finding at CT [58]. It has been used to correctly diagnose simultaneous volvulus and ileo-ileal intussusceptions [59].

32.7.5.2 Limitations

The radiation exposure limits its application in neonates and young children: the younger the infant, the greater the long-term risk. In addition, 10/100 control patients have an inverted SMA/SMV relationship (10% false positive rate) and 11/38 patients with malrotation had an apparently normal SMA/SMV relationship (27% false

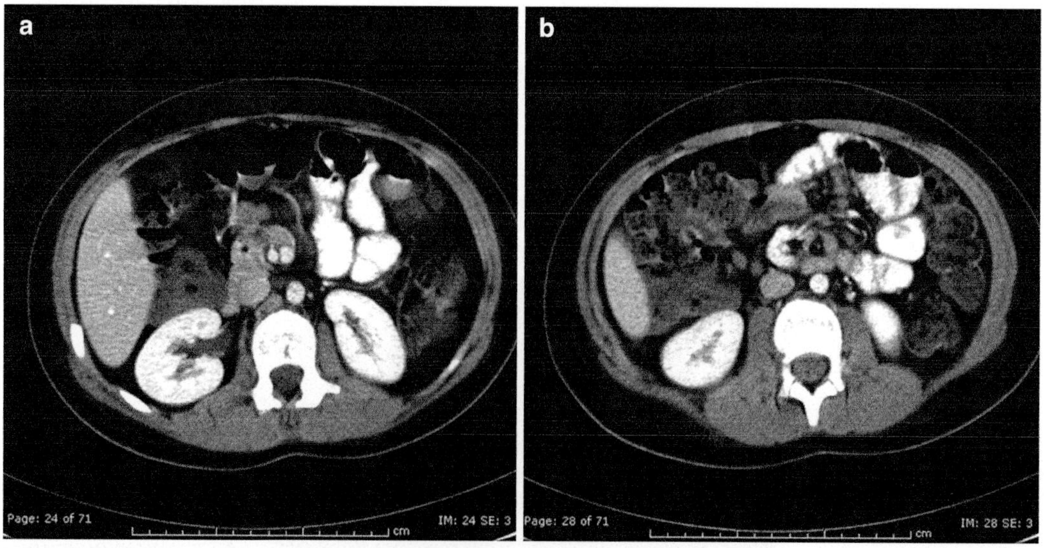

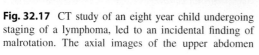

Fig. 32.17 CT study of an eight year child undergoing staging of a lymphoma, led to an incidental finding of malrotation. The axial images of the upper abdomen reveal an abnormal orientation of the superior mesenteric vessels at the root of the mesentery, with the ileocolic valve and caecum in the right upper quadrant

negative rate) [57], which suggests that this diagnostic criterion should not be used in isolation.

32.7.5.3 Role

This investigation is used rarely in neonates because of the high radiation exposure. In children and adults it occasionally reveals malrotation as an unexpected or incidental finding [58] (Fig. 32.17).

32.7.6 MRI

The role of MRI in the diagnosis of malrotation is yet to be established. A prospective non-randomised observational investigation into whether MRI could provide an alternative to contrast imaging (and thus avoid radiation) is being conducted [60].

32.8 Management

32.8.1 Initial Resuscitation (Table 32.7)

The paediatric surgical service should be notified as soon as a diagnosis of malrotation with volvulus is made: this diagnosis represents one of the few critical emergencies in paediatric surgery.

These children range from having relatively few signs initially to being profoundly shocked and unstable. Initial clinical examination determines whether there is evidence of compromised bowel perfusion: distended tender abdomen with guarding, tachycardic, or shocked and unresponsive. An intravenous line should be inserted through which fluid and electrolyte deficiencies are corrected, broad spectrum antibiotics effective against bowel organisms are administered, and vasopressor medication given to manage hypotensive shock. Oral feeds are stopped and a nasogastric tube inserted. Where the blood supply to the bowel is suspected to be compromised, an exploratory laparotomy or laparoscopy should be performed as quickly as possible, even if it means omitting imaging or other investigations beforehand.

Table 32.7 Key points for the initial management of malrotation with volvulus

• Immediate involvement of paediatric surgical service
• Insertion of intravenous line
• Take blood for haematology, blood culture, electrolyte, acid-base balance and for cross-match
• Correct fluid and electrolyte deficits
• Nil orally and nasogastric tube insertion
• Antibiotics effective against bowel organisms
• Dopamine (if required, as infusion 3 mcg/kg/min)
• Urgent surgical intervention:
– Careful discussion with family
– Consent covering all likely operative scenarios
– Do NOT delay surgery for imaging or other investigations if patient has evidence of compromised gut

32.8.2 Indications for Surgery

Emergency surgery is always indicated where volvulus causing compromised blood flow to the small bowel is suspected. The sooner the surgery, the better the outcome for the child. Even in the absence of signs of peritonitis, surgical intervention is urgent where imaging has demonstrated volvulus.

Where the history has been suggestive of malrotation with intermittent volvulus, but there is no current volvulus, surgery should still be performed reasonably promptly, before any further episode of volvulus occurs—because the next volvulus may cause irreversible vascular compromise to the bowel.

Where malrotation has been discovered incidentally in a child who is otherwise asymptomatic there has been less agreement on whether, and how urgently, surgery should be performed. Uncertainty has related to the relative risk of surgical morbidity (from a Ladd procedure) and of later volvulus if left untreated. It is the author's opinion that the consequences of volvulus are so potentially catastrophic that all children with diagnosed malrotation, even if completely asymptomatic, should undergo a Ladd procedure. This is supported by a review of a national database of 219 children older than one year undergoing a Ladd procedure which emphasized the importance of surgery in all children with incidentally found malrotation [61]. A Markov decision analysis review of quality of life adjusted life expectancy with and without a Ladd procedure in asymptomatic patients with malrotation showed the highest advantage of surgery was in children under 1 year of age, with a declining advantage up to the age of 20 years, after which observation alone may be more appropriate [62]. However, many patients assumed to be asymptomatic have significant non-specific symptoms, or symptoms wrongly attributed to other conditions during adulthood [63]. Inability to predict who will later suffer the serious consequences of volvulus further justifies surgical intervention in all patients where a diagnosis of malrotation has been made [33].

The essential goals of surgery are to:

1. untwist any volvulus to re-establish circulation to the bowel, and assess bowel viability
2. broaden the mesenteric attachment of the small bowel to reduce the chances of subsequent volvulus

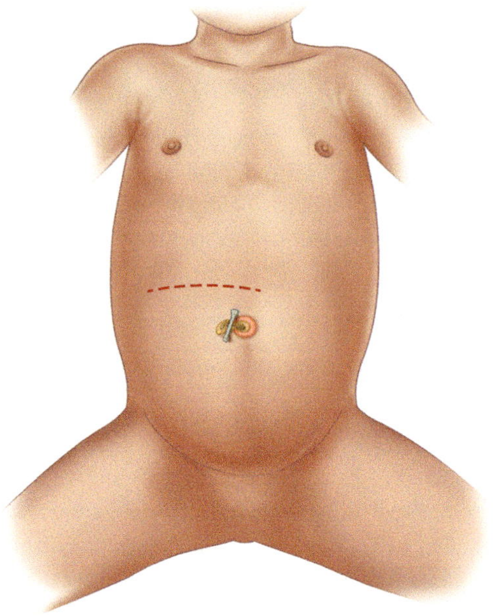

Fig. 32.18 The open approach to a Ladd procedure is performed through a supra-umbilical, predominantly right-sided transverse muscle-cutting incision

32.8.3 Surgical Approach

Traditionally, surgery for malrotation has been performed through an open approach, although recent refinements in laparoscopic techniques in infants and children now mean that the laparoscopic approach can be considered a legitimate alternative approach for selected patients. A laparoscopic approach may have a specific advantage when imaging has been inconclusive [64].

32.8.3.1 Open Approach

Currently, this is the preferred approach when there is concern about the viability of the midgut or there is marked abdominal distension. A transverse superumbilical muscle cutting incision is employed (Fig. 32.18). The peritoneum is opened, and in the neonate the falciform ligament is divided between ligatures.

32.8.3.2 Laparoscopic Approach

Laparoscopy represents an alternative surgical approach, with the choice of trocar size determined according to the size of the child. Three trocars of 3.5 mm can be used for infants [65]. Normally the scope is introduced through the umbilicus with two working ports in the mid to lower abdomen on either side (Fig. 32.19). The patient is supine near the foot of the table so the surgeon can stand between the legs. The reverse Trendelenberg position improves visualisation of the duodenum.

A laparoscopic approach may be most appropriate in the absence of volvulus, where imaging has suggested the diagnosis of malrotation in the absence of ongoing symptoms [50, 65, 66], and sometimes when imaging has not been able to exclude the diagnosis in a child with suspicious symptoms [64]. Laparoscopic derotation of volvulus in neonates and infants may be difficult and potentially dangerous where the small bowel is markedly distended or the bowel viability is marginal, and for this reason some caution its use in this situation [50]. Nevertheless, it has been performed laparoscopically with success in neonates where volvulus has not progressed to infarction [67].

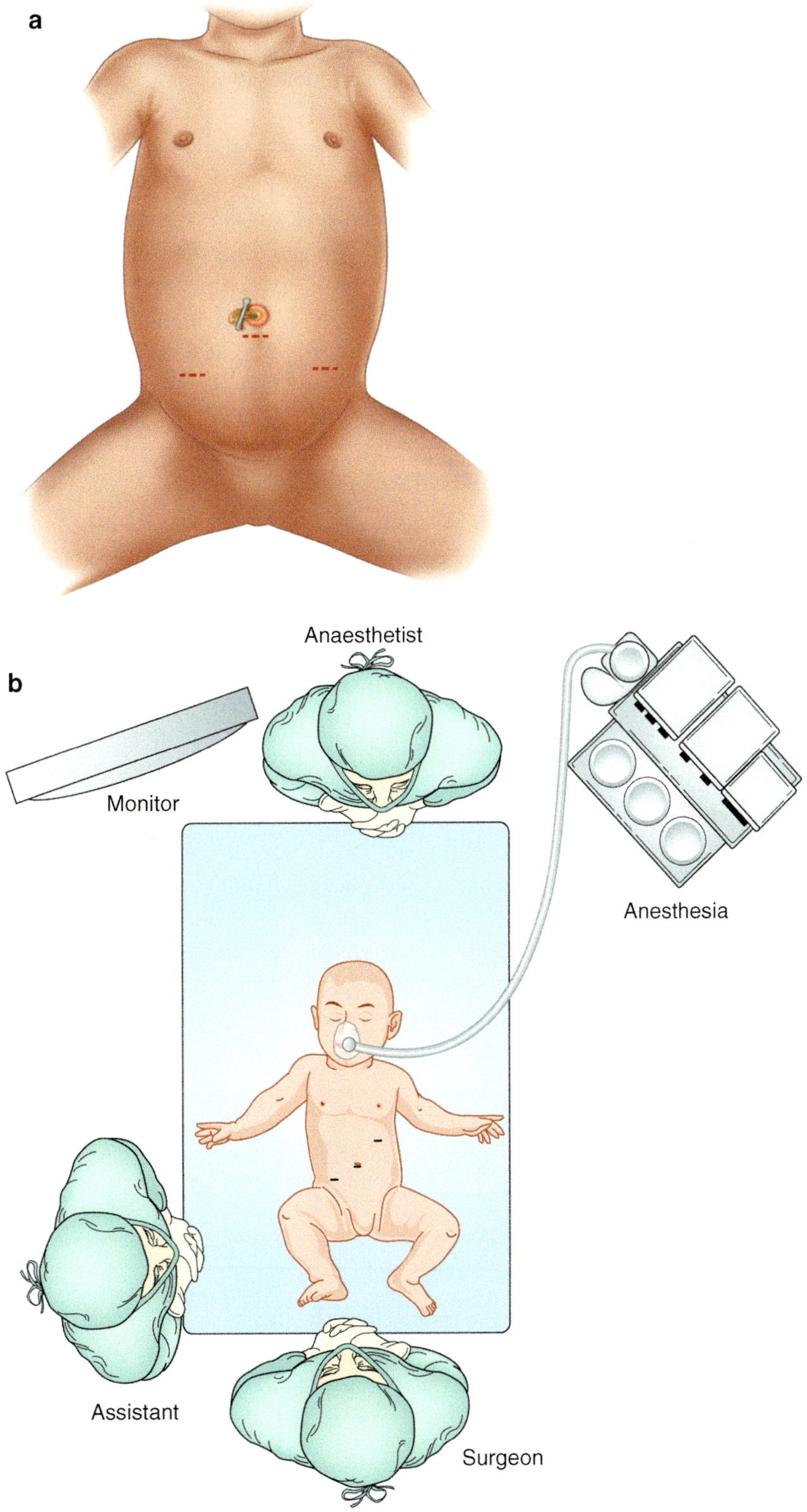

Fig. 32.19 The laparoscopic approach to a Ladd procedure is performed using an umbilical incision and usually two working ports, although sometimes a third working port (to elevate the liver edge) can be helpful

It would be reasonable to expect that in about 25–33% of cases conversion to an open procedure may be necessary [66, 68] although one report of 36 laparoscopic procedures had a conversion rate of 8.3% [69]. Rothenberg has advocated conversion to an open procedure where the dilated loops of bowel are clearly ischaemic to avoid undue delay and bowel injury [64]. Successful application of the procedure in older children with midgut volvulus has also been reported [70]. Operative times average about one hour [65], and are similar to that of the open approach [69].

32.8.4 Initial Operative Assessment

32.8.4.1 Deliver Bowel

In the open approach, once the peritoneal cavity has been opened, free fluid is aspirated, and the midgut is delivered through the wound (Fig. 32.20). The wound must be of sufficient size that this can be done without causing trauma to bowel which may already be friable. Evisceration of the small bowel is required to assess the root of the mesentery (Fig. 32.21). With the laparoscopic approach this is not possible, so the features that must be looked for to assess rotation are: the curve of the duodenum as it runs from right to left behind the superior mesenteric vessels, evidence of peritoneal condensations (Ladd bands) crossing in front of the duodenum, the location and fixation of the ligament of Treitz (which should be to the left of the superior mesenteric vessels) and the fixation of the caecum and right colon.

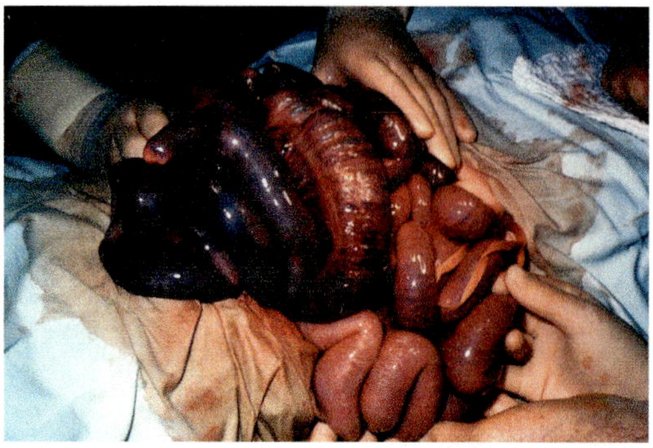

Fig. 32.20 In the open approach, the first step is to deliver the small bowel into the wound. This allows its viability to be assessed, as well as facilitates inspection of the root of the small bowel mesentery

32.8.4.2 Untwist the Small Bowel Mesentery

Where volvulus is confirmed (Fig. 32.21), the bowel is rotated in a counter clockwise direction to untwist it (Fig. 32.22). Examination of the root of the mesentery will confirm that it has been fully detorted. In the laparoscopic approach this may be easier to perform once the duodenum has been mobilised, and involves "walking" the bowel from proximal to distal.

32.8.4.3 Assess Bowel Viability

Once the volvulus has been untwisted the entire small bowel is inspected carefully (Fig. 32.23). It should be realised that assessment of the viability of ischemic neonatal bowel can be difficult, especially in the neonate. Sometimes the bowel is less

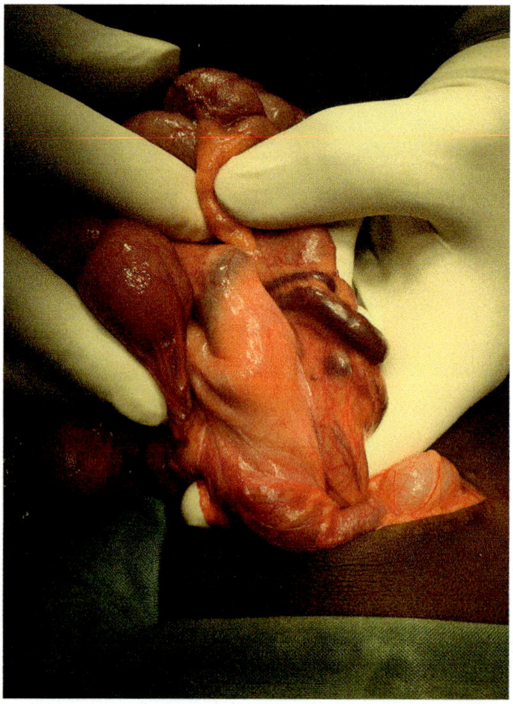

Fig. 32.21 The second step is to inspect the root of the small bowel mesentery and confirm volvulus, evident by the twisting of the bowel around the mesentery

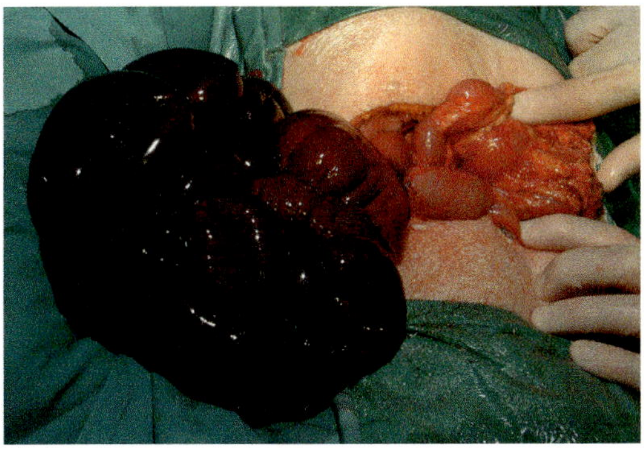

Fig. 32.22 An example of the operative appearance of ischaemic midgut due to malrotation where the blood flow through the superior mesenteric vessels has been compromised by volvulus. Only 20 cm of jejunum remained viable, but after a prolonged period of total parenteral nutrition the bowel adapted and the child survived (Courtesy P. Losty)

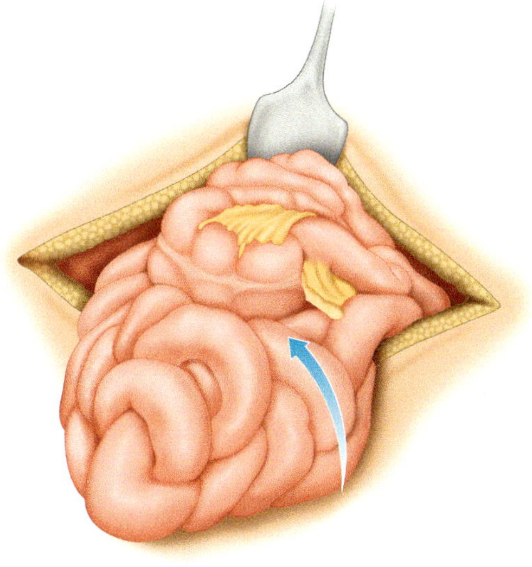

Fig. 32.23 Untwisting of midgut volvulus occurs in a counter-clockwise direction

damaged than it may appear to be on initial macroscopic inspection. A conservative approach in these patients is essential to minimise the risk of short bowel syndrome: bowel that may appear to be of marginal viability, and has not undergone full thickness necrosis is preserved and left in situ.

Where there is any ongoing doubt about the viability of bowel following detorsion of the volvulus, a second look laparotomy 1–2 days later is indicated. By then, bowel that is recoverable will have become more clearly demarcated from that in which irreversible damage has occurred. Only where there is definite full thickness bowel necrosis is resection indicated. At the edges of resection bowel viability is often precarious, for which reason primary anastomosis is not always indicated, and it may be better to fashion a temporary stoma at the lines of resection. Preferably, any stomas are placed close together at one end of the wound, to facilitate subsequent closure.

Occasionally, much of, or the entire small bowel is found to be gangrenous at the time of surgery (Figs. 32.20 and 32.23), and a decision has to be made whether it is in the infant's best interests to simply close the abdomen (leaving the bowel in situ) or whether to excise the necrotic bowel, usually with construction of stomas, with a view to long term TPN. Where the bowel is left in situ the infant usually dies from sepsis and shock within a day or two.

Operative decision-making also needs to take into account a number of other factors which include: whether there is sufficient length for potential long term bowel adaption; the availability and appropriateness of long term TPN; resources for eventual home-based TPN; whether subsequent small bowel transplantation is an option; the nature of associated abnormalities; the importance of informed parental involvement in decision making, and consideration of the likely quality of life of the patient.

It is important to involve the family fully in any discussion on management options. This should be done in conjunction with a neonatologist, social worker, and a support person(s) for the family. Preferably these discussions have started preoperatively (on the basis of the clinical features and their interpretation), which gives the surgeon an advantage should extensive necrosis be identified at surgery.

32.8.4.4 Broaden the Mesentery

In non rotation, the caecum and ascending colon are in apposition to the duodenum and proximal jejunum. There are fascial peritoneal bands between the two. These need to be divided to broaden the mesentery (Fig. 32.24).

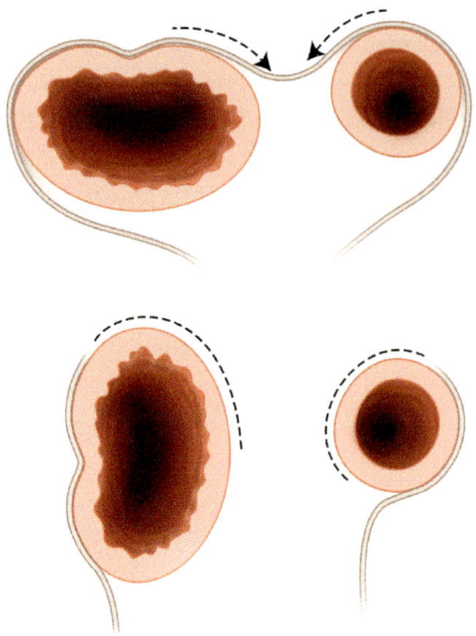

Fig. 32.24 Schematic representation of how the root of the small bowel mesentery is broadened by dissection between the duodenum and caecum, as viewed from inferiorly

Incision of the peritoneal condensations between the caecum/ascending colon on the left, and the duodenum/proximal jejunum on the right (Figs. 32.25 and 32.26), allows the small bowel mesentery to be broadened. The tight peritoneal bands extending over and to the right of the duodenum (often referred to as "Ladd bands") are divided first (Fig. 32.25) as this "straightens out the duodenum, making expansion of the mesenteric attachment between the caecum and duodenum easier (Fig. 32.26). The incision of the mesentery is extended peripherally until the mesentery is broad. Once completed, the bowel is returned to the abdominal cavity, with the small bowel predominantly to the right, and the large bowel predominantly to the left.

32.8.4.5 "en passant" Appendicectomy

Appendicectomy is usually undertaken because of the diagnostic difficulties that subsequent appendicitis produces, as the appendix is located on the left side of the abdomen with the caecum and colon. The morbidity of appendicectomy in this situation is negligible, and prophylactic antibiotics effective against bowel organisms are usually administered at the time of surgery.

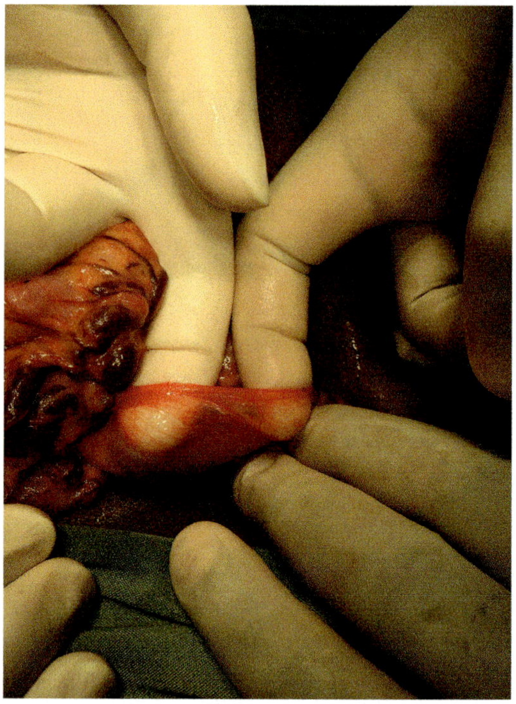

Fig. 32.25 Division of Ladd bands (which run across the duodenum and obstruct it in non-rotation with volvulus) straightens the duodenum, facilitating broadening of the root of the small bowel mesentery

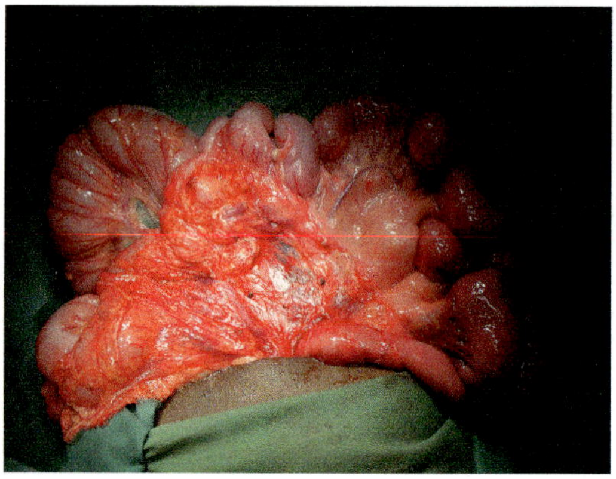

Fig. 32.26 Division of the fascial condensations between the caecum and duodenum opens up and broadens the root of the small bowel mesentery, reducing the risk of subsequent volvulus

32.9 Complications and Results (Table 32.8)

32.9.1 Early Complications

There is surprisingly little information about the complications and subsequent morbidity after surgery for malrotation and volvulus, perhaps because of the rarity of the condition and the relatively small numbers of patients any single institution treats. A number of problems can be encountered in the first days after surgery:

- Reperfusion injury effects and haemo-instability. Restoration of a blood supply to critically damaged bowel may produce a sequence of events with both metabolic and circulatory consequences. These infants must be cared for in a tertiary neonatal unit which has the capacity to provide cardio-respiratory support and prolonged mechanical ventilation. They often need inotropic support, antibiotics, and careful fluid, electrolyte and haematological monitoring.
- Prolonged ileus. This occurs because of dissection close to the root of the small bowel mesentery and duodenum, and is exacerbated if there has been any ischaemic compromise to the small bowel from volvulus. Post-operative ileus for up to a week is not uncommon. Signs that it is resolving include: decrease in the volume of nasogastric aspirates, a softer and less distended abdomen, and the passage of flatus and stools. The older child will start to feel hungry. If an ileus continues for more than a week it needs to be distinguished from ongoing obstruction due to mechanical causes such as recurrence of volvulus, adhesive obstruction and intussusception. A laparoscopic approach may be associated with shorter times to starting feeds and to attaining full feeds [69], perhaps indicating that less ileus occurs with this approach.
- Post-operative intussusception. This is rare after a Ladd procedure, but must always be considered where features of worsening obstruction occur after any retroperitoneal or complex intra-abdominal procedure [71]. Causative factors may include the appendiceal stump acting as a leadpoint, and non-fixation of the ileocaecal mesentery [72]. In one series, 5 of 159 patients undergoing the Ladd procedure suffered post-operative intussusception [73], significantly more common than post-operative intussusceptions after laparotomies for other conditions ($P < 0.001$).
- Wound infection and dehiscence. These are more likely to occur after open surgery, and contributing factors include bacteraemia/septicaemia, and a tight distended abdomen (e.g. from ileus) post-operatively. The incidence can be minimized by perioperative antibiotics and meticulous wound closure (good bites of tissue, not pulled too tightly). Improvements in antibiotics, surgical technique and suture materials mean these complications are now rare.
- Dysmotility. Dysmotility often persists after surgery for malrotation [74], but its causes are poorly understood and difficult to quantify. Some have suggested that it may be due to defective intrinsic enteric innervation [74, 75] or from damage sustained at the time of volvulus. It may be prolonged.
- Laparoscopic results. The difficult view often afforded on laparoscopy, loss of orientation, a

Table 32.8 Sequelae and complications of surgery for malrotation with volvulus

Early	• Septicaemia • Reperfusion injury effects • Haemodynamic instability • Prolonged ileus
Late	• Adhesive bowel obstruction • Recurrence of volvulus • Short gut syndrome – malabsorption – failure to thrive – complications of TPN • Motility disturbance
Death	• Secondary to extensive loss of midgut or complications of subsequent supportive management e.g. TPN, small bowel transplantation

limited working space (especially when the bowel is distended), the requirement for extensive bowel manipulation and problems with interpretation (e.g. is the mesentery narrowed to a degree that predisposes to volvulus and therefore should be broadened?) all have the potential to cause two problems: (1) injury to the bowel wall; and (2) inadequate broadening of the mesentery. Post-operative obstruction may indicate an incomplete Ladd procedure or be due to adhesions [64].

A laparoscopic approach, particularly in the absence of volvulus, produces similar results to those involving an open approach. Basically, while the surgical approach is different, the operation within the peritoneal cavity is essentially the same. Operative times in the absence of volvulus or compromised bowel are similar [69]. There is some indication that a laparoscopic approach may allow for earlier feeds and have a decreased hospital stay [69].

Laparoscopy may be difficult where volvulus has supervened, particularly if there is marked distension or dilatation of the small bowel, because of compromised operative vision.

32.9.2 Late Results and Complications

A number of problems can be encountered weeks or years after the Ladd procedure for malrotation:

- Adhesive bowel obstruction. This is the most common cause of readmission after surgery to correct malrotation [27]. In one series [76], 11 of 46 (24%) patients were readmitted within 6 months of surgery with an acute bowel obstruction, of which six required surgical division of their adhesions, and one patient died. Six patients had multiple admissions for small bowel obstruction. In the nine patients (of 161 in the series) who developed an adhesive bowel obstruction reported by El-Gohary et al. [32], five required operative adhesiolysis following failure of conservative management
- Recurrence of volvulus. This is a well recognised phenomenon, and in some cases may result from inadequate expansion of the root of the small bowel mesentery at the time of the original surgery, or in other cases there is a more localised volvulus in the presence of adhesions. It is reasonably rare: occurring once in 161 cases reported by El-Gohary [32]
- Persistent gastro-intestinal symptoms. This affects about 25% of patients. Symptoms include: vomiting, anorexia, constipation or diarrhoea and chronic abdominal pain. Often their exact cause is difficult to establish with certainty.
- Short gut syndrome. The intrinsic capacity for further adaption and lengthening of the small bowel as the infant grows is substantial, and continues to occur over many months and years. However, despite this, some children simply have insufficient bowel for adequate absorption of nutrients. All the therapeutic options are less than satisfactory and have significant morbidity in their own right. Most commonly, long-term home TPN is employed, but there are various other options available, including serial transverse enteroplasty (STEP) procedure [77], and small bowel transplantation. Not all are readily available treatment options and they all carry with them significant morbidity.
- Complications of total parenteral nutrition. Many of these patients require a central venous line for extended periods of time, and are subject to all their complications: line sepsis, dislodgement of lines, fracturing of lines, displaced tips, and the consequences of catheter tip perforation of vessels. In one series of 27 patients, 2 died of sepsis related to parenteral nutrition [63]. These patients are also subject to all the metabolic complications of long-term parenteral nutrition.

32.9.3 Mortality

Overall, the mortality rate for malrotation undergoing surgery is less than 10% [78, 79], and declining, reflecting improvements in neonatology and paediatric anaesthesia, as well as in the management of short bowel syndrome. Mortality is primarily due to extensive midgut infarction secondary to volvulus (Table 32.9). Prematurity and associated abnormalities also influence mortality [79, 80]. The survival of

Table 32.9 Factors influencing mortality in malrotation with volvulus

Key determinant	Volvulus causing extensive small bowel necrosis
Other factors	Prematurity Associated abnormalities e.g. congenital heart disease

those who are left with short bowel syndrome after extensive resection has improved in recent years as a result of refinements in intensive neonatal care, parenteral nutrition, and perhaps small bowel transplantation.

Where volvulus is producing ischemic damage to the small bowel, mortality is reduced by early diagnosis and immediate surgical intervention. In short, the main determinants of outcome are: (1) high index of suspicion of malrotation with volvulus; (2) early diagnosis; and (3) prompt treatment.

Despite this, the greatest delay in instituting treatment is between first presentation to a medical practitioner and diagnosis. This highlights the importance of educating medical practitioners to have a high index of suspicion of the possibility of malrotation with volvulus in any infant who presents with bile stained vomiting or unexplained abdominal tenderness.

32.10 The Future

32.10.1 Genetics of Malrotation

As more is learnt about the genetics of malrotation and the molecular events surrounding development of the dorsal mesentery and rotation of the bowel, it may be possible to test at risk families. New technologies are becoming available, such as high resolution chromosome analysis by DNA microarrays which are much more sensitive in detecting chromosomal imbalances than earlier techniques. Similarly, improvements in sequencing technology may facilitate the detection of previously unrecognised mutations [1]. Increasingly, the clinical geneticist is likely to become involved in the management of all patients with malrotation who have coexisting abnormalities or features suggestive of a syndrome.

32.10.2 Antenatal Intervention

If malrotation predisposing to volvulus could be identified with greater accuracy on antenatal ultrasonography, or if volvulus can be identified as soon as it occurs, the potential exists for antenatal surgical intervention (and in the former situation, deliberate early induction of labour before volvulus occurs). However, this is unlikely to be achieved in the foreseeable future because of the lack of sensitivity and specificity of diagnosis on antenatal imaging and the inability to predict accurately the true risk of volvulus prior to birth for each case. Where volvulus has been identified antenatally, additional issues relate to the delay between ischaemia occurring and its recognition on imaging, and the risk to both fetus and mother of any intervention.

32.10.3 Management of Short Gut Syndrome

Therapeutic options are limited where midgut volvulus has caused extensive necrosis of the small bowel, and none is entirely satisfactory. The amount of adaption of small bowel that occurs with time in young children is extraordinary, but there remain a difficult group of patients who, even with adaption, are simply left with insufficient bowel for adequate enteral nutrition. For these patients, the options range from long-term total parenteral nutrition [81] to intestinal transplantation. A long sequence of surgical techniques to increase the length or absorptive capacity of the small bowel have been described, tried, and mostly abandoned. Where the proximal bowel is markedly dilated, longitudinal infolding plication may be beneficial (as is used in jejunal atresia) and has the advantage that no bowel is incised or resected, with virtually no complications: peristalsis is improved and there is no loss of absorptive area. The Bianchi and STEP procedures [77] are much more invasive: although popular in a few hands, they are of arguable benefit. Survival after intestinal transplantation is now about 78% at one year, and 65% at three years, although some high-volume centres are reporting even better survival rates, up to 74% at three years [82]. Nevertheless, significant ongoing problems after small bowel transplantation include: the need for immunosuppression; graft rejection; cost; and the limited availability of donor organs [83], such that in most parts of the world this is not considered a realistic alternative. Despite this, it is likely that there will be ongoing improvements in surgical interventions designed to improve gut motility and absorptive area, with a consequent reduction in morbidity.

There is another option on the horizon which has the potential also of improving the plight of children with short gut syndrome; this is tissue engineering of the small bowel to enable regeneration and restoration of small bowel function using the patient's own cells [84]. The process begins with generation of induced pluripotent stem cells (iPSCs) from somatic cells using a combination of four retrovirally transduced transcription factors: Oct3/4, Sox2, Klf4, and c-Myc [85]. The iPSCs resemble embryonic stem cells in many respects, such as their capacity for self-renewal and because they can differentiate into a variety of other cells. These characteristics make them useful for customized rejection-free cell transplant therapy by controlling their differentiation into smooth muscle sheets with peristalsis-like contraction and into intestinal epithelial cells [86, 87]. In addition, iPSCs overcome the ethical issues surrounding the use of fertilized eggs. Further refinements to improve the techniques of iPSC tissue engineering gut following volvulus are a prerequisite for its clinical application in short bowel syndrome.

References

1. Martin V, Shaw-Smith C. Review of the genetic factors in intestinal malrotation. Pediatr Surg Int. 2010;26(8):769–81.
2. Mahlapuu M, Ormestad M, Enerback S, Carlsson P. The forked transcription factor Foxf1 is required for differentiation of extra-embryonic and lateral plate mesoderm. Development. 2001;2:155–66.
3. Davis NM, Kurpois NA, Sun X, Gros J, Martin JF, Tabin CJ. The chirality of gut rotation derives from left-right asymmetric changes in the architecture of the dorsal mesentery. Dev Cell. 2008;1:134–45.
4. McVay MR, Kokoska ER, Jackson RJ, Smith SD. The changing spectrum of intestinal malrotation: diagnosis and management. Am J Surg. 2007;6:712–7.
5. Warner BW. Malrotation. In: Oldham KT, Colombani PM, Foglia RP, editors. Surgery of Infants and Children: Scientific Principles and Practice. Philadelphia: Lippincott-Raven Publishers; 1997. p. 1229–40.
6. Larsen WJ. Human embryology. New York: Churchill Livingstone; 1993. p. 205–34.
7. Grosfeld JL, Rescorla FJ. Duodenal atresia and stenosis: reassessment of treatment and outcome based on antenatal diagnosis, pathologic variance and long-term follow-up. World J Surg. 1993;17:301–9.
8. Gabra HOS, Stewart RJ, Nour S. Madgut malrotation and associated Hirschsprung's disease: a diagnostic dilemma. Pediatr Surg Int. 2007;23(7):703–5.
9. Brereton RJ, Taylor B, Hall C. Intussusception and intestinal malrotation in infants: Brit. J Surg. 1986;73:55–7.
10. Inan M, Aydiner CY, Ayvaz S. Malrotation as a preparing ground for intussuception. Pediatr Surg Int. 2003;19:616.
11. Moore SW, Kirsten M, Muuller EW, Numanoglu A, Chitnis M, Le Grange E, Banieghbal B, Hadley GP. Retrospective surveillance of intussusceptions in South Africa, 1998–2003. J Infect Dis. 2010;202(Suppl 1):S156–61.
12. Burke TE, Fitzgerald RJ. Intussusception, volvulus and malrotation. Aust NZ J Surg. 1985;55(1):73–4.
13. Smith SL. Familial midgut volvulus. Surgery. 1972;3:420–6.
14. Chappell L, Gorman S, Campbell F, Ellard S, Rice G, Dobbie A, Crow Y. A further example of a distinctive autosomal recessive syndrome comprising neonatal diabetes mellitus, intestinal atresias and gall bladder agenesis. Am J Med Genet A. 2008;13:1713–7.
15. Guttman FM, Braun P, Garance PH, Blanchard H, Collin PP, Dallaire L, Desjardins JG, Perreault G. Multiple atresias and a new syndrome of hereditary multiple atresias involving the gastrointestinal tract from stomach to rectum. J Pediatr Surg. 1973;5:633–40.
16. Erez I, Reish O, Kovalivker M, Lazar L, Raz A, Katz S. Congenital short-bowel and malrotation: clinical presentation and outcome of six affected offspring in three related families. Eur J Pediatr Surg. 2001;5:331–4.
17. Anneren G, Meurling S, Olsen L. Megacystis-microcolon-intestinal hypoperistalsis syndrome (MMIHS), an autosomal recessive disorder: clinical reports and review of the literature. Am J Med Genet. 1991;2:251–4.
18. Farag TI, al-Awadi SA, el-Badramany MH, Usha R, el-Ghanem M. Second family with "apple peel" syndrome affecting four siblings: autosomal recessive inheritance confirmed. Am J Med Genet. 1993;1:119–21.
19. Brisset S, Joly G, Ozilou C, Lapierre JM, Gosset P, Le Lorc'h M, Raoul O, Turleau C, Vekemans M,

Romana SP. Molecular characterization of partial trisomy 16q24.1-qter: clinical report and review of the literature. Am J Med Genet. 2002;4:339–45.
20. Shanske A, Ferreira JC, Leonard JC, Fuller P, Marion RW. Hirschsprung disease in an infant with a contiguous gene syndrome of chromosome 13. Am J Med Genet. 2001;3:231–6.
21. Skandalakis JE, Gray SW, Ricketts R, et al. The small intestines. In: Skandalakis JE, Gray SW, editors. Embryology for surgeons. 2nd ed. Baltimore: Williams & Wilkins; 1994. p. 184.
22. Kantor JL. Anomalies of the colon: their roentgen diagnosis and clinical significance. Resume of 10 years' study. Radiology. 1934;23:651.
23. Torres AAM, Ziegler MM. Malrotation of the intestine. World J Surg. 1993;17:326–31.
24. Parish A, Hartley R. Intestinal malrotation. In Pediatrics: gastroenterology articles; 2006. E-medicine: http:/www.emedicine.com/ped/gastroenterology.htm
25. Smith VL, Long F, Nwomeh BC. Monozygotic twins with discordant intestinal rotation. Pediatr Radiol. 2006;26:1–3.
26. Aslanabadi S, Ghalehgolab-Behbahan A, Jamshidi M, Veisi P, Zarrintan S. Intestinal malrotations: a review and report of thirty cases. Folia Morphol (Warsz). 2007;66(4):277–82.
27. Spigland N, Brandt ML, Yazbeck S. Malrotation presenting beyond the neonatal period. J Pediatr Surg. 1990;25(11):1139–42.
28. Beasley SW, de Campo J. Pitfalls in the radiological diagnosis of malrotation. Australasian Radiol. 1987;31:376–83.
29. Maxson RT, Franklin PA, Wagner CW. Malrotation in the older child: surgical management, treatment and outcome. Am Surg. 1995;61:135–8.
30. El Gohari MA, Cook RC. Intestinal malrotation beyond the neonatal period. Z Kinderchir. 1984;39:237–41.
31. Durkin ET, Lund DP, Shaaban AF, Schurr MJ, Weber SM. Age-related differences in diagnosis and morbidity of intestinal malrotation. J Am Coll Surg. 2008;206(4):658–63.
32. El-Gohary Y, Alagtal M, Gillick J. Long-term complications following operative intervention for intestinal malrotation: a 10 year review. Pediatr Surg Int. 2010;26:203–6. https://doi.org/10.1007/s00383-009-2483-y.
33. Penco JM, Murillo JC, Hernandez A, De La Calle PU, Masioan DF, Acelituno FR. Anomalies of intestinal rotation and fixation: consequences of late diagnosis beyond two years of age. Pediatr Surg Int. 2007;23(8):723–30.
34. Cassart M, Massez A, Lingier P, Absil AS, Donner C, Avni F. Sonographic prenatal diagnosis of malpositioned stomach as a feature of uncomplicated intestinal malrotation. Pediatr Radiol. 2006;36(4):358–60.
35. Rajab KE, Al Juffairi Z, Issa AA. Antenatal diagnosis and management of fetal midgut volvulus. Bahrain Med Bull. 2007;29(3):106–8.
36. De Felice C, Massafra C, Di Maggio G, Tota G, Bracci R. Relationship between intrauterine midgut volvulus without malrotation and preterm delivery. Acta Obstet Gynaecol Scand. 1997;76:386.
37. Thomas D, Goolaerts JP, Watkins L, Autin C, Barlow P. Gastrointestinal anomalies, spleen and abdominal wall. http://www.sonoworld.com/TheFetus/page.aspx?id=1036
38. Miyakoshi K, Tanaka M, Miyazaki T, et al. Prenatal ultrasound diagnosis of small bowel torsion. Obstet Gynecol. 1998;91:802–3.
39. Shimanuki Y, Aihara T, Takano H. Clockwise whirlpool sign at color Doppler US: an objective and definitive sign of midgut volvulus. Radiol. 1996;199(1):261–4.
40. Hertzberg BS, Bowie JD. Fetal gastrointestinal abnormalities. Radiol Clin Nth Am. 1990;28(1):101–14.
41. Teele RT, Pease PWB, Rowley RSH. Malrotation in newborns following antenatal diagnosis of intra-abdominal cyst. Pediatr Radiol. 1998;28:717–21.
42. Biyyam DR, Dighe M, Siebert JR. Antenatal diagnosis of intestinal malrotation on fetal MRI. Pediatr Radiol. 2009;39:847–9.
43. Klzo L, Zizka J, Hodik K, Juttnerova V, Elias P, et al. Liver meconium, haemorrhage: the value of T1-weighted images in fetal MRI. Pediatr Radiol. 2006;36(8):792–801.
44. Miyakoshi K, Ishimoto H, Tanigaki S, Minegishi K, Tanaka M, Miyazaki T. Prenatal diagnosis of midgut volvulus by sonography and magnetic resonance imaging. Am J Perinatol. 2001;18(8):447–50.
45. Criscera CA, Ginsburg HB, Gittes GK. Fetal midgut volvulus presenting at term. J Pediatr Surg. 1999;34(8):1280–1.
46. Spitz L, Orr JD, Harries JT. Obstructive jaundice secondary to chronic midgut volvulus. Arch Dis Child. 1983;58(5):383–5.
47. Yanez R, Spitz L. Intestinal malrotation presenting outside the neonatal period. Arch Dis Childhood. 1986;61:682–5.
48. Applegate KE, Anderson JM, Klatte EC. Intestinal malrotation in children: a problem-solving approach to the upper gastrointestinal series. Radiographics. 2006;26(5):1485–500.
49. Yousefzadeh DK. The position of the duodenojejunal junction: the wrong horse to bet on in diagnosing or excluding malrotation. Pediatr Radiol. 2009;39(2):172–7.
50. Gross E, Chen MK, Lobe TE. Laparoscopic evaluation and treatment of intestinal malrotation in infants. Surg Endoscopy. 1996;10(9):936–7.
51. Brandt M, et al. Intestinal malrotation. UpToDate. http//www.uptodate.com/contents/intestinal-malrotation. Accessed 8 June 2011.
52. Chao HC, King MS, Chen JY, Lin SJ, Lin JN. Sonographic features related to volvulus in neonatal intestinal malrotation. JUM. 2000;19(6):371–6.
53. Pracos JP, Sann L, Genin G. ultrasound diagnosis of midgut volvulus: the "whirlpool sign". Pediatr Radiol. 1992;22(1):18–20.
54. Reid JR. 2011. http://emedicine.medscape.com/article/411249-overview

55. Weinberger E, Winters WD, Liddell RM, et al. Sonographic diagnosis of intestinal malrotation in infants: importance of the relative positions of the superior mesenteric vein and artery. Am J Radiol. 1992;159:825.
56. Boudiaf M, Soyer P, Terem C, Pelage JP et al. CT evaluation of small bowel obstruction. 2001. http://radiographics.rsna.org/content/21/3/613.full
57. Taylor GA. CT appearance of the duodenum and mesenteric vessels in children with normal and abnormal bowel rotation. Pediatr Radiology. 2011;41(11):1378–83.
58. Zissin R, Rathaus V, Oscadchy A, Kots E, Gayer G, Shapiro-Feinberg M. Intestinal malrotation as an incidental finding on CT in adults. Abdom Imaging. 1999;24:550–5.
59. Dawrant MJ, Lee JC, Ho CP, De Caluwe D. Complex presentation of intussusceptions in childhood. Pediatr Surg Int. 2005;21(9):730–2.
60. http://www.controlled-trials.com/ISRCTN55042368
61. Malek MM, Burd RS. Surgical treatment of malrotation after infancy: a population-based study. J Pediatr Surg. 2005;40(1):285–9.
62. Malek MM, Burd RS. The optimal management of malrotation diagnosed after infancy: a decision analysis. Am J Surg. 2006;191(1):45–51.
63. Cohen Z, Kleiner O, Finlay R, Mordehal J, Newman N, Kurtzbart E, Mares AJ. How much of a misnomer is "asymptomatic" intestinal malrotation? Isr Med Assoc J. 2003;5(3):172–4.
64. Rothenberg SS. Malrotation. In: Najmaldin A, Rotheberg SS, DCG C, Beasley SW, editors. Operative endoscopy and endoscopic surgery in infants and children. London: Hodder Arnold; 2005. p. 263–7.
65. Bass KD, Rothenberg SS, Chang JHT. Laparoscopic Ladd's procedure in infants with malrotation. J Pediatr Surg. 1998;33(2):279–81.
66. Fraser JD, Aguayo P, Sharp SW, Ostlie DJ, St Peter SD. The role of laparoscopy in the management of malrotation. J Surg Res. 2009;156(1):80–2.
67. Adikibi BT, Strachan CL, MacKinlay GA. Neonatal laparoscopic Ladd's procedure can be safely performed even if the bowel shows signs of ischaemia. J Laparoendosc Surg Tech A. 2009;19(Suppl 1):S167–70.
68. Hagendoorn J, Viera-Travassos D, Van dee Zee D. Laparoscopic treatment of intestinal malrotation in neonates and infants: retrospective study. Surg Endoscopy. 2011;25(1):217–20.
69. Stanfill AB, Pearl RH, Kalvakuri K, Wallace LJ, Vegunta RK. Laparoscopic Ladd's procedure: treatment of choice for midgut malrotation in infants and children. J Laparoendoscopic Surg Tech. 2010;20(4):369–72.
70. Yamashita H, Kato H, Uyama S, Kanata T, Nishizawa F, Kotegawa H. Laparoscopic repair of intestinal malrotation complicated by midgut volvulus. Surg Endosc. 1999;13:1160–2.
71. Bodycomb J, Beasley SW, Auldist AW. Postoperative intussusception. Pediatr Surg Int. 1987;2(2): 108–9.
72. Tatekawa Y, Muraji T, Nishijima E, Tsugawa C, Matamoros MA, Mouri N, Sato S, Moriuchi T. Postoperative intussusceptions after surgery for malrotation and appendicectomy in a newborn. Pediatr Surg Int. 1998;14(3):171–2.
73. Kidd J, Jackson R, Wagner CW, Smith SD. Intussusception following the Ladd procedure. Arch Surg. 2000;135:713–5.
74. Devane SP, Coombes R, Smith VV, Bisset WM. Booth IW et al Persistent gastrointestinal symptoms after correction of malrotation. Arch Dis Child. 1992;67:218–21.
75. Coombs RC, Buick RG, Gornall PG, et al. Intestinal malrotation: the role of small intestinal dysmotility in the cause of persistent symptoms. J Pediatr Surg. 1991;26(5):553–6.
76. Murphy FL, Sparnon AL. Long-term complications following intestinal malrotation and Ladd's procedure: a 15 year review. Pediatr Surg Int. 2006;22(4):326–9.
77. Modi BP. First report of the international serial transverse enteroplasty data registry: indications, efficacy and complications (International STEP Data Registry). J Am Coll Surg. 2007;204(3):365–71.
78. Andrassy RJ, Mahour GH. Malrotation of the midgut in infants and children: a 25-year review. Arch Surg. 1981;116(2):158–60.
79. Messineo A, MacMillan JH, Palder SB, et al. Clinical features affecting mortality in children with malrotation of the intestine. J Pediatr Surg. 1992;27: 1343.
80. Kouwenberg M, Severijnen RSVM, Kapusta L. Congenital cardiovascular defects in children with intestinal malrotation. Pediatr Surg Int. 2008;24(3):257–63.
81. Sala D, et al. Long-term outcomes of short bowel syndrome requiring long-term/home intravenous nutrition compared in children with gastroschisis and those with volvulus. Transplant Proc. 2010;42(1):5–8. https://doi.org/10.1016/j.trasnproceed.2009.12.033.
82. http://www.chp.edu/CHP/Survival+Rates+Transplantation. Accessed 25 Sept 2011.
83. Perez A, Grikscheit TC, Blumberg RS, et al. Tissue-engineered small intestine: ontogeny of the immune system. Transplantation. 2002;74:619–23.
84. Yoshida A, Chitcholtan K, Evans JJ, Nock VA, Beasley SW. In vitro tissue-engineering of smooth muscle sheets with peristalsis using a murine induced pluripotent stem cell line. J Pediatr Surg. 2012;47(2):329–35.
85. Takahashi K, Yamanaka S. Induction of pluripotent stem cells from mouse embryonic and adult fibroblast cultures by defined factors. Cell. 2006;126:663–76.
86. See "peristalsis sheet" at http://www.otago.ac.nz/christchurch/research/surgery/index.html#paediatric
87. http://www.youtube.com/user/PaedSurgUOC#p/a/u/1/T2yXdaJhl-I).
87. Orzech N, Navarro OM, Langer JC. Is ultrasonography a good screening test for malrotation? J Pediatri. Surg. 2006;41:1005–9.

Jejuno-Ileal Atresia and Stenosis

33

Alastair J.W. Millar and Alp Numanoglu

Abstract

Successful outcome after surgery for atresia of the small intestine is still sometimes accompanied by significant complications. An understanding of the aetiology and the realization that the proximal blind ending dilated bulbous atretic bowel was the cause of most of these complications and resection of this segment with primary anastomosis of proximal to distal bowel led to a dramatic improvement in outcomes from a mortality of 90—100% to a survival of over 80% in the 1950's. Subsequent improvement in some technical aspects of bowel anastomosis and neonatal perioperative care along with advances in nutrition both parenteral and enteral have made current treatment one of the many success stories of neonatal surgery.

Keywords

Intestinal atresia • Aetiology • Pathogenesis • Classification • Surgery Outcomes

33.1 Introduction

Successful outcome after surgery for atresia of the small intestine is still sometimes accompanied by significant complications [1, 2]. An understanding of the aetiology and the realization that the proximal blind ending dilated bulbous atretic bowel was the cause of most of these complications and resection of this segment with primary anastomosis of proximal to distal bowel led to a dramatic improvement in outcomes from a mortality of 90–100% to a survival of over 80% in the 1950s [3–8]. Subsequent improvement in some technical aspects of bowel anastomosis and neonatal perioperative care along with advances

A.J.W. Millar, FRCS, FRACS(Paed Surg) (✉)
Emeritus Professor of Paediatric Surgery, University of Cape Town, Red Cross War Memorial Children's Hospital, Cape Town, South Africa
e-mail: alastair.millar@uct.ac.za

A. Numanoglu, MBChB(Turkey), FCS(SA)
Charles F.M. Saint Professor of Paediatric Surgery, Division of Paediatric Surgery, Red Cross War Memorial Children's Hospital, University of Cape Town, Cape Town, South Africa
e-mail: alp.numanoglu@uct.ac.za

P.D. Losty et al. (eds.), *Rickham's Neonatal Surgery*, https://doi.org/10.1007/978-1-4471-4721-3_33

in nutrition both parenteral and enteral have made current treatment one of the many success stories of neonatal surgery [9–16].

33.2 History

Intestinal atresia has long been recognized as a cause of neonatal bowel obstruction and is well described in the literature [3, 17, 18]. The first description of ileal atresia was credited to Goeller in 1684. In 1911, Fockens of Rotterdam reported the first successfully treated case of small intestinal atresia [19]. Up until 1952, however, the mortality rate of atresia of the small intestine remained very high, even at the best pediatric surgical centers [3, 20]. Late presentation, dysmotility of the dilated bowel proximal to the atresia after end to end anastomosis, the blind loop syndrome, malnutrition, infections, prematurity, and associated congenital abnormalities contributed to this high mortality. In a comprehensive review of the world literature up to 1950, Evans could find reports of only 39 successfully treated cases of jejunoileal atresia [3]. In 1952, Louw published results of an investigation of 79 patients treated at Great Ormond Street Hospital, London from 1925 recording a mortality of up to 100% in the more distal ileal atresias [20]. Due to delayed presentation his overriding impression was that of ischaemia of the proximal bulbous blind end which resulted from prolonged raised intraluminal pressure. He supported the proposal by Spriggs that jejuno-ileal atresia was probably due to a vascular accident rather than being the result of inadequate recanalization, as had previously been commonly accepted [3, 21, 22]. The findings of bile pigment, lanugo hairs and squames distal to the atresia seemed to confirm this hypothesis.

At his instigation, Barnard perfected an experimental model in pregnant mongrel bitches and reproduced all types of atresia found in humans [23]. This not only confirmed Louw's hypothesis, but also provided the opportunity to improve the technical aspects of corrective surgery, which involved resection of the dilated proximal blind ending bowel and primary end-to-end anastomosis. These factors, along with advances in neonatal care, have achieved survival rates greater than 90% in the current era [4–6]. Interestingly, Nixon had come to the same conclusion i.e. that resection of the bulbous blind end was necessary as he had observed marked dysmotility with ineffective peristalsis of this dilated segment if primary end to end anastomosis without resection had been done. He suggested that this was the prime reason for poor results. He also proved this hypothesis experimentally [7, 8]. He also advocated resection of the most dilated bowel with end to end anastomosis. Thus occurred a great leap forward in the outcomes of treatment for intestinal atresia.

33.3 Classification

The accepted classification is Grosfeld's modification of that described by Bland Sutton. The most proximal atresia or stenosis determines whether it is classified as jejunal or ileal [10, 17] (Fig. 33.1).

Stenosis [10%]: The proximal dilated and distal collapsed segments of intestine are in continuity with an intact mesentery but at the junction there is a short, narrow, somewhat rigid segment with a minute lumen which may mimic atresia type I. The small intestine is of normal length.

Atresia Type 1 [24%]: (Fig. 33.2) The dilated proximal and collapsed distal segments of intestine are in continuity and the mesentery is intact. The obstruction is caused by a membrane with intestinal mucosa on both proximal and distal sides. The pressure in the proximal intestine may expand the membrane into the distal intestinal lumen, so that the transition from distended to collapsed intestine is conical in appearance; the 'windsock' effect. The distal intestine is completely collapsed but the bowel immediately distal to a 'windsock' may be dilated by the windsock. The small intestine is of normal length.

Atresia Type II [9%]: Blind ends joined by a short fibrous cord. The proximal intestine terminates in a bulbous blind end that is grossly distended and hypertrophied for several centimeters but more proximally assumes a normal appearance. This dilated blind end often has poor prograde peristalsis. The distal completely collapsed intestine commences as a blind end that is occasionally bulbous, owing to the remains of a fetal intussusception. The

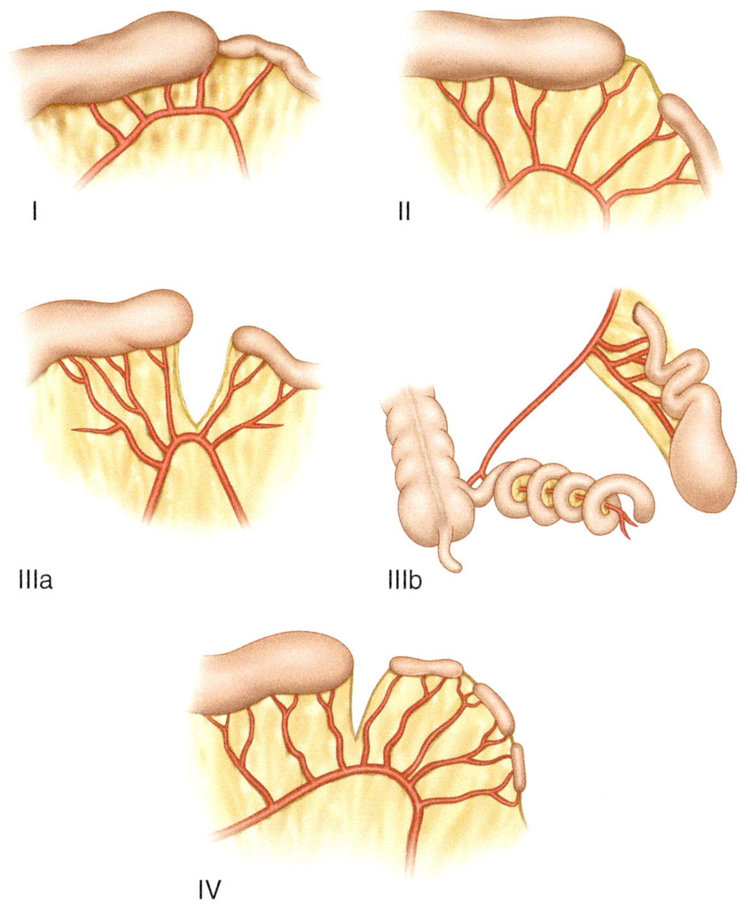

Fig. 33.1 Classification of Intestinal Atresia. From Grosfeld JL et al., Operative Management of Intestinal Atresia and Stenosis based on pathological findings. J Pediatric Surg 1979; 14: 368; used with permission

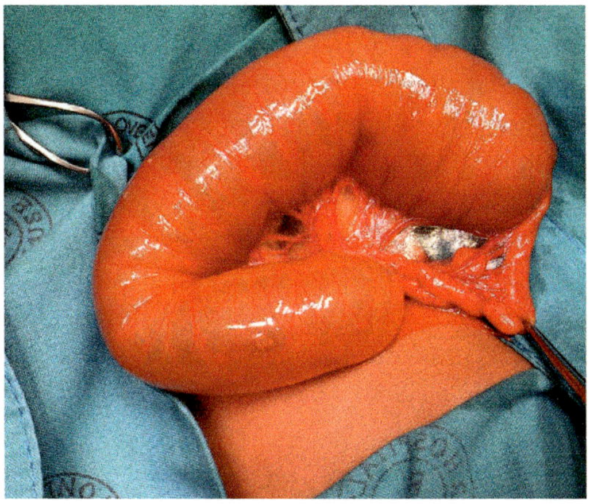

Fig. 33.2 Type I jejunal atresia. Abdominal radiograph had shown a triple bubble of dilated gas filled bowel proximal to the atresia (see Fig. 33.10) which was confirmed at laparotomy showing the typical dilated proximal jejunum and adjacent distal collapsed worm-like bowel

two blind ends are joined by a thin fibrous band, with the corresponding intestinal mesentery intact. The small intestinal length is usually normal.

Atresia Type IIIa [15%]: The appearance is similar to that in type II, but the blind ends are completely separate. There is always a mesenteric defect of varying size and the proximal intestine may, as a secondary event, undergo torsion or become over-distended with resultant increase in intraluminal pressure leading to necrosis and perforation. The total length of intestine is reduced to a varying extent.

Type IIIb [19%] ['Apple Peel' or 'Christmas Tree' deformity]: (Figs. 33.3, 33.4, and 33.5) As in type IIIa, the blind ends are unconnected and the mesenteric defect is large. The atresia is usually localized in the proximal jejunum near the ligament of Treitz, with absence of the superior mesenteric artery beyond the origin of the middle

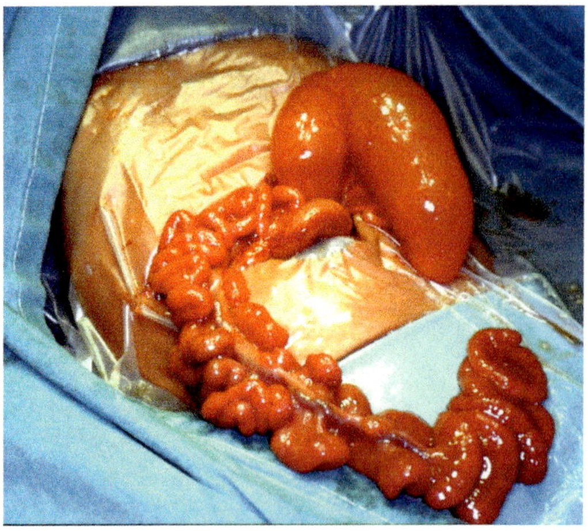

Fig. 33.3 Typical type IIIb 'apple peel' atresia with a dilated blind ending jejunum and loss of proximal mesentery. The single vascular arcade to the distal ileum arising from the right and middle colic arteries is evident. Malrotation is present with a central lying caecum

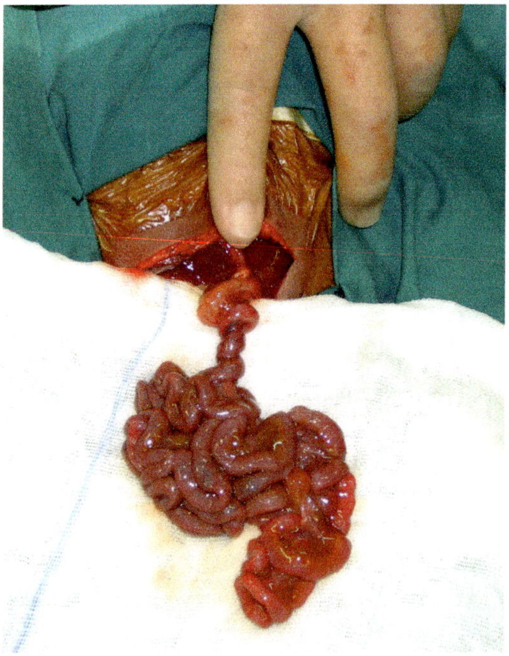

Fig. 33.4 Type IIIb jejunal atresia with tenuous blood supply and 720° anti-clockwise volvulus [unusual]

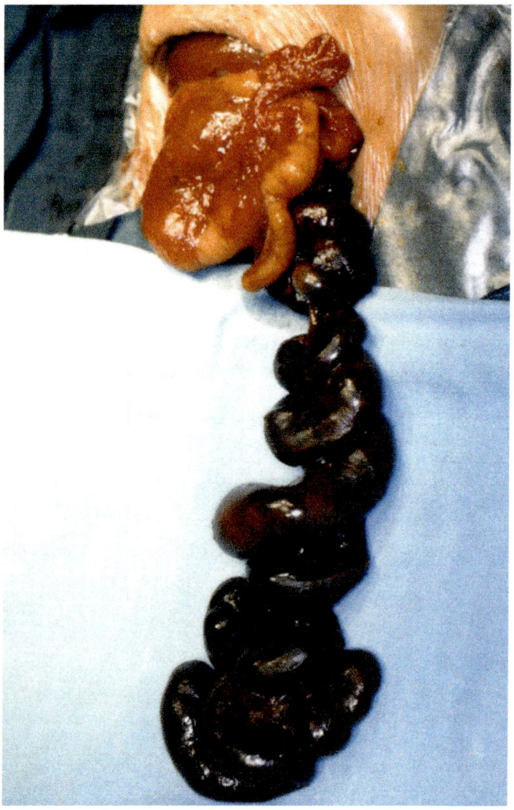

Fig. 33.5 An established type IIIb atresia where the remaining bowel has undergone ischaemic infarction from torsion shortly before birth

colic branch and absence of the dorsal mesentery. The distal intestine assumes a helical configuration around an attenuated single artery of blood supply arising from the ileocolic or right colic arcade. Occasionally further atresias of type I or II are found in the distal intestine, usually close to the blind end. There is always a significant reduction in intestinal length. Vascularity of the distal intestine may be impaired and secondary volvulus of the 'apple peel' may occur resulting in very short lengths of surviving bowel.

Type IV [23%] [multiple atresias]: (Figs. 33.6, 33.7 and 33.8) Multiple atresias can be combinations of types I–III and often present morphologically as a string of sausages. Multiple atresias are often localized to a short segment of intestine. The site of the most proximal atresia determines whether it is classified as jejunal or ileal.

33.3.1 Prognosis

The prognosis for all types of intestinal atresia is currently excellent with most recent series reporting long term survival of greater than 90% [12, 24]. A small number may succumb from

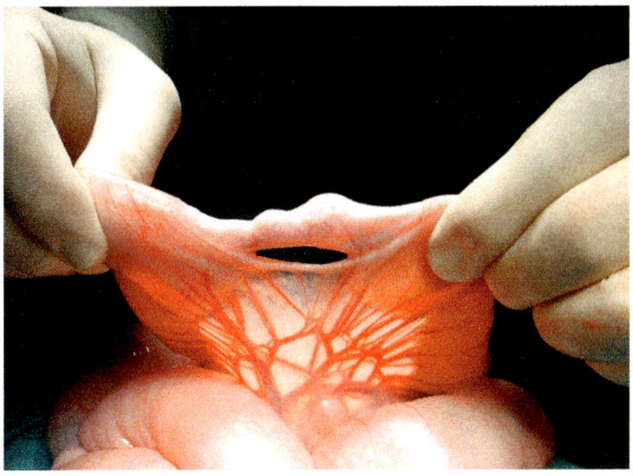

Fig. 33.6 Segment of stenotic jejunum but showing deficient mesentery in a type IV atresia

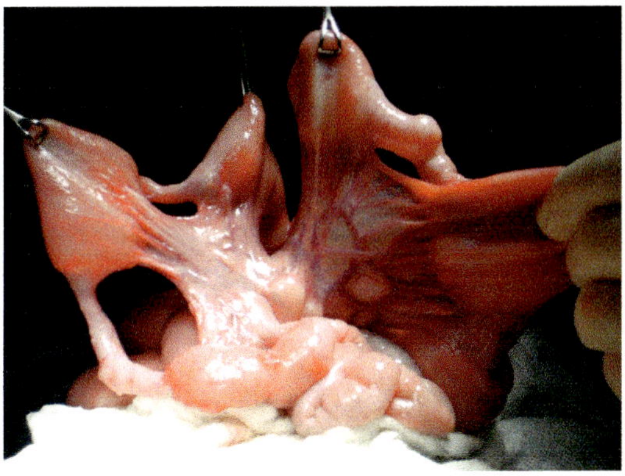

Fig. 33.7 Type IV atresia with evidence of multiple mesenteric defects

prematurity, associated abnormalities, which are rare outside the gastrointestinal tract, ultra-short gut syndrome and complications of either parenteral nutrition (liver disease or central line related) or occasionally as a consequence of complications from bowel transplant in those few in whom enteral autonomy cannot be established [2, 12, 25–28].

33.4 Epidemiology

The prevalence of jejunoileal atresia widely varies among different countries and geographical areas. In France, the prevalence is 2.25 cases per 10,000 live births [29, 30]. The overall prevalence of small intestinal atresia in Spain and Latin America is 1.3 cases per 10,000 live births and in Africa 1 per 3000 live births [31]. There

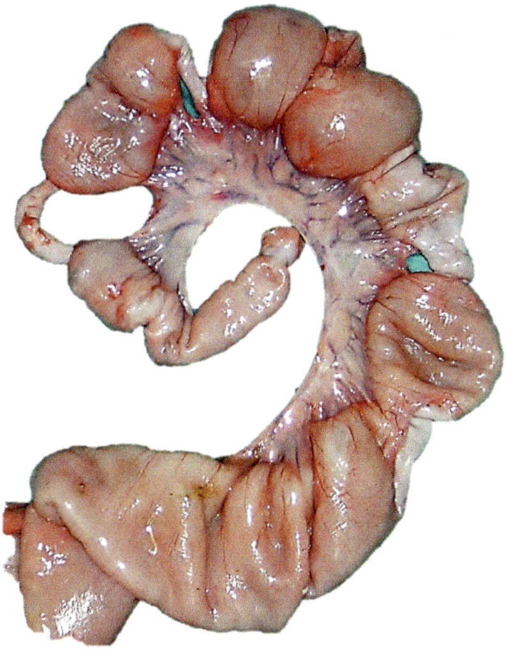

Fig. 33.8 Resected specimen of Type IV atresia (Fig. 33.7) with multiple sacular segments of bowel with types I, II and II atresias

also appears to be an increased incidence in twin pregnancies at 7.3 per 10,000 live births [32].

Intestinal atresia accounts for about one third of all cases of neonatal intestinal obstruction. In West Africa, intestinal atresia is the fourth most common cause of neonatal intestinal obstruction after anorectal malformations, Hirschsprung disease, and strangulated inguinal hernias [31, 33]. In an 11-year retrospective review of 500 children in India, intestinal atresias were found to be the most common cause of intestinal obstruction in newborns and the second most common cause (11.8%) after intussusception (20.8%) in all age groups [33]. Boys and girls are equally affected [34].

33.5 Aetiology and Genetics

Our present understanding of the etiology of intestinal atresias is based upon the classic experimental work of Louw and Barnard reported in 1955 [23]. These investigators observed that ligating mesenteric vessels and causing strangulated obstruction in fetal dogs resulted in atretic lesions of the small intestine that were similar to those observed clinically in human neonates. Thus, atresias and stenoses of the small intestine are believed to be due to an ischemic insult. This etiologic mechanism explains the frequent association of atresias with mesenteric defects and with other conditions that may cause strangulated obstruction of the intestinal tract (e.g. volvulus, intussusception, internal hernias and gastroschisis) [35–39]. Ischaemic experimental animal models in lambs, rabbits, rodents and chick embryos have replicated the work of Louw and Barnard confirming the ischaemic aetiology of most cases [40–43]. This etiology may also explain why intestinal atresia is associated with maternal smoking and vasoconstrictor drug exposure during pregnancy and thrombophilic diatheses [44]. Inherited thrombophilia has been shown to be present with increased frequency in infants with congenital atresia suggesting that in-utero thrombotic events may play a role in the aetiology [40, 44–47]. There have also been several case series reported of familial small bowel atresia most frequently type IV lesions [48]. More recently some of the established concepts have been questioned [49]. However the localized nature of the vascular accident occurring late in fetal life would explain the low incidence (less than 10%) of coexisting abnormalities of extra-abdominal organs. It is proposed that the ischaemic segment is absorbed with proximal and distal healing. Ongoing proximal peristaltic activity results in the typical bulbous dilatation of the bowel immediately adjacent to the atresia. The proximal bowel may perforate in utero leading to meconium peritonitis. If the insult has occurred later in gestation, evidence of the cause eg. intussusception, volvulus may be observed. The anomaly is usually not genetically determined although affected monozygotic twins and siblings have been described. A genetic basis however has been established for type III b and IV multiple atresias [48, 50–55]. However, most cases are sporadic with no familial history [56].

33.6 Associated Anomalies

Associated anomalies outside the gastrointestinal tract are rare, however there is a < 1% incidence of association of proximal jejunal atresia with duodenal atresia and several reported cases of an association with biliary atresia [46]. Also there are specific immunodeficiency syndromes decribed with multiple atresias in addition to epidermolysis bullosa [57–59]. There is a well-known association with cystic fibrosis and less frequently ileal atresia may be seen with total colonic aganglionosis [31, 60, 61].

33.7 Antenatal Presentation

Fetal diagnosis is now possible in many cases of jejuno-ileal atresia which may show polyhydramnios, dilated echogenic and thickened bowel on ultrasound scanning [62] (Fig. 33.9). This may be clearly advantageous, as delivery can be planned at or near a specialist centre with full neonatal surgical capability. Counseling is essential by a multidisciplinary team (obstetrician, paediatric surgeon, neonatologist) and a careful search for associated anomalies is important. However prenatal detection rates vary widely in fetal medicine centres (9–24%), and there appears to be a high rate of false positive scans with the more distal atresias being less likely to be diagnosed [43, 62, 63].

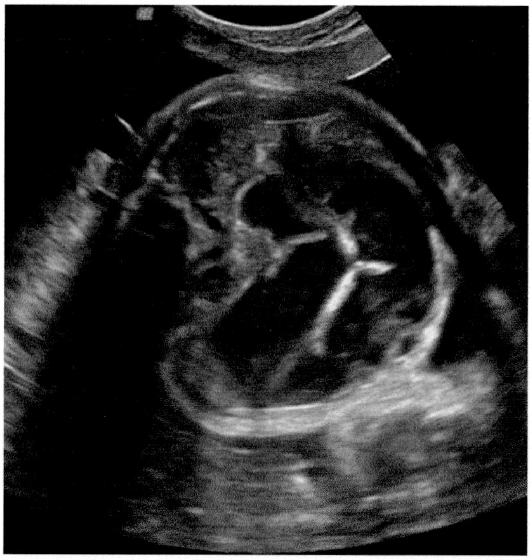

Fig. 33.9 Antenatal ultrasound scan showing dilated hyperechoic loops of fluid filled bowel

33.8 Clinical Presentation and Diagnosis

Intestinal atresia should be suspected in any newborn showing evidence of bowel obstruction (bilious vomiting, abdominal distension and failure to pass meconium) [1, 13, 64]. Many are born prematurely or small for gestational age presumably due to failure to absorb nutrient from ingested amniotic fluid or when in association with the abdominal wall abnormalities of gastroschisis and exomphalos [65]. Aspiration via a naso-gastric tube of more than 25 ml of fluid from the stomach in a newborn is very suggestive of obstruction. Antenatal ultrasound scanning as noted may show dilated loops of bowel with vigorous peristalsis, which is diagnostic of obstruction. Polyhydramnios may develop but is more commonly seen in duodenal and oesophageal obstructions [62, 63, 66]. The more distal the atresia the more generalized the abdominal distension and the lower the incidence of polyhydramnios. After aspiration of gastric contents the abdomen will be less distended and visible peristalsis may be observed. There is a failure to pass meconium and typically small volume grey mucoid stools are passed. Abdominal tenderness or peritonitis only develops with complications of ischaemia or perforation. This commonly occurs with delay in diagnosis and is due to either increased intraluminal pressure from swallowed air or secondary volvulus of the bulbous blind ending bowel above the level of the first obstruction [6, 24]. In most patients a simple abdominal x-ray with antero-posterior and either cross-table or left lateral decubitus projection are adequate to make the diagnosis based upon the presence of dilated air-filled intestinal loops and air-fluid levels [67] (Figs. 33.2 and 33.10). In addition, plain abdominal x-rays will suggest the level of obstruction based upon the number of dilated bowel loops. The presence of multiple dilated bowel loops of varying calibre without air-fluid levels suggests the possibility of meconium ileus, particularly if the intestinal content has a 'ground glass' appearance. A single very dilated loop with a large fluid level is often indicative of a distal atresia in ileum or colon [61, 68, 69].

The differential diagnosis includes other causes of intestinal obstruction in the neonate [24]. In patients with evidence of a proximal complete obstruction, the differential diagnosis is limited and no additional diagnostic studies are required. In patients with multiple dilated bowel loops suggesting a distal obstruction, the differential diagnosis includes several conditions for which surgical intervention may not be required. Therefore, in these patients a contrast enema may

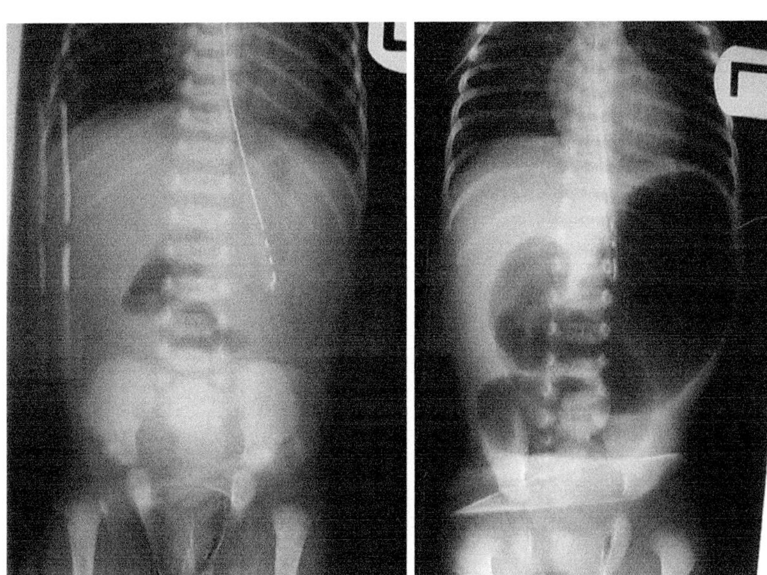

Fig. 33.10 Abdominal radiographs of an infant with jejunal atresia before aspiration via the nasogastric tube and after injection of air as contrast

be helpful to look for evidence of meconium plug or meconium ileus which may respond to non-operative managements. In addition, a contrast enema may demonstrate findings suggestive of Hirschsprung's disease which would direct initial management toward obtaining confirmatory tests for this disease. A contrast enema showing a patent colon is also helpful in that demonstration of colonic patency by injection of saline at operation, a sometimes tedious procedure, is not required (Fig. 33.11).

In patients with intestinal stenosis diagnosis is frequently delayed as the obstruction is incomplete. Plain abdominal x-rays may demonstrate proximal bowel dilation, however in most patients a gastrointestinal contrast meal or enema is required to confirm and locate the site of partial obstruction. The classical appearance of the colon distal to jejuno-ileal atresia is an unused or microcolon. Malrotation may also be observed in 10–30% of babies with jejuno-ileal atresia [24] (Fig. 33.12). Occasionally dystrophic intraperitoneal calcification of meconium peritonitis may be seen on plain radiograph, signifying intrauterine bowel perforation. If the atresia has formed late in intrauterine life, the bowel distal to the atresia may assume the calibre of a used colon.

33.9 Surgical Management

All patients should receive judicious fluid hydration prior to operative intervention. In addition, a nasogastric or orogastric tube should be passed to

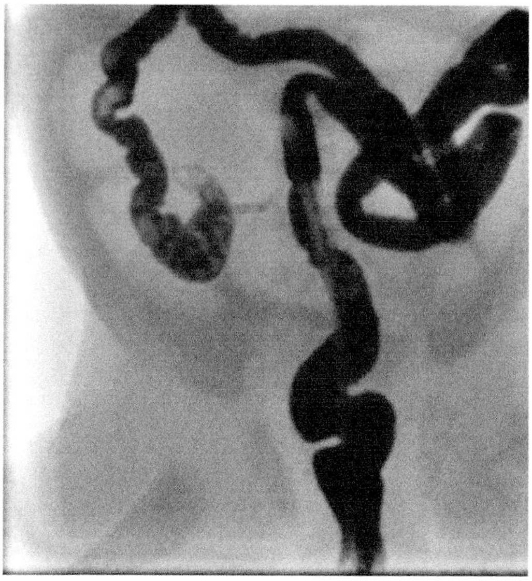

Fig. 33.12 Contrast enema in infant with Type IIIb atresia. Note large air filled loops indicating a proximal atresia with a patent 'unused' colon ending in the right upper quadrant suggesting malrotation or possible right sided colonic atresia

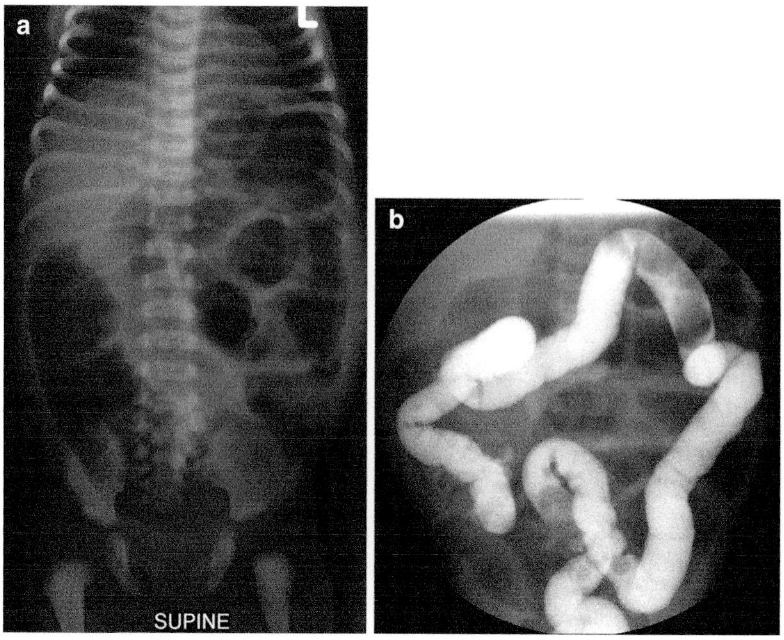

Fig. 33.11 (**a**) Abdominal radiograph of infant with ileal atresia. Note multiple dilated gas-filled loops of bowel and one large loop in the right lower abdomen. (**b**) Contrast enema in the same patient shows a patent normal colon of good size indicating a possible late in-utero event causing the atresia

empty the stomach and decrease the risk of vomiting and aspiration. In general, patients with intestinal atresias have a low risk of associated cardiac anomalies, so that preoperative special investigation is not required unless the patient has clinical evidence of a serious cardiac defect. Adequate operative exposure is obtained through a supra-umbilical, transverse incision transecting the rectus muscles 1–2 cm. above the umbilicus. However, increasingly minimally invasive techniques are used with small circum-umbilical incisions or even laparoscopic techniques and extra-corporial anastomosis [70–73]. At exploration, the site of the most proximal atresia is readily identified by the marked change in intestinal caliber. The outer wall of the intestine at the site of obstruction may appear intact, ischaemic and congested or there may be an associated defect in continuity of the intestine and the mesentery (type III). The intestine proximal to the obstruction which is dilated and hypertrophied frequently has a cyanosed appearance and may have some necrotic areas either from sustained intraluminal pressure or secondary volvulus, especially if there has been a delay in presentation. Perforation may have developed antenatally, leading to meconium peritonitis or may occur as a postnatal event, especially if diagnosis is delayed. The peristaltic movements in this segment are subnormal and ineffective, and histologic and histochemical abnormalities can be observed up to 20 cm cephalad to the atretic segment [8, 74–76]. In contrast, the distal bowel is unused and worm-like in appearance, but potentially normal in length and function. Generally, surgical treatment requires excision of the ends of the intestine involved in the atresia. It is also essential to look for distal sites of obstruction, which can occur in up to 20% of patients and may not be immediately obvious due to lack of calibre change beyond the proximal atresia [24]. These distal points of obstruction can be identified by flushing the distal intestinal lumen with saline to confirm intestinal continuity to the level of the ileocaecal valve or rectum if a preoperative enema showing colon patency has not been performed. After resection of the atretic segment, the surgeon is faced with the task of re-establishing continuity between intestinal segments often with marked lumen size discrepancies. This is best achieved by end-to-end extra-mucosal single layer anastomosis with larger gaps between interrupted sutures on the dilated segment. Discrepancies in size of bowel lumen of up to 8:1 have been accommodated using this technique. Another consideration is the potential dysmotility of the proximal markedly dilated segment which may result in delayed intestinal function and problems with bacterial overgrowth [4, 77]. Therefore, in patients with a relatively short segment of severely dilated proximal intestine, resection of the dilated segment with reestablishment of continuity by end-to-end anastomosis is the best option. However, in patients with long segments of proximal intestine that are significantly dilated, or loss of intestinal length eg. Type III a and b, resection of the whole involved segment may result in inadequate remaining intestinal length to allow absorption of enteric nutrients (i.e. short-bowel syndrome). Therefore, these patients frequently are treated by either imbrication or tapering enteroplasty of the proximal dilated segment [78]. To date, no randomized studies have compared the outcomes in patients with intestinal atresias with or without the addition of an enteroplasty or plication however some benefit appears evident [77, 79–82].

In patients with jejunal atresia just distal to the ligament of Treitz duodenal derotation and tapering duodeno-jejunoplasty is advocated [82]. It is important to be careful to avoid cutting back too far such that the pancreas and ampulla of Vater are protected [83]. Passage of a trans-anastomotic feeding tube for early commencement of enteral feeding is a useful adjunct to post-operative nutrient support particularly if delay in restoration of foregut function is expected due to gross dilatation of the proximal bowel and if parenteral nutrition is not available, a situation still common in many parts of the world. The trans-anastomotic tube can either be passed via the nasogastric route or via a Stamm gastrostomy performed on the anterior aspect of the stomach. The total residual length of bowel should be measured with a tape and recorded as this gives some guidance as to prognosis.

Patients who have multiple atresias (type IV) or an apple-peel deformity (type IIIb) are particularly challenging management problems [77, 78, 84–87]. These patients may require multiple anastomoses and frequently will experience long-term delays in return of intestinal function [86]. In addition, many of these patients will have short-bowel syndrome due to inadequate residual intestinal length. In type IIIb atresias the blood supply to the remaining small bowel (closer to the distal blind end) may have a particularly precarious blood supply (see Figs. 33.3, 33.4 and 33.5). The bowel should be displayed in a position of non-rotation keeping the free mesenteric border in sight and restrictive fibrotic bands along this free edge should be divided prior to primary anastomosis to enhance blood supply and venous drainage. The mesentery from any resected bowel is retained and may assist in closure of mesenteric defects [24]. This technique is very helpful and prevents kinking or distortion of the anastomosis. Furthermore, the potential for kinking the single marginal artery and vein requires careful placement of the bowel into the peritoneal cavity at the completion of the anastomosis. Multiple atresias are often localized to a short segment of intestine, and resection with one anastomosis is preferred if sufficient intestinal length remains. If the bowel length is critical, multiple anastomoses should be performed [25, 85]. In type IV atresias with multiple segments of bowel it is useful to pass a nasogastric tube through these segments consecutively like a string of beads. This facilitates performing the multiple anastomoses and may even act as a stent during the post-operative period [56, 85, 88].

In general the formation of stomas is unnecessary and should be avoided as dilated bowel does not reduce in calibre and fluid and electrolyte losses may be severe (vide infra). In infants with congenital short bowel, lengthening procedures such as the serial transverse enteroplasty procedure (STEP) and lengthening and tailoring procedures (LILT, Bianchi) have no defined place at the initial operation although sporadic reports have appeared in the literature [89–92]. It would seem wiser to perform a primary end-to-end anastomosis and allow for adaptation to progress before intervening surgically when a plateau of enteral tolerance has been achieved and the infant is well grown and outside the neonatal period. The fashioning of stomas, e.g. Bishop–Koop, Santulli, Rehbein or double barrel, as practiced by some, is not routinely advocated unless there is gross intraperitoneal contamination, making a primary anastomosis unsafe [34, 38, 93, 94]. The Bishop-Koop stoma seems to be particularly associated with an increased incidence of complications [12]. Jejuno-ileal atresia associated with a gastroschisis is treated by resection and primary anastomosis if there is limited oedema and matting from amniotic peritonitis. If there is marked oedema and matting initial reduction of the eviscerated bowel with the atresia intact and primary closure of the abdominal wall defect, if possible, is preferred [95]. After allowing for disappearance of the oedema (10–14 days), a second laparotomy is performed with resection of the atretic segment and primary anastomosis. In the long term there is up to 20% incidence of prolonged dysmotility which may benefit from surgical interventions of tapering or imbrication [74, 81, 96–98]. So-called 'closing gastroschisis' may be associated with the both exit and entry level atresias with loss of intestinal length. Serial antenatal ultrasound scanning may show increasing bowel dilatation which should prompt early preterm delivery [99].

Postoperative care requires nasogastric decompression for several days after the operation (longer for high jejunal atresias). Therapeutic antibiotics are usually continued for 5–7 days or longer directed by culture of gastric aspirate and enteric content, and an oral antifungal agent is given prophylactically. Gavage feeding can begin as soon as there is evidence of bowel peristalsis. If a trans-anastomotic tube has been placed, hourly feedings can commence in small volumes from the day following surgery. Oral intake is commenced when the neonate is alert, sucks well, and there is evidence of prograde gastrointestinal function, i.e., clear gastric effluent of low volume, a soft abdomen and stools have been passed. Surveillance should continue until the infant has established normal gastrointestinal function. If at any time there is suspicion of a leak at the anastomosis (suggested by ileus, abdominal distension, vomiting and peritonitis), a plain radiograph of the abdomen should be taken. If this reveals free air in the abdomen more than 24 h after operation, laparotomy should be performed immediately and the leaking site sutured or the anastomosis redone. Parenteral nutrition is given initially and weaned slowly as enteral feeding is increased as per protocols. There is increasing evidence that keeping the daily fat load to 1 g/kg body weight and the use of fish oil containing lipid will reduce the incidence and severity of parenteral nutrition associated liver disease [100, 101].

33.10 Complications and Special Considerations

Although a survival rate of more than 90% can be expected, complications are not infrequent [24, 36, 56, 102]. These include anastomotic leaks and stricture formation, ischemia of the bowel due to the delicate blood supply, especially in type IIIb, adhesive bowel obstruction, the short bowel syndrome, infections related to the wound, intravenous access, chest, septicemia and bacterial overgrowth with blind loop syndrome or episodes of gram negative central line infections from bacterial translocation. In predicting the ultimate functional outcome, the following factors must be taken into consideration: the ileum adapts to a greater degree than the jejunum, the neonatal small intestine still has a period of maturation and growth ahead of it, and the actual residual small intestinal length is difficult to determine accurately at the time of the initial surgery. The proximal obstructed bowel segment is dilated and its functional potential may be overestimated, while that of the distal unused collapsed bowel may be underestimated. Of some importance is an intact ileocecal valve, which allows for accelerated intestinal adaptation with shorter residual jejunoileal length. The absence of the ileocecal valve may also lead to an increased transit-time, malabsorption, diarrhea and increased bacterial contamination of the small bowel. The full management of the short bowel syndrome is beyond the scope of this chapter [103].

33.10.1 Outcome

Before 1952 the mortality rate for congenital atresias of the small intestine even in the best centres was around 90% [3, 20]. Between 1952 and 1955, there was moderate improvement in outcome due to improved neonatal care [16]. At that stage most were treated by primary anastomosis without resection. With liberal resection of the blind ends and end-to-end anastomosis, the survival rate increased to 78% during 1955–1958 in one centre [4–6].

During the 25 year period from 1990 to 2015, 160 patients with jejuno-ileal atresias and stenoses were admitted to the pediatric surgical service at the Red Cross War Memorial Children's Hospital. There were 13 deaths (92% survival). Factors contributing to the mortality rate were: type of atresia (type III), proximal bowel infarction with peritonitis (delayed presentation), anastomotic leaks, missed distal atresia, the short bowel syndrome with PN associated liver disease, sepsis and more recently HIV infections [104]. The morbidity of patients with intestinal atresia is directly related to the length of the bowel if there is gross insufficiency (short bowel syndrome) as well as any degree of dysmotility which is particularly prevalent in babies with gastroschisis.

Infants with Ultra-short bowel [less than 10% of expected length] are usually infants with type III or IV atresia [24, 105].

33.11 Quality of Life and Long-Term Outcome

The quality of life in the long-term is dependent on the length of residual bowel, associated disease, [2, 12, 102, 106, 107] (Table 33.1) e.g., Cystic fibrosis, dysmotility especially with gastroschisis and the medical management of the short bowel syndrome. Increasingly, with appropriate medical and surgical management, most of these children can achieve enteral autonomy. A few may require life-long parenteral nutritional supplementation or may develop irreversible intestinal failure associated liver disease requiring

Table 33.1 Jejunal atresia and stenosis: Red Cross Children's Hospital—Experience 1959–2015

Type	Jejunum	Ileum	Total	(%)
Stenosis	22	14	36	10
Type I	68	18	86	24
Type II	22	14	36	10
Type IIIa	28	27	55	15
Type IIIb	68	1	69	19
Type IV	67	14	81	22
Total	275	88	363	100
Mortality related to type of atresia[a]				
Type	Patients	Mortality	%	
Stenosis	36	0	0	
Type I	86	4	6	
Type II	36	4	11	
Type IIIa	53	8	15	
Type IIIb	68	10	16	
Type IV	81	12	15	
Total	363	36	10	

[a]Last 25 year survival (1990–2015) 147/160 (92%)

either bowel or bowel and liver transplant. There are some who may require parenteral nutritional support from time to time in childhood during periods of enteric stress as they have little or no reserve. All children with short bowel are at risk of subclinical vitamin and micro-nutrient deficiency and can be divided into four main clinical categories: (a) those with normal alimentary function; (b) those with adequate function for growth and development but little or no reserve; (c) those with adequate function for survival after a prolonged period of adaptation and parenteral nutrition support and (d) those with uncorrectable intestinal insufficiency.

In those patients in group c) it is remarkable how far one can go with very little bowel using all the surgical and medical techniques available. In our own series, there are two infants with presenting lengths of 11 and 14 cm (ileocaecal valve intact 1 cm and 2 cm ileum respectively). Both have achieved full enteral autonomy at 13 months and 20 months of age after Bianchi procedures were done at around 6 months of age when a plateau of 80% enteral tolerance was reached without surgical intervention apart from the initial end to end anastomosis without resection. Neither of these have any evidence of liver disease using SMOF [a soya, medium chain triglyceride, olive oil and fish oil balanced fat emulsion lipid] as the preferred parenteral nutritional formula along with all other modalities of short bowel syndrome care [108].

References

1. de Lorimier A. Congenital atresia and stenosis of the jejunum and ileum. Surgery. 1969;65:819.
2. Stollman TH, de Blaauw I, Wijnen MH, van der Staak FH, et al. Decreased mortality but increased morbidity in neonates with jejunoileal atresia; a study of 114 cases over a 34-year period. J Pediatr Surg. 2009;44(1):217–21.
3. Evans CH. Atresias of the gastrointestinal tract. Int Abstr Surg. 1951;92(1):1–8.
4. Louw JH. Congenital atresia and stenosis of the small intestine. The case for resection and primary end-to-end anastomosis. S Afr J Surg. 1966;4(2):57–64.
5. Louw JH. Resection and end-to-end anastomosis in the management of atresia and stenosis of the small bowel. Surgery. 1967;62(5):940–50.
6. Louw JH. Congenital jejunoileal atresia: observations on its pathogenesis and treatment. Z Kinderchir. 1980;33(1):3–17.
7. Nixon HH. Intestinal obstruction in the newborn. Arch Dis Child. 1955;30(149):13–22.
8. Nixon HH. An experimental study of propulsion in isolated small intestine, and applications to surgery in the newborn. Ann R Coll Surg Engl. 1960;27:105–24.
9. Cywes S, Davies MR, Rode H. Congenital jejuno-ileal atresia and stenosis. S Afr Med J. 1980;57(16):630–9.
10. Grosfeld JL, Ballantine TV, Shoemaker R. Operative mangement of intestinal atresia and stenosis based on pathologic findings. J Pediatr Surg. 1979;14(3):368–75.
11. Lloyd DA. J.H. Louw Memorial Lecture. From puppy dogs to molecules: small-bowel atresia and short-gut syndrome. S Afr J Surg. 1999;37(3):64–8.
12. Kumaran N, Shankar KR, Lloyd DA, Losty PD. Trends in the management and outcome of jejuno-ileal atresia. Eur J Pediatr Surg. 2002;12(3):163–7.
13. Hays, D., Intestinal atresia and stenosis. 1969.
14. Burjonrappa SC, Crete E, Bouchard S. Prognostic factors in jejuno-ileal atresia. Pediatr Surg Int. 2009;25(9):795–8.
15. Dalla Vecchia LK, Grosfeld JL, West KW, Rescorla FJ, Scherer LR, Engum SA. Intestinal atresia and stenosis: A 25 year experience with 277 cases. Arch Surg. 1998;133(5):490–6.
16. Benson CD. Resection and primary anastomosis of the jejunum and ileum in the newborn. Ann Surg. 1955;142(3):478–85.
17. Bland Sutton J. Imperforate ileum. Am J Med Sci. 1889;98:457.

18. Davis D. Congenital occlusions of the intestine. SGO. 1922;34:12.
19. Fockens P. Operativ geheilter Fall von kongenitaler Dunndarmatresie. Zentralbl Chir. 1911;38:532.
20. Louw JH. Congenital intestinal atresia and severe stenosis in the newborn; a report on 79 consecutive cases. S Afr J Clin Sci. 1952;3(3):109–29.
21. Spriggs N. Congenital intestinal occlusion. Guys Hosp Rep. 1912;66:143.
22. Tandler J. Zur Entwicklungsgeschichte des menschlichen duodenum in fruhen Embryonalstadien. Morphol Jahrb. 1900;29:187–219.
23. Louw JH, Barnard CN. Congenital intestinal atresia; observations on its origin. Lancet. 1955;269(6899):1065–7.
24. Millar A. Intestinal atresia and stenosis. Pediatric Surgery. 3rd ed; 2000.
25. Goulet OJ, et al. Neonatal short bowel syndrome. J Pediatr. 1991;119(1 (Pt 1)):18–23.
26. Gupte GL, et al. Current issues in the management of intestinal failure. Arch Dis Child. 2006;91(3):259–64.
27. Hoehner JC, Ein SH, Kim PC. Management of gastroschisis with concomitant jejuno-ileal atresia. J Pediatr Surg. 1998;33(6):885–8.
28. Smith GH, Glasson M. Intestinal atresia: factors affecting survival. Aust N Z J Surg. 1989;59(2):151–6.
29. Francannet C, Robert E. Epidemiological study of intestinal atresias: central-eastern France Registry 1976–1992. J Gynecol Obstet Biol Reprod (Paris). 1996;25(5):485–94.
30. Best KE, Tennant PWG, Rankin J. Small intestinal atresia in europe: prevalence, associated anomalies and pregnancy outcomes. Arch Dis Childhood Fetal Neonatal Ed. 2011;96(1):Fa56–7.
31. Adeyemi D. Neonatal intestinal obstruction in a developing tropical country: patterns, problems, and prognosis. J Trop Pediatr. 1989;35(2):66–70.
32. Cragan JD, Louise Martin M, Moore CA, Khoury MJ. Descriptive epidemiology of small intestinal atresia, Atlanta, Georgia. Teratology. 1993;48(5):441–50.
33. Ratan SR, et al. Surgically treated gastro-intestinal obstruction in children: causes and implications. Indian J Gastroenterol. 2006;25(6):320–2.
34. Bishop HC, Koop CE. Management of meconium ileus; resection, Roux-en-Y anastomosis and ileostomy irrigation with pancreatic enzymes. Ann Surg. 1957;145(3):410–4.
35. Haller JA Jr, et al. Intestinal atresia. Current concepts of pathogenesis, pathophysiology, and operative management. Am Surg. 1983;49(7):385–91.
36. Nixon HH, Tawes R. Etiology and treatment of small intestinal atresia: analysis of a series of 127 jejunoileal atresias and comparison with 62 duodenal atresias. Surgery. 1971;69(1):41–51.
37. Nguyen D. In utero intussusception producing ileal atresia and meconium peritonitis with and without free air. Pediatr Surg Int. 1995;10:406.
38. Santulli TV, Blanc WA. Congenital atresia of the intestine: pathogenesis and treatment. Ann Surg. 1961;154:939–48.
39. Todani T, Tabuchi K, Tanaka S. Intestinal atresia due to intrauterine intussusception: analysis of 24 cases in Japan. J Pediatr Surg. 1975;10(4):445–51.
40. Graham JM-P, Marin-Padilla M, Hoefnagel D. Jejunal Atresia Associated with Cafergot® Ingestion During Pregnancy. Clin Pediatr. 1983;22(3):226–8.
41. Kaga Y. Intestinal atresia in fetal dogs produced by localised ligation of mesenteric vessels. J Pediatr Surg. 1975;10:949.
42. Moutsouris C. The "solid stage" and congenital intestinal atresia. J Pediatr Surg. 1966;1(5):446–50.
43. Patricolo M, Noia G, Rossi L, Zangari A, Pomini F, Catesini C, Filippetti R, Galli T, Iacobelli BD, Capuano LG, Romano D, Mancuso S, Rivosecchi M. An experimental animal model of intestinal obstruction to simulate in utero therapy for jejunoileal atresia. Fetal Diagn Ther. 1998;13(5):298–301.
44. de Chadarevian JP, et al. Terminal ileal atresia, total colonic aganglionosis, and thrombophilia. Pediatr Dev Pathol. 2009;12(5):394–7.
45. Gluer S. Intestinal Atresia Following Intraamniotic Use of Dyes. European Journal of Pediatric Surgery: Official Journal of Austrian Association of Pediatric Surgery. Z Kinderchir. 1995;5(4):240–2.
46. Yanagihara J, Nakamura J, Shimotake T, Deguchi E, Iwai N. An Association of Multiple Intestinal Atresia and Biliary Atresia: A Case Reportb. European Journal of Pediatric Surgery: Official Journal of Austrian Association of Pediatric Surgery. Z Kinderchir. 1995;5(6):372–4.
47. Johnson SM, Meyers RL. Inherited thrombophilia: a possible cause of in utero vascular thrombosis in children with intestinal atresia. J Pediatr Surg. 2001;36(8):1146–9.
48. Mishalany HG, Najjar FB. Familial jejunal atresia: three cases in one family. J Pediatr. 1968;73(5):753–5.
49. Nichol PF, Reeder A, Botham R. Humans, mice, and mechanisms of intestinal atresias: a window into understanding early intestinal development. J Gastrointest Surg. 2011;15(4):694–700.
50. Blyth H, Dickson JA. Apple peel syndrome (congenital intestinal atresia): a family study of seven index patients. J Med Genet. 1969;6(3):275–7.
51. Guttman FM, et al. Multiple atresias and a new syndrome of hereditary multiple atresias involving the gastrointestinal tract from stomach to rectum. J Pediatr Surg. 1973;8(5):633–40.
52. Kimble R. Jejuno-ileal atresia, An inherited condition? Pediatr Surg Int. 1995;10:400.
53. Puri P, Fujimoto T. New observations on the pathogenesis of multiple intestinal atresias. J Pediatr Surg. 1988;23(3):221–5.
54. Shorter NA, Georges A, Perenyi A, Garrow E. A proposed classification system for familial intestinal atresia and its relevance to the understanding of the etiology of jejunoileal atresia. J Pediatr Surg. 2006;41(11):1822–5.
55. Herman TEA, Mc Alister WH. Familial type 1 jejunal atresias and renal dysplasi. Pediatr Radiol. 1995;25(4):272–4.

56. Baglaj M, Carachi R, Lawther S. Multiple atresia of the small intestine: A 20 year review. Eur J Pediatr Surg. 2008;18(1):13–8.
57. Bass J. Pyloric atresia associated with multiple intestinal atresias and immune difficiency. J Pediatr Surg. 2002;37(6):941–2.
58. Cole C, Freitas A, Clifton MS, Durham MM. Hereditary multiple intestinal atresias: 2 new cases and review of the literature. J Pediatr Surg. 2010;45(4):E21–4.
59. Walker MW, Lovell MA, Kelly TE, Golden W, Saulsbury FT. Multiple areas of intestinal atresia associated with immunodeficiency and posttransfusion graft-versus-host disease. J Pediatr. 1993;123(1):93–5.
60. Roberts HE, Cragan JD, Cono J, Khoury MJ, Weatherly MR, Moore CA. Increased frequency of cystic fibrosis among infants with jejunoileal atresia. Am J Med Genet. 1998;78(5):446–9.
61. Gaillard D, Bouvier R, Scheiner C, Nessmann C, Delezoide AL, Dechelotte P, Leheup B, Cordier MP, Carles D, Lallemand A. Meconium ileus and intestinal atresia in fetuses and neonates. Pediatr Pathol Lab Med. 1996;16(1):25–40.
62. Wax JR, Hamilton T, Cartin A, Dudley J, Pinette MG, Blackstone J. Congenital jejunal and ileal atresia: natural prenatal sonographic history and association with neonatal outcome. J Pediatr Surg. 2009;44(1):71–4.
63. Ruiz MJ, Thatch KA, Fisher JC, Simpson LL, Cowles RA. Neonatal outcomes associated with intestinal abnormalities diagnosed by fetal ultrasound. Fetal Diagn Ther. 1998;13(5):298–301.
64. Tibboel D, Molenaar JC, Van Nie CJ. New perspectives in fetal surgery: the chicken embryo. J Pediatr Surg. 1979;14(4):438–40.
65. Lopez de Torre B, Tovar JA, Uriarte S, Aldazabal P. The nutrition of the fetus with intestinal atresia: studies in the chick embryo model. J Pediatr Surg. 1992;27(10):1325–8.
66. Tam PK, Nicholls G. Implications of antenatal diagnosis of small-intestinal atresia in the 1990s. Pediatr Surg Int. 1999;15(7):486–7.
67. Tongsong T, Chanprapaph P. Triple bubble sign: a marker of proximal jejunal atresia. Int J Gynecol Obstet. 2000;68(2):149–50.
68. Touloukian RJ. Intestinal atresia. Clin Perinatol. 1978;5(1):3–18.
69. Touloukian RJ. Diagnosis and treatment of jejunoileal atresia. World J Surg. 1993;17(3):310–7.
70. Baniеghbal B, Beale PG. Minimal access approach to jejunal atresia. J Pediatr Surg. 2007;42(8):1362–4.
71. Lima M, et al. Evolution of the surgical management of bowel atresia in newborn: laparoscopically assisted treatment. Pediatr Med Chir. 2009;31(5):215–9.
72. Yamataka A, et al. Laparoscopy-assisted surgery for prenatally diagnosed small bowel atresia: simple, safe, and virtually scar free. J Pediatr Surg. 2004;39(12):1815–8.
73. St. Peter SD, Little DC, Barsness KA, Copeland DR, Calkins CM, Yoder S, Rothenberg SS, Islam S, Tsao K, Ostlie DJ. Should We Be Concerned About Jejunoileal Atresia During Repair of Duodenal Atresia? J Laparoendosc Adv Surg Tech. 2010;20(9):773–5.
74. Doolin EJ, H.S. Ormsbee, and J.L. Hill, Motility abnormality in intestinal atresia. J Pediatr Surg. 1987;22(4):320–4.
75. Masumoto K, et al. Abnormalities of enteric neurons, intestinal pacemaker cells, and smooth muscle in human intestinal atresia. J Pediatr Surg. 1999;34(10):1463–8.
76. Ozguner IF, Savas C, Ozguner M, Candir O. Intestinal atresia with segmental musculature and neural defect. J Pediat Surg. 2005;40(8):1232–7.
77. Millar AJ, Rode H, Cywes S. A method of derotation and duodeno-jejunostomy for high jejunal atresia. J Pediatr Surg. 2001;36(5):833–4.
78. Yamataka A, Koga H, Shimotakahara A, Kobayashi H, Lane GJ, Miyano T. Novel procedures for enhancing high jejunal atresia repair: bilateral side-plication and plication before anastomosis. Pediatr Surg Int. 2005;21(11):907–10.
79. Cowles RA, et al. Serial transverse enteroplasty in a newborn patient. J Pediatr Gastroenterol Nutr. 2007;45(2):257–60.
80. Luo CC, Ming YC, Chao HC, Chu SM. Duodenal Derotation and Extent Tapering Jejunoplasty as Primary Repair for Neonates With High Jejunal Atresia. Pediat Neonatol. 2010;51(5):269–72.
81. Takahashi A, Suzuki N, Ikeda H, Kuroiwa M, Tomomasa T, Tsuchida Y, Kuwano H. Results of bowel plication in addition to primary anastomosis in patients with jejunal atres. J Pediatr Surg. 2001;36(12):1752–6.
82. Kling K, et al. A novel technique for correction of intestinal atresia at the ligament of Treitz. J Pediatr Surg. 2000;35(2):353–5. discussion 356.
83. Dewan PA, Guiney EJ. Duodenoplasty in the management of duodenal atresia. Pediatr Surg Int. 1990;5(4):253–4.
84. Chaet MS, Warner BW, Sheldon CA. Management of multiple jejunoileal atresias with an intraluminal SILASTIC stent. J Pediatr Surg. 1994;29(12):1604–6.
85. Federici S, Domenichelli V, Antonellini C, Dòmini R. Multiple intestinal atresia with apple peel syndrome: successful treatment by five end-to-end anastomoses, jejunostomy, and transanastomotic silicone stent. Pediatr Surg. 2003;38(8):1250–2.
86. Honzumi M, Okuda A, Suzuki H. Duodenal motility after tapering duodenoplasty for high jejunal and multiple intestinal atresia. Pediatr Surg Int. 1993;8(2):116–8.
87. Smith MB, Smith L, Wells W, Shapira E, Hendrickson M, Moynihan PC. Concurrent jejunal atresia with "apple peel" deformity in premature twins. Pediatr Surg Int. 1991;6(6):425–8.

88. Yardley I, Khalil B, Minford J, Morabito A. Multiple jejunoileal atresia and colonic atresia managed by multiple primary anastomosis with a single gastroperineal transanastomotic tube without stomas. J Pediatr Surg. 2008;43(11):45–6.
89. Dutta S. The STEP procedure: defining its role in the management of pediatric short bowel syndrome. J Pediatr Gastroenterol Nutr. 2007;45(2):174–5.
90. Ehrlich PF, Mychaliska GB, Teitelbaum DH. The 2 STEP: an approach to repeating a serial transverse enteroplasty. J Pediatr Surg. 2007;42(5):819–22.
91. Morikawa N, Kuroda T, Kitano Y, Tanaka H, Takayasu H, Fujino A, Shibata Y, Tanemura H, Muto M, Honna T. Repeat STEP procedure to establish enteral nutrition in an infant with short bowel syndrome. Pediatr Surg Int. 2009;25(11):1007–11.
92. Wales PW, Dutta S. Serial transverse enteroplasty as primary therapy for neonates with proximal jejunal atresia. J Pediatr Surg. 2005;40(3):E31–4.
93. Rehbein F. The double tube technique for the treatment of meconium ileus and small bowel atresia. J Pediatr Surg. 1968;3:723.
94. Rosenmann J. A reappraisal of the Mikulicz enterostomy in infants and children. Surgery. 1982;91:34.
95. van Hoorn WA, Hazebroek FW, Molenaar JC. Gastroschisis associated with atresia—a plea for delay in resection. Z Kinderchir. 1985;40(6):368–70.
96. Phillips JD, Raval M, Redden C, Weiner TM. Gastroschisis, atresia, dysmotility: surgical treatment strategies for a distinct clinical entity. J Pediatr Surg. 2008;43(12):2208–12.
97. Piper HG, Alesbury J, Waterford SD, Zurakowski D, Jaksic T. Intestinal atresias: factors affecting clinical outcomes. J Pediat Surg. 2008;43(7):1244–8.
98. Ellaway C, Beasley SW. Bezoar formation and malabsorption secondary to persistent dilatation and dysmotility of the duodenum after repair of proximal jejunal atresia. Pediatr Surg Int. 1997;12(2–3):190–1.
99. Houben C, et al. Closing gastroschisis: diagnosis, management, and outcomes. J Pediatr Surg. 2009;44(2):343–7.
100. Hess RA, et al. Survival outcomes of pediatric intestinal failure patients: analysis of factors contributing to improved survival over the past two decades. J Surg Res. 2011;170(1):27–31.
101. Nehra D, Fallon EM, Puder M. The prevention and treatment of intestinal failure-associated liver disease in neonates and children. Surg Clin North Am. 2011;91(3):543–63.
102. Grosfeld JL, O'Neill J, Coran A. Jejunoileal atresia and stenosis. Paediatr Surg. 2006;2:6.
103. Thompson JS, et al. Current management of the short bowel syndrome. Surg Clin North Am. 2011;91(3):493–510.
104. Karpelowsky JS, et al. Outcomes of human immunodeficiency virus-infected and -exposed children undergoing surgery—a prospective study. J Pediatr Surg. 2009;44(4):681–7.
105. Shakya VC, Agrawal C, Shrestha P, Poudel P, Khaniya S, Adhikary S. Management of jejunoileal atresias: an experience at eastern Nepal. BMC Surg. 2010;26(10):35.
106. Danismend EN, Frank JD, Brown S. Morbidity and Mortality in Small Bowel Atresia. Jejuno-ileal Atresia. European Journal of Pediatric Surgery: Official Journal of Austrian Association of Pediatric Surgery. Z Kinderchir. 1987;42(1):17–8.
107. Dicken BJ, et al. Medical management of motility disorders in patients with intestinal failure: a focus on necrotizing enterocolitis, gastroschisis, and intestinal atresia. J Pediatr Surg. 2011;46(8):1618–30.
108. Kelly DA. Preventing parenteral nutrition liver disease. Early Hum Dev. 2011;86(11):683–7.

Duplications of the Alimentary Tract

34

Antti I. Koivusalo and Risto J. Rintala

Abstract

Duplications of the alimentary tract are cystic or tubular structures most often in close proximity with a section of the alimentary tract. The most common location is abdomen and the most common location is small intestine. Duplications possess a surrounding muscular layer, an inside mucosal layer, intrinsic nerves and peristalsis. Approximately 10% of duplications are multiple and there is a high prevalence of coexisting malformations of vertebral column, intestines and urinary tract and genitals. A diagnosed duplication should always warrant for search of others and the coexisting malformations. Duplications may contain heterotropic gastric or other kind of mucosa.

Duplications are increasingly often diagnosed antenatally. One third of foregut and midgut duplications present during infancy whereas hindgut duplications without an external sign of duplicated anus or genitalia may remain undiagnosed longer. In an infant the most common symptom is vomiting from gastric outlet obstruction by a large cystic duplication, alternatively duplication may cause intestinal volvulus or intussusception. Duplications in the mouth, oropharynx, neck and thorax may cause airway obstruction. Heterotropic gastric mucosa in duplication may ulcerate and cause haemorrhage or perforation. Because of the risk of significant complications and the risk of eventual malignant transformation surgical removal of duplication is practically always indicated.

Keywords

Alimentary tract duplications • Embryology • Surgery • Outcomes

34.1 Introduction

Duplications of the alimentary tract can occur anywhere from oropharynx to anus. Depending on their embryonic origin duplications can be

A.I. Koivusalo, MD, PhD • R.J. Rintala, MD, PhD (✉)
Section of Paediatric Surgery, Children's Hospital, University Central Hospital, University of Helsinki, PO BOX 281, Helsinki 00029 HUS, Finland
e-mail: risto.rintala@hus.fi

P.D. Losty et al. (eds.), *Rickham's Neonatal Surgery*, https://doi.org/10.1007/978-1-4471-4721-3_34

divided to foregut, midgut and hindgut duplications, all of which have a characteristic presentation and a pattern of associated malformations.

Approximately two thirds of all intestinal duplications are discovered within the first two years of life, with one third identified in the newborn period. Although duplications may have a protean modes of presentation the most common symptoms are associated with the tendency of the duplications to occupy space and compress hollow viscus and the tendency to haemorrhage from the heterotrophic gastric mucosa. Duplications can be diagnosed antenatally and in some cases intrauterine or immediate postnatal interventions are indicated. Neonatal emergencies associated with duplications are high airway obstruction, respiratory distress, haemorrhage and intestinal obstruction. Alimentary tract duplications are associated with potentially fatal complications and when diagnosed surgical treatment is always indicated. With time malignant transformation of the duplications can occur.

34.2 Definition, Etiology, Epidemiology and Anatomical Characteristics

Early criteria by Ladd required the alimentary tract duplications to possess (I) a well-defined coat of smooth muscle, (II) an epithelial lining representing some portion of the intestinal tract (III) intimate anatomic association with some portion of the gastrointestinal tract [1]. More recently it has been found that duplications may contain several kinds of heterotropic mucosa, respiratory epithelium, bronchogenic cartilage [2–4] and duplications may be located far apart from the section of the alimentary tract from which their mucosal lining is derived. The muscular wall of duplications possesses intrinsic innervation and exerts peristalsis [5, 6].

The embryologic origin of alimentary tract duplications has remained somewhat obscure. The theories of the etiology of alimentary tract duplications include those of abortive or partial twinning, split notochord and anomalous adhesions [7], diverticula and canalization defect [8] and environmental factors [9]. Although these theories may explain long doubled segments of intestine and anal opening, dorsal location with tethering to the vertebral column and occurrence of associated anomalies, no single theory explains the anatomical and histological variations found in alimentary tract duplications. It is assumed that duplications occur early in fetal life and develop after the formation of the notochord after the third gestation week. There is some evidence that expression of the sonic hedgehog gene by the notochord affects the Shh-GLi signalling pathway and may contribute to a spectrum of bronchopulmonary, alimentary tract and associated anomalies [10]. Foregut duplications and lesions in foregut derived respiratory tract such as bronchogenic cyst and congenital pulmonary airway malformations (CPAM) and other foregut malformations such as oesophageal atresia may actually share a common etiology [11–14]. Thoracoabdominal duplications may interfere with the development of diaphragm, vena cava and the portal vein [15–18]. Despite the obscure genetic and embryological origin it has become practical to refer to foregut, midgut and hindgut derived duplications. Thus duplications from the pharynx to the papilla of Vater are considered foregut derived, duplications of the third and fourth part of duodenum, jejunum, ileum and little over the middle portion of the transverse colon midgut derived and duplications of rest of the colon, rectum and anus hindgut derived.

Alimentary tract duplications have a reported incidence of 1 in 4500 fetal and neonatal autopsies [19]. There is a slight overall male preponderance [6].

Approximately 20% of duplications are located in the mediastinum, 1–2% are cervical or oral and 2% are thoracoabdominal, whereas rest of the locations are abdominal including gastric (2%), duodenal (6%), jejunal and ileal (53%), colonic (13%) and rectal (4%) [20].

Rectal duplications may have a fistulous vaginal or cutaneous opening [6, 21]. Duplications of pancreas, gallbladder and the extrahepatic biliary tract [22–24] and even gastrointestinal triplications [25, 26] have been reported. Of alimentary tract duplications 75–85% are cystic which predominantly lack communication with their adjacent intestine, whereas the remaining duplications are tubular that may or may not have one or more direct communications across the common septum [27, 28]. Duplications are typically located in the dorsal aspect of the adjacent intestine. According to Li and colleagues 75% lie parallel to the mesentery receiving a main artery from one leaf of mesentery whereas 25% are intramesenteric and receive arteries from both mesenteric leaves, [29], but occasionally separate duplications with vascular pedicle occur [30]. Some duplications are located retroperitoneally completely isolated without contact from their organ of derivation [31].

Enteric duplications are multiple in 10–20% of patients, and detection of one duplication indicates search for other noncontiquous duplications [6] and also CPAM lesions [11]. Of all alimentary tract duplications 35–70% contain heterotropic gastric mucosa, the occurrence being highest in foregut and small bowel and lowest in hindgut duplications [6, 27]. Ulceration with subsequent haemorrhaging of the heterotopic gastric mucosa within duplication is a typical manifestation in 10–20% of patients [6, 32–34]. Other types of heterotropic tissue in duplications include those derived of pancreas, thyroid, lung, bronchi and adrenal cortex [6, 32, 35]. Children with enteric duplications have a relatively high incidence of associated anomalies. Vertebral anomalies including malformed vertebraes, spina bifida occulta, anterior meningocele, scoliosis and tethetring connections to the spinal canal can occur in 50% of thoracic and thoracoabdominal lesions whereas midgut duplications are associated with intestinal atresias, intestinal malrotation, and hindgut duplications with genital and urinary tract anomalies [6, 32, 35]. The presence of multiple noncontiguous duplications increase the probability of associated malformations to 100% [6]. Duplication cysts which extend into the spinal cord are referred as neurenteric cysts.

34.3 Clinical Presentation

Clinical presentation of alimentary tract duplications depend on their anatomic level, mass effect and space occupying capacity and specific complications related especially with the heterotopic mucosa. Often duplications are found incidentally in routine imaging or in prenatal ultrasound. Duplications can cause symptoms in a fetus. An intrathoracal duplication with mediastinal shift and hydrops in a fetus [36] and bleeding fetal oesophageal duplication [37] have been reported. Approximately two thirds of all intestinal duplications are discovered within the first two years of life, with at least one third identified in the newborn period [6, 20, 27, 33, 38]. As much as 30% of abdominal duplications are detected prenatally [28].

Duplications of mouth, mandible, oral cavity and tongue are often evident immediately after birth and large duplication cysts in the oropharyngeal region can cause congenital high airway obstruction syndrome (CHAOS) [39, 40]. Cervical and thoracic enlarged foregut duplications, primarily oesophageal duplications and bronchogenic cysts, may begin to compress oesophagus and bronchi and cause cough, wheezing, dyspnoea, and respiratory infection [10, 30, 33, 41]. Ulceration of gastric mucosa in the duplication can cause haemoptysis [10].

The most common symptoms in a neonate with an abdominal duplication is vomiting and abdominal distention [28, 38, 41]. Gastric, pyloric, duodenal or pancreatic duplications can cause gastric outlet or duodenal obstruction with the resulting copious vomiting and compression of the common bile tract by a duplication cyst may cause jaundice and recurrent pancreatitis [6, 10, 32, 35].

Duplications of the small and large bowel present as intestinal obstruction caused either by mechanical obstruction of the enlarged duplication, or, a duplication may cause intussusception or volvulus [28, 32] Ulcerated haemorrhaging gastric mucosa in small bowel duplication can cause an enlarged mass in the intestinal wall with the resulting perforation, peritonitis or melena [6, 32]. Hindgut duplications may present as a second opening in the perineum or in females into the back wall of vagina [6]. In addition, the mass effect of hindgut duplications may cause abdominal distention, constipation and obstruction of the urinary tract [6].

34.4 Diagnosis

Fetal ultrasound screening [28, 42, 43] and fetal MRI [39, 44] have improved significantly the detection and diagnosis of the alimentary tract duplications. In antenatally detected abdominal duplications as high as 24% incidence of volvulus has been reported [28], arguing for early surgical intervention or close postnatal observation in neonates with antenatally diagnosed duplication in the abdomen. Fetal ultrasound and MRI imaging of duplications at risk of causing airway obstruction are crucial in determining whether an intervention for CHAOS is indicated [39].

In neonatal diagnostics ultrasound scan is the most common imaging modality. Ultrasound scan has, however, limitations in the evaluation of thoracic duplications. In MRI most duplications have low signal intensity in T1 images and very high intensity in T2 images, whereas in CT duplication is sharply marginated and has homogenous a near water attenuation. In CT scan the image of a duplication may be confused with that of an abscess with a similar the enchanging rim and cystic appearance, but the lack of septic symptoms in an infant should suggest duplication. Lack of gas in the duplication indicates non-communication with the neighboring part of the alimentary tract [45].

In neonates half of the abdominal cystic duplications present as a palpable mass. In ultrasound examination at least 50% of duplications can be detected as a fluid—filled structure with the characteristic echogenic signal of the mucosal layer surrounded by a dense layer representing the surrounding smooth muscle. This double-layered appearance is usually not circumferential as the layers are not uniform in thickness [45] (Fig. 34.1). This characteristic wall structure is not present in lymphatic malformations, cystic hamartomas, ovarian cysts, and mesenteric or omental cysts, but these structures as well as Meckel's diverticulum can cause false positive findings [46]. Other radiologic studies including plain radiographs, gastrointestinal contrast studies and MRI will further assist the diagnosis, and associated malformations and simultaneously occurring other duplications may be detected simultaneously. In an evaluation of a child with abdominal pains and anaemia a technetium 99 pertechnate scan for Meckel's diverticulum may detect heterotropic gastric mucosa in a duplication [47, 48]. Duplications are sometimes difficult to diagnose radiologically and it is not rare that a duplication is diagnosed at the operation.

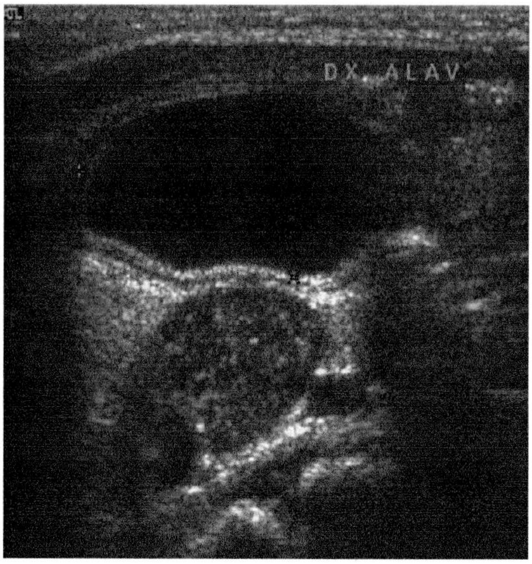

Fig. 34.1 A typical ultrasound scan of a cystic duplication of the terminal ileum, markings indicate the characteristic multi-layered wall

34.4.1 Duplications of Oropharynx

Duplications of oropharynx may be of similar etiology than those of the more distal gastrointestinal tract. Theories of etiology include duplications of the prosenccephalon, olfactory placodes, stomatoideal plate and branchial arches and split notochord. Duplications of mouth, floor of the mouth, lips, and mandible may require complex surgery. Lingual duplications and duplications at the floor of the oral cavity may cause feeding problems, but sometimes even cause high airway obstruction and may require immediate intubation or extrauterine intrapartum (EXIT) intervention [39, 49].

34.4.2 Cervical Oesophageal Duplications

Cervical oesophageal duplications are exceedingly rare and approximately 20 cases have been reported [50–52]. The most common presentation is respiratory distress, which can be life threatening. Rapid intubation, imaging with CT or MRI and surgical excision are indicated. If the lesion cannot be completely excised, stripping of the mucosa will result in obliteration of the cyst cavity. Differential diagnosis includes lymphatic malformations, bronchogenic cysts, laryngeal and tracheobronchial retention cysts and branchial and thyroglossal cysts [50].

34.4.3 Thoracic and Thoracoabdominal Duplications

Thoracic and thoracoabdominal duplications represent 20% of all alimentary tract duplications. Most common location is in the lower half of the posterior mediastinum with the predominance of the right side, but the lesions may protrude into either hemithorax. Thoracic duplications are predominatly cystic and often located within the oesophageal wall without communication into the oesophageal lumen. Thoracal duplications are often associated with vertebral anomalies and may possess a tethering adhesion with the vertebral column [10, 12, 27, 35, 38]. Thoracic and thoracoabdominal cysts may present as neurenteric cysts which are duplications which extend into spinal canal. Neurenteric cyst presents often with neurological symptoms and if radiological imaging suggests a neurenteric cyst, a neurosurgeon is included in the team which perform the evaluation and the ultimate treatment [27, 53]. Bronchogenic cyst is a variant of alimentary tract duplication with cartilagenous wall and ciliated respiratory epithelium. Bronchogenic cyst is noncommunicating and often located near the tracheal bifurcation but can occur anywhere along the alimentary canal [10, 12].

Appropriate imaging of the duplication and spinal column with ultrasound, CT or MRI (Fig. 34.2) is mandatory. Differential diagnostics include neurogenic tumors, anterior mediastinal masses such as lymphoma, teratoma and pericardial cyst, CPAM and cystic structures of the diaphragm. Treatment consists of excision of the lesion either via thoracotomy or thoracoscopically. A duplication cyst of the oesophagus may be resected without entering the mucosal lumen of the oesophagus. After excision it is recommendable to instil air or fluid into oesophagus to ascertain that no inadvertent perforation of the oesophageal wall remain unregocnized.

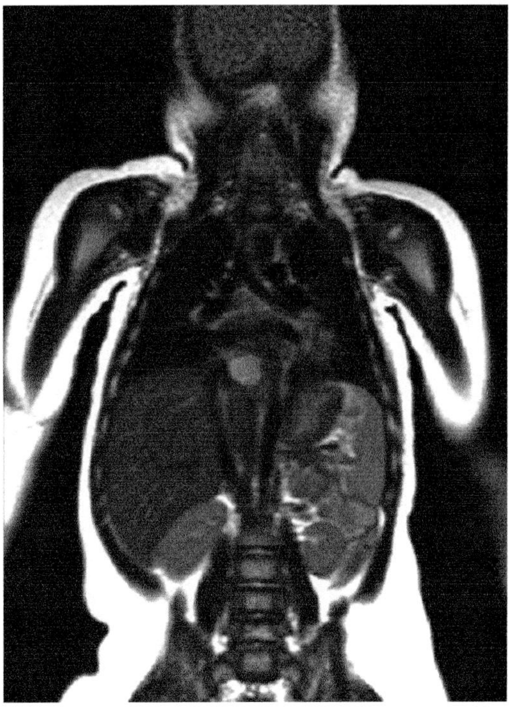

Fig. 34.2 Oesophageal duplication (between *black line*) in mediastinal MRI scan

34.4.4 Thoracoabdominal Duplications

Foregut duplications can expand from thorax to abdomen through the diaphragm or hiatus. It is not unusual that they adhere to several of adjacent organs such as oesophagus, stomach, duodenum and pancreas and may contain tissue from mixed sources [35, 53, 54]. Associated anomalies of vertebral column occur frequently. Thorough preoperative imaging of the lesion and the surrounding structures is of paramount importance. Large duplications may distort the anatomy of the mesenteric vasculature unexpectedly. Surgical approach requires combination of thoracotomy and abdominal incision but sometimes combined thoracoscopic and laparoscopic resection can be made. Sometimes all extensions of thoracoabdominal duplications may be difficult to detect and incomplete extension with missed neurenteric or abdominal components have led to fatal meningeal and abdominal infections [54, 55].

34.4.5 Gastric Duplications

Gastric duplications occur most often on the greater curvature. They are predominantly cystic and may grow relatively large, and are often seen in antenatal ultrasound. Symptoms begin often at the first months of life. Mass effect of the duplication cause gastric outlet obstruction and abdominal distension and symptoms include vomiting, gastrooesophageal reflux and abdominal pain. A palpable mass can often be felt. Differential diagnostics include duodenal duplication, choledochal cyst, mesenteric cyst, cystic lesions of the liver, and cystic neurogenic tumours and in older children pancreatic pceudocyst In rare occasions the duplication is located at the pylorus [56]. Communication to pancreatic or biliary ductal systems is usually seen in duodenal duplications but may occur also in gastric duplications [57, 58]. The treatment of gastric duplication is resection whenever possible. In some cases segmental resection of the stomach or a partial resection of the duplication with mucosal stripping are required. Small duplications may be resected laparoscopically.

34.4.6 Duplications of the Duodenum and the Pancreas

Duodenal duplications are predominantly cystic, usually located in the second and third part of the duodenum on the posteromedial aspect and often in close proximity with the papilla of Vater and biliary and pancreatic ducts. Approximately 30% communicate with the pancreaticobiliary system and aberrant ducts to pancreatic head may occur. In some cases the main pancreatic and biliary ducts drain into the duplication. The symptoms include those of gastric outlet obstruction, abdominal pain, recurrent pancreatitis jaundice and haemorrhage. Approximately 10% of cases present before the age of one year, most often the presentation is during the first decade of life [59, 60]. In a neonate differential diagnostics include choledochal cyst, cystic variant of biliary atresia and cystic lesions of the liver.

The most common treatment for symptomatic duodenal duplications in children is open surgical resection. The proximity to pancreaticobiliary ducts and common wall between duplication cyst and duodenum adds difficulties to complete resection. Appropriate imaging of the relationship and anatomy of the duplication and the pancreaticobiliary system with MR cholangiogram or ERCP or with operative cholangiogram is highly recommendable [10]. Complete resection or partial resection with mucosectomy of the duplication is possible in most of the cases. In some cases the best option is drainage of the cyst into duodenum with mucosal stripping or if complete mucosal stripping may injure pancreaticobiliary tract the absence of gastric mucosa may be ascertained with intraoperative frozen sections [54]. In intraluminal duodenal duplications which do not contain gastric heterotropic tissues internal endoscopic drainage may be another treatment option [60]. In duodenal duplications involving the pancreatic head and biliary tract pancreaticoduodenectomy is the treatment of choice [61].

Duplications of the pancreatic head pose similar diagnostic and therapeutic challenges as duodenal duplications and before surgical excision is attempted a thorough imaging is mandatory. Surgical treatment may include complete excision or local excision with stripping of the mucosa with or without drainage to Roux-Y jejunal loop, or pancreaticoduodenectomy [10, 22, 62]. Duplications of the tail of the pancreas may be treated with spleen saving distal open or laparoscopic pancreatectomy [10, 62]. Because the high risk of complications and the possibility of malignant transformation incidentally diagnosed or asymptomatic gastric duodenal and duplications should be evaluated for prophylactic surgical treatment. Gastric mucosa in gastric, duodenal and pancreatic duplications have been reported to cause hypergastrinemia with the presentation of recalcitrant gastrooesophageal reflux and gastric ulcers [22, 23].

34.4.7 Duplicated Liver, Common Bile Duct and Gallbladder

These lesions are rare and often present as properly developed functioning structures rather than attached non-communicating cysts. A boy with central diaphragmatic defect has been reported to possess a fully duplicated liver [23]. Also a case of intrahepatic location of an ileal duplication cyst has been reported [63]. There are many reported anatomic variations in the human biliary tree and they include a few cases of the duplications of the common bile duct [64, 65] Gallbladder duplications may present as a bilobed or bifid gallbladder or two gallbladders may have separate cystic ducts or share a Y or H shaped cystic duct [66].

34.4.8 Duplications of the Small Bowel

Duplications of the small intestine are the most common duplications of the alimentary tract. Small bowel duplications occur most often in the ileum and 50% are found near the ileocolic junction. Their shape may be tubular or cystic and typical location is in the mesenteric side of the intestine. Duplications of the small bowel are increasingly diagnosed with antenatal ultrasound.

The duplication shares often a common wall with the neighbouring intestine. Communication with the neighbouring intestine is not common but has implications into the clinical presentation. A proximal communication into a tubular duplication may allow accumulation of intestinal contents and subsequent dilatation of the duplication, whereas a distal communication allows drainage into the neighbouring intestine. Small cystic duplications may function as a leading point for volvulus or intussusception. Of small bowel duplications 20–50% contain gastric mucosa [27, 67] that can cause ulceration, bleeding and perforation and be diagnosed with technetium scan. Ten percent of patients with small bowel duplications have concomitant intestinal atresias, and approximately 10–20% may have a coexisting abdominal or thoracic duplication [6].

Symptoms from small bowel include intestinal obstruction caused by dilatation of a cyst obstructing the neighbouring intestine or intestinal volvulus or intussusception, or melaena and anaemia from a bleeding duplication [32, 67]. Antenatal complications are rare [43].

Optimal treatment is excision of the duplication. In duplications of convenient size laparoscopy or a small umbilical laparotomy may be used. A cystic duplication may be removed by excising the duplication with a small section of the neighbouring intestine. If there is a risk of resecting the ileocaecal valve a local resection of the cystic duplication with stripping of the mucosa is often adequate. In the case of long tubular duplications excision together with the neighbouring intestine may lead to excess loss of functional small bowel and intestinal failure. In some cases it is possible to open the muscular wall of the duplication and remove the mucosa. Some duplications may be amenable for resection by using the split mesentery technique by Bianchi [68]. Creating communications from the duplication to the neighbouring intestine retains the risk of bleeding from heterotropic gastric tissue, but may function as a temporary drainage if for example it is estimated that in a growing infant the lengthening of small bowel will allow resection of the lesion at a later date without a risk of intestinal failure. Infants with asymptomatic small bowel duplications need not to be operated in the neonatal period but should undergo evaluation for prophylactic resection within a few months [67].

34.4.9 Duplications of the Colon and Rectum

Duplications of the colon and rectum are much less common than duplications of the small bowel [28]. They constitute 17% of all gastrointestinal tract duplications. However, they are more commonly complex and the spectrum ranges from simple duplication cyst to partial or complete hindgut duplications that may be associated with complex anorectal and cloacal anomalies. Hindgut duplications are also not uncommon in patients with cloacal exstrophy. Most common type of duplication in the colon and rectum is a cystic duplication, these constitute more than half of the cases [28, 69]. Although cystic duplications can be found throughout colon and rectum, the most common site is cecum. Rectal cystic duplications are usually situated low in the rectum but unlike midgut duplications they almost always rise from the posterior rectal wall. Some of these low rectal duplications cysts may prolapse through the anus. Tubular duplications are more common in the colon and rectum than in other parts of the gastrointestinal tract. In the colon the tubular duplication usually resides, as midgut duplications, in the mesentery. However, rectal tubular duplications usually lie between rectum and sacrum; this suggests a different pathogenetic mechanism. Anterior duplications are extremely rare [70]. The extreme form of tubular duplication is the duplication of most or whole length of colon and rectum. These are commonly associated with genitourinary, vertebral and spinal anomalies. These duplications are usually side-to-side with the colon and rectum. The duplicated colon and rectum may end as a rectourethral or rectovaginal fistula, may end blindly or as a double anus. There is usually a communication between both colons. These long colorectal duplications are sometimes associated with duplicated genitalia and rarely with duplicated urinary bladder.

The duplications of colon and rectum may not be symptomatic in the newborn unless there is an obstruction. Some of the duplications present as a cystic mass that may have been detected already antenatally. The long tubular duplications that are associated with anorectal or urogenital malformations usually present in the newborn. In case one of communication to the urogenital tract the presenting symptom is meconium or stool passing from the urethra in males or vagina in females. Rectal cystic duplications commonly present in early infancy, a typical finding is a mass prolapsing partially or completely through the anus. If there is no obstruction of the bowel continuity the diagnosis of simple colonic and rectal duplications is usually delayed. Later symptoms may include constipation, vague abdominal pain, failure to thrive and bleeding [70, 71]. The bleeding source may be ectopic gastric mucosa that may be present in colon and rectum duplications, too [28].

The diagnosis of duplications of the colon and rectum may be difficult. Intra-abdominal duplications are commonly visualised by echography. Echography, however, does not necessarily provide exact anatomical localization of the lesion. MRI studies, especially MRI enterography, exactly delineate the anatomy of duplications. MRI is especially useful in rectal duplications that may not be detected by echography. MRI shows the extent of the lesion and its relationship to sacrum, rectum and urinary tract. Long tubular duplications that have an ectopic opening in the urogenital tract or perineum may be studied by retrograde contrast injections.

The optimal treatment of duplications of colon and rectum is surgical removal. Cystic lesions and short tubular colonic lesions are easily treated by limited resection of colon with the duplication. In long duplications innovative surgical techniques may need to be applied. If the length of the duplication is not too long, the mucosa may be stripped from the entire length of the duplication. Another option is to create a wide window between the duplication and the native bowel in both ends of duplication. Short rectal tubular duplications and cystic duplication well above the anal canal may be removed by a posterior sagittal approach. The duplications share a common muscular wall with the rectum, usually the intergrity of the native rectal mucosa can be preserved thus avoiding bowel diversion. If the duplication has been infected and drained before, the definitive surgery should be performed under colostomy cover because scar formation around the duplication may preclude removal without resection of the full-thickness posterior rectal wall. Longer rectal duplications may be managed by creating a long side-to-side anastomosis with staplers applied both through rectum and transabdominally, openly or laparoscopically. If a colorectal duplication is associated with an anorectal malformation, the best policy is to retain the anus that is in its normal position and resect the distal part of the bowel that ends as a rectourogenital fistula. The drainage of the duplicated colon and rectum to normal bowel has to be ascertained. If both bowel terminations end as fistulae to perineum or urogenital tract, innovative surgical solutions have to be used that may need to include pull-through of the distal bowel and reconstruction of sphincter complex.

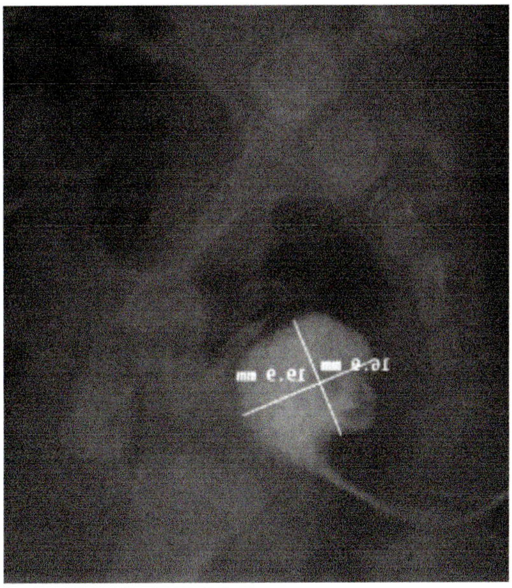

Fig. 34.4 Lateral contrast X-ray of the anal canal duplication

34.4.10 Duplication of the Anal Canal

Duplication of the anal canal is a specific entity that comprises of a duplicated anus and anal canal that lie posteriorly to the normal anus. Over 40 cases have been reported in the literature [72]. The anus is small in size (Fig. 34.3) but has a separate voluntary sphincter system. The proximal extension is variable but usually not more than a couple of centimetres (Fig. 34.4). This anomaly occurs almost extensively in females. Communication with the native anal canal is very uncommon. Anal canal duplication is sometimes associated with presacral mass or teratoma, and sacral deformities consistent with Currarino syndrome [72–74].

Diagnosis can be made by clinical inspection only, further useful studies are contrast fistulography through the duplicated anus and MRI that detects the possibly associated presacral and sacral abnormalities. The treatment of anal canal duplication is straightforward; the lesion may be excised through a posterior perineal approach in most cases. Care must be taken as the proximal part of the duplicated anal canal share a common muscular wall with the normal anal canal. Longer proximal extension or associated presacral mass may require the use of a formal posterior sagittal approach. The functional prognosis following removal is excellent as the sphincter system of the native anus is normal.

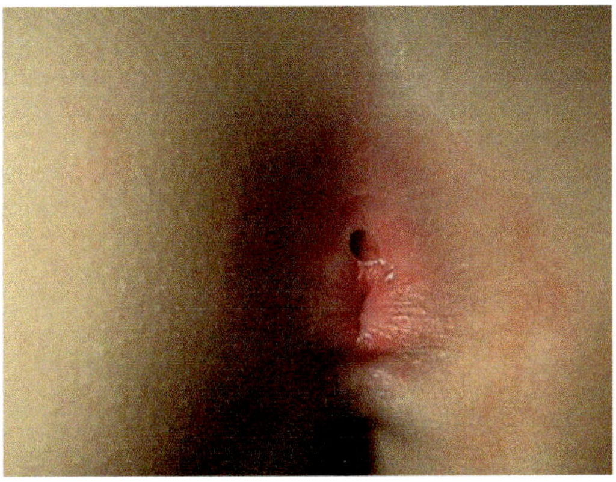

Fig. 34.3 Posterior anal canal duplication

34.5 Complications and Long-Term Results

Recurrence and complications may occur because of incomplete resection, missed transdiaphragmatic duplication tract, missed neurenteric component, loss of small bowel due to missed volvulus or excessive resection of small bowel and or haemorrhage from inadvertently retained heterotropic gastric mucosa. Following surgery for duplications mortality rate may be as high as 8%. Highest mortality is associated with thoracoabdominal duplications. After appropriate surgical resection the long-term outcomes are, however, excellent.

Untreated duplications may bleed, perforate [75] and become colonized by bacteria [76, 77]. In addition several cases of malignancy in duplications has been reported [78–80]. These have occurred especially in rectal duplications [80]. Surgical resection of a diagnosed duplications is therefore always warranted.

References

1. Ladd WE. Duplications of the alimentary tract. South Med J. 1937;30:363.
2. Gorsler C, Schier F, Danzer E. Ciliated epithelium in a midgut enteric duplication: a case report. Eur J Pediatr Surg. 2001;11:136–8.
3. McNally J, Charles AK, Spicer RD, Grier D. Mixed foregut cyst associated with esophageal atresia. J Pediatr Surg. 2001;36:939–40.
4. Kim DH, Kim JS, Nam ES, Shin HS. Foregut duplication cyst of the stomach. Pathol Int. 2000;50:142–5.
5. Simonovský V. Jejunal duplication cyst displaying peristalsis and a five-layered appearance of the wall: a preoperative ultrasound diagnosis. Eur Radiol. 1996;6:153–5.
6. Ildstad ST, Tollerud DJ, Weiss RG, Ryan DP, McGowan MA, Martin LW. Duplications of the alimentary tract. Clinical characteristics, preferred treatment, and associated malformations. Ann Surg. 1988;208(2):184–9.
7. Bentley JF, Smith JR. Developmental posterior enteric remnants and spinal malformations: the split notochord syndrome. Arch Dis Child. 1960;35:76–86.
8. Bremer JL. Diverticula and duplications o f the intestinal tract. Arch Pathol. 1952;38:132.
9. Mellish RWP, Koop CE. Clinical manifestations of the duplication of the bowel. Pediatrics. 1961;27:397.
10. Azzie G, Beasley S. Diagnosis and treatment of foregut duplications. Semin Pediatr Surg. 2003;12:46–54.
11. Langston C. New concepts in the pathology of congenital lung malformations. Semin Pediatr Surg. 2003;12:17–37.
12. Nobuhara KK, Gorski YC, La Quaglia MP, Shamberger RC. Bronchogenic cysts and esophageal duplications: common origins and treatment. J Pediatr Surg. 1997;32:1408–13.
13. McNally J, Charles AK, Spicer RD, Grier D. Mixed foregut cyst associated with esophageal atresia. Pediatr Surg. 2001;36:939–40.
14. Qi B, Beasley SW, Williams AK. Evidence of a common pathogenesis for foregut duplications and esophageal atresia ith tracheo-esophageal fistula. Anat Rec. 2001;264:3–100.
15. Smith M, Madan S, Christoph L, Set P, D'Amore A. Congenital pulmonary malformations associated with oesophageal duplication and teratoma: prenatal to postnatal management. J Pediatr Surg. 2008;43:E31–3.
16. Danzer E, Paek BW, Farmer DL, Poulain FR, Farrell JA, Harrison MR, Albanese CT. Congenital diaphragmatic hernia associated with a gastroesophageal duplication cyst: a case report. J Pediatr Surg. 2001;36:626–8.
17. Hishiki T, Ohsone Y, Tatebe S, Kawarasaki H, Mizuta K, Saito T, Terui E, Muramatsu T. A neonatal case of thoracoabdominal duplication associated with right congenital diaphragmatic hernia, absent inferior vena cava, and congenital portoazygous shunt: etiopathogenesis and surgical management. J Pediatr Surg. 2006;41:E21–4.
18. Bhat NA, Agarwala S, Wadhwa S, Gupta AK, Bhatnagar V. Thoracoabdominal intestinal duplication with absent inferior vena cava. Pediatr Surg Int. 2001;17:540–2.
19. Potter EL. Pathology of the Fetus and Newborn. Arnold Edward; 1961. Ann Surg. 1988;208:184–9.
20. Heiss K. Intestinal Duplications. In: Oldham KT, Colombani PM, Foglia RP, editors. Surgery of infants and children, scientific principles and practice. Philadelphia: Lippincot-raven; 1997.
21. Banu T, Chowdhury TK, Hogue M, Hannan MJ. Congenital double anus with total colon duplication: a case report. J Pediatr Surg. 2007;42:E1–2.
22. Siddiqui AM, Shamberger RC, Filler RM, Perez-Atayde AR, Lillehei CW. Enteric duplications of the pancreatic head: definitive management by local resection. J Pediatr Surg. 1998;33:1117–20. discussion 1120–1.
23. Khan MH, Yaqub N, Ashraf M. Complete liver duplication with right central diaphragmatic defect. J Coll Physicians Surg Pak. 2004;14:504–5.
24. Paraskevas G, Papaziogas B, Ioannidis O, Kitsoulis P, Spanidou S. Double common bile duct: a case report. Acta Chir Belg. 2009 Jul-Aug;109(4):507–9.
25. Queizán A, Hernandez F, Rivas S, Herrero F. Prenatal diagnosis of gastric triplication. Eur J Pediatr Surg. 2006;16:52–4.
26. Gisquet H, Lemelle JL, Lavrand F, Droulle P, Schmitt M. Colonic triplication associated with anorectal malformation: case presentation of a rare embryological disorder. J Pediatr Surg. 2006;41:e17–9.
27. Holcomb GW 3rd, Gheissari A, O'Neill JA Jr, Shorter NA, Bishop HC. Surgical management of alimentary tract duplications. Ann Surg. 1989;209:167–74.
28. Puligandla PS, Nguyen LT, St-Vil D, Flageole H, Bensoussan AL, Nguyen VH, Laberge JM. Gastrointestinal duplications. J Pediatr Surg. 2003;38:740–4.

29. Li L, Zhang JZ, Wang YX. Vascular classification for small intestinal duplications: experience with 80 cases. J Pediatr Surg. 1998;33:1243–5.
30. Srivastava P, Gangopadhyay AN, Kumar V, Upadhyaya VD, Sharma SP, Jaiman R, Hasan Z. Noncommunicating isolated enteric duplication cyst in childhood. J Pediatr Surg. 2009;44:e9–e10.
31. Okamoto T, Takamizawa S, Yokoi A, Satoh S, Nishijima E. Completely isolated alimentary tract duplication in a neonate. Pediatr Surg Int. 2008; 24:1145–7.
32. Iyer CP, Mahour GH. Duplications of the alimentary tract in infants and children. J Pediatr Surg. 1995;30:1267–70.
33. Kleinhaus S, Boley SJ, Winslow P. Occult bleeding from a perforated gastric duplication in an infant. Arch Surg. 1981;116:122.
34. Wardell S, Vidican DE. Ileal duplication cyst causing massive bleeding in a child. J Clin Gastroenterol. 1990;12:681–4.
35. Bower RJ, Sieber WK, Kiesewetter WB. Alimentary tract duplications in children. Ann Surg. 1978;188:669–74.
36. Martínez Ferro M, Milner R, Voto L, Zapaterio J, Cannizzaro C, Rodríguez S, Bonifacino G, Sanchez JM, Adzick NS. Intrathoracic alimentary tract duplication cysts treated in utero by thoracoamniotic shunting. Fetal Diagn Ther. 1998;13:343–7.
37. Peiper M, Lambrecht W, Kluth D, Huneke B. Bleeding esophageal duplication detected in utero. Ann Thorac Surg. 1995;60:1790–1.
38. Grosfeld JL, O'Neill JA Jr, Clatworthy HW Jr. Enteric duplications in infancy and childhood: an 18-year review. Ann Surg. 1970;172:83–90.
39. Hall NJ, Ade-Ajayi N, Peebles D, Pierro A. Antenatally diagnosed duplication cyst of the tongue: modern imaging modalities assist perinatal management. Pediatr Surg Int. 2005;21:289–91.
40. Chiu HH, Hsu WC, Shih JC, Tsao PN, Hsieh WS, Chou HC. The EXIT (ex utero intrapartum treatment) procedure. J Formos Med Assoc. 2008;107:745–8.
41. Carachi R, Azmy A. Foregut duplications. Pediatr Surg Int. 2002;18:371–4.
42. Correia-Pinto J, Tavares ML, Monteiro J, Moura N, Guimarães H, Estevão-Costa J. Prenatal diagnosis of abdominal enteric duplications. Prenat Diagn. 2000;20: 163–7.
43. Chen M, Ho WK, Hsieh TC, Lee CS, Hsiao CC, Chang SP, Lee DJ, Yang AD. Huge duplication cyst of small intestine: ultrasonographic features and prenatal aspiration. Prenat Diagn. 2006;26:86–8.
44. Rangasami R, Chandrasekharan A, Archana L, Santhosh J. Case report: Antenatal MRI diagnosis of esophageal duplication cyst. Indian J Radiol Imaging. 2009;19:75–7.
45. Hur J, Yoon CS, Kim MJ, Kim OH. Imaging features of gastrointestinal tract duplications in infants and children: from oesophagus to rectum. Pediatr Radiol. 2007;37:691–9.
46. Cheng G, Soboleski D, Daneman A, Poenaru D, Hurlbut D. Sonographic pitfalls in the diagnosis of enteric duplication cysts. AJR Am J Roentgenol. 2005;184:521–5.
47. Torgerson CL, Young DW, Vaid YN, Georgeson KE, Kelly DR. Intestinal Duplication: Imaging With Tc-99m Sodium Pertechnetate. Clin Nucl Med. 1996;21:968.
48. Kiratli PO, Aksoy T, Bozkurt MF, Orhan D. Detection of ectopic gastric mucosa using 99mTc pertechnate: review of the literature. Ann Nucl Med. 2009;23: 97–105.
49. Suhaili DN, Somasundaram S, Lau SH, Ajura AJ, Roslan AR, Ramli R. Duplication of lower lip and mandible—a rare diprosopus. Int J Pediatr Otorhinolaryngol. 2011;75:131–3. Epub 2010 Nov 9.
50. Nguyen LH, Nguyen VH, Daniel SJ, Emil S. Cervical esophageal duplication cyst: case report and review of the literature. Nayan S, J Pediatr Surg. 2010;45:e1–5.
51. Nazem M, Amouee AB, Eidy M, Khan IA, Javed HA. Duplication of cervical oesophagus: a case report and review of literatures. Afr J Paediatr Surg. 2010;7(3):203–5.
52. McCullagh M, Bhuller AS, Pierro A, Spitz L. Antenatal identification of a cervical oesophageal duplication. Pediatr Surg Int. 2000;16:204–5.
53. Cai C, Shen C, Yang W, Zhang Q, Hu X. Intraspinal neurenteric cysts in children. Can J Neurol Sci. 2008;35:609–15.
54. Stringer MD, Spitz L, Abel R, Kiely E, Drake DP, Agrawal M, Stark Y, Brereton RJ. Management of alimentary tract duplication in children. Br J Surg. 1995;82:74–8.
55. Martinez-Ferro M, Laje P, Piaggio L. Combined thoraco-laparoscopy for trans-diaphragmatic thoraco-abdominal enteric duplications. J Pediatr Surg. 2005;40:e37–40.
56. Chin AC, Radhakrishnan RS, Lloyd J, Reynolds M. Pyloric duplication with communication to the pancreas in a neonate simulating hypertrophic pyloric stenosis. J Pediatr Surg. 2011;46:1442–4.
57. Oeda S, Otsuka T, Akiyama T, Ario K, Masuda M, Taguchi S, Shono T, Kawazoe S. Recurrent acute pancreatitis caused by a gastric duplication cyst communicating with an aberrant pancreatic duct. Intern Med. 2010;49:1371–5.
58. Kaneko K, Ando H, Watanabe Y, Seo T, Harada T, Ito F. Gastric duplication communicating with the left hepatic duct: a rare case of recurrent hemobilia in a child. J Pediatr Surg. 1999;34:1539–40.
59. Chen JJ, Lee HC, Yeung CY, Chan WT, Jiang CB, Sheu JC. Meta-analysis: the clinical features of the duodenal duplication cyst. J Pediatr Surg. 2010;45:1598–606.
60. Romeo E, Torroni F, Foschia F, De Angelis P, Caldaro T, Santi MR, di Abriola GF, Caccamo R, Monti L, Dall'Oglio L. Surgery or endoscopy to treat duodenal duplications in children. J Pediatr Surg. 2011;46:874–8.

61. Tang SJ, Raman S, Reber HA, Bedford R, Roth BE. Duodenal duplication cyst. Endoscopy. 2002;34:1028–9.
62. Stephen TC, Bendon RW, Nagaraj HS, Sachdeva R. Antral duplication cyst: a cause of hypergastrinemia, recurrent peptic ulceration, and hemorrhage. J Pediatr Gastroenterol Nutr. 1998;26:216–8.
63. Seidman JD, Yale-Loehr AJ, Beaver B, Sun CC. Alimentary duplication presenting as an hepatic cyst in a neonate. Am J Surg Pathol. 1991;15:695–8.
64. Paraskevas G, Papaziogas B, Ioannidis O, Kitsoulis P, Spanidou S. Double common bile duct: a case report. Acta Chir Belg. 2009;109:507–9.
65. Bender EA, Springhetti S, Shemisa K, Wittenauer J. Left-sided gallbladder (sinistroposition) with duplication of the common bile duct. JSLS. 2007;11:148–50.
66. Kothari PR, Kumar T, Jiwane A, Paul S, Kutumbale R, Kulkarni B. Unusual features of gall bladder duplication cyst with review of the literature. Pediatr Surg Int. 2005;21:552–4. Epub 2005 May 12.
67. Laje P, Flake AW, Adzick NS. Prenatal diagnosis and postnatal resection of intraabdominal enteric duplications. J Pediatr Surg. 2010;45:1554–8.
68. Bianchi A. Intestinal loop lengthening—a technique for increasing small intestinal length. J Pediatr Surg. 1980;15:145–51.
69. Macpherson RI. Gastrointestinal tract duplications: clinical, pathologic, etiologic, and radiologic considerations. Radiographics. 1993;13:1063–80.
70. Rajah S, Ramanujam TM, Anas SR, Jayaram G, Baskaran P, Ganesan J, Tin M. Duplication of the rectum: report of four cases and review of the literature. Pediatr Surg Int. 1998;13:373–6.
71. La Quaglia MP, Feins N, Eraklis A, Hendren WH. Rectal duplications. J Pediatr Surg. 1990;25:980–4.
72. Koga H, Okazaki T, Kato Y, Lane GJ, Yamataka A. Anal canal duplication: experience at a single institution and literature review. Pediatr Surg Int. 2010;26:985–8.
73. Jacquier C, Dobremez E, Piolat C, Dyon JF, Nugues F. Anal canal duplication in infants and children—a series of 6 cases. Eur J Pediatr Surg. 2001;11:186–91.
74. Lisi G, Illiceto MT, Rossi C, Broto JM, Jil-Vernet JM, Lelli CP. Anal canal duplication: a retrospective analysis of 12 cases from two European pediatric surgical departments. Pediatr Surg Int. 2006;22:967–73.
75. Hwang IK, Namkung S, Kim BS, Kim HC, Lee IS, Hwang WC. Perforated ileal duplication cyst with haemorrhagic pseudocyst formation. Pediatr Radiol. 2003;33:489–91. Epub 2003 Apr 24.
76. Jancelewicz T, Simko J, Lee H. Obstructing ileal duplication cyst infected with Salmonella in a 2-year-old boy: a case report and review of the literature. J Pediatr Surg. 2007;42:E19–21.
77. Trojan J, Mousset S, Caspary WF, Hoepffner N. An infected esophageal duplication cyst in a patient with non-Hodgkin's lymphoma mimicking persistent disease. Dis Esophagus. 2005;18:287–9.
78. Kim TH, Kim JK, Jang EH, Lee JH, Kim YB. Papillary adenocarcinoma arising in a tubular duplication of the jejunum. Br J Radiol. 2010;83:e61–4.
79. Kusunoki N, Shimada Y, Fukumoto S, Iwatani Y, Ohshima T, Arahi E, Miyazaki N, Maeda S. Adenocarcinoma arising in a tubular duplication of the jejunum. J Gastroenterol. 2003;38:781–5.
80. Michael D, Cohen CR, Northover JM. Adenocarcinoma within a rectal duplication cyst: case report and literature review. Ann R Coll Surg Engl. 1999;81:205–6.

Meconium Ileus

35

Andrea Conforti and Pietro Bagolan

*"Woe is the child who tastes salty from a kiss on the brow,
for he is cursed, and soon must die,"*

17th Century German Children's Song

Abstract

Baron Carl von Rokitansky in late nineteenth century observed "a case of foetal death due to meconium peritonitis", while Landstainer firstly described meconium ileus (MI) in 1905, when thickened meconium was noted in a newborn with pathologic changes of the pancreas (Landsteiner, Zentralbl Allg Pathol 16:903–907, 1905). An unknown enzyme deficiency was supposed to cause both fibrotic changes of the pancreas and meconium inspissation. In 1936, the term cystic fibrosis of the pancreas (CF) was coined by Fanconi to describe the association between chronic pulmonary disease and pancreatic insufficiency (Zigler, Curr Probl Surg 31:441–444, 1994). Nonetheless, it was only two years later that Anderson described the connection between MI and CF reporting similar pattern of hystologic pancreatic abnormalities in both CF and MI newborns, suggesting a causative link between CF, abnormal intestinal mucus secretion and the abnormally viscid nature of meconium in MI infants (Anderson, Am J Dis Child 56:344–399, 1938). However, it was only in 1996 when Rozmahel et al. firstly reported a modifier locus for MI on chromosome 7 in a murine CF model (cfm1) (Rozmahel et al., Nat Genet. 12:280–287, 1996).

Keywords

Meconium ileus • Newborn intestinal obstruction • Gastrograffin enema
Cystic fibrosis • Surgery • Stoma

35.1 History

Baron Carl von Rokitansky in late nineteenth century observed "a case of foetal death due to meconium peritonitis", while Landstainer firstly described meconium ileus (MI) in 1905, when thickened meconium was noted in a newborn with pathologic changes of the pancreas

A. Conforti, MD • P. Bagolan, MD (✉)
Department of Medical and Surgical Neonatology,
Bambino Gesù Children's Research Hospital,
4, P.zza S.Onofrio, 00165 Rome, Italy
e-mail: pietro.bagolan@opbg.net

P.D. Losty et al. (eds.), *Rickham's Neonatal Surgery*, https://doi.org/10.1007/978-1-4471-4721-3_35

[1]. An unknown enzyme deficiency was supposed to cause both fibrotic changes of the pancreas and meconium inspissation. In 1936, the term cystic fibrosis of the pancreas (CF) was coined by Fanconi to describe the association between chronic pulmonary disease and pancreatic insufficiency [2]. Nonetheless, it was only two years later that Anderson described the connection between MI and CF reporting similar pattern of hystologic pancreatic abnormalities in both CF and MI newborns, suggesting a causative link between CF, abnormal intestinal mucus secretion and the abnormally viscid nature of meconium in MI infants [3] (Fig. 35.1). However, it was only in 1996 when Rozmahel et al. firstly reported a modifier locus for MI on chromosome 7 in a murine CF model (cfm1) [4]

In 1941, Rasor and Stevenson first described mechanical intestinal obstruction due to inspissated stool in patients beyond neonatal period [5]. This condition, known as meconium ileus equivalent, as well as MI was invariably lethal up to late '40s, when Hyatt and Wilson reported the first series of five consecutive patients survived, treated with enemas though enterotomies [6].

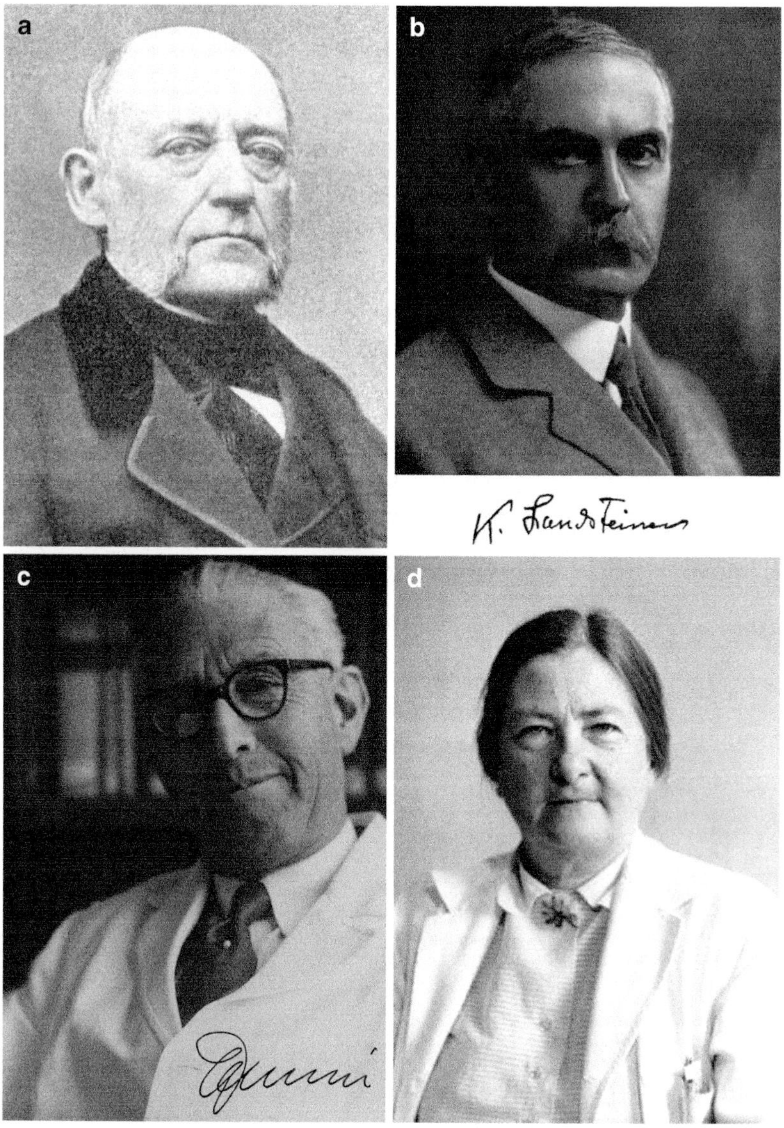

Fig. 35.1 (**a**) Baron Carl von Rokitansky; (**b**) Karl Landstainer; (**c**) Guido Fanconi; (**d**) Dorothy Hansine Anderson

About 20 years later, in 1969 Noblett introduces a novel therapy applying hyperosmolar diatrizoate enema (Gastrografin ®) in uncomplicated patients [7]. Since the introduction of non-operative management of MI, the first-line approach was progressively shifted from surgery to intervention radiology. During mid 70', neonatal screening for CF was gradually introduced and became common practice [8].

Actually survival rate of MI newborns is approaching 100% in developed countries, depending mostly on management of CF complications.

35.2 Definition and Classification

Meconium ileus (MI) is defined as a foetal/neonatal intestinal obstruction caused by ispissated meconium at the level of the terminal ileum. It can be classified into two categories: *uncomplicated* (or simple) and *complicated (or complex)* [9]. Later in life presentation is usually referred as meconium ileus equivalent or distal ileal obstruction syndrome (DIOS).

Uncomplicated meconium ileus should be diagnosed prenatally (hyperechoic bowel, bowel loop dilatation), however it is usually recognized after birth in term newborn admitted for distal small bowel obstruction causing abdominal distension. Classically, vomiting (bilious) and failure to stool highlights abdominal obstruction. Characteristic inspissated meconium is found at surgery. Prenatal suspicious should arise in case of confirmatory genetic findings or suggestive intestinal dilatation associated with echogenic bowel. Nonetheless latter sign have poor prognostic value due to its a-specificity [10].

Conversely, *complicated meconium ileus* has high prenatal detection rate due to the evidence of complications (intestinal perforation and/or necrosis, ascites, volvulus) discovered during in utero evaluations. Calcifications are frequently presented and may be found either prenatally (as hyper-echogenic spots or loop dilatation or foetal ascites) or postnatally at abdominal plain x-rays. Signs of peritonitis (including erythematous and edematous abdominal skin) should be present.

35.3 Epidemiology

The meconium syndromes occur primarily in Caucasians and in the past they were considered closely linked to cystic fibrosis (CF), one of the most common serious genetic diseases in whites, given that 80–90% of new-borns with meconium ileus (MI) were believed to have CF [11]. This opinion has changed since it was observed that more than 20% up to 40% of the population with MI are not affected by CF [12, 13]. The pathogenesis of MI in the absence of CF is not yet clear, even though it is assumed that both the immaturity of the myenteric plexus and the interstitial cells of Cajal may predispose to MI as it has been recently reported [14, 15]. However MI and CF remain closely linked in most of the patients.

Cystic fibrosis is transmitted as autosomal recessive disease, thus both parents must be heterozygotes for the gene and each offspring has one in four chance of developing the disease. The highest heterozygote frequency is reported in whites (1/29 births) while it is much less common in non-Caucasian population (1/17.000 births in blacks and 1/90.000 births in Asians). As a consequence the incidence of homozygous condition (just CF) in whites is 1/1150 to 2500 live birth [16, 17].

MI is the first clinical manifestation of CF in 10–20% of affected infants. In families with a first child affected by CF with MI the risk rate of a subsequent child with the identical clinical presentation of CF and MI is 30% compared with 6% in families in which the first child with CF did not have MI [18]. The number of males and females affected is similar. It has been estimated that number of cases with CF is constantly rising, from 3500 at the end of 1980s to more than 7000 by the millennium [19].

35.4 Etiology and Pathophysiology

Two pathogenetic events appear to begin in utero and result in an intraluminal accumulation of highly viscid and tenacious meconium: (1) the pancreatic exocrine enzyme deficiency; (2) the secretion of hyperviscous mucus by pathologically abnormal intestinal glands.

Other common manifestations of cystic fibrosis (CF) include azospermia in nearly all patients, pancreatic insufficiency in 90%, diabetes mellitus in 20%, obstructive biliary disease in 15–20%, and meconium ileus in 10–20%. Abnormally thick and viscous mucus secretions are responsible for bowel, pancreatic duct and airways in the lung obstructions. Exocrine glands throughout the body are affected by an abnormal function of chloride transport. Pathologic data suggest that the intestinal glandular disease plays a primary role in the pathogenesis of MI associated with CF while pancreatic disease plays a secondary one [16]. Two main explanations of secretion changes have been proposed: A) the hyper-permeability to water loss of an already viscid secreted mucus, thus further concentrating secretions; B) the impairment of fluid movement to and from the extravascular space, preventing the normal dilution of material of the cellular lumen that becomes toxic to those cells laden with the product [20]. The analysis of meconium in infants affected by CF shows a low water, minerals (sodium potassium and magnesium are almost the half in concentration when compared with meconium of controls), protein-bound carbohydrate and trypsin content. On the other hand samples of meconium from patients with CF show a greater amount of albumin, mucoproteins and calcium. The meconium hyperviscosity is probably due to the increased concentration of proteins (neonates with MI and CF have a protein content of 80–90%, compared with 7% in normal infants) [21] and to the simultaneous decreased concentration of carbohydrates [22].

The mutated gene of CF that encodes for the cell membrane protein, termed the Cystic Fibrosis Transmembrane Regulator (CFTR) was identified in 1989 by F. Collins [23] and more than 1000 different CF mutations have been identified until now. The locus was located on the long arm of chromosome 7, band q31 [24]. The most common mutation (ΔF508) is responsible for approximately 70% of clinical cases. It acts through the CFTR protein degradation in the endoplasmic reticulum prior to folding and trafficking. Functionally the gene encodes a protein that is primarily responsible for regulating the opening and closing of chloride channels. The defect affects all epithelial-lined structures. The mutation of the CFTR leads to an abnormal chloride transport in the apical membrane of epithelial cells (preventing excretion) and sodium (up-regulating the absorption). The biological normal function of CFTR differs according to its tissue location: in its location on the apical membrane of epithelial cells of sweat glands it is responsible for reabsorption of chloride and sodium, thus its deficient function lead to an abnormally high content of both electrolytes in the sweat of affected infants (Fig. 35.2). Similarly, there are

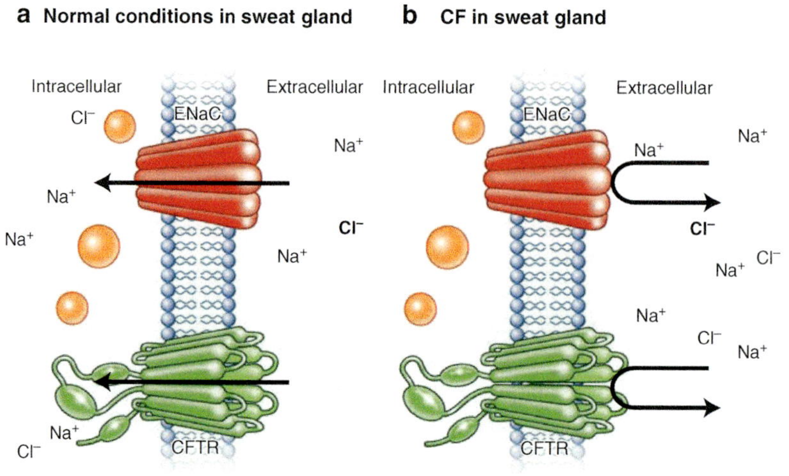

Fig. 35.2 (**a**) Normal CFTR channels in the sweat gland: CFTR channels transport chloride in epithelial tissue to maintain salt and fluid balance. (**b**) CFTR dysfunction leads to pronounced abnormalities in the sodium chloride homeostasis (loss of chloride ion reabsorption). the result is a higher concentration of chloride in the sweat test

also alterations of the water and electrolyte component of the mucociliary clearance mechanism in the respiratory tract resulting in an increasingly viscous mucous [19]. The precise manner in which the deficient chloride (and sodium) transport leads to the manifestations of CF is not well known. All tubular structures lined by the affected epithelia (respiratory, gastrointestinal, biliary, pancreatic and reproductive system) will be characterized by desiccation and reduced clearance of their secretion. Patients who are homozygotes for this mutation typically develop pancreatic insufficiency but may have variable pulmonary disease.

The occurrence of MI in patients with CF is clearly influenced by genetic factors as it was reported in a large twin study that showed a greater concordance for MI in monozygous twins compared with dizygous ones [25]. The variation might be explained by the CFTR genotype. In fact the homozygosity for most common CFTR mutation (ΔF508) in infants with CF is strongly associated with MI [19]. Nevertheless also non-CFTR genes (so called "modifier genes") may influence the risk for developing MI. In 1996 Rozmahel et al. [4] firstly reported a modifier locus for MI on chromosome 7 in a murine CF model (cfm1). Subsequently several markers on human chromosome 19 (the region syntenic to the mouse locus) showed significant linkage with the presence of MI in 185 sibling pairs [26]. Recently Van der Doef et al. reported an association between a variant in the CLCA1 gene and meconium ileus in European CF patients [27]. The causal role between human modifier genes CFM1, CLCA1 and others recently provided as new candidates, such as ADIPOR2 and SLC4A4 [28], and MI has yet to be discovered.

Because the small intestinal mucus glands produce thick secretion even in utero, the meconium is abnormally viscid, sticky and adherent. Typically in new-born babies affected by MI, the proximal ileum is greatly dilated and contains this abnormal meconium, the distal ileum is obstructed by thickly packed, round, mucus plug that resemble a rosary crown. Colon is collapsed and small because not used ("ex non usu"). Infants born with this clinical form have the so-called "simple" MI. However it may progress, even in utero, toward a "complicated" MI. In these cases the massively dilated proximal bowel may volvulize and/or perforate. When this happens early in gestation, one or more intestinal atresia may be produced while infants may present either free or encysted meconium peritonitis when perforation arrives late in gestation. Each of these presentations has different clinical and radiological manifestations and needs specific therapeutic considerations.

No much is known neither about the differences of MI in newborns with and without CF, nor about the specific genetic basis of MI in patients affected by CF [13]. Patients with MI and CF generally have mild pancreatic involvement and more severe intestinal glandular disease. In contrast those with CF without MI have a pattern of progressive pancreatic involvement with age. At birth, the lungs are normal in CF patients. However progressive and diffuse pulmonary disease develops as a result of mucus plugging of the small airways and secondary infections. The sweat sodium and chloride levels are elevated from birth in patients with CF but unrelated to the severity or distribution of organ involvement [29]. Different clinical characteristics have been recently reported in patients affected by MI without and with CF. Complex meconium ileus (including meconium peritonitis), prematurity and low birth weight are more frequently associated with MI without CF and this also implies that in preterm infants, especially presenting with complex MI, counselling of the parents in the first days of life should take into account the relatively low risk that their child is affected by CF [13].

35.5 Diagnosis

35.5.1 Prenatal Detection

Complicated MI is usually detected during pregnancy: ultrasonographic evaluations may reveal dilated hyperechoic bowel loops, abdominal calcifications possibly associated with ascites [30]. In some cases signs of meconium periorchitis (rare disorder caused by foetal meconium peritonitis with subsequent spillage of meconium into the scrotal sac) may be detected [31]. Nonetheless, complicated MI represents a minority of cases.

More frequently during routinely performed second trimester ultrasonographic examination, the presence of hyperechogenic foetal bowel loops associated or not with bowel dilatation and/or polyhydramnios, and or giant pseudocysts may raise suspicion of MI (Fig. 35.3). Hyperechogenic bowel is a relatively common event (detected in 0.04—1.80% of fetuses) and it is not pathologic in itself, however it may be an indicator of different disorders (hypothyroidism, chromosome abnormalities, infections, gastrointestinal disorders, foetal growth restriction, intra-amniotic bleeding, etc.) [32, 33]. Familial history of CF (reported in up to 33% of patients with MI), coupled with in utero amniocentesis with restriction fragment length polymorphism analysis and prenatal sonographic findings, allow accurate prediction of intestinal obstruction due to MI and CF [34]. Different algorithm have been reported as the one showed in Fig. 35.4. It is well established that all types of intestinal obstructions, included all types of intestinal atresia, should be associated to CF with various frequencies [35]. In all cases of supposed intestinal obstruction (especially if MI is suspected) during foetal life, parental genetic screenings as well as amniocentesis are warranted [35].

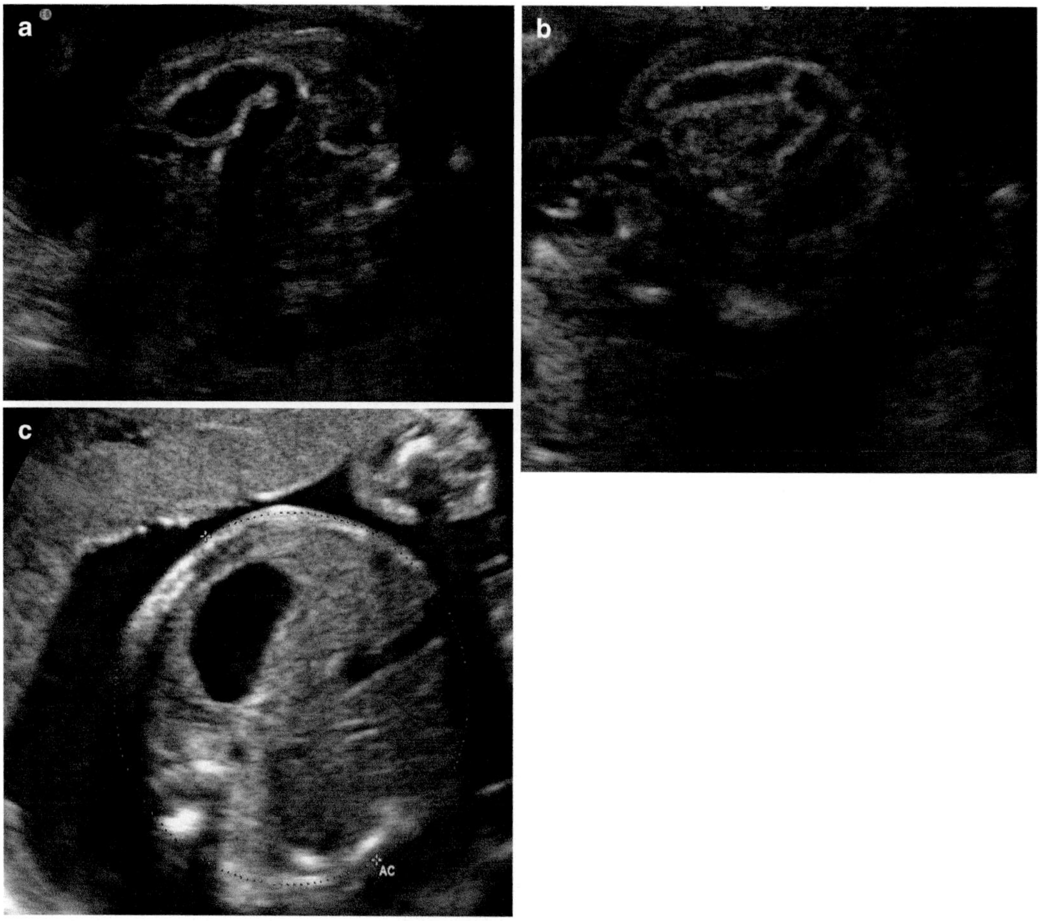

Fig. 35.3 (**a**) Intestinal hyperechogenicity; (**b**) Diffuse hyperechogenicity; (**c**) Prenatal pseudocyst

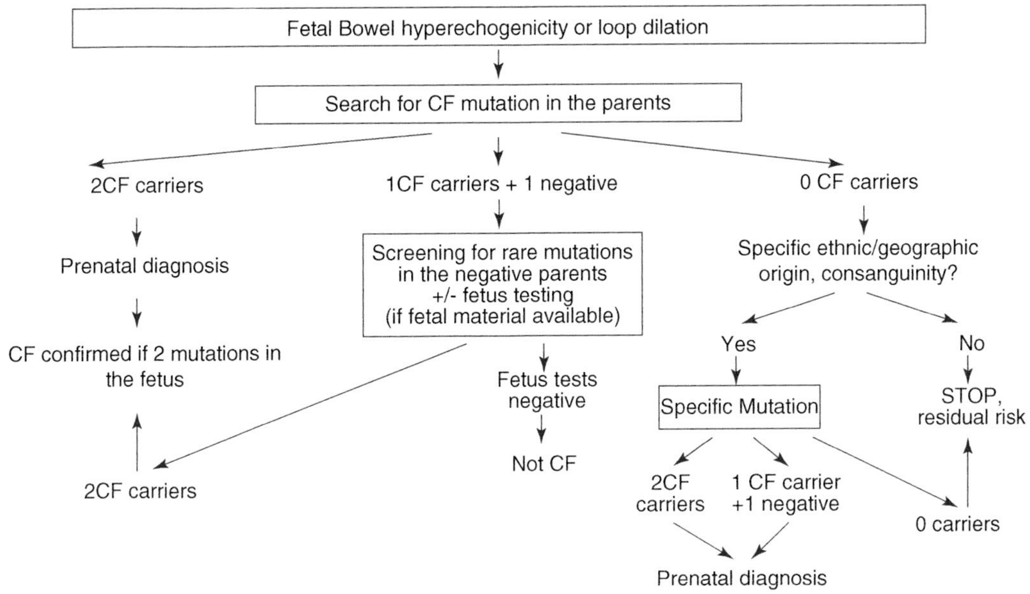

Fig. 35.4 Diagnostic testing in fetal bowel hyperechogenicity or loop dilatation. Modified from: Dequeker E, Stuhrmann M, Morris MA et al.: Best practice guidelines for molecular genetic diagnosis of cystic fibrosis and CFTR-related disorders – updated European recommendations. Eur J Hum Gen 2009; 17: 51–65.

35.5.2 Postnatal Presentation

Newborn affected by MI frequently present abdominal distension at birth before air swallows. Failure to pass meconium usually leads to progressive small bowel over-distension and bilious vomiting. Visible peristaltic waves are often present as well as palpable, thick, malleable bowel loops. Classical clinical sign report on the "putty sign" when finger pressure over a firm loop of bowel conduct to intestine indentation. No signs of peritoneal irritation are present at birth in case of uncomplicated MI. Rectal examination is usually unremarkable and classically no meconium is expelled on withdrawal of the examining finger/rectal tube.

In case of complicated MI, prenatal bowel perforation lead to abdominal pseudocyst arrangement. Classically, intestinal occlusion develops due to the pseudocyst creation, with bile stained gastric fluid, bile or faecal vomiting, abdominal distension, and impossibility of meconium passage. A palpable abdominal swelling is usually present on clinical examination at birth, as well as signs of peritoneal irritation (not mandatory) and skin discoloration. Hypovolemic shock and sepsis may rapidly rise, and clinical and radiological signs (free abdominal air, air-fluid levels within the pseudocyst or in the bowel loops) of intestinal perforation can be detected.

Less frequently, when prenatal intestinal perforation spontaneously heals, intestinal continuity could be re-established and no intestinal occlusion is detected at birth. In those cases the only findings is the presence of calcification on abdominal X-rays or US.

35.5.3 Imaging

Radiological findings in case of uncomplicated MI demonstrate typical abdominal obstruction, with air-fluid levels. Singleton's (granular "soap bubble") and/or Neuhauser's (ground-glass appearance) signs should be frequently detected in the right lower abdominal quadrant. Nonetheless, those features are not exclusively diagnostic for MI, even if collectively they strongly suggest it [35, 36] (Fig. 35.5a). A confirmative study is the contrast enema with water-soluble contrast agent

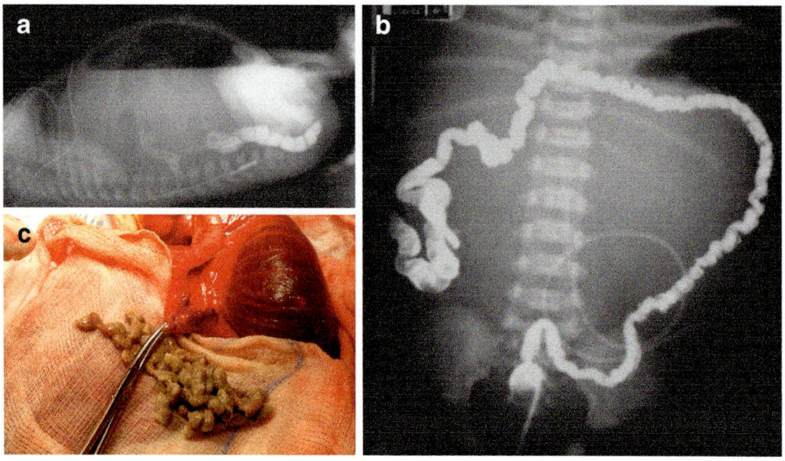

Fig. 35.5 (**a**) Plain abdominal X-ray: note the appearance of abdominal obstruction, with diffuse air-fluid levels; (**b**) Contrast enema with water-soluble contrast agent: normally positioned colon characterized by small calibre (microcolon); (**c**) Meconium pellets

whether hyper or iso-osmolar (to prevent mucosal damage). Contrast enema (Fig. 35.5b) will reveal a normally positioned colon characterized by small calibre, the so-called "microcolon" or "unused" colon. It may be empty or it may contain pellets of thickened meconium. If contrast enema refluxes through ileo-cecal valve, meconium pellets should be observed in the terminal ileum. Furthermore, refluxes of contrast enema in the more proximal ileum may reveal a transition zone to dilated proximal loops. The passage of contrast into the terminal ileum may results in pellets evacuation (Fig. 35.5c), with complete or partial resolution of intestinal obstruction. Contrast studies have to be followed under fluoroscopy to prevent possible unexpected colonic perforation [34, 37].

Frequently, contrast fails to reflux to terminal ileum neither confirming the diagnosis of MI nor excluding the level of the occlusion. Therefore, surgical intervention is required for therapeutic and diagnostic purposes.

35.5.4 Laboratory Test

Even when strong suspicion of MI may raise from clinical history, physical examination as well as imaging, definitive diagnosis of CF should be obtained only with the sweat test. Sweat is collected from infant's skin and pilocarpine ionophoresis is applied to quantify chloride and sodium. The accuracy of sweat test is strictly linked to the minimum amount of sweat to be collected (100 mg) and therefore it is commonly believed that it is really significant in newborn-infants weighted 3.0, 3.5 Kg or more A measured concentration of sweat chloride more than 60 mEq/L is diagnostic for CF. The discovery of CFTR confirmed the role of electrolyte transport in the etiology of CF and gave a molecular rationale to the sweat test for diagnosing CF. Although the ability to test for CFTR gene mutations gives a new dimension to diagnosing CF, the sweat chloride test remains the standard procedure to confirm a CF diagnosis [38, 39]. Despite the potential usefulness of the information, acquiring a CF genotype can be difficult. Although currently available mutation screening panels can identify 90% of CFTR mutations, 9.7% of genotyped individuals in the Cystic Fibrosis Foundation Patient Registry have at least 1 un-identified mutation. Furthermore, the consequences of the vast majority of CFTR mutations remain unknown, even if the genotype is identified [39].

Historically, a number of tests have been developed to support the diagnosis of MI in CF patients: an increase albumin level (>20 mg/g) in faecal specimen as well as a decrease in trypsin concentration (<80 mg/g) were reported to be a good indicator for MI [34]. Nonetheless, due to the low specificity and sensitivity of those tests, all current protocols rely on immunoreactive trypsin (IRT) test as the primary screening test and on sweat test for confirming or excluding the diagnosis of CF. [39] The elevation of immunoreactive trypsin (IRT) in the blood of neonates with CF and its measurement in dried blood spots was first described in 1979, [40, 41]. Since then it gradually became the gold standard first-line screening for diagnosis of CF.

35.6 Differential Diagnosis

MI should be the earliest manifestation of CF, with a frequency reported as high as 10–20% of neonatal cases affected by CF. MI is reported to account for 10–25% of all cases of neonatal intestinal obstruction [34, 35]. As a result, major causes of differential diagnosis reside within the multiplicity of conditions resulting in neonatal intestinal obstruction. The foremost conditions to be investigated and excluded are: intestinal atresia, midgut volvulus, Hirschsprung disease, meconium plug syndrome, neonatal small left colon, hypothyroidism and prematurity.

35.6.1 Intestinal Atresia

Intestinal atresia is usually associated with upper abdominal distension. Characteristically, newborns affected by upper jejunal atresia present bilious vomiting, increasing abdominal distension, failure to pass meconium. A plain abdominal x-ray may reveal thumb-sized intestinal loops ("rule of thumb") and air-fluid levels. The site of the atresia frequently appears as a larger loop with significant air-fluid level, with no air beyond that point.

Proximal jejunal atresia may be associated with upper abdominal distension, while a more generalized distension usually denotes a distal bowel obstruction. Severe enlargement of intestinal loops may lead to respiratory distress as a result of diaphragmatic elevation. At physical examination visible veins and intestinal patterning, characterized by visible bowel loops can be present.

Definitive diagnosis may require laparotomy.

35.6.2 Midgut Volvulus

Acute midgut volvulus represents the classical neonatal surgical emergency, with sudden onset of bilious vomiting in a previously healthy infant. Infants with complete obstruction rapidly develop intestinal ischemia with a firm distended abdomen, hypovolemia and shock.

Prenatal volvulus may lead to intestinal atresia, associated with MI, presenting as complicated MI. Prenatal US reveal intestinal distension associated with calcification secondary to complicated MI, while postnatal radiological findings include sign of intestinal occlusion associated or not with signs of meconium peritonitis [42, 43].

35.6.3 Hirschsprung Disease

HD should be considered in any child who has a history of constipation. Classically, patients affected by HD have a history of delayed passage of meconium within the first 48 h of life. Physical examination often demonstrates abdominal distension that was absent at birth. Rectal examination of newborn infant with HD reveals a tight anus that may be incorrectly diagnosed as anal stenosis. Rectal examination usually leads to emission of gas and faecal matter under pressure. Contrast enema should be useful to detect the classical transition zone (passage from a narrow, spastic intestinal segment to a dilated proximal segment), while rectal biopsies allow definitive diagnosis [42, 43]. Exclusion of ano-rectal malformations (mainly low-lying imperforate anus) is a cornerstone of differential diagnosis of constipation.

35.6.4 Meconium Plug Syndrome and Neonatal Small Left Colon

Meconium plug syndrome (MPS) and neonatal small left colon syndrome (SLCS) are diagnoses to be excluded. MPS was firstly described in 1956 as a distinct condition characterized by transient large bowel obstruction relieved by the passage of meconium plugs. Conversely, SLCS was firstly described in 1974 as a neonatal obstructive condition reported in infants of diabetic mothers in whom contrast enema showed a narrow left colon. Recent reports are less prone to consider those as specific diagnoses, due to the high incidence of overlapping between MPS and SLCS and others well-defined diseases (e.g. Hirschsprung's disease and Cystic Fibrosis) that impose discrimination [44, 45].

35.6.5 Hypothyroidism

Hypothyroidism is not a surgical challenge, however it may became evident during neonatal period as a delayed passage of meconium beyond 24–48 h of life, with subsequent sub-occlusive characteristics. Dosage of thyroid hormones allows a correct diagnosis and substitutive therapy.

35.6.6 Prematurity

Functional gastrointestinal dysmotility is a common condition that affects premature infants. Delay in achievement of full enteral nutrition results in dependence on prolonged parenteral nutrition, predisposing to adverse outcomes. Intestinal immaturity is believed to be responsible for this condition, which may require surgical intervention to treat possible complications such as necrotising enterocolitis and spontaneous perforations. Even if no definitive data are available, intestinal dismotility in preterm babies should be related to some degree of depletion of interstitial cells of Cajal [46].

35.7 Treatment

Even though there are many operative considerations in CF such as jejunoileal atresia, intussusceptions, fibrosing colonopathy, inguinal hernias, bronchiectasis, pneumothorax, hepatobiliary and pancreatic disease and rectal prolapse, none are associated so intimately with CF as MI [47]. MI was considered pathognomonic for CF of which is the first clinical manifestation and it is also now recognised that patients with MI (and with CF) probably represent a different phenotype with earlier presentation and worse pulmonary function [48, 49]. However MI has been described also in association with rare conditions such as pancreatic aplasia and total colonic aganglionosis [50]. As previously said, in neonates with MI meconium is extremely viscid and sticky causing multiple intraluminal plugs leading to a complete obstruction of the terminal ileum. Approximately half of these newborn babies are affected by a simple uncomplicated obstruction while the remaining present typical complications of MI including volvulus, gangrene, atresia, perforation which may result in giant cystic meconium peritonitis. Therefore management of MI is greatly different depending on the presence of a simple (uncomplicated) or a complex (complicated) clinical presentation.

35.7.1 Nonoperative Management (Simple MI)

Hypertonic enema washout has become the initial non-surgical procedure for diagnosis and treatment of infants with uncomplicated MI and it is nowadays considered the procedure of choice for solubilising and washing out obstructing plugs of meconium in those selected cases [51]. As a consequence the surgeon has to examine always the patient to define the real indications and rule out possible contraindications to enema. In her original paper Noblett reported the main rules for the successful use of non operative management of MI: (1) rule out other types of neonatal intestinal obstruction (by a preliminary enema); (2) exclude cases with complicated MI; (3) attend as a neonatal surgeon to the procedure; (4) always perform the technique under fluoroscopic control; (5) give fluids to the baby (one to three times maintenance) and administer prophylactic antibiotic therapy; (6) be, the patient and surgeon, prepared for possible emergent operation should complications arrive [7].

The contrast material used must be water soluble to loosen the inspissated pellets of meconium and to be safer than barium in case a perforation occurs during the study. These enemas break up the plug by two mechanisms: (1) on the contact, the enema acts as a direct solvent; (2) the greater osmolality of the agent results in the shift of fluid into the bowel lumen, which hydrates and softens the inspissated meconium. Preliminary management includes naso-gastric decompressive tube and intravenous fluids to replace pre-existing deficits or ongoing losses (because of the hyperosmotic nature of the enema). Broad spectrum antibiotics should be administered and blood culture obtained to rule out sepsis. The most frequently used agent is Gastrografin®. Thanks to its hyperosmolar (meglumine diatrizoate 1900 mOsm per L), and emulsifying (0.1% polysorbate 80) properties, Gastrografin® is able to draw liquid into the intestinal lumen inducing an osmotic diarrhoea (and a putative osmotic dieresis) until the contrast is passed. Many radiologists today are used to dilute the gastrografin to 25–50% or to increasingly use new dilute contrast agents to reduce serious fluid derangements and potential complications (hypovolemic shock, colonic mucosal and submucosal inflammation, intestinal perforation and ischemic enterocolitis). Perforations secondary to contrast enema has been reported to occur from 2.7% more recently to 23% of patients in the past [52]. Nonetheless in recent experimental studies, Gastrografin® resulted the most efficacious agent for the in vivo relief of obstruction and for reducing viscosity without intestinal mucosal damage [53]. A comparative study also found a significantly increased rate of success when using Gastrografin® compared to other agents [38]. Risks can be minimized if care is taken to avoid overdistension of the bowel, such as with the use of fluoroscopy for administration.

Thus the solution (50% Gastrografin®) is gently infused under fluoroscopic observation through an enema-tip non-balloon catheter (the buttocks taped together around the catheter) into the rectum, the microcolon, till the terminal ileum. The injudicious non use of both fluoroscopic control or non-balloon catheter have been reported as potentially responsible for bowel injury leading to intestinal perforation [20]. When the contrast medium reaches the dilated meconium-impacted ileum, the study is terminated. An abdominal radiograph should be repeated in 8–12 h to rule out perforations and determine whether the obstruction has been relieved. When the evacuation is obtained but obstructions persists, more than one contrast hyperosmolar enemas may be performed with the same method [7] provided that the patient does not show any signs of deterioration or complications [29]. N-acetylcysteine has also a role in non-operative management of MI even though, because of its delay in effectiveness, it is not recommended as a first line therapy [53]. Warm saline enemas containing 1% N-acetylcysteine can be administered to facilitate complete evacuation upon returning to the neonatal unit. Moreover N-acetylcysteine (5–10 mL of 5%–10%) can be administered per nasogastric tube every 6 h to clearing meconium from above [54]. Heart rate, systemic blood pressure and urine output have to be carefully observed before, during and after the procedure. Usually, passage of meconium pellets followed by semiliquid meconium occurs within the first 12 h. About 30% up to 50% of patients with simple MI may be managed this way, but the success varies widely in reported series. Recent report [52] show that early studies treating MI with Gastrografin reported higher success rate (63–83%) [55] when compared with more recent studies [56] despite the same enema agent has been used. The explanations for the discrepancies may be possibly two: the more cautious approach of radiologists to these patients resulting in a low complication rate that is inversely related to a high failure rate and the use of different and less osmotically active than Gastrografin contrast agents. When either non evacuation occurs after a successfully refluxing enema or the contrast agent cannot be refluxed in the dilated ileum, the non operative technique should be abandoned and operative intervention planned [20].

35.7.2 Operative Management 1 (Unresponsive to Medical Treatment)

Infants that can't be successfully managed by hyperosmolar contrast enema require operative management. Nearly one half to two thirds of infants need operative management of their MI intestinal occlusion due either to a failed non-operative management with MI or to the presence of complications (intestinal atresia, volvulus with or without gangrene, perforation, giant meconium cysts formation, or a combination of these) (Fig. 35.6) [57]. The aims of operation are: (1) the complete relief of the meconium impaction (unsuccessful non-operative manage-

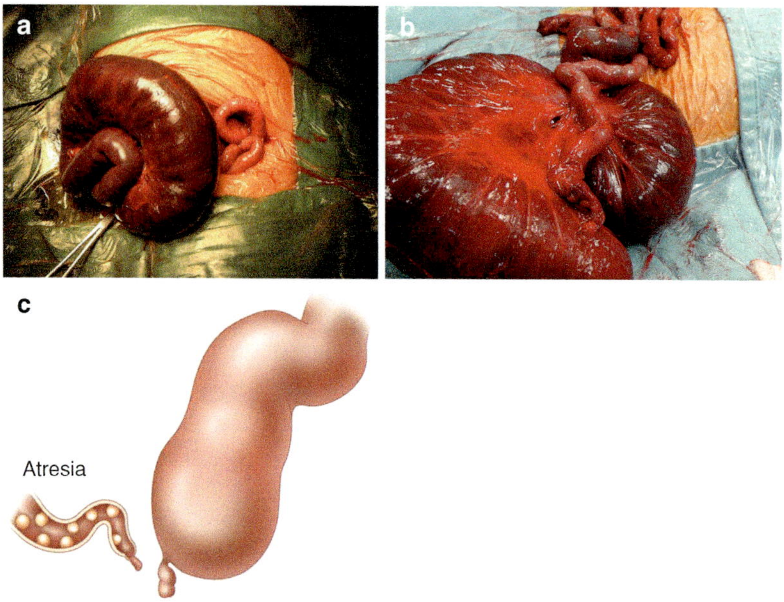

Fig. 35.6 Intestinal Atresia: intraoperative findings (**a**, **b**) and explicative diagram (**c**). Ileal atesia is usually suggested by a distal bowel obstruction pattern on plain radiograph with associated presence of air-fluid levels. Meconium ileus can be associated with ileal atresia, and at operation, the findings of sticky meconium should raise suspicions

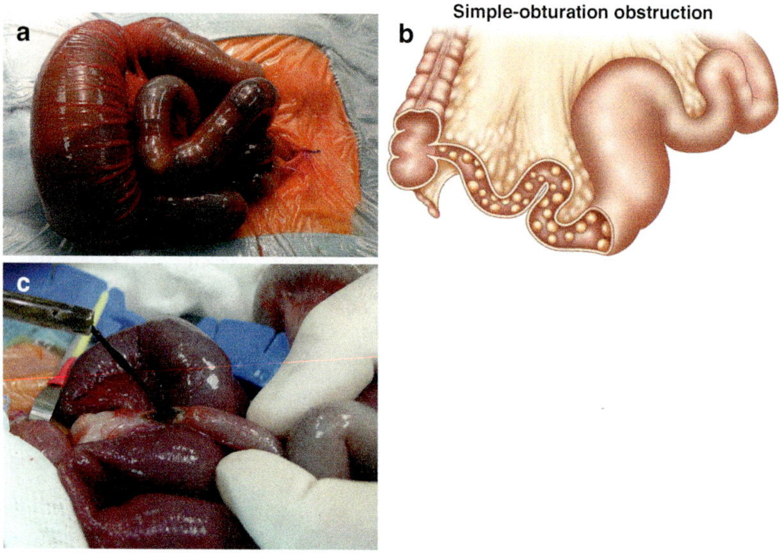

Fig. 35.7 Uncomplicated Meconium Ileus. (**a**) Characteristic meconium pearls at surgery; (**b**) Explicative drawing: distended terminal ileus, inspissated meconium forming meconium pearls and the typical unused microcolon; (**c**) Sticky meconium at surgery

ment); (2) The removal of the specific surgical complication (patients with complicated MI); (3) The complete restoration of bowel continuity when possible.

Several operative procedure have been proposed to surgically remove impacted meconium: enterotomy and irrigation, limited resection with irrigation, different types of obstruction-relieving stoma with or without partial resection; tube enterostomy; tube decompressive stoma plus irrigating tube, primary resection and anastomosis. Intraoperative irrigation of impacted meconium is always required, so enterotomy and intraoperative irrigation for mechanical separation of the pellets from the bowel wall and evacuation of the meconium is the recommended technique currently (Fig. 35.7). Several irrigating solution can be used such as warmed saline, 50% (or more) diatrizoate solution, 2–4% N-acetylcysteine (the most commonly used) [58]. The irrigating agent is introduced through a minimal enterotomy and the meconium, once solubilised, is gently milked distally (into the colon) or evacuated proximally (through the enterostomy).

A tube (simple or "T" shaped) enterostomy can be created soon after terminal ileum has been disimpacted. Leaving this tube in place, generally located at the junction of the proximal dilated ileum with distal collapsed one (were surgeon has just removed intraluminal meconium pearls) ensures a route for the continuous local instillation of solubilising agent beginning on the first postoperative days. The aforementioned tube enterostomy also avoids the need for reoperation and stoma closure once the obstruction will be definitively relieved on 10th–15th postoperative day. A pursestring suture is placed on the antimesenteric border of the dilated ileum near the transition from large to small caliber ileum. A small (8 French), soft pluri-windowed catheter is inserted through the enterotomy and gently advanced in the distal ileum (Fig. 35.8). It is then used to irrigate by manual mixing of the solubilising agent with the thick meconium and meconium pearls. The meconium is removed through the enterotomy and pellets are either manually removed or flushed into the colon. By the 14th–15th days the catheter can be removed stated that any irrigant (milk included) pass freely into the colon and the obstruction is definitely relieved. Appendectomy, irrigation with gastrografin through the appendix stump followed by gentle expression of the meconium has been proposed as an alternative technique to evacuate meconium avoiding enterotomy, enterostomy or bowel resection [59]. Nowadays enterotomy with irrigation is the treatment of choice for patients with uncomplicated MI that couldn't be successfully managed with non-operative management.

A temporary obstruction-relieving stoma (with or without resection) may be an alternative surgical strategy. The stoma can be fashioned in different ways as shown in the Fig. 35.9.

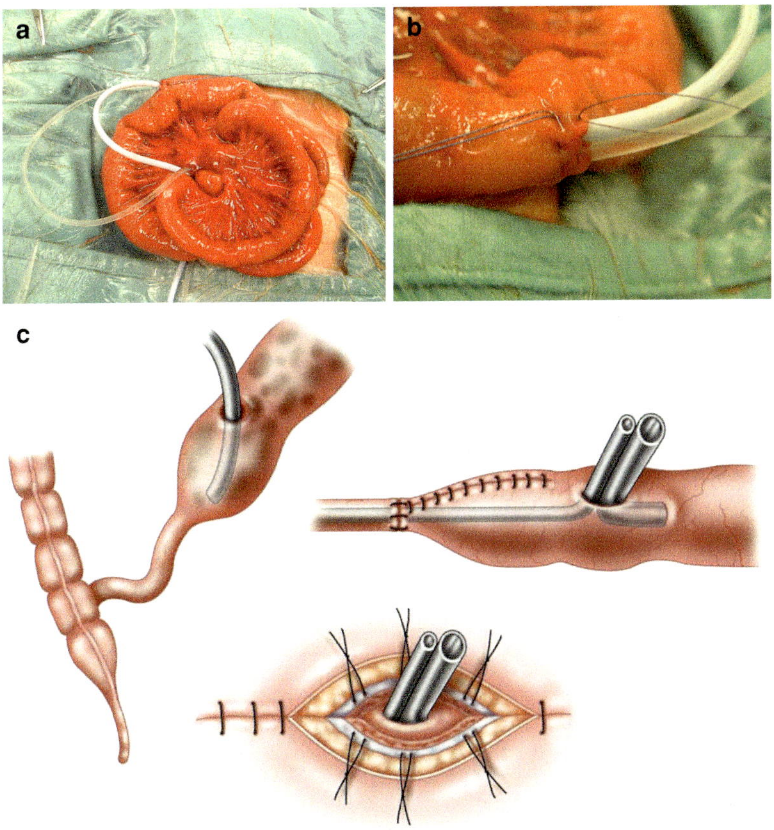

Fig. 35.8 (**a**) Tube ileostomy in the proximal ileus (usually a 10 Ch tube is inserted through the enterotomy); a second 5–7 Ch tube is inserted into the distal narrow ileus and/or microcolon for constant irrigation with increasing amount of fluids, promoting enlargement of the distal intestine. (**b**) Intraoperative picture and (**c**) explicative diagrams

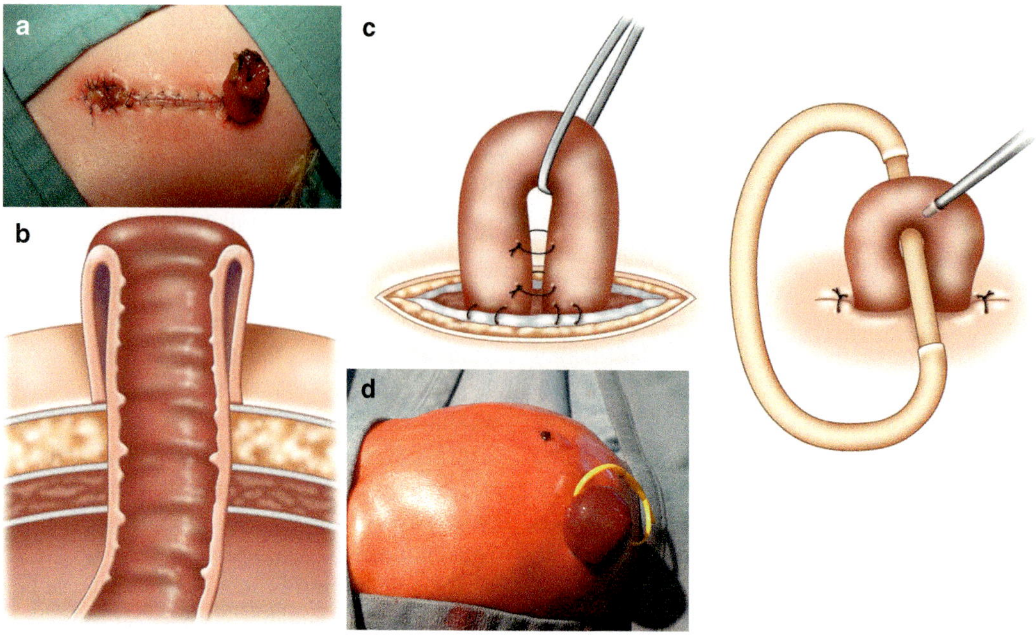

Fig. 35.9 (**a**) Ileostomy: note the discrepancy between the proximal and distal ileus; (**b**) Ileostomy diagram; (**c**) Loop ileostomy diagram; (**d**) Intraoperative view

Classic Mikulitz side-by-syde enterostomy quick to perform and without the necessity of intraoperative meconium evacuation, thereby minimizing intraperitoneal contamination;

Bishop-Koop end (proximal)-to-side (distal) anastomosis and distal loop ostomy: the dilated intestinal loop with inspissated meconium is resected, an appropriately sized end (proximal ileum) to side (distal ileum) anastomosis peformed, approximately 4–5 cm. From distal open and close to the anterior abdominal wall. The distal ileum is exited to assume the function of decompressive stoma of proximal ileum while the distal one is persistently obstructed. In the immediate post-operative period (12–24 h), the stoma should be used as a catheter access to instil solubilising agents to remove meconium pearls in the distal ileum, relieving obstruction. The initial large enterostomy output will diminish once the distal obstruction is relieved due to the passage of stool through the end-to-side anastomosis, into the terminal ileum and microcolon. This technique enhances irrigation of distal ileum while the more enlarged loop of the proximal one (filled with inspissated meconium) is resected to create an appropriately sized end to be anastomosed to the distal one. A second surgical procedure is always required to close the ostomy.

Santulli side (proximal)-to-end (distal) anastomosis and proximal loop ostomy, the reverse of Bishop-Koop technique. The distal ileum is end-to-side anastomosed to the proximal one that is also exited without resection as an end enterostomy. The proximal ileal loop is easily decompressed without a mandatory resection and its irrigation enhanced. The catheter for the postoperative distal intestinal loop instillation of solubilising agents has to be passed through the stoma intraoperatively.

Because of the high output of ileal temporary stoma, it is always necessary to close such a stoma as soon as possible to avoid excessive liquid and electrolytes losses. Thus a second surgical procedure is always required.

35.7.3 Operative Management 2 (Complicated MI)

By definition, complicated MI includes infants with intestinal atresia, bowel gangrene and volvulus (Fig. 35.10) or perforation with varying degrees of meconium peritonitis. Complicated MI

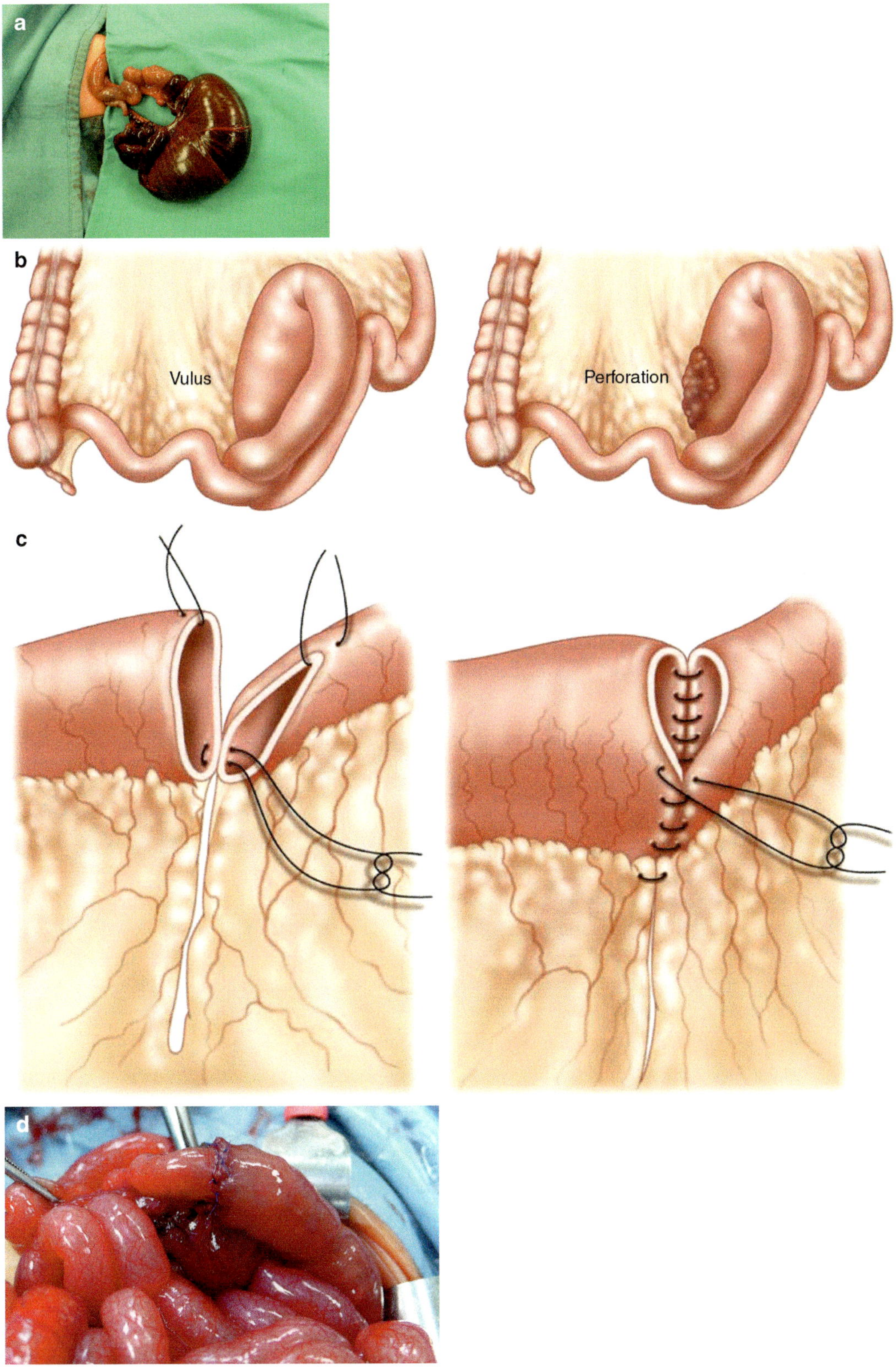

Fig. 35.10 (**a**) Complicated Meconium Ileus: intraoperative view of volvulus; (**b**) Explicative drawings; (**c**) End-to-end ileal anastomosis: diagrams and intraoperative view (**d**)

with prenatal volvulus of ileum may lead to ischemic necrosis, intestinal perforation and foetal peritonitis, intestinal atresia, or combination of these events. CF has been observed in 6–12% of neonates with jejunoileal atresia [35, 60]. The treatment of complicated MI requires operation in most patients. An exception to this rule is the rare baby where a prenatal perforation has left extraluminal intraperitoneal calcified meconium after a spontaneously self-sealed perforation without interruption of intestinal continuity. Sterile meconium extruded after foetal perforation may be partially reabsorbed (and trace amounts becoming calcified) or lead to several surgical appearances: meconium pseudocyst (a membrane into which the perforated bowel empties), adhesive meconium peritonitis (perforation for weeks before delivery), meconium ascites and absence of calcifications (perforation only few days before delivery), bacterially infected ascites (colonization by intestinal organisms from the neonatal perforated intestine). In cases with complicated meconium ileus, surgical procedure has to be adapted to the specific operative findings. The dissection may be bloody and difficult because of dense vascular adhesions. Resection of atretic or necrotic intestinal loop, bowel irrigation, and primary end-to-end anastomosis are sufficient in most neonates with jejuno-ileal atresia without compromised bowel and volvulus. In cases with atresia the blind proximal dilated pouch is frequently atonic if left in place, so it should be sacrificed when it still an adequate bowel length can be ensured. Short gut prevention is always a guiding principle. In patients with inadequate bowel length and significant bowel dilatation, consideration should be given to preserve sufficient intestinal length by tapering enteroplasty or leaving the dilated bowel in place for subsequent bowel elongation. Most neonates require peritoneal drainage and temporary diversion that can then be closed three to 6 weeks after the first laparotomy [61].

35.8 Outcomes

A number of authors reported a decrease in morbidity and mortality for MI patients in recent years [56, 62, 63]. This is consistent with the observed improvement of overall survival in patients affected by CF [64, 65] Even if, newborn screening for CF offers the opportunity for early medical and nutritional intervention that can lead to improved outcomes, there is a paucity of evidence on the care of infants diagnosed with CF. To fulfil this gap, in 2009 Borowitz and colleagues, on behalf of the Cystic Fibrosis Foundation developed recommendations based on a systematic review of the evidence and expert opinion. These guidelines encompass "monitoring and treatment recommendations for infants diagnosed with CF". Guidelines were intended to help guide families, primary care providers, and specialty care centres in the care of infants with CF [66]. To this purpose a routine monitoring and care recommendations for the infant diagnosed with CF was developed.

A CF care team at a dedicated centre should see patients at least once every 3 months [66, 67]. At each visit, patients should have a history and physical examination performed by a specialised CF physician. Furthermore, a nutritionist or registered dietician should also evaluate patients with speciality care in CF, and if possible, patients should perform spirometry to monitor lung function. On a yearly basis or when clinical symptoms dictate, a chest X-ray, blood work, and full pulmonary function testing (including measurement of lung volumes and diffusing capacity) should be performed.

Intravenous aminoglycosides are commonly used to treat lung infections. Aminoglycoside levels should be monitored while the patient is on therapy. Hearing screens should be performed at least annually on all CF patients receiving aminoglycosides. Levels of nephrotoxic antibiotics should be monitored while the patient is on therapy. Serum creatinine levels should be checked weekly in these patients and antibiotic doses should be adjusted accordingly. Immunisation for influenza should be carried out in all children who are eligible [66].

Different authors have also studied the impact of neonatal meconium obstruction in patients affected by CF at late follow-up. MI in patients with CF was not associated to higher risk for late clinical deterioration or decreased survival. Some investigators suggest that adequate initial

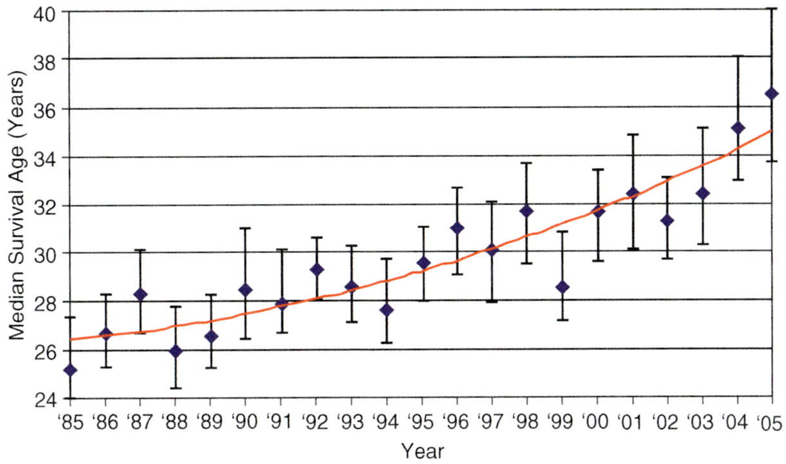

Fig. 35.11 This represents the age by which half of the current CF registry population would be expected to be dead, given the ages of the patients in the registry and the mortality distribution of the deaths in 2005. The whiskers represent the 95% confidence intervals for the survival estimates, so the 2005 median predicted survival is between 33.7 and 40.0 years. From: Strausbough SD and Davis PB Cystic fibrosis: a review of epidemiology and pathobiology. Clin Chest Med 2007; 28: 279–288

nutritional and medical management of MI allows further similar nutritional status and pulmonary function tests compared to other early-diagnosed CF patients [57, 68]. However, Escobar and colleagues found in their 32-year evaluation of outcomes of surgically treated CF patients, an increased risk for late complications including meconium ileus equivalent and fibrosing colonopathy (actually cumulatively addressed as DIOS) [47]. Nevertheless, epidemiological studies have demonstrated striking improvement in outcomes for patients affected by CF in the last 30 years, with an actual median survival now approaching the fifth decade of life [69] (Fig. 35.11).

References

1. Landsteiner K. Darmverschluss durch eingeductes meconium pankreatitis. Zentralbl Allg Pathol. 1905;16:903–7.
2. Zigler MM. Meconium ileus. Curr Probl Surg. 1994;31:441–4.
3. Anderson DH. Cystic fibrosis, of the pancreas and its relation to celiac disease. Am J Dis Child. 1938;56:344–99.
4. Rozmahel R, Wilschansky M, Matin A, et al. Modulation of disease severity in cystic fibrosis transmembrane conductance regulator deficient mice by a secondary genetic factor. Nat Genet. 1996;12:280–7.
5. Rasor GB, Stevenson W. Meconium ileus equivalent. Rocky Mount Med J. 1941;38:218–20.
6. Hiatt RB, Wilson PE. Celiac syndrome: Therapy of meconium ileus: report of eight cases with review of the literature. Surg Gynecol Obstet. 1948;87:317–27.
7. Noblett HR. Treatment of uncomplicated meconium ileus by Gastrografin enema: a preliminary report. J Pediatr Surg. 1969;4:190–7.
8. Lambotte C. Neonatal diagnosis of hereditary metabolic diseases. Rev Med Liege. 1973;28:837–51.
9. Ziegler MM. Meconium ileus. Curr Pro Surg. 1994;32:731–77.
10. MacGregor SN, Tamura R, Sabbagha R, et al. Isolated hyperechoic fetal bowel: significance and implications for management. Am J Obstet Gynecol. 1995;173:1254–8.
11. Rudolph CD. Meconium diseases of infancies. In: Rudolph CD, Rudolph AM, Hoestetter MK, et al., editors. Rudolph's of Pediatrics. 21st ed. New York: McGraw-Hill; 2001. p. 1407–9.
12. Fakhoury K, Durie PR, Levison H, et al. Meconium ileus in the absence of cystic fibrosis. Arch Dis Child. 1992;67:1204–6.
13. Gorter RR, Karimi A, Sleeboom C, et al. Clinical and genetic characteristics of meconium ileus in newborn with and without cystic fibrosis. JPGN. 2010;5:569–72.
14. Toyosaka A, Tomimoto Y, Nose K, et al. Immaturity of the myenteric plexus is the aetiology of meconium ileus without mucoviscidosis: a istopathologic study. Clin Autonom Res. 1994;4:175–83.
15. Yoo SY, Jung SH, Eom M, et al. Delayed maturation of interstitial cells of Cajal in meconium obstruction. J Ped Surg. 2002;37:1758–61.
16. Thomaidis TS, Arey JB. The intestinal lesions in cystic fibrosis of the pancreas. J Pediatr. 1963;63:444.
17. Karem BS, Rommens JM, Buchana JA, et al. Identification of the cystic fibrosis gene: genetic analysis. Science. 1989;245:1073.

18. Karem E, Corey M, Kerem B, et al. Clinical and genetic comparisons of patients with cystic fibrosis, with or without meconium ileus. J Pediatr. 1989;114:767–73.
19. Davenport M. Cystic fibrosis: surgical consideration. In: Stringer M, editor. Pediatric Surgery and Urology: Long term outcomes. 1st ed. London: W.B. Sunders Company LTD; 1998.
20. Zigler MM. Meconium Ileus. In: Grosfeld JL, editor. Pediatric Surgery. 6th ed. Philadelphya: Mosby Elsevier; 2006.
21. Shutt WH, Isles TE. Protein in meconium from meconium ileus. Arch Dis Child. 1968;43:178.
22. Welsh MJ. Cystic fibrosis. In: Scriver CR, Beaudet AL, Sly WS, et al., editors. The metabolic and molecular basis of inherit diseases. 7th ed. New York: McGraw-Hill; 1994.
23. Riordan JR, Rommens JM, Kerem BS, et al. Identification of the cystic fibrosis gene: Cloning and characterization of complementary DNA. Science. 1989;245:1066–73.
24. Knowlton RG, Cohen-Haguenauer O, Van Cong N, et al. A polymorphic DNA marker linked to cystic fibrosis is located on chromosome 7. Nature. 1985;318:380–2.
25. Blackman SM, Deering-Brose R, McWilliams R, et al. Relative contribution of genetic and non genetic modifiers to intestinal obstruction in cystic fibrosis. Gastroenterology. 2006;131:1030–9.
26. Zialenski J, Corey M, Rozmahel R, et al. Detection of a cystic fibrosis modifier locus for meconium ileus on human chromosome 19q13. Nat Genet. 1999;22:128–9.
27. Van der Doef HP, Slieker MG, Staab D, et al. Association of the CLCA1 p.S357N variant with meconium ileus in European patients with cystic fibrosis. J Pediatr Gastroenterol Nutr. 2010;50:347–9.
28. Dorfman R, Li W, Suun L, et al. Modifier gene study of meconium ileus in cystic fibrosis: statistical considerations and gene mapping results. Hum Genet. 2009;126(6):763–78.
29. Walker SR, Barksdale EM Jr. Meconium syndromes and cystic fibrosis. In: Oldham KT, editor. Principles and Practice of Pediatric Surgery. 1st ed. Philadelphya: Lippincott W and W; 2005.
30. Chan LK, Tang HY, Tse HY, et al. Meconium peritonitis: prenatal diagnosis, postnatal management and outcome. Prenat Diagn. 2005;25:676–82.
31. Regev RH, Markovich O, Arnon S, et al. Meconium periorchitis: intrauterine diagnosis and neonatal outcome: case reports and review of the literature. J Perinatol. 2009;29:585–7.
32. Penna L, Bower S. Hyperechogenic bowel in the second trimester fetus: a review. Prenat Diagn. 2000;20:909–13.
33. Scotet V, De Braekeleer M, Audrezet MP, et al. Prenatal detection of cystic fibrosis by ultrasonography: a retrospective study of more than 346000 pregnancies. J Med Genet. 2002;39:443–8.
34. Culling B, Ogle R. Genetic counselling issues in cystic fibrosis. Pediatr Respir Rev. 2010;11:75–9.
35. Casaccia G, Trucchi A, Nahom A, et al. The impact of cystic fibrosis on neonatal intestinal obstruction: the need for prenatal/neonatal screening. Pediatr Surg Int. 2003;19:75–8.
36. Hussain SM, Meradj M, Robbin SGF, et al. Plain film diagnosis in meconium plug syndrome, meconium ileus and neonatal Hirschsprung's disease. Pediatr Radiol. 1991;21:556–9.
37. Leonidas JC, Berton WE, Baker DH, et al. Meconium ileus and its complication: a reappraisal of plain film roentgen diagnostic criteria. Am J Roentgenol. 1970;108:598–609.
38. Kao SCS, Franken EA Jr. Non operative treatment of simple meconium ileus: A survey of the Society for Pediatric Radiology. Pediatr Radiol. 1995;25:97–100.
39. Farrell PM, Rosenstein BJ, White TB, et al. Guidelines for diagnosis of cystic fibrosis in newborns through older adults: Cystic Fibrosis Foundation consensus report. J Pediatr. 2008;153:S4–S14.
40. Castellani C, Southern KW, Brownlee K, et al. European best practice guidelines for cystic fibrosis neonatal screening. J Cyst Fibros. 2009 May;8(3):153–73.
41. Crossley JR, Elliott RB, Smith PA. Dried-blood spot screening for cystic fibrosis in the newborn. Lancet. 1979;1:472–4.
42. De la Hunt MN. The acute abdomen in the newborn. Semin Fetal Neonat Med. 2006;11:191–7.
43. Hajivassiliou CA. Intestinal obstruction in neonatal/pediatric surgery. Sem Pediatr Surg. 2003;12:241–53.
44. Burge D, Drewett M. Meconium plug obstruction. Pediatr Surg Int. 2004;20:108–10.
45. Keckler SJ, St. Peter SD, Spilde TL, et al. Current significance of meconium plug syndrome. J Pediatr Surg. 2008;43:896–8.
46. Williams A. Early enteral feeding of the preterm infant. Arch Dis Child Fetal Neonatal Ed. 2000;83:F219–20.
47. Escobar MA, Grosfeld JL, Burdick JJ, et al. Surgical considerations in cystic fibrosis: a 32-year evaluation of outcomes. Surgery. 2005;138:560–71. discussion 571-2.
48. Li Z, Kosorok MR. Longitudinal pulmonary status of cystic fibrosis children with meconium ileus. Pulmonol. 2004;38:277–84.
49. Mornet E, Serre JL, Farrrel M, et al. Genetic differences between cystic fibrosis with and without meconium ileus. Lancet. 1988;1:376–8.
50. Stringer MD, Brereton RJ, Drake DP, Kiely EM, Agrwal M, Mouriquand PDE, et al. Meconium ileus due to extensive intestinal aganglionosis. J Pediatr Surg. 1994;23:501–3.
51. Karimi A, Gorter RR, Sleeboom C, et al. Issues in the management of simple and complex meconium ileus. Pediatr Surg Int. 2011;9:963–8. Epub 2011 Apr 22.
52. Copeland DR, St. Peter SD, Sharp SW. Diminishing role of contrast enema in simple meconium ileus. J Pediatr Surg. 2009;44:2130–2.

53. Burke MS, Ragi JM, Hratch L, et al. New strategies in nonoperative management of meconium ileus. J Pediatr Surg. 2002;37:760–4.
54. Meeker IA, Kincannon WN. Acetylcystein to liquefy inspissated meconium causing intestinal obstruction in the newborn. Surgery. 1964;56:419–25.
55. Rowe MI, Furst AJ, Altman DH, et al. The neonatal response to Gastrografin enema. Pediatrics. 1971;48:29–35.
56. Del Pin CA, Czyrko C, Ziegler MM, et al. Management and survival of meconium ileus: a 30-year review. Ann Surg. 1992;215:179–18557.
57. Munck A, Gerardin M, Alberti C, et al. Clinical outcome of cystic fibrosis presenting with or without meconium ileus: a matched cohort study. J Pediatr Surg. 2006;41:1556–60.
58. Shaw A. Safaty of N-Acetylcysteine in treatment of meconium obstruction of the newborn. J Pediatr Surg. 1969;13:475–9.
59. Fitzgerald R, Conlan K. Use of the appendix stump in the treatment of meconium ileus. J Pediatr Surg. 1989;24:899–900.
60. Farrel PM. improving the health of patients with cystic fibrosis through newborn screening. Adv Pediatr Infect Dis. 2000;47:79–115.
61. Mychaliska GB. Introduction to neonatal intestinal obstruction. In: Oldham KT, editor. Principles and Practice of Pediatric Surgery. 1st ed. Philadelphya: Lippincott W and W; 2005.
62. Fuchs JR, Langer JC. Long-term outcome after neonatal meconium obstruction. Pediatrics. 1998;101:e1–7.
63. Mabogunje OA, Wang CI, Mahour GH. Improved survival of neonates with meconium ileus. Arch Surg. 1982;117:37–40.
64. George PM, Banya W, Pareek N, et al. Improved survival at low lung function in cystic fibrosis: cohort study from 1990 to 2007. BMJ. 2011;342:d1008.
65. Debray D, Kelly D, Houwen R, et al. Best practice for the diagnosis and management of cystic fibrosis-associated liver disease. J Cyst Fibros. 2011;10(suppl. 2):S29–36.
66. Borowitz D, Robinson KA, Rosenfeld M, et al. Cystic fibrosis foundation evidence-based guidelines for management of infants with cystic fibrosis. J Pediatr. 2009;155:S73–93.
67. Eigen H, Rosenstein BJ, Fitz Simmons S, et al. A multicenter study of alternate-day prednisone therapy in patients with cystic fibrosis. Cystic Fibrosis Foundation Prednisone Trial Group. J Pediatr. 1995;126:515–23.
68. Efrati O, Nir J, Fraser D, et al. Meconium ileus in patients with cystic fibrosis is not a risk factor for clinical deterioration and survival: the Israeli multicenter study. JPGN. 2010;50:173–8.
69. Strausbough SD, Davis PB. Cystic fibrosis: a review of epidemiology and pathobiology. Clin Chest Med. 2007;28:279–88.

Ascites in the Newborn

36

Stavros P. Loukogeorgakis and Paolo De Coppi

Abstract

Ascites (Greek: ascos; "baglike") is a gastroenterological term that describes the accumulation of fluid, which may consist of transudates (low protein count) or exudates (high protein count). The incidence of ascites in paediatric patients is unknown, but the condition is rare. Ascites may be present in the fetus, and there are significant differences in its aetiology between neonates and older children.

Keywords

Newborn ascites • Aetiology • Pathogenesis • Surgery • Peritoneo-venous shunts

36.1 Overview

36.1.1 Background

Ascites (Greek: *ascos*; "baglike") is a gastroenterological term that describes the accumulation of fluid, which may consist of transudates (low protein count) or exudates (high protein count). The incidence of ascites in paediatric patients is unknown, but the condition is rare. Ascites may be present in the fetus, and there are significant differences in its aetiology between neonates and older children.

Fetal ascites has been associated with a wide variety of conditions and may occur in isolation or in conjunction with hydrops both immunological (secondary to alloimmune haemolytic disease or Rhesus isoimmunisation) and non-immunological (intra-uterine infections, chromosomal abnormalities, fetal tumours including sacro-coccygeal teratoma, cardiac anomalies, twin-to-twin transfusion) [1]. Neonatal ascites can be classified broadly in chylous, biliary and urinary. Ascites may be present at birth (associated with fetal ascites) or develop in the early post-natal period. In older paediatric patients, ascites can be secondary to trauma, infection, cancer, as well as gastrointestinal, hepatobiliary or pancreatic disease. Geographic and socio-economic factors have a significant impact on the aetiology of ascites. Trauma and infection (e.g. tuberculosis) are more common causes of paediatric ascites in developing counties, whereas neoplasms, and conditions

S.P. Loukogeorgakis, MBBS, BSc, PhD, MRCS
P. De Coppi, MD, PhD (✉)
Surgery Unit, Institute of Child Health,
30 Guildford Street, London WC1 N1EH, UK
e-mail: p.decoppi@ucl.ac.uk

P.D. Losty et al. (eds.), *Rickham's Neonatal Surgery*, https://doi.org/10.1007/978-1-4471-4721-3_36

affecting the gastrointestinal and hepatobiliary systems are more frequent in developed countries [2]. Ascites after major surgery is also a well-recognised entity in paediatric patients of all ages, and usually appears as a consequence of major retroperitoneal dissection. The latter is typically associated to neuroblastoma resection and requires early intervention [3, 4].

36.1.2 Clinical Presentation

Neonates and infants with ascites usually present with abdominal distension; clinical examination reveals a fluid "thrill" (sensitivity 20–80%; specificity 82–100%) [2], shifting dullness on percussion (sensitivity 60–88%; specificity 56–90%) [2], and hepatosplenomegaly. Jaundice may be present but this is dependent on the underlying cause. Moreover, patients with gross ascites may present with increased work of breathing (intercostal recession, raised respiratory rate) and hypoxia/hypercapnia due to diaphragmatic "splinting". There may be evidence of sepsis including temperature instability, hypo−/hyperglycaemia, and raised inflammatory markers. Peritoneal irritation (pain and guarding on palpation) is uncommon in neonates with ascites, but is often observed in older infants and children. Its presence is determined by the primary aetiology.

36.1.3 Investigations

An abdominal X-ray is often performed as part of the initial patient assessment. Characteristic features include diffusely increased density of the abdomen, poor definition of soft tissue shadows, medial displacement of bowel and solid viscera, and increased separation of bowel loops (Fig. 36.1a). Definitive radiological diagnosis of ascites is made with trans-abdominal ultrasound (first line radiological investigation) (Fig. 36.1b), and/or computerised tomography (CT; more sensitive for small amounts of intra-peritoneal fluid) (Fig. 36.1c). With the advent of attempts to reduce ionising radiation exposure, magnetic resonance imaging could play a more important role in the detection of free fluid in the peritoneal cavity [2].

Abdominal paracentesis and laboratory analysis of the intra-peritoneal fluid may be required for specific diagnosis when the cause of ascites is not apparent. Paracentesis can usually be performed quickly, inexpensively, and safely [2, 5]. Traditional classification of the causes of ascites has been based on measurement of protein content and specific gravity of intra-peritoneal fluid [Transudate (low protein content, specific gravity <1.0): due to portal hypertension of any cause; e.g. cirrhosis, fulminant liver failure, Budd-Chiari syndrome, portal vein thrombosis; Exudate (high protein content, specific gravity >1.0): non-portal hypertensive aetiology; e.g. infection, neoplasia, biliary leak, nephrotic syndrome]. However, this has now been superseded by measurement of the serum-ascites albumin gradient (SAAG), which has been shown to be a better discriminant compared to older measures (SAAG >1.1 g/dL: equivalent to transudate; SAAG <1.1 g/dL: equivalent to exudates) [6]. Depending on the differential diagnosis, ascitic fluid collected from paracentesis should also be submitted for white blood cell count (and differential), as well as bilirubin, amylase, triglyceride, urea and creatinine measurements. Moreover, bedside inoculation of blood culture bottles with ascitic fluid should be performed if indicated.

36.2 Fetal Ascites

Isolated fetal ascites is defined as fluid accumulation in the abdominal cavity without accumulation in other body cavities or sub-cutaneous tissue (hydrops fetalis). The natural history of isolated ascites remains unclear, but several investigators have reported that it is often caused by in-utero infection (e.g. cytomegalovirus; CMV) [7], cardiac (e.g. arrhythmia, heart failure) [8, 9], renal (e.g. polycystic kidney disease) [10], gastrointestinal (e.g. intestinal atresia, meconium peritonitis) [11, 12], hepatobiliary (e.g. biliary atresia, portal venous malformations) [13], and metabolic disorders (e.g. Niemann-Pick disease) [14] (see Table 36.1 for summary of causes). Isolated fetal

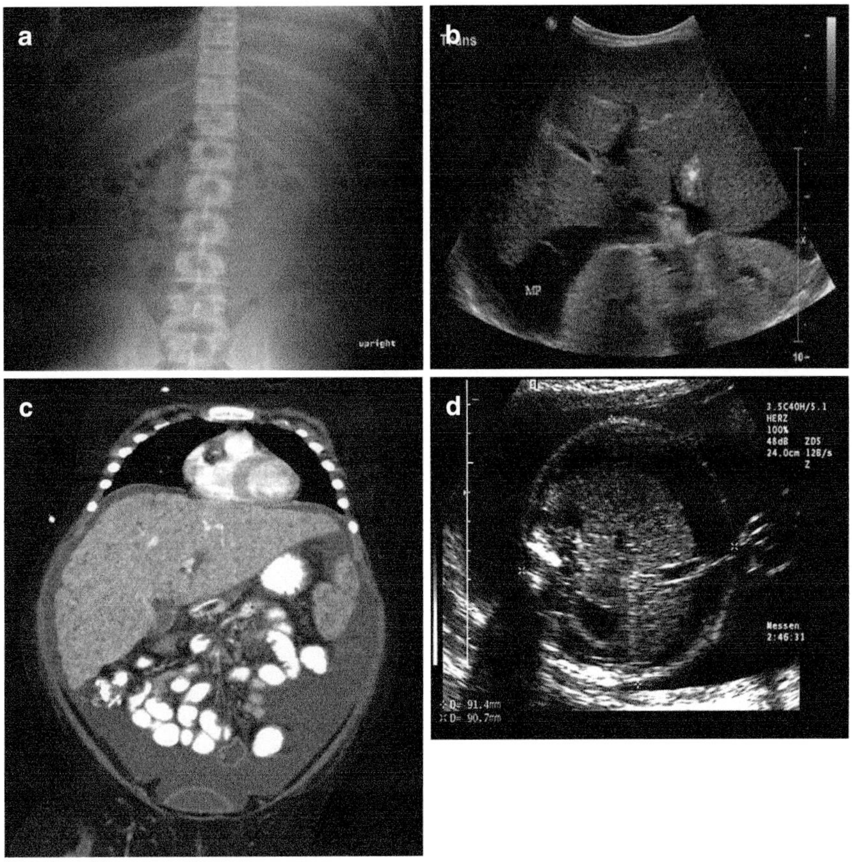

Fig. 36.1 Radiological investigations of fetal and neonatal ascites. (**a**) Abdominal X-ray of patient with ascites. (**b**) Ultrasound image of ascites visible in the hepato-renal fossa. (**c**) Ascites on computerised tomography (CT) with contrast. (**d**) Isolated fetal ascites on prenatal ultrasound at 29 weeks gestation. Adapted from Giefer et al. JPGN 2011; 52 [5] 503–513 and Schmider et al. Fetal Diagn Ther 2003; 18,230–236; used with permission

ascites occasionally occurs primarily without an identifiable cause (idiopathic fetal ascites). Although the mechanisms of idiopathic fetal ascites are not fully understood, in many of these fetuses there is chylous ascites after birth secondary to congenital lymphatic abnormalities [15].

Fetal ascites is usually a radiological diagnosis detected prenatally during imaging of the fetus with ultrasound (Fig. 36.1d), typically performed at gestational age between 21 and 30 weeks [2], and it is often associated with poly- or oligohydramnios [16, 17].

The prognosis for fetuses with isolated ascites is mostly favourable, and survival rates as high as 94% have been reported [18]. Gestational age at onset of ascites has been shown to be the most significant prognostic factor (onset during early gestation associated with worse outcomes) [19]. A large patient series focusing on fetal ascites has shown that ascites accompanied by hydrops fetalis had less favourable prognosis compared to isolated fetal ascites [20]. However, close monitoring after identification of fetal ascites is recommended since isolated ascites can also be the first sign of hydrops fetalis and thus these conditions are not mutually exclusive. The presence of isolated fetal ascites is a rare diagnosis and work-up should be followed to ensure identification of an underlying cause, as most of the cases are associated with other abnormalities [1, 18, 19].

Fetal abdominal paracentesis (FAP) has been advocated by some authors as a potential prenatal intervention for gross fetal ascites to reduce abdominal circumference [21]. Recent studies

Table 36.1 Causes of fetal and neonatal ascites

Type of disorder	Fetus	Neonate
Hepatobiliary	Biliary atresia Portal venous malformations	Cirrhosis Alpha-1-antitrypsin deficiency Budd-Chiari syndrome Biliary atresia Biliary perforation Portal venous malformations
Gastrointestinal	Meconium peritonitis Malrotation (+/− Volvulus) Intestinal atresia Intussusception Cystic Fibrosis	Intestinal perforation Malrotation (+/− Volvulus) Intestinal atresia Necrotising enterocolitis Pancreatitis
Genitourinary	Hydronephrosis Polycystic kidney disease Urinary obstruction Cloaca	Obstructive uropathy: Posterior urethral valves Ureterocele Ureteral stenosis/atresia Bladder perforation (iatrogenic) Nephrotic syndrome
Lymphatic	Congenital lymphatic abnormality (unspecified)	Congenital lymphatic abnormality (unspecified)
Cardiac	Arrhythmia Heart failure	Arrhythmia Heart failure
Metabolic	Niemann-Pick (Type C) Glycosylation disorders Lysosomal storage disorders	Niemann-Pick (Type C) Glycosylation disorders Lysosomal storage disorders
Haematological	Haemolytic anaemia Haemochromatosis	Haemochromatosis
Infection	Cytomegalovirus Parvovirus Syphillis Toxoplasmosis	Appendicitis Acute hepatitis
Chromosomal	Turner syndrome Trisomy 21	
Other	Maternal/fetal abuse Idiopathic	Abdominal trauma Idiopathic

Adapted from Giefer et al. JPGN 2011; 52 [5] 503–513; used with permission

however have shown that FAP has no long-term effect on preventing an enlarged abdomen because of rapid fluid re-accumulation [22] while it may still have a therapeutic role according to others since FAP may reduce the rate of caesarean section and ensure the safe delivery of the baby due to a short-term reduction in fetal abdominal size [21]. Abdominal-amniotic shunting (AAS) has also been proposed [23–25] for the management of fetal ascites, though its efficacy has been debated. Indeed, the benefits of AAS have been limited by high complication rates; some authors have reported shunt displacement and/or malfunction in up to 30% of cases.

36.3 Neonatal Ascites

The aetiology of neonatal ascites is similar to that of ascites in the fetus (see Table 36.1 for summary of the causes), although many congenital diseases do not typically manifest with ascites until after birth [2]. The three main types of neonatal ascites that come to the attention of paediatric surgical teams (chylous, biliary, and urinary) are described below. In addition, there are multiple iatrogenic causes of ascites in the newborn, including extravasation of parenteral nutrition from femoral or umbilical venous catheters [26], and gastric perforation from gastric catheters and/or feeding tubes. Treatment of the latter usually requires explorative laparoscopy and/or laparotomy, drainage of the leaked content, and (when possible) repair of the injury. Ascites may also be a post-operative complication of procedures involving major retroperitoneal dissection (e.g. resection of neuroblastoma) [27].

36.3.1 Chylous Ascites

36.3.1.1 Aetiology

Chylous ascites occurs in neonates with a slight male predominance and is generally rare [28, 29]. Neonatal chylous ascites is almost always idiopathic, and congenital lymphatic abnormalities are thought to be the usual underlying cause [30]. Moreover, conditions causing external compression of lymphatics (e.g. malrotation, hernia, intussusception, and tumours) can also result in chylous ascites in neonates [31]. Trauma with disruption of lymphatic ducts is another cause, but it is more common in infants and older children. Anecdotally, chylous ascites has been found in patients undergoing laparoscopic procedures (e.g. hernia repair), subsequently diagnosed with malrotation and volvulus [32, 33].

36.3.1.2 Diagnosis

Neonates with chylous ascites present with increased abdominal girth and non-specific symptoms such as irritability and poor feeding. Recent weight gain despite reduced oral intake may also be present. Following detailed history and clinical examination, ultrasonography and/or CT scanning may confirm the chylous fluid (unique biphasic fat-fluid level in the supine patient) [34], and may help rule out underlying causes. The gold standard for diagnosis of chylous ascites is abdominal paracentesis. Laboratory analysis reveals lymphocytosis (>75% of cells seen in microscopy), and markedly elevated triglyceride content (>1500 mg/dL).

36.3.1.3 Management

Conservative and symptomatic management is usually the treatment of choice once surgical causes (e.g. malrotation, neoplasia) have been excluded. Surgery is considered only when conservative therapy fails. Medical therapy aims to decrease the rate of chyle formation, promoting damaged lymphatics to seal as well as the development of alternate lymphatic pathways [35]. Standard treatment comprises dietary modification combined with diuretics (spironolactone) and paracentesis [36]. In particular high protein and low fat combined with medium-chain triglycerides are usually effective in transient conditions such as inflammation or leaky lymphatics [37]. However, stopping of enteral feeding and parenteral nutrition it is usually a more effective treatment and allows maintenance of calorie intake [38]. The somatostatin analogue octreotide has also been successfully used to reduce ascites in less-responsive cases [39]. These non-operative techniques however may take weeks to work and have limited success [27, 36, 37]. Treatment of the ascites using a permanent drain may initially be effective but it is not recommended; the fluid discarded not only rapidly re-accumulates in most cases but also is rich in electrolytes, protein, and white cells [35].

When all the conservative options have failed, surgical intervention may have a role. Various methods have been used to identify the site of leakage intra-operatively including the use of dyes (e.g. Sudan dye), a high-fat pre-operative meal, pre-operative lymphangiography and lymphoid scintigraphy [40]. The first reported surgical cure by direct ligation of a leaking lacteal was in 1977 by Pearl and colleagues [41]. More recently laparoscopic ligation of the lymphatic trunk has been successfully adopted and while it may difficult to locate the exact point of leakage, direct suturing of the leaking area is usually successful [40].

If direct repair fails, a peritoneovenous shunt (PVS) may be needed [4, 35]. Use of early shunts was limited by high failure rates secondary to blockage [42]. Introduction of the LeVeen and Denver

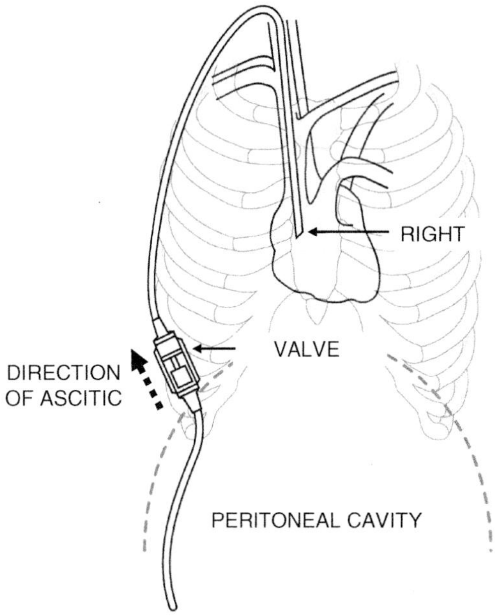

Fig. 36.2 The Denver shunt. Adapted from Rahman et al. JPS 2011; 46: 315–319; used with permission

shunts renewed interest in this form of management [35, 43]. These shunts allow ascitic fluid to flow down a pressure gradient from the peritoneal cavity to the venous circulation, and have a valve mechanism that prevents backflow of blood if the venous pressure rises above the intra-abdominal pressure. The advantage of the Denver shunt (Fig. 36.2) is that the valve chamber lies in the subcutaneous tissue and therefore can be manually compressed to relieve blockage and promote flow [35].

Use of PVS in our institution has resulted in resolution of persistent chylous ascites in the overwhelming majority of patients (>90% response to treatment) [4, 35]. The use of the Denver shunt has reduced the number of shunt failures owing to shunt blockage, as the shunt chamber can be pumped to relieve blockage, and flushed percutaneously if necessary. Blockage should be suspected if there is re-accumulation of ascitic fluid. Shunt infections may respond to intravenous antibiotics, but removal may be necessary [4, 35]. Other complications that have been reported include cardiac congestion, disseminated intravascular coagulation, sepsis, nephritis, dissemination of malignant cells, and perforation of the coronary sinus [44].

36.3.2 Biliary Ascites

36.3.2.1 Aetiology

Biliary ascites in neonates is typically an isolated finding probably related to congenital bile duct malformations [45]. The almost universal site of perforation is at the junction of the cystic duct with the common bile duct, but spontaneous rupture of the intrahepatic duct has been also reported (especially the left intrahepatic bile duct) [46, 47]. The pathophysiology of these "spontaneous" bile duct perforations is currently unclear, but congenital weakness and/or vascular insufficiency of the bile duct wall, elevated intra-ductal pressure from a long common channel and pancreatic reflux have been implicated. Biliary atresia and perforation of a choledochal cyst can also be causative [48, 49]. Biliary ascites is occasionally observed in association with sepsis and ABO blood group incompatibility.

36.3.2.2 Diagnosis

Neonates with biliary ascites present with abdominal distension and jaundice (conjugated hyperbilirubinaemia) [50]. Usually, there are no symptoms and signs of peritonitis. Ultrasonography is used to confirm the presence of ascites and may detect biliary congenital anomalies or obstructing lesions. Cholescintigraphy (Hepatobiliary Imino-Diacetic Acid scan; HIDA scan) may also be useful in demonstrating a biliary leak; following intravenous injection of ^{99}Tc-IDA, radio-nuclide is detected outside the biliary tree and within the peritoneal cavity [46, 51]. Diagnostic paracentesis reveals elevated bilirubin levels in the intra-peritoneal fluid [51].

36.3.2.3 Management

The mainstay of treatment for biliary ascites in the newborn is surgical drainage [45, 47]. This can be achieved with open (laparotomy) or laparoscopic procedures. At operation, sterile bile ascites and bile staining of the peritoneal cavity are found. An intra-operative cholangiogram should be performed through the gallbladder and a drain should be placed at the site of perforation [45, 47, 49]. Lesions are usually self-limiting, and the perforation seals with drainage [45, 47, 49].

Aggressive surgical intervention is not indicated because the congenitally weakened bile duct may be further damaged during attempts at anastomosis.

36.3.3 Urinary Ascites

36.3.3.1 Aetiology

Neonatal urinary ascites is most commonly due to bladder or ureteric perforation secondary to distal obstruction of the urinary system. Posterior urethral valves (PUV) are the most common cause [52–54], and as a result the incidence of urinary ascites in greater male newborns. Moreover, some newborns with PUV present with upper tract perforation (forniceal rupture or parenchymal "blow-out"); the resulting urinary extravasation may lead to peri-renal urinoma formation and in some cases urinary ascites [55, 56]. Other factors predisposing to urinary ascites include the presence of a ureterocele, congenital bladder diverticuli or intra-peritoneal bladder [57, 58]. Iatrogenic urinary ascites is frequently observed, due to trauma to the dome of the bladder or a patent urachus during umbilical arterial catheterisation [59, 60]. Complex urinary anomalies (e.g. cloaca) may allow reflux of urine through the genital tract into the peritoneal cavity, without the presence of a perforation [61].

36.3.3.2 Diagnosis

Neonates with urinary ascites present with gross abdominal distension and associated respiratory embarrassment due to diaphragmatic elevation. In advanced cases the Potter sequence may also be present (oligohydramnios associated with congenital abnormalities in the urinary system resulting in physical deformities including characteristic facies, and lower extremity anomalies). Patients may also present with a history of failure to thrive, lethargy and recurrent urinary tract infections (with or without sepsis). Baseline biochemical tests may reveal deranged renal function, electrolyte abnormalities (due to urinary re-absorption), and acidosis [62]. Evaluation of urinary ascites begins with ultrasonography, and micturating cysto-urethrography (MCUG) should also be performed. The latter will aid in the diagnosis of PUV, but may not always demonstrate the site of perforation [58, 63]. Renal scintigraphy (^{99}Tc-MAG3 scan) may be useful in the diagnosis of upper tract perforations [64]. Biochemical analysis of ascitic fluid reveals concentrations of urea and creatinine higher than in the serum [58, 63].

36.3.3.3 Management

Initial treatment is usually directed at decompressing the bladder and upper urinary tract by trans-urethral insertion of a 5- or 8-Fr feeding tube into the bladder. This may be sufficient to stop leakage of urine in the peritoneal cavity. Rehydration, correction of electrolyte abnormalities, and administration of antibiotics should also be performed. In the case of PUV, cystoscopic ablation should be performed as soon as possible to ensure permanent relief of distal urinary tract obstruction [53]. Therapeutic paracentesis may be indicated in cases of gross urinary ascites with respiratory compromise, worsening renal function and electrolyte imbalance, infection and/or hypertension. If MCUG demonstrates bladder rupture, a cutaneous vesicostomy may be necessary [54, 65]. If leak from a hydronephrotic kidney occurs, insertion of a percutaneous nephrostomy often solves the problem. Unfortunately, with forniceal rupture the kidney is typically decompressed. In these cases, the involved kidney should be explored through a small flank incision, and a temporary cutaneous pyelostomy or ureterostomy may be formed. However, in most cases, mobilizing the kidney, separating it from the adjacent peritoneum, and leaving a drain in the retroperitoneal space will allow the leak to resolve, provided that the distal urinary tract has been decompressed.

Table 36.2 summarises the aetiology, clinical characteristics and management of the major types of neonatal ascites.

Table 36.2 Major types of neonatal ascites

	Chylous	Biliary	Urinary
Cause	Idiopathic Congenital lymphatic anomalies External lymphatic compression Trauma	Bile duct perforation Choledochal cyst perforation Biliary atresia	Obstructive uropathy: PUV Ureterocele Ureteral stenosis/atresia Bladder perforation (iatrogenic) Cloaca
Clinical Presentation	Abdominal distension Irritability/Lethargy Poor feeding	Abdominal distension Jaundice (conjugated) Irritability/Lethargy Poor feeding	Gross abdominal distension Respiratory compromise UTI/Urosepsis Electrolyte derangement Renal failure Irritability/Lethargy Poor feeding
Diagnosis	USS (CT/MRI) Raised lymphocytes in AF Raised triglycerides in AF	USS (CT/MRI) HIDA Intra-op. cholangiogram Raised bilirubin in AF	USS (CT/MRI) MCUG ^{99}Tc-MAG3 Raised urea and creatinine in AF
Management	Medium chain triglycerides (diet) Diuretics (spironolactone) Therapeutic paracentesis Octreotide Direct surgical repair Peritoneovenous shunt	Surgical drainage (open/lap.)	Urinary catheterisation Therapeutic paracentesis PUV ablation Vesicostomy Ureterostomy Pyelostomy

Adapted from Giefer et al. JPGN 2011; 52 [5] 503–513; used with permission
USS ultrasound, *CT* computerised tomography, *MRI* magnetic resonance imaging, *AF* ascitic fluid, *HIDA* hepatobiliary imino-diacetic acid scan, *PUV* posterior urethral valves, *MCUG* micturating cysto-urethrography

References

1. Schmider A, Henrich W, Reles A, Kjos S, Dudenhausen JW. Etiology and prognosis of fetal ascites. Fetal Diagn Ther. 2003;18:230–6.
2. Giefer MJ, Murray KF, Colletti RB. Pathophysiology, diagnosis, and management of pediatric ascites. J Pediatr Gastroenterol Nutr. 2011;52:503–13.
3. Chung CJ, Bui V, Fordham LA, Hill J, Bulas D. Malignant intraperitoneal neoplasms of childhood. Pediatr Radiol. 1998;28:317–21.
4. Sooriakumaran P, McAndrew HF, Kiely EM, Spitz L, Pierro A. Peritoneovenous shunting is an effective treatment for intractable ascites. Postgrad Med J. 2005;81:259–61.
5. Runyon BA. Paracentesis of ascitic fluid. A safe procedure. Arch Intern Med. 1986;146:2259–61.
6. Runyon BA, Montano AA, Akriviadis EA, Antillon MR, Irving MA, McHutchison JG. The serum-ascites albumin gradient is superior to the exudate-transudate concept in the differential diagnosis of ascites. Ann Intern Med. 1992;117:215–20.
7. Sun CC, Keene CL, Nagey DA. Hepatic fibrosis in congenital cytomegalovirus infection: with fetal ascites and pulmonary hypoplasia. Pediatr Pathol. 1990;10:641–6.
8. Richards DS, Wagman AJ, Cabaniss ML. Ascites not due to congestive heart failure in a fetus with lupus-induced heart block. Obstet Gynecol. 1990;76:957–9.
9. Ojala TH, Hornberger LK. Fetal heart failure. Front Biosci (Schol Ed). 2010;2:891–906.
10. Machin GA. Diseases causing fetal and neonatal ascites. Pediatr Pathol. 1985;4:195–211.
11. Voss LM, Hadden W, Pease PW, Clarkson PM. Neonatal ascites due to congenital jejunal obstruction. Aust Paediatr J. 1988;24:260–1.
12. Patton WL, Lutz AM, Willmann JK, Callen P, Barkovich AJ, Gooding CA. Systemic spread of meconium peritonitis. Pediatr Radiol. 1998;28:714–6.
13. Achiron R, Gindes L, Kivilevitch Z, et al. Prenatal diagnosis of congenital agenesis of the fetal portal venous system. Ultrasound Obstet Gynecol. 2009;34:643–52.
14. Manning DJ, Price WI, Pearse RG. Fetal ascites: an unusual presentation of Niemann-Pick disease type C. Arch Dis Child. 1990;65:335–6.
15. Chereau E, Lejeune V, Gonzales M, Carbonne B. Voluminous fetal chylous ascites: a case of complete spontaneous prenatal regression. Fetal Diagn Ther. 2007;22:81–4.

16. Pelizzo G, Codrich D, Zennaro F, et al. Prenatal detection of the cystic form of meconium peritonitis: no issues for delayed postnatal surgery. Pediatr Surg Int. 2008;24:1061–5.
17. Shono T, Taguchi T, Suita S, Nakanami N, Nakano H. Prenatal ultrasonographic and magnetic resonance imaging findings of congenital cloacal anomalies associated with meconium peritonitis. J Pediatr Surg. 2007;42:681–4.
18. Zelop C, Benacerraf BR. The causes and natural history of fetal ascites. Prenat Diagn. 1994;14:941–6.
19. Nose S, Usui N, Soh H, et al. The prognostic factors and the outcome of primary isolated fetal ascites. Pediatr Surg Int. 2011;27:799–804.
20. Favre R, Dreux S, Dommergues M, et al. Nonimmune fetal ascites: a series of 79 cases. Am J Obstet Gynecol. 2004;190:407–12.
21. de Crespigny LC, Robinson HP, McBain JC. Fetal abdominal paracentesis in the management of gross fetal ascites. Aust N Z J Obstet Gynaecol. 1980;20:228–30.
22. Okawa T, Soeda S, Watanabe T, Sato K, Sato A. Repeated paracentesis in a fetus with meconium peritonitis with massive ascites: a case report. Fetal Diagn Ther. 2008;24:99–102.
23. Seeds JW, Herbert WN, Bowes WA Jr, Cefalo RC. Recurrent idiopathic fetal hydrops: results of prenatal therapy. Obstet Gynecol. 1984;64:30S–3S.
24. Bernaschek G, Deutinger J, Hansmann M, Bald R, Holzgreve W, Bollmann R. Feto-amniotic shunting—report of the experience of four European centres. Prenat Diagn. 1994;14:821–33.
25. Fung TY, Fung HY, Lau TK, Chang AM. Abdomino-amniotic shunting in isolated fetal ascites with polyhydramnios. Acta Obstet Gynecol Scand. 1997;76:706–7.
26. Shareena I, Khu YS, Cheah FC. Intraperitoneal extravasation of total parental nutrition infusate from an umbilical venous catheter. Singap Med J. 2008;49:e35–6.
27. Leibovitch I, Mor Y, Golomb J, Ramon J. The diagnosis and management of postoperative chylous ascites. J Urol. 2002;167:449–57.
28. Karagol BS, Zenciroglu A, Gokce S, Kundak AA, Ipek MS. Therapeutic management of neonatal chylous ascites: report of a case and review of the literature. Acta Paediatr. 2010;99:1307–10.
29. Chye JK, Lim CT, Van der Heuvel M. Neonatal chylous ascites—report of three cases and review of the literature. Pediatr Surg Int. 1997;12:296–8.
30. Man DW, Spitz L. The management of chylous ascites in children. J Pediatr Surg. 1985;20:72–5.
31. Seltz LB, Kanani R, Zamakhshary M, Chiu PP. A newborn with chylous ascites caused by intestinal malrotation associated with heterotaxia syndrome. Pediatr Surg Int. 2008;24:633–6.
32. Shariff FU, Curry J, De CP, Drake DP. Laparoscopic finding of chylous ascites and intestinal malrotation in an infant presenting with left inguinal hernia. J Laparoendosc Adv Surg Tech A. 2008;18:651–3.
33. Zarroug AE, Srinivasan SK, Wulkan ML. Incidental chylous fluid during hernia repair may be a harbinger of malrotation. J Pediatr Surg. 2010;45:E17–8.
34. Hibbeln JF, Wehmueller MD, Wilbur AC. Chylous ascites: CT and ultrasound appearance. Abdom Imaging. 1995;20:138–40.
35. Rahman N, De CP, Curry J, et al. Persistent ascites can be effectively treated by peritoneovenous shunts. J Pediatr Surg. 2011;46:315–9.
36. Aalami OO, Allen DB, Organ CH Jr. Chylous ascites: a collective review. Surgery. 2000;128:761–78.
37. Cochran WJ, Klish WJ, Brown MR, Lyons JM, Curtis T. Chylous ascites in infants and children: a case report and literature review. J Pediatr Gastroenterol Nutr. 1985;4:668–73.
38. Asch MJ, Sherman NJ. Management of refractory chylous ascites by total parenteral nutrition. J Pediatr. 1979;94:260–2.
39. Huang Y, Zhuang S, Li Y, Liu M, Chen H, Du M. Successful management of congenital chylous ascites in a premature infant using somatostatin analogue. Indian J Pediatr. 2011;78:345–7.
40. Kuroiwa M, Toki F, Suzuki M, Suzuki N. Successful laparoscopic ligation of the lymphatic trunk for refractory chylous ascites. J Pediatr Surg. 2007;42:E15–8.
41. Pearl J, Joyner J, Collins DL. Chylous ascites: the first reported surgical cure by direct ligation. J Pediatr Surg. 1977;12:687–91.
42. Smith AN. The application of the Holter valve to the treatment of resistant ascites. Gut. 1963;4:192.
43. Leveen HH, Christoudias G, Ip M, Luft R, Falk G, Grosberg S. Peritoneo-venous shunting for ascites. Ann Surg. 1974;180:580–91.
44. Herman R, Kunisaki S, Molitor M, Gadepalli S, Hirschl R, Geiger J. The use of peritoneal venous shunting for intractable neonatal ascites: a short case series. J Pediatr Surg. 2011;46:1651–4.
45. Banani SA, Bahador A, Nezakatgoo N. Idiopathic perforation of the extrahepatic bile duct in infancy: pathogenesis, diagnosis, and management. J Pediatr Surg. 1993;28:950–2.
46. Haller JO, Condon VR, Berdon WE, et al. Spontaneous perforation of the common bile duct in children. Radiology. 1989;172:621–4.
47. Chilukuri S, Bonet V, Cobb M. Antenatal spontaneous perforation of the extrahepatic biliary tree. Am J Obstet Gynecol. 1990;163:1201–2.
48. Ando H, Ito T, Watanabe Y, Seo T, Kaneko K, Nagaya M. Spontaneous perforation of choledochal cyst. J Am Coll Surg. 1995;181:125–8.
49. Ando K, Miyano T, Kohno S, Takamizawa S, Lane G. Spontaneous perforation of choledochal cyst: a study of 13 cases. Eur J Pediatr Surg. 1998;8:23–5.
50. Davenport M, Betalli P, D'Antiga L, Cheeseman P, Mieli-Vergani G, Howard ER. The spectrum of surgical jaundice in infancy. J Pediatr Surg. 2003;38:1471–9.
51. Kasat LS, Borwankar SS, Jain M, Naregal A. Spontaneous perforation of the extrahepatic bile duct in an infant. Pediatr Surg Int. 2001;17:463–4.

52. Scott TW. Urinary ascites secondary to posterior urethral valves. J Urol. 1976;116:87–91.
53. Gurgoze MK, Yildirmaz S, Dogan Y, Ozel K, Gun O. A rare cause of ascites in a newborn: posterior urethral valve. Pediatr Int. 2010;52:154–5.
54. Sahdev S, Jhaveri RC, Vohra K, Khan AJ. Congenital bladder perforation and urinary ascites caused by posterior urethral valves: a case report. J Perinatol. 1997;17:164–5.
55. Garrett RA, Franken EA Jr. Neonatal ascites: perirenal urinary extravasation with bladder outlet obstruction. J Urol. 1969;102:627–32.
56. Yerkes EB, Cain MP, Padilla LM. In utero perinephric urinoma and urinary ascites with posterior urethral valves: a paradoxical pop-off valve? J Urol. 2001;166:2387–8.
57. Murphy D, Simmons M, Guiney EJ. Neonatal urinary ascites in the absence of urinary tract obstruction. J Pediatr Surg. 1978;13:529–31.
58. Morrell P, Coulthard MG, Hey EN. Neonatal urinary ascites. Arch Dis Child. 1985;60:676–8.
59. Dmochowski RR, Crandell SS, Corriere JN Jr. Bladder injury and uroascites from umbilical artery catheterization. Pediatrics. 1986;77:421–2.
60. Hepworth RC, Milstein JM. The transected urachus: an unusual cause of neonatal ascites. Pediatrics. 1984;73:397–400.
61. Adams MC, Ludlow J, Brock JW III, Rink RC. Prenatal urinary ascites and persistent cloaca: risk factors for poor drainage of urine or meconium. J Urol. 1998;160:2179–81.
62. Printza N, Ververi A, Bandouraki M, Vargiami E, Gidaris D, Papachristou F. Life-threatening hyponatremia and acute renal failure due to iatrogenic neonatal bladder rupture. Urol Int. 2012;88:238–40.
63. Tank ES, Carey TC, Seifert AL. Management of neonatal urinary ascites. Urology. 1980;16:270–3.
64. Boughattas S, Hassine H, Chatti K, Salem N, Essabbah H. Scintigraphic findings in a case of bilateral urinomas and ascites secondary to posterior urethral valves. Clin Nucl Med. 2003;28:923–5.
65. Arora P, Seth A, Bagga D, Aneja S, Taluja V. Spontaneous bladder rupture secondary to posterior urethral valves in a neonate. Indian J Pediatr. 2001;68:881–2.

37 Neonatal Bowel Obstruction

Alexander M. Turner, Basem A. Khalil,
and James Bruce

Abstract

The purpose of this chapter is to introduce the concepts of neonatal bowel obstruction to the reader and outline its presentation, effects upon the child, investigation, and general principles of treatment. Common causes are described in detail elsewhere in the book, but rare causes and miscellany are discussed here in more detail.

Keywords

Newborn intestinal obstruction • Classification • Diagnosis and management

37.1 Introduction

The purpose of this chapter is to introduce the concepts of neonatal bowel obstruction to the reader and outline its presentation, effects upon the child, investigation, and general principles of treatment. Common causes are described in detail elsewhere in the book, but rare causes and miscellany are discussed here in more detail.

Neonatal bowel obstruction occurs when the normal passage of meconium or milk from mouth to anus is interrupted by physical forces or by bowel dysfunction. Its presentation may be acute or chronic, affect proximal or distal gut and have variable effects on the neonate, which will determine overall outcome. The classical surgical sieve to define the causes of bowel obstruction apply; extrinsic, intra-mural (intrinsic) or luminal. Obstruction may also be partial, intermittent or complete. Use of the term "sub-clinical obstruction" should be avoided, as any level of obstruction will have consequences to the gut and become clinically apparent, otherwise there is no obstruction. Functional bowel obstruction describes the scenario where bowel dysfunction contributes to the development of meconium or milk bolus stasis, which then leads on to physical luminal obstruction. However, it is perhaps better to approach classification of obstruction as to how it relates to presentation, because this is how the diagnosis is made.

A.M. Turner, BSc, MB, ChB, FRCS(Paeds), PhD
Department of Paediatric Urology, Leeds Children's Hospital, Leeds, UK

B.A. Khalil, MPH, PhD, FRCS(Paed)
Department of Pediatric Surgery, SIDRA, Doha, Qatar

J. Bruce, MB, ChB, FRCS(Ed), FRACS (✉)
Department of Paediatric Surgery, Central Manchester Children's Hospital, Manchester, UK
e-mail: James.bruce@mft.nhs.uk

P.D. Losty et al. (eds.), *Rickham's Neonatal Surgery*, https://doi.org/10.1007/978-1-4471-4721-3_37

37.2 Key Features

A normal, term neonate can begin feeding immediately after birth. This has advantages not only in terms of nutrition, but also for the development of normal feeding and bowel reflexes, immunological defence and psychological benefits for mother and child alike. Premature infants should also be fed, but with caution in the context of gestational age and weight, also in terms of co-existing morbidities. Specific problems that can arise in feeding the preterm infant are discussed later.

The suspicion for bowel obstruction can be raised either antenatally, where polyhydramnios or intrauterine growth retardation may have been a feature, with or intrauterine without other findings associated with obstruction, such as increased nuchal thickness to suggestive of trisomy 21 and thus duodenal atresia. Alternatively, and more commonly, it is the symptoms and signs the neonate displays after birth which prompt investigation. The key features of bowel obstruction are progressive vomiting, abdominal signs such as tenderness or distension, constipation and, later, radiological evidence. Further signs may include irritability, or abnormal physiological parameters, such as tachy/bradycardia or tachy/bradypnoea, which represent responses to the primary insult. For a neonate, these require interpretation.

37.2.1 Vomiting

Quite distinct from the complex, centrally mediated action of vomiting, regurgitation of feed should be recognised as a separate entity in the neonate, although its presence instead of vomiting should not reassure the clinician into a false sense of security. Generally, neonatal regurgitation of recently ingested feed, provided it does not represent the entire feed after every feed, usually does not represent serious or surgical pathology. However, if the initial feed results in regurgitation with distress especially if accompanied by coughing or choking, apnoea or bradycardia, then investigation should commence towards exploring the diagnosis of oesophageal atresia. This is normally confirmed on plain chest X-ray where the nasogastric tube (NGT) is seen coiling in the upper oesophagus, with the presence of distal abdominal gas identifying the presence of a tracheo-oesophageal fistula. Congenital oesophageal stenosis, an extremely rare condition is caused by either intramural ectopic tracheobronchial elements or fibromuscular hypertrophy or a luminal membrane typically affecting the distal oesophagus [1]. Endoscopic dilatation or surgical options such as resection of the affected segment with primary anastamosis or myotomy have been described. Affecting as few as 1 in 50,000 live births, presentation may only occur when solid food is commenced [1].

Vomit produced by a neonate should be classified carefully into one of three groups:

(a) Non-bilious vomit: Colourless or luminous yellow, contains enteric juice from the stomach and may be clear in the absence of feed, or milky if a feed has been taken.
(b) Bilious vomit: Dark green, akin to mint sauce. Freshly produced bile of golden colour has been acted upon by stomach acid to produce the green colour.
(c) Non-bilious vomit developing into bilious vomit: Often after prolonged vomiting, the colour may change from milky to lime green to dark green. Conversely, an improving obstruction for example may produce vomit or aspirate that lightens in colour from dark green to clear, again via a lime green stage.

In relation to bowel obstruction, interruption of flow proximal to the ampulla of Vater will produce non-bilious vomit. Depending upon the distance of the obstruction distal to the ampulla, vomit may be immediately bilious, or become bilious after non-bilious vomiting.

Persistent non-bilious, milky vomiting of the entire feed, permanent hunger and stomach distension raises the possibility of an early presentation of pyloric stenosis, which is not a congenital abnormality and usually presents between 2 and 6 weeks of life, or pyloric atresia, a rare cause of gastric outlet obstruction. The latter occurs in 1 in 100,000 live births and can exist, in descending order of frequency, as a membrane (Type I), a solid core of tissue (Type II) or complete atresia where there is a gap between the stomach and duodenum [2]. Its most frequent association is epidermolysis bullosa, but may also co-exist with other intestinal atresias. Treatment is surgical, with either excision of the web, pyloroplasty or gastroduodenostomy [2] where, as an isolated problem, prognosis is good.

Neonatal bilious vomiting should be considered to be a surgical emergency until proved otherwise. Physical obstruction to the gut requires rapid assessment and occasionally immediate surgery after resuscitation. The type and site of obstruction cannot be hypothesised without consideration of other presenting features.

37.2.2 Abdominal Tenderness and Distension

A neonate who handles poorly, with labile physiological responses to abdominal palpation, or who appears to be in pain, often intermittently (colicky), should be considered to have an intra-abdominal pathology, especially in the presence of bilious vomiting. The presence or absence of abdominal distension is moot in such cases, except to allow the clinician to consider what type of insult is evolving. Proximal small bowel obstruction may largely result in stomach distension whereas distal large bowel obstruction may result in massive pan-gut distension. The level of distension can only reflect the most proximal obstruction, so one cannot exclude multiple obstructions or duel pathology on this basis.

37.2.3 Constipation

A term neonate should pass meconium within 24 h of life. As feed is introduced, the stool changes to a lighter colour, often yellow and seedy, and this confirms continuity of the bowel. Clearly, when confronted with a neonate who is vomiting bile and has abdominal signs, the relevance of constipation can only be assessed in hindsight, and it is common for babies to pass meconium despite bowel obstruction. The presence of meconium throughout the gut implies that continuity has at one stage existed, and so the bowel obstruction has been a late event. The consistency of the meconium may indicate the length of time gut stasis has occurred or may reflect an inherent increased viscosity of the bowel mucus as seen in cystic fibrosis. The absence of meconium distal to the obstruction implies an insult early in gestation such as duodenal atresia, and the lack of conditioning of this segment by the flow of amniotic fluid of can lead to secondary problems such as small calibre gut, which may be dysmotile.

37.2.4 Abdominal Radiology

Whilst resuscitating the child, arrangements should be made to image the abdomen. The simplest and most informative radiological procedure is the plain chest and abdominal X-ray. From this one investigation, confirmation of the hypothesis of bowel obstruction can be achieved, with some information about the level of the obstruction.

The X-ray should be interrogated for signs in the chest, such as position of the endotracheal tube (if any), adequacy and clarity of the lung fields in cases of grossly distended abdomen and respiratory embarrassment, and to predict the need for ventilation. The presence of gut in the chest should also be sought. The course of the NG tube should be studied and interpreted with the clinical findings.

In the abdomen, the information to be gleaned should be the extent and position of bowel gas, whether there is gas present in the rectum and if there are distended loops, to what degree and at what level. Air fluid levels may be seen. Widely spaced bowel loops, thickened bowel wall or mucosal inflammation are signs of pathology. Necrotising enterocolitis can be implied from gut demonstrating wall pneumatosis, with or without evidence of portal venous gas. Evidence of free gas would confirm perforation. On a supine antero-posterior film this may be identified with the so-called "football sign", an incongruous gas shadow overlying the liver and epigastrium that could not be contained in a bowel loop. The outline of the falciform ligament may also be seen. Rigler's sign, where both the inner and outer lines of end-on bowel are seen clearly is also suggestive, but composite shadowing of overlying bowel loops should not confuse the issue. If there is doubt, a lateral decubitus film with the right side uppermost should be used to see air above the liver. Calcification of meconium implies long-standing stasis and may be identifiable outside of the bowel loops, which would suggest previous perforation.

Just as important is analysis of areas of paucity of gas, suggestive that the gut either contains no gas or there is a significant quantity of ascites or space occupying lesion causing the loops to "float" centrally or be pushed to one side respectively. Finally, the bony structures should be examined, particularly an assessment of the sacral spine.

In the case of a neonate with bilious vomiting (where Hirschsprung's disease, anorectal malformation or other lower GI anomalies are unlikely), it is essential to perform upper gastrointestinal contrast studies, to establish primarily whether the gut is normally rotated. Subtle abnormality in the position of the fourth part of duodenum relative to the pylorus is just as valid a sign for malrotation as the characteristic corkscrew appearance in midgut volvulus. Once diagnosed laparotomy should occur as a matter of urgency. If the diagnosis of volvulus is suspected but not confirmed by these modalities, ultrasonography may help with assessment of the superior mesenteric arterial and venous axis. In normal individuals the artery should lie to the left of the vein, but in volvulus it may be anterior or even to the right. Ultrasound showing a normal mesenteric axis does not exclude volvulus. As such, where in doubt despite investigations, a diagnostic laparotomy remains the safest option.

In other types of intestinal obstruction, the contrast study is also important in identifying the level and type of obstruction, in terms of partial or complete obstruction, but in the latter, only the most proximal obstruction will be identified. In cases of inspissated meconium, the contrast study, by virtue of its high osmolarity, can act both as diagnostic and therapeutic tool, but there should be awareness of the hypovolaemic effect of significant fluid shifts from the neonatal circulation into the gut and remedies should be in place before treatment.

37.3 Management

Principles of management of the neonate with bowel obstruction begin as with any other clinical case, with assessment of the airway, breathing and circulation. Consideration of co-morbidities should be made, especially when considering surgical options. The overall state of the child will depend upon the aetiology, but the following principles should be observed. The child should receive no enteral input. Adequate intravenous access should be secured and blood taken for assessment of renal function (bearing in mind time after birth), haematological parameters, clotting and for potential transfusion. Blood gas analysis should take place to assess the overall condition of the child and the extent of any metabolic acidosis. Although non-specific, if the bowel is thought to be at risk of ischaemia, elevated blood gas lactate levels may add to this concern [3]. However, it should be noted that a normal lactate does not exclude bowel necrosis/ischaemia. As the child is not feeding, regular blood sugar levels should be taken. Crystalloid intravenous fluid should be given according to local guidelines. If the child is shocked or is suspected to have large third space losses of fluid into the gut, deficit fluid boluses should be administered. A NG tube should be passed and its position checked with aspiration of fluid onto Litmus paper or by X-ray. All fluid aspirated this way should be replaced volume for volume. Extra potassium may need to be given to account for these losses.

Should a child need assisted ventilation, full intubation is preferable, as external positive-pressure ventilation will cause the gut to inflate, exacerbating the obstructive symptoms and risking respiratory embarrassment.

During this time, some progress should have been made towards confirming the diagnosis. Depending upon the type of obstruction and the condition of the child, a plan for surgical inter-

Table 37.1 Causes of physical intestinal obstruction in the neonatal period

Gastric	Early pyloric stenosis Pyloric web or atresia Epidermolysis bullosa pyloric atresia syndrome
Duodenum	Stenosis Atresia Malrotation Annular pancreas
Jejunum	Stenosis Atresia
Ileum	Stenosis Atresia Malrotation Meconium ileus Vitello-intestinal duct remnant Intussusception Milk curd obstruction
Colonic	Stenosis Atresia Imperforate anus Poorly developed colon e.g. megacystis microcolon intestinal hypoperistalsis syndrome
Global	Duplication anomalies Internal hernia or inguinal hernia Volvulus with or without (e.g. about a Meckel's band) malrotation Neoplasm

vention can be made. Neonatal bowel obstruction may be *physical* or *functional* in nature. Physical obstructions are caused by intrinsic, extrinsic or luminal compromise of the gut, usually occurring at a specific level which can be determined in advance radiologically, or at surgery. The common types are discussed elsewhere. Table 37.1 shows the causes of physical neonatal intestinal obstruction related to intestinal level. Where the symptoms and signs of bowel obstruction are present without physical obstruction, be it from within the gut or without, it is said to be functional obstruction. This occurs when peristalsis fails to propel bowel content toward the anus and may in turn lead to physical obstruction by excessive absorption of water and desiccation of meconium.

Mature intestinal motility depends upon the coordinated contraction and relaxation of the gut resulting in segmentation and peristalsis of bowel content from mouth to anus. The development of an intact neuronal pathway to control and effect these motor actions is essential. Development of the enteric nervous system occurs in a cephalocaudal direction, as does maturation of the ganglion cells. Incomplete population by ganglion cells renders the distal gut aganglionic and so a term neonate who has not passed meconium within 24 h of birth should be observed closely for signs of obstruction and be considered for rectal biopsy to determine the presence or absence of ganglion cells. Hirschprung's disease will be discussed in detail in a later chapter.

In a premature infant of very or extremely low birth weight (VLBW <1.5 kg; ELBW <1 kg), meconium may not be passed for a number of days but does not immediately warrant such investigation because of immaturity of the enteric nervous system. The motor patterns associated with mature gut cannot be assumed to occur in these infants. Abnormal consistency of meconium can also exacerbate the effect of immature gut in pre-term bowl obstruction [4]. It has been suggested that the consistency of the bowel content may determine the extent of propulsion the gut utilises at a given level (reviewed by [5]). For example, liquid matter may only require peristalsis just proximal to the bolus, whereas more solid material may also require distal relaxation. In E/VLBW infants, where the gut would expect to propel liquid meconium, any increased viscosity in the bowel such as that resulting from milk ingestion or a pathological processes such as cystic fibrosis [6], may render the gut unable to prevent obstruction. This is particularly pertinent to the use of formula milk and milk fortifiers, designed to enhance the nutritional status of feed given to premature or small for gestation infants. It is recognised that human milk is not enough for adequate growth in these infants and so formula +/− fortifier is used. Both are often rich in calcium and fat, and also contain proteins, carbohydrate, minerals and other electrolytes. Growth is enhanced, more so in small for gestation compared to appropriate for gestation VLBW neonates [7]. For the reasons stated above, the immature gut may not be able to propel liquids of high viscosity, stasis occurs and obstruction develops. Milk curd obstruction usually occurs at the terminal ileum and analysis of material removed at laparotomy has revealed a precipitate of calcium and fatty acid [8, 9]. Once suspected, feeds should be stopped and gastrograffin enema can be performed as a diagnostic and therapeutic measure; established obstruction with inspissated milk may require laparotomy. In the absence of an obvious cause of obstruction in E/VLBW infants, it should not be assumed that insufficient peristaltic activity is purely attributable to immaturity; those undergoing laparotomy for intestinal obstruction or perforation should also have full-thickness biopsies sent for histological analysis to exclude rarer causes such as muscular dysplasia or aplasia, possibly occurring as a result of ischaemic insult [10, 11].

If gut immaturity can be responsible for functional obstruction in VLBW infants, then it follows that delayed maturation of ganglion cells in a term infant may lead to failure to pass meconium and intestinal obstruction. This condition should be considered where ganglion cells are present on rectal biopsy but they appear small and nuclear morphology and cytoplasmic immunohistochemistry is abnormal [12]. Another group of patients with signs and symptoms of Hirschprung's disease but with normal rectal biopsy have been identified [13]. Labelled as benign transient non-organic ileus, neonates displayed abdominal gaseous distension with X-ray features similar to Hirschprung's disease but with a normal ano-rectal reflex. Both these groups (which may have significant overlap) by their nature are self-limiting problems, which may respond to anal stimulation, rectal washout or enema, and so they are important to recognise prior to what may be unnecessary surgical intervention.

A rare cause of functional bowel obstruction in combination with a non-obstructed, distended urinary bladder is the megacystis microcolon intestinal hypoperistalsis syndrome (MMIHS). This severe, often fatal congenital condition is characterised by reduced or absent peristaltic bowel activity, microcolon and malrotation. The huge, lax bladder fails to empty and without drainage by catheterisation or vesicostomy, upper tract damage persists. A number of aetiological theories have been postulated, which centre upon the role of the mesenchyme in terms of muscular, neurological and endocrine function (reviewed by [14]). Observations of degeneration in smooth muscle with vacuolation, coupled with the presence of excessive connective tissue were fortified with the finding that expression of collagen type I was markedly increased and smooth muscle actin, desmin and dystrophin muscle proteins were decreased in MMIHS detrusor compared to normal controls [15]. Furthermore, the finding that MMIHS small bowel lacked nicotinic acetylcholine receptor subunit 3 may suggest a neurogenic background to the disorder [16]. Affecting females predominantly, outcomes are poor; a systematic review of 227 cases between 1976 and 2011 revealed 80% mortality, the majority of the survivors being entirely reliant upon total parenteral nutrition (TPN) [17], although multivisceral transplantations have occurred with some success [18].

The development of functional bowel obstruction can be anticipated in certain cases, with knowledge of maternal medical history. Already susceptible by virtue of being a neonate, further immunosuppression as a result of haematological disease or human immunodeficiency virus (HIV) for example increases the risk of neonatal infection, especially when carried by the mother. Cytomegalovirus (CMV), the most common congenital viral infection [19], is responsible for most developmental disabilities attributable to infection [20] and may be transmitted during pregnancy or by breast milk. Although the spectrum of damage caused by CMV does not classically include the gut, the effects of gastrointestinal infection are well described (reviewed by [21]). Although the infection itself may cause inflammation, diarrhoea, or haemorrhage, its link as a primary causative agent in surgical pathology of the gut is not as clear. The presence of typical nuclear inclusion bodies in resected gut and mesentery may only prove co-existence of CMV with a primary pathology, but nevertheless it has been suggested that both functional and physical bowel obstruction may be caused by the infection. The mechanism by which CMV may be involved in cases of necrotizing enterocolitis, Hirschprung's disease, intestinal perforation or even atresia has not been established. It follows, however, that inflammation and vasculitis in the developing mesentery and gut could lead to ischaemic damage and thus the spectrum of atresias and their complications; intrauterine parvovirus B19 has been implicated in the same way [22]. CMV is an aetiological factor in enteric ganglioneuronitis in children with HIV infection [23] and so it follows that an insult to the developing enteric nervous system by the infection could result in a disease clinically similar to Hirschprung's. Interestingly, the use of antiretroviral therapy in neonates of mothers with HIV has itself been implicated in the development of functional distal bowel obstruction; this resolved once the drug was stopped and no surgical intervention was necessary [24].

The scenario of a neonate with the signs and symptoms of bowel obstruction and a mother with diabetes mellitus (DM), should raise the suspicion of the rare small left colon syndrome [25]. Characteristic contrast enema appearances of a narrow descending colon and sharp transitional zone at the splenic flexure is seen in these patients, up to 50% of whom have mothers with DM. Clearly, with such appearances Hirschprung's disease must be excluded, but when positively identified, bowel washouts and the contrast enema is sufficient to relive the obstruction with no further problems being encountered [25]. The pathogenesis of this condition is unclear, although it may relate to the balance of autonomic stimulation upon the developing bowel in the presence of fluctuating levels of glycaemia.

37.4 Summary

Early recognition of neonatal bowel obstruction is essential for the rapid resuscitation and homeostasis. Delay in treatment may result in dehydration, shock, profound electrolyte imbalance, sepsis, loss of gut or death. The three key signs of bilious vomiting, delayed or absent stooling and abdominal distension or tenderness should be heeded and transfer to a specialist centre arranged immediately for further investigation. Radiological assessment of the abdomen with and without contrast agents is a critical tool in determining the level and type of obstruction. Treatment is almost universally surgical, with the aim to restore continuity of the gut, either with a primary procedure or staged approach with the use of stomas.

References

1. Romeo E, Foschia F, de Angelis P, Caldaro T, Federici di Abriola G, Gambitta R, Buoni S, Torroni F, Pardi V and Dall'oglio L. Endoscopic management of congenital esophageal stenosis. J Pediatr Surg. 2011;46:838–41.
2. Okoye BO, Parikh DH, Buick RG, Lander AD. Pyloric atresia: five new cases, a new association, and a review of the literature with guidelines. J Pediatr Surg. 2000;35:1242–5.
3. Tanaka K, Hanyu N, Iida T, Watanabe A, Kawano S, Usuba T, Iino T, Mizuno R. Lactate levels in the detection of preoperative bowel strangulation. Am Surg. 2012;78:86–8.
4. Dimmitt RA, Moss RL. Meconium diseases in infants with very low birth weight. Semin Pediatr Surg. 2000;9:79–83.
5. Burns AJ, Roberts RR, Bornstein JC, Young HM. Development of the enteric nervous system and its role in intestinal motility during fetal and early postnatal stages. Semin Pediatr Surg. 2009;18:196–205.
6. Chaudry G, Navarro OM, Levine DS, Oudjhane K. Abdominal manifestations of cystic fibrosis in children. Pediatr Radiol. 2006;36:233–40.
7. Mukhopadhyay K, Narnag A, Mahajan R. Effect of human milk fortification in appropriate for gestation and small for gestation preterm babies: a randomized controlled trial. Indian Pediatr. 2007;44:286–90.
8. Flikweert ER, La Hei ER, De Rijke YB, Van de Ven K. Return of the milk curd syndrome. Pediatr Surg Int. 2003;19:628–31.
9. Quinlan PT, Lockton S, Irwin J, Lucas AL. The relationship between stool hardness and stool composition in breast- and formula-fed infants. J Pediatr Gastroenterol Nutr. 1995;20:81–90.
10. Miserez M, Barten S, Geboes K, Naulaers G, Devlieger H, Penninckx F. Surgical therapy and histological abnormalities in functional isolated small bowel obstruction and idiopathic gastrointestinal perforation in the very low birth weight infant. World J Surg. 2003;27:350–5.
11. Oretti C, Bussani R, Janes A, Demarini S. Multiple segmental absence of intestinal musculature presenting as spontaneous isolated perforation in an extremely low-birth-weight infant. J Pediatr Surg. 2010;45:E25–7.
12. Burki T, Kiho L, Scheimberg I, Phelps S, Misra D, Ward H, Colmenero I. Neonatal functional intestinal

obstruction and the presence of severely immature ganglion cells on rectal biopsy: 6 year experience. Pediatr Surg Int. 2011;27:487–90.
13. Yamauchi K, Kubota A, Usui N, Yonekura T, Kosumi T, Nogami T, Ohyanagi H. Benign transient non-organic ileus of neonates. Eur J Pediatr Surg. 2002;12:168–74.
14. Puri P, Shinkai M. Megacystis microcolon intestinal hypoperistalsis syndrome. Semin Pediatr Surg. 2005;14:58–63.
15. Rolle U, Puri P. Structural basis of voiding dysfunction in megacystis microcolon intestinal hypoperistalsis syndrome. J Pediatr Urol. 2006;2:277–84.
16. Richardson CE, Morgan JM, Jasani B, Green JT, Rhodes J, Williams GT, Lindstrom J, Wonnacott S, Thomas GA, Smith V. Megacystis-microcolon-intestinal hypoperistalsis syndrome and the absence of the alpha3 nicotinic acetylcholine receptor subunit. Gastroenterology. 2001;121:350–7.
17. Gosemann JH, Puri P. Megacystis microcolon intestinal hypoperistalsis syndrome: systematic review of outcome. Pediatr Surg Int. 2011;27:1041–6.
18. Raofi V, Beatty E, Testa G, Abcarian H, Oberholzer J, Sankary H, Grevious M, Benedetti E. Combined living-related segmental liver and bowel transplantation for megacystis-microcolon-intestinal hypoperistalsis syndrome. J Pediatr Surg. 2008;43:e9–e11.
19. Boeckh M, Geballe AP. Cytomegalovirus: pathogen, paradigm, and puzzle. J Clin Invest. 2011;121:1673–80.
20. Din ES, Brown CJ, Grosse SD, Wang C, Bialek SR, Ross DS, Cannon MJ. Attitudes toward newborn screening for cytomegalovirus infection. Pediatrics. 2011;128:e1434–42.
21. Bonnard A, Le Huidoux P, Carricaburu E, Farnoux C, Berrebi D, Aigrain Y, de Lagausie P. Cytomegalovirus infection as a possible underlying factor in neonatal surgical conditions. J Pediatr Surg. 2006;41:1826–9.
22. Schild RL, Hansmann M. Small bowel atresia: antenatal intestinal vascular accident or parvovirus B19 infection? Ultrasound Obstet Gynecol. 1998;11:227.
23. Anderson VM, Greco MA, Recalde AL, Chandwani S, Church JA, Krasinski K. Intestinal cytomegalovirus ganglioneuronitis in children with human immunodeficiency virus infection. Pediatr Pathol. 1990;10:167–74.
24. Brindley NM. Antiretroviral agents mimicking functional neonatal bowel obstruction: a case report. Eur J Pediatr Surg. 2006;16:276–8.
25. Ellis H, Kumar R, Kostyrka B. Neonatal small left colon syndrome in the offspring of diabetic mothers-an analysis of 105 children. J Pediatr Surg. 2009;44:2343–6.

Necrotising Enterocolitis

38

Nigel J. Hall, Simon Eaton, and Agostino Pierro

Abstract

Necrotising enterocolitis (NEC) is a devastating disease of infants and the commonest gastrointestinal emergency in the newborn period. It is a condition characterised by intestinal necrosis affecting the ileum and/or colon. There is a wide spectrum of clinical manifestations. In the least severe cases there may be mild inflammation of the intestinal wall in a baby with mild abdominal distension and minimal systemic upset. The most severely affected cases, however, may show evidence of full thickness intestinal necrosis with perforation, respiratory and cardiovascular collapse, multi-system organ failure and in some cases death

Keywords

Necrotising enterocolitis (NEC) • Bell's classification • Staging • Peritoneal drainage • Surgery • Stomas • RCTs

38.1 Introduction

Necrotising enterocolitis (NEC) is a devastating disease of infants and the commonest gastrointestinal emergency in the newborn period. It is a condition characterised by intestinal necrosis affecting the ileum and/or colon. There is a wide spectrum of clinical manifestations. In the least severe cases there may be mild inflammation of the intestinal wall in a baby with mild abdominal distension and minimal systemic upset. The most severely affected cases, however, may show evidence of full thickness intestinal necrosis with perforation, respiratory and cardiovascular collapse, multi-system organ failure and in some cases death.

The term 'necrotizing enterocolitis' first appeared in the European literature in the 1950s when Schmid and Quaiser described infants dying from necrotic lesions of the gastrointestinal tract [1]. However, it was not until the 1960s, when Santulli

N.J. Hall, PhD, MRCPCH, FRCS(Paed) (✉)
University Surgery Unit, Faculty of Medicine, University of Southampton, Southampton UK
e-mail: n.j.hall@soton.ac.uk

S. Eaton, PhD
Developmental Biology and Cancer Programme, UCL Institute of Child Health and Great Ormond Street Children's Hospital, London, UK

A. Pierro, MD, FRCS(Eng), OBE
Division of General and Thoracic Surgery, The Hospital for Sick Children, Toronto, ON, Canada

P.D. Losty et al. (eds.), *Rickham's Neonatal Surgery*, https://doi.org/10.1007/978-1-4471-4721-3_38

et al. reported a series of 64 infants with NEC that it became recognized as a distinct clinical entity [2]. Since then, the condition has been increasingly recognised, at least partly due to the advances made in neonatal care in the past 40 years and the increasing survival of infants at the extremes of prematurity creating a larger population at risk of developing NEC.

Currently, the reported incidence of NEC varies from 0.5 to 5 per 1000 live births [3] but NEC is predominantly a disease of preterm infants and those of low birth weight. The incidence is as high as 10–14% in infants less than 1000 g [4, 5] and more than 90% of affected infants are born prematurely [6]. Despite several decades of active research in the field of NEC, the mortality rate remains unchanged [7] and is over 30% in infants weighing less than 1000 g [8]. New treatments are desperately needed to improve outcome from this devastating condition.

38.2 Pathogenesis and Risk Factors

Several theories and mechanisms of injury have been proposed to explain the aetiology of NEC. However, despite over 30 years of research the aetiology remains unclear and no single mechanism at present can account for the pathogenesis in all cases. The interaction of multiple factors is likely to be responsible in the majority of cases. Several risk factors have been shown to be associated with NEC, and others implicated by strong association. Intestinal immaturity of premature infants, particularly those of extremely low birth weight, is thought to be central to the pathogenesis, although the precise nature of this immaturity and the mechanisms by which disease ensues are unclear. Proposed risk factors are summarised in Table 38.1.

38.2.1 Peripartum Events

There are several risk factors related to pre- and peri- natal events which are associated with NEC. Absent or reversed end diastolic blood flow in the umbilical artery has been reported as a predisposing factor [9] most likely due to creating a degree of chronic relative intestinal ischaemia. In addition there is an association with maternal eclampsia, fetal distress and premature rupture of membranes. In the immediate postnatal period, risk factors include asphyxia, hypothermia, respiratory distress syndrome, apnoeic episodes, cyanotic congenital heart disease, persistent fetal circulation, persistent ductus arteriosus and sepsis. In addition, there is some evidence that NEC may be associated with red blood cell transfusion [10]. It is likely that all result at least in part in a degree of relative intestinal ischaemia or hypoxia perhaps predisposing the infant to developing NEC in the presence of subsequent risk factors.

Table 38.1 Proposed risk factors for NEC

Peripartum events
Absent or reversed end diastolic umbilical artery blood flow
Maternal eclampsia
Fetal distress
Premature rupture of membranes
Delivery by caesarean section
Perinatal asphyxia
Perinatal hypothermia
Neonatal period
Respiratory distress syndrome
Apnoeic episodes
Congenital heart disease
Persistent fetal circulation
Persistent ductus arteriosus (PDA)
Sepsis
Umbilical catheterisation
Exchange transfusion
Nsaid treatment of PDA
Feeding regimen
Formula feed (as opposed to breast milk)
High density milk formulae
Early enteral feeding
Rapid advancement of enteral feeding
Bacterial involvement
Precise role unclear (intraluminal bacteria probably essential for the development of NEC)

38.2.2 Feeding Regimen

The majority of infants who develop NEC have been fed enterally. There is often pressure to provide feeds of increased calorific density in order to meet the growth requirements of the premature neonate. Such feeds are often hyperosmolar and may result in mucosal damage in the pre-existing immature intestine and thereby contributing to the development of NEC. Breast milk appears to offer some protection against NEC, probably as a result of its immunologically active components including immunoglobulins, cytokines and complement proteins [11, 12]. An association between the development of NEC and the administration of milk containing bovine derived proteins has also been proposed.

38.2.3 Altered Blood Supply

NEC has been associated with a number of predisposing factors which are believed to result in intestinal vascular insufficiency and subsequent selective mesenteric ischaemia. The causes of this vascular insufficiency include pre- and perinatal stress (e.g. reversed umbilical arterial blood flow, maternal pre-eclampsia), umbilical catheterization, exchange transfusion, congenital cardiac disease and indomethacin treatment. This results in the loss of the protective mucosal barrier, autodigestion and presents an opportunity for bacterial invasion. In addition to these associations, evidence for a vascular component in the aetiology of NEC comes from an experimental animal model in which a disease like NEC is observed following an intestinal ischaemia reperfusion injury [13].

38.2.4 Bacterial Involvement

While the precise role of bacterial agents in the development of NEC is unclear, several factors suggest their involvement. Occasionally NEC is seen to occur in clusters, in which a higher than expected number of cases are observed in one centre [14]. Identical organisms are grown from babies within these clusters and the initiation of infection control measures has been shown to control such outbreaks [15]. However, different organisms are grown from separate outbreaks so it cannot be claimed that a single organism is involved in development of NEC. Bacterial involvement in the pathogenesis of NEC is also implicated by association; endotoxaemia [16, 17] and positive blood cultures are common in infants with NEC and the gastrointestinal pneumatosis found in NEC contains 30% hydrogen, a gas produced solely by bacterial metabolism [18]. Furthermore, in experimental animals, an NEC-like illness can be inuced by ingestion of *Clostridium* species [19] and administration of bacterial endotoxin [20, 21]. Recent advances in pyrosequencing techniques to identify the intestinal microbiome have led to a surge in interest in examining the development of NEC in relation to the intestinal microflora. Although a precise bacterial signature has not been identified, it seems that development of NEC is immediately preceded by a loss in bacterial diversity [22]. Microbial triggering of the hyper-inflammatory cascade of NEC involves the toll-like receptor family, and other recent work is dissecting the molecular events involved in the initiation of mucosal damage [23].

38.3 Prevention

A variety of interventions have been proposed to prevent NEC. This is the most logical approach to combating a disease for which there are no specific therapies. Given the multifactorial aetiology of the disease any intervention decreasing the incidence of one of the recognized risk factors may be decrease the incidence of NEC. Although interventions such as immunoglobulin administration [24] or prophylactic enteral antibiotics have been shown to reduce incidence of NEC in individual studies, subsequent reviews and concerns over adverse effects have precluded their widespread usage [25, 26].

Other novel agents have been suggested for the prevention of NEC including lactoferrin [27], recombinant erythropoietin [28], glutamine [29] and arginine [30]. Whilst there is some evidence to support a reduction in incidence of NEC with these compounds, the mechanisms of action are unclear and may be attributable to other secondary effects. None is in current widespread use, although further studies of these and other agents are warranted.

The most robust evidence for interventions to prevent development of NEC exists for the administration of probiotics (reviewed [31]) and modulation of feeding regimes in infants at highest risk of NEC. The role of bacteria in the pathogenesis of NEC has led investigators to determine the effect of probiotics on the incidence on NEC. Several randomised controlled trials have demonstrated a significant reduction in incidence of NEC following routine probiotic administration [32, 33] and meta-analysis of these studies appears to confirm this [34]. However, the population at highest risk, i.e. those born at <30 weeks gestation and/or <1000 g birthweight, have been notably underrepresented in randomised controlled trials and therefore the meta-analyses, and a recent large randomised controlled trial in the UK showed no benefit of probiotic administration [35]. Furthermore, there remain unanswered questions as to which probiotic should be used and at what dose [36].

There is little doubt that one of the most important preventative measures is that of feeding infants at risk of NEC with breast milk as opposed to formula milk. This effect has been known for more than 20 years [11], but despite changes in infant formula, breast milk still appears to offer significant protection [12, 37]. Quigley et al., in a Cochrane review, demonstrated a significantly lower incidence of NEC in human milk-fed infants [38]. If fortification of breast milk is necessary to achieve adequate growth then a fortifier based on human milk appears to lower the incidence of NEC (and NEC requiring surgery) compared to a cow's milk based fortifier [37]. However, availability of either human milk and/or human milk based products is problematic.

In addition to this it has been a long held belief that the time at which enteral feeds are first introduced and the rate at which they are increased may affect the incidence of NEC. In an attempt to demonstrate this definitively, several groups have recently published results of well-designed randomised controlled trials investigating the effect of early versus delayed enteral feeding in infants at risk of NEC [39, 40]. Whilst both demonstrated a trend towards reduction in incidence of NEC with delayed enteral feeding, neither study in isolation demonstrated a statistically significant effect, and current meta-analyses do not support the use of a delayed introduction or slower rate of enteral feeds to prevent NEC.

Clusters of cases of NEC have been described, and anecdotally there is marked geographic variation in prevalence between countries and/or centres. How much of this is due to differences in feeding practise or other aspects of neonatal care, and how much of it may be due to genetic or environmental factors is unknown. Although there is some evidence that certain genotypes may predispose infants to NEC [41–43], the effects of these genotypes are not strong and most of the studies have been relatively small-scale.

38.4 Clinical Features and Diagnosis

Infants with NEC usually display both specific and non-specific gastrointestinal signs. In the early stages of the disease, abdominal distension with or without tenderness, feeding intolerance with increased gastric residuals, vomiting and occult blood in the stools may all be present. These findings may become more severe as the disease progresses to include abdominal wall oedema, erythema and ascites. A small proportion of infants with NEC present with a palpable abdominal mass (usually due to matted loops of bowel around an area of gangrene or perforation) and/or persistent intestinal obstruction.

In addition to these gastrointestinal signs, generalized non-specific signs indicative of systemic deterioration or sepsis are often present. In their mildest form, these include temperature instability, hypovolaemia, tachycardia, and mild respiratory distress. In more advanced disease, clinical features of a systemic inflammatory response frequently develop including hypotension requiring inotropes, respiratory failure requiring ventilatory support, coagulopathy and renal failure.

Whilst there are no defining laboratory parameters of use in the diagnosis of NEC, a number of haematological and biochemical abnormalities may be observed including raised or depressed white cell count, thrombocytopenia, metabolic acidosis, glucose instability and elevated C-reactive protein levels [17, 44–46], although none of these are universally present in all cases. There also potentially some other more specific markers of intestinal damage, such as intestinal fatty-acid binding protein [47, 48], but these are not yet suitable for routine clinical use. Urinary and plasma proteomics has identified other potential markers, but again translation to the clinical scenario may take some years [49, 50].

Radiographic imaging is essential in the diagnosis of NEC. The pathognomonic radiological finding is that of pneumatosis intestinalis (Fig. 38.1) representing gas within the wall of the bowel, which is believed to originate from pathogenic bacteria. If this gas becomes absorbed into the mesenteric circulation it may result in the presence of portal venous gas seen as a narrow,

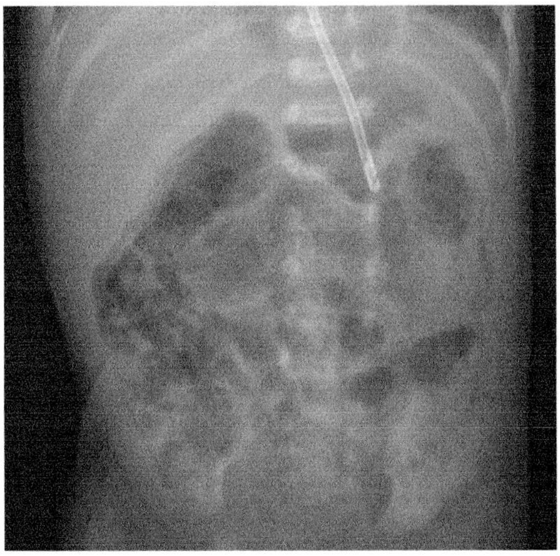

Fig. 38.1 Plain AXR demonstrating pneumatosis intestinalis in an infant with suspected NEC

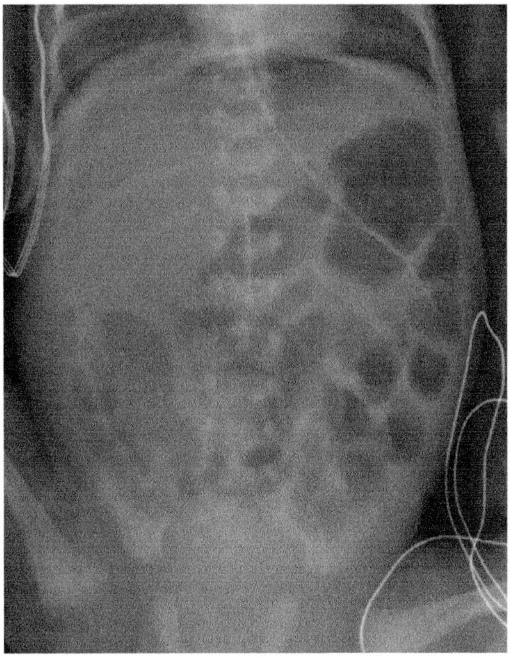

Fig. 38.2 Plain AXR demonstrating pneumoperitoneum in an infant with NEC

linear air-dense area in the hepatic region on X-ray. The most significant radiological finding is that of pneumoperitoneum (Fig. 38.2) resulting from intestinal perforation, as this is a clear indication that surgery is required. Free air may be seen in a number of ways including:

- The football sign (free gas outlining the falciform ligament and umbilical arteries)
- As a triangular gas shadow clearly not within the intestinal lumen often bordered by the subhepatic space and hepatorenal fossa
- As Rigler's sign, in which there is clear visualization of the outer as well as the inner wall of a loop of bowel

In many cases the identification of perforation is challenging and a lateral decubitus or lateral shoot through radiograph may be useful (Fig. 38.3). There are cases in which intestinal perforation may be represented by a completely gasless abdomen and it is not unusual to find a sealed perforation at laparotomy in the absence of free air on the abdominal radio-

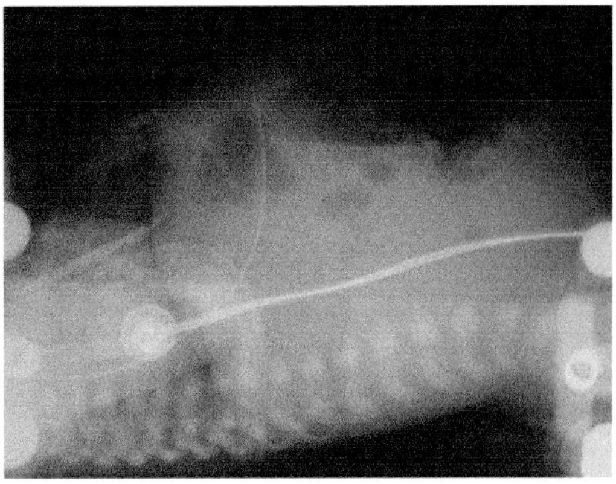

Fig. 38.3 Lateral shoot-through AXR in an infant with NEC demonstrating pneumoperitoneum

graph. An abdominal ultrasound scan may be helpful for diagnosis in these cases. Colour doppler ultrasound has been advocated in some centres, but this requires specific training [51–53] and has the disadvantage of being very operator dependent.

38.5 Staging

This combination of clinical features, laboratory indices and radiological findings have been grouped together to form a staging system (Table 38.2) for NEC known as Bell's staging [54]. The use of such a staging system has been used by some surgeons to select the most appropriate treatment but its value is probably greatest in defining severity of disease in determining the effectiveness of therapy on survival and outcome. Some authors have attempted to define staging on the basis of only radiographic findings [55], but this has not found widespread usage.

38.6 Clinical Management

38.6.1 Medical Management

Most infants with suspected (Bell's Stage I) or less advanced (Stage IIA or B) NEC are managed non-surgically although they may require intensive medical care. This may be described as predominantly supportive as there are no specific treatments for NEC. This supportive treatment includes appropriate ventilatory support, adequate fluid resuscitation, inotropic support as required and correction of acid–base imbalance, coagulopathy, and thrombocytopenia. The intestine is rested and decompressed with a nasogastric tube and broad spectrum antibiotics are given usually for 7–10 days. Antibiotics may be modified appropriately in light of microbiological culture results.

Although there are no specific therapies for NEC, various therapeutic agents or manoeuvres have been tested in experimental models of NEC. These include captopril [56], platelet activating factor antagonists [57], moderate controlled hypothermia [58], and stem cells [59, 60]. However, because of the experimental models studied, it is not clear whether some of these agents are effective at prevention or as therapy. Of note, moderate therapeutic hypothermia was found to be feasible and safe in infants with NEC [61] and a randomised controlled trial to test effectiveness is currently in progress (CoolNEC).

Serial clinical and radiological examination is of extreme importance to monitor progression of disease and detect any evidence of intestinal perforation or other indication for surgical intervention. In the absence of such indication, medical management should continue for 7–10 days depending on severity of illness. Following this, feeds may be slowly reintroduced paying particular attention to feed intolerance suggestive of a repeat episode of NEC or intestinal stricture. From the time of diagnosis to re-establishment of full enteral feeds it is essential to maintain nutritional input with parenteral nutrition (PN) adequate for tissue healing and repair, and body growth.

38.6.2 Surgical Management

Despite aggressive medical treatment, a proportion of infants with NEC require acute surgical intervention. Surgeons differ over indications for surgery since there is the potential to cause serious harm by operating on a fragile, critically unwell preterm infant [62]. Indications for surgery are listed in Table 38.3.

Table 38.2 Modified Bell staging criteria for NEC

Stage	I	IIA	IIB	IIIA	IIIB
Description	Suspected NEC	Mild NEC	Moderate NEC	Severe NEC	Severe NEC
Systemic signs	Temperature instability, apnoea, bradycardia	Similar to stage I	Mild acidosis, thrombocytopenia	Respiratory and metabolic acidosis, mechanical ventilation, hypotension, oliguria, DIC	Further deterioration and shock
Intestinal signs	Increased gastric residuals, mild abdominal distension, occult blood in the stool	Marked abdominal distension ± tenderness, absent bowel sounds, grossly bloody stools	Abdominal wall oedema and tenderness ± palpable mass	Worsening wall oedema with erythema and induration	Evidence of perforation
Radiographic signs	Normal or mild ileus	Ileus, dilated bowel loops, focal pneumatosis	Extensive pneumatosis, early ascites ± PVG	Prominent ascites, fixed bowel loop, no free air	Pneumoperitoneum

Modified from Walsh MC, Kliegman RM. Necrotizing enterocolitis: treatment based on staging criteria. Pediatr Clin North Am 1986;33:179–201; used with permission
DIC disseminated intravascular coagulopathy, *PVG* portal venous gas

Table 38.3 Indications for surgery in acute NEC

Absolute indications
Pneumoperitoneum
Clinical deterioration despite maximal medical treatment
Abdominal mass with persistent intestinal obstruction
Relative indications
Increased abdominal tenderness, distension and/or discolouration
Portal vein gas

The principles of surgical treatment for acute NEC are to remove necrotic intestine and control intra-abdominal sepsis whilst preserving as much intestinal length as possible. Within these principles, a number of surgical options exist and the procedure of choice is somewhat contentious. The traditional surgical approach to NEC has been to perform a laparotomy, resect all areas of necrotic intestine and exteriorize the bowel to allow adequate time for healing and growth before restoring intestinal continuity at a later stage. However, stomas, and in particular ileostomies are poorly tolerated by preterm infants as they may predispose to nutritional and metabolic disturbances and poor growth as a consequence of fluid and electrolyte depletion. Some surgeons therefore advocate primary anastomosis following intestinal resection for NEC wherever possible and this is feasible even in small, critically unwell infants [63]. However, there is no good evidence to support one approach over the other. In children who are unstable during surgery or have intra-operative complications such as haemorrhage the quickest approach is usually preferable; this is usually to fashion a stoma.

Some children have more than one section of bowel affected by NEC, so-called multifocal disease. For this a number of operations have been proposed including multiple resections and multiple primary anastomoses. A 'clip and drop' approach may also be useful in multifocal disease followed 24–48 h later by a 'second-look' laparotomy [64].

Unfortunately a number of infants present at laparotomy with extensive or panintestinal NEC. Surgical options in this scenario are limited and many surgeons would consider withdrawing care faced with an infant with panintestinal gangrene (NEC totalis). However, some infants with very extensive disease may benefit from a high diverting jejunostomy [65].

A final surgical manoeuvre used in infants with perforated NEC is placement of a peritoneal drain. Primary peritoneal drainage (PPD) was initially proposed as a method of stabilizing infants with intestinal perforation prior to definitive surgical treatment [66]. Subsequently, it was reported as definitive treatment for intestinal perforation as some infants required no further surgical treatment [67, 68]. There have been two recent prospective randomised controlled trials investigating the use of PPD in infants with perforated NEC compared to laparotomy [69, 70]. Neither definitely demonstrated an advantage of either PPD or laparotomy over the other, and this was also true when a meta-analysis of the two trials was performed ([69]; Fig. 38.4). However, one study concluded that PPD was not an effective definitive procedure for perforated NEC as its use was followed by a rescue laparotomy in approximately ¾ of the infants [69]. Whether there remains a role for PPD in the stabilisation of a critically unwell child with perforated NEC and respiratory compromise prior to transfer to another centre for a laparotomy remains unclear [71].

The authors' proposed surgical management of NEC is illustrated in Fig. 38.5.

38.7 Outcome

Despite intensive medical and surgical treatment a number of infants do not survive the acute episode of NEC. These fall broadly into two groups: those who have panintestinal disease whose intestine cannot be salvaged and those who have surgically and medically and treatable disease but who develop a significant inflammatory response syndrome resulting in multi-organ dysfunction syndrome. Whilst overall mortality from NEC is may be as high as 35%, birth weight is a significant determinant predictor of mortality such that the mortality from NEC is as high as 42% in infants

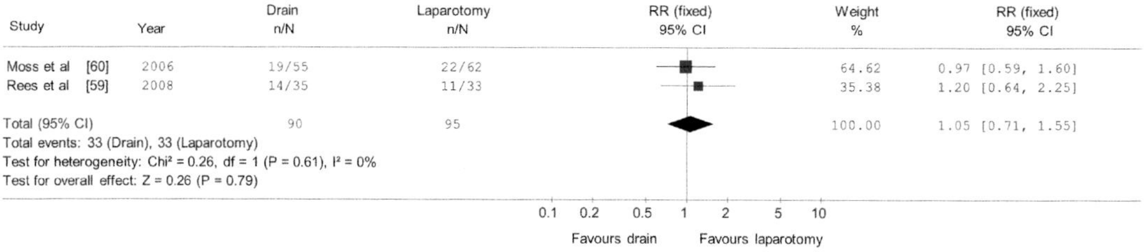

Fig. 38.4 Meta-analysis of primary peritoneal drainage vs. primary laparotomy for NEC. Outcome is mortality. [59, 60]

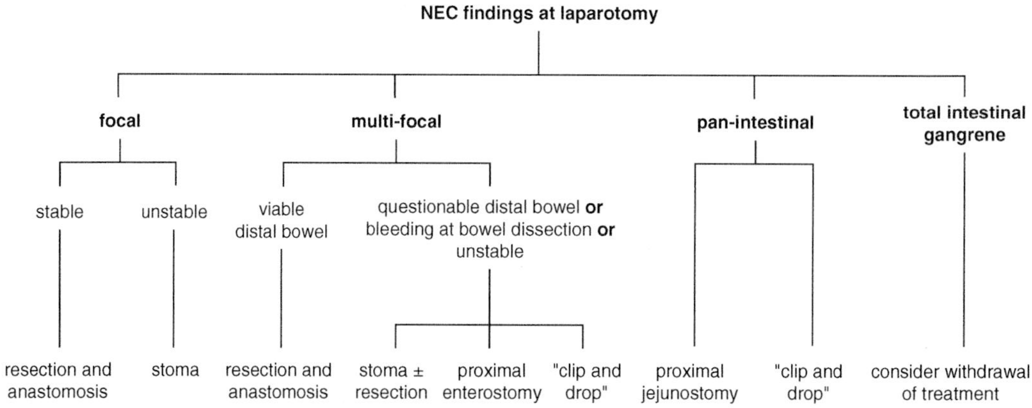

Fig. 38.5 Proposed surgical strategy for NEC. Modified from Pierro A, Hall N. Surgical treatment of infants with necrotizing enterocolitis. Semin Neonatol 2003;8:223–32

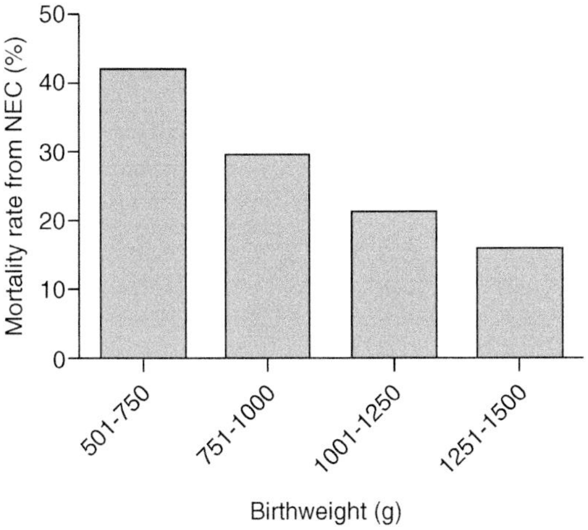

Fig. 38.6 Mortality of NEC by birthweight category [8]

born <750 g [8]. With increasing birth weight, mortality from NEC decreases (Fig. 38.6). However, the mortality of those infants requiring surgery does not seem to be birth weight dependent [7].

In those who survive the acute episode of NEC, a proportion will develop an intestinal stricture either related to medically treated NEC or at the site of a previous anastomosis. Surgical resection of such strictures is usually necessary. Longer term outcome is related to remaining intestinal length and its capacity for adequate nutrient absorption. Malabsorption may result from a variety of factors including gut dysmotility, enzyme deficiency, abnormal intestinal mucosa, bacterial overgrowth, decreased bowel length and vitamin B12 deficiency secondary to ileal resection. Short bowel syndrome is the most serious gastrointestinal complication associated with NEC and great efforts are taken to avoid resection of more bowel length than is absolutely necessary. Supporters of resection and primary anastomosis cite this as one of the advantages over stoma formation.

PN-related complications are commonly encountered in infants with NEC and include sepsis, suppression of the immune response and impairment of liver function. Standard strategies to minimise the risk of these complications are used aggressively as some of these infants may have a long term PN dependency.

In addition to the intestinal sequelae of NEC, it is being increasingly recognised that NEC has a deleterious neurodevelopmental effect, the mechanisms of which are not understood [72, 73]. Whilst it is recognised that many preterm infants suffer from neurodevelopmental impairment, neurodevelopmental outcome appears worse in infants who have had NEC. In addition to the intestinal function following NEC it is essential that this important outcome measure is monitored as we strive towards novel therapeutic strategies that are desperately needed.

References

1. Schmid KO, Quaiser K. Über eine besonders schwer verlaufende Form von Enteritis beim Säugling. Österreichische Zeitschrift für Kinderchirurgie. 1953;114
2. Barlow B, Santulli TV, Heird WC, Pitt J, Blanc WA, Schullinger JN. An experimental study of acute neonatal enterocolitis—the importance of breast milk. J Pediatr Surg. 1974;9:587–95.
3. Lin PW, Stoll BJ. Necrotising enterocolitis. Lancet. 2006;368:1271–83.
4. Rees CM, Eaton S, Pierro A. National prospective surveillance study of necrotizing enterocolitis in neonatal intensive care units. J Pediatr Surg. 2010;45: 1391–7.
5. Lemons JA, Bauer CR, Oh W, Korones SB, Papile LA, Stoll BJ, et al. Very low birth weight outcomes of the National Institute of Child Health and Human Development Neonatal Research Network, January 1995 through December 1996. Pediatrics. 2001;107:art-e1.
6. Ahle M, Drott P, Andersson RE. Epidemiology and Trends of Necrotizing Enterocolitis in Sweden: 1987–2009. Pediatrics. 2013;132:e443–51.
7. Thyoka M, De Coppi P, Eaton S, Hall NJ, Khoo AK, Curry JI, et al. Advanced necrotizing enterocolitis part 1: mortality. Eur J Pediatr Surg. 2012;22(1):8–12.
8. Fitzgibbons SC, Ching Y, Yu D, Carpenter J, Kenny M, Weldon C, et al. Mortality of necrotizing enterocolitis expressed by birth weight categories. J Pediatr Surg. 2009;44:1072–5.
9. Malcolm G, Ellwood D, Devonald K, Beilby R, Henderson-Smart D. Absent or reversed end diastolic flow velocity in the umbilical artery and necrotising enterocolitis. Arch Dis Child. 1991;66:805–7.
10. Sayari AJ, Tashiro J, Sola JE, Perez EA. Blood transfusions, increased rates of surgical NEC, and lower survival: a propensity score-matched analysis. J Pediatr Surg. 2016;51:927–31.
11. Lucas A, Cole TJ. Breast milk and neonatal necrotising enterocolitis. Lancet. 1990;336:1519–23.

12. Meinzen-Derr J, Poindexter B, Wrage L, Morrow AL, Stoll B, Donovan EF, et al. Role of human milk in extremely low birth weight infants' risk of necrotizing enterocolitis or death. J Perinatol. 2009;29:57–62.
13. Vejchapipat P, Eaton S, Fukumoto K, Parkes HG, Spitz L, Pierro A. Hepatic glutamine metabolism during endotoxemia in neonatal rats. Nutrition. 2002;18:293–7.
14. van Acker J, de Smet F, Muyldermans G, Bougatef A, Naessens A, Lauwers S. Outbreak of necrotizing enterocolitis associated with Enterobacter sakazakii in powdered milk formula. J Clin Microbiol. 2001;39:293–7.
15. Rotbart HA, Levin MJ. How contagious is necrotizing enterocolitis? Pediatr Infect Dis. 1983;2:406–13.
16. Scheifele DW. Role of bacterial toxins in neonatal necrotizing enterocolitis. J Pediatr. 1990;117:S44–6.
17. Scheifele DW, Olsen EM, Pendray MR. Endotoxinemia and thrombocytopenia during neonatal necrotizing enterocolitis. Am J Clin Pathol. 1985;83:227–9.
18. Engel RR. Origin of mural gas in necrotizing neterocolitis. Pediatr Res. 1973;7:292.
19. Lawrence G, Bates J, Gaul A. Pathogenesis of neonatal necrotising enterocolitis. Lancet. 1982;1:137–9.
20. Caplan MS, Hsueh W. Necrotizing enterocolitis: role of platelet activating factor, endotoxin, and tumor necrosis factor. J Pediatr. 1990;117:S47–51.
21. Zani A, Cordischi L, Cananzi M, De Coppi P, Smith VV, Eaton S, et al. Assessment of a Neonatal Rat Model of Necrotizing Enterocolitis. Eur J Pediatr Surg. 2008;18:423–6.
22. Warner BB, Deych E, Zhou Y, Hall-Moore C, Weinstock GM, Sodergren E, et al. Gut bacteria dysbiosis and necrotising enterocolitis in very low birthweight infants: a prospective case-control study. Lancet. 2016;387:1928–36.
23. Nino DF, Sodhi CP, Hackam DJ. Necrotizing enterocolitis: new insights into pathogenesis and mechanisms. Nat Rev Gastroenterol Hepatol. 2016;13(10):590–600.
24. Eibl MM, Wolf HM, Furnkranz H, Rosenkranz A. Prevention of necrotizing enterocolitis in low-birth-weight infants by IgA-IgG feeding. N Engl J Med. 1988;319:1–7.
25. Foster J, Cole M. Oral immunoglobulin for preventing necrotizing enterocolitis in preterm and low birth-weight neonates. Cochrane Database Syst Rev 2004;CD001816.
26. Bury RG, Tudehope D. Enteral antibiotics for preventing necrotizing enterocolitis in low birthweight or preterm infants. Cochrane Database Syst Rev 2001;CD000405.
27. Manzoni P, Rinaldi M, Cattani S, Pugni L, Romeo MG, Messner H, et al. Bovine lactoferrin supplementation for prevention of late-onset sepsis in very low-birth-weight neonates: a randomized trial. JAMA. 2009;302:1421–8.
28. Ledbetter DJ, Juul SE. Erythropoietin and the incidence of necrotizing enterocolitis in infants with very low birth weight. J Pediatr Surg. 2000;35:178–81.
29. Tubman TR, Thompson SW, McGuire W. Glutamine supplementation to prevent morbidity and mortality in preterm infants. Cochrane Database Syst Rev 2008;CD001457.
30. Amin HJ, Zamora SA, McMillan DD, Fick GH, Butzner JD, Parsons HG, et al. Arginine supplementation prevents necrotizing enterocolitis in the premature infant. J Pediatr. 2002;140:425–31.
31. Fleming P, Hall NJ, Eaton S. Probiotics and necrotizing enterocolitis. Pediatr Surg Int. 2015;31:1111–8.
32. Lin HC, Hsu CH, Chen HL, Chung MY, Hsu JF, Lien RI, et al. Oral probiotics prevent necrotizing enterocolitis in very low birth weight preterm infants: a multicenter, randomized, controlled trial. Pediatrics. 2008;122:693–700.
33. Samanta M, Sarkar M, Ghosh P, Ghosh J, Sinha M, Chatterjee S. Prophylactic probiotics for prevention of necrotizing enterocolitis in very low birth weight newborns. J Trop Pediatr. 2009;55:128–31.
34. AlFaleh K, Anabrees J. Probiotics for prevention of necrotizing enterocolitis in preterm infants. Evid Based Child Health. 2014;9:584–671.
35. Costeloe K, Hardy P, Juszczak E, Wilks M, Millar MR. Bifidobacterium breve BBG-001 in very preterm infants: a randomised controlled phase 3 trial. Lancet. 2016;387:649–60.
36. Soll RF. Probiotics: are we ready for routine use? Pediatrics. 2010;125:1071–2.
37. Sullivan S, Schanler RJ, Kim JH, Patel AL, Trawoger R, Kiechl-Kohlendorfer U, et al. An exclusively human milk-based diet is associated with a lower rate of necrotizing enterocolitis than a diet of human milk and bovine milk-based products. J Pediatr. 2010;156:562–7.
38. Quigley MA, Henderson G, Anthony MY, McGuire W. Formula milk versus donor breast milk for feeding preterm or low birth weight infants. Cochrane Database Syst Rev 2007;CD002971.
39. Leaf A. Alimentazione del neonato pretermine IUGR: studio multicentrico ADEPT (Abnormal Doppler Enteral Prescription Trial). (Feeding the IUGR premature newborn infant: the multicenter ADEPT study). Minerva Pediatr. 2010;62:31–3.
40. Karagianni P, Briana DD, Mitsiakos G, Elias A, Theodoridis T, Chatziioannidis E, et al. Early versus delayed minimal enteral feeding and risk for necrotizing enterocolitis in preterm growth-restricted infants with abnormal antenatal Doppler results. Am J Perinatol. 2010;27:367–73.
41. Moonen RM, Paulussen AD, Souren NY, Kessels AG, Rubio-Gozalbo ME, Villamor E. Carbamoyl Phosphate Synthetase Polymorphisms as a Risk Factor for Necrotizing Enterocolitis. Pediatr Res. 2007;62:188–90.
42. Treszl A, Tulassay T, Vasarhelyi B. Genetic basis for necrotizing enterocolitis—risk factors and their relations to genetic polymorphisms. Front Biosci. 2006;11:570–80.
43. Sampath V, Le M, Lane L, Patel AL, Cohen JD, Simpson PM, et al. The NFKB1 (g.-24519delATTG) Variant is Associated with Necrotizing Enterocolitis (NEC) in Premature Infants. J Surg Res. 2011;169:E51–7.
44. Ragazzi S, Pierro A, Peters M, Fasoli L, Eaton S. Early full blood count and severity of disease in neonates with necrotizing enterocolitis. Pediatr Surg Int. 2003;19:376–9.

45. Ververidis M, Kiely EM, Spitz L, Drake DP, Eaton S, Pierro A. The clinical significance of thrombocytopenia in neonates with necrotizing enterocolitis. J Pediatr Surg. 2001;36:799–803.
46. Evennett NJ, Alexander N, Petrov M, Pierro A, Eaton S. A systematic review of serologic tests in the diagnosis of necrotizing enterocolitis. J Pediatr Surg. 2009;44:2192–201.
47. Derikx JP, Evennett NJ, Degraeuwe PL, Mulder TL, van Bijnen AA, van Heurn LW, et al. Urine based detection of intestinal mucosal cell damage in neonates with suspected necrotising enterocolitis. Gut. 2007;56:1473–5.
48. Evennett NJ, Hall NJ, Pierro A, Eaton S. Urinary intestinal fatty acid-binding protein concentration predicts extent of disease in necrotizing enterocolitis. J Pediatr Surg. 2010;45:735–40.
49. Ji J, Ling XB, Zhao Y, Hu Z, Zheng X, Xu Z, et al. A data-driven algorithm integrating clinical and laboratory features for the diagnosis and prognosis of necrotizing enterocolitis. PLoS One. 2014;9:e89860.
50. Sylvester KG, Ling XB, Liu GY, Kastenberg ZJ, Ji J, Hu Z, et al. Urine protein biomarkers for the diagnosis and prognosis of necrotizing enterocolitis in infants. J Pediatr. 2014;164:607–12.
51. Faingold R, Daneman A, Tomlinson G, Babyn PS, Manson DE, Mohanta A, et al. Necrotizing enterocolitis: assessment of bowel viability with color doppler US. Radiology. 2005;235:587–94.
52. Silva CT, Daneman A, Navarro OM, Moore AM, Moineddin R, Gerstle JT, et al. Correlation of sonographic findings and outcome in necrotizing enterocolitis. Pediatr Radiol. 2007;37:274–82.
53. Yikilmaz A, Hall NJ, Daneman A, Gerstle JT, Navarro OM, Moineddin R, et al. Prospective evaluation of the impact of sonography on the management and surgical intervention of neonates with necrotizing enterocolitis. Pediatr Surg Int. 2014;30:1231–40.
54. Walsh MC, Kliegman RM. Necrotizing enterocolitis: treatment based on staging criteria. Pediatr Clin North Am. 1986;33:179–201.
55. Coursey CA, Hollingsworth CL, Wriston C, Beam C, Rice H, Bisset G III. Radiographic predictors of disease severity in neonates and infants with necrotizing enterocolitis. AJR Am J Roentgenol. 2009;193:1408–13.
56. Zani A, Eaton S, Leon FF, Malerba A, Hall NJ, De Coppi P, et al. Captopril reduces the severity of bowel damage in a neonatal rat model of necrotizing enterocolitis. J Pediatr Surg. 2008;43:308–14.
57. Lu J, Pierce M, Franklin A, Jilling T, Stafforini DM, Caplan M. Dual roles of endogenous platelet-activating factor acetylhydrolase in a murine model of necrotizing enterocolitis. Pediatr Res. 2010;68:225–30.
58. Stefanutti G, Pierro A, Parkinson EJ, Smith VV, Eaton S. Moderate hypothermia as a rescue therapy against intestinal ischemia and reperfusion injury in the rat. Crit Care Med. 2008;36:1564–72.
59. Tayman C, Uckan D, Kilic E, Ulus AT, Tonbul A, Murat HI, et al. Mesenchymal stem cell therapy in necrotizing enterocolitis: a rat study. Pediatr Res. 2011;70:489–94.
60. Zani A, Cananzi M, Eaton S, Pierro A, De Coppi P. Stem cells as a potential treatment of necrotizing enterocolitis. J Pediatr Surg. 2009;44:659–60.
61. Hall NJ, Eaton S, Peters MJ, Hiorns MP, Alexander N, Azzopardi DV, et al. Mild Controlled Hypothermia in Preterm Neonates With Advanced Necrotizing Enterocolitis. Pediatrics. 2010;125:e300–8.
62. Rees CM, Hall NJ, Eaton S, Pierro A. Surgical strategies for necrotizing enterocolitis: a survey of practice in the United Kingdom. Arch Dis Child. 2005;90:F152–5.
63. Hall NJ, Curry J, Drake DP, Spitz L, Kiely EM, Pierro A. Resection and primary anastomosis is a valid surgical option for infants with necrotizing enterocolitis who weigh less than 1000 g. Arch Surg. 2005;140:1149–51.
64. Ron O, Davenport M, Patel S, Kiely E, Pierro A, Hall NJ, et al. Outcomes of the "clip and drop" technique for multifocal necrotizing enterocolitis. J Pediatr Surg. 2009;44:749–54.
65. Thyoka M, Eaton S, Kiely EM, Curry JI, Drake DP, Cross KM, et al. Outcomes of diverting jejunostomy for severe necrotizing enterocolitis. J Pediatr Surg. 2011;46:1041–4.
66. Book LS, Herbst JJ, Atherton SO, Jung AL. Necrotizing enterocolitis in low-birth-weight infants fed an elemental formula. J Pediatr. 1975;87:602–5.
67. Lessin MS, Luks FI, Wesselhoeft CW Jr, Gilchrist BF, Iannitti D, DeLuca FG. Peritoneal drainage as definitive treatment for intestinal perforation in infants with extremely low birth weight (<750 g). J Pediatr Surg. 1998;33:370–2.
68. Rovin JD, Rodgers BM, Burns RC, McGahren ED. The role of peritoneal drainage for intestinal perforation in infants with and without necrotizing enterocolitis. J Pediatr Surg. 1999;34:143–7.
69. Rees CM, Eaton S, Kiely EM, Wade AM, McHugh K, Pierro A. Peritoneal drainage or laparotomy for neonatal bowel perforation? A randomized controlled trial. Ann Surg. 2008;248:44–51.
70. Moss RL, Dimmitt RA, Barnhart DC, Sylvester KG, Brown RL, Powell DM, et al. Laparotomy versus peritoneal drainage for necrotizing enterocolitis and perforation. N Engl J Med. 2006;354:2225–34.
71. Pierro A, Eaton S, Rees CM, De CP, Kiely EM, Peters MJ, et al. Is there a benefit of peritoneal drainage for necrotizing enterocolitis in newborn infants? J Pediatr Surg. 2010;45:2117–8.
72. Rees CM, Pierro A, Eaton S. Neurodevelopmental outcomes of neonates with medically and surgically treated necrotizing enterocolitis. Arch Dis Child Fetal Neonatal Ed. 2007;92:F193–8.
73. Hintz SR, Kendrick DE, Stoll BJ, Vohr BR, Fanaroff AA, Donovan EF, et al. Neurodevelopmental and growth outcomes of extremely low birth weight infants after necrotizing enterocolitis. Pediatrics. 2005;115:696–703.

Neonatal Intestinal Failure and Transplantation

39

Mikko P. Pakarinen and Antonino Morabito

Abstract

Neonatal intestinal failure is a devastating condition which carries a significant morbidity and mortality. The most important causes of intestinal failure include short bowel syndrome, motility disorders and rare mucosal enteropathies. The management of these complex patients is challenging and requires a multidisciplinary approach for optimal outcomes. Multidisciplinary coordinated efforts are aimed to optimize nutritional, surgical and medical therapy. The main goals of the treatment include assuring adequate growth and development, optimal utilization of the adaptation potential of the remaining bowel in order to achieve intestinal autonomy and effective prevention and treatment of complications. Survival and successful adaptation depends on an early institution of intestinal rehabilitation which consist of liver-sparing parenteral nutrition, careful central venous feeding line management to avoid and control infections and to maintain venous access sites, individualized enteral nutrition, optimal medical management and carefully planned surgical procedures as well as social integration. Recent refinements in surgical, nutritional and medical treatment have been associated with significant reductions in morbidity and improvements in survival. Autologous gastrointestinal reconstruction is a valuable option in selected patients from the very beginning in the planned management of these patients. The resultant reduction in parenteral nutrition requirement limits the extent of the side effects improving both patients' prognosis and quality of life. The great majority of neonates with short bowel syndrome can be weaned from par-

M.P. Pakarinen, MD, PhD (✉)
Children's Hospital, Section of Pediatric and Pediatric Transplantation Surgery,
University Central Hospital, University of Helsinki,
P.O.Box 281, Helsinki 00029, Finland
e-mail: mikko.pakarinen@hus.fi

A. Morabito, MD, FRCS(Ed), FRCS(Eng), FICS
Department of Pediatric Surgery,
University of Florence, Florence, Italy

P.D. Losty et al. (eds.), *Rickham's Neonatal Surgery*, https://doi.org/10.1007/978-1-4471-4721-3_39

enteral nutrition while liver-intestinal transplantation serves as a salvage therapy for those who develop life-threatening complications such as liver failure, central vein thrombosis or recurrent catheter-associated bloodstream infections.

Keywords
Autologous intestinal reconstruction • Intestinal failure • Intestinal transplantation • Neonates • Longitudinal intestinal lengthening and tailoring • Parenteral nutrition • Short bowel syndrome • STEP

39.1 Introduction

Neonatal intestinal failure (IF) refers to any intrinsic intestinal disease leading to an inability to sustaining growth by adequate enteric absorption of fluids, electrolytes and energy. IF carries a significant morbidity and mortality as well as economical burden. The most important causes of IF include short bowel syndrome (SBS), motility disorders and rare mucosal enteropathies. The management of these complex patients is challenging and requires a multidisciplinary approach for optimal outcomes. Recent refinements in surgical management, medical treatment and delivery of parenteral nutrition (PN) have been associated with significant reductions in morbidity and improvements in survival. The great majority of neonates with IF can be weaned from PN while intestinal transplantation serves as a salvage therapy for those who develop life-threatening complications such as liver failure or recurrent catheter-associated bloodstream infections.

39.2 Epidemiology and Mortality

The exact incidence and prevalence figures are difficult to define due to variable definitions of IF but number of patients appears to be increasing. A recent nationwide Italian study reported 0.1% occurrence rate of IF out of 30,353 newborns [1]. Incidence of neonatal IF was 0.05% in a prospective nationwide study covering all of Finland with 60,430 newborns corresponding 46 per 100,000 live births [2]. IF was defined as the need for PN for longer than 4 weeks in both abovementioned studies [1, 2]. A population-based survey from Canada estimated the incidence of surgically treated SBS to be 25 per 100,000 live births [3]. The occurrence of SBS increases along with decreased birth weight and prematurity being 0.7% among low birth weight preterm infants and 1.1% among very low birth weight infants [4].

Before the advent of PN in 1968 IF was a fatal condition [5]. Since then mortality rates have markedly declined and survival rates may currently reach 90% [1, 2, 6–10]. Establishment of special multidisciplinary care teams for neonates with IF appears to be the major contributor for the improved survival rates [11, 12]. During the first 2 years of life the overall and the disease-specific mortality of neonatal SBS is three and five times higher in relation to control cohort with comparable underlying disease characteristics [3]. IF associated mortality has a bimodal distribution [12]. Most of the deaths occur during the first years of life due to underlying disease or surgery associated complications [11, 13]. Recently, a multicenter follow-up of 272 infants reported 73% 5-year survival rate [85]. Delayed complications of IF such as intestinal failure associated liver disease (IFALD) and sepsis due to catheter-associated bloodstream infections and bacterial translocation from the intestine continue to cause mortality among long-term survivors requiring PN [84]. A 5 years survival rate of

95% has been reported for IF patients weaned from PN by the age of 2.5 years as opposed to 52% for those not weaned [14]. In addition to weaning off PN, occurrence of cholestasis (conjugated bilirubin > 2.5 mg/dL) and short age-adjusted small bowel length (< 10% of normal) is the major predictors of mortality in pediatric SBS [11, 15]. The overall mortality is higher in neonates with severe motility disorders and mucosal enteropathies as the underlying cause for IF in relation to those with SBS [16].

39.3 Definition

Neonatal IF is defined as any intrinsic intestinal disease leading to an inability to sustain hydration, electrolyte, nutrient and energy balance, growth and development by adequate enteric absorption. The definition may also be based on the absolute or age-adjusted length and anatomy of the remaining bowel, the extent and duration of PN requirement, factual intestinal absorptive capacity or fecal energy loss [12, 15, 17]. In the literature, the duration of PN requirement signifying IF usually ranges from 28 to 42 days and from two to 6 months [1, 2, 8, 10, 11, 13]. The percentage of normal age-adjusted bowel length may be a stronger predictor of weaning from PN than absolute length of the remaining intestine, which depends on gestational age of a neonate [15, 18]. Age-specific norms for intestinal length in children are available [18]. A commonly used limit for neonatal SBS is a residual small intestinal length less than 25% of predicted for gestational age [3, 10, 13]. Citrulline is a nonessential amino acid that is principally synthesized by small bowel enterocytes. Serum citrulline concentration reflects small intestinal mucosal mass and enteral feeding tolerance and may be used as a biomarker to define the degree of IF [19–21]. Among pediatric IF patients a serum citrulline positively correlates with the length of the remaining small intestine and a level below 12 μmol/L is strongly predictive of permanent dependence of PN [19–21].

By definition, IF results in prolonged dependence of PN regardless of the underlying intestinal disease which greatly modulates the natural history on IF. PN may be partial or total and temporary or permanent. Most neonates with IF can be weaned from PN whereas others require partial or total PN for several years or even permanently. Some patients develop complications especially during long-term PN including liver failure and catheter-related sepsis. These patients may be considered as candidates for intestinal transplantation.

39.4 Causes of Intestinal Failure

The causes of IF and their relative frequencies are outlined in Table 39.1. The frequency distribution of the underlying intestinal diseases varies by different centers while SBS, severe motility disorders and mucosal enteropathies account for the majority of cases [1, 2, 14, 17, 22]. Different etiologies may coexist in one patient. Clearly, the most common cause for neonatal IF is SBS characterized by reduction of functional gut mass (or length) below the minimal amount necessary for

Table 39.1 Etiology of neonatal intestinal failure

Short bowel syndrome (70–90%)
Necrotizing enterocolitis
Malrotation midgut volvulus
Adhesive volvulus
Small intestinal atresia
Gastroscihis
Operative complications
Severe intestinal motility disorders (5–20%)
Chronic intestinal pseudo-obstruction
Extensive aganglionosis (Hirschsprung)
Intestinal neuronal dysplasia
Autoimmune
Mitochondrial cytopathies
Epithelial diseases of the small intestine (5–10%)
Epithelial dysplasia
Mikrovillus atrophy
Autoimmune enteropathy

adequate digestive and absorptive capacity associated with rapid intestinal transit. SBS may result from resection, disease related intestinal loss or congenital short bowel. The primary etiologies of neonatal SBS include necrotizing enterocolitis, intestinal atresia, gastroschisis and malrotation with mid-gut volvulus [1–3, 12].

Severe intestinal motility disorders result in recurrent or chronic intestinal obstruction in the absence of mechanical occlusion due to impaired motor activity and peristalsis. Of these total colonic aganglionosis (Hirschsprung disease) with extended jejuno-ileal involvement and chronic intestinal pseudo-obstruction are relatively common causes of IF [1, 2, 10, 14, 22]. Chronic intestinal pseudo-obstruction is very heterogenous condition including neuropathic and myopathic forms with or without urinary tract involvement [23, 24]. Megacystis microcolon intestinal hypoperistalsis syndrome represents a rare and severe form of dysmotile intestinal obstruction in the newborn resulting in IF in the vast majority of cases [24].

Mucosal enteropathies, which often result in IF include congenital diseases of enterocyte development such as microvillus atrophy and intestinal epithelial dysplasia [17]. Autoimmune enteropathy is characterized by a defect in regulatory T-cells and immune dysregulation and may respond to immunosuppressive therapy [17].

39.5 Pathophysiology

39.5.1 Adaptation

With time the majority of neonates with SBS can be weaned from PN which is the mainstay of treatment. Weaning from parenteral to full enteral nutrition is possible due to intestinal adaptation which refers to structural and functional changes following resection resulting in a gradual increase in absorptive capacity of the remaining bowel. The adaptation process is well characterized in experimental animals [25]. Enlargement of diameter and length of the remaining bowel as well as increase in villus height and crypt depth result in enlargement of intestinal absorptive surface both at macroscopic and microscopic level [25]. These adaptation mechanisms appear to occur also in human neonates [26], although systematic studies are missing. Clinically, postresectional adaptation-related bowel dilatation often occurs to an extent which impairs intestinal peristaltic function predisposing to bacterial overgrowth, malabsorption and unprogressive weaning from PN.

The amount, anatomy and functional state of the remaining intestine as well as the etiology of IF essentially influences the possibility of achieving intestinal autonomy. Predictors of prolonged PN dependence are shown in Table 39.2. The chances for weaning off PN are markedly worse in children with severe intestinal dysmotility disorders or congenital enteropathies when compared to those with SBS as an underlying cause for IF [10, 16, 22–24, 86]. While the majority neonates with SBS achieve intestinal autonomy, most of those with intestinal dysmotility or microvillus atrophy and intestinal epithelial dysplasia remain dependent on PN [16, 22, 86]. In SBS the remaining bowel is most often functionally intact enabling adaptation, whereas primarily and permanently diseased intestine in motility disorders and enteropathies rarely improves with time and is highly resistant to various modes of medical and surgical treatment.

Among neonates with SBS, the length of the remaining small intestine is strongly correlated with PN dependence being the most important single predictor of PN dependence [6, 16, 27–29]. In general, the presence of ileocecal valve (ICV) and residual colon or ileum are associated with shorter duration of PN and improved chances of weaning off PN [6, 15,

Table 39.2 Predictors of prolonged PN duration in neonatal intestinal failure

Remaining small intestinal length <40 cm <10% of age adjusted
Resected ileocecal valve
No remaining ileum
No or short remaining colon
End ostomy
Dysmotility or epithelial disorder as etiology

27–29]. The vast majority of neonates with more than 35–40 cm of small bowel remaining eventually achieve intestinal autonomy [6, 27, 28]. In a material of 135 neonates with SBS, 40% of those with less than 40 cm residual small bowel and without ICV remained dependent on PN after 8 years, whereas 80% of those with 40–80 cm residual small bowel and an intact ICV were weaned off PN within 1 year [30]. Among 272 infants with a mean residual small intestinal length of 41 cm 47% weaned off PN by 5 years [85]. However, a wide variance exists and some neonates wean off PN with as little as 10 cm of small intestine below the ligament of Treitz [31]. Some of this variance may be explained by rapid in utero growth of small intestinal length, doubling during the last trimester of gestation [18]. Accordingly, instead of the absolute length, the percentage of normal age-adjusted bowel length may be a more accurate determinant of weaning from PN [15, 18]. Functional destruction of the remaining intestine may prolong PN despite favorable anatomy. For example, motility of the remaining bowel may be impaired due to ischemic injury and scarring in necrotizing enterocolitis.

Retained ICV restrains colonization of the small intestinal lumen by colonic bacteria and subsequent development of bacterial overgrowth and is beneficial by slowing transit. Because the presence of ICV in the clinical setting is almost invariably associated with partly retained ileum, some of the beneficial functional effects of ICV may be, in fact, mediated by the residual ileum. Even a short segment of preserved ileum is advantageous in several ways. Active absorption of conjugated bile acids and vitamin B_{12} is confined to the distal ileum. Interruption of the enterohepatic circulation of bile acids results in impaired micelle formation and malabsorption of fat and fat-soluble vitamins. In children with SBS significant malabsorption of bile acids continues after weaning off PN being markedly more severe among those without any remaining ileum [32]. The ileum is capable of acquiring absorption functions that occur in the proximal small intestine under physiological conditions, such as absorption of cholesterol [33]. In addition to its ability to absorb water and electrolytes, residual colon has been shown to significantly increase energy absorption in adults with SBS by metabolizing carbohydrates to short chain fatty acids which are effectively absorbed from the colon [34].

39.5.2 Bacterial Overgrowth

In children with SBS, PN dependence is prolonged by development of bacterial overgrowth [12, 17, 35]. Bacterial overgrowth exacerbates intestinal malabsorption by causing mucosal injury, by metabolizing intraluminal nutrients and by deconjugating bile acids [36]. Deconjugation interferes absorption of bile acids, which leads to disruption of digestion and absorption of lipids (see above). Moreover, bacterial overgrowth predisposes to bacterial translocation through inflamed and damaged intestinal epithelium with increased permeability and may thereby contribute to development of IFALD [36, 37, 87]. D-Lactic acidosis is relatively common consequence of bacterial overgrowth as a result of the production of D-lactic acid by gram-positive anaerobes [12, 16, 36]. Signs of D-lactic acidosis in neonates include an anion gap acidosis with low L-lactate combined with neurological symptoms such as ataxia and altered level of consciousness.

Bacterial overgrowth is a frequent complication occurring in up to 60% of children with SBS [35]. It is associated with abdominal distension, vomiting, increased intestinal excretions, diarrhea and poor progression of enteral feedings. Bacterial overgrowth may involve a single episode, but often become a recurrent chronic problem. The first diagnosis is most often made by the second year of life [35]. Ideally, the diagnosis should be based on direct cultures of small intestinal aspirates or hydrogen breath test. However, interpretation of these methods has significant limitations in SBS [36] and may be impossible to perform among neonates.

A dilated small intestinal segment with impaired motility, resection of ICV and an intestinal stricture causing partial occlusion predispose to bacterial overgrowth. Symptomatic dilatation of the small bowel or stricture should undergo prompt surgical treatment after radiological confirmation. If this is not possible, intermittent enteral antimicrobial therapy including metronidazole, amoxicillin-clavulanic acid, trimethoprim-sulfamethoxazole or fluconazole is usually effective [10, 35, 36]. Instead of bacterial eradication, the goal of antibiotic treatment is to modify bacterial flora enough to improve symptoms. The use of broad-spectrum antibiotic should be as limited as possible in order to avoid development of multiresistant strains. Restriction of dietary carbohydrates is advisable to decrease fermentative diarrhea and to prevent D-lactic acidosis [38]. Currently, the use of probiotics is controversial because they are capable of translocating into blood stream and causing sepsis [12].

39.5.3 Intestinal Failure Associated Liver Disease

Depending on definition, IFALD occurs in up to 60–80% of neonates with IF, who require prolonged PN [1, 2, 13, 39]. Biochemical signs include conjugated hyperbilirubinemia associated with increased gamma glutamyl transferase and aminotransferases. Histology of IFALD in neonates involves cholestasis, periportal inflammation, and steatosis, and may progress to bile duct proliferation, fibrosis and biliary cirrhosis leading to liver failure [40]. Biochemical cholestasis is not well correlated with the presence or degree of histologically observed liver fibrosis, which a common finding after long-term PN despite well preserved biochemical liver function [41, 42, 88]. Despite resolution of cholestasi and portal inflammation, liver fibrosis and steatosis persists in about half of the patients after weaning off PN [88, 89]. Although laboratory markers of liver function usually normalize after weaning off PN liver histology remains abnormal for years in the majority of patients. At present, the clinical significance of persistent histological changes of the liver remains unclear, but clearly point to ongoing need to follow up these children also after weaning off PN.

Jaundice is the hallmark and usually the first clinical sign of IFALD. Cholelithiasis may occur in form of biliary sludge especially among neonates. Portal hypertension and associated esophageal varices with splenomegaly and hyperpslenism as well as decrease in liver-derived coagulation factors as a sign of impaired hepatic synthetic capacity are usually observed late in the disease course. Neonates who develop jaundice or signs of IFAL require full biochemical work up with hepatobiliary ultrasound examination and liver biopsy if any diagnostic uncertainty remains.

The cause of IFALD is multifactorial and still incompletely understood [40]. Etiological factors are displayed in Table 39.3. Bacterial overgrowth and increased intestinal permeability may provide mechanisms causing and maintaining IFALD [88]. In mice, PN-induced increase in permeability promotes Toll-like receptor dependent Kupffer cell activation and liver injury, presumably due to bacterial translocation [87]. In children with SBS, infections, loss of the ileocecal valve, bowel dilatation and impaired motility are know risk factors of bacterial overgrowth and histological liver injury [88]. A plant sterol, stigmasterol, a component of soy and olive oil PN lipid emulsions, promotes cholestasis, hepatic macrophage activation and liver injury in mice [90]. In neonates, serum stigmasterol content parallels the amount and duration of PN and correlates positively with direct bilirubin concentration [2]. Immaturity of liver function in neonates may explain their susceptibility to IFALD over

Table 39.3 Risk factors of intestinal failure associated liver disease

Short intestinal remnant
Duration of parenteral nutrition
Lack of enteral feeding
Interrupted enterohepatic circulation
Prematurity and low-birth weight
Recurrent sepsis
Bacterial overgrowth
Excess parenteral glucose
Excess parenteral fat
Excess parenteral plant sterols
Soy bean based parenteral fat emulsion
Lack of parenteral ω[omega]-3 fatty acids

older children. Preventive measures consist of avoiding excessive parenteral energy especially as intravenous fat infusions, cyclic PN infusions, enteral feeding, avoidance and prompt treatment of infectious complications and management of bacterial overgrowth. Delivery of parenteral fat may be restricted to every other day or discontinued especially during episodes of sepsis. Neonates tolerate well interruption of PN infusion for up to several hours without hypoglycemia as long as enteral feedings are continued during the break. Routine assessment of liver function is mandatory in neonatal IF. Ursodeoxycholic acid 10–30 mg/kg/day may improve biochemical signs of cholestasis and jaundice [43]. Optimal dosing, duration of therapy and effect on outcomes concerning IFALD remain unclear.

With progression of enteral feedings or modification of PN, biochemical cholestasis resolves in majority of patients. This is first reflected by a normalization of bilirubin followed by a delayed resolution of aminotransferases. On the other hand, persistent elevation of bilirubin has an adverse prognosis and it is an independent predictor of liver failure in neonatal SBS [40, 44]. The probability of liver failure is at least 36% for a total bilirubin level of 6 mg (102 μmol/L) between 3 and 6 months age [44].

39.6 Management of Intestinal Failure

Neonatal IF is currently managed by multidisciplinary coordinated efforts aimed to optimize nutritional, surgical and medical therapy. The main goals of the treatment include assuring adequate growth and development, optimal utilization of the adaptation potential of the remaining bowel in order to achieve intestinal autonomy and effective prevention and treatment of complications. Survival depends on an early (at diagnosis) institution of intestinal rehabilitation which consist of liver-sparing PN, careful central venous feeding line management to avoid and control infections and to maintain venous access sites, individualized enteral nutrition, optimal medical management and carefully planned non-transplant surgery as well as social integration. Expertise on liver and intestinal transplantation should be readily available for a small proportion of children who develop potentially fatal complications during their management.

39.6.1 Parenteral Nutrition

PN is used to compensate for intestinal fluid loses and to provide adequate nutritional intake of energy, vitamins and micronutrients for normal growth while minimizing adverse effects [12, 17, 30]. It should ensure positive energy balance, sufficient protein synthesis and adaptation of the remaining bowel while preventing nutritional deficiencies [30]. PN is tailored for individual requirements while amount and composition of parenteral energy is adjusted based on weight gain, head circumference, growth and liver function. Excessive parenteral energy either as fat (>1 g/kg/day) or glucose (>12–14 g/kg/day) should be avoided. Stable neonates with IF seldom require parenteral energy over 80–90 kcal/kg/day for adequate growth. Fat and water soluble vitamins and trace elements are routinely supplemented as a part of PN.

Soy oil-based lipid emulsion has been identified as a risk factor of cholestatic liver disease, putatively due to its high omega-6 fatty acid and plant sterol, especially stigmasterol, content [40]. As omega-3 fatty acids are associated with reversal of cholestasis, use of fish oil, which is devoid of plant sterols and high in omega-3 fatty acids may be beneficial. A number of studies have reported beneficial properties of fish oil either alone or in combination with other lipids [45]. These studies indicate that use of fish oil emulsion as PN lipid source among neonates with IF is associated with decreased occurrence of cholestasis as well as faster and higher rate of recovery from IFALD [45–48]. It is plausible that benefits of fish oil are mediated by reduced lipid and plant sterol administration rather than omega-3 fatty acids [90, 91]. Although exact dosing and optimal combination with other lipid sources are currently unclear, fish oil emulsions appear to be beneficial in the treatment of IF and should be considered at least for patients with anticipated prolonged duration of PN and for those who develop PN associated cholestasis [46]. Fish oil is not an universal solution for IFALD and an optimally balanced lipid product remains to be established. Both olive oil based lipid preparations and SMOF have less omega-6 fatty acids and plant sterols in relation to soy oil. In relation to soy base emulsions, olive oil is rich in omega-9 fattyacids and an antioxidant α-tocopherol and poor in omega-6 fattyacids and plant sterols. Combination of fish oil with olive oil based lipid emulsion may be especially beneficial in neonates with SBS by providing sufficiently energy, omega-3 fatty acids and α-tocopherol and lesser amounts of plant sterols and omega-6 fatty acids [2, 49].

39.6.2 Catheter-Related Sepsis and Thrombosis

Patients with IF and dependent on PN require a reliable central venous (CV) access to survive. Four main routes are available for CV catheter insertion: subclavian, external jugular, internal jugular and femoral vein. The superior vena cava is the preferred location which should always be confirmed by radiologic evaluation. Regardless of the method of insertion, every effort avoiding contamination and preserving the vessel used for insertion should be made. Despite careful care, complications are common including infections, mechanical complications and trombosis.

Central line-associated bloodstream infection is a too common complication of central line use and strict protocols to maintain CV catheter should be implemented. With any suspicion of infection a blood culture at least through the central line should be taken. The single most common organism isolated is coagulase-negative Staphylococci followed by Enterococci, Staphylococcus aureus and Candida sp. The catheter should be replaced if the patients' condition does not improve after 24–48 h therapy with broad-spectrum antibiotics or if signs of cardiovascular instability develop. Antimicrobial therapy is narrowed according to antibiotic sensitivity. Effective prevention central line infections is possible with antibiotic, taurolidine or ethanol locks [50]. Ethanol and taurolidine avoids the problem of antibiotic resistance and over four-fold reduction of central line infection rate has been reported by ethanol lock therapy administered 3 days per week [51].

Fibrin deposition, which is also a source for microbial colonization, is the most common cause of central line occlusion [52]. Ultrasonography is combined with venography if diagnostic uncertainty remains. Catheters occluded by a fibrin sheet or intraluminal blood clot usually reopens by fibrinolytic agents such as alteplase. Venous thrombosis related to CV catheter requires anticoagulation with subcutaneous low molecular weight heparin or intravenous unfractioned heparin [52]. After initial therapy both K-vitamin antagonists and low molecular weight heparin can be used to prevent recurrent venous thrombosis and loss of central venous access sites. A blockage secondary to drug precipitate or PN components often responds to 70% ethanol solution left in the catheter's lumen for 1 h. This procedure can be repeated on a daily basis.

39.6.3 Enteral Nutrition and Medical Treatment

Enteral nutrition is essential in the management of neonatal SBS. As much nutrition as possible should be provided via the intestine while overfeeding should be avoided [92]. In addition to promoting intestinal adaptation, enteral nutrition prevents IFALD by stimulating hepatobiliary axis and by preventing translocation of enteric bacteria by supporting mucosal integrity. An optimal formula for enteral nutrition in pediatric IF has not been established. Most of those who achieve intestinal autonomy continue to require a significant surplus of dietary energy up to 50% above normal requirement combined with supplementations of fat-soluble vitamins (A,D,E,K) and vitamin B_{12} trace elements such as zinc, selenium and magnesium according to their serum concentrations. Close and long-term follow-up of these children is mandatory.

Enteral feedings are started as soon as possible and advanced gradually as tolerated. PN is tapered proportionally to increased enteral intake. Advancement of enteral feeds may be based on a predetermined limit of intestinal excretions such as 50 mL/kg/day. Other prerequisites include positive fluid balance, adequate growth and an absence of perineal rash due to excessive diarrhea. To assure optimal water absorption and to control high-volume intestinal excretions, enteral sodium supplementation may be used with a starting dose of 4 mmol/kg/day to an extent to keep urinary sodium above 30 mmol/L. Oral feeding is important in order to establish prerequisite for development of eating skills and to avoid food aversion. It may also promote intestinal adaptation by stimulating secretion of salivary epidermal growth factor and pancreaticobiliary secretion. At leas a part of enteral feeds should be given orally whenever possible. If progression of enteral bolus feeds fails, continuous enteral feeding is an effective way to increase mucosal contact time and intestinal absorption [30, 53]. Initially a significant portion of enteral nutrition is often delivered via nasogastric tube or, preferentially, via percutaneous endoscopic feeding gastrostomy. Excessive tube feeding may aggravate bowel dilatation and bacterial overgrowth especially in patients with dysmotile intestine [84, 92]. Transgastric or open feeding jejunostomies are reserved for those with impaired gastric emptying. To improve intestinal adaptation in newborns with SBS, breast milk is incorporated to enteral formulas that mainly consist of preparations containing hydrolyzed protein and medium chain triglycerides. Breast milk contains beneficial immunomodulatory factors as well as growth hormone and epidermal growth factor, which may promote intestinal adaptation [54]. Solid foods are started at the age of 4–6 months to improve eating skills while enteral formula may be changed to a more energy-dense low osmolar whole protein preparation.

Composition of enteral feeds is modified individually according to tolerance and anatomy of the remaining intestine. For example, in patients with colon in continuity soluble fibers such as pectin may be beneficial [30]. Soluble fibers are fermented into short chain fatty acids which are absorbed in the colon providing energy [34]. Because short chain fatty acids stimulate electrolyte and water absorption soluble fibers can be expected to increase stool consistency in patients with remaining colon [10, 30]. Gastric hypersecretion of acid and fluid following massive small intestinal resection is a result of decreased intestinal gastrin catabolism and hypergastrinemia. Increased gastric fluid secretion contributes to increased intestinal water and electrolyte loses while increased acid secretion decreases luminal pH leading to bile acid precipitation and subsequently impaired micelle formation as well as inactivation of pancreatic enzymes impairing lipid absorption. Gastric acid hypersecretion responds to proton pump inhibitors and adequate lipid digestion can be ascertained with enteral pancreatic enzyme substitution. Rapid intestinal transit associated with SBS may be treated empirically with antimotility agents such as loperamide and clonidine. However, their use may exacerbate abdominal distension and symptoms of bacterial overgrowth.

Proadaptive medication aims to pharmacologically enhance intestinal adaptation beyond physiological level by improving absorptive function and growth of the intestinal remnant. Glucagon-like-peptide 2 have been show to decrease PN requirement and increase villus height among adults with SBS [55]. Beneficial proadaptive effects have been described for recombinant human growth hormone and epidermal growth factor in small pilot studies of children with SBS [56, 57]. Unfortunately, sustained treatment effect requires continuing therapy and clinical value of currently available pharmacological proadative regimens in pediatric SBS remains unclear.

39.6.4 Surgical Principles and Initial Operative Management

The main principles in surgical treatment of SBS include bowel preservation, recruitment of all available absorptive surface into intestinal continuity, bowel lengthening surgery and intestinal transplantation. Possible intestinal strictures and fistulas are treated according to standard surgical principles.

At the initial operation every effort is made in order the conserve as much viable bowel as possible. In cases of uncertain bowel viability only frankly necrotic bowel is removed and a second look operation is performed after 24–48 h following resuscitation. During this time the margins of intestinal necrosis delineate more clearly facilitating the decision making for additional resections. The anatomy and length of the remaining bowel should be recorded in detail to guide later treatment. Continuity of the entire intestinal tract is established without any unnecessary delay after stabilization of general status and confirmation of adequate pulmonary function. Re-establishment of intestinal continuity brings all remaining bowel to contact with luminal chyme, which is the most important single factor promoting intestinal adaptation.

The inherent predisposition for dilatation can be exploited by generating controlled expansion of the remaining bowel as part of the initial management of short bowel among neonates with less than 45 cm of the remaining small bowel with the poorest changes of spontaneous adaptation [58, 59, 94]. A large tube is passed into the end of proximal and distal bowel and brought out onto the abdominal wall (Fig. 39.1). The proximal tube is clamped for an increasing period of time for achieving controlled bowel obstruction driven dilatation. Proximal stoma effluent is recycled via tube into the distal intestine. In 20–24 weeks time the remaining bowel dilates enough to perform a lengthening procedure.

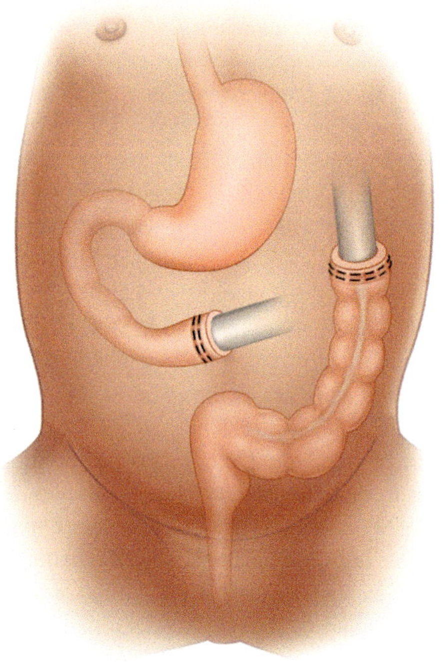

Fig. 39.1 The inherent predisposition for dilatation can be exploited by generating controlled expansion of the remaining bowel as part of the initial management of short bowel among neonates with less than 45 cm of the remaining small bowel. A large tube is passed into the end of proximal and distal bowel and brought out onto the abdominal wall. The proximal tube is clamped for an increasing period of time for achieving controlled bowel obstruction driven dilatation. Clamping is performed at each oral feed aiming to have the tube closed between feeds e.g. for 3–4 h. Proximal stoma effluent is recycled via tube into the distal intestine. In 20–24 weeks the remaining bowel dilates enough to perform a lengthening procedure

Neonates with a rare form of Hirschsprung disease where aganlionosis extends to or beyond the duodenojejunal flexure are very difficult to manage. Removal of the entire aganglionic bowel would result in intractable short bowel without changes for adaptation. These patients can be salvaged by myectomy-myotomy of the retained proximal jejenum as initially described by Ziegler [60]. After histological confirmation of the transitional zone by multilevel biopsies, the entire aganglionic bowel is resected excluding 40 cm of the proximal jejunum which is brought to the abdominal as a jejunostomy. Few weeks later antimesenteric myectomy-myotomy of the aganglionic segment is performed. In addition to providing perquisite for stable PN without massive stomal fluid losses, the operation facilitates significant enteral tolerance preventing development of liver disease [60, 86]. Maintenance of abdominal domain by distending small bowel also aids in preparation for intestinal transplantation [86].

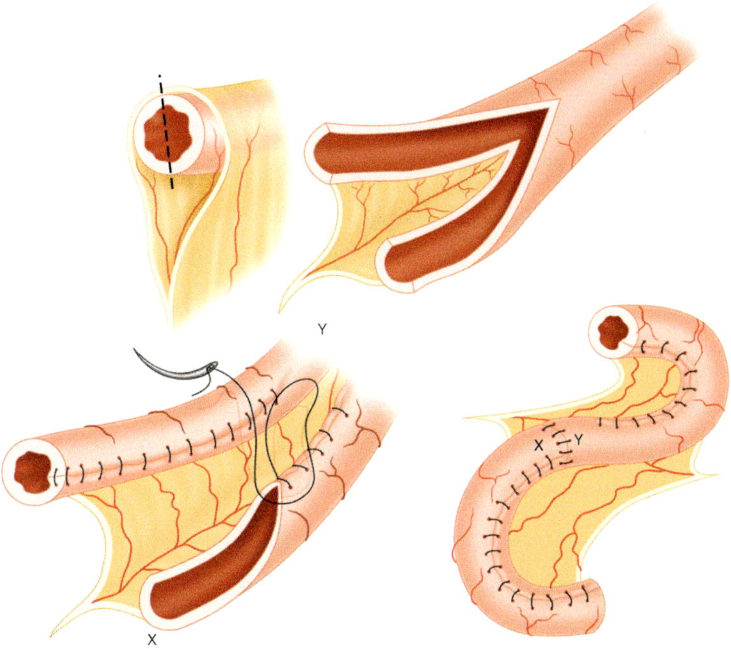

Fig. 39.2 In the LILT procedure the mesentery supplying the dilated small bowel segment is bluntly dissected into two leaves. The bowel is then divided longitudinally between the two leaves, preserving with each half the associated mesentery and blood supply. Each half is remodeled into a tube either by performing longitudinal division of the bowel with a surgical stapler or by suturing. These two hemi-loops of bowel, each with half of the original diameter, are then anastomosed end to end in an isoperistaltic fashion, doubling the length of the dilated segment

39.6.5 Autologous Intestinal Reconstruction

Non-transplant surgery or bowel lengthening may be regarded as a process, potentially involving more than one procedure, aiming to achieve enteral autonomy [58, 61]. This process is better known as autologous gastrointestinal reconstruction (AGIR), which is used as adjunct to medical management for a selected group of children with SBS who reach a plateau in advancement of their enteral nutrition, develop bowel dilatation and bacterial overgrowth [58, 61, 93]. The goal of AGIR is to improve intestinal absorption and facilitate enteral autonomy by manipulation of existing dilated bowel remnant [58, 61]. The resultant reduction in PN requirement limits the extent of the side effects improving both patients' prognosis and quality of life. The principle of AGIR relies on postresectional adaptation-induced bowel dilatation, which often occurs beyond physiological level impairing intestinal function by causing impaired motility, obstruction, stasis and bacterial overgrowth. The most widely used AGIR procedures in children today include longitudinal intestinal lengthening and tailoring (LILT) and serial transverse enteroplasty (STEP). Operations such as colonic interposition, intestinal segment reversal, recirculating loops, artificial valves and the Iowa procedure are associated with less predictable outcomes and are more rarely used.

The modern era of AGIR started after Bianchi published his LILT procedure in 1980 [62]. The mesentery supplying the dilated bowel segment is bluntly dissected into two leaves (Fig. 39.2). The bowel is then divided longitudinally between the two leaves, preserving with each half the associated mesentery and blood supply. Each half is remodeled into a tube either by performing longitudinal division of the bowel with a surgical stapler or by suturing. These two hemi-loops of bowel, each with half of the original diameter, are then anastomosed end to end in an isoperistaltic fashion, doubling the length of the dilated segment.

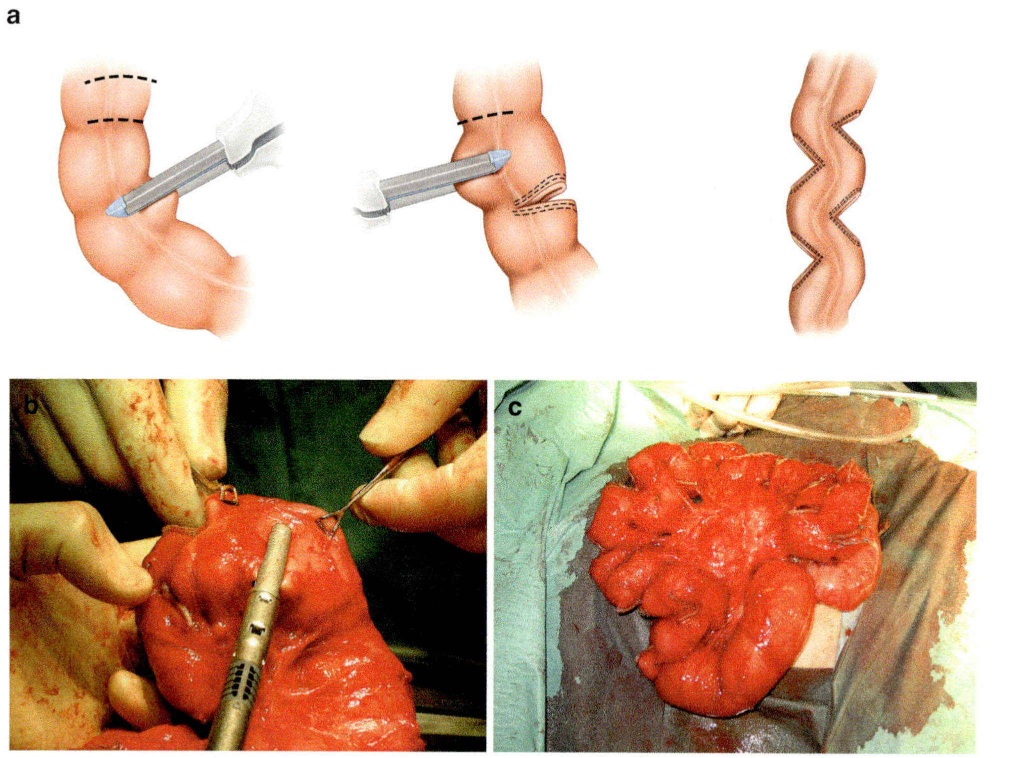

Fig. 39.3 (**a**) The STEP procedure is performed by firing linear staplers alternatively from the mesenteric and anti-mesenteric edge perpendicular to the long axis of the dilated small bowel. (**b**) Small openings in the mesentery are created at each point of stapler application. The distance between subsequent firings of the stapler is guided by the normal diameter of the small bowel being approximately 2 cm. (**c**) The length of the dilated bowel segment increases depending on the degree of dilatation. In this case of combined small bowel atresia and gastroschisis the length doubled after STEP performed at the age of 8 months. The initial length of the remaining proximal small bowel was 30 cm with an absent ileocecal valve. The patient weaned off parenteral nutrition at the age of 3 years 5 months after repeat STEP procedure

Kim et al. initially described the STEP procedure in 2003 [63]. The operation is performed by firing linear staplers alternatively from the mesenteric and anti-mesenteric edge perpendicular to the long axis of the dilated small bowel (Fig. 39.3). Small openings in the mesentery are created at each point of stapler application. The distance between subsequent firings of the stapler is guided by the normal diameter of the small bowel being approximately 2 cm. The length of the dilated bowel segment increases depending on the degree of dilatation even more than 100% [64]. The STEP can be performed on both symmetrical and asymmetrical bowel for example after previous LILT surgery.

Patient selection for AGIR surgery has clarified during the recent years. Autologous gastrointestinal reconstruction is not the last resort in the treatment of short bowel, but valuable option from the very beginning in the planned management of these patients. The main indication is persistent dependency of PN without evidence of further adaptation (progression of enteral nutrition) despite optimized medical therapy with the presence of dilated remaining small intestine. In addition to a radiological gastrointestinal contrast study, magnetic resonance imaging enterography provides useful information in preoperative assessment of the remaining bowel. The STEP is an effective surgical treatment for recalcitrant bacterial overgrowth with or without d-lactic acidosis in the setting of SBS and in neonatal bowel obstruction associated with marginal small bowel length that would be further compromised by simple tapering such as intestinal atresia [61, 65]. Patient assessment for AGIR should be performed before development of liver disease. End-stage liver failure is a clear contraindication for bowel lengthening procedures [66, 67], although the presence of jaundice and mild hepatic fibrosis without concurrent portal hypertension or decreased hepatic synthetic function may not decrease overall survival [64]. Reversal of liver disease occurs in the great majority of patients who are weaned off PN after intestinal lengthening [64, 67]. In patients with complicated cirrhosis including coagulopathy, ascites or portal hypertension the preferred initial treatment is intestinal transplantation.

The current follow-up times extend to decades after LILT, but are still limited to few years after STEP [58, 61, 64–72]. In these reports survival rates after LILT range between 30% and 100% [58, 64, 66, 68–70] being 77% in the largest single center report of 53 children [64], and around 90% in two recent series [66, 70]. Comparable survival between 79 and 100% has been reported after STEP [64, 65, 71, 72, 95]. The main causes of mortality after both procedures are liver failure and septic complications [64–66, 70, 72]. Variance in patient selection strongly modifies outcomes after AGIR surgery both in terms of survival and rate of weaning PN. Combining the available data on bowel lengthening, PN requirement decreases almost invariably while 40–70% of children including non-survivors achieve enteral autonomy mostly during the first postoperative year without significant differences between LILT and STEP. The final length of the remaining small intestine is the main predictor of achieving enteral autonomy after AGIR surgery [64, 66]. The great majority of patients are operated on between the age of 6 months and 2 years.

The main surgical complications of AGIR procedures include anastomotic leakage, adhesive bowel obstruction, inter-loop fistulae, bacterial sepsis, stricture, gastrointestinal bleeding from the stapler or suture line and bowel redilation. Bowel redilation after intestinal lengthening prevents achievement of intestinal autonomy in a significant proportion of patients [73, 74]. Excluding case reports two series have addressed the efficiency of repeat bowel lengthening with the STEP procedure among children with bowel redilation [73, 74]. An average time to redilation was about 12–24 months and 13–43% weaned off PN after repeat STEP regardless of type of initial bowel lengthening. Despite inferior results in relation to primary bowel lengthening, repeat STEP is a valuable treatment among patients, who remain dependent on PN with stable liver function not precluding the possibility of intestinal transplantation [73].

39.7 Transplantation

39.7.1 Indications and Timing

Intestinal transplantation (ITx) is well established and the only remedial treatment for patients with irreversible IF who develop life-threatening complications during long-term PN [75]. Failure of PN may result from liver failure, recurrent catheter related sepsis, thrombosis of major central venous accesses or intractable water and electrolyte losses associated with recurrent severe dehydration [17]. Dependence on PN alone is not indication to ITx, because most children with IF including those with the shortest remaining bowel can be managed successfully by other means [96–98]. Scarcity of appropriate size donor organs increases waiting list mortality among very young pediatric patients [76]. Progression of above mentioned complications of PN during long waiting times may hamper performance and recovery from transplantation thereby decreasing the changes of survival. To ascertain the best possible changes of success specific guidelines regarding assessment for ITx have been published [17, 75, 77]. These include bilirubin level over 3 mg/dL or complications of portal hypertension, thrombosis of two or more central veins, two or more episodes of central line related sepsis per year or one episode of line fungemia and frequent episodes of intractable dehydration. Essentially, all intestinal failure programs should have active collaborative connections to centers performing liver and intestinal transplantation [77]. Optimization of medical treatment and nutrition as well as confirmation of unfeasibility of autologous intestinal lengthening procedures before transplantation is mandatory. The decision to proceed with ITx must be discussed extensively among multidisciplinary team including pediatric transplant surgeons and gastroenterologists and the changes of survival carefully balanced with the risks of transplantation. The parents must be fully informed about these issues.

39.7.2 Type of Transplant and Technical Considerations

The type of transplant is planned individually for each recipient based on liver function, the underlying disease for IF, for example SBS versus dysmotility, and physical condition and anatomy of the remaining intestine and vasculature. Broad categories of ITx include isolated intestinal, liver-intestinal and multivisceral transplantation (Fig. 39.4). The right colon is often included in the intestinal allograft in patients without native colon in order to improve absorption of water and electrolytes. Careful assessment of liver function before transplantation is essential. Although significant hepatic fibrosis and liver disease may regress following isolated ITx [64, 78], patients with complicated portal hypertension and deranged synthetic function require additional liver replacement. In practice, very young pediatric patients have most often concomitant irreversible hepatic and intestinal failure being potential candidates for combined liver-intestinal transplantation. In some children liver cirrhosis and advanced portal hypertension may hinder intestinal adaptation and prevent potentially achievable weaning off PN. In these patients enteral autonomy is achievable following isolated liver transplantation with or without additional autologous intestinal reconstructive surgery [79].

In intestinal or liver-intestinal transplantation nonfunctional recipient intestine is removed all the way to the very proximal jejunum. In isolated ITx the donor portal vein extending to the superior mesenteric vein or the inferior vena may be utilized for graft venous outflow (Fig. 39.4). In children with SBS the superior mesenteric vein may be inaccessible due to multiple previous laparotomies leaving the inferior vena cava the most feasible option. The arterial inflow is obtained either from the superior mesenteric artery or

Fig. 39.4 (**a**) In isolated ITx the donor portal vein extending to the superior mesenteric vein or the inferior vena may be utilized for graft venous outflow. The arterial inflow is obtained either from the superior mesenteric artery or infrarenal aorta. In order to avoid tension and twisting of the vascular anastomoses, interposition grafts are sutured to the chosen vessels before the graft is brought to the field. (**b**) Liver-intestinal transplantation in most commonly performed using en bloc allograft with preserved duodenum, biliary tract and portal vein. The recipient portal vein is anostomosed to the inferior vena cava in order to drain retained native splanchnic circulation. The suprahepatic vena vaca of the allograft is connected to the common ostium of the hepatic veins and a Carrel patch including the hepatic and the superior mesenteric artery is anastomosed to the aorta. The intestinal continuity is restored and a direct access to the proximal graft for postoperative nutrition and medication is ascertained by a feeding jejunostomy. A temporary ileostomy for endoscopic monitoring is performed

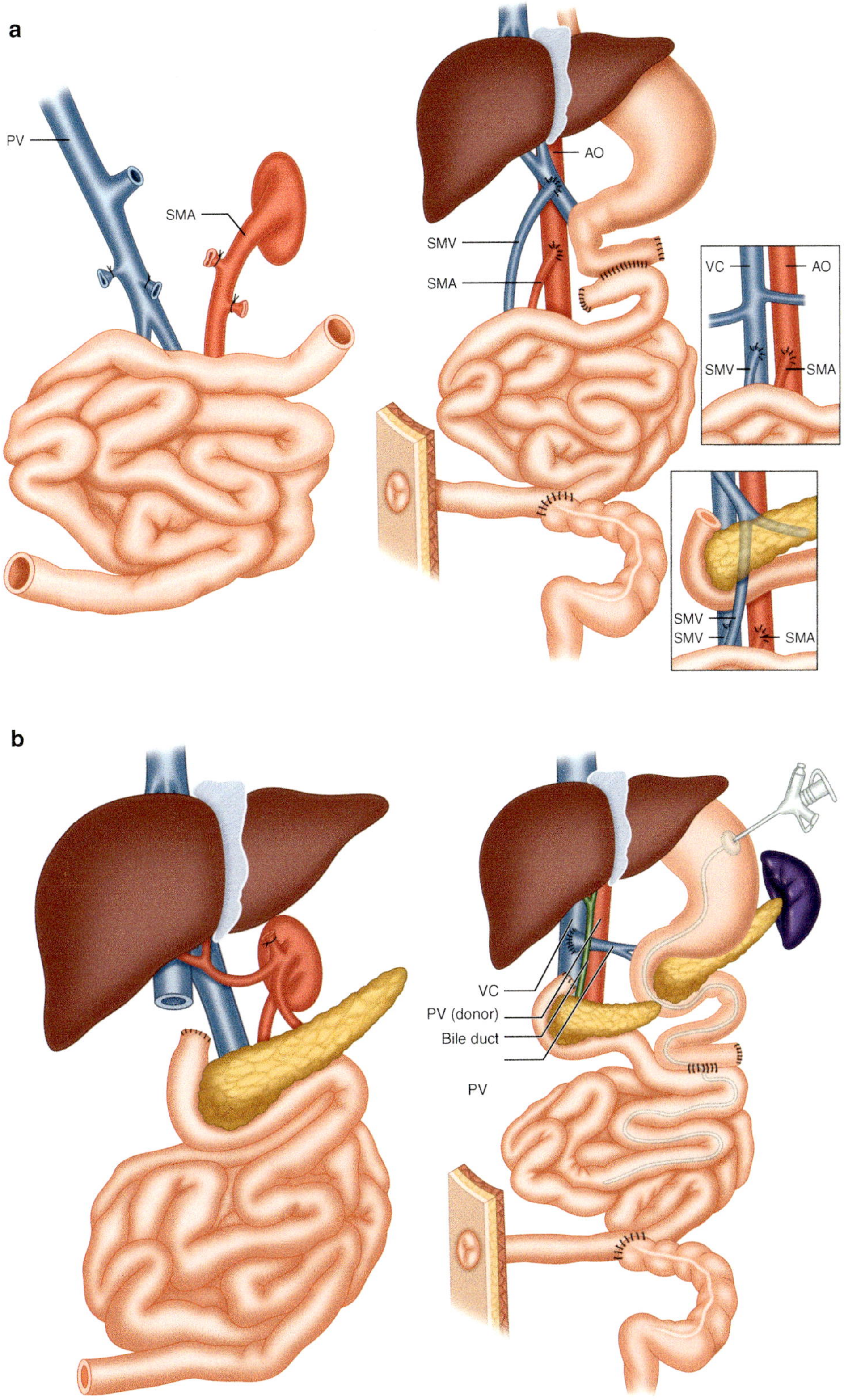
a
PV
SMA
AO
SMV
SMA
VC
AO
SMV
SMA
SMV
SMV
SMA
b
VC
PV (donor)
Bile duct
PV

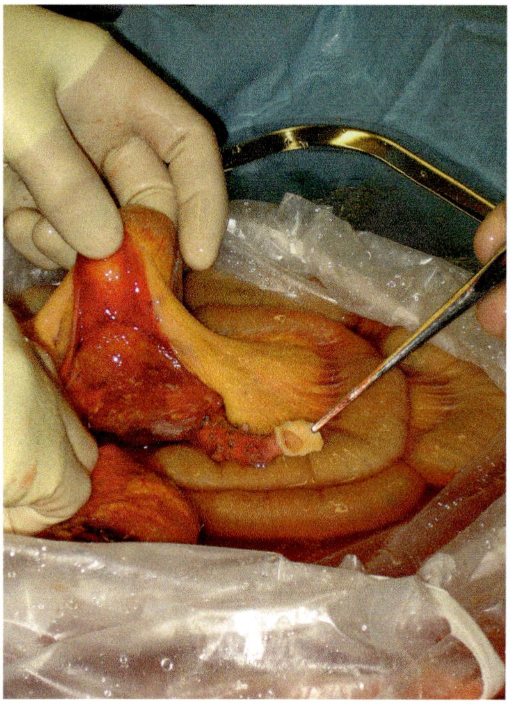

Fig. 39.5 Perfused intestinal graft including the ascending colon ready for implantation. The superior mesenteric artery (in forceps) was anastomosed to the infrarenal aorta

infrarenal aorta (Fig. 39.5). In order to avoid tension and twisting of the vascular anastomoses, interposition grafts are sutured to the chosen vessels before the graft is brought to the field. Liver-intestinal transplantation in most commonly performed using en bloc allograft with preserved duodenum biliary tract and portal vein. After removal of the liver, the recipient portal vein is anostomosed to the inferior vena cava in order to drain retained native splanchnic circulation. The suprahepatic vena caca of the allograft is connected to the common ostium of the hepatic veins and a Carrel patch including the hepatic and the superior mesenteric artery is anastomosed to the aorta. The intestinal continuity is restored and a direct access to the proximal graft for postoperative nutrition and medication is ascertained by a feeding jejunostomy. A temporary ileostomy for endoscopic monitoring is performed.

39.7.3 Outcomes

Most patients regain full enteral autonomy in few months after ITx. Although intestinal transplant contains significant amounts of donor lymphocytes, graft versus host disease is uncommon. Despite different tacrolimus-based immunosuppression protocols and frequent graft monitoring with endoscopically guided biopsies, acute rejection occur in 60% of children [80, 81]. Other common complications include bacterial and viral infections. Cytomegalovirus prophylaxis is continued for several months together with routine surveillance of Cytomegalo- and Epstein-Barr viral load. Infection or reactivation of Epstein-Barr virus predisposes to post transplantation lymphoproliferation disease, which may proceed to monoclonal B-cell lymphoma without treatment (Fig. 39.6). Overall, post transplantation lymphoproliferation occurs in 10% of cases [80, 81]. Renal insufficiency due to calcineurin inhibitor toxicity and other complications of high-dose immunosuppression are major concerns while chronic graft rejection necessitating retransplantation especially following isolated ITx continues to cause delayed graft losses [80].

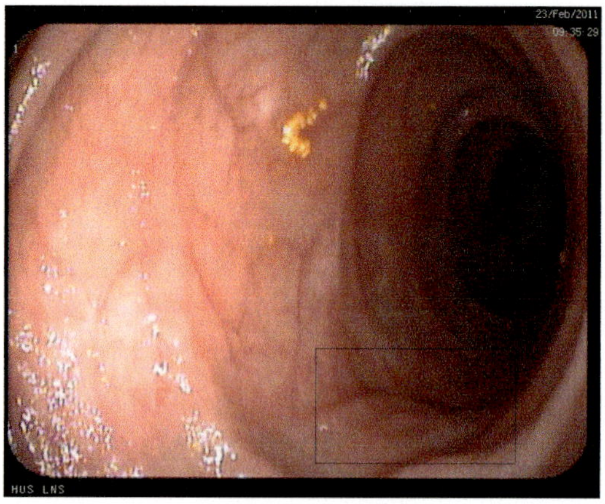

Fig. 39.6 An endoscopic view of the ileum 3 months after transplantation. The *black rectangle* high lights a mucosal nodule with a central depression, which demonstrated Epstein-Barr virus-positive polyclonal lymphoproliferation. Complete resolution occurred after reduction of immunosuppression and anti-CD20 antibody treatment

Currently, 1 and 5 year graft survival after combined liver-intestinal transplantation reaches 90% and 80% in large centers [80]. Although patient survival is higher after isolated ITx due to feasibility of graft enterectomy and re-transplantation, five-year graft survival remains around 60% as a result of more frequent chronic rejection in relation to combined liver-intestinal transplantation [80, 81]. In a large registry-based report of 852 children from US 50% were alive 10 years after isolated ITx [82]. Importantly, normal growth and good quality of life are achievable following ITx and long-term intestinal autonomy is possible in the majority of patients [80, 83]. During the recent years the rate of intestinal and especially combined intestinal liver transplantation among children has decreased. This most likely reflects advancements in surgical and medical therapy of SBS as well as increased awareness of liver protecting strategies in neonatal IF.

References

1. Salvia G, Guarino A, Terrin G, et al. Neonatal onset intestinal failure: an Italian multicenter study. J Pediatr. 2008;153:674–6.
2. Kurvinen A, Nissinen MJ, Andersson S, et al. Parenteral plant sterols and intestinal failure -associated liver disease in neonates. J Pediatr Gastroenterol Nutr. 2012;54:803–11.
3. Wales PW, de Silva N, Kim J, Lecce L, To T, Moore A. Neonatal short bowel syndrome: population-based estimates of incidence and mortality rates. J Pediatr Surg. 2004;39:690–5.
4. Cole CR, Hansen NI, Higgins RD, Ziegler TR, Stoll BJ. Very low birth weight preterm infants with surgical short bowel syndrome: incidence, morbidity and mortality, and growth outcomes at 18 to 22 months. Pediatrics. 2008;122:e573–82.
5. Wilmore DW, Dudrick SJ. Growth and development of an infant receiving all nutrients exclusively by vein. JAMA. 1968;203:860–4.
6. Goulet O, Baglin-Gobet S, Talbotec C, et al. Outcome and long-term growth after extensive small bowel resection in the neonatal period: a survey of 87 children. Eur J Pediatr Surg. 2005;15:95–101.
7. Torres C, Sudan D, Vanderhoof J, et al. Role of intestinal rehabilitation program in the treatment of advanced intestinal failure. J Pediatr Gastroenterol Nutr. 2007;45:204–12.
8. Modi BP, Langer M, Ching YA, et al. Improved survival in a multidisciplinary short bowel syndrome program. J Pediatr Surg. 2008;43:20–4.
9. Javid PJ, Malone FR, Reyes J, Healey PJ, Horslen SP. The experience of a regional pediatric intestinal failure program: successful outcomes from intestinal rehabilitation. Am J Surg. 2010;199:676–9.
10. Pakarinen MP, Koivusalo AI, Rintala RJ. Outcomes of intestinal failure—a comparison between children with short bowel and dysmotile intestine. J Pediatr Surg. 2009;44:2139–44.
11. Hess RA, Welch KB, Brown PI, Teitelbaum DH. Survival outcomes of pediatric intestinal failure patients: analysis of factors contributing to improved survival over the past two decades. J Surg Res. 2011;170:27–31.
12. Gutierrez IM, Kang KH, Jaksic T. Neonatal short bowel syndrome. Semin Fetal Neonatal Med. 2011;16:157–63.
13. Wales PW, de Silva N, Kim JH, Lecce L, Sandhu A, Moore AM. Neonatal short bowel syndrome a cohort study. J Pediatr Surg. 2005;40:755–62.
14. Nucci A, Cartland Burns R, Armah T, et al. Interdisciplinary management of pediatric intestinal failure: a 10-year review of rehabilitation and transplantation. J Gastrointest Surg. 2008;12:429–36.
15. Spencer AU, Neaga A, West B, et al. Pediatric short bowel syndrome; redefining predictors of success. Ann Surg. 2005;242:403–12.
16. Diamanti A, Sole Basso M, Castro M, et al. Irreversible intestinal failure: prevalence and prognostic factors. J Pediatr Gastroenterol Nutr. 2008;47:450–7.
17. Goulet O, Ruemmele F. Causes and management of intestinal failure in children. Gastroenterology. 2006;130:S16–28.
18. Struijs M-C, Diamond IR, de Silva N, Wales PW. Establishing norms for intestinal length in children. J Pediatr Surg. 2009;44:933–8.
19. Rhoads JM, Plunkett E, Galanko J, et al. Serum citrulline levels correlate with enteral tolerance and bowel lenght in infants with short bowel syndrome. J Pediatr. 2005;146:542–7.
20. Fitzgibbons S, Ching YA, Valim C, et al. Relationship between serum citrulline levels and progression to parenteral nutrition independence in children with short bowel syndrome. J Pediatr Surg. 2009;44:928–32.
21. Bailly-Botuha C, Colomb V, Thioulouse E, et al. Plasma citrulline concentration reflects enterocyte mass in children with short bowel syndrome. Pediatr Res. 2009;65:559–63.
22. Guarino A, De Marco G. Natural history of intestinal failure, investigated through a national network-based approach. J Pediatr Gastroenterol Nutr. 2003;37:136–41.
23. Heneyke S, Smith VV, Spitz L, Milla PJ. Chronic intestinal pseudo-obstruction: treatment and long term follow up of 44 patients. Arch Dis Child. 1999;81:21–7.

24. Gosemann J-H, Puri P. Megacystis microcolon intestinal hypoperistalsis syndrome: systematic review of outcome. Pediatr Surg Int. 2011;27(10):1041–6. [Epub ahead of print].
25. Dowling RH. Small bowel adaptation and its regulation. Scand J Gastroenterol. 1982;17(Suppl 74):53–74.
26. Rossi L, Kadamba P, Hugosson C, De Vol EB, Habib Z, Al-Nassar S. Pediatric short bowel syndrome: adaptation after massive small bowel resection. J Pediatr Gastroenterol Nutr. 2007;45:213–21.
27. Andorsky DJ, Lund DP, Lillehei CW, et al. Nutritional and other postoperative management of neonates with short bowel syndrome correlates with clinical outcomes. J Pediatr. 2001;139:27–33.
28. Georgeson KE, Breaux CW Jr. Outcome and intestinal adaptation in neonatal short-bowel syndrome. J Pediatr Surg. 1992;27:344–50.
29. Wilmore DW. Factors correlating with a successful outcome following extensive intestinal resection in newborn infants. J Pediatr. 1972;80:88–95.
30. Goulet O, Ruemmele F, Lacaille F, Colomb V. Irreversible intestinal failure. J Pediatr Gastroenterol Nutr. 2004;38:250–69.
31. Kurkchubasche AG, Rowe MI, Smith SD. Adaptation in short-bowel syndrome: reassessing old limits. J Pediatr Surg. 1993;28:1069–71.
32. Pakarinen MP, Kurvinen A, Gylling H, et al. Cholesterol metabolism in pediatric short bowel syndrome after weaning off parenteral nutrition. Dig Liver Dis. 2010;42:554–9.
33. Pakarinen MP, Miettinen TA, Lauronen J, et al. Adaptation of cholesterol absorption after proximal resection of porcine small intestine. J Lipid Res. 1996;37:1766–75.
34. Nordgaard I, Hansen BS, Mortensen PB. Importance of colonic support for energy absorption as small-bowel failure proceeds. Am J Clin Nutr. 1996;64:222–31.
35. Kaufman SS, Loseke CA, Lupo JV, et al. Influence of bacterial overgrowth and intestinal inflammation on duration of parenteral nutrition in children with short bowel syndrome. J Pediatr. 1997;131:356–61.
36. Eamonn M, Quigley M, Quera R. Small intestinal bacterial overgrowth: roles of antibiotics, prebiotics and probiotics. Gastroentrology. 2006;130:S78–90.
37. Sondheimer JM, Asturias E, Cadnapaphornchai M. Infection and cholestasis in neonates with intestinal resection and long-term parenteral nutrition. J Pediatr Gastroenterol Nutr. 1998;27:131–7.
38. Kocoshis SA. Medical management of pediatric intestinal failure. Semin Pediatr Surg. 2010;19:20–6.
39. Diamond IR, de Silva N, Pencharz PB, Kim JH, Wales PW. Neonatal short bowel syndrome outcomes after the establishment of the first Canadian multidisciplinary intestinal rehabilitation program: preliminary experience. J Pediatr Surg. 2007;42:806–11.
40. Kelly DA. Preventing parenteral nutrition liver disease. Early Hum Dev. 2010;86:683–7.
41. Fitzgibbons SC, Jones BA, Hull MA, et al. Relationship between biopsy-proven parenteral nutrition-associated liver fibrosis and biochemical cholestasis in children with short bowel syndrome. J Pediatr Surg. 2010;45:95–9.
42. Kurvinen A, Nissinen MJ, Gylling H, et al. Effects of long-term parenteral nutrition on serum lipids, plant sterols, cholesterol metabolism, and liver histology in pediatric intestinal failure. J Peadiatr Gastroenterol Nutr. 2011;53:440–6.
43. San Luis VA, Btaiche IF. Ursodiol in patients with parenteral nutrition-associated cholestasis. Ann Pharmacother. 2007;41:1867–72.
44. Kaufman SS, Pehlivanova M, Fennelly EM, et al. Predicting liver failure in parenteral nutrition-dependent short bowel syndrome of infancy. J Pediatr. 2010;156:580–5.
45. Koletzko B, Goulet O. Fish oil containing intravenous lipid emulsions in parenteral nutrition-associated cholestatic liver disease. Curr Opin Clin Nutr Metab Care. 2010;13:321–6.
46. Puder M, Valim C, Meisel JA, et al. Parenteral fish oil improves outcomes in patients with parenteral nutrition-associated liver injury. Ann Surg. 2009;250:395–402.
47. Goulet O, Antebi H, Wolf C, et al. A new intravenous fat emulsion containing soybean oil, medium-chain triglycerides, olive oil, and fish oil: a single-center, double-blind randomized study on efficacy and safety in pediatric patients receiving home parenteral nutrition. J Parenter Enteral Nutr. 2010;34:485–95.
48. Tomsits E, Pataki M, Tölgyesi A, Fekete G, Rischak K, Szollar L. Safety and efficacy of a lipid emulsion containing a mixture of soybean oil, medium-chain triglycerides, olive oil, and fish oil: a randomised, double-blind clinical trial in premature infants requiring parenteral nutrition. J Pediatr Gastroenterol Nutr. 2010;51:514–21.
49. Lilja HE, Finkel Y, Paulsson M, Lucas S. Prevention and reversal of intestinal failure-associated liver disease in premature infants with short bowel syndrome using intravenous fish oil in combination with omega-6/9 lipid emulsions. J Pediatr Surg. 2011;46:1361–7.
50. Le HD, Fallon EM, de Meijer VE, et al. Innovative parenteral and enteral nutrition therapy for intestinal failure. Semin Pediatr Surg. 2010;19:27–34.
51. Jones BA, Hull MA, Richardson DS, et al. Efficacy of ethanol locks in reducing central venous catheter infections in pediatric patients with intestinal failure. J Pediatr Surg. 2010;45:1287–93.
52. van Ommen CH, Tabbers MM. Catheter-related thrombosis in children with intestinal failure and long-term parenteral nutrition: how to treat and to prevent? Thromb Res. 2010;126:465–70.
53. Joly F, Dray X, Corcos O, Barbot L, Kapel N, Messing B. Tube feeding improves intestinal absorption in short bowel syndrome patients. Gastroenterology. 2009;136:824–31.

54. Olieman JF, Penning C, Ijsselstijn H, et al. Enteral nutrition in children with short-bowel syndrome: current evidence and recommendations for the clinician. J Am Diet Assoc. 2010;110:420–6.
55. Jeppesen PB, Pertkiewicz M, Messing B, et al. Teduglutide reduces need for parenteral support among patients with short bowel syndrome with intestinal failure. Gastroenterology. 2012;143:1473–81.
56. Sigalet DL, Martin GR, Butzner JD, Buret A, Meddings JB. A pilot study of the use of epidermal growth factor in pediatric short bowel syndrome. J Pediatr Surg. 2005;40:763–8.
57. Goulet O, Dabbas-Tyan M, Talbotec C, et al. Effect of recombinant human growth hormone on intestinal absorption and body composition in children with short bowel syndrome. J Parenter Enteral Nutr. 2010;34:513–20.
58. Bianchi A. From the cradle to enteral autonomy: the role of autologous gastrointestinal reconstruction. Gastroenterology. 2006;130:S138–S46.
59. Murphy F, Khalil BA, Gozzini S, King B, Bianchi A, Morabito A. Controlled tissue expansion in the initial management of the short bowel state. World J Surg. 2011;35:1142–5.
60. Ziegler MM, Royal RE, Brandt J, Drasnin J, Martin LW. Extended myectomy-myotomy. A therapeutic alternative for total intestinal aganglionosis. Ann Surg. 1993;218:504–11.
61. Jones BA, Hull MA, Kim HB. Autologous intestinal reconstruction surgery for intestinal failure management. Curr Opin Organ Transplant. 2010;15:341–5.
62. Bianchi A. Intestinal loop lengthening-a technique for increasing small intestine length. J Pediatr Surg. 1980;15:145–51.
63. Kim HB, Fauza D, Garza J, et al. Serial transverse enteroplasty (STEP): a novel bowel lengthening procedure. J Pediatr Surg. 2003;38:425–9.
64. Sudan D, Thompson J, Botha J, et al. Comparison of intestinal lengthening procedures for patients with short bowel syndrome. Ann Surg. 2007;246:593–604.
65. Modi BP, Javid PJ, Jaksic T, et al. First report of the international serial transverse enteroplasty data registry: indications, efficacy, and complications. J Am Coll Surg. 2007;204:365–71.
66. Reinshagen K, Kabs C, Wirth H, et al. Long-term outcome in patients with short bowel syndrome after longitudinal intestinal lengthening and tailoring. J Pediatr Gastroenterol Nutr. 2008;47:573–8.
67. Reinshagen K, Zahn K, von Buch C, et al. The impact of longitudinal intestinal lengthening and tailoring on liver function in short bowel syndrome. J Pediatr Surg. 2008;18:249–53.
68. Weber TR. Isoperistaltic bowel lengthening for short bowel syndrome in children. Am J Surg. 1999;178:600–4.
69. Walker SR, Nucci A, Yaworski JA, Barksdale EM Jr. The Bianchi procedure: a 20-year single institution experience. J Pediatr Surg. 2006;41:113–9.
70. Khalil BA, Ba'ath ME, Aziz A, et al. Intestinal rehabilitation and bowel reconstructive surgery: improved outcomes in children with short bowel syndrome. J Pediatr Gastroenterol Nutr. 2012;54(4):505–9. [Epub ahead of print].
71. Ching YA, Fitzgibbons S, Valim C, et al. Long-term nutritional and clinical outcomes after serial transverse enteroplasty at a single institution. J Pediatr Surg. 2009;44:939–43.
72. Wales PW, de Silva N, Langer JC, Fecteau A. Intermediate outcomes after serial transverse enteroplasty in children with short bowel syndrome. J Pediatr Surg. 2007;42:1804–10.
73. Andres AM, Thompson J, Grant W, et al. Repeat surgical bowel lengthening with the STEP procedure. Transplantation. 2008;85:1294–9.
74. Miyasaka EA, Brown PI, Teitelbaum DH. Redilation of bowel after intestinal lengthening procedures—an indicator for poor outcome. J Pediatr Surg. 2011;46:145–9.
75. Fishbein TM. Intestinal transplantation. N Engl J Med. 2009;361:998–1008.
76. Mian SI, Dutta S, Le B, Esquivel CO, Davis K, Castillo RO. Factors affecting survival to intestinal transplantation in the very young pediatric patient. Transplantation. 2008;85:1287–9.
77. Beath S, Pironi L, Gabe S, et al. Collaborative strategies to reduce mortality and morbidity in patients with chronic intestinal failure including those who are referred for small bowel transplantation. Transplantation. 2008;85:1378–84.
78. Fiel MI, Sauter B, Wu H-S, et al. Regression of hepatic fibrosis after intestinal transplantation in total parenteral nutrition liver disease. Clin Gastroenterol Hepatol. 2008;6:926–33.
79. Dell-Olio D, Beath SV, de Ville de Goyet J, et al. Isolated liver transplant in infants with short bowel syndrome: insights into outcomes and prognostic factors. J Pediatr Gastroenterol Nutr. 2009;48:334–40.
80. Nayyar N, Mazariegos G, Ranganathan S, et al. Pediatric small bowel transplantation. Semin Pediatr Surg. 2010;19:68–77.
81. Kato T, Tzakis AG, Selvaggi G, et al. Intestinal and multivisceral transplantation in children. Ann Surg. 2006;243:756–66.
82. Lao OB, Healey PJ, Perkins JD, Horslen S, Reyes JD, Goldin AB. Outcomes in children after intestinal transplant. Pediatrics. 2010;125:e550–8.
83. Lacaille F, Vass N, Sauvat F, et al. Long-term outcome, growth and digestive function in children 2 to 18 years after intestinal transplantation. Gut. 2008;57:455–61.
84. D'Antiga GO. Intestinal failure in children: the European view. J Pediatr Gastroenterol Nutr. 2013;56:118–26.
85. Squires RH, Duggan C, Teitelbaum DH, et al. Natural history of pediatric intestinal failure: initial report from the Pediatric Intestinal Failure Consortium. J Pediatr. 2012;161:723–8.

86. Pakarinen MP, Kurvinen A, Koivusalo AI, Ruuska T, Mäkisalo H, Jalanko H, Rintala RJ. Surgical treatment and outcomes of severe pediatric intestinal motility disorders requiring parenteral nutrition. J Pediatr Surg. 2013;48:333–8.
87. El Kasmi KC, Anderson AL, Devereaux MW, et al. Toll-like receptor 4-dependent Kupffer cell activation and liver injury in a novel mouse model of parenteral nutrition and intestinal injury. Hepatology. 2012;55:1518–28.
88. Mutanen A, Lohi J, Heikkilä P, Koivusalo AI, Rintala RJ, Pakarinen MP. Persistent abnormal liver fibrosis after weaning off parenteral nutrition in pediatric intestinal failure. Hepatology. 2013;58: 729–38.
89. Mutanen A, Heikkilä P, Lohi J, Raivio T, Jalanko H, Pakarinen MP. Serum FGF21 increases with hepatic fat accumulation in pediatric onset intestinal failure. J Hepatol. 2014;60:183–90.
90. El Kasmi KC, Anderson AL, Devereaux MW, et al. Phytosterols promote liver injury and Kupffer cell activation in parenteral nutrition-associated liver disease. Sci Transl Med. 2013;5(206):206ra137. doi: https://doi.org/10.1126/scitranslmed.3006898.
91. Cober MP, Killu G, Brattain A, Welch KB, Kunisaki SM, Teitelbaum DH. Intravenous fat emulsions reduction for patients with parenteral nutrition-associated liver disease. J Pediatr. 2012;160:421–7.
92. Goulet O, Olieman J, Ksiazyk J, et al. Neonatal short bowel syndrome as a model of intestinal failure: physiological background for enteral feeding. Clin Nutr. 2013;32:162–71.
93. Pakarinen MP, Kurvinen A, Koivusalo AI, Iber T, Rintala RJ. Long-term controlled outcomes after autologous intestinal reconstruction surgery in treatment of severe short bowel syndrome. J Pediatr Surg. 2013;48:339–44.
94. Khalil BA, Ba'ath ME, Aziz A, et al. Intestinal rehabilitation and bowel reconstructive surgery: improved outcomes in children with short bowel syndrome. J Pediatr Gastroenterol Nutr. 2012;54:505–9.
95. Jones BA, Hull MA, Potanos KM, et al. Report of 111 consecutive patients enrolled in the International Serial Transverse Enteroplasty (STEP) Data Registry: a retrospective observational study. J Am Coll Surg. 2013;216:438–46.
96. Infantino BJ, Mercer DF, Hobson BD, et al. Successful rehabilitation in pediatric ultrashort small bowel syndrome. J Pediatr. 2013;163:1361–6.
97. Sanchez SE, Javid PJ, Healey PJ, Reyes J, Horslen SP. Ultrashort bowel syndrome in children. J Pediatr Gastroenterol Nutr. 2013;56:36–9.
98. Diamanti A, Conforti A, Panetta F, et al. Long-term outcome of home parenteral nutrition in patients with ultra-short bowel syndrome. J Pediatr Gastroenterol Nutr. 2014;58(4):438–42. [Epub ahead of print].

Hirschsprung's Disease

40

Prem Puri and Florian Friedmacher

Abstract

Hirschsprung's disease (HD) is a relatively common cause of intestinal obstruction in newborn infants. It is characterized by the absence of ganglion cells in the distal bowel, which begins at the level of the internal anal sphincter and extends proximally for varying distances. The absence of ganglion cells has been attributed to the failure of migration of neural crest cells.

Keywords

Hirschsprung disease • Aetiology and pathogenesis • Surgery • Outcomes

40.1 Introduction

Hirschsprung's disease (HD) is a relatively common cause of intestinal obstruction in newborn infants. It is characterized by the absence of ganglion cells in the distal bowel, which begins at the level of the internal anal sphincter and extends proximally for varying distances. The absence of ganglion cells has been attributed to the failure of migration of neural crest cells.

P. Puri, MS, FRCS, FRCS(ED), FACS (✉)
F. Friedmacher, MD, MSc
National Children's Research Centre, Our Lady's Children's Hospital, Crumlin, Dublin 12, Ireland
e-mail: prem.puri@ncrc.ie

40.1.1 Historical Background

In 1691, the Dutch anatomist Ruysch [1] described a 5-year old girl with abdominal pain who finally died from an intestinal bowel obstruction. More than 200 years later, Jacobi [2] described two newborns with intestinal bowel obstruction that may have been attributable to congenital megacolon. The Danish pediatrician Hirschsprung described in 1887 two cases of infant boys who had died from constipation due to dilatation and hypertrophy of the colon [3]—a condition that later bore his name. In 1901, Tittel [4] noted the absence of ganglion cells in the distal colon of a child with HD. The Swedish pediatric surgeon Ehrenpreis [5] recognized in 1946 the aganglionosis as the cause of congenital megacolon in newborns. Whitehouse and Kernohan [6] presented in

P.D. Losty et al. (eds.), *Rickham's Neonatal Surgery*, https://doi.org/10.1007/978-1-4471-4721-3_40

1948 a series of 11 cases, which demonstrated that the aganglionosis within the distal colon is the cause of functional obstruction in infants with HD. In 1948, Swenson and Bill [7] recommended recto-sigmoidectomy with preservation of the sphincters as the optimal treatment for HD. Since then, neonatal diagnosis of HD and improvements in surgical techniques have resulted in an evolution towards one-stage pull-through operations with minimal invasive access. All these advances have resulted in a significantly improved morbidity and mortality in newborns with HD [8].

40.1.2 Classification

While the internal anal sphincter is the constant inferior limit [9], HD can be classified as classical recto-sigmoid HD when the aganglionic segment does not extend beyond the upper sigmoid colon, long-segment HD when aganglionosis extends to the splenic flexure or transverse colon, and total colonic aganglionosis when the aganglionic segment involves the entire colon with a short segment of terminal ileum (total colonic aganglionosis [TCA]) [10–12]. Table 40.1 shows the relative frequency of different forms of HD. Total intestinal aganglionosis with absence of ganglion cells from the duodenum to the rectum is the rarest form of HD and associated with high morbidity and mortality rates [13, 14]. Ultrashort-segment HD is a rare condition, characterized by an aganglionic segment of 1–3 cm length [15–17]. "Zonal aganglionosis" is a phenomenon involving a zone of aganglionosis occurring within a normally inverted intestine [18–20]. Skip segment HD (SSHD) involves a "skip area" of normally ganglionated intestine, surrounded proximally and distally by aganglionosis [21–23]. The occurrence of SSHD has no clear embryological explanation. To date, 24 cases of SSHD have been reported in the literature [24].

Table 40.1 Forms of Hirschsprung's disease (HD) and frequency

Form of HD	Level of aganglionosis	Frequency (%)
Recto-sigmoid	Sigmoid colon	72–88
Long-segment	Splenic flexure or transverse colon	9–24
Total colonic aganglionosis	Terminal ileum	3–13

40.1.3 Epidemiology

Several demographic studies have shown a remarkably constant incidence of HD, which is approximately 1:5000 live births [25–27]. However, significant interracial differences in the incidence of HD have been reported: 1:10,000 in Hispanic subjects, 1:6000 in white subjects, 1:4761 in black subjects, and 1:3571 Asian subjects [28]. Different levels of consanguinity may explain some of these differences, but recent genetic studies point to different frequencies of HD-associated mutations within different ethnic populations [29]. With a male-to-female ratio of 4:1, HD is far more common in boys [11, 30]. Interestingly, the male preponderance is less evident in long-segment HD, where the male-to-female ratio is 1.5–2:1 [25–27]. In TCA, the gender distribution even seems to be reversed with a reported male-to-female ratio of 0.8:1 [31].

40.2 Etiology

40.2.1 Failure of Neural Crest Cell Migration

The enteric nervous system (ENS) is the largest and most complex division of the peripheral nervous system, containing about 100 million neurons [32]. Embedded within the walls of the gastrointestinal tract, it represents a unique network of innervations, which functions largely independently of the central nervous system. Most of the neurons are located either in myenteric or submucosal ganglia and only a few are scattered within the mucosa. One of the main functions of the ENS is to coordinate the normal bowel motility and secretory activities.

It is generally accepted that the enteric ganglion cells primarily originate from the vagal neural crest cells (NCCs) [33–35]. The embryonic neural crest arises in the neural tube, originating within the central nervous system, but NCCs detach from this tissue via reduction of cell-cell and cell-matrix adhesion. The epithelio-mesenchymal transformation allows NCCs to migrate along pathways. Pathway selection is most likely achieved by balanced combinations of molecules that promote and reduce adhesion [36, 37]. Several investigators have suggested that the enteric neurons follow a dual gradient of development from each end of the gut toward the midline, with vagal NCCs providing the main source of enteric neurons [38]. Furthermore, animal studies have shown that sacral NCCs also contribute to the hindgut ENS [39, 40]. However, to which extent the sacral NCCs contribute to the ENS in humans is less clear. Failure of the vagal-derived NCCs to colonize the hindgut results in failure of ENS development in this region, suggesting an interaction between sacral and vagal enteric NCCs may be necessary for sacral NCC contribution to the ENS [38].

In the human fetus, neural crest-derived neuroblasts first appear in the developing esophagus at 5 weeks, and then migrate down to the anal canal in a cranio-caudal direction during the 5th–12th week of gestation [41]. The NCCs first form the myenteric plexus just outside the circular muscle layer. The mesenchymally derived longitudinal muscle layer then forms, sandwiching the myenteric plexus after it has been formed in the 12th week of gestation. In addition, after the cranio-caudal migration has ended, the submucous plexus is formed by the neuroblasts, which migrate from the myenteric plexus across the circular muscle layer and into the submucosa; this progresses in a cranio-caudal direction during the 12th–16th weeks of gestation [35]. The submucosal plexus can be divided into an outer plexus (Schabadasch's plexus), which is located in the submucosal layer adjacent to the circular muscle layer, and an inner submucous plexus (Meissner's plexus), located close to the muscularis mucosae [42]. The absence of ganglion cells in HD has been attributed to a failure of migration of NCCs. The earlier the arrest of migration, the longer the aganglionic segment is.

40.2.2 Genetic Factors

Evidence for a role of genetic factors in the etiology of HD is indicated by an increased risk of recurrence for siblings of affected individuals compared with the general population: an unbalanced sex-ratio, the association of HD with other genetic diseases (including chromosomal anomalies and congenital malformation syndromes), and the existence of several animal models of colonic aganglionosis showing specific Mendelian modes of inheritance [43]. HD is known to occur in families. The reported incidence of familial cases in recto-sigmoid HD varies between 3.6 and 7.8%. In TCA, a familial incidence of 15–21% has been observed and in the rare total intestinal aganglionosis an incidence of 50% [44, 45].

The recurrence risk in siblings is dependent upon the sex of the affected person and the extent of aganglionosis. Badner et al. [30] calculated the risk of HD transmission to relatives and found that the recurrence risk to siblings increases as the aganglionosis becomes more extensive. The brothers of patients with recto-sigmoid HD have a higher risk (4%) than sisters (1%). Much higher risks are observed in cases of long-segment HD. The brothers and sons of affected female individuals have a 24 and 29% risk of being affected, respectively [8]. Besides that, a different reproductive rate between male and female carriers could contribute to the parental transmission asymmetry seen in HD [46].

Although HD occurs as an isolated phenotype in at least 70% of cases, associations with various chromosomal anomalies, hereditary syndromes and congenital malformations have been frequently reported. Trisomy 21 (Down syndrome) is by far the most frequent chromosomal anomaly, occurring in 2–15% of all HD cases [47–50]. As individuals with Down syndrome display a 40-fold greater risk of HD than the general population, chromosome 21 is clearly involved in the etiology of HD [51, 52].

Other chromosomal anomalies that have been described in association with HD include interstitial deletion of distal 13q, partial deletion of 2p, reciprocal translocation, and trisomy 18 mosaic [8]. Numerous syndromes and coexisting anomalies (including multiple endocrine neoplasia type 2 and familial medullary thyreoid carcinoma, neuroblastoma, congenital central hypoventilation syndrome, Waardenburg syndrome and related pigmentary anomalies) are associated with HD. Other syndromes and malformations with HD as a frequent feature are: Mowat-Wilson syndrome, Goldberg-Shprintzen syndrome, Bardet-Biedl syndrome, McKusick-Kauffman syndrome, Smith-Lemli-Opitz syndrome, Cartilage-hair hypoplasia syndrome, and distal limb anomalies [53, 54].

During the past 15 years, several genes have been identified that control the morphogenesis and differentiation of the ENS. It has been demonstrated that mutations or deletions of these genes interfere with the development of the ENS. So far, at least 18 susceptibility genes are known to be involved in the development of HD [55–88] (Table 40.2). Of these genes, the RET gene (encoding a tyrosine-kinase receptor) is the major gene causing HD [89, 90]. Mutations in the coding region of RET are responsible for 50% of familial HD cases and 15% of sporadic ones [69, 91]. Thus, both rare and common mutations contribute to the multifactorial HD liability [92]. As all known genes that have been implicated in the development of HD together only account for 20% of all HD cases [72, 84, 93, 94], further genes may also be involved in the development of HD.

Table 40.2 Genes involved in the development of Hirschsprung's disease

Gene	Locus	Reference
RET	11q11.2	[6, 48, 109]
GDNF	5p13.1-p12	[4, 53]
NRTN	19p13.3	[23]
GFRA1	10q26.11	[97]
EDNRB	13q22	[2, 68, 116]
EDN3	20q13.2-q13.3	[10, 141]
ECE1	1p36.1	[47]
SOX10	22q13.1	[44, 113, 136, 139]
PHOX2B	4p12	[18, 32]
HOXB5	17q21.3	[18, 34, 74, 164]
NKX2.1	14q13	[33]
ZFHX1B	2q22.3	[31, 57, 155]
TCF4	18q21.1	[127]
KIAA1279	10q22.1	[12]
NRG1	8p12	[35, 146, 147]
NRG3	10q23.1	[145]
L1cam	Xq28	[153, 157]

40.3 Pathophysiology

The underlying pathophysiologic feature in HD is the functional intestinal obstruction caused by a narrowed distal aganglionoic colon that prevents the propagation of peristaltic waves. However, the pathophysiology of HD is still poorly understood. It has long been recognized that the obstructive symptoms in HD are secondary to the abnormal motility of the distal narrow segment, but there is still no clear explanation for the occurrence of the spastic or tonically contracted aganglionic segment of the bowel [95]. Several abnormalities have been described to explain the basis for the motility dysfunction in the contracted bowel.

40.3.1 Cholinergic Hyperinnervation

There is a marked increase in cholinergic nerve fibers in the intermuscular zone and submucosa of the aganglionic segment in HD. These fibers appear as thick nerve trunks and correspond to extrinsic preganglionic parasympathetic nerves [96–100]. The continuous acetylcholine release from the axons of these parasympathetic nerves results in an excessive accumulation of the enzyme acetylcholinesterase (AChE) that is typically found in the lamina propria mucosae, muscularis mucosae, and circular muscle with histochemical staining techniques. Both, the thick nerve trunks and the increased AChE activity are most pronounced in the most distal aganglionic rectum and progressively diminish proximally as normal bowel is approached [101]. The proximal extent of increased cholinergic activity does not necessarily correspond to the extent of the aganglionosis, which usually extends more proximally to a variable degree. Pharmacologic investigations of the colon in HD have demonstrated a higher acetylcholine release in the aganglionic segment at rest and after stimulation compared with the proximal ganglionic bowel [102, 103]. AChE concentration has also found to be higher in the serum and erythrocytes of children suffering from HD [104]. Since acetylcholine is the main excitatory neurotransmitter, cholinergic nerve hyperplasia has been proposed as the cause of spasticity of the aganglionic segment. However, the aganglionic bowel still appears narrow after the application of benzalkonium chloride or corrosive sublimate in experimental animal models of aganglionosis and animals exhibit typical obstructive symptoms [105, 106]. Therefore, the cholinergic hyperinnervation does not seem to be a prerequisite to the appearance of a narrow spastic segment.

40.3.2 Adrenergic Innervation

Fluorescent-histochemical studies for localization of adrenergic nerves have demonstrated a numerically increase and chaotic distribution in the aganglionic segement of HD. They are also present in the circular and longitudinal muscle layers as well as in the mucosa, whereas they are almost never found in normal ganglionic bowel [107–109]. However, despite the elevated number of adrenergic fibers in the aganglionic colon, the sensitivity to epinephrine is apparently not increased [110, 111]. The tissue concentration of norepinephrine is 2–3 times higher in the aganglionoc bowel than in the normal colon. Furthermore, there is also a corresponding increase in tyrosine hydroxylase, an enzyme that regulates the norepinephrine biosynthesis [109]. Because adrenergic nerves normally act to relax the bowel, it is unlikely that the adrenergic hyperactivity is responsible for the increased tone in the aganglionic segment [8].

40.3.3 Nitrergic Innervation

Nitric oxide (NO) is considered to be one of the most important neurotransmitters involved in relaxation of the smooth muscle of the gut [112]. It is synthesized in a reaction catalyzed by nitric oxide synthase (NOS) using L-arginine and molecular oxygen as co-substrates to form L-citrulline and NO. When NO binds to cytosolic guanylate cyclase, it increases the production of 3′5'-cyclic guanosine monophosphate (GMP) with subsequent relaxation of smooth muscle [37]. NOS has been shown to colocalize with reduced nicotine adenine dinucleotide phosphate (NADPH) diaphorase, which has been demonstrated to have identical functions [113, 114]. Several investigators have studied NOS distribution in the ganglionic and aganglionic bowel in patients with HD using NOS immunohistochemistry or NADPH diaphorase histochemistry [115–119]. In normal and ganglionic colon from patients with HD, there is a strong NADPH diaphorase staining of the submucous and myenteric plexuses and a large number of positive nerve fibers in the circular and longitudinal muscle as well as in the muscularis mucosae [37]. However, in the aganglionic segment are no ganglia present and there is an absence or marked reduction of NADPH diaphorase positive nerve fibers in both muscle layers and in the muscularis mucosae. The typical hypertrophied nerve trunks appear weakly stained [37]. Kusafuka and Puri [120] examined the expression of neural NOS mRNA in the aganglionic segment from seven patients with HD and demonstrated that NOS mRNA expression was decreased at least 1/50–1/100 of the level of expressed in ganglionic bowel. These findings indicate that there is an impaired NO synthesis in the aganglionic segment and this deficiency could prevent smooth muscle relaxation, thereby causing the lack of peristalsis in HD. In an interesting experiment, Bealer et al. [121] compared the effect of an exogenous source of NO, S-nitroso-*N*-acetylpenicillamine (SNAP) on the isometric tension of smooth muscle strips from aganglionic bowel and demonstrated a 70% reduction of resting tension. These results suggest that the defective distribution of nerves containing NOS may be involved in the pathogenesis of HD.

40.3.4 Interstitial Cells of Cajal

Interstitial cells of Cajal (ICC) form a network of mesenchymal cells that are widely distributed within the submucosal, intra- and intermuscular layers of the gastrointestinal tract. ICCs act as the pacemaker cells of the gut, which are electrically coupled to the smooth muscle cells by generating slow waves [122]. Abnormalities of ICCs have been described in several disorders of human intestinal motility including HD. Vanderwinden et al. [119] using a c-kit immunohistochemistry first described that ICCs were scarce and its network appeared disrupted in aganglionic segments of HD whereas the distribution of ICCs in the ganglionic bowel of HD was similar to that observed in controls. Yamataka et al. [123, 124] found few c-kit positive cells in the muscle layers in HD and a moderate number around the thick nerve bundles in the space between the two muscle layers in the aganglionic bowel. Horisawa et al. [125] reported no differences in c-kit immunopositive cells in aganglionic segments compared with corresponding area of ganglionic bowel. Using a whole-mount and frozen sections stained with c-kit immunohistochemistry preparations, Rolle et al. [126] showed an altered distribution of ICCs in the entire resected bowel of HD patients and not only in the aganglionic segment. Moreover, gap junctions connecting ICCs were immunolocalized by anti-Connexin 43 antibody and found to be absent in the aganglionic part and highly reduced in the transition zone [127]. Rolle et al. [126] furthermore proposed that persistent dismotility problems after pull-through operation in HD may be due to altered distribution and impaired function in ICCs. Investigating the tissue distribution of Ca^{2+}-activated K^{+} channels 2 and 3 (SK2 and SK3) in ICCs, Piotrowska et al. [128] found a strong expression in normal human colon with a markedly decreased expression of SK3 channels in aganglionic bowel, which may also contribute to the motility dysfunction in HD.

40.3.5 Enteroendocrine Cells

Using the generic enteroendocrine cell immunohistochemical markers chromogranin A and synaptophysin, Soeda et al. [129] demonstrated that the number of enteroendoccrine cells in the aganglionic colon in patients with HD were significantly increased compared with the number in the normal ganglionic segment. The increase of enteroendocrine cells in the mucosa of aganglionic colon may well influence sustained contraction of the bowel wall mainly mediated by the release of 5-hydroxytryptamine [8].

40.3.6 Smooth Muscle Cells

Since smooth muscle cells (SMCs) are the final effector for bowel motility, it is likely that they could also be abnormal in HD. The cytoskeleton of SMCs consists of proteins whose primary function is to serve as a structural framework that surround and support the contractile apparatus of actin and myosin filaments in the body of these cells. Nemeth et al. [130] studied the distribution of cytoskeleton in SMCs of HD bowel by means of immunohistochemistry and found that dystrophin, vinculin, and desmin immunoreactivity was either absent or weak in aganglionic bowel, whereas it was moderate to strong in the normal ganglionic bowel from patients with HD. Neural cell adhesion molecule (NCAM) is a cell surface glycoprotein involved in cell-cell adhesion during development that has been suggested to play an important role in development and maintenance of the neuromuscular system [131–133]. NCAM is present in the innervation of normal infant bowel and, less densely, in some components of the enteric smooth muscle. Contradictory results have been published regarding the NCAM expression in the smooth muscle of aganglionic bowel. Kobayashi et al. [117] described a lack of expression of NCAM in the muscularis propria of the aganglionic bowel compared with the ganglionic segment, whereas Romanska et al. [134] have found an increased NCAM expression in muscle, particularly in the muscularis mucosae. In any case, both authors agree that there is a strong expression of NCAM in the hypertrophic nerve trunks from the aganglionic segment.

40.3.7 Extracellular Matrix

Although extracellular matrix (EM) abnormalities have been described mainly related to the pathogenesis of HD, they could also have an influence on its pathophysiology. The lethal spotted mouse, an animal model which develops aganglionosis in its distal bowel, displays an abnormal distribution of EM components including laminin, collagen type IV, glycosaminoglycans and proteoglycans in the smooth muscle layer [135, 136]. Parikh et al. [137] demonstrated that the laminin concentration in aganglionic bowel was twice as high as in the ganglionic bowel of HD and three times higher than in age-matched controls. Moreover, by means of immunohistochemistry, they found an uneven distribution of laminin and collagen type IV in the muscularis propria of aganglionic bowel, being more intensely expressed in the circular layer than in the longitudinal layer [138]. The same authors have described that EM components tenascin and fibronectin are more intensely expressed in aganglionic bowel from patients with HD [139].

40.4 Pathology

The characteristic gross pathological feature in HD is the dilatation and hypertrophy of the proximal colon with an abrupt or gradual transition to narrowed distal bowel (Fig. 40.1b). Although the degree of dilatation and hypertrophy increases with age, the cone-shape transition zone from dilated to narrow bowel is usually evident in the newborn.

Histologically, HD is characterized by the absence of ganglionic cells in the myenteric and submucous plexuses and the presence of hypertrophied non-myelinated nerve trunks in the space normally occupied by the ganglionic cells

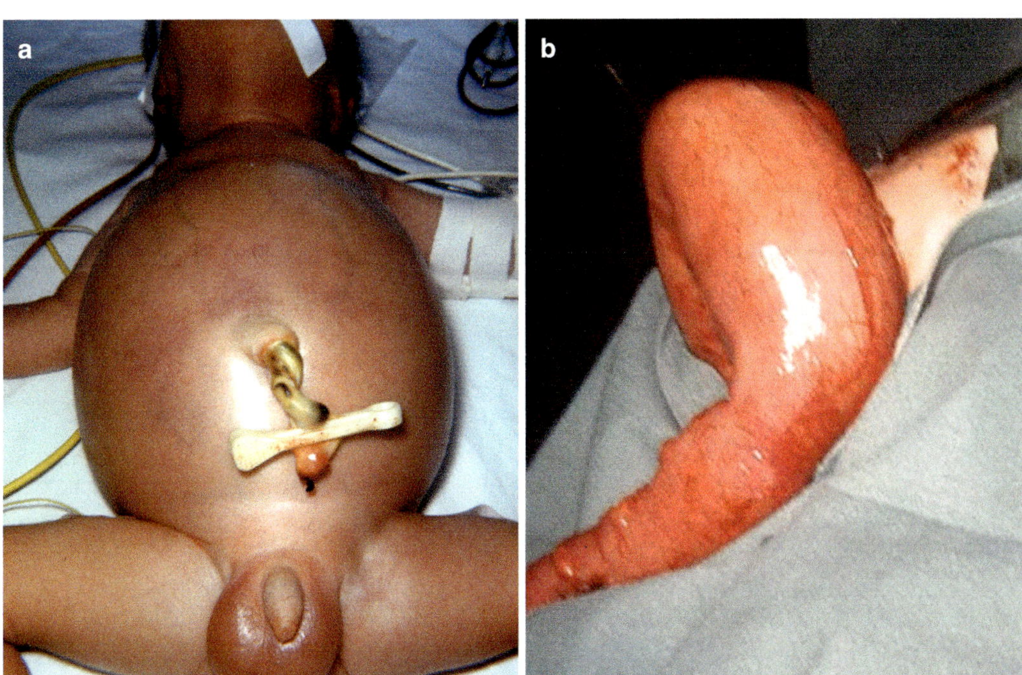

Fig. 40.1 Two-day-old newborn with Hirschsprung's disease presenting with marked abdominal distension and failure to pass meconium (**a**). Typical gross pathology in Hirschsprung's disease showing dilatation and hypertrophy of the proximal colon with transitional zone at recto-sigmoid level (**b**)

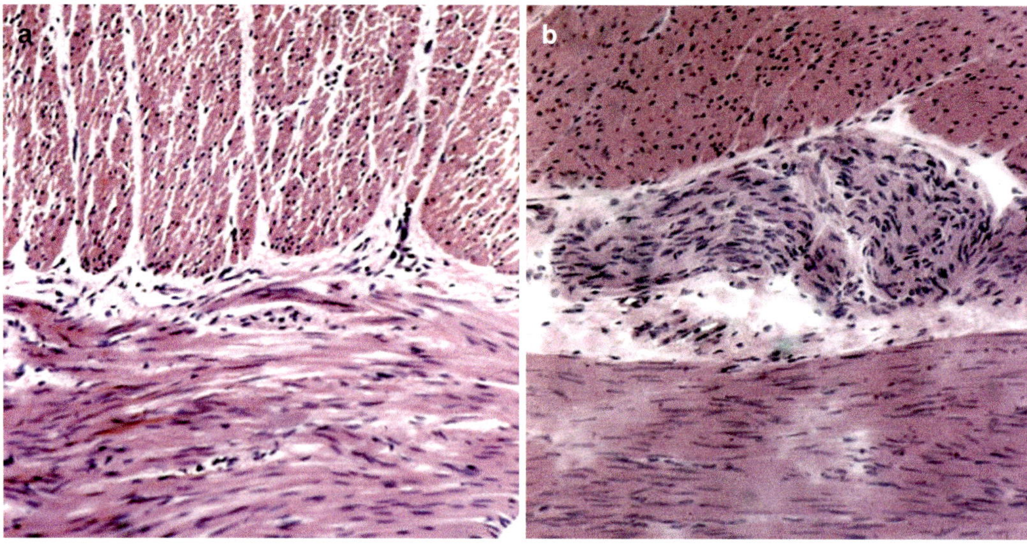

Fig. 40.2 Rectal biopsies showing presence of ganglionic cells in the myenteric and submucous plexuses of normal bowel (**a**), and absence with replacement by hypertrophied nerve trunks in a patient with Hirschsprung's disease (**b**)

(Fig. 40.2b). The aganglionic segment of bowel is followed proximally by a hypoganglionic segment of varying length. This hypoganglionic zone is characterized by a reduced number of ganglion cells and nerve fibers in myenteric and submucous plexuses.

40.5 Diagnosis

The diagnosis of HD is usually based on clinical history, radiological studies, anorectal manometry, and in particular on histological examination of the rectal wall biopsy specimens.

40.5.1 Clinical Features

80–90% of all patients with HD have clinical symptoms and are diagnosed during the neonatal period. Delayed passage of meconium is the cardinal symptom in neonates with HD. Over 90% of affected patients fail to pass meconium in the first 24 h of life. The usual presentation of HD in the neonatal period is with constipation, abdominal distension, and vomiting during the first few days of life (Fig. 40.1a). About 20% of the babies with HD present with diarrhea. Diarrhea in HD is always a symptom of Hirschsprung's associated enterocolitis (HAEC), which represents the most common cause of death in patients with HD. HAEC usually resolves under adequate therapy or may result in life-threatening toxic megacolon, which is characterized by a sudden onset of marked abdominal distension, bile stained vomiting, fever, signs of dehydration, sepsis, and shock. Rectal examination or introduction of a rectal tube results in the explosive evacuation of gas and foul-smelling stools. In older children, the main symptom is persistent constipation and chronic abdominal distension.

40.5.2 Radiological Evaluation

In newborns with HD, a plain abdominal X-ray film will show dilated loops of bowel with fluid levels and airless pelvis. Occasionally, one may be able to see a small amount of air in the undistended rectum and dilated colon above it raising the suspicion of HD (Fig. 40.3a). Plain abdominal X-ray films obtained in patients with TCA may show characteristic signs of ileal obstruction with air-fluid levels or simple gaseous distension of small intestinal loops. In patients with HAEC,

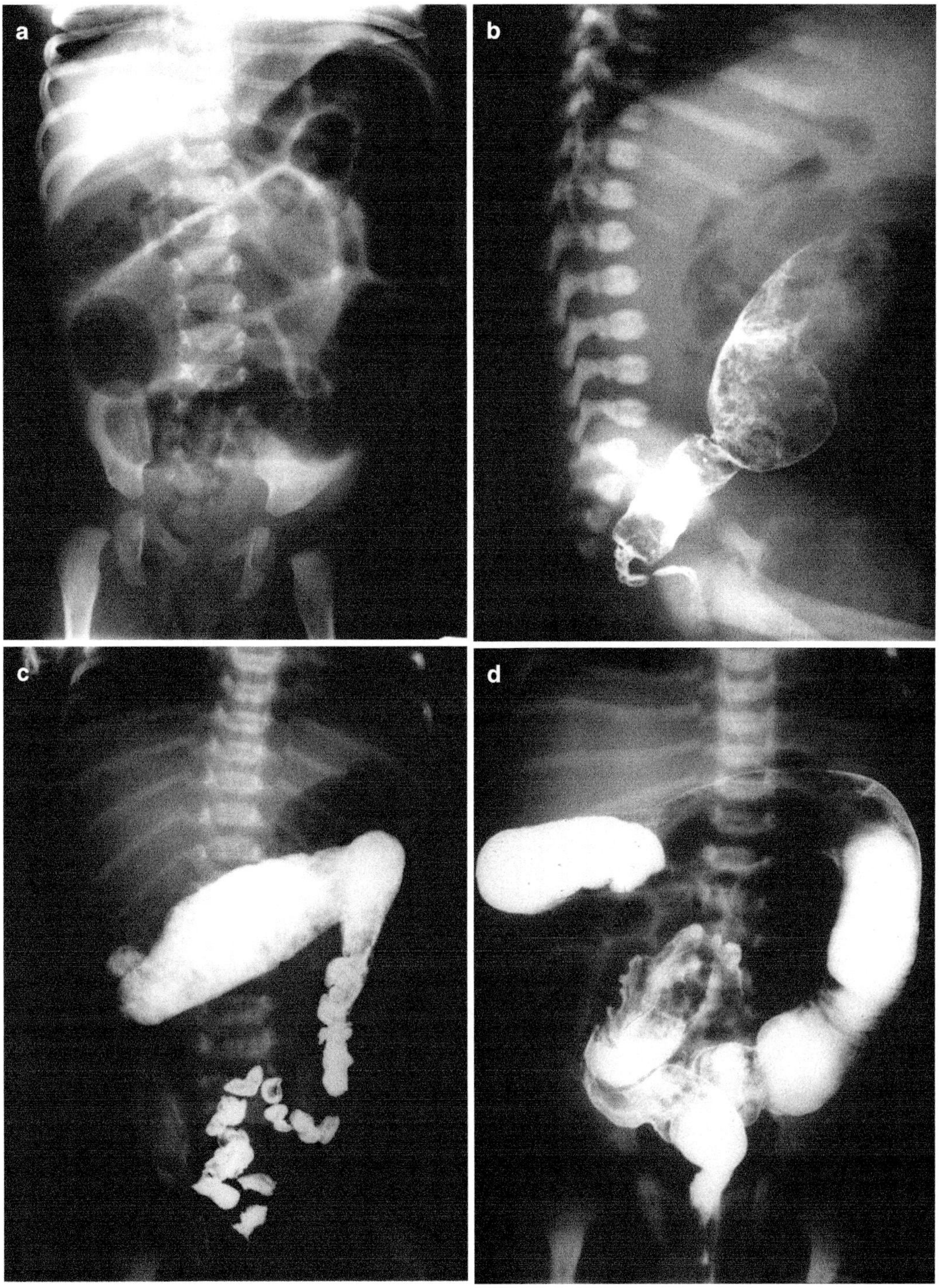

Fig. 40.3 Radiological evaluations for Hirschsprung's disease: Plain abdominal X-ray film in a 4-day-old newborn showing marked dilatation of large and small bowel loops with gas in the undilated rectum (**a**). A barium enema in this patient revealed the transition zone at the recto-sigmoid level (**b**). Delayed 24-h film in lateral position showing barium retention with accentuated transition at splenic fixture in a 10-day-old newborn (**c**). Enterocolitis complicating Hirschsprung's disease: Spasm at recto-sigmoid level with fine mucosal ulceration and mucosal edema giving cobblestone appearance (**d**)

plain abdominal X-ray films may show thickening of the bowel wall with mucosal irregularity or a grossly dilated colon loop, indicating toxic megacolon. A pneumoperitoneum may be found in those with perforation. Spontaneous perforation of the intestinal tract has been reported in 3% of patients with HD [140]. Using a careful technique, a barium enema performed by an experienced radiologist, should achieve a high degree of reliability in diagnosing HD in newborns. It is important that the infant should not have rectal washouts or even digital examinations prior to barium enema, as such interference may distort the transition zone appearance and give a false-negative diagnosis. A soft rubber catheter is inserted into the lower rectum and held in position with firm strapping across the buttocks. Due to the risk of perforation and the possibility of distorting a transition zone by distension, a balloon catheter should not be used. The barium should be injected slowly in small amounts under fluoroscopic control with the baby in the lateral position. A typical case of HD will demonstrate flow of barium from the undilated rectum through a cone-shaped transition zone into dilated colon (Fig. 40.3b). Some cases may show an abrupt transition between the dilated proximal colon and the distal aganglionic segment, leaving the diagnosis in little doubt. In some cases, findings on the barium enema are uncertain and a delayed abdominal X-ray film at 24 h may confirm the diagnosis by demonstrating the retained barium and often accentuating the appearance of the transition zone (Fig. 40.3c). In the presence of)HAEC, a barium enema can demonstrate spasm, mucosal edema, and ulceration (Fig. 40.3d). In TCA, the contrast enema is not pathognomonic and may not provide a definitive diagnosis. The colon in TCA is of normal caliber in 25–77% of cases [141].

40.5.3 Anorectal Manometry

In normally innervated bowel, distension of the rectum produces relaxation of the recto-sphincteric reflex. In normal individuals, upon distending the rectal balloon with air, the rectum immediately responds with a transient rise in pressure lasting 15–20 s. At the same time, the rhythmic activity of the internal anal sphincter (IAS) is depressed or abolished and its pressure falls by 15–20 cm. The duration of relaxation coincides with the rectal wave (Fig. 40.4a). In patients with HD, the rectum often shows spontaneous waves of varying amplitude and frequency in the resting phase. The rhythmic activity of the IAS is more pronounced. However, there is a complete absence of IAS relaxation upon rectal distension. (Fig. 40.4b). Failure to detect the recto-sphincteric reflex in premature and term infants is believed to be due to technical difficulties and not to immaturity of ganglion cells. Light sedation, particularly in infants and small children, may overcome technical difficulties encountered in this age group.

40.5.4 Rectal Biopsy

The diagnosis of HD is usually confirmed by examination of rectal biopsy specimens. The introduction of histochemical staining techniques for the detection of AChE activity in rectal suction biopsies (RSBs) has resulted in a reliable and simple method for the diagnosis of HD [142–144]. A rapid technique for performing AChE histochemistry in only 6 min has also been developed [145]. A full-thickness RSB is rarely indicated for the diagnosis of HD except in TCA. In normal individuals, barely detectable AChE activity is observed within the lamina propria and muscularis mucosa. On the other hand, the submucosal ganglion cells show strong staining for AChE (Fig. 40.5a). In HD, there is a marked increase in AChE activity in the lamina propria mucosae and muscularis mucosae, which is associated with the hypertrophied extrinsic nerve fibers of the aganglionic segment [145–149] (Fig. 40.5b). In TCA, AChE activity in RSB presents an atypical pattern, different from the classical one. Positive AChE fibers can be found in the lamina propria as well as the muscularis mucosae. However, cholinergic fibers present a lower density than in classical HD. Furthermore, it has been shown that NADPH diaphorase histochemi-

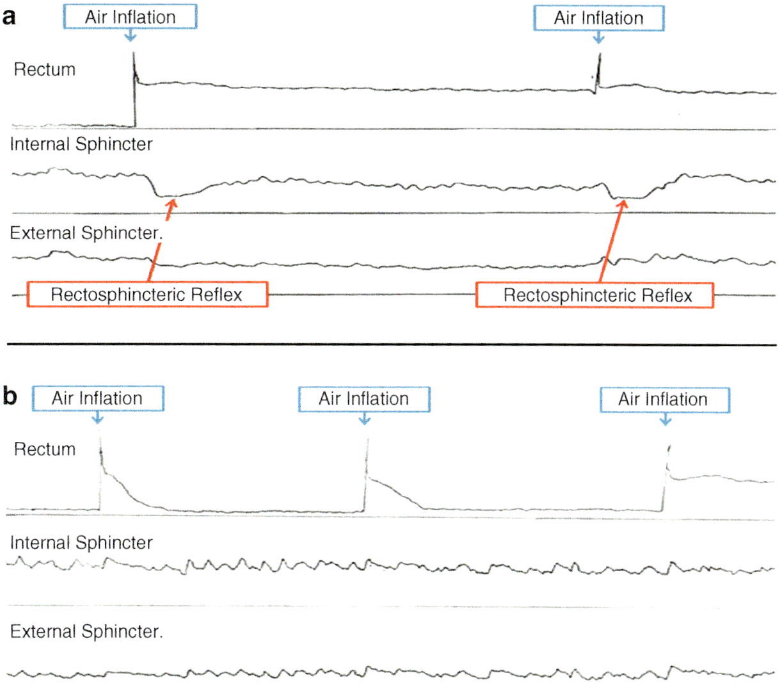

Fig. 40.4 Anorectal manometry showing evidence of the normal internal anal sphincter (IAS) recto-sphincteric reflex on rectal balloon inflation (**a**), and absence of IAS relaxation and presence of marked rhythmic activity of the IAS in a patient with Hirschsprung's disease (**b**)

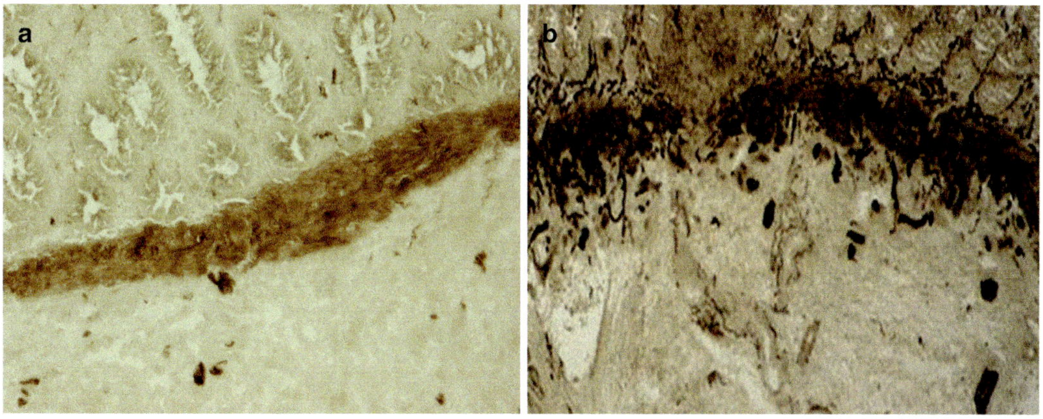

Fig. 40.5 Normal rectum showing minimal acetylcholinesterase (AChE) staining in mucosa, lamina propria, and muscularis mucosae (**a**). Hirschsprung's disease is characterized by a marked increase in AChE-positive nerve fibers in the lamina propria and muscularis mucosae (**b**)

cal staining may be an important additional technique for diagnosing HD [150].

40.5.5 Differential Diagnosis

Several conditions must be considered when an infant is being evaluated for HD. Table 40.3 provides a list of common differential diagnosis. Colonic atresia gives similar plain abdominal X-ray film findings as in HD, but is readily excluded with barium enema showing complete mechanical obstruction. Distal small bowel atresia shows gross distension of the bowel loop immediately proximal to the obstruction with the widest fluid level in it. In meconium ileus the

Table 40.3 Differential diagnosis of Hirschsprung's disease

Location	Differential diagnosis
Small intestine	Small bowel obstruction
	Malrotation, volvulus
	Intestinal atresia
	Meconium ileus
Colon	Colonic atresia
	Meconium plug syndrome
	Small left colon syndrome
	Anorectal malformation
Other causes	Intestinal motility disorders
	Pseudo-obstruction
	Necrotizing enterocolitis
	Sepsis
	Electrolyte abnormalities
	Hypothyroidism
	Drugs

typical mottled thick meconium may be seen. Also, clear, sharp fluid levels are not a feature in erect or lateral decubitus views. However, HD can sometimes simulate meconium ileus in plain abdominal X-ray films and may give equivocal findings on Gastrografin or barium enema. Meconium plugs obstructing the colon can present as HD with strongly suggestive history and plain abdominal X-ray films. Small left colon syndrome with marked distension proximal to narrowed descending colon also simulates HD at the left colonic flexure. These two conditions usually resolve with Gastrografin enema, but a minority of these cases will actually have HD which should be excluded clinically.

40.6 Surgical Management

A number of different surgical techniques have been described for the treatment of HD. The four most commonly used procedures are the recto-sigmoidectomy developed by Swenson and Bill, the retrorectal approach developed by Duhamel, the endorectal procedure developed by Soave, and deep anterior colorectal anastomosis developed by Rehbein [8, 151]. The basic principle in all these procedures is to bring the ganglionic bowel down to the anus. The long-term results of any of these operations are satisfactory if they are performed correctly.

In recent years, the vast majority of cases of HD are diagnosed in the neonatal period. Many centers are now performing one-stage pull-through operations in the newborn with minimal morbidity rates and encouraging results. The advantages of operating on the newborn are that the colonic dilation can be quickly controlled by washouts and at operation the caliber of the pull-through bowel is near normal, allowing for an accurate anastomosis that minimizes leakage and cuff infection. A number of investigators have described and advocated a variety of one-stage pull-through procedures for newborn with HD using minimal invasive laparoscopic techniques. More recently, a transanal endorectal pull-through (TERP) operation performed without opening the abdomen has been used with excellent results in recto-sigmoid HD.

40.6.1 Preoperative Management

Preoperatively, a good barium enema study is essential for this technique. A typical case of recto-sigmoid HD usually demonstrates flow of barium from undilated rectum through a cone-shaped transition zone into dilated sigmoid colon. Once the diagnosis of HD has been confirmed by RSB, the newborn should be prepared for surgery. Rectal irrigations are carried out twice a day for 2–3 days prior surgery. Intravenous gentamicin and metronidazole are started on the morning of operation. If the newborn has HAEC, correction of dehydration and electrolyte imbalance by infusion of appropriate fluids will be required. It is essential to decompress the bowel as early as possible in these babies. Deflation of the intestine may be carried out by rectal irrigations, but some babies may require colostomy.

40.6.2 Transanal One-Stage Endorectal Pull-through Operation

A one-stage pull-through operation can be successfully performed in these patients using a transanal endorectal approach without opening the abdomen. This procedure is associated with excellent clinical results and permits early post-operative feeding, early hospital discharge, no visible scars, and low incidence of enterocolitis [152, 153]. Most pediatric surgeons prefer the TERP operation for managing patients with classical segment recto-sigmoid HD.

40.6.2.1 Operative Technique

The patient is positioned on the operating table in the lithotomy position. The legs are strapped over sandbags. A Foley catheter is inserted into the bladder. An anal retractor is placed to retract perianal skin. The rectal mucosa is circumferentially incised using the cautery with a fine-tipped needle, approximately 5 mm from the dentate line, and the submucosal plane is developed. The proximal cut edge of the mucosal cuff is held with multiple fine silk sutures, which are used for traction (Fig. 40.6). The endorectal dissection is then carried out proximally, staying in the submucosal plane.

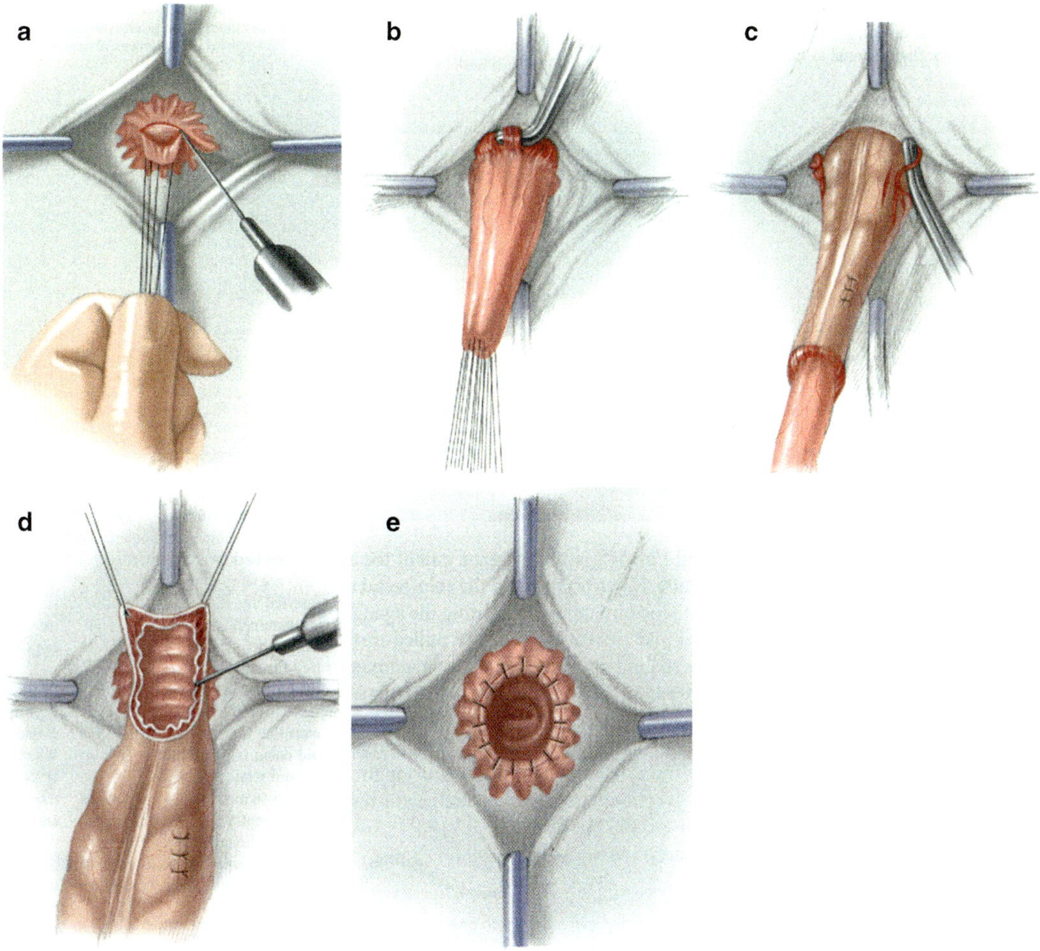

Fig. 40.6 Transanal endorectal pull-through operation: Rectal mucosa is circumferentially incised using the needle-tip cautery approximately 5 mm above the dentate line and the submucosa plane is developed (**a**). When the submucosal dissection is extended proximally for about 3 cm, the muscle is divided circumferentially, and the full-thickness of the rectum and sigmoid colon is mobilized out through the anus (**b**). On reaching the transition zone, full-thickness rectal biopsies are taken for frozen section to confirm ganglion cells (**c**). The colon is divided several centimeters above the most proximal biopsy site (**d**). A standard Soave-Boley anastomosis is performed (**e**)

When the submucosal dissection has extended for about 3 cm, the rectal muscle is divided circumferentially, and the full thickness of the rectum and sigmoid colon is mobilized out through the anus. This requires division of rectal and sigmoid vessels, which can be done under direct vision using cautery.

When the transition zone is encountered, full-thickness biopsy sections are taken, and frozen section confirmation of ganglion cells is obtained. The rectal muscular cuff is split longitudinally either anteriorly or posteriorly. The colon is then divided several centimeters above the most proximal normal biopsy site, and a standard Soave-Boley anastomosis is performed. No drains are placed. The patient is started on oral feeds after 24 h and discharged home on the third postoperative day. Digital rectal examination is performed 2 weeks after the operation. Routine rectal dilatation is not performed unless there is evidence of a stricture.

40.6.3 Postoperative Complications

Early postoperative complications which can occur after any type of pull-through operation include wound infections, anastomotic leakage, anastomotic stricture, retraction or necrosis of the neorectum, intestinal adhesions, and ileus. Late complications include constipation, enterocolitis, incontinence, anastomotic problems, adhesive bowel obstruction, and urogenital complications.

40.6.3.1 Anastomotic Leakage

The most dangerous early postoperative complication following the definitive abdomino-perineal pull-through operation is leakage at the anastomotic suture line. Factors responsible for anastomotic leakage include ischemia of the distal end of the colonic pull-through segment, tension on the anastomosis, incomplete anastomotic suture lines, and inadvertent rectal manipulation. If a leak is recognized in a patient without a colostomy, it is imperative to perform a diverting colostomy promptly, to administer intravenous antibiotics and to irrigate the rectum with antibiotic solution a few times daily. Delay in establishing fecal diversion is likely to result in an extensive pelvic abscess which may require laparotomy and transabdominal drainage.

40.6.3.2 Retraction of Pull-through

Retraction of a portion or of the entire colonic segment from the anastomosis can occur and is usually seen within 3 weeks after the operation. Evaluation under general anesthesia is generally necessary. In occasional patients, resuturing the anastomosis may be feasible transanally. For those with separation of less than 50% of the anastomosis, but with adequate vascularity of the colon, a diverting colostomy for approximately 3 months is necessary. For patients with wide separation at the anastomosis, early transabdominal reconstruction of the pull-through is recommended.

40.6.3.3 Perianal Excoriation

Perianal excoriations occur in nearly half of the patients undergoing pull-through operations, but generally resolve within 3 months with local therapy and resolution of diarrhea. It is helpful to begin placing a barrier cream on the perianal each movement for the first few weeks. Resolution of diarrhea will often hasten the clearance of perianal skin irritation.

40.6.3.4 Constipation

Constipation is common after definitive repair of HD and can be due to residual aganglionosis and high anal tone. Repeated and forceful anal dilations combined with botulinum toxin injection into the IAS under general anesthesia may resolve the problem. In some patients, a myectomy of the IAS may be needed. In patients with scarring, stricture, or intestinal neuronal dysplasia proximal to aganglionic segment, treatment consists of treating the underlying cause.

40.6.3.5 Enterocolitis

HAEC is a significant complication of HD both in the pre- and postoperative periods [140, 154]. It can occur at any time from the neonatal period onwards to adulthood and can be independent of the medical management and surgical procedure performed. The incidence of HAEC ranges from 20 to 58% [140]. Fortunately, the mortality rate has declined over the last 30 years from 30 to 1%. This decrease in mortality is related to earlier diagnosis of HD and HAEC, rectal decompression, appropriate vigorous resuscitation, and antibiotic therapy. It has been reported that routine postoperative rectal washouts decrease both the incidence and the severity of the episodes of HAEC following definitive surgery. In episodes of recurrent HAEC, which can develop in up to 56% of patients, anal dilatations have been recommended. However, prior to commencing a treatment regime, a contrast enema should be performed to rule out a mechanical obstruction. Patients with a normal rectal biopsy may require a sphincterotomy.

40.6.3.6 Fecal Soiling

Soiling is fairly common after all types of pull-through operation. However, the precise incidence primarily dependent on how assiduously the investigator looks for it. The reported incidence of soiling ranges from 10 to 30% [8]. The attainment of normal postoperative defecation is clearly dependent on intensity of bowel training, social background, and respective intelligence of the patients. Mental handicap (including Down syndrome) is invariably associated with long-term incontinence [155]. Those patients with preoperative HAEC would also seem to have a marginally higher long-term risk of incontinence. In some patients in who soiling is intractable and a social problem, a Malone procedure may be needed to stay clean.

40.7 Long-Term Outcome

Most patients who underwent pull-through operation for HD generally have a satisfactory long-term outcome [141, 153, 156, 157]. A recent large multicenter study showed no significant differences in continence and stooling patterns after transanal compared with transabdominal approach [153]. However, some children have persistent postoperative problems such as constipation, enterocolitis, and soiling [158–160]. In order to identify and provide early treatment options for these problems, it is important to follow these patients closely, at least until they are through the toilet training process. The vast majority of residual bowel problems can be managed by non-surgical treatment such as laxatives, enemas or intrasphincteric botulinum toxin injection [157, 161, 162]. In one-third of all patients with HD, which require a redo pull-through operation, a retained aganglionic segment or transition zone bowel is the underlying cause for persistent abdominal distension and recurrent bowel symptoms [163]. But overall, adolescents and adults with HD usually have a relatively good quality of life, social satisfaction and sexual function [156, 164].

References

1. Ruysch F. Observationum anatomico-chirurgicarum centuria. Amsterdam; 1691.
2. Jacobi A. On some important causes of constipation in infants. Am J Obstet Gynecol. 1869;2:96–113.
3. Hirschsprung H. Stuhlträgheit Neugeborener in Folge von Dilatation und Hypertrophie des Colons. Jahrb f Kinderheilkunde. 1888;27:1–7.
4. Tittel K. Über eine angeborene Missbildung des Dickdarms. Wien Klin Wochenschr. 1901;14:903–7.
5. Ehrenpreis T. Megacolon in the newborn: a clinical and roentgenological study with special regard to the pathogenesis. Acta Chir Scand Suppl. 1946;112:94.
6. Whitehouse FR, Kernohan JW. Myenteric plexuses in congenital megacolon: study of 11 cases. Arch Intern Med. 1948;82:75–111.
7. Swenson O, Bill AH. Resection of rectum and rectosigmoid with preservation of the sphincter for benign spastic lesions producing megacolon. Surgery. 1948;24:212–20.
8. Puri P. Hirschsprung's disease. In: Puri P, editor. Newborn Surgery. London: Hodder Arnold; 2011. p. 554–65.
9. Haricharan RN, Georgeson KE. Hirschsprung disease. Semin Pediatr Surg. 2008;17:266–75.
10. Kleinhaus S, et al. Hirschsprung's disease: a survey of the members of the Surgical Section of the American Academy of Pediatrics. J Pediatr Surg. 1979;14:588–97.
11. Sherman JO, et al. A 40-year multinational retrospective study of 880 Swenson procedures. J Pediatr Surg. 1989;24:833–8.

12. Suita S, et al. Hirschsprung's disease in Japan: analysis of 3852 patients based on a nationwide survey in 30 years. J Pediatr Surg. 2005;40:197–201.
13. Senyuz OF, et al. Total intestinal aganglionosis with involvement of the stomach. Pediatr Surg Int. 1988;3:74–5.
14. Sharif K, et al. New perspective for the management of near-total or total intestinal aganglionosis in infants. J Pediatr Surg. 2003;38:25–8.
15. Meier-Ruge W. Ultrashort segment Hirschsprung disease: an objective picture of the disease substantiated by biopsy. Z Kinderchir. 1985;40: 146–50.
16. Meier-Ruge WA, et al. Diagnosis and therapy of ultrashort Hirschsprung's disease. Eur J Pediatr Surg. 2004;14:392–7.
17. Neilson IR, Yazbeck S. Ultrashort Hirschsprung's disease: myth or reality. J Pediatr Surg. 1990;25: 1135–8.
18. Haney PJ, Hill JL, Sun CCJ. Zonal colonic aganglionosis. Pediatr Radiol. 1982;12:258–61.
19. MacIver AG, Whitehead R. Zonal colonic aganglionosis, a variant of Hirschsprung's disease. Arch Dis Child. 1972;47:233–7.
20. Seldenrijk CA, et al. Zonal aganglionosis: an enzyme and immunohistochemical study of two cases. Virchows Arch A Pathol Anat Histopathol. 1986;410:75–81.
21. Kapur RP, et al. Hypothesis: pathogenesis of skip areas in long-segment Hirschsprung's disease. Pediatr Pathol Lab Med. 1995;15:23–37.
22. Martin LW, et al. Hirschsprung's disease with skip area (segmental aganglionosis). J Pediatr Surg. 1979;14:686–7.
23. Sprinz H, Cohen A, Heaton LD. Hirschsprung's disease with skip area. Ann Surg. 1961;153:143–8.
24. O'Donnell AM, Puri P. Skip segment Hirschsprung's disease: a systematic review. Pediatr Surg Int. 2010;26:1065–9.
25. Orr JD, Scobie WG. Presentation and incidence of Hirschsprung's disease. BMJ. 1983;287:1671–1.
26. Passarge E. Genetics of Hirschsprung's disease: evidence for heterogeneous etiology and a study of 63 families. N Engl J Med. 1967;276:138–43.
27. Spouge D, Baird PA. Hirschsprung disease in a large birth cohort. Teratology. 1985;32:171–7.
28. Torfs C (1998) An epidemiological study of Hirschsprung's disease in a multiracial Californian population. Paper presented at the Third International Meeting: Hirschsprung's disease and related neurocristopathies, Evian, France.
29. Emison ES, et al. A common sex-dependent mutation in a RET enhancer underlies Hirschsprung disease risk. Nature. 2005;434:857–63.
30. Badner JA, et al. A genetic study of Hirschsprung's disease. Am J Hum Genet. 1990;46:568–80.
31. Ikeda K, Goto S. Diagnosis and treatment of Hirschsprung's disease in Japan. An analysis of 1628 patients. Ann Surg. 1984;199:400–5.
32. Paran TS, Rolle U, Puri P. Enteric nervous system and developmental abnormalities in childhood. Pediatr Surg Int. 2006;22:945–59.
33. Gershon MD. Functional anatomy of the enteric nervous system. In: Holschneider AM, Puri P, editors. Hirschsprung's disease and allied disorders. Heidelberg: Springer; 2008. p. 21–49.
34. Gershon MD, Chalazonitis A, Rothman TP. From neural crest to bowel: development of the enteric nervous system. J Neurobiol. 1993;24:199–214.
35. Puri P, Rolle U. Development of the enteric nervous system. In: Holschneider AM, Puri P, editors. Hirschsprung's disease and allied disorders. Heidelberg: Springer; 2008. p. 13–20.
36. Puri P, Ohshiro K, Wester T. Hirschsprung's disease: a search for etiology. Semin Pediatr Surg. 1998;7:140–7.
37. Rolle U, Nemeth L, Puri P. Nitrergic innervation of the normal gut and in motility disorders of childhood. J Pediatr Surg. 2002;37:551–67.
38. Burns AJ, et al. Development of the enteric nervous system and its role in intestinal motility during fetal and early postnatal stages. Semin Pediatr Surg. 2009;18:196–205.
39. Burns AJ, Le Douarin NM. The sacral neural crest contributes neurons and glia to the post-umbilical gut: spatiotemporal analysis of the development of the enteric nervous system. Development. 1998;125:4335–47.
40. Le Douarin NM, Teillet MA. Migration of neural crest cells to wall of digestive tract in avian embryo. J Embryol Exp Morphol. 1973;30:31–48.
41. Puri P, Shinkai T. Pathogenesis of Hirschsprung's disease and its variants: recent progress. Semin Pediatr Surg. 2004;13:18–24.
42. Furness JB, Costa M. Structure of the enteric nervous system. In: Furness JB, editor. The enteric nervous system. Oxford: Blackwell; 2006. p. 1–28.
43. Tam PK, Garcia-Barcelo M. Genetic basis of Hirschsprung's disease. Pediatr Surg Int. 2009;25: 543–58.
44. Caniano DA, et al. Total intestinal aganglionosis. J Pediatr Surg. 1985;20:456–60.
45. Nemeth L, et al. Three-dimensional morphology of gut innervation in total intestinal aganglionosis using whole-mount preparation. J Pediatr Surg. 2001;36:291–4.
46. Jannot AS, et al. Male and female differential reproductive rate could explain parental transmission asymmetry of mutation origin in Hirschsprung disease. Eur J Hum Genet. 2012;20:917–20.
47. Caniano DA, Teitelbaum DH, Qualman SJ. Management of Hirschsprung's disease in children with trisomy 21. Am J Surg. 1990;159: 402–4.
48. Goldberg E. An epidemiological study of Hirschsprung's disease. Int J Epidemiol. 1985;13:479–85.
49. Moore SW. Down syndrome and the enteric nervous system. Pediatr Surg Int. 2008;24:873–83.

50. Quinn FMJ, Surana R, Puri P. The influence of trisomy 21 on outcome in children with Hirschsprung's disease. J Pediatr Surg. 1994;29:781–3.
51. Arnold S, et al. Interaction between a chromosome 10 RET enhancer and chromosome 21 in the Down syndrome-Hirschsprung disease association. Hum Mutat. 2009;30:771–5.
52. Moore SW, Zaahl MG. Intronic RET gene variants in Down syndrome-associated Hirschsprung disease in an African population. J Pediatr Surg. 2012;47:299–302.
53. Amiel J, et al. Hirschsprung disease, associated syndromes and genetics: a review. J Med Genet. 2008;45:1–14.
54. Wallace AS, Anderson RB. Genetic interactions and modifier genes in Hirschsprung's disease. World J Gastroenterol. 2011;17:4937–44.
55. Amiel J, et al. Heterozygous endothelin receptor B (EDNRB) mutations in isolated Hirschsprung disease. Hum Mol Genet. 1996;5:355–7.
56. Angrist M, et al. Germline mutations in glial cell line-derived neurotrophic factor (GDNF) and RET in a Hirschsprung disease patient. Nat Genet. 1996;14:341–4.
57. Attié T, et al. Diversity of RET proto-oncogene mutations in familial and sporadic Hirschsprung disease. Hum Mol Genet. 1995;4:1381–6.
58. Bidaud C, et al. Endothelin-3 gene mutations in isolated and syndromic Hirschsprung disease. Eur J Hum Genet. 1997;5:247–51.
59. Brooks AS, et al. Homozygous nonsense mutations in KIAA1279 are associated with malformations of the central and enteric nervous systems. Am J Hum Genet. 2005;77:120–6.
60. Carter TC, et al. Hirschsprung's disease and variants in genes that regulate enteric neural crest cell proliferation, migration and differentiation. J Hum Genet. 2012;57:485–93.
61. Doray B, et al. Mutation of the RET ligand, neurturin, supports multigenic inheritance in Hirschsprung disease. Hum Mol Genet. 1998;7:1449–52.
62. Garavelli L, et al. Hirschsprung disease, mental retardation, characteristic facial features, and mutation in the gene ZFHX1B (SIP1): confirmation of the Mowat-Wilson syndrome. Am J Med Genet A. 2003;116A:385–8.
63. Garcia-Barcelo M, et al. Association study of PHOX2B as a candidate gene for Hirschsprung's disease. Gut. 2003;52:563–7.
64. Garcia-Barcelo MM, et al. Evaluation of the NK2 homeobox 1 gene (NKX2–1) as a Hirschsprung's disease locus. Ann Hum Genet. 2008;72:170–7.
65. Garcia-Barcelo MM, et al. Correlation between genetic variations in Hox clusters and Hirschsprung's disease. Ann Hum Genet. 2007;71:526–36.
66. Garcia-Barcelo MM, et al. Genome-wide association study identifies NRG1 as a susceptibility locus for Hirschsprung's disease. Proc Natl Acad Sci U S A. 2009;106:2694–9.
67. Herbarth B, et al. Mutation of the Sry-related Sox10 gene in dominant megacolon, a mouse model for human Hirschsprung disease. Proc Natl Acad Sci U S A. 1998;95:5161–5.
68. Hofstra RM, et al. A loss-of-function mutation in the endothelin-converting enzyme 1 (ECE-1) associated with Hirschsprung disease, cardiac defects, and autonomic dysfunction. Am J Hum Genet. 1999;64:304–8.
69. Hofstra RMW, et al. RET and GDNF gene scanning in Hirschsprung patients using two dual denaturing gel systems. Hum Mutat. 2000;15:418–29.
70. Ivanchuk SM, et al. De novo mutation of GDNF, ligand for the RET/GDNFR-alpha receptor complex, in Hirschsprung disease. Hum Mol Genet. 1996;5:2023–6.
71. Jiang Q, et al. Copy number variants in candidate genes are genetic modifiers of Hirschsprung disease. PLoS One. 2011;6:e21219.
72. Kusafuka T, Wang YP, Puri P. Novel mutations of the endothelin-B receptor gene in isolated patients with Hirschsprung's disease. Hum Mol Genet. 1996;5:347–9.
73. Lui VC, et al. Perturbation of hoxb5 signaling in vagal neural crests down-regulates ret. leading to intestinal hypoganglionosis in mice. Gastroenterology. 2008;134:1104–15.
74. Myers SM, et al. Investigation of germline GFR alpha-1 mutations in Hirschsprung disease. J Med Genet. 1999;36:217–20.
75. Pasini B, et al. Loss of function effect of RET mutations causing Hirschsprung disease. Nat Genet. 1995;10:35–40.
76. Pingault V, et al. Human homology and candidate genes for the dominant megacolon locus: a mouse model of Hirschsprung disease. Genomics. 1997;39:86–9.
77. Puffenberger EG, et al. A missense mutation of the endothelin-B receptor gene in multigenic Hirschsprung's disease. Cell. 1994;79:1257–66.
78. Rosenfeld JA, et al. Genotype-phenotype analysis of TCF4 mutations causing Pitt-Hopkins syndrome shows increased seizure activity with missense mutations. Genet Med. 2009;11:797–805.
79. Southard-Smith EM, Kos L, Pavan WJ. Sox10 mutation disrupts neural crest development in Dom Hirschsprung mouse model. Nat Genet. 1998;18:60–4.
80. Stanchina L, et al. Genetic interaction between Sox10 and Zfhx1b during enteric nervous system development. Dev Biol. 2010;341:416–28.
81. Svensson PJ, et al. A heterozygous frameshift mutation in the endothelin-3 (EDN-3) gene in isolated Hirschsprung's disease. Pediatr Res. 1999;45:714–7.
82. Tang CS, et al. Genome-wide copy number analysis uncovers a new HSCR Gene: NRG3. PLoS Genet. 2012;8:e1002687.

83. Tang CS, et al. Mutations in the NRG1 gene are associated with Hirschsprung disease. Hum Genet. 2012;131:67–76.
84. Tang CSM, et al. Fine mapping of the NRG1 Hirschsprung's disease locus. PLoS One. 2011;6:e16181.
85. Wakamatsu N, et al. Mutations in SIP1, encoding Smad interacting protein-1, cause a form of Hirschsprung disease. Nat Genet. 2001;27:369–70.
86. Wallace AS, et al. L1cam acts as a modifier gene during enteric nervous system development. Neurobiol Dis. 2010;40:622–33.
87. Wallace AS, et al. L1cam acts as a modifier gene for members of the endothelin signalling pathway during enteric nervous system development. Neurogastroenterol Motil. 2011;23:e510–22.
88. Zhu J, et al. HOXB5 cooperates with NKX2–1 in the transcription of human RET. PLoS One. 2011;6:e20815.
89. Edery P, et al. Mutations of the RET proto-oncogene in Hirschsprung's disease. Nature. 1994;367:378–80.
90. Romeo G, et al. Point mutations affecting the tyrosine kinase domain of the RET proto-oncogene in Hirschsprung's disease. Nature. 1994;367:377–8.
91. Sancandi M, et al. Incidence of RET mutations in patients with Hirschsprung's disease. J Pediatr Surg. 2000;35:139–42.
92. Emison ES, et al. Differential contributions of rare and common, coding and noncoding Ret mutations to multifactorial Hirschsprung disease liability. Am J Hum Genet. 2010;87:60–74.
93. Alves MMM, et al. Mutations in SCG10 are not involved in Hirschsprung's disease. PLoS One. 2010;5:e15144.
94. Kusafuka T, Wang YP, Puri P. Mutation analysis of the RET, the endothelin-B receptor, and the endothelin-3 genes in sporadic cases of Hirschsprung's disease. J Pediatr Surg. 1997;32:501–4.
95. Dasgupta R, Langer JC. Hirschsprung disease. Curr Probl Surg. 2004;41:942–88.
96. Kakita Y, et al. Selective demonstration of mural nerves in ganglionic and aganglionic colon by immunohistochemistry for glucose transporter-1: prominent extrinsic nerve pattern staining in Hirschsprung disease. Arch Pathol Lab Med. 2000;124:1314–9.
97. Kobayashi H, Obriain DS, Puri P. Nerve growth factor receptor immunostaining suggests an extrinsic origin for hypertrophic nerves in Hirschsprung's disease. Gut. 1994;35:1605–7.
98. Payette RF, et al. Origin and morphology of nerve fibers in the aganglionic colon of the lethal spotted (ls/ls) Mutant Mouse. J Comp Neurol. 1987;257:237–52.
99. Tam PKH, Boyd GP. Origin, course, and endings of abnormal enteric nerve fibers in Hirschsprung's disease defined by whole-mount immunohistochemistry. J Pediatr Surg. 1990;25:457–61.
100. Watanabe Y, et al. Spatial distribution and pattern of extrinsic nerve strands in the aganglionic segment of congenital aganglionosis: stereoscopic analysis in spotting lethal rats. J Pediatr Surg. 1995;30:1471–6.
101. Weinberg AG. Hirschsprung's disease: a pathologist's view. Perspect Pediatr Pathol. 1975;2:207–39.
102. Frigo GM, et al. Some observations on intrinsic nervous mechanism in Hirschsprung's disease. Gut. 1973;14:35–40.
103. Vizi ES, et al. Characteristics of cholinergic neuroeffector transmission of ganglionic and aganglionic colon in Hirschsprung's disease. Gut. 1990;31:1046–50.
104. Boston VE, Cywes S, Davies MRQ. Serum and erythrocyte acetylcholinesterase activity in Hirschsprung's disease. J Pediatr Surg. 1978;13: 407–10.
105. Imamura K, et al. Pathophysiology of aganglionic colon segment: experimental study on aganglionosis produced by a new method in rat. J Pediatr Surg. 1975;10:865–73.
106. Sato A, et al. Pathophysiology of aganglionic colon and anorectum: an experimental study on aganglionosis produced by a new method in the rat. J Pediatr Surg. 1978;13:399–435.
107. Garrett JR, Howard ER, Nixon HH. Autonomic nerves in rectum and colon in Hirschsprung's disease: a cholinesterase and catecholamine histochemical study. Arch Dis Child. 1969;44:406–17.
108. Nirasawa Y, et al. Hirschsprung's disease: catecholamine content, alpha-adrenoceptors, and the effect of electrical stimulation in aganglionic colon. J Pediatr Surg. 1986;21:136–42.
109. Touloukian RJ, Aghajanian G, Roth RH. Adrenergic hyperactivity of aganglionic colon. J Pediatr Surg. 1973;8:191–5.
110. Hiramoto Y, Kiesewet WB. Response of colonic muscle to drugs: in-vitro study of Hirschsprung's disease. J Pediatr Surg. 1974;9:13–20.
111. Wright PG, Shepherd JJ. Some observations on response of normal human sigmoid colon to drugs in vitro. Gut. 1966;7:41–51.
112. Bult H, et al. Nitric oxide as an inhibitory nonadrenergic noncholinergic neurotransmitter. Nature. 1990;345:346–7.
113. Dawson TM, et al. Nitric oxide synthase and neuronal NADPH diaphorase are identical in brain and peripheral tissues. Proc Natl Acad Sci U S A. 1991;88:7797–801.
114. Hope BT, et al. Neuronal NADPH diaphorase is a nitric oxide synthase. Proc Natl Acad Sci U S A. 1991;88:2811–4.
115. Bealer JF, et al. Nitric oxide synthase is deficient in the aganglionic colon of patients with Hirschsprung's disease. Pediatrics. 1994;93:647–51.
116. Guo RS, et al. The distribution and co-localization of nitric oxide synthase and vasoactive intestinal polypeptide in nerves of the colons with Hirschsprung's disease. Virchows Arch. 1997;430:53–61.
117. Kobayashi H, Obriain DS, Puri P. Lack of expression of NADPH diaphorase and neural cell adhe-

sion molecule (NCAM) in colonic muscle of patients with Hirschsprung's disease. J Pediatr Surg. 1994;29:301–4.
118. Larsson LT, et al. Lack of neuronal nitric oxide synthase in nerve fibers of aganglionic intestine: a clue to Hirschsprung's disease. J Pediatr Gastroenterol Nutr. 1995;20:49–53.
119. Vanderwinden JM, et al. Interstitial cells of Cajal in human colon and in Hirschsprung's disease. Gastroenterology. 1996;111:901–10.
120. Kusafuka T, Puri P. Altered mRNA expression of the neuronal nitric oxide synthase gene in Hirschsprung's disease. J Pediatr Surg. 1997;32:1054–8.
121. Bealer JF, et al. Effect of nitric oxide on the colonic smooth muscle of patients with Hirschsprung's disease. J Pediatr Surg. 1994;29:1025–9.
122. Mostafa RM, Moustafa YM, Hamdy H. Interstitial cells of Cajal, the Maestro in health and disease. World J Gastroenterol. 2010;16:3239–48.
123. Yamataka A, et al. A lack of intestinal pacemaker (C-Kit) in aganglionic bowel of patients with Hirschsprung's disease. J Pediatr Surg. 1995;30:441–4.
124. Yamataka A, et al. Intestinal pacemaker C-KIT+ cells and synapses in allied Hirschsprung's disorders. J Pediatr Surg. 1997;32:1069–74.
125. Horisawa M, Watanabe Y, Torihashi S. Distribution of c-kit immunopositive cells in normal human colon and in Hirschsprung's disease. J Pediatr Surg. 1998;33:1209–14.
126. Rolle U, et al. Altered distribution of interstitial cells of Cajal in Hirschsprung disease. Arch Pathol Lab Med. 2002;126:928–33.
127. Nemeth L, Maddur S, Puri P. Immunolocalization of the gap junction protein Connexin43 in the interstitial cells of Cajal in the normal and Hirschsprung's disease bowel. J Pediatr Surg. 2000;35:823–8.
128. Piotrowska AP, Solari V, Puri P. Distribution of Ca^{2+}-activated K channels, SK2 and SK3, in the normal and Hirschsprung's disease bowel. J Pediatr Surg. 2003;38:978–83.
129. Soeda J, Obriain DS, Puri P. Mucosal neuroendocrine cell abnormalities in the colon of patients with Hirschsprung's disease. J Pediatr Surg. 1992;27:823–7.
130. Nemeth L, Rolle U, Puri P. Altered cytoskeleton in smooth muscle of aganglionic bowel. Arch Pathol Lab Med. 2002;126:692–6.
131. Covault J, Sanes JR. Distribution of N-CAM in synaptic and extrasynaptic portions of developing and adult skeletal muscle. J Cell Biol. 1986;102: 716–30.
132. Moore SE, Walsh FS. Specific regulation of N-CAM/D2-CAM cell adhesion molecule during skeletal muscle development. EMBO J. 1985;4: 623–30.
133. Thiery JP, et al. Cell adhesion molecules in early chicken embryogenesis. Proc Natl Acad Sci U S A. 1982;79:6737–41.
134. Romanska HM, et al. Increased expression of muscular neural cell adhesion molecule in congenital aganglionosis. Gastroenterology. 1993;105:1104–9.
135. Payette RF, et al. Accumulation of components of basal laminae: association with the failure of neural crest cells to colonize the presumptive aganglionic bowel of ls/ls mutant mice. Dev Biol. 1988;125:341–60.
136. Tennyson VM, et al. Distribution of hyaluronic acid and chondroitin sulfate proteoglycans in the presumptive aganglionic terminal bowel of Ls/Ls fetal mice: an ultrastructural analysis. J Comp Neurol. 1990;291:345–62.
137. Parikh DH, et al. Quantitative and qualitative analysis of the extracellular matrix protein, laminin, in Hirschsprung's disease. J Pediatr Surg. 1992;27:991–6.
138. Parikh DH, et al. Abnormalities in the distribution of laminin and collagen Type IV in Hirschsprung's disease. Gastroenterology. 1992;102:1236–41.
139. Parikh DH, et al. The extracellular matrix components, tenascin and fibronectin, in Hirschsprung's disease: an immunohistochemical study. J Pediatr Surg. 1994;29:1302–6.
140. Murphy F, Menezes M. Enterocolitis complicating Hirschsprung's disease. In: Holschneider AM, Puri P, editors. Hirschsprung's disease and allied disorders. Heidelberg: Springer; 2008. p. 133–43.
141. Menezes M, et al. Long-term clinical outcome in patients with total colonic aganglionosis: a 31-year review. J Pediatr Surg. 2008;43:1696–9.
142. Lake BD, et al. Hirschsprung's disease: appraisal of histochemically demonstrated acetylcholinesterase activity in suction rectal biopsy specimens as an aid to diagnosis. Arch Pathol Lab Med. 1978;102:244–7.
143. Meier-Ruge W, Bruder E. Histopathological diagnosis and differential diagnosis of Hirschsprung's disease. In: Holschneider AM, Puri P, editors. Hirschsprung's disease and allied disorders. Heidelberg: Springer; 2008. p. 185–98.
144. Meier-Ruge W, et al. Acetylcholinesterase activity in suction biopsies of rectum in diagnosis of Hirschsprung's disease. J Pediatr Surg. 1972;7:11–7.
145. Kobayashi H, et al. A new rapid acetylcholinesterase staining kit for diagnosing Hirschsprung's disease. Pediatr Surg Int. 2007;23:505–8.
146. Kobayashi H, et al. A rapid technique of acetylcholinesterase staining. Arch Pathol Lab Med. 1994;118:1127–9.
147. Martucciello G, et al. Controversies concerning diagnostic guidelines for anomalies of the enteric nervous system: a report from the fourth International Symposium on Hirschsprung's disease and related neurocristopathies. J Pediatr Surg. 2005;40:1527–31.
148. Montedonico S, et al. Histochemical staining of rectal suction biopsies as the first investigation in patients with chronic constipation. Pediatr Surg Int. 2008;24:785–92.

149. Moore SW, Johnson G. Acetylcholinesterase in Hirschsprung's disease. Pediatr Surg Int. 2005;21:255–63.
150. Miyazaki E, Ohshiro K, Puri P. NADPH-diaphorase histochemical staining of suction rectal biopsies in the diagnosis of Hirschsprung's disease and allied disorders. Pediatr Surg Int. 1998;13:464–7.
151. Puri P. Hirschsprung's disease. In: Puri P, Höllwarth M, editors. Pediatric surgery. Heidelberg: Springer; 2006. p. 275–88.
152. De La Torre L, Langer JC. Transanal endorectal pull-through for Hirschsprung disease: technique, controversies, pearls, pitfalls, and an organized approach to the management of postoperative obstructive symptoms. Semin Pediatr Surg. 2010;19:96–106.
153. Kim AC, et al. Endorectal pull-through for Hirschsprung's disease-a multicenter, long-term comparison of results: transanal vs transabdominal approach. J Pediatr Surg. 2010;45:1213–20.
154. Murphy F, Puri P. New insights into the pathogenesis of Hirschsprung's associated enterocolitis. Pediatr Surg Int. 2005;21:773–9.
155. Menezes M, Puri P. Long-term clinical outcome in patients with Hirschsprung's disease and associated Down's syndrome. J Pediatr Surg. 2005;40:810–2.
156. Jarvi K, et al. Bowel function and gastrointestinal quality of life among adults operated for Hirschsprung's disease during childhood: a population-based study. Ann Surg. 2010;252:977–81.
157. Menezes M, Corbally M, Puri P. Long-term results of bowel function after treatment for Hirschsprung's disease: a 29-year review. Pediatr Surg Int. 2006;22:987–90.
158. Heij HA, et al. Long-term anorectal function after Duhamel operation for Hirschsprung's disease. J Pediatr Surg. 1995;30:430–2.
159. Marty TL, et al. Gastrointestinal function after surgical correction of Hirschsprung's disease: long-term follow-up in 135 patients. J Pediatr Surg. 1995;30:655–8.
160. Polley TZ Jr, Coran AG, Wesley JR. A ten-year experience with ninety-two cases of Hirschsprung's disease. Including sixty-seven consecutive endorectal pull-through procedures. Ann Surg. 1985;202:349–55.
161. Levitt MA, et al. Hirschsprung disease and fecal incontinence: diagnostic and management strategies. J Pediatr Surg. 2009;44:271–7.
162. Minkes RK, Langer JC. A prospective study of botulinum toxin for internal anal sphincter hypertonicity in children with Hirschsprung's disease. J Pediatr Surg. 2000;35:1733–6.
163. Friedmacher F, Puri P. Residual aganglionosis after pull-through operation for Hirschsprung's disease: a systematic review and meta-analysis. Pediatr Surg Int. 2011;27:1053–7.
164. Moore SW, Albertyn R, Cywes S. Clinical outcome and long-term quality of life after surgical correction of Hirschsprung's disease. J Pediatr Surg. 1996;31:1496–502.

Anorectal Malformations

41

Marc A. Levitt and Richard J. Wood

Abstract

Anorectal malformations (ARM) present across a range of defects, from isolated malformations with a good functional prognosis to complex malformations with associated defects, and a poor functional prognosis. The potential for bowel control can be predicted even in the newborn, which is the information that the parents are most concerned about.

Keywords

Imperforate anus • Anorectal malformations • Classification • Surgery Bowel management • Outcomes

Anorectal malformations (ARM) present across a range of defects, from isolated malformations with a good functional prognosis to complex malformations with associated defects, and a poor functional prognosis. The potential for bowel control can be predicted even in the newborn, which is the information that the parents are most concerned about.

A newborn with ARM has no anal opening (Fig. 41.1) or has a visible fistula (Figs. 41.2 and 41.3). In males, meconium in the urine indicates a recto-urinary fistula, the most common defect. Usually there is no prenatal clue to an ARM diagnosis, but occasionally a dilated viscus is seen (Figs. 41.4 and 41.5) [1].

Associated problems such as cardiac conditions, esophageal atresia, duodenal atresia, urologic, and spinal defects, should be investigated in the first 24 h. The baby should remain NPO, and on IV fluids. A nasogastric tube manages gastric distension and also checks for patency of the esophagus. The newborn evaluation should include: an echocardiogram, an abdominal X-ray to check for duodenal atresia, AP and lateral films of the sacrum to assess sacral development (Fig. 41.6), a kidney ultrasound to check for hydronephrosis or absent kidney, a pelvic ultrasound in females with a single perineal orifice

M.A. Levitt, MD
Center for Colorectal and Pelvic Reconstruction, Nationwide Children's Hospital, 700 Children's Drive, Columbus, OH 43205, USA
e-mail: Marc.Levitt@nationwidechildrens.org

R.J. Wood, MD
Associate Director, Center for Colorectal and Pelvic Reconstruction, Nationwide Children's Hospital, 700 Children's Drive, Columbus, OH 43205, USA

Assistant Professor of Surgery, The Ohio State University, 700 Children's Drive, Columbus, OH 43205, USA
e-mail: richard.Wood@nationwidechildrens.org

P.D. Losty et al. (eds.), *Rickham's Neonatal Surgery*, https://doi.org/10.1007/978-1-4471-4721-3_41

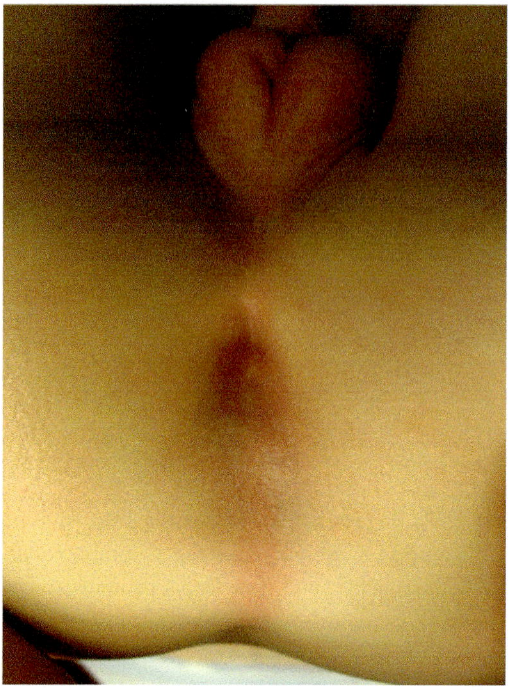

Fig. 41.1 Newborn male with ARM and no anal opening

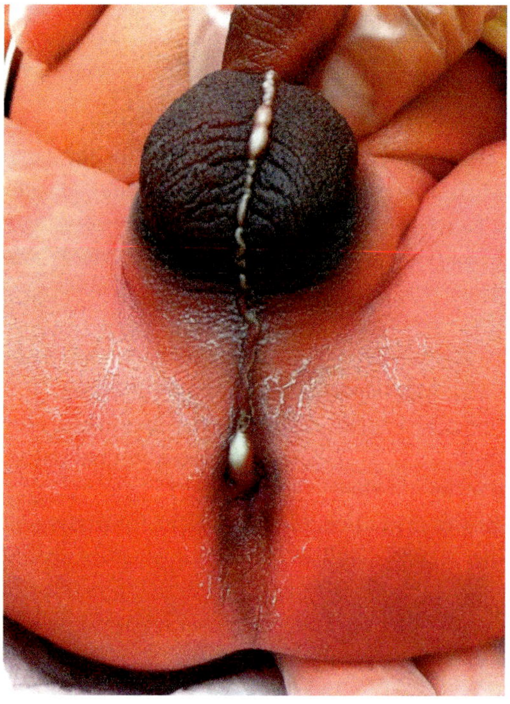

Fig. 41.2 Newborn male with ARM and visible fistula Seen as subepithelial mucous. From Peña A. Anorectal Anomalies. Sprincer Science + Business Media 2009; ebook; used with permission

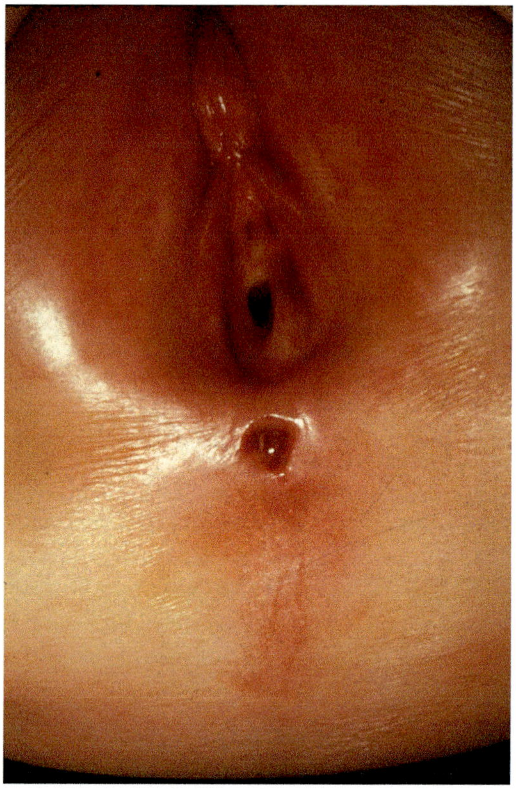

Fig. 41.3 Newborn female with ARM and visible fistula in the perineum, anterior to the center of the Sphincter. From Peña A: Anorectal Malformations. Seminars in Pediatric Surgery 4(1):35–47, 1995; Copyright Elsevier 1995; used with permission

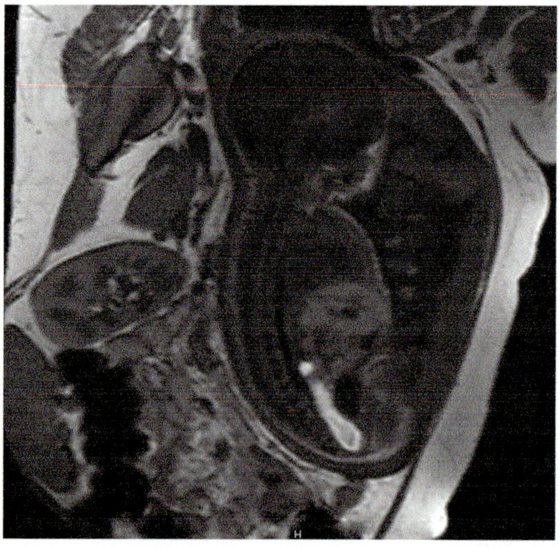

Fig. 41.4 Prenatal images on a fetal MRI of a dilated rectosigmoid in a patient with ARM. Levitt MA, Pena A. Ashcraft's Pediatric Surgery. Elsevier Ltd., Oxford UK; 2010, pp.:468–490. Copyright Elsevier 2010; used with permission

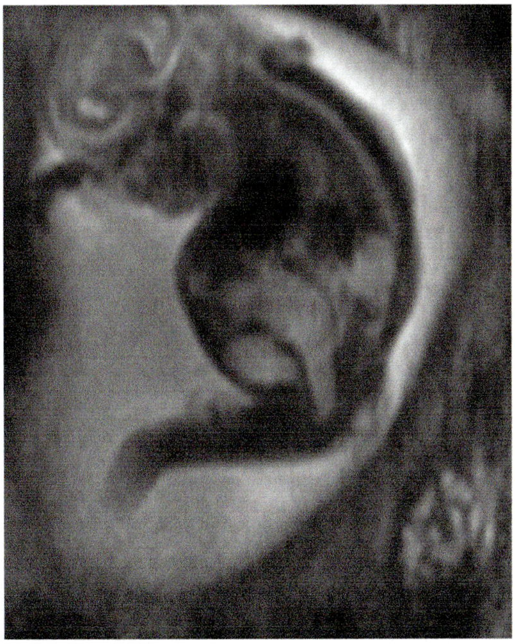

Fig. 41.5 Prenatal image of a cloaca with hydrocolpos

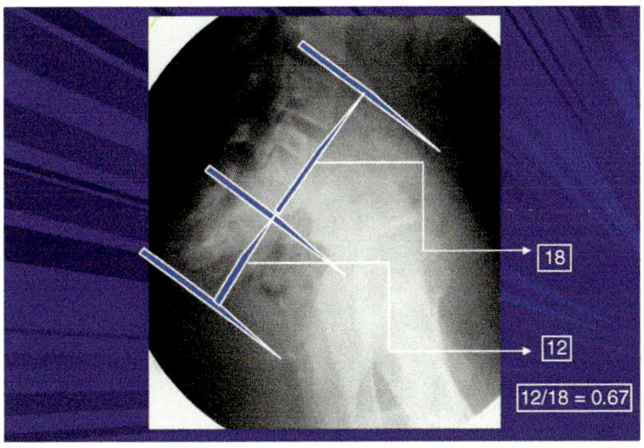

Fig. 41.6 Sacral ratio-lateral image of sacrum with sacral ratio measurements. The development of the sacrum is predictive of continence potential. It is ideally calculated after three months of age

to check for hydrocolpos, and a spinal ultrasound to evaluate for the presence of a tethered cord.

After 24 h, if no meconium is identified on the perineum or in the urine, in male patients, a cross fire film with the baby in prone position (Fig. 41.7) can show the gas of the distal rectum. Prior to 24 h, the bowel is not yet distended, and the rectum is therefore collapsed by the surrounding sphincter mechanism, so radiologic evaluations that are done too early will most likely show a falsely high rectum.

The next key decision for the surgeon is whether or not the newborn needs a colostomy.

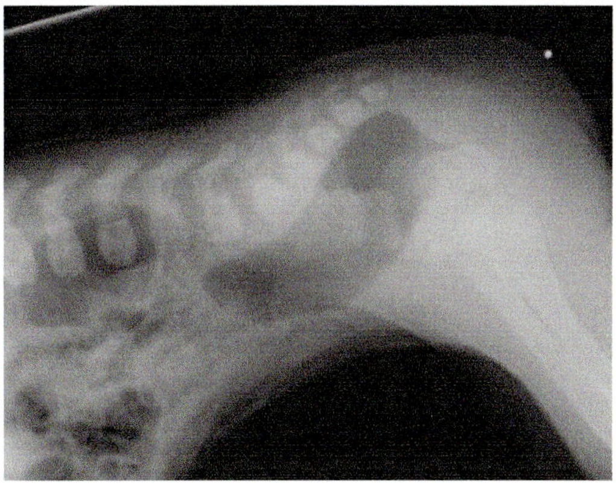

Fig. 41.7 Cross-fire film showing the height of rectal air column. In this case the distal rectum is too far away to reach in a newborn operation so a colostomy is indicated. From Peña A. Atlas of surgical management of anorectal malformations, Springer Verlag, New York 1989; used with permission

Figures 41.8 and 41.9 show the decision making algorithm for the newborn with ARM.

41.1 Males

41.1.1 Rectoperineal Fistula

With careful inspection of the perineum in this malformation, a perineal fistula is visible (Fig. 41.2). This is the lowest type of anorectal malformation. If the patient is stable and the surgeon has experience with this repair, a primary anoplasty can be done in the newborn period. If the patient is premature or has respiratory or cardiac issues, or if the surgeon choses to delay the repair, the fistula can be dilated and the surgical repair can be done within the first few months of life. This malformation has excellent prognosis for bowel control provided the patient receives a good operation, and the sacrum and spine are normal (Fig. 41.10). Associated malformations are rare in such cases. Constipation is common postoperatively and should be proactively treated [2].

41.1.2 Rectobulbar and Rectoprostatic Urethral Fistulae

Patients with rectourethral fistula might have meconium in the urine that can be identified

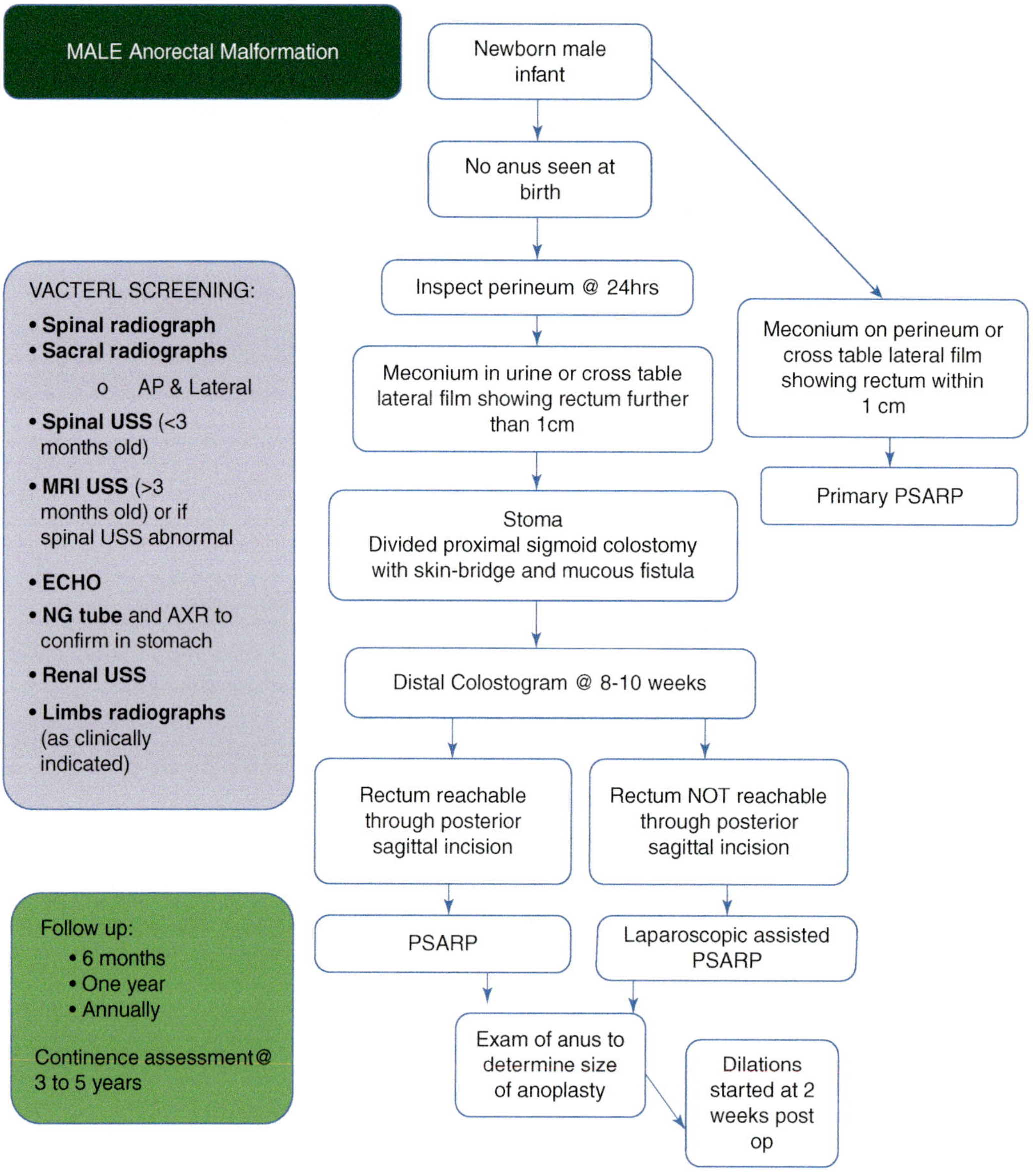

Fig. 41.8 Treatment algorithm for the newborn male ARM patient

on urinalysis or by placing a piece of gauze on the tip of the penis. There are two types: bulbar (Fig. 41.11) and prostatic (Fig. 41.12). Both require a colostomy in the newborn period, mainly because the precise location of the fistula can only be determined with a distal colostogram [3]. Without such a study a perineal exploration is risky and other midline whitish structures (bladder neck, vas deferens, seminal vesicles) can be found and injured.

Patients with rectobulbar fistula in general have excellent potential for bowel control, and patients with rectoprostatic fistula have a slightly lower chance of bowel control.

Characteristics in favor of a good prognosis for bowel control are: a lower malformation, a well-formed sacrum (sacral ratio >0.7), and the absence of a tethered cord or other spinal anomalies. Characteristics that indicate poor prognosis in terms of bowel control are: a higher malformation, poorly developed sacrum (sacral ratio <0.4), and the presence of a tethered cord or other spinal anomalies. These factors comprise the ARM continence index scorecard (Fig. 41.10).

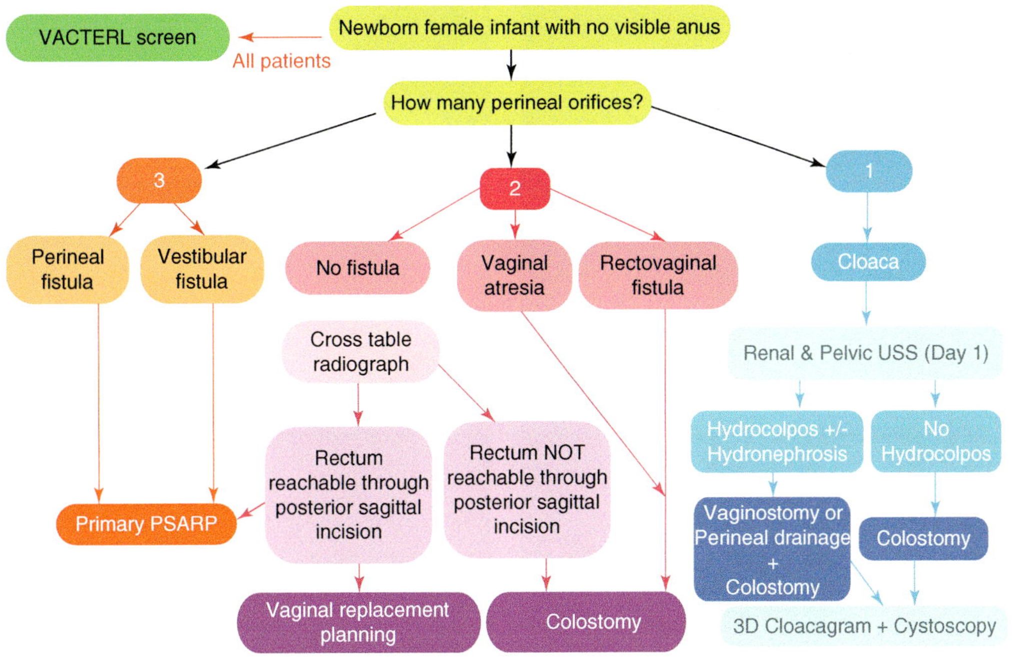

Fig. 41.9 Treatment algorithm for the newborn female ARM patient

1. ARM type –		
	Rectal perineal fistula	
	Rectal stenosis	
	Rectal atresia	
	Recto bulbar fistula	
	Recto vestibular fistula	
	Imperforate anus without fistula	
	Cloaca <3 cm common channel	
	Recto prostatic fistula	
	Recto vaginal fistula	
	Recto bladder neck fistula	
	Cloaca >3 cm common channel	
	Covered exstrophy	
	Cloacal exstrophy	

3. Sacrum –		
Sacral Ratio		
	Great than 0.7	
	Between 0.4 and 0.69	
	Less than 0.4	
Hemisacrum		
Presacral mass		
Sacral hemivertebra		

2. Spine –		
Termination (end) of the conus		
	Normal	
	Abnormally low termination	
Myelomeningocele		
	Yes	
	No	
Filum appearance		
	Normal	
	Abnormal - fatty thickening	
	Myelomeningocele	

Fig. 41.10 ARM continence index

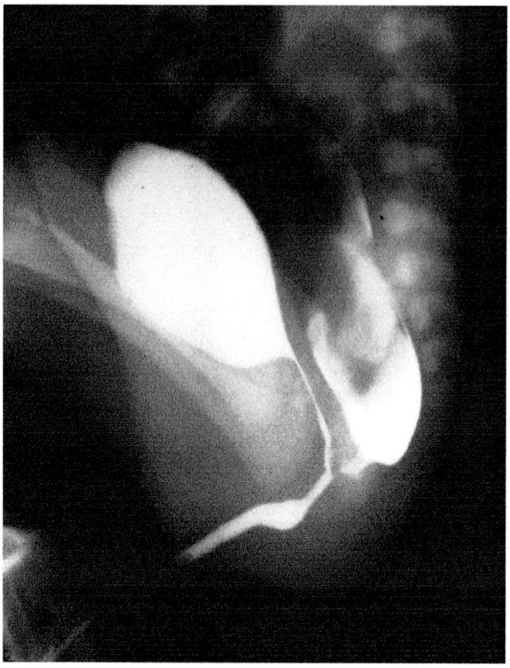

Fig. 41.11 Distal colostogram of a rectobulbar fistula. From Peña A. Atlas of surgical management of anorectal malformations, Springer Verlag, New York 1989, used with permission

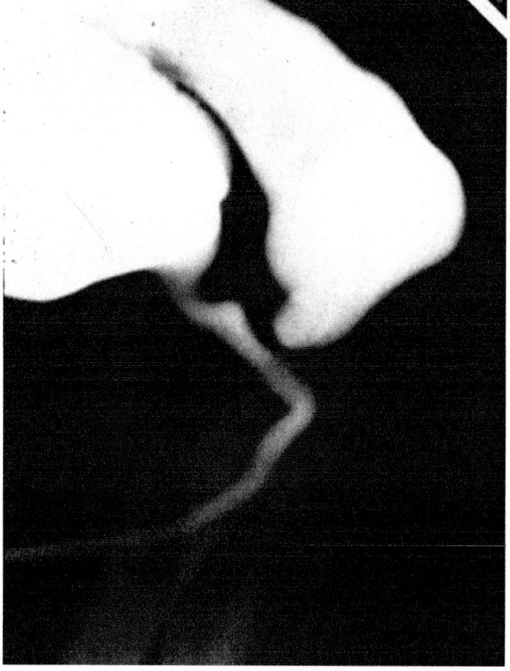

Fig. 41.12 Distal colostogram of a rectoprostatic fistula. From Peña A. Atlas of surgical management of anorectal malformations, Springer Verlag, New York 1989; used with permission

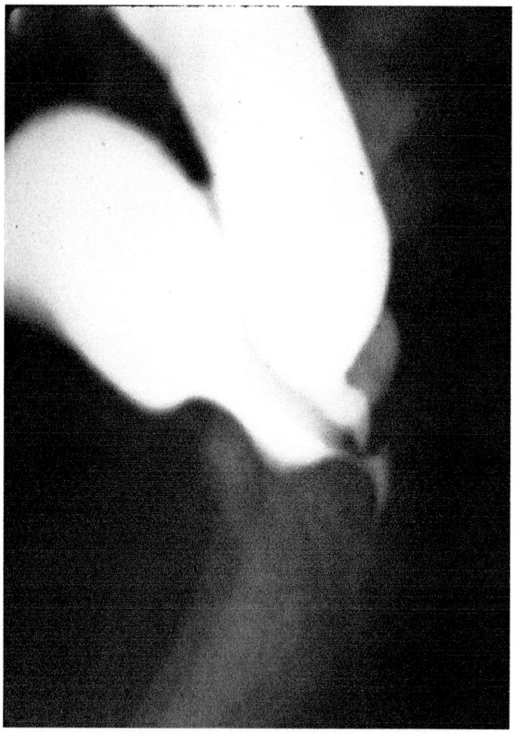

Fig. 41.13 Distal colostogram of a rectobladderneck fistula. From Levitt MA, Pena A. Ashcraft's Pediatric Surgery. Elsevier Ltd., Oxford UK; 2010, pp.:468–490. Copyright Elsevier 2010; used with permission

41.1.3 Rectobladderneck Fistula

The highest type of anorectal malformation in male patients is a rectobladder neck fistula (Fig. 41.13) which comprises 10% of cases. The prognosis for bowel control is usually poor. A colostomy is also required during the newborn period. Associated defects are common, particularly urologic. Delineation of these different types of urethral fistulas are represented by the schematic depicted in Fig. 41.14. The deltoid represents the location of a rectobladderneck fistula, the triceps represents the rectoprostatic fistula, and the elbow of the urethra or below marks the location of a rectobulbar fistula.

41.1.4 Imperforate Anus with No Fistula

In this type of malformation the rectum is blind and almost always is found at the level of the bulbar urethra. Rarely, the blind rectum is found in the pelvis. The functional prognosis is similar to

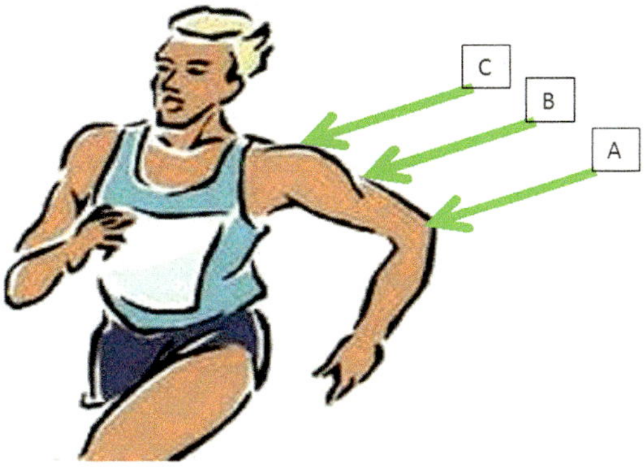

Fig. 41.14 Schematic of the three types of recto urethral fistula in males

that of rectourethral bulbar fistula cases. If the air column on a cross table lateral film is within 1 cm of the perineum, a newborn repair could be done, however the surgeon might not be able to differentiate this defect from a recto bulbar fistula case without a distal colostogram, and therefore, a colostomy is the safest first step. This malformation is particularly common in children with Down syndrome.

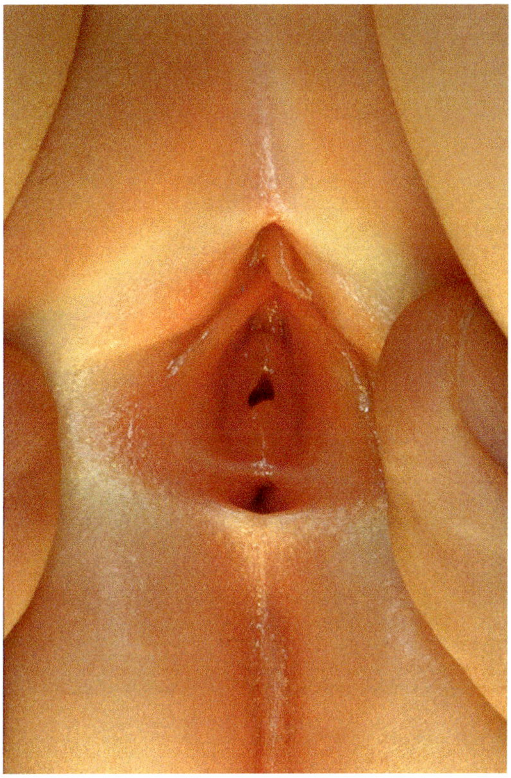

Fig. 41.15 Rectovestibular fistula

41.2 Females

41.2.1 Rectoperineal Fistula

In females, as in males, rectoperineal fistula (Fig. 41.3) is the lowest type of anorectal malformation. Potential for bowel control is excellent provided the patient receives a good operation, has a normal sacrum (sacral ratio >0.7) and no tethered cord or spinal anomalies. An anoplasty can be performed during the newborn period if the patient is stable; or Hegar dilation of the fistula can be done and the repair deferred for later, but best done prior to 3 months of age. Associated defects are rare. Confirmation of the presence of a vagina is vital and checked for visually by pulling out and separating the labia.

41.2.2 Rectovestibular Fistula

This is the most common defect seen in females and is one in which the rectum opens in the vestibule just below the posterior vaginal wall (Fig. 41.15) With a good operation, a normal sacrum (sacral ratio >0.7) and no tethered cord or spinal anomalies, potential for bowel control is excellent. A primary repair can be done in the newborn period or within the first 3 months. It is important to confirm the presence of a vagina and check whether there is a vaginal septum (which occurs in 5% of patients with vestibular fistula) [4].

41.2.3 Cloaca

When the urethra, vagina, and rectum join together as a common channel that opens as a single orifice in the perineum, at the same location of the normal urethra, this malformation is called a cloaca. The newborn must be evaluated for hydronephrosis and a hydrocoplos (a distended vagina filled with urine and mucus) [5]. The hydrocolpos can compress the trigone of the bladder, and cause ureterovesical obstruction, megaureters, and hydronephrosis (Fig. 41.16). It can also get infected (pyocolpos) and can perforate. If detected during ultrasound

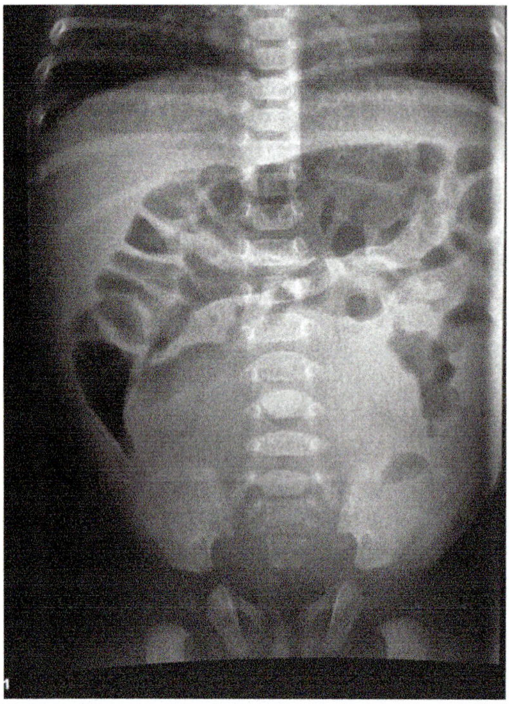

Fig. 41.16 Dilated vagina (hydrocolpos) seen as a pelvic mass on plain abdominal X-ray

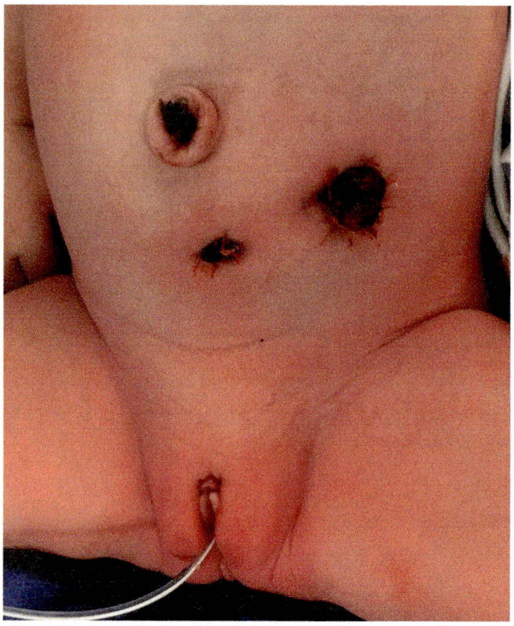

Fig. 41.17 Colostomy in a patient with ARM (Cloaca)

examination, it should be drained with perineal catheterization or with a trans-abdominal indwelling pigtail catheter or sutured to the abdominal wall as a tubeless vaginostomy.

This drainage should remain in place until the definitive cloacal repair. When draining a hydrocolpos if there is bilaterality, a window can be created through the common wall, allowing for a single tube to drain both hemivaginas.

These patients do not have a disorder of sexual development although this is erroneously suspected sometimes given the appearance of the genitalia. A prominent clitoris or phallus-like structure, in a patient with a single perineal orifice is a cloaca, needs to be contrasted with the same situation in a patient with an urogenital sinus and normal anus; who could have congenital adrenal hyperplasia.

The functional prognosis in patients with cloaca is related to the length of the common channel which can be anywhere from 0.5 to 7 cm. The operative plan is based on this length and also the length of the urethra from the urethral take off to the bladderneck [6]. Cloacas with a common channel less than 3 cm with good sacrum (sacral ratio >0.7), and normal spine have good prognosis for bowel and urinary control. A common channel longer than 3 cm usually suggests a more complex defect with less favorable prognosis, and is one that often needs complex maneuvers for urethral and vaginal reconstruction [7]. Duplication of the Mullerian structures (hemi-vaginas, a vaginal septum and two cervices) happens in about half of patients with cloaca [4].

Almost all patients with cloaca have an associated urological defect. If after draining the hydrocolpos the bladder still does not empty well and the hydronephrosis does not improve, then a vesicostomy is needed. All patients need a newborn colostomy (Fig. 41.17).

41.2.4 Imperforate Anus with No Fistula

The rectum ends blindly in this type of malformation at approximately 1–2 cm deep to the perineal skin, and is common in patients with Down syndrome. The prognosis is very good and a primary repair or colostomy during the newborn period are both appropriate options.

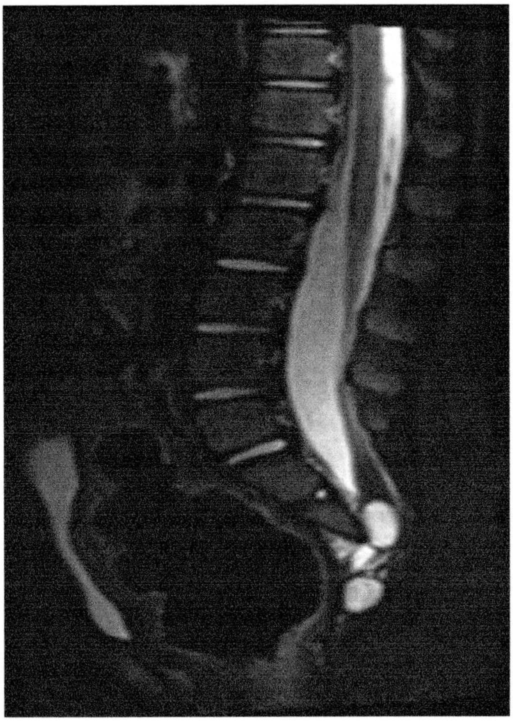

Fig. 41.18 MRI showing a presacral mass associated with anal stenosis

41.2.5 Rectal Atresia and Stenosis

These are rare defects occurring in only 1% of cases of anorectal malformations with the same characteristics in both genders. Unique to this defect is the presence of a normal anal canal. The obstruction or narrowing is located about 1–2 cm above the skin level. These patients have excellent prognosis for bowel control since the sphincter mechanism is normal as well as the anal canal. About one third of these patients have an associated presacral mass (Fig. 41.18). A colostomy is needed during the newborn period [8].

41.3 Colostomy

A colostomy decompresses the GI tract and diverts the stool. To avoid fecal contamination of the urinary system, the stoma is ideally completely diverting (Fig. 41.17). The proximal end is best located in the mobile portion of the descending colon, taking advantage of its attachments to the retroperitoneum, which helps to avoid stomal prolapse. Enough distal bowel must be left for the future pullthrough (Fig. 41.19). The proximal stoma should be matured and placed in the flat portion of the left quadrant equidistant from last left rib, the umbilicus, and the iliac crest (Fig. 41.17). This allows a colostomy bag to easily adapt to the abdominal wall. The distal stoma should be separated enough from the proximal one so that a stoma bag will not cover it, or the distal limb can be pursestringed closed until the time of the distal colostogram. In addition, the mucous fistula should be made small and flat to avoid prolapse, since it is only used for injection of contrast material. An important step during the creation of the colostomy is to irrigate the distal segment of the colon with saline until it is completely clean of meconium. Leaving meconium behind can lead to a fecaloma and contamination of the urine when there is a fistula between the rectum and the urinary tract.

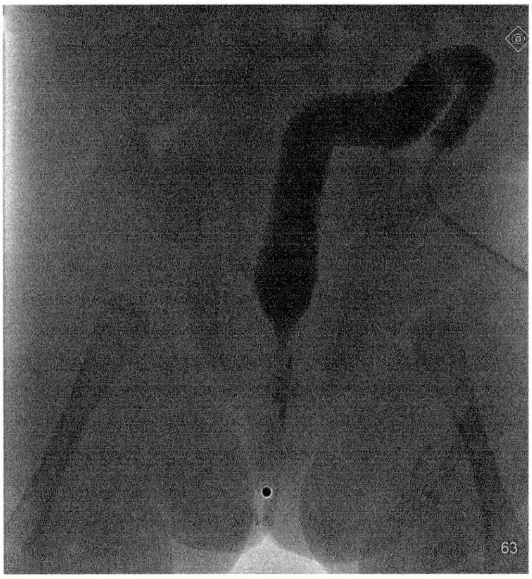

Fig. 41.19 Contrast study through an ideally located colostomy in the proximal sigmoid

41.4 Primary Repair for Females

In perineal fistulas and imperforate anus with no fistula the rectum is adjacent to the posterior vagina; in vestibular fistulas, the rectum shares a common wall with the vagina.

The operation proceeds with the patient in prone position, and the pelvis elevated [9]. Multiple silk sutures are placed around the fistula if one is present to exert uniform traction. A posterior sagittal incision (usually not much more posterior than the most posterior point of the sphincter mechanism) is made through the skin, subcutaneous tissue and the parasagittal fibers. The sphincter mechanism is divided in the midline. A white fascia surrounding the rectum is dissected, starting with the lateral walls and then anteriorly to the contiguous or common wall between rectum and vagina. The anterior plane is visualized by seeing the dissection already performed on the lateral planes. The rectum is lifted superiorly and the wall between rectum and vagina is completely dissected until the two structures are separated from each other and an areolar plane of separation is reached. If there is need to gain rectal length, the dissection is done as close as possible to the rectal wall, ligating with cautery the attachments and vessels on the posterior and lateral walls until the rectum reaches the perineum without tension. The perineal body is closed up to the anterior limit of the sphincter mechanism that is delineated with the use of an electric stimulator. The rectum is tacked to the posterior edge of the muscle complex up to the level of the skin. The reconstruction of the posterior sagittal incision reapproximates the ischiorectal fat, parasagittal fibers, subcutaneous tissue and skin and an anoplasty is performed with interrupted long-term absorbable sutures.

41.5 Primary Repair in Males

In perineal fistulas and imperforate anus with no fistula, the rectum is adjacent to the urethra. A Foley catheter is inserted, the patient is placed prone on the operating table with the pelvis elevated. Multiple silk stiches are placed in the fistula, if present, at the mucocutaneous junction. A midline posterior sagittal incision is made, staying perfectly in the midline, dividing the skin, subcutaneous tissue, parasagittal fibers, and muscle complex. The posterior rectal wall is identified. Silk stitches are placed in the posterior rectal wall which is then opened in the midline. More silk stitches are placed in the rectal wall edges as the rectum continues to be opened. The contiguous wall between the rectum and the urethra is carefully dissected, maintaining traction on the rectum. The lateral walls of the rectum should be cleaned in order to help to define the anterior plane. Once the rectum is completely separated from the urethra, rectal bands and vessels need to be ligated with cautery in order to gain length for a perineal anoplasty without tension. The posterior and anterior limits of the sphincter are delineated with the stimulator. The perineal body is then reconstructed up to the anterior limit of the sphincter, and the levator muscle edges are closed to each other. Sutures are placed in the posterior edge of the muscle complex, incorporating the posterior wall of the rectum. The posterior sagittal incision is closed up to the skin and an anoplasty is performed with long-term interrupted absorbable sutures. For bladderneck and high prostatic fistula cases, the repair begins with a laparoscopic dissection of the distal rectum. The rest of the operation is similar but is done supine.

References

1. Livingston J, Elicevik M, Crombleholme T, Peña A, Levitt M. Prenatal diagnosis of persistent cloaca: a 10 year review of prenatal diagnosis. J Ultrasound Med. 2012;31:403–7.
2. Levitt MA, Kant A, Peña A. The morbidity of constipation in patients with anorectal malformations. J Pediatr Surg. 2010;45:1228–33.
3. Wood R, Levitt MA. Pediatric anal and colorectal problems. Clin Colon Rectal Surg. [In Press]
4. Breech L. Gynecologic concerns in patients with anorectal malformations. Semin Pediatr Surg. 2010;19:139–45.
5. Levitt MA, Peña A. Pitfalls in the management of newborn cloacas. Pediatr Surg Int. 2005;21:264–9.
6. Wood RJ, Reck-Burneo CA, Dajusta D, Ching C, Jayanthi R, Bates DG, Fuchs ME, McCracken K, Hewitt G, Levitt MA. Cloaca reconstruction: a new algorithm which considers the role of urethral length in determining surgical planning. J Pediatr Surg. 2017 Oct 12. pii: S0022-3468(17)30644-9.
7. Levitt MA, Peña A. Cloacal malformations: lessons learned from 490 cases. Semin Pediatr Surg. 1997;32:58–61.
8. Lane VA, Wood RJ, Reck C, Skerritt C, Levitt MA. Rectal atresia and anal stenosis: the difference in the operative technique for these two distinct congenital anorectal malformations. Tech Coloproctol. 2016;20:249–54.
9. Peña A, Devries PA. Posterior sagittal anorectoplasty: important technical considerations and new applications. J Pediatr Surg. 1982;17:796–811.

Part V

Liver, Biliary Tract, Pancreas

Biliary Atresia

42

Mark Davenport

Abstract

The first clear documented case of biliary atresia in English was reported in 1891 by the Edinburgh physician John Thompson. The child was jaundiced and was noted to have clay-coloured stool and dark urine throughout and ultimately died from liver failure or sepsis at a few months of age. The post-mortem drawings showed a normally formed but empty gallbladder two small bile filled cysts in the porta hepatis and an absence of the common hepatic duct.

Keywords

Biliary atresia • Classification • Aetiology and pathogenesis Portoenterostomy • Variant anomalies • Outcomes

42.1 History

The first clear documented case of biliary atresia in English was reported in 1891 by the Edinburgh physician John Thompson [1]. The child was jaundiced and was noted to have clay-coloured stool and dark urine throughout and ultimately died from liver failure or sepsis at a few months of age. The post-mortem drawings showed a normally formed but empty gallbladder two small bile filled cysts in the porta hepatis and an absence of the common hepatic duct.

Early reports of surgical intervention were unconvincing until William Ladd published a series in 1928 of 11 cases he had operated upon [2]. Though not all of these were biliary atresia, some appearing to be choledochal cysts and luminal blockages with inspissated bile, he was able to clear the jaundice in a majority using biliary reconstruction techniques such as hepaticojejunostomy with a Roux loop. However, as surgical experience increased with newborn surgical jaundice then it was realised that biliary atresia was actually usually "uncorrectable" by conventional means as no proximal bile-containing lumen could ever be identified.

Morio Kasai, working in Sendai, Japan in the late 1950s, adopted a much more radical approach to the biliary dissection, advocating complete excision of the extrahepatic biliary tree and anastomosis of the Roux loop to the denuded, transected,

M. Davenport, ChM, FRCS(Eng), FRCPS(Glas)
Department of Paediatric Surgery, King's College Hospital, Denmark Hill, London SE5 9RS, UK
e-mail: Markdav2@ntlworld.com

P.D. Losty et al. (eds.), *Rickham's Neonatal Surgery*, https://doi.org/10.1007/978-1-4471-4721-3_42

albeit "solid" porta hepatis [3]. He recognised that actually most retained some communication with the intrahepatic bile ducts via microscopic biliary channels and exposure of these could restore bile flow in a proportion. This operation, now known as a Kasai portoenterostomy (KPE) does still fail in a high proportion but is still the main initial procedure in most and the only alternative to try and salvage the native liver.

The first liver transplant for a child with biliary atresia was attempted in 1963 in Denver, Colorado by Thomas Starzl [4]. Though unsuccessful as she died on-table from uncontrollable bleeding, it did mark a historical milestone. Liver transplant programmes emerged throughout the world in the 1960s, but all wilted in the face of ineffective immunosuppression and invariable recipient demise. Only with the discovery of cyclosporine at the end of the 1970s as an effective immunosuppressive agent did liver transplantation become a viable proposition for children with BA. The UK liver transplant programme for children began in the mid-1980s as the Kings College Hospital—Cambridge collaboration led by Sir Roy Calne and Alex Mowat.

42.2 Introduction

Biliary atresia (BA) remains a somewhat elusive disease, confined as it is to infancy but yet with its origin essentially unknown. It is potentially fatal; certainly if left to run its natural course, but can be treated effectively by expeditious surgery in a high proportion. For the remainder, liver transplantation is an option and indeed BA remains the single most common cause for this in the paediatric age-group.

42.3 Pathophysiology

BA is an *occlusive pan-ductular cholangiopathy* and thus affects both intra- and extrahepatic bile ducts [5]. The commonest classification divides BA into three types based on the most proximal level of occlusion of the extrahepatic biliary tree (Fig. 42.1). In Types 1 and 2 where there is a degree of preservation of structure of the intrahepatic bile ducts there is still blunting, irregularity and pruning (and absence of dilatation, even when obstructed). In the commonest, Type 3, the intrahepatic bile ducts are grossly abnormal with myriad small ductules coalescing at the porta hepatis. Where retrograde cholangiography is possible this is seen as a "cloud". In about 5% of cases, extrahepatic cyst formation (containing clear mucus or bile) can occur in the otherwise occluded biliary tree. Such cystic biliary atresia [6] is distinguishable clinical and histologically from simple obstruction in a cystic choledochal malformation, where there is preservation of an epithelial lining and retention of a normal and often dilated intrahepatic biliary tree.

42.3.1 Etiological Heterogeneity

BA is not a single disease, certainly not one with a single cause. In all probability it is a phenotype resulting from a number of different aetiologies [5]. Four groups can be defined clinically:

i. Biliary Atresia Splenic Malformation (BASM) syndrome [7, 8]
ii. Cystic BA [6]
iii. CMV IgM IgM +ve BA [9]
iv. Isolated BA

Other entities are fewer in number, but there seems to be a relationship with other gastrointestinal anomalies such as oesophageal atresia and jejunal atresia in a small proportion (<1% of large series) and occasional cases with a defined chromosomal abnormality (e.g. cat-eye syndrome and chromosome 22 aneuploidy [10].

Developmental biliary atresia is a term which we have used and includes (i) and (ii), where the onset is almost certainly prenatal, and evident by the time of birth [11]. The onset of occlusion in (iv) is much more contentious and some authorities hold that the bile duct can be normal and patent at the time of birth becoming occluded secondarily (by virally-mediated damage for instance).

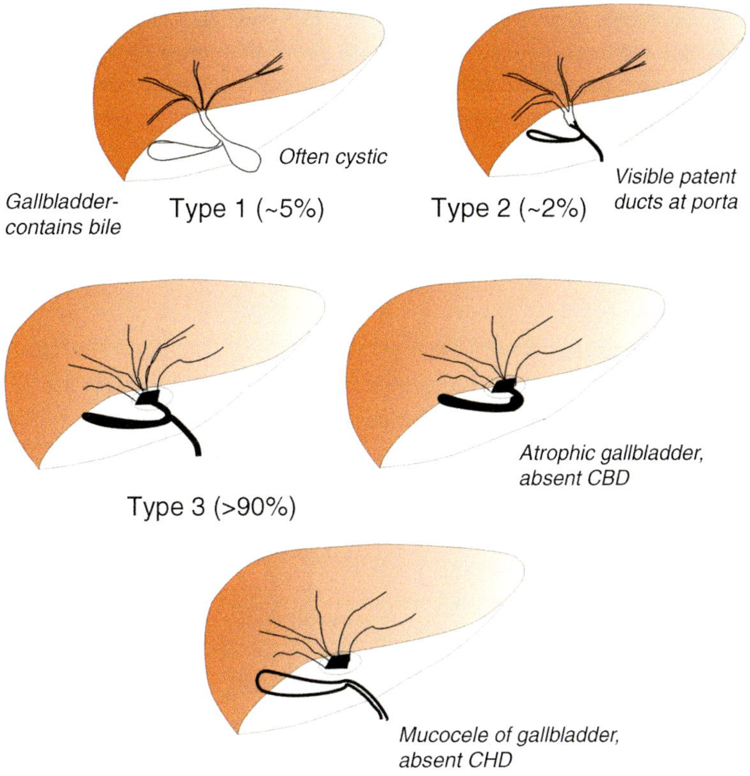

Fig. 42.1 Schematic illustration of biliary atresia classification

42.3.2 Biliary Atresia Splenic Malformation (BASM) Syndrome

While the association of BA with polysplenia had been recognised for some time, clarification of what constitutes BASM is only relatively recent [7]. The constellation of other anomalies is peculiar and the reasons for this still obscure. The common embryological insult may simply be timing (30–35 days) rather than a specific genetic defect. There are key genes which are important in both bile duct development (e.g. *JAG1* [12], *HNF-6*), and visceral and somatic symmetry (e.g. inv. [13], *CFC-1*), although correlation with the human condition is patchy. A possible genetic link has recently been reported by a French group who found an increased frequency of mutations in the *CFC-1* gene (on Chromosome 2), compared to controls [14].

42.3.3 Pathology

The macroscopic appearance of the extrahepatic biliary tree ranges from being inflamed, hypertrophic yet intact to an atrophic negligible remnant with absent parts. In about 20% of those with type 3 BA, there will be a patent CBD and relatively normal looking gallbladder containing clear mucus—a mucocele. In some, particularly those with the BASM syndrome the CBD will be completely absent and the gallbladder no more than a shrunken, atrophic remnant (Fig. 42.1).

The histological appearance within the liver appears more stereotypical, even reactive, with a time-dependent sequence to overt macronodular cirrhosis. BA is not simply a mechanical biliary obstruction (in which case there would be dilatation of the intrahepatic bile ducts) and there is a marked inflammatory component. Histologically, there is early portal tract inflammation and an obvious mononuclear cell infiltrate; and later there appears to be bile-ductule plugging and re-duplication.

There is abnormal expression of Class II antigen and increased expression of the cell adhesion molecules, ICAM-1 and VCAM-1, on sinusoidal and biliary epithelium in BA infants [15, 16]. This is believed to facilitate the infiltration of circulating mononuclear cells which then become activated *in situ*. The mononuclear infiltrate is believed by a number of authors to be the specific destructive element of BA targeted at bile duct epithelium and therefore cholangiodestructive [16, 17]. Its composition can be ascertained by immunohistochemistry and appears predominantly CD4+ T lymphocytes (specifically Th1 and CD56+ (natural killer) NK cells). Infiltrating CD8+ cells do occur but some studies have suggested that they lack the normal markers of activation (e.g. perforin, granzyme B and Fas ligand) [18]. Most recently, increases in the Th17 (IL-17+) subset have been identified; principally in the mouse model [19] but also in clinical cases [20]. It is known that biliary epithelial cells possess an innate immune system consisting of the Toll-like receptor family and are able to recognize pathogen-associated molecular patterns (PAMPs). In some adult auto-immune diseases such as primary biliary cirrhosis, Th17 cells are implicated in the cholangiopathy and this too appears to be the case in BA [20].

The Th1 subset, regulatory T cells (Tregs) may also play a part in aetiology and defects have been shown in the mouse model [21, 22] although human evidence is patchy [20, 23]. The hypothesis is that there is an early perinatal absence of regulatory T-regs which are believed essential for suppressing and inhibiting NK cell expansion and which allows viral exposure to initiate a sequence of (auto) immune mediated bile duct damage.

That there is a potent systemic inflammatory process is reinforced by increased expression of the cytokines, sICAM-1 and sVCAM-1 in the circulation [24, 25], as is seen in other immunologically-mediated liver diseases such as primary biliary cirrhosis and sclerosing cholangitis; with levels of the sVCAM-1 at least being shown to be prognostic [25]. Increasing levels of various other cytokines (e.g. IL-2, TNFα and IL-18), can also be shown post-operatively but most discriminate poorly between those who would clear their jaundice or not, although, conversely some (e.g. IL-2, IFNγ, IL-4, IL-10, TNFα and sICAM-1) were better predictors of subsequent need for early transplantation [26].

Resident (Kupffer cells) or systemic/recruited macrophages seem to play a dual role in BA; as both the presenters of antigenic material in the first place and latterly as the initiating force for fibrosis in the development of chronic liver disease. Tracy et al. [27] first showed increases in resident macrophages (CD68+) with marked expression of the lipopolysaccharide receptor, CD14+. Increased levels of both CD68+ cells and its circulating markers (TNFα and IL-18) have also been shown impair prognosis post-KPE [26, 28].

42.3.4 Viruses and Biliary Atresia

It is possible to reproduce histological BA in particular strains of mice (Balb/c) by exposing the newly born pups to particular strains of hepatotropic viruses (e.g. Rhesus Rotavirus (RRV)) [29]. A group from Hannover has recently shown that this can be prevented by vaccination of the dams against RRV using either of two vaccines (RotaTeq® and Rotarix®) [30]. Thus although most offspring still developed cholestasis there was little subsequent development of actual BA.

Many groups have tried to identify either viruses or at least a trace of a virus in human BA. Initially serological techniques were used [31] but latterly increasingly sophisticated PCR techniques have been applied. The most comprehensive study has been that of Rauschenfels et al. [32], who looked at a panel of hepatotropic viruses in a series of 74 cases of BA at the time of diagnosis. The commonest viruses, identified by presence of DNA/RNA were reovirus type III (33%) and cytomegalovirus (11%). Interestingly, some children had PCR evidence of multiple viruses leaving the authors actually unconvinced that viruses really played any aetiological role, rather they suggested they were innocent bystanders in cholestatic infants.

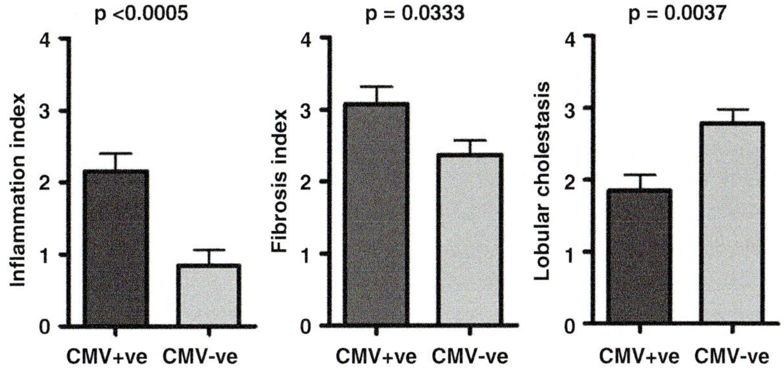

Fig. 42.2 Comparison of liver histology in infants with biliary atresia—CMV IgM +ve (n = 13) *versus* CMV IgM −ve (n = 54). Semiquantitive score (0–4) for inflammation, fibrosis and lobular cholestasis. [reproduced with permission from Zani A, Quaglia A, Hadzic N, Zuckerman M, Davenport M. Cytomegalovirus-associated biliary atresia: An aetiological and prognostic subgroup. J Pediatr Surg 2015; 50: 1739–45.]

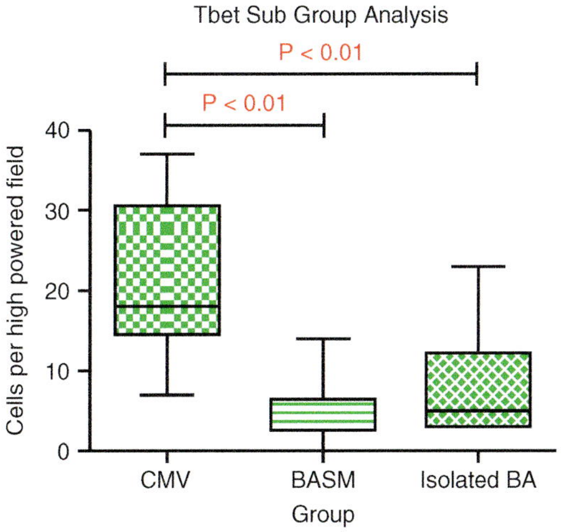

Fig. 42.3 Box and whisker chart showing significantly larger Th-1 cell (T_{bet} +ve) infiltrate in CMV patients compared with BASM (P < 0.01) and Isolated BA (P < 0.01) groups. (Reproduced with permission from Hill R, Quaglia A, Hussain M, Hadzic N, Mieli-Vergani G, Vergani D, et al. Th-17 cells infiltrate the liver in human biliary atresia and are related to surgical outcome. J Pediatr Surg 2015; 50:1297–303)

We have recently focused on those infants who have IgM +ve serological evidence of cytomegalovirus to try and prove a clinical link with viral exposure [9]. It is possible to differentiate these from infants with isolated BA (but CMV IgM−ve) both clinically (higher serum AST and bilirubin values, larger spleen sizes and a poor response to surgery), histologically (Fig. 42.2) and in terms of the composition of infiltrating mononuclear cells [9, 20] (Fig. 42.3).

42.3.5 (Auto)immune Response and Inflammation in Biliary Atresia

That there is a potent inflammatory reaction within the livers of infants with BA is unquestioned. Several groups have tried to link this presumably detrimental process with perinatal viral exposure though this has been based more on work in mice than in humans [33, 34]; with one group showing that adoptive transfer of hepatic T cells from BA mice into naïve immunodeficient recipients produces bile duct specific inflammation and injury [35]. In human tissue it has been shown that biliary epithelial cells have the potential to mount an antiviral response and to initiate apoptotic pathways in response to a synthetic double stranded RNA analog [36]. A recent intriguing observation has been of an increased prevalence of α-enolase antibodies in infants with BA, identified from work in the mouse model, with the speculation that there is a degree of molecular mimicry between antigens of viral origin and cholangiocyte antigens [37].

42.3.6 Biliatresone

There had been observations made that in certain circumstances sheep (to a lesser extent cattle) could develop biliary atresia by maternal grazing on land colonized by certain strains of weed (Red

Crumbweed, *Dysphania glomulifera*). Later work by Michael Pack in Pennsylvania isolated an isoflavonoid compound (now termed **biliatresone**) which retained the property of biliary tropism and consistently caused failure of bile duct development in both a zebrafish and a mouse model [38]. The relationship to human BA has not been shown but it does reiterate the concept of aetiological heterogeneity and allow the possibility of an environmental cause of this disease.

42.4 Clinical Features

The key features of BA are conjugated jaundice persisting beyond 14 days of age, acholic stools, and dark urine in an otherwise healthy term neonate. Indeed there is some evidence that conjugated jaundice is present from day 1 and 2 of life in most infants who later turn out to have BA [39]. Birth there is no difference in gestational age or birth weight between those with developmental compared to isolated BA and both cohorts demonstrate failure to thrive by the time they are admitted [11]. Fat malabsorption is the presumed mechanism for this and will also cause deficiency of the fat-soluble vitamins D, A, E and most importantly K. As a result some infants will present with a bleeding tendency and even an intracranial haemorrhage. Vitamin D is also remarkably low at presentation and even more so if they are of a non-Caucasian background, at least in those born in the UK [40].

Some infants with cystic BA will present with an abnormal maternal ultrasound scan, typically at around 20 weeks gestation [6, 41]. Clinicians need to recognise BA as a possibility for this scenario and facilitate a post-natal US and timely referral rather than assume these most all be choledochal cysts and that surgery can wait.

Liver fibrosis and cirrhosis are time-dependent features which seem to begin perinatally even in those infants with developmental BA [42]. Features such as obvious ascites, marked hepatosplenomegaly and a macronodular liver should therefore be late signs not seen before 80–90 days or so.

42.4.1 Diagnostic Workup

Liver biochemistry will show a conjugated hyperbilirubinemia, modestly raised transaminases (AST and ALT), and significantly raised γ-glutamyl transpeptidase (GGT) [5]. Protein and albumin levels are usually normal. Haemoglobin and white cell counts are normal although the platelet count may be raised. We now calculate an AST to Platelet ratio index (APRi), and use it as a surrogate marker of liver fibrosis. It does have a degree of long-term prognostic value but only if it is low (Fig. 42.4). Table 42.1 illustrates the medical and surgical differential of a conjugated jaundice [43].

The ultrasound examination is a key part of the protocol as it usually excludes other possible surgical diagnoses (e.g. choledochal malformation, inspissated bile syndrome etc.). All are characterised by intrahepatic or common bile duct dilatation. Ultrasound may be suggestive of BA as a diagnosis by showing an atrophic gallbladder with no evidence of filling between feeds. A more specific, albeit controversial, sign is the so-called "triangular cord sign" which was first identified

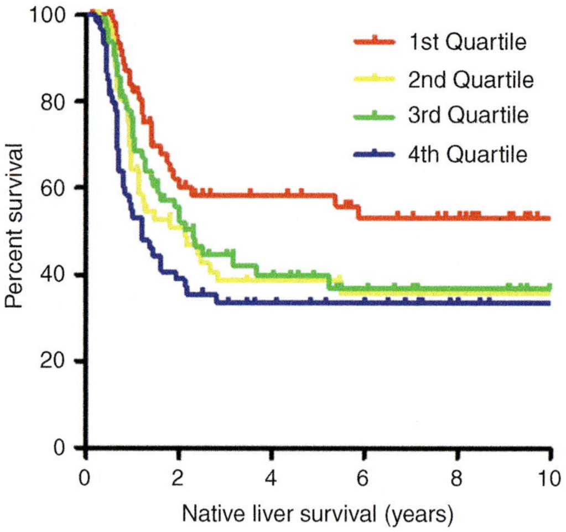

Fig. 42.4 Native liver actuarial survival curves of patients with biliary atresia based on AST-to-Platelet Ratio index (APRi) quartiles. Higher values suggest more liver fibrosis. 1st quartile: < 0.4; 2nd quartile 0.4–0.7; 3rd quartile 0.7–1.1; 4th quartile 1.1–11. (Reproduced with permission from Grieve A, Makin E, Davenport M. Aspartate Aminotransferase-to-Platelet Ratio index (APRi) in infants with biliary atresia: Prognostic value at presentation. J Pediatr Surg 2013; 48: 789–795)

Table 42.1 Differential diagnosis of conjugated hyperbilirubinaemia

Medical	Key investigation	Surgical	Key investigation
"TORCH" infections toxoplasma, cytomegalovirus, hepatitis, syphilis	Serology	Choledochal malformation	US and MRCP
α-1-Antitrypsin deficiency	Protein electrophoresis (PiMM is normal, PiZZ denotes A-1AT)	Inspissated bile syndrome	US and percutaneous transhepatic cholangiogram
Alagille's syndrome	Facies, echocardiography, Vertebral x-rays	Spontaneous perforation of bile duct	US and radio-isotope scan
Cystic fibrosis	Sweat test	Tumours	US and CT scan
Parenteral nutrition associated cholestasis	History, liver biopsy		
Progressive familial intrahepatic cholestasis	Liver biopsy, genetic analysis		
Metabolic causes e.g. galactosaemia	Gal-1-PUT level		

US ultrasound, *MRCP* magnetic cholangiopancreatography, *CT* computed tomography

by Park et al. in 1997 [44] and purports to represent the sonographic appearance of the solid proximal biliary remnant in front of the bifurcation of the portal vein. Some authors believe it to be highly accurate and specific for BA [45].

Radio-isotope (Technitium (Tc) labelled iminodiacetic acid derivatives) hepatobiliary imaging was formerly quite popular in showing absence of biliary excretion. However, it is rarely specific and there is considerable overlap with neonatal hepatitis.

Percutaneous liver biopsy, looking for histological features of "large-duct obstruction" as against those of "neonatal hepatitis", is safe and well-tolerated but needs an experienced pathologist to interpret. Currently it is this diagnostic method of choice in two out of the three English BA centres.

Direct cholangiography is certainly possible, either using ERCP [46] or at laparoscopy [47]. ERCP is technically challenging even with the right equipment, but can avoid laparotomy in larger infants. Laparoscopy and direct puncture of the gallbladder is relatively straightforward as an access point for a cholangiogram, though whether it is really advantageous is a moot point given you still have to surgical access the abdominal cavity for the umbilical camera port.

In some centres, particularly in Asia, simple placement of a naso-duodenal tube and luminal content aspiration over 24 h is the principle method of making the diagnosis. It has never caught on in North America or Europe.

42.4.2 Screening for Biliary Atresia

In order to diminish the time to definitive surgery, some countries have adopted a screening programme. The most well-developed has been that in Taiwan [48], where mothers are issued with colour coded cards and asked to compare their infant's stool. Recognition of pale stool prompts further investigation and referral. This certainly has lowered the time to surgery in that country but to no lower than we would expect in the UK where there is no such co-ordinated programme. Interestingly they do manage to avoid the very old infant with BA and overt cirrhosis which is still seen here in the UK.

42.5 Surgery: Kasai Portoenterostomy

The operation can be divided into various sections.

Confirmation of diagnosis: a limited (1 cm) right-upper quadrant muscle-cutting incision allows access to the gallbladder and a cholangiogram (if possible). If there is no lumen then that, in itself, is evidence for BA. The cholangiogram should show the complete biliary tree and drain into the duodenum to exclude BA.

Mobilization of Liver: our practice suggests that complete porta hepatis dissection requires full mobilization of the liver by dividing the falciform, and left triangular ligaments. This allows it to be everted outside of the abdominal cavity. The anaesthetist needs to be aware of this manoeuvre as it reduces venous return and requires intravenous volume support. Alternatively, some surgeons leave the liver *in-situ* but sling the right and left vascular pedicles and use traction to expose the porta hepatis. There is a small risk of portal vein thrombosis with this technique.

Portal Dissection: The gallbladder is mobilized from its bed and the distal CBD divided and then dissected back towards the porta hepatis (Fig. 42.5 and Fig. 42.6). Ligate and divide small veins to the porta plate which facilitates downwards traction of the portal vein confluence and exposes the caudate lobe. On the left side, there is often an isthmus of liver parenchyma (from segment III to IV) which may need division by coagulation diathermy to open up the recessus of Rex (where the umbilical vein becomes the left portal vein). On the right side, the division of right vascular pedicle into anterior and posterior should be visualized. The "width" of the transected portal plate should extend from this bifurcation and a small inominate fossa on the extreme right to the point where umbilical vein joins the left portal vein.

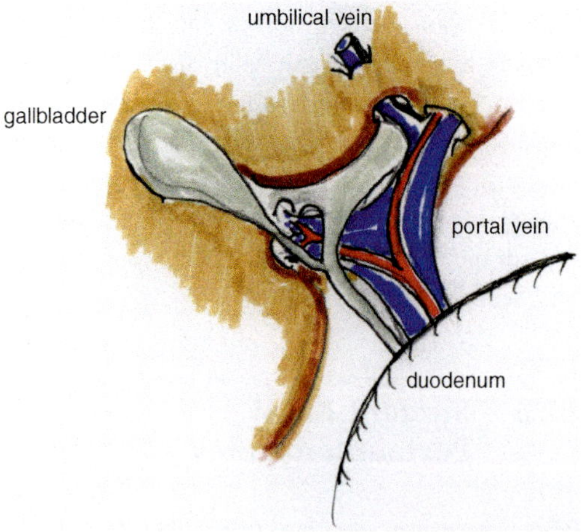

Fig. 42.5 Kasai portoenterostomy: anatomy of the region

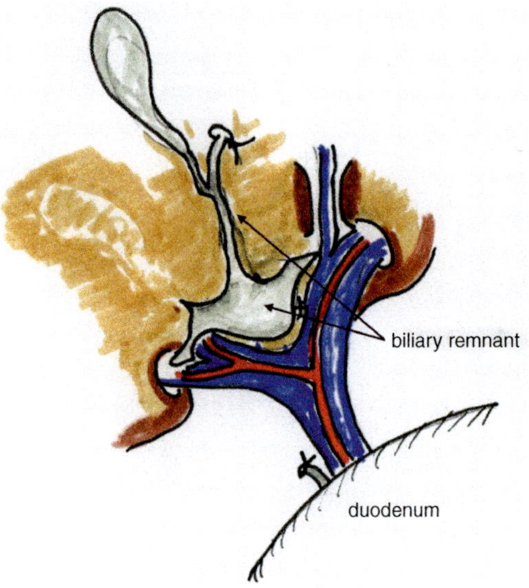

Fig. 42.6 Kasai portoenterostomy: division of common bile duct and mobilisation of gallbladder

Porta Hepatis transection: Excise remnants flush with the liver capsule by developing a plane between solid white biliary remnant and the underlying liver starting at the gallbladder fossa. Excising liver parenchyma itself does not seem to improve bile drainage and so-called "deep coring" adds absolutely nothing. All of the denuded area now needs to be incorporated into the Roux loop.

Roux Loop and Portoenterostomy: A standard retrocolic Roux loop measuring 40–45 cm should be constructed. The jejunojejunostomy lies about 10 cm from the ligament of Trietz and can be stapled or sutured. The proximal anastomosis must be wide (~2 cm) and end-to-side is appropriate. Fine precise, suturing (e.g. 6/0 PDS®) at the edge of the portal plate are satisfactory but remember most remnant ductules are concentrated in the right and left recesses of the dissection (Fig. 42.7).

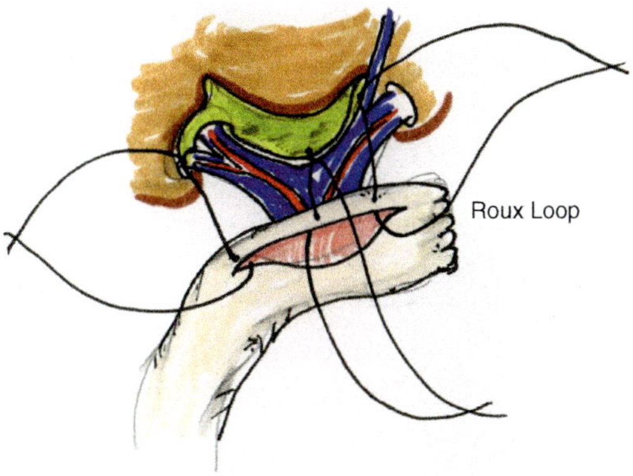

Fig. 42.7 Kasai portoenterostomy: resection of biliary remnants and anastomosis with Roux loop

42.5.1 Options and Alternatives

Patency of the native gallbladder and common bile duct might tempt one to consider a portocholecystostomy, as it does have the advantage of abolishing post-operative cholangitis. However, the anastomosis is not as flexible as a standard Roux loop and revisions for repeated biliary obstruction have been described with a poorer long-term outcome compared to a standard Roux loop [49].

Laparoscopic Kasai operations have been reported by minimally invasive enthusiasts [50] but this has not been taken up by the larger centres performing the standard KPE on a regular basis. It has become apparent that laparoscopic Kasai surgery doesn't offer anything advantageous to the child beyond a better scar and an adhesion-free abdominal cavity for the transplant surgeon. Results are certainly not better and rarely comparable and centres for instance in China and Germany have reverted to the standard open approach [51, 52]. This is likely to be due to the difficulties with portal plate dissection using currently available laparoscopic instruments. Radical resection of all extrahepatic biliary remnants from all biliary sectors and a wide portoenterostomy encompassing all the margins of that resection are the key features to maximize results and it can be a difficult, delicate dissection in the open without the constraints of videosurgery.

In some circumstances, the anatomy of the less common type 1 and 2 BAs, typically manifest as cystic biliary atresia, will allow a hepaticojejunostomy to be performed as there is still a bile duct to join to. However, this is tenuous at best and though these groups do have a better long-term outcome [53, 54] it is probably more sensible to dissect it higher and clear the portal plate as in a standard KPE.

42.5.2 Adjuvant Therapy for Biliary Atresia

Although a number of drugs have the potential to improve the outcome of KPE, there has been little published in the way of scientific data to provide unquestioned evidential support for any. Nonetheless two classes of drug deserve exposition.

42.5.2.1 Corticosteroids

Small, uncontrolled series have suggested benefit in terms of increased bile flow post KPE [55, 56] and post-operative steroids became popular. Our first prospective, double-blind, randomized, placebo-controlled trial using a low-dose of prednisolone (2 mg/kg/day) was published in 2007 [57]. This showed a significant increased rate of jaundice clearance (especially in young livers) in the steroid group but did not translate to a reduced need for transplant or improved overall survival. We followed this with an open-label designed study using contemporaneous controls and a higher dose (5 mg/kg/day) regimen [58]. This now showed statistical improvement in clearance of jaundice and correction of liver enzyme abnormalities but no change in need for transplant. A further randomized, placebo controlled trial (the START trial) from the USA failed to show a statistically significant difference in measures of outcome although the principle measure of jaundice clearance was the same as the aforementioned UK experience (15% improvement with steroids) [58, 59]. The most recent evaluation of the evidence has concluded steroid benefit [60]. All three UK centres continue to use high-dose steroids albeit different ones and for different durations.

42.5.2.2 Ursodeoxycholic Acid (UDCA)

This is widely thought to be beneficial, but only if surgery has already restored bile flow to a real degree. UDCA "enriches" bile and has a choleretic effect, increasing hepatic clearance of supposedly toxic endogenous bile acids and may confer a cytoprotective effect on hepatocytes. Willot et al. [61] assessed the effect of UDCA on liver function in children >1 year post-KPE in a crossover study in 16 children with BA who had undergone 'successful' surgery defined by resolution of jaundice 6 months after surgery. These patients were all treated with UDCA (25 mg/kg/day in three divided doses) for 18 months at which point treatment was stopped and their clinical and biochemical status monitored. Six months later only one had worsened clinically with recurrence of jaundice however, all but two had sustained significant worsening in liver enzymes. These were all then restarted on UDCA and 6 months later all of these had significant diminution in their liver enzymes.

42.5.3 Post-operative Complications

Ineffectiveness of the KPE and continuation of the natural history of BA is the most common problem leading to end-stage liver disease. Jaundice will worsen accompanied by abdominal distension and ascites with failure to thrive and malnutrition. Such infants require urgent consideration of liver transplantation. There are some specific complications which can occur independently of this process though.

42.5.3.1 Cholangitis

Restoration of a bilio-intestinal link predisposes to ascending cholangitis and is seen in up to 50% of large series [53, 62, 63]. This is much more likely to occur in those with BA compared to the those with choledochal malformations as the latter's bile flow is so much better than even the best KPE. The risk is apparent in the first 2 years post-surgery although the reason for this is obscure. Presumably there is some time-dependent change in local immunological defense.

Most children will present with pyrexia, worsening jaundice and a change in liver biochemistry and should be treated aggressively with broad-spectrum intravenous antibiotics effective against Gram−ve organisms (e.g. gentamicin, meropenem, Tazocin (piperacillin/tazobactam)).

42.5.3.2 Portal Hypertension and Oesophageal Varices

Portal venous pressure, when measured at KPE, is abnormally high in about 70% of BA infants and is caused by increasing liver fibrosis and correlates with age at KPE, bilirubin level and ultrasound measured spleen size [64]. It, however, is a poor predictor of outcome either in terms of response to KPE or even in those who will develop varices. This confirms the results of a previous study from King's College Hospital where original liver histology at KPE was graded and compared with variceal formation as assessed endoscopically in 77 children, some 2–4 years later [65]. The implication from both is that it is the result of the KPE in terms of clearance of jaundice and more importantly the abbreviation and perhaps attenuation of the hepatic fibrotic process, rather than the early state of the liver which determines variceal formation.

Varices take time to develop and bleeding is unusual before 9 months of age and usually occurs from 2—3 years. Using endoscopic surveillance about 60% of children surviving beyond 2 years will have definite varices and of these about 20–30% will bleed [66, 67]. Emergency treatment of bleeding varices specifically includes the use of vasopressin (e.g. terlipressin) or somatostatin analogues (e.g. octreotide) sometimes even a Sengstaken-pattern tube [68]. Most are treated endoscopically with banding or in the very young injection sclerotherapy. In those with reasonable restoration of liver function this should be all that is necessary; however those who are still jaundiced require transplant assessment. The role of propranolol in BA children with portal hypertension particularly those with cirrhosis has not been formalized.

42.5.3.3 Ascites

This is related to and caused by portal hypertension in part, but other contributory factors include hypoalbuminaemia and hyponatraemia. It predisposes to spontaneous bacterial peritonitis. Conventional treatment includes a low-salt diet, fluid restriction and the use of diuretics particularly spironolactone. Often seen in settings of malnutrition, due consideration should be given to naso-gastric feeding to try and increase calorie and protein intake.

42.6 Outcome and Results

According to the latest survey of outcome of the results of KPE in England and Wales, in 424 infants there was clearance of jaundice (to a bilirubin of ≤20 μmol/L) in 55%. As a consequence, the five and 10-year native liver survival estimate was 47 and 43%; with the overall survival estimate at 10 years being 90% [69] (Fig. 42.8). This compares well with data from other national surveys (e.g. Japan [70] France [71], Switzerland [72] and Canada [73].

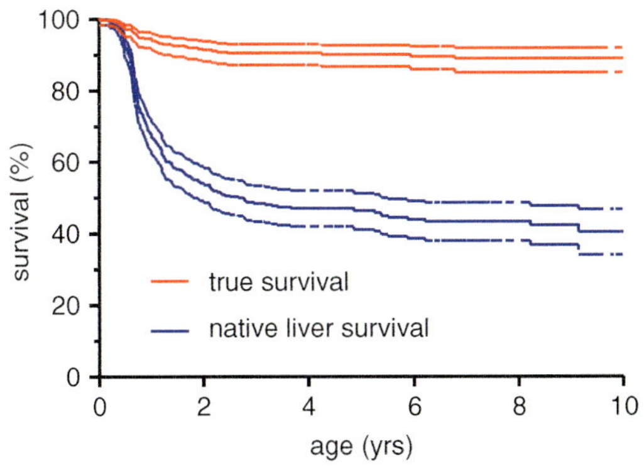

Fig. 42.8 Actuarial true and native liver survival curves [median (±95% CI)] for biliary atresia (n = 443) in England and Wales (1999—2009). (Reproduced with permission from Davenport M, Ong E, Sharif K, et al. Biliary atresia in England and Wales: results of centralization and new benchmark. J Pediatr Surg 2011; 46: 1689–94)

42.6.1 Prognostic Factors

The results of surgery of BA are largely unpredictable in individual cases though a number of factors can be identified as important.

42.6.1.1 Age at Kasai Portoenterostomy

The effect of age on outcome following KPE is still a contentious, complex issue—although not in its simplest expression. That is, if a bile-obstructed liver is left alone then delayed surgery will be associated with less good results; the liver ultimately becoming cirrhotic and unsalvageable.

But the effect is neither simple nor linear. For example, infants coming to KPE at King's College Hospital in the 1980s and 1990s were divided into age by quartiles and their subsequent native liver survival calculated. Only the oldest quartile had a worse outcome [74], even then not reaching statistical significance. However, when 225 infants from the 1990s, and 2000s were divided into specific age cohorts and by their putative aetiological group then a significant effect on outcome was shown but only for those where the BA was considered developmental (BASM and Cystic BA). For all those remaining infants with isolated BA, there was barely any discernable effect up until about 100 days of age [74]. Certainly there were no cut-offs. Dogmatic assertions that something specific happens at 6 or 8 weeks or 10 weeks really should be confined to the history books.

42.6.1.2 Surgical Experience

It has previously been shown in the UK that the more KPEs you do (as a centre, and arbitrarily >5/year), the better the outcome [75, 76]. This led to superspecialisation in England and Wales (and later Denmark [77] and Finland [78]) and an awareness of the need to improve collaboration and communication between centres in others (e.g. France, USA, Canada) [54, 73]).

42.6.1.3 Liver Histology and Biliary Remnant

There is improved outcome in types 1 and 2 compared to type 3 BA; and cystic BA compared to non-cystic BA [6, 53, 54]. Almost certainly this is due to improved preservation of the connections between the intra and extrahepatic bile ducts and ductules. Infants with BASM also have a worse prognosis and appear at risk of sudden death in the first year following KPE. Whether this is due to an intrinsically worse liver disease, a smaller biliary remnant tissue or the effect of other anomalies (e.g. cardiac) is not known. Prospective evaluation of the macroscopic features of the hepatobiliary elements (hardness of the liver, presence of ascites etc.) was relatively poorly predictive of outcome with only actual size of resected biliary remnants being really discriminatory [79]. Microscopic examination of the transected bile duct remnant will show a varying amount of residual ductules. Older series suggested that only those showing large ductules (>300 μm) had a distinctly better outcome [80] but a later evaluation showed that minimal or no ductules in the remnant was also predictive of lack of effect of KPE [81].

Conclusion

In conclusion, although the cause of biliary atresia remains enigmatic a complementary system of surgical treatment has evolved over the past 35 years, which has improved the overall survival to adulthood in affected infants from a dismal 10 to about 90%. Not many surgical diseases can claim such a remarkable change in outlook.

References

1. Thomson J. On congenital obliteration of the bile ducts. Edinb Med J. 1891;37:523–31.
2. Ladd WE. Congenital atresia and stenosis of the bile ducts. JAMA. 1928;91:1082–5.
3. Kasai M, Suzuki S. A new operation for "non-correctable" biliary atresia—portoenterostomy. Shijitsu. 1959;13:733–9.
4. Starzl TM, Marchioro TL, Von Kaulia KN, et al. Homotransplantation of the liver in humans. Surg Gynecol Obstet. 1963;117:659–76.
5. Hartley JL, Davenport M, Kelly DA. Biliary atresia. Lancet. 2009;374(9702):1704–13.
6. Caponcelli E, Knisely AS, Davenport M. Cystic biliary atresia: an etiologic and prognostic subgroup. J Pediatr Surg. 2008;43:1619–24.
7. Davenport M, Savage M, Mowat AP, Howard ER. The biliary atresia splenic malformation syndrome. Surgery. 1993;113:662–8.
8. Davenport M, Tizzard SA, Underhill J, Mieli-Vergani G, Portmann B, Hadzić N. The biliary atresia splenic malformation syndrome: a 28-year single-center retrospective study. J Pediatr. 2006;149:393–400.
9. Zani A, Quaglia A, Hadzic N, Zuckerman M, Davenport M. Cytomegalovirus-associated biliary atresia: an aetiological and prognostic subgroup. J Pediatr Surg. 2015;50:1739–45.
10. Allotey J, Lacaille F, Lees MM, Strautnieks S, Thompson RJ, Davenport M. Congenital bile duct anomalies (biliary atresia) and chromosome 22 aneuploidy. J Pediatr Surg. 2008;43:1736–40.
11. Livesey E, Cortina Borja M, Sharif K, Alizai N, McClean P, Kelly D, Hadzic N, Davenport M. Epidemiology of biliary atresia in England and Wales (1999–2006). Arch Dis Child Fetal Neonatal Ed. 2009;94:F451–5.
12. Kohsaka T, Yuan ZR, Guo SX, et al. The significance of human jagged 1 mutations detected in severe cases of extrahepatic biliary atresia. Hepatology. 2002; 36:904–12.
13. Shimadera S, Iwai N, Deguchi E, Kimura O, Fumino S, Yokoyama T. The inv mouse as an experimental model of biliary atresia. J Pediatr Surg. 2007;42:1555–60.
14. Davit-Spraul A, Baussan C, Hermeziu B, Bernard O, Jacquemin E. CFC1 gene involvement in biliary atresia with polysplenia syndrome. J Pediatr Gastroenterol Nutr. 2008;46:111–2.
15. Dillon PW, Belchis D, Minnick K, Tracy T. Differential expression of the major histocompatibility antigens and ICAM-1 on bile duct epithelial cells in biliary atresia. Tohoku J Exp Med. 1997;181:33–40.
16. Davenport M, Gonde C, Redkar R, Koukoulis G, Tredger M, Mieli-Vergani G, Portmann B, Howard ER. Immunohistochemistry of the liver and biliary tree in extrahepatic biliary atresia. J Pediatr Surg. 2001;36:1017–25.
17. Mack CL, Falta MT, Sullivan AK, Karrer F, Sokol RJ, Freed BM, Fontenot AP. Oligoclonal expansions of CD4+ and CD8+ T-cells in the target organ of patients with biliary atresia. Gastroenterology. 2007;133:278–87.
18. Ahmed AF, Ohtani H, Nio M, et al. CD8+ T cells infiltrating into bile ducts in biliary atresia do not appear to function as cytotoxic T cells: a clinicopathological analysis. J Pathol. 2001;193:383–9.
19. Harada K, Nakanuma Y. Biliary innate immunity: function and modulation. Mediators Inflamm 2010;2010. pii: 373878. Epub 2010 Jul 27.
20. Hill R, Quaglia A, Hussain M, Hadzic N, Mieli-Vergani G, Vergani D, et al. Th-17 cells infiltrate the liver in human biliary atresia and are related to surgical outcome. J Pediatr Surg. 2015;50:1297–303.
21. Tucker RM, Feldman AG, Fenner EK, Mack CL. Regulatory T cells inhibit Th1 cell-mediated bile duct injury in murine biliary atresia. J Hepatol. 2013;59:790–6.

22. Lages CS, Simmons J, Chougnet CA, Miethke AG. Regulatory T cells control the CD8 adaptive immune response at the time of ductal obstruction in experimental biliary atresia. Hepatology. 2012;56:219–27.
23. Brindley SM, Lanham AM, Karrer FM, Tucker RM, Fontenot AP, Mack CL. Cytomegalovirus-specific T-cell reactivity in biliary atresia at the time of diagnosis is associated with deficits in regulatory T cells. Hepatology. 2012;55:1130–8.
24. Minnick KE, Kreisberg R, Dillon PW. Soluble ICAM-1 (sICAM-1) in biliary atresia and its relationship to disease activity. J Surg Res. 1998;76:53–6.
25. Davenport M, Gonde C, Narayanaswamy B, Mieli-Vergani G, Tredger JM. Soluble adhesion molecule profiling in preoperative infants with biliary atresia. J Pediatr Surg. 2005;40:1464–9.
26. Narayanaswamy B, Gonde C, Tredger JM, Hussain M, Vergani D, Davenport M. Serial circulating markers of inflammation in biliary atresia—evolution of the post-operative inflammatory process. Hepatology. 2007;46:180–7.
27. Tracy TF, Dillon P, Fox ES, et al. The inflammatory response in pediatric biliary disease: macrophage phenotype and distribution. J Pediatr Surg. 1996;31:121–5.
28. Kobayashi H, Puri P, O'Briain S, et al. Hepatic overexpression of MHC Class II antigens and macrophage-associated antigens (CD68) in patients with biliary atresia of poor prognosis. J Pediatr Surg. 1997;32:596–3.
29. Petersen C, Biermanns D, Kuske M, Schäkel K, Meyer-Junghänel L, Mildenberger H. New aspects in a murine model for extrahepatic biliary atresia. J Pediatr Surg. 1997;32:1190–5.
30. Turowski C, Leonhardt J, Teichmann B, Heim A, Baumann U, Kuebler JF, Petersen C. Preconceptional oral vaccination prevents experimental biliary atresia in newborn mice. Eur J Pediatr Surg. 2010;20:158–63.
31. Morecki R, Glaser JH, Cho S, Balistreri WF, Horwitz MS. Biliary atresia and reovirus type 3 infection. N Engl J Med. 1982;307:481–4.
32. Rauschenfels S, Krassmann M, Al-Masri AN, Verhagen W, Leonhardt J, Kuebler JF, Petersen C. Incidence of hepatotropic viruses in biliary atresia. Eur J Pediatr. 2009;168:469–76.
33. Miethke AG, Saxena V, Shivakumar P, Sabla GE, Simmons J, Chougnet CA. Post-natal paucity of regulatory T cells and control of NK cell activation in experimental biliary atresia. J Hepatol. 2010;52:718–26.
34. Shivakumar P, Sabla G, Mohanty S, McNeal M, Ward R, Stringer K, Caldwell C, Chougnet C, Bezerra JA. Effector role of neonatal hepatic CD8+ lymphocytes in epithelial injury and autoimmunity in experimental biliary atresia. Gastroenterology. 2007;133:268–77.
35. Mack CL, Tucker RM, Lu BR, et al. Cellular and humoral autoimmunity directed at bile duct epithelia in murine biliary atresia. Hepatology. 2006;44:1231–9.
36. Harada K, Sato Y, Itatsu K, et al. Innate immune response to double stranded RNA in biliary epithelial cells is associated with the pathogenesis of biliary atresia. Hepatology. 2007;46:1146–54.
37. Lu BR, Brindley SM, Tucker RM, Lambert CL, Mack CL. α-Enolase autoantibodies cross-reactive to viral proteins in a mouse model of biliary atresia. Gastroenterology. 2010;139:1753–61.
38. Davenport M. Biliary atresia: from Australia to the zebrafish. J Pediatr Surg. 2016;51:200–5.
39. Harpavat S, Finegold MJ, Karpen SJ. Patients with biliary atresia have elevated direct/conjugated bilirubin levels shortly after birth. Pediatrics. 2011;128:e1428–33.
40. Ng J, Paul A, Wright N, Hadzic N, Davenport M. Vitamin D Levels in infants with biliary atresia: pre and post Kasai portoenterostomy. J Pediatr Gastroenterol Nutr 2016. ;62(5):746–50. [Epub ahead of print].
41. Hinds R, Davenport M, Mieli-Vergani G, Hadzic N. Antenatal presentation of biliary atresia. J Pediatr. 2004;144:43–6.
42. Makin E, Quaglia A, Kvist N, Petersen BL, Portmann B, Davenport M. Congenital biliary atresia: liver injury begins at birth. J Pediatr Surg. 2009;44:630–3.
43. Davenport M, Betalli P, D'Antiga L, et al. The spectrum of surgical jaundice in infancy. J Pediatr Surg. 2003;38:1471–9.
44. Park WH, Choi SO, Lee HJ, et al. A new diagnostic approach to biliary atresia with emphasis on the ultrasonographic triangular cord sign: comparison of ultrasonography, hepatobiliary scintigraphy, and liver needle biopsy in the evaluation of infantile cholestasis. J Pediatr Surg. 1997;32:1555–9.
45. Humphrey TM, Stringer MD. Biliary atresia: US diagnosis. Radiology. 2007;244:845–51.
46. Shanmugam NP, Harrison PM, Devlin J, Peddu P, Knisely AS, Davenport M, Hadžić N. Selective use of endoscopic retrograde cholangiopancreatography in the diagnosis of biliary atresia in infants younger than 100 days. J Pediatr Gastroenterol Nutr. 2009;49:435–41.
47. Nose S, Hasegawa T, Soh H, Sasaki T, Kimura T, Fukuzawa M. Laparoscopic cholecystocholangiography as an effective alternative exploratory laparotomy for the differentiation of biliary atresia. Surg Today. 2005;35:925–8.
48. Hsiao CH, Chang MH, Chen HL, Lee HC, Wu TC, Lin CC, et al. Universal screening for biliary atresia using an infant stool color card in Taiwan. Hepatology. 2008;47:1233–40.
49. Zhao R, Li H, Shen C, Zheng S, Xiao X. Hepatic portocholecystostomy (HPC) is ineffective in the treatment of biliary atresia with patent distal extrahepatic bile ducts. J Investig Surg. 2011;24:53–8.
50. Dutta S, Woo R, Albanese CT. Minimal access portoenterostomy: advantages and disadvantages of standard laparoscopic and robotic techniques. J Laparoendosc Adv Surg Tech A. 2007;17:258–64.
51. Wong KK, Chung PH, Chan KL, Fan ST, Tam PK. Should open Kasai portoenterostomy be performed for biliary atresia in the era of laparoscopy? Pediatr Surg Int. 2008;24:931–3.

52. Ure BM, Kuebler JF, Schukfeh N, Engelmann C, Dingemann J, Petersen C. Survival with the native liver after laparoscopic versus conventional Kasai portoenterostomy in infants with biliary atresia: a prospective trial. Ann Surg. 2011;253:826–30.
53. Davenport M, Kerkar N, Mieli-Vergani G, Mowat AP, Howard ER. Biliary atresia: the King's College Hospital experience (1974–1995). J Pediatr Surg. 1997;32:479–85.
54. Superina R, Magee JC, Brandt ML, et al. The anatomic pattern of biliary atresia identified at time of Kasai hepatoportoenterostomy and early postoperative clearance of jaundice are significant predictors of transplant-free survival. Ann Surg. 2011;254:577–85.
55. Meyers RL, Book LS, O'Gorman M, et al. High dose steroids, ursodeoxycholic acid and chronic intravenous antibiotics improve bile flow after Kasai procedure in infants with biliary atresia. J Pediatr Surg. 2004;38:406–11.
56. Kobayashi H, Yamataka A, Koga H, Okazaki T, Tamura T, Urao M, et al. Optimum prednisolone usage in patients with biliary atresia post-portoenterostomy. J Pediatr Surg. 2005;40:327–30.
57. Davenport M, Stringer MD, Tizzard SA, McClean P, Mieli-Vergani G, Hadzic N. Randomized, double-blind, placebo-controlled trial of corticosteroids after Kasai portoenterostomy for biliary atresia. Hepatology. 2007; 46: 1821–7.
58. Davenport M, Parsons C, Tizzard S, Hadzic N. Steroids in biliary atresia: single surgeon, single centre, prospective study. J Hepatol. 2013;59:1054–8.
59. Bezerra JA, Spino C, Magee JC, Shneider BL, Rosenthal P, Wang KS, et al. Use of corticosteroids after hepatoportoenterostomy for bile drainage in infants with biliary atresia: the START randomized clinical trial. JAMA. 2014;311:1750–9.
60. Chen Y, Nah SA, Chiang L, Krishnaswamy G, Low Y. Postoperative steroid therapy for biliary atresia: systematic review and meta-analysis. J Pediatr Surg. 2015;50:1590–4.
61. Willot S, Uhlen S, Michaud L, et al. Effect of ursodeoxycholic acid on liver function in children after successful surgery for biliary atresia. Pediatrics. 2008;122:e1236–41.
62. Ecoffey C, Rothman E, Bernard O. Bacterial cholangitis after surgery for biliary atresia. J Pediatr. 1987;111:824–9.
63. Rothenberg SS, Schroter GP, Karrer FM, Lilly JR. Cholangitis after the Kasai operation for biliary atresia. J Pediatr Surg. 1989;24:729–32.
64. Shalaby A, Makin E, Davenport M. Portal venous pressure in biliary atresia. J Pediatr Surg. 2012;47:363–6.
65. Kang N, Davenport M, Driver M, Howard ER. Hepatic histology and the development of esophageal varices in biliary atresia. J Pediatr Surg. 1993;28:63–6.
66. Stringer MD, Howard ER, Mowat AP. Endoscopic sclerotherapy in the management of esophageal varices in 61 children with biliary atresia. J Pediatr Surg. 1989;24:438–42.
67. Duché M, Ducot B, Tournay E, et al. Prognostic value of endoscopy in children with biliary atresia at risk for early development of varices and bleeding. Gastroenterology. 2010;139:1952–60.
68. Eroglu Y, Emerick KM, Whitington PF, Alonso EM. Octreotide therapy for control of acute gastrointestinal bleeding in children. J Pediatr Gastroenterol Nutr. 2004;38:41–7.
69. Davenport M, Ong E, Sharif K, et al. Biliary atresia in England and Wales: results of centralization and new benchmark. J Pediatr Surg. 2011;46:1689–94.
70. Nio M, Ohi R, Miyano T, Saeki M, Shiraki K, Tanaka K. Five- and 10-year survival rates after surgery for biliary atresia: a report from the Japanese Biliary Atresia Registry. J Pediatr Surg. 2003;38:997–1000.
71. Serinet MO, Broué P, Jacquemin E, Lachaux A, Sarles J, Gottrand F, et al. Management of patients with biliary atresia in France: results of a decentralized policy 1986–2002. Hepatology. 2006;44:75–84.
72. Wildhaber BE, Majno P, Mayr J, Zachariou Z, Hohlfeld J, Schwoebel M, et al. Biliary atresia: Swiss national study, 1994–2004. J Pediatr Gastroenterol Nutr. 2008;46:299–307.
73. Schreiber RA, Barker CC, Roberts EA, Martin SR, Alvarez F, Smith L, et al. Biliary atresia: the Canadian experience. J Pediatr. 2007;151:659–65.
74. Davenport M, Caponcelli E, Livesey E, Hadzic N, Howard E. Surgical outcome in biliary atresia: etiology affects the influence of age at surgery. Ann Surg. 2008;247:694–8.
75. McClement JW, Howard ER, Mowat AP. Results of surgical treatment for extrahepatic biliary atresia in United Kingdom 1980–2. Br Med J. 1985;290:345–7.
76. McKiernan PJ, Baker AJ, Kelly DA. The frequency and outcome of biliary atresia in the UK and Ireland. Lancet. 2000;355:25–9.
77. Kvist N, Davenport M. Thirty-four years' experience with biliary atresia in Denmark: a single center study. Eur J Pediatr Surg. 2011;21:224–8.
78. Lampela H, Ritvanen A, Kosola S, et al. National centralization of biliary atresia care to an assigned multidisciplinary team provides high-quality outcomes. Scand J Gastroenterol. 2012;47:99–107.
79. Davenport M, Howard ER. Macroscopic appearance at portoenterostomy—a prognostic variable in biliary atresia. J Pediatr Surg. 1996;31:1387–90.
80. Howard ER, Driver M, McClement J, Mowat AP. Results of surgery in 88 consecutive cases of extrahepatic biliary atresia. J R Soc Med. 1982;75:408–13.
81. Tan CE, Davenport M, Driver M, Howard ER. Does the morphology of the extrahepatic biliary remnants in biliary atresia influence survival? A review of 205 cases. J Pediatr Surg. 1994;29:1459–64.

Choledochal Cyst

43

Naomi Iwai

Abstract

A choledochal cyst (congenital dilatation of the bile duct) shows extra and/or intrahepatic dilatation of the bile duct, and mainly cystic dilatation of the common bile duct. Although the etiology is unknown, it might be congenital. In 1936, Yotsuyanagi suggested a new etiological theory based on unequal epithelial proliferation at the stage of the physiological occlusion of the primitive choledochus. Thereafter, Babbit proposed an abnormal relationship between the common bile duct and pancreatic duct. However, Rustad and Lilly suggested that this abnormal relationship was simply a malformation associated with a choledochal cyst. Therefore, the etiology has not yet been established.

Keywords

Congenital disorders biliary tract • Choledochal cyst • Surgery • Outcomes

43.1 Introduction

A choledochal cyst (congenital dilatation of the bile duct) shows extra and/or intrahepatic dilatation of the bile duct, and mainly cystic dilatation of the common bile duct. Although the etiology is unknown, it might be congenital. In 1936, Yotsuyanagi [1] suggested a new etiological theory based on unequal epithelial proliferation at the stage of the physiological occlusion of the primitive choledochus. Thereafter, Babbitt [2] proposed an abnormal relationship between the common bile duct and pancreatic duct. However, Rustad and Lilly [3] suggested that this abnormal relationship was simply a malformation associated with a choledochal cyst. Therefore, the etiology has not yet been established. The estimated incidence in Western countries varies between 1 in 100,000 and 1 in 150,000 [4]. The incidence is higher in Asia and more prevalent in women, with a male to female ratio of 1:4.

With advancements in diagnostic imaging early diagnosis can be achieved within the infantile period. A surgical technique, Roux-en-Y hepaticojejunostomy after excision of the cyst, is feasible for the treatment of a choledochal cyst. The prognosis is favorable. However, long-term follow-up including the possibility of carcinogenesis is needed.

N. Iwai, MD, PhD
Department of Surgery, Meiji University of Integrative Medicine, Kyoto, Japan
e-mail: niwai@koto.kpu-m.ac.jp

P.D. Losty et al. (eds.), *Rickham's Neonatal Surgery*, https://doi.org/10.1007/978-1-4471-4721-3_43

43.2 Classification

In 1959 Alonso-Lej et al. [5] proposed three types of choledochal cyst:

- Type I: cystic or diffuse fusiform dilatation of the extrahepatic bile duct
- Type II: diverticulum of the extrahepatic bile duct
- Type III: the distal end of the common bile duct dilates cystically, which presses into the duodenum (called a choledochocele)

Type I is the most common, and Type II and III are extremely rare.

Since then, Todani et al. [6] further classified choledochal cysts mainly into five types, based on analyses of cholangiographic findings (Fig. 43.1).

- Type I. Common type: (a) choledochal cyst in a narrow sense; (b) segmental choledochal dilatation; and (c) diffuse or cylindrical dilatation.
- Type II: Diverticulum type in the whole extrahepatic duct.
- Type III: Choledochocele
- Type IV-A: Multiple cysts at the intra- and extrahepatic ducts
- Type IV-B: Multiple cysts at the extrahepatic duct only
- Type V: Intrahepatic bile duct cyst (single or multiple)

Type I is divided into three subtypes in view of morphologic findings and surgical treatment. Type IV is also divided into two subtypes. Type IV-A comprises multiple cysts that involve intra- and extrahepatic bile duct cysts, and Type IV-B also involves multiple cysts, but confined to the extrahepatic bile duct alone. Multiple intrahepatic cysts coexisting with fibrosis of the liver is referred to as Caroli's disease [7]. However, the etiology or pathophysiology is different from that of choledochal cysts.

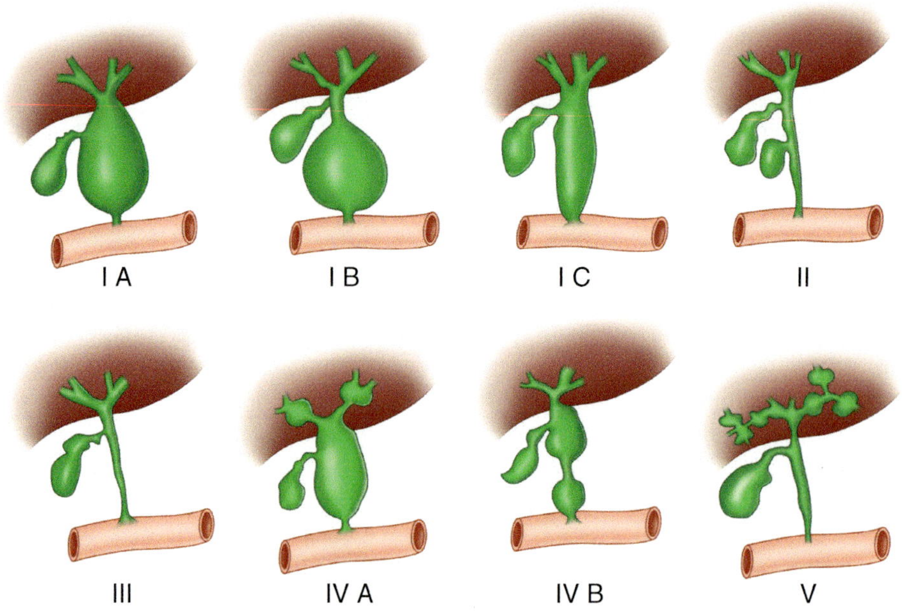

Fig. 43.1 Todani's classification of congenital bile duct cysts (choledochal cysts)

43.3 Prognosis

The prognosis after the excision of a choledochal cyst followed by hepaticojejunostomy with Roux-en-Y anastomosis is mostly favorable [8, 9]. Before resorting to cyst excision, carcinoma of the biliary tract occurred in 18 of 108 patients (16.6%) after internal drainage by cyst enterostomy [10]. After the excision of a choledochal cyst, we [11] encountered a case of local recurrence of adenocarcinoma arising from the distal end of the cyst 2 years postoperatively. Therefore, long-term follow-up is required, especially for the possibility of carcinogenesis.

In cases of preoperative hyperbilirubinemia, bile drainage with a T-tube is needed to relieve the symptom, and definitive surgery can be performed electively after the establishment of a favorable condition. Even after the successful excision of a choledochal cyst, Hori et al. [12] encountered six cases of liver transplantation for refractory hyperbilirubinemia caused by liver fibrosis, with good results.

43.4 Prenatal Diagnosis

Fetal diagnosis is possible by ultrasonography or magnetic resonance imaging in cases of choledochal cyst [13, 14]. Prenatal diagnosis using ultrasound has been performed at various intervals, ranging from 15 to 37 weeks. A cystic lesion at the hepatic portal region detected by ultrasonography commonly suggests the diagnosis of a choledochal cyst. Of these cystic lesions, however, we seldom encounter cases of Type-I cystic biliary atresia (Noncorrectable cystic type) [15].

A question regarding the optimal timing of definitive surgery has been raised when the prenatal diagnosis of a choledochal cyst is made by ultrasonography. As operative management in early infancy is safe, the early excision of a choledochal cyst is recommended. However, the precise timing of definitive surgery is different among investigators. Howell [16] and Lee [17] insisted that the early excision of a cyst in the newborn period was optimal because the grade of liver fibrosis increases with age and excision in the newborn period poses less of a risk to the patient than delayed surgery. On the contrary, Foo [18] reported that they performed definitive surgery at the age of 4 months as early excision of a choledochal cyst. Lugo-Vicente [19] also suggested that elective excision at 6 weeks of age was appropriate unless the patient was symptomatic. Therefore, no consensus has been reached on the best timing of definitive surgery when the diagnosis of a choledochal cyst is made prenatally. Accordingly, I would suggest that definitive surgery should be conducted within 2 months of age because there is a possibility not only of choledochal cyst but also of cystic biliary atresia, for which definitive surgery should be carried out within 2 months of age [20].

43.5 Clinical Presentation

Clinical signs and symptoms are highly dependent on two factors: the age at onset and reflux of pancreatic juice into the bile duct through the pancreaticobiliary maljunction [21]. Todani [22] reported the characteristics of a choledochal cyst in early infancy, aged less than 24 months. They are usually of the cystic type, and a huge abdominal mass and jaundice with acholic stools are typically found. Also, no symptom suggesting acute pancreatitis is observed. Davenport [23] also reported that choledochal cyst children with pancreatitis are older than those with painless jaundice (4.2 versus 1.5 years, respectively; $p = 0.005$).

In children aged more than 2 years with a choledochal cyst, they mainly complain of abdominal pain accompanied by nausea or vomiting, which might be confused with cyclic vomiting. The pattern of abdominal pain is similar to that of recurrent pancreatitis, and is examined based on the serum amylase level. Jaundice in this age group is intermittent and usually associated with pain in the epigastrium or in the right hypochondrium.

Jaundice is caused by inadequate bile drainage into the duodenum because of cholangitis. However, the jaundice is usually transient. Further, cholangitis occasionally causes liver dysfunction associated with elevations of AST and ALT, in which biliary obstruction is complete at the papilla of Vater

43.6 Diagnostic Images

An abdominal plain film should be taken first, in which a diffuse shadow corresponding to a choledochal cyst might be found. Abdominal ultrasonography serves as an important tool for the differentiation of obstructive jaundice and abdominal pain in children [24]. Abdominal CT is further conducted after ultrasonography if it shows an abdominal cyst. ERCP (Endoscopic Retrograde Cholangiopancreatography) or MRCP (Magnetic Resonance Cholangiopancreatography) may be preoperatively employed to detect a pancreaticobiliary maljunction in a choledochal cyst. However, sedation or general anesthesia is required to perform ERCP or MRCP. Hepatobiliary scintigraphy is not necessarily mandatory for a preoperative diagnosis. However, it is useful for follow-up to observe bile flow after the operation.

43.6.1 Ultrasonography

Abdominal ultrasonography is a good initial screening method when diagnosing a choledochal cyst [25]. Such ultrasonography is noninvasive and can be performed at bed side without any sedation. It can provide us with information on the presence or absence of biliary and pancreatic ductal dilatation in addition to the status of the liver in terms of the density (Fig. 43.2).

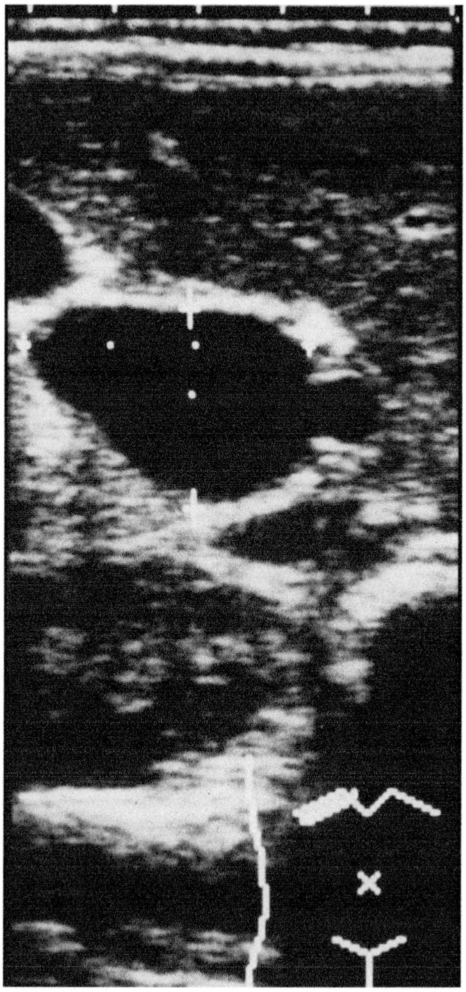

Fig. 43.2 Abdominal ultrasonography showing a cystic dilatation of the common bile duct in a 4-year-old girl

43.6.2 CT

The findings shown by abdominal CT are similar to those of abdominal ultrasonography. CT shows relationships among the biliary tract, pancreas, and gallbladder in the same slice. CT also provides an accurate diagnosis of a choledochal cyst with intrahepatic involvement (Fig. 43.3).

Computed tomography cholangiography (CTC) is also a noninvasive method for evaluation of the biliary system aside from radiation [26]. Bile duct imaging obtained using contrast material,

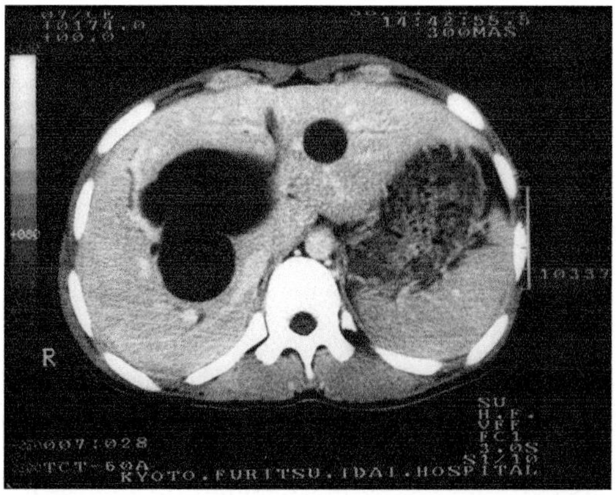

Fig. 43.3 CT of the abdomen in a 12-year-old girl at the hepatic hilum. The main locular lesion is a cystic dilatation of the common bile duct and the others are dilatations of the intrahepatic bile ducts

Biliscopin, yields extensive anatomical detail (Fig. 43.4). The emergence of multidetector-row CT (MDCT) is a major technological breakthrough that has markedly changed conventional CT.

43.6.3 ERCP

Otto et al. [27] and Paris et al. [28] reported an appraisal of ERCP for pancreaticobiliary disease in children, and that ERCP was useful and safe even in children. ERCP is capable of directly showing not only the dilatation of the bile duct, but also the presence or absence of an abnormal pancreaticobiliary maljunction (Fig. 43.5). Accordingly, ERCP is an essential investigative method in choledochal cyst management [29]. However, ERCP requires general anesthesia, and experience of ERCP for younger pediatric patients remains limited. Therefore, intraoperative cholangiography is occasionally done instead of preoperative ERCP to provide accurate anatomical information on the biliary ductal system, especially in younger pediatric patient.

43.6.4 MRCP

MRCP is widely used for hepatobiliary and pancreatic disease even in children. It allows the noninvasive and accurate detection of pancreaticobiliary maljunction without irradiation and avoids the life-threatening complications of ERCP. MRCP is capable of visualizing the pancreatic duct and pancreaticobiliary junction (Fig. 43.6). Therefore, this modality can be a viable alternative to ERCP in children with choledochal cysts [30]. However, MRCP in children is limited due to the need for sedation, high cost, and long scanning time required.

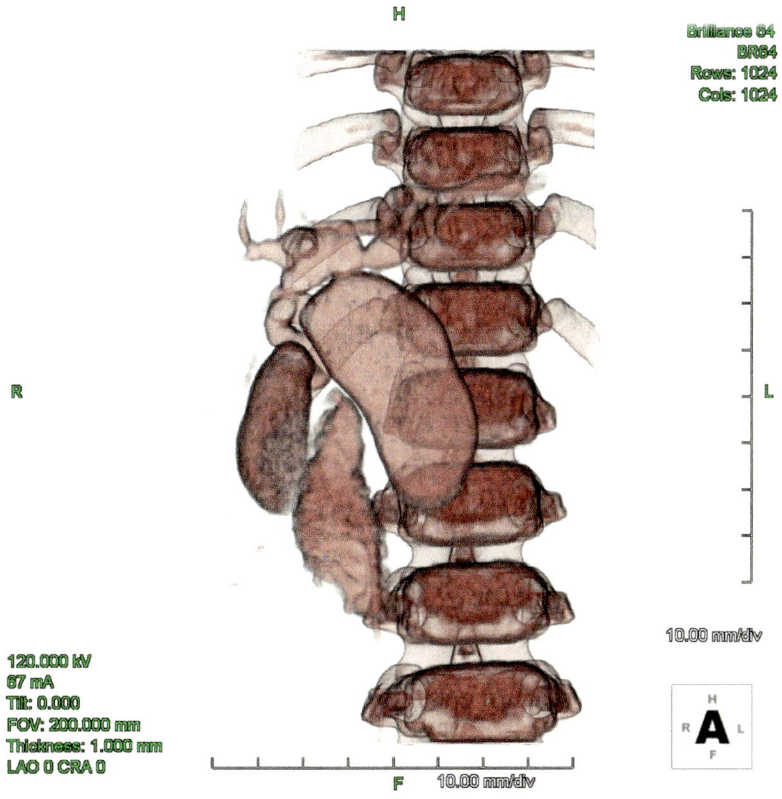

Fig. 43.4 CTC image of the biliary duct in a 2-year-old boy with choledochal cyst, providing a more anatomical detail of the biliary duct

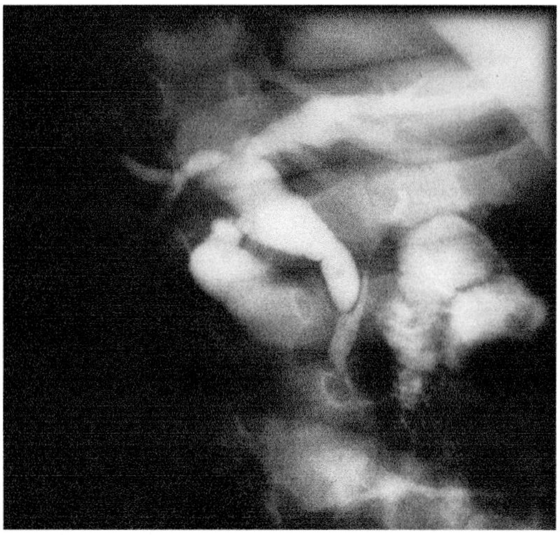

Fig. 43.5 ERCP image in a 3-year-old boy with the fusiform type of choledochal cyst, showing the presence of a pancreaticobiliary maljunction

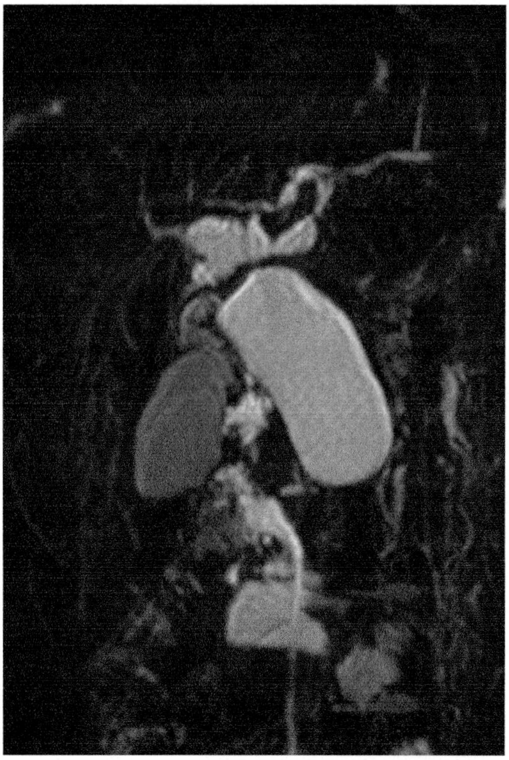

Fig. 43.6 MRCP image in a 2-year-old boy, showing cystic dilatation of the common bile duct and the presence of a pancreaticobiliary maljunction

43.7 Surgical Management

Before 1970, internal drainage without cyst excision was the norm. However, it became evident that the longer such patients were followed, the greater the number of complications, such as pancreatitis [31], calculus formation [32], or carcinogenesis [33]. In 1970, Kasai et al. [34] and Ishida et al. [35] reported favorable results of cyst excision with hepaticojejunostomy. Thereafter, choledochal cyst excision with subsequent hepaticojejunostomy has been widely accepted for this condition. Lilly [36] described a technique for total cyst excision using a plane of dissection between the inner and outer layers of the cyst. With the advancement of early diagnosis, we [37] have not recently experienced cases of severe pericystic inflammation to necessitate Lilly's technique, especially in infantile cases.

To decrease the incidence of ascending cholangitis, Todani et al. [38] suggested that a wide anastomosis at the hepatic hilum, allowing the free drainage of bile, is necessary in all patients with or without intrahepatic involvement to prevent cholangitis or stone formation. On the contrary, Miyano et al. [8] reported that hepaticojejunostomy at the hepatic hilum was indicated in only selected cases such as those with intrahepatic involvement. However, there was no significant difference in the morbidity associated with any of the procedures.

After cyst excision, we employ two biliary reconstructive procedures, Roux-en-Y hepaticojejunostomy or hepaticoduodenostomy. Most surgeons [39–41] prefer performing Roux-en-Y hepaticojejunostomy because, after this procedure, there is a low incidence of ascending cholangitis or stone formation. On the other hand, Todani et al. [42] and Santore et al. [43] preferred performing hepaticoduodenostomy after cyst excision. They suggested that hepaticoduodenostomy was more physiological and technically easier. However, hepaticoduodenostomy has been unexpectedly shown to often lead to bile reflux gastritis, so it is now superseded by Roux-en-Y hepaticojejunostomy [44].

Spontaneous perforation is a rare complication of a choledochal cyst which is difficult to diagnose due to its nonspecific clinical presentation [45, 46]. Vomiting and abdominal pain are the most common complaints. In cases of biliary pseudocyst formation, however, there is no overt sign of peritonitis [47]. The surgical treatment can be either single-staged cyst excision or a two-staged procedure with initial drainage followed by delayed cyst excision. The treatment strategy is based on the stability of the patient and grade of peritonitis.

The management of congenital dilatation of the intrahepatic bile ducts such as Caroli's disease [48] is difficult. The spontaneous course of this disease is dominated by biliary infection: cholangitis, septicemia, and intrahepatic and subphrenic abscesses. Ultrasonography and CT are useful for diagnosis and follow-up. Treatments consist of symptomatic treatment of cholangitis with antibiotics, and some endoscopic and surgical drainage procedures [49]. Partial hepatic lobectomy could be employed when the disease is localized and amenable to resection. The prognosis is fairly favorable unless recurrent cholangitis is present. Liver transplantation is the final treatment for this disease, and Hori et al. [12] reported that patients with refractory symptoms and complications secondary to liver failure are appropriate for liver transplantation.

43.8 Special Considerations

43.8.1 Carcinogenesis

Todani et al. [6] warned that cases of cancer arising from choledochal cysts were increasing. Ten percent of adults patients with an established diagnosis have malignancy of the biliary tract. We [11] encountered the youngest case of 12-year-old girl in whom an adenocarcinoma arose from the distal part of the choledochal cyst. According to the histopathological findings [50], papillary adenocarcinoma frequently occurs in the choledochal cyst wall. Therefore, we need to perform careful checks of children with choledochal cysts from the viewpoint of carcinogenesis.

A choledochal cyst is almost always associated with pancreaticobiliary maljunction, and is sometimes associated with biliary carcinoma. Ono et al. [51] pointed out that pancreaticobiliary maljunction was a major risk factor for biliary malignancy, and he also reported that hyperplastic change of the biliary epithelium leading to malignant degeneration had been triggered by chronic inflammation because of the reflux of pancreatic juice into the biliary tract in patients with pancreaticobiliary maljunction. In addition, Imazu et al. [52] reported that the incidence of mucosal hyperplasia of the gallbladder was significantly higher in the fusiform type than in the cystic type of choledochal cysts.

Bile duct cancer could develop even after the excision of a choledochal cyst. Ono et al. [53] reported the development of bile duct cancer 26 years after the resection of a choledochal cyst, and Watanabe et al. [54] also reported that the intervals between cyst excision and cancer detection ranged from 1 to 19 years (average: 9 years).

Therefore, patients must be followed up because of late complications such as malignant degeneration even after choledochal cyst excision. At each postoperative visit, the liver function and amylase levels in serum and urine must be checked. Ultrasonography of the liver and pancreas are also useful for follow-up. Those patients require close monitoring so that any recurrent carcinoma of the remnant bile duct can be found early.

43.8.2 Pancreaticobiliary Maljunction Without Choledochal Cyst

Recently, the presence of pancreaticobiliary maljunction without a choledochal cyst has attracted attention [55, 56]. However, the precise definition of a dilated common bile duct in children has not been fully established [57]. Miyano et al. [58] defined a nondilated type common bile duct as less than 8 mm in diameter (patients aged

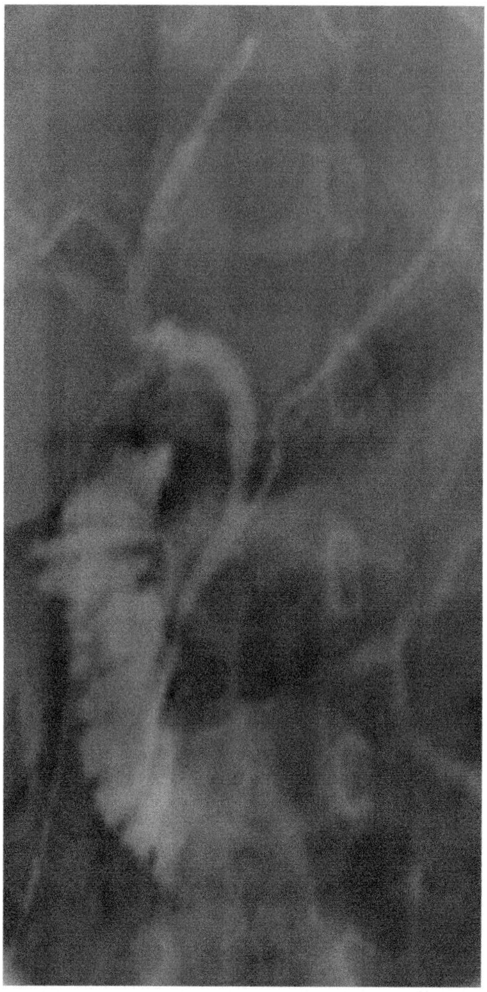

Fig. 43.7 Intraoperative cholangiopancreatography showing the presence of pancreatobiliary maljunction without choledochal cyst in a 2-year-old boy

1–7 years). According to our experience (Fig. 43.7) clinical symptoms are abdominal pain, vomiting, or jaundice, which are not different from those of a choledochal cyst [59].

Surgical indications in pancreaticobiliary maljunction in the absence of biliary dilatation are controversial. Some investigators [60, 61] have insisted that prophylactic cholecystectomy is sufficient, especially in adult patients. On the contrary, Miyano and Ando [62] adovocated excision of the common bile duct in addition to cholecystectomy for the prevention of pancreatic juice reflux into the bile duct. It is now suggested that the extrahepatic bile duct should be excised in pediatric patients with the nondilated type of pancreaticbiliary maljunction as well as in those with the dilated type (choledochal cyst).

43.9 Long Term Results

Most patients with a choledochal cyst have a favorable prognosis when diagnosed and treated early. Nonetheless, late complications and the long-term results of a series of patients who are older than 10 years after cyst excision with hepaticojejunostomy have scarcely been reported.

Our own series consisted of 56 patients with choledochal cysts and over a 10-year postoperative follow-up [63]. The dilatation of intrahepatic bile ducts persisted in the first 10 years, but all returned to normal thereafter.

Recurrent abdominal pain was encountered in two, one had pancreas divisum with a pancreatic stone, and one had adhesive small bowel obstruction. Two patients developed biliary tract malignancy even after excision of the choledochal cyst. Event-free and overall survival rates were 89% (50/56) and 96% (54/56), respectively. Saing et al. [64] reported the late results of 41 patients who underwent cyst excision with hepaticojejunostomy, and there was no mortality and they are all enjoying a good quality of life. Takeshita et al. [65] also reported two death cases out of the 137 with cyst excision as a long-term result. One died because of biliary cirrhosis and the other developed intrahepatic cholangiocarcinoma. Accordingly, long-term surveillance for the development of malignancy is still essential, especially if there is ongoing dilatation of the intrahepatic bile duct or biliary stone.

From the viewpoints of convenience and reliability, a combination of ultrasonography and CT once per year on an outpatient basis is therefore considered to be suitable for successive follow-up in patients with a choledochal cyst after excision of the cyst with hepaticojejunostomy [51].

43.10 Laparoscopic Surgery

Laparoscopic surgery for the resection of a choledochal cyst was initially reported by Ure et al. [66]. The laparoscopic technique included excision of the cyst and a Roux-en-Y anastomosis was constructed after exteriorization of the small bowel via the infraumbilical trocar incision. Thereafter, laparoscopic surgery for children with a choledochal cyst has been gaining in popularity [67]. In some cases, however, conversion to open surgery was required due to oozing on cyst dissection. Urushihara et al. [68] reported total laparoscopic surgery comprising excision of the cyst and wide Rouex-en-Y hepaticojejunostomy with ductoplasty for a patient with stricture near the confluence of the hepatic ducts. Diao et al. [69] and Nguyen et al. [70] reported intermediate-term results of laparoscopic surgery for choledochal cysts and they concluded that the intermediate-term results were comparable to open surgery, and laparoscopic surgery was feasible and a safe procedure for a choledochal cyst.

However, none of those investigators reported the results of a series older than 10 years after laparoscopic cyst excision with hepaticojejunostomy, especially from the point of biliary tract malignancy. Therefore, the long-term follow-up of patients undergoing laparoscopic surgery is needed.

References

1. Yotsuyanagi S. Contribution to the etiology and pathology of idiopathic cystic dilatation of the common bile duct, with report of three cases. Gann. 1936;30:601–53.
2. Babbitt DP. Congenital choledochal cyst: new etiological concept based on an anomalous relationship on the common bile duct and pancreatic bulb. Ann Radiol. 1968;12:231–40.
3. Rustad DG, Lilly JR. Letter to the editor. Surgery. 1987;101:250.
4. Lu S. Biliary cysts and strictures. In: Kaplowitz N, editor. Liver and biliary diseases. Baltimore: Williams & Wilkins, 1996. p. 739–53.
5. Alonso-Lej RWB, Passagno DJ. Congenital choledochal cyst, with a report of two and an analysis of 94 cases. Int Abstr Surg. 1959;108:1–30.
6. Todani T, Watanabe Y, Naruse M, et al. Congenital bile duct cyst. Classification, operative procedures, and review of thirty-seven cases including cancer arising from choledochal cyst. Am J Surg. 1977;134:263–9.
7. Caroli J, Soupault R, Kossakowski J, et al. La dilatation polykystique congenital des voices biliares intrahepatiques. Semin Hop. 1958;34:488–95.
8. Miyano T, Yamataka A, Kato Y, et al. Hepaticoenterostomy after excision of choledochal cyst in children: a 30-year experience with 180 cases. J Pediatr Surg. 1996;31:1417–21.
9. She WH, Chung HY, Lan LC, et al. Management of choledochal cyst: 30-year experience and results in a single center. J Pediatr Surg. 2009;44:2307–11.
10. Shi LB, Peng SY, Meng XK, et al. Diagnosis and treatment of congenital choledochal cyst: 20 year's experience in China. World J Gastroenterol. 2001;7:732–4.
11. Iwai N, Deguchi E, Yanagihara J, et al. Cancer arising in a choledochal cyst in a 12-year-old girl. J Pediatr Surg. 1990;25:1261–3.
12. Hori T, Oike F, Ogura Y, et al. Liver transplantation for congenital biliary dilatation: a single-center experience. Dig Surg. 2010;27:492–501.
13. Ruiz-Elizalde AR, Cowels RA. A practical algorithm for accurate diagnosis and treatment of perinatally identified biliary ductal dilatation: three cases that underscore the importance of an individualized approach. J Matern Fetal Neonatal Med. 2009;22:622–8.
14. Mackenzie TC, Rowel LJ, Flake AW, et al. Management of prenatally diagnosed choledochal cysts. J Pediatr Surg. 2001;36:1241–3.
15. Iwai N, Deguchi E, Sasaki Y, et al. Antenatal diagnosis of biliary atresia (noncorrectable cyst type). Eur J Pediatr Surg. 1999;9:340–2.
16. Howell CG, Templeton JM, Weiner S, et al. Antenatal diagnosis and early surgery for choledochal cyst. J Pediatr Surg. 1983;18:387–93.
17. Lee SC, Kim HY, Se J, et al. Is excision of choledochal cyst in the neonatal period necessary ? J Pediatr Surg. 2006;41:1984–6.
18. Foo DC, Wong KK, Lon LC, et al. Impact of prenatal diagnosis on choledochal cysts and the benefits of early excision. J Pediatr Surg. 2009;45:28–30.
19. Lugo-Vicente HI. Prenatally diagnosed choledochal cysts: observation or early surgery? J Pediatr Surg. 1995;30:1288–90.
20. Kasai M. Advances in treatment of biliary atresia. Jpn J Surg. 1983;13:265–76.
21. Okada A, Nakamura T, Higaki J, et al. Congenital dilatation of the bile duct in 100 instances and its relationship with anomalous junction. Surg Gynecol Obstet. 1990;171:291–8.
22. Todani T, Urushihara N, Morotomi Y, et al. Characteritics of choledochal cysts in neonates and early infants. Eur J Pediatr Surg. 1995;5:143–5.
23. Davenport M, Stringer MD, Howard ER. Biliary amylase and congenital choledochal dilatation. J Pediatr Surg. 1995;30:474–7.
24. Gubernick JA, Rosenberg HK, Ilaslan H, et al. US approach to jaundice in infants and children. Radiographics. 2000;20:173–95.
25. Kim JE, Lee JK, Lee KT, et al. The clinical significance of common bile-duct dilatation in patients without biliary symptoms or causative lesions on ultrasonography. Endoscopy. 2001;33:495–500.
26. Fumino S, Ono S, Iwai N, et al. Diagnostic impact of computed tomography cholangiography and magnetic resonance cholangiopancreatography on pancreaticobiliary maljunction. J Pediatr Surg. 2011;46:1373–8.

27. Otto AK, Neal MD, Slivka AN, et al. An appraisal of endoscopic retrograde cholangiopancreatography (ERCP) for pancreaticobiliary disease in children: our institutional experience in 231 cases. Surg Endosc. 2011;25:2536–40.
28. Paris C, Bejjani J, Beaunoyer M, et al. Endoscopic retrograde cholangiopancreatography is useful and safe in children. J Pediatr Surg. 2010;45:938–42.
29. Sharma AK, Wakhlu A, Sharma SS. The role of endoscopic retrograde cholangiopancreatography in the management of choledochal cyst in children. J Pediatr Surg. 1995;30:65–7.
30. Chavhan GB, Babyn PS, Manson D, et al. Pediatric MR cholangiopancreatography: principles, technique, and clinical applications. Radiographics. 2008;28:1951–62.
31. Karjoo M, Bishop HG, Borns P, et al. Choledochal cyst presenting as recurrent pancreatitis. Pediatrics. 1973;51:289–91.
32. Matsumoto Y, Uchida K, Nakase A, et al. Congenital cystic dilatation of the common bile duct as a cause of primary bile stone. Am J Surg. 1977;134:346–52.
33. Tsuchiya R, Harada N, Ito T, et al. Malignant tumors in choledochal cysts. Ann Surg. 1977;186:22–8.
34. Kasai M, Asakura Y, Taira Y. Surgical treatment of choledochal cyst. Ann Surg. 1970;172:844–51.
35. Ishida M, Tsuchida Y, Saito S, et al. Primary excision of choledochal cysts. Surgery. 1970;68:884–8.
36. Lilly JR. Total excision of choledochal cyst. Surg Gynecol Obstet. 1978;146:254–6.
37. Iwai N, Yanagihara J, Tokiwa K, et al. Congenital choledochal dilatation with emphasis on pathophysiology of the biliary tract. Ann Surg. 1992;215:27–30.
38. Todani T, Watanabe Y, Urushihara N, et al. Biliary complication after excisional procedure for choledochal cyst. J Pediatr Surg. 1995;30:478–81.
39. Okada A, Nakamura T, Okumura K, et al. Surgical treatment of congenital dilatation of bile duct (choledochal cyst) with technical consideration. Surgery. 1987;101:238–43.
40. Stringer MD, Dhawan A, Davenport M, et al. Choledochal cysts: lessons from a 20 year experience. Arch Dis Child. 1995;73:528–31.
41. Shimotakahara A, Yamataka A, Yanai T, et al. Roux-en-Y hepaticojejuno stomy or hepaticoduodenostomy for biliary reconstruction during the surgical treatment of choledochal cyst: which is better? Pediatr Surg Int. 2005;21:5–7.
42. Todani T, Watanabe Y, Mizuguchi T, et al. Hepaticoduodenostomy at the hepatic hilum after excision of choledochal cyst. Am J Surg. 1981;142:584–7.
43. Santore MT, Behar BJ, Blinman TA, et al. Hepaticoduodenostomy vs hepaticojejunostomy for reconstruction after resection of choledochal cyst. J Pediatr Surg. 2011;46:209–13.
44. Okada A, Hasegawa T, Oguchi Y, et al. Recent advances in patho physiology and surgical treatment of congenital dilatation of the bile duct. J Hepatobiliary Pancreat Surg. 2002;9:342–51.
45. Chiang L, Chui CH, Low Y, et al. Perforation: a rare complication of choledochal cysts in children. Pediatr Surg Int. 2011;27:823–7.
46. Ando K, Miyano T, Kohno S, et al. Spontaneous perforation of choledochal cyst: a study of 13 cases. Eur J Pediatr Surg. 1998;8:23–5.
47. Fumino S, Iwai N, Deguchi E, et al. Spontaneous rupture of choledochal cyst with pseudocyst formation-report on 2 cases and literature review. J Pediatr Surg. 2006;41:e19–21.
48. Madjov R, Chervenkov P, Madjova V, et al. Caroli's disease. Report of 5 cases and review of literature. Hepatogastroenterology. 2005;52:606–9.
49. Yonem O, Bayraktar Y. Clinical characteristics of Caroli's syndrome. World J Gastroenterol. 2007;13:1934–7.
50. Kamisawa T, Okamoto A, Tsuruta K, et al. Carcinoma arising in congenital choledochal cysts. Hepatogastroenterology. 2008;55:329–32.
51. Ono S, Fumino S, Iwai N. Diagnosis and treatment of pancreaticobiliary maljunction in children. Surg Today. 2011;41:601–5.
52. Imazu M, Iwai N, Tokiwa K, et al. Factors of biliary carcinogenesis in choledochal cysts. Eur J Pediatr Surg. 2001;11:24–7.
53. Ono S, Sakai K, Iwai N, et al. Development of bile duct cancer in a 26-year-old man after resection of infantile choledochal cyst. J Pediatr Surg. 2008;43:E17–9.
54. Watanabe Y, Toki A, Todani T. Bile duct cancer developed after cyst excision for choledochal cyst. J Hepaticobiliary Pancreat Surg. 1999;6:207–12.
55. Ohta T, Nakagawa T, Ueno K, et al. Clinical experience of biliary tract carcinomas associated with anomalous union of the pancreaticobiliary ductal system. Jpn J Surg. 1990;20:36–43.
56. Todani T, Watanabe Y, Urushihara N, et al. Choledochal cyst, pancreatobiliary malunion and cancer. J Hepatobilary Pancreat Surg. 1994;1:247–51.
57. Witcombe JB, Cremin BJ. The width of the common bile duct in childhood. Pediatr Radiol. 1978;7:147–9.
58. Miyano T, Ando K, Yamataka A, et al. Pancreatobiliary maljunction associated with nondilatation or minimal dilatation of the common bile duct in children: diagnosis and treatment. Eur J Pediatr Surg. 1996;6:334–7.
59. Iwai N, Fumino S, Tsuda T, et al. Surgical treatment for anomalous arrangement of the pancreaticbiliary duct with nondilatation of the common bile duct. J Pediatr Surg. 2004;39:1794–6.
60. Yamauchi S, Koga A, Matsumoto S, et al. Anomalous junction of pancreaticobiliary duct without congenital choledochal cyst: a possible risk factor for gallbladder cancer. Am J Gastroenterol. 1987;82:20–4.
61. Tanaka K, Nishimura A, Yamada K, et al. Cancer of the gallbladder associated with anomalous junction of the pancreaticobiliary duct system without bile duct dilatation. Br J Surg. 1993;80:622–4.
62. Ando H, Ito T, Nagaya M, et al. Pancreaticobiliary maljunction without choledochal cysts in infants

and children: clinical features and surgical therapy. J Pediatr Surg. 1995;30:1658–62.
63. Ono S, Fumino S, Iwai N, et al. Long-term outcomes after hepatico jejunostomy for choledochal cyst: a 10- to 27-year follow-up. J Pediatr Surg. 2010;45:376–8.
64. Saing H, Han H, Chan KL, et al. Early and late results of excision of choledochal cysts. J Pediatr Surg. 1997;32:1563–8.
65. Takeshita N, Ota T, Yamamoto M. Forty-year experience with flow diversion surgery for patients with congenital choledochal cyst with pancreaticobiliary maljunction at a single institution. Ann Surg. 2011;254:1050–3.
66. Ure B, Schier F, Schmidt AL, et al. Laparoscopic resection of congenital choledochal cyst, choledochojejunostomy, and extraabdominal Roux-en-Y anastomosis. Surg Endosc. 2005;19:1055–7.
67. Palanivelu C, Rangarajun M, Parthasarathi R, et al. Laparoscopic management of choledochal cysts: technique and outcomes- a retrospective study of 35 patients from a tertiary center. J Am Coll Surg. 2008;207:839–46.
68. Urushihara N, Fukuzawa H, Fukumoto K, et al. Totally laparoscopic management of choledochal cyst: Roux-en-Y jejunostomy and wide hepaticojejunostomy with hilar ductoplasty. J Laparoendosc Adv Surg Tech A. 2011;21:361–6.
69. Diao M, Li L, Cheng W. Laparoscopic versus open Roux-en-Y hepatojejunostomy for children with choledochal cysts: intermediate-term follow-up results. Surg Endosc. 2010;25:1587–73.
70. Nguyen Thanh L, Hien PD, Dung le A, et al. Laparoscopic repair for choledochal cyst: lessons from 190 cases. J Pediatr Surg. 2010;45:540–4.

44 Spontaneous Biliary Perforation, Liver Cysts, and Abscesses

Mark Davenport

Abstract

This is a peculiar condition which seems limited to the first few weeks of life whereby perforation occurs in the extrahepatic bile duct typically leading to bile in the peritoneal cavity, abdominal distension and jaundice. It should be distinguished from spontaneous perforation in a pre-existing choledochal malformation, said to occur in about 5–10% of all large series.

Keywords

Spontaneous biliary perforation • Liver cysts • Liver abscess

44.1 Spontaneous Perforation of the Bile Duct

This is a peculiar condition which seems limited to the first few weeks of life whereby perforation occurs in the extrahepatic bile duct typically leading to bile in the peritoneal cavity, abdominal distension and jaundice. It should be distinguished from spontaneous perforation in a pre-existing choledochal malformation, said to occur in about 5–10% of all large series [1].

Although at one time it was stated [2] to be the second commonest cause of surgical jaundice (after biliary atresia) this is clearly not the case. In our review of 171 consecutive infants with surgical jaundice, spontaneous perforation of the bile duct only accounted for about 2% of cases [3]. By comparison, infants with choledochal malformation (7%) and inspissated bile syndrome (8%) were much more commonly seen.

44.1.1 History

Dijkstra from the Netherlands first reported a case of spontaneous perforation of the bile duct in infancy in 1932 [4]. Thereafter only individual reports followed with the first real series of six cases being published in 1991 from King's College Hospital, London [5] and 11 infants seen over a 22 year period by Chardot et al. from Bicetre Hospital, Paris [6].

44.1.2 Anatomy and Pathogenesis

Why there should be spontaneous perforation in what appears to be a normal bile duct is not

M. Davenport, ChM, FRCS(Eng), FRCPS(Glas)
Department of Paediatric Surgery, King's College Hospital, Denmark Hill, London SE5 9RS, UK
e-mail: Markdav2@ntlworld.com

P.D. Losty et al. (eds.), *Rickham's Neonatal Surgery*, https://doi.org/10.1007/978-1-4471-4721-3_44

known. Characteristically the perforation occurs at the junction of the cystic duct and common hepatic duct and this may be because it is structurally the weakest part of the extrahepatic biliary tree. Usually it is anterior and the bile then floods into the general peritoneal cavity. Occasionally it can be posterior and is therefore somewhat constrained with bile leaking into the lesser sac. Most authors assume there has been some obstruction in the bile duct leading to an acute rise in biliary pressure as the precipitating factor but actual evidence of this is rare.

The second commonest site of perforation appears to occur in the cystic duct [6].

44.1.3 Clinical Features

Most infants present from 1 to 16 weeks with insidious abdominal distension due to the accumulation of bile ascites. They are also usually jaundiced, possibly because of the biliary obstruction but also because of peritoneal reabsorption of bilirubin. Ascites often prompts development of a hydrocele or hernia and this leads to the characteristic sign of greenish discolouration of the skin overlying hernia (umbilical or inguinal) or hydrocele (Fig. 44.1). Vomiting will usually occur simply due to distension. In those with the posterior variant then symptoms can be vague and ill-defined. Sometimes the lesser sac only fills with bile leading to vomiting and at this age some have been explored on the basis of a diagnosis of pyloric stenosis [7].

44.1.4 Investigations

All infants should show a conjugated hyperbilirubinaemia with elevated mild elevations of the AST and γGT. Ultrasonography should show free fluid in most infants and probably some kind of ill-defined complex cyst or mass at the porta hepatis. Intrahepatic bile ducts may or may not be dilated. The diagnostic procedure of choice is the radioisotope scan which should show bile leakage into the peritoneal cavity. In those few centres with the capacity for ERCP, this may also be considered,

44.1.5 Management

All infants require resuscitation to a greater or lesser extent depending on the length of history. Usually the bile is sterile but intravenous antibiotic cover is essential from diagnosis through to definitive treatment.

There have been isolated cases where simple peritoneal drainage alone has been performed [8] however this is usually inadequate and most should come to laparotomy [5, 6]. There have been a number of surgical options put forward but invariably experience will be limited. On-table cholangiography is a key part of the assessment and should show whether there is any on-going distal obstruction. If there is no obvious occlusion then oversewing of the perforation can be contemplated. Alternatively a T tube (e.g. 6Fg) may be fashioned to lie within the bile duct

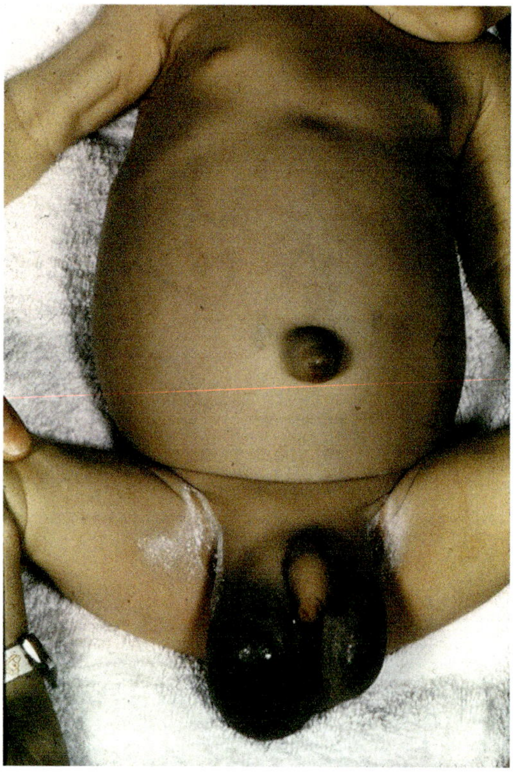

Fig. 44.1 Three-week old infant with spontaneous biliary perforation showing an obvious umbilical hernia and hydroceles. Skin pigmentation due to leaching of bile from peritoneal cavity

and provide a controlled biliary fistula to the skin [5]. It is then left in-situ for 2/3 weeks and if cholangiogram confirms biliary patency then it can be removed.

Dissection may show that there has been disintegration of the duct and in which case, cholecystectomy and hepaticojejunostomy should be performed as a biliary reconstruction. This is not an easy option because it's a relatively small duct to anastomose onto and the tissues will be oedematous and swollen. For those posterior perforations so far encountered we have chosen this option in the absence of an effective alternative and had good outcomes. Theoretically it might be possible to insert some kind of indwelling stent at ERCP to reflect the commonest option in adults. We have tried this and a percutaneous drain in one infant but the results was unconvincing and we resorted to laparotomy to correct it definitively.

Perforation confined to the cystic duct is relatively straightforward and should be treated by cholecystectomy.

44.1.6 Complications

Most post-operative complications, including death, revolve around failure to establish safe biliary drainage and on-going biliary obstruction leading to liver fibrosis and eventually cirrhosis. Some cases of what appear later to be an acquired form of biliary atresia may arise as a consequence of a sealed biliary perforation, periductal inflammation and stenosis [9]. Unlike typical biliary atresia these infants will have had a defined jaundice-free interval after birth.

Portal vein thrombosis appears to be a particular hazard for the posterior perforation and may simply be due to the irritant effects of leaking bile upon the neighbouring portal vein [7]. Usually this is only apparent some months after the acute event perhaps with increasing splenomegaly. Some authors have described a more acute presentation with early ascites [10] but this appears atypical. Chylous ascites is also possible and presumed to be due to damage to the periductal lymphatics ascending to the porta hepatis [11].

Post-operative follow-up should include serial liver biochemistry and ultrasonography at minimum but ideally would include a radio-isotope scan to show restoration of a normal biliary excretion pattern.

44.2 Parenchymal Liver Cysts

Congenital cysts arising within the parenchyma of the liver can be divided morphologically (unilocular or multilocular), histologically (simple parenchymal, mesenchymal hamartoma or rarely teratoma), or on the basis of content (typically bile-containing or not) [12].

The incidence is not known but one large Australian centre with 22,000 births per year identified three cysts of liver origin over 10 years [13]. In adults the incidence of simple liver cysts is much higher (3–18%) [14, 15].

Isolated intrahepatic bile cysts may be choledochal malformations but occur rarely and are not necessarily part of Caroli's syndrome [16]. Most can be left alone unless showing evidence of secondary infection, bile duct obstruction or stone formation.

The usual presentation for most liver cysts is antenatal detection in the second or third trimester and following birth can be shown to be entirely without symptoms. Occasionally cysts can be so large as to be palpable but it is rare that they obstruct either the bile flow (and hence become jaundiced) or the gastrointestinal tract [17].

Figure 44.2 suggests an appropriate diagnostic algorithm including ultrasound, CT & MR scan together with radio-isotope excretion imaging [18].

44.2.1 Management

Those adjudged to be simple parenchymal cysts can be left alone and followed up by serial US. The expectation is that they will diminish relatively in size over the years (Fig. 44.3). Those that appear to be mesenchymal hamartomas or teratomas require surgical excision. This usually involves partial hepatectomy although teratoma often have a thick-walled capsule which facilitates

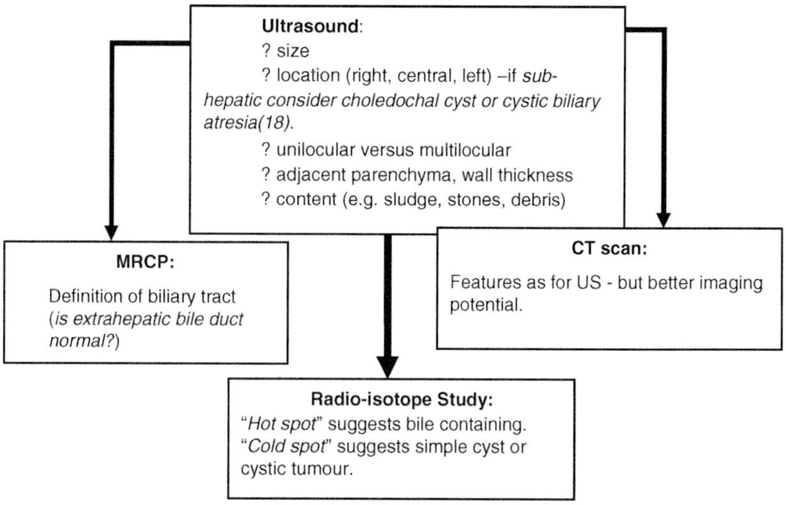
Ultrasound:
? size
? location (right, central, left) –if *sub-hepatic consider choledochal cyst or cystic biliary atresia(18).*
? unilocular versus multilocular
? adjacent parenchyma, wall thickness
? content (e.g. sludge, stones, debris)
MRCP:
Definition of biliary tract
(*is extrahepatic bile duct normal?*)
CT scan:
Features as for US - but better imaging potential.
Radio-isotope Study:
"*Hot spot*" suggests bile containing.
"*Cold spot*" suggests simple cyst or cystic tumour.

Fig. 44.2 Diagnostic approach to antenatally detected liver cyst

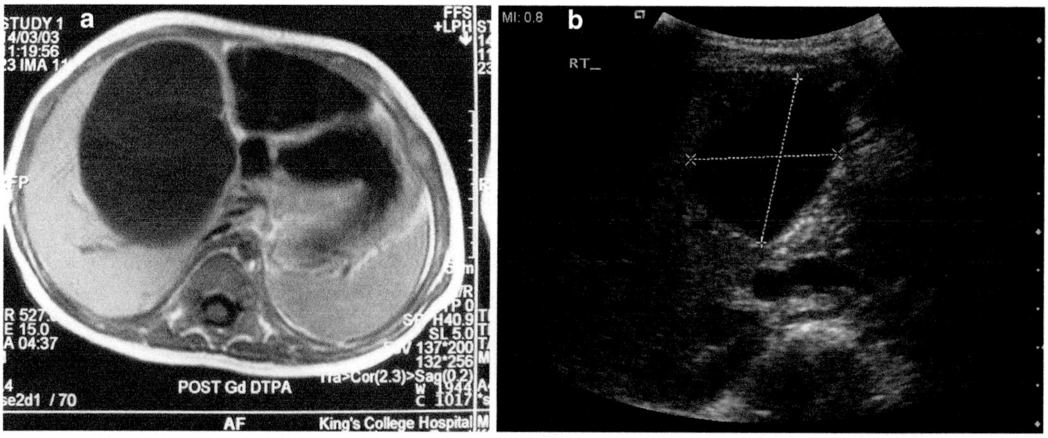

Fig. 44.3 Antenatally detected parenchymal liver cyst: measured at 22 mm diameter during CT scan in first week of life (**a**) and reaching 40 × 50 mm by ultrasound at 9 years (**b**)

enucleation. Simple aspiration of cysts either antenatally or postnatally has been reported [19, 20], however recurrence is highly likely. Large cysts may need to be treated and occasionally fenestration or marsupialisation could be considered if anatomically suitable. This can be achieved using a laparoscopic approach [21].

44.3 Parenchymal Liver Abscess

Infection and abscess formation within the liver are not commonly seen in the neonatal period, indeed less than 100 cases have been reported in the literature. Nevertheless it is certainly possible and may follow generalized sepsis, umbilical catheterization or ascending omphalitis. Other predisposing conditions included necrotizing enterocolitis, maternal infection and being an infant of diabetic mother or a immunodeficiency state such as HIV [22–24]. The problem is more often found in the preterm and those of low birth weight.

One well-described mechanism is the misplaced or infected umbilical vein catheter. This may lacerate portal vein or ductus venosus resulting in an intrahepatic haematoma or inadvertent intravenous fluid (typically high osmolar glucose solution) collection which becomes secondarily infected.

There is a wide spectrum of pathogenic organisms including bacteria (staphylococcal *spp.*, enterobacter, Klebsiella *spp.* and E. coli) and fungi (Candida *spp.*) [24]. In some countries, tuberculosis has been reported as a pathogen in neonatal liver abscesses [23].

Investigations will show a neutrophil leucocytosis, raised C-reactive protein levels and abnormal liver biochemistry. A careful ultrasound should distinguish abscess from cyst although CT scan may be needed to show the contrast-enhancing rim of peri-abscess tissue. Percutaneous aspiration should be considered to identify organism and deduce sensitivities and can also be therapeutic.

Pyogenic liver abscess may also become complicated and discharge into adjacent spaces such as the pleura, peritoneum and even the pericardium. Later, venous thrombosis involving the portal vein (or more rarely the hepatic veins) may occur leading to portal hypertension and splenomegaly.

44.3.1 Management

Management is initially directed at the sepsis and is primarily aggressive broad-spectrum antibiotic (occasionally antifungal) therapy, which should be continued for at least 3–4 weeks. This is the only realistic option in multifocal abscesses (probably the majority) but in solitary collections other options may be considered. Lee et al. from Toronto described aspiration and/or catheter drainage (5Fg pigtail) in eight neonates with excellent results. Occasionally for solitary abscesses open surgery may be contemplated if there is no radiological alternative available. In which case, the key aim is to drain the contents of the cavity without initiating liver damage or inducing haemorrhage.

Infants with resolving collections require long-term serial ultrasonography to monitor resolution and detect any suggestion of portal vein thrombosis.

References

1. Ando K, Miyano T, Kohno S, Takamizawa S, Lane G. Spontaneous perforation of choledochal cyst: a study of 13 cases. Eur J Pediatr Surg. 1998;8:23–5.
2. Holland RM, Lilly JR. Surgical jaundice in infants: other than biliary atresia. J Pediatr Surg. 1992;1:125–9.
3. Davenport M, Betalli P, D'Antiga L, Cheeseman P, Mieli-Vergani G, Howard ER. The spectrum of surgical jaundice in infancy. J Pediatr Surg. 2003;38:1471–9.
4. Dikjstrat CH. Graluistorting in de buikholte bij een zuigeling. Maandschr Kindegeneeskd. 1932;1:409–14.
5. Davenport M, Heaton ND, Howard ER. Spontaneous perforation of the bile duct in infancy. Br J Surg. 1991;78:1068–70.
6. Chardot C, Iskandarani F, De Dreuzy O, Dusquesne B, Pariente D, Bernard O, et al. Spontaneous perforation of the biliary tract in infancy: a series of 11 cases. Eur J Pediatr Surg. 1996;6:41–6.
7. Livesey E, Davenport M. Spontaneous perforation of the biliary tract and portal vein thrombosis in infancy. Pediatr Surg Int. 2008;24:357–9.
8. Lilly JR, Weintraub WH, Altman RP. Spontaneous perforation of the extrahepatic bile ducts and bile peritonitis in infancy. Surgery. 1974;75:664–73.
9. Davenport M, Saxena R, Howard E. Acquired biliary atresia. J Pediatr Surg. 1996;31:1721–3.
10. Moore TC. Massive bile peritonitis in infancy due to spontaneous bile duct perforation with portal vein occlusion. J Pediatr Surg. 1975;10:537–8.
11. Hyde GA. Spontaneous perforation of bile ducts in early infancy. Pediatrics. 1965;35:453–7.
12. Charlesworth PB, Ade-Ajayi N, Davenport M. Natural history and long-term follow-up of antenatally-detected liver cysts. J Pediatr Surg. 2007;42:494–9.
13. Foley PT, Sithasanan N, McEwing R, et al. Enteric duplications presenting as antenatally detected abdominal cysts. Is delayed resection appropriate? J Pediatr Surg. 2003;38:1810–3.
14. Gaines PA, Sampson MA. The prevalence and characterization of simple hepatic cysts by ultrasound examination. Br J Radiol. 1989;289(62):335–7.
15. Carrim ZI, Murchison JT. The prevalence of simple renal and hepatic cysts detected by spiral computed tomography. Clin Radiol. 2003;53:626–9.
16. Yonem O, Bayraktar Y. Clinical characteristics of Caroli's syndrome. World J Gastroenterol. 2007;13:1934–7.
17. Shankar SR, Parelkar SV, Das SA, et al. An antenatally-diagnosed solitary, non-parasitic hepatic cyst with duodenal obstruction. Pediatr Surg Int. 2000;16:214–5.
18. Caponcelli E, Knisely AS, Davenport M. Cystic biliary atresia: an etiologic and prognostic subgroup. J Pediatr Surg. 2008;43:1619–24.
19. Ito M, Yoshimura K, Toyoda N, et al. Aspiration of a giant hepatic cyst in the fetus in utero. Fetal Diagn Ther. 1997;12:221–5.
20. Artzt W, Stock M, Yaman C. Prenatal diagnosis and therapy of fetal hepatic cyst in the second trimester. Geburtshilfe Frauenheilkd. 1998;58:129–31.
21. Kathouda N, Mavor E, Gugenheim J, et al. Laparoscopic management of benign cystic lesions of the liver. J Hepato-Biliary-Pancreat Surg. 2000;7:212–7.

22. Moss TJ, Pysher TJ. Hepatic abscess in neonates. Am J Dis Child. 1981;135:726–8.
23. Simeunovic E, Arnold M, Sidler D, Moore SW. Liver abscess in neonates. Pediatr Surg Int. 2009;25:153–6.
24. Filippi L, Poggi C, Gozzini E, Meleleo R, Mirabile L, Fiorini P. Neonatal liver abscesses due to Candida infection effectively treated with caspofungin. Acta Paediatr. 2009;98:906–9.

45 Surgery for Congenital Hyperinsulinism

N. Scott Adzick and Pablo Laje

Abstract

Transient hypoglycemia in the newborn period is common and generally associated either with immaturity of the glucose regulatory pathways (which responds to frequent feeds and resolves spontaneously within hours), or with stress-associated hyperinsulinism (which responds well to hyperglycemic drugs and resolves spontaneously within the first few weeks or months of life). Congenital Hyperinsulinism (HI) is the most frequent cause of persistent, long-term hypoglycemia in newborns and infants, and can lead to severe and irreversible brain damage and developmental delay. It is a rare congenital disorder of the glucose metabolism that has an estimated incidence of 1–1.4 cases per 50,000 live births, leading to about 80–120 new cases in the United States each year. An incidence as high as 1 in 2500 live births has been reported in populations with high consanguinity like Arabians and Ashkenazi Jews. Inappropriate oversecretion of insulin is the hallmark of HI, and the genetic background is quite variable. Depending on the genetic mutation, babies with HI may be treated medically or may require surgery either as a palliative treatment or as a definitive cure.

Keywords

Congenital pancreatic disease • Congenital hyperinsulinism • Surgery

45.1 Introduction

Transient hypoglycemia in the newborn period is common and generally associated either with immaturity of the glucose regulatory pathways (which responds to frequent feeds and resolves spontaneously within hours), or with stress-associated hyperinsulinism (which responds well to hyperglycemic drugs and resolves spontaneously within the first few weeks or months of

N.S. Adzick, MD, MMM (✉) • P. Laje, MD
Department of Surgery, The Children's Hospital of Philadelphia, 34th and Civic Center Boulevard, Philadelphia, PA 19104, USA
e-mail: adzick@email.chop.edu

P.D. Losty et al. (eds.), *Rickham's Neonatal Surgery*, https://doi.org/10.1007/978-1-4471-4721-3_45

life). Congenital Hyperinsulinism (HI) is the most frequent cause of persistent, *long-term* hypoglycemia in newborns and infants, and can lead to severe and irreversible brain damage and developmental delay. It is a rare congenital disorder of the glucose metabolism that has an estimated incidence of 1–1.4 cases per 50,000 live births, leading to about 80–120 new cases in the United States each year [1, 2]. An incidence as high as 1 in 2500 live births has been reported in populations with high consanguinity like Arabians and Ashkenazi Jews. Inappropriate oversecretion of insulin is the hallmark of HI, and the genetic background is quite variable. Depending on the genetic mutation, babies with HI may be treated medically or may require surgery as either a palliative treatment or as a definitive cure.

45.2 History

Congenital hyperinsulinism was first described by McQuarrie in 1954, who initially termed it "syndrome of idiopathic hypoglycemia of infants" [3]. At that time, assays for the accurate measurement of plasma insulin were not available. However, he suggested that there could be an association between the disease and a state of hyperinsulinism, and he also highlighted the "high incidence of a familial or genetic trait of the disease". The first pancreatectomy performed on a child with HI was reported in 1934 by Evarts Graham, 20 years before the disease was described. The pancreas was explored searching for an adenoma, but since no evidence of an adenoma was found, a near-total pancreatectomy [~90%] was performed, and the patient's hypoglycemia resolved [4]. The revolutionary development of an insulin radioimmunoassay in the late 1950s by Nobel Prize laureate Rosalyn Yalow confirmed that insulin oversecretion was crucial to the pathophysiology of HI [5]. For decades it was believed that insulin was secreted by an excessive number of islets resulting from *nesidioblastosis*, an abnormal postnatal budding of endocrine cells off the pancreatic ducts ("nesidion" = island). This theory, proposed by Yakovac et al. at the Children's Hospital of Philadelphia (CHOP), came from the histologic analysis of pancreatic specimens from HI cases stained with insulin-specific techniques. Later studies in the 1980s showed that nesidioblastosis was in fact a normal neonatal phenomenon, and the term "nesidioblastosis" has been abandoned [6, 7]. Advances in molecular biology and genetics led to our current understanding of the disease, which occurs due to a variety of genetic derangements that alter the regulatory mechanisms of glucose homeostasis.

45.3 Pathophysiology

Glucose homeostasis is complex and is influenced by a large number of factors. Plasma glucose levels are maintained within the normal range by mechanisms that respond to the postprandial and fasting states in opposite directions. During the postprandial state, the liver accumulates glucose in the form of glycogen (glycogenogenesis), while during the fasting state, the liver releases glucose by glycogenolysis. Multiple hormones and factors promote glycogenolysis and hyperglycemia: glucocorticoids, glucagon, catecholamines, somatostatin and others. However, insulin is the only endogenous hormone that reduces plasma glucose levels. Insulin inhibits glucose release from the liver and promotes glucose uptake in peripheral tissues. When the plasma glucose level rises, glucose enters the beta cell's cytoplasm through the high-capacity GLUT-2 transporter, which is followed by an increase in intracellular glucose metabolism. As a consequence, the intracellular concentration of ATP increases (as does the ATP/ADP ratio), and the ATP-dependent potassium channels (K-ATP channel) located in the cytosolic membrane of the beta cell become inactive and close. Potassium accumulates on the inner surface of the cytoplasmic membrane and depolarizes it. The depolarization generates the activation of voltage-dependent calcium channels and calcium accumulates in the cytoplasm, which eventually triggers a calcium-dependent insulin exocytosis (Fig. 45.1). When the K-ATP channel located in the cytoplasmic membrane is defective due to *loss-of-function*

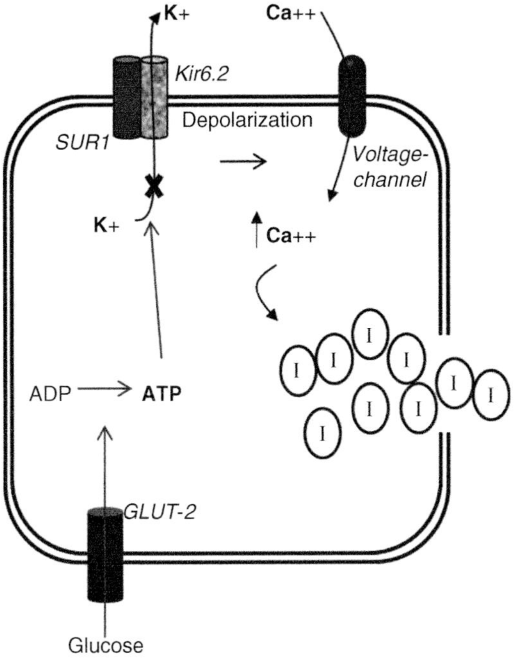

Fig. 45.1 Insulin release as a physiologic response to hyperglycemia. The ATP/ADP ratio increases as a consequence of the glucose metabolism. The ATP-sensitive potassium channel reacts to this by closing. The accumulation of potassium in the cytoplasmic surface of the beta-cell membrane depolarizes it. This event triggers an influx of calcium through voltage-sensitive calcium channels, which in turn generates a calcium-dependent insulin release. *SUR1* sulfonylurea receptor 1, *Kir6.2* inward-rectifier potassium ion channel 6.2, *ATP* adenosine triphosphate, *ADP* adenosine diphosphate, *GLUT-2* glucose transporter 2, *I* insulin

genetic mutations, it remains inactivated at all times, regardless of the plasma glucose level, generating a non-regulated, persistent, insulin release that leads to unregulated hypoglycemia. This is the most common pathophysiologic mechanism of HI. The insulin levels, however, are never strikingly elevated in HI. The K-ATP channel is composed of 2 subunits: SUR1 (a sulfonylurea receptor, the regulatory subunit) and Kir6.2 (the ion pore), which are encoded by adjacent genes located in the short arm of chromosome 11. Less commonly, HI occurs due to genetic defects in other enzymes. Pancreatic glutamate dehydrogenase (GDH) is a mitochondrial enzyme that catalyzes the reversible oxidation of glutamate to alpha-ketoglutarate (and ammonia), which after a series of intermediate steps through the tricarboxylic acid cycle results in an elevation of the intracellular ATP/ADP ratio and consequently an insulin release. *Gain-of-function* mutations in the GDH gene lead to HI and hyperammonemia ("hyperinsulinism/hyperammonemia [HI/HA] syndrome") [8, 9]. Pancreatic glucokinase (GK) produces the phosphorylation of intracellular glucose to glucose-6-phosphate (G6-P), which is the first step of the glycolytic pathway that will ultimately increase the production of ATP and stimulate insulin release. GK has a low affinity for glucose and is not self-regulated by its end product G6-P. Gain-of-function mutations in the GK gene increase the affinity of GK for glucose so that more insulin is released at any given plasma glucose level, which in turn leads to HI (although most of these cases have a mild clinical course) [10, 11]. More recently, deficiencies in the mitochondrial fatty acid beta-oxidation enzyme "short-chain hydroxyacyl-CoA dehydrogenase" (SCHAD) have been identified as a rare cause of HI, and the mechanism appears to be a loss of the natural inhibitory effect that SCHAD exerts on the mitochondrial GDH [12].

45.4 Diagnosis

The diagnosis of HI is confirmed when all of the following metabolic criteria are present: (1) fasting *and* postprandial hypoglycemia with unsuppressed hyperinsulinism (neonatal hypoglycemia is generally defined as a glucose plasma level of <50 mg/dL after the first 24 h of life with an insulin level >36 pmol/L), (2) suppression of lipolysis and suppression of ketogenesis at the time of the hypoglycemia (lipolysis and hepatic ketogenesis are part of the normal physiologic response to hypoglycemia, and are physiologically inhibited by insulin), and (3) a positive hyperglycemic response to a dose of glucagon, which is a direct insulin antagonist (glucose must increase by 30–50 mg/dL after 0.25–1 mg of intravenous glucagon). Additionally, these criteria must be present for a prolonged period of time and outside certain clinical circumstances such as perinatal stress.

45.5 Classification

45.5.1 Histological Classification

There are two major histological forms of HI: *focal* and *diffuse*, which have a different genetic background and a different management strategy. Focal disease consists of a single focus of adenomatous islet cell hyperplasia surrounded by normal lobular pancreatic tissue. Focal lesions respect the limits of the pancreatic lobules, as opposed to insulinomas which are well demarcated and do not respect the limits of pancreatic lobules. The beta cells within the focal lesion have an enlarged cytoplasm and typically normal nuclei, although some can have nucleomegaly. They accumulate in central clusters, surrounded by non-beta islet cells. The proliferated endocrine cells in the focal lesions push the exocrine components toward the periphery, but there are always some exocrine acinar cells intermixed within the endocrine cells [13]. The size of a focal lesion is variable, from a few millimeters in diameter to much greater than a centimeter. It can be located in the surface of the pancreas, or deep within the organ. Superficial lesions can often be identified visually by subtle differences in color and/or by palpation, since focal lesions tend to be firmer than the normal pancreas. In our experience we have been able to identify the focal lesion by visualization and/or palpation in approximately two-thirds of the cases. Focal lesions can be located anywhere in the pancreas. In our series of more than 140 focal lesions treated by partial pancreatectomy, the distribution was 45% in the pancreatic head, 25% in the neck/body, 15% in the tail, and 15% had "other location", which included focal lesions unusually large that extended beyond a single pancreatic segment, and very rarely lesions that were present within ectopic pancreatic tissue [14]. In the diffuse form of the disease, most, if not all, beta cells are abnormal throughout the organ. The hallmark feature of the beta cells in diffuse HI is the nucleomegaly, which is defined as nuclei that occupy an area three times larger than the nuclei of the adjacent non-beta endocrine cells or four times larger than the nuclei of the adjacent acinar cells. Other nuclear abnormalities (e.g. abnormal shape, pseudoinclusions) may also be present. The total number of endocrine cells in pancreases with diffuse HI is not different than in pancreases from euglycemic age-match individuals. The distribution of the abnormal cells is not always homogeneous. In some cases, cells with clear nucleomegaly can be very concentrated in one area and very sparse in another area of the same specimen, intermixed with beta islet cells that do not look histologically abnormal [15].

Of *all* patients with HI, 30–40% have focal disease and 60–70% have diffuse disease. Among patients who have required surgery at CHOP (which represent approximately 60% of all HI patients), approximately 50% have focal disease and 50% have diffuse disease.

45.5.2 Therapeutic Classification

From a management standpoint, HI is divided in two groups: diazoxide-*responsive* and diazoxide-*resistant*. The initial drug in the management of HI is diazoxide, which inhibits insulin secretion by activating the K-ATP channel. Diazoxide binds to the SUR1 subunit of the channel, but in order to be effective both subunits must be structurally normal and functional. Since the most common causes of HI involve defects in the SUR1/Kir6.2 genes, the majority of HI patients do not respond to diazoxide and the only ones that do are those with mutations in the GK, GDH, SCHAD, or other genes. In our experience with more than 450 patients with HI, only 33% were diazoxide-*responsive,* whereas 67% were diazoxide-*resistant*. Most of diazoxide-*resistant* patients underwent surgery, although some were deemed not candidates for surgery due to a variety of reasons and were managed with different medical strategies [16].

45.6 Genetics

The development of genetic testing and diagnosis has allowed identification of a large number of mutations in patients with HI. To date, about 50%

of patients with HI have a known genetic mutation. The most frequent mutations cause a loss of function in the K-ATP channel of the cytoplasmic membrane of the pancreatic beta cells. This channel is composed of the subunits SUR1 and Kir6.2, which are encoded by two genes located next to each other in the p15.4 region of the chromosome 11: ABCC8 and KCNJ11. The *diffuse* form of HI occurs most frequently as a consequence of mutations of the SUR1/Kir6.2 complex inherited in a recessive manner [17]. There are currently more than 200 known mutations in the ABCC8 and KCNJ11 genes, and some of them have a remarkably high prevalence within certain populations [18]. Very rare mutations of the SUR1 gene inherited in a dominant manner have been identified as a cause of diffuse HI, but the clinical presentation of these patients is milder than patients with recessive disease and they respond partially to diazoxide. In addition, compound heterozygous mutations in the ABCC8/KCNJ11 genes have also been identified as a cause of diffuse HI, but their clinical course is milder [19–21]. Diffuse disease can also occur due to mutations in other genes. Gain-of-function mutations in the GK gene (located in the p15.3-p15.1 region of chromosome 7) inherited in a dominant manner can lead to diffuse HI. Several mutations have been identified already and all affect the same region of the enzyme [10, 11, 22, 23]. A variety of dominant gain-of-function, missense, single-nucleotide mutations in the GDH gene (GLUD1, chromosome 10, region q23.3) have been identified in patients with diffuse HI. These mutations in the GLUD1 gene, as a group, represent the second most frequent cause of HI. All identified mutations affect the GTP-binding site of the enzyme (GTP is the most potent GDH inhibitor) which makes the enzyme work at a higher basal rate [8, 9]. Diffuse HI has also been described as a consequence of recessive mutations in the mitochondrial enzyme short-chain L-3-hydroxyacyl-CoA dehydrogenase (SCHAD) gene located in the q22–26 region of chromosome 4. The mutations affect different regions of the protein which explains the heterogeneous clinical presentation of these cases [12, 24]. Over the last few years, cases of diffuse HI have been linked to mutations in three new genes: HNF4A (encoding the hepatocyte nuclear factor 4a; chromosome 20q12–13.1; dominant inheritance), SLC16A1 (encoding the monocarboxylate transporter; chromosome 1p13.2–p12; gain-of-function mutations; dominant inheritance), and UCP2 (encoding the mitochondrial uncoupling protein 2; chromosome 11, region q13; dominant inheritance). Their pathophysiologic mechanisms are not yet well understood, and their age at onset and clinical presentation is variable [25–28].

The *focal* form occurs when an individual with a constitutional paternally inherited mutation in the SUR1/Kir6.2 complex loses the normal maternal allele (an event called "loss of heterozygosity") in a group of pancreatic beta cells (a "two-hit" phenomenon), which not only will oversecrete insulin but will also develop an adenomatous hyperplastic proliferative pattern. The 11p15 region has several genes subject to genomic imprinting. The loss of the maternal 11p15 not only affects the expression of the ABCC8/KCNJ11 genes (not imprinted), but also affects the expression of the maternal tumor suppressor gene H19 and the cell cycle regulator $p57^{kip2}$ (region 11p15.5). The tumor suppressor gene H19 (strongly imprinted and of exclusively maternal monoallelic expression) exerts an antagonistic effect on the insulin-like growth factor 2 (IGF2) expressed exclusively from the paternal allele. The imbalance between IGF2 and H19 is the reason for the adenomatous proliferation of the affected cells. The loss of the maternal allele in a focal lesion can be evidenced by genetic testing and immunohistochemistry (decreased $p57^{kip2}$ staining within the focal lesion) [29]. With regard to the ABCC8/KCNJ11 genes, some cases have only the single abnormal paternal allele, whereas some patients have a duplication of the paternal abnormal allele, which is called uniparental paternal isodisomy.

When a baby is diagnosed with HI in the absence of a family history, the parents and the patient must undergo genetic testing. In cases of diazoxide-*responsive* disease, the genetic testing is not urgent and even with the newest technology can take several weeks. In diazoxide-*resistant* cases, which theoretically have a mutation in the

SUR1/Kir6.2 complex, the genetic testing becomes more critical because it can help in the differential diagnosis of diffuse versus focal disease, determine the need for imaging studies, and provide prognostic information.

45.7 Prenatal Diagnosis and Counseling

The prenatal diagnosis of HI based on the genetic analysis of known mutations in family members is possible, allowing immediate medical management at the time of birth. The genetic mutations that cause diffuse HI respond to the Mendelian inheritance laws with the exception of the *de novo* mutations. For the recessive forms of the HI, the chance of developing the disease in the offspring (homozygous for the affected allele) is 25% for each individual, whereas in cases of dominant inheritance the chance is 50%. Prenatal screening of all known mutations in all HI-involved genes in the general population is not justified by the overall low incidence of the disease, but prenatal diagnosis is justified and currently available for families with previously affected children [30]. While the inheritance of an abnormal ABCC8/KCNJ11 gene from paternal origin does respond to Mendelian laws, the occurrence of focal disease in subsequent siblings of an affected individual is unpredictable given the fact that the second event in the pathogenesis of the disease (the loss of the normal maternal allele) occurs as a random event in somatic cells. The likelihood of this occurrence is extremely low, but it has been described [31].

45.8 Medical Management

The first step in the treatment of newborns with HI is to provide enough glucose to maintain normoglycemia. This is usually achieved by a combination of a high-concentration glucose intravenous infusion plus frequent enteral feeds. The required glucose infusion rate (GIR), calculated as % dextrose × IV rate × 0.169/Wt in kg, can be as high as 25 mg/kg/min which is nearly three times higher than the physiological hepatic glucose release during fasting periods in newborns. Along with supportive glucose management, HI-specific drugs must be initiated. The first line drug is diazoxide. Diazoxide is an agonist of the K-ATP channel and is not effective in patients with recessively inherited mutations in the ABCC8/KCNJ11 complex and severe HI, but it is effective at variable levels in patients with dominant mutations in the ABCC8/KCNJ11 complex, patients with compound heterozygous ABCC8/KCNJ11 mutations, syndromic HI cases (e.g. Beckwith-Wiedeman syndrome) and patients with mutations in most of the other HI-related genes of dominant inheritance known to date. The dose of diazoxide is 5–20 mg/kg/day divided in three oral doses. After 5 days of treatment the response to diazoxide is evaluated by a fasting test, off intravenous glucose and off any other hyperglycemic medications (Fig. 45.2). Patients with the ability to maintain a plasma glucose level >70 mg/dL for at least 12 h are considered diazoxide-*responsive*. For these patients, an adequate feeding regimen is established and they are discharged home on long-term diazoxide treatment. The adverse effects of diazoxide are sodium and fluid retention which can be problematic in patients with concomitant pulmonary or cardiac diseases but can be controlled with the simultaneous administration of diuretics, and hypertrichosis which can be disturbing for the parents but is a benign condition. Patients who cannot maintain glucose levels above 70 mg/dL for 12 h are presumed to have recessively-inherited disease and are considered diazoxide-*resistant*. In these patients, diazoxide is discontinued, the glucose infusion is re-established immediately, and preoperative planning starts. A variety of alternative drugs can be tried in these patients, but mainly as stabilizing agents prior to surgical intervention. Octreotide is a synthetic long-acting somatostatin analog that inhibits insulin secretion by a direct inhibition of voltage-dependent calcium channels. It is generally administered subcutaneously every 6–8 h, but can also be given in a continuous intravenous infusion. The starting dose is 2 μg/kg/day, but it must always be titrated up due to rapid tachyphylaxis. The maximum dose is 15 μg/kg/day. Patients with a partial response to diazoxide

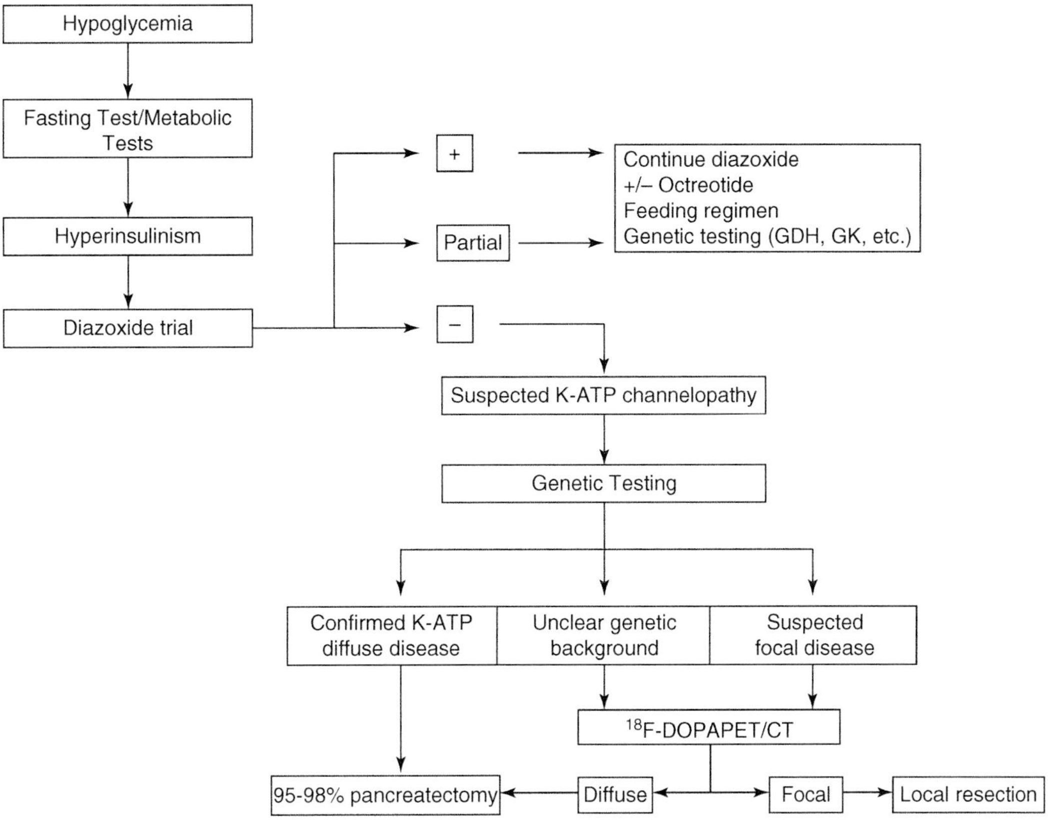

Fig. 45.2 Current algorithm for the management of patients with hyperinsulinism

and some patients with persistent hypoglycemia after a near-total pancreatectomy have been successfully managed at home by a combination of long-term subcutaneous octreotide (twice daily) and a very strict feeding regimen via a gastrostomy. However, octreotide is not recommended for long-term treatment due to its many potential adverse effects (some of which can be life-threatening [e.g. necrotizing enterocolitis]) and its rapid desensitization [32]. Glucagon is a natural insulin antagonist that elevates the plasma glucose levels by activating the enzyme phosphorilase A, which catalyzes the degradation of glycogen. It can be used preoperatively as a continuous intravenous infusion to help maintaining adequate glucose levels or as an intravenous bolus to rescue patients from severe hypoglycemic episodes, but it is not suitable for long-term management. Other drugs, like the calcium channel blocker nifedipine, have been used in the past in the long-term management of patients with HI but their effectiveness is very limited and their use is currently not recommended.

45.9 Preoperative Management

The most relevant aspect of the preoperative planning in patients with diazoxide-*resistant* HI is to differentiate between *diffuse* and *focal* disease, because the surgical strategy is radically different between the two, as is the clinical outcome. Genetic testing is the first step. In the ideal situation, two K-ATP channel mutations are found (one from each parent) confirming diffuse disease, or only one mutation of paternal origin is found, possibly consistent with focal disease. There are situations, however, in which the genetic analysis is difficult to interpret. Sometimes no mutation is found, or in other instances an identified genetic variant is not disease-causing but simply a rare polymorphism. Additionally, the identification of a mutation in the paternal line does not exclude the possibility of a disease-causing postzygotic mutation on the maternal line (resulting in diffuse HI) not reflected in peripheral blood leukocytes [33].

Patients with genetically confirmed recessive K-ATP-related diffuse disease do not need preoperative imaging and should undergo a near-total pancreatectomy if they cannot be safely managed with medical therapy. The resection of less than 95% of the pancreas is associated with a higher need for another resection and is not recommended [34]. All other patients need preoperative imaging to localize the suspected focal lesion or to help in the differential diagnosis of focal versus diffuse disease when the genetic background is unknown or unclear.

45.10 Imaging Studies

All conventional non-invasive image studies (ultrasound, computerized tomography, magnetic resonance) have been used to try to distinguish between focal and diffuse disease or to localize genetically suspected focal lesions, but these radiologic tests are not helpful. Invasive interventional tests were developed in the late 1980s and were used until 2004 [35, 36]. The Arterial Stimulation with Venous Sampling (ASVS) test measures insulin in the hepatic veins after injecting calcium (a stimulant of insulin release) selectively in the arteries that supply the different regions of the pancreas. An immediate rise in insulin from stimulation in only one artery suggests focal HI in the corresponding area of the pancreas (gastroduodenal artery: pancreatic head; superior mesenteric artery: uncinate process and neck; splenic artery: pancreatic body or tail), whereas an insulin rise in all three areas suggests diffuse HI. The Transhepatic Portal Venous Sampling of the pancreatic veins (THPVS) measures insulin levels in the small pancreatic veins that drain the different regions of the organ to determine if there is an area of higher concentration, consistent with focal disease, or not, consistent with diffuse disease. These techniques take several hours to be performed, are technically very demanding, and their sensitivity and specificity for distinguishing between focal and diffuse disease are limited [37]. They have been largely replaced by what is now considered the gold-standard imaging study: ^{18}fluoro-L-3–4 dihydroxyphenylalanine positron emission tomography merged with a low-radiation computerized tomography (^{18}FPET/CT). The study was originally developed in the late 1990s for the detection of tumors of neuroendocrine origin in adults, and has been used in HI patients since 2004 [38–40]. Islet cells of the pancreas, like all other neuroendocrine cells, take up L-dihydroxyphenylalanine (L-DOPA), convert it to L-dopamine by the enzyme DOPA decarboxylase, and store it in vesicles. Similarly, these cells can take up ^{18}fluoro-L-3–4 dihydroxyphenylalanine (18FDOPA), convert it into ^{18}fluoro-dopamine and store it in vesicles that can be tracked by their gamma radiation. At CHOP, the isotope ^{18}FDOPA is administered in children under an FDA-approved Investigational New Drug (IND) protocol and the approval of the Institutional Review Board. The isotope has a half-life of 110 min, so it is manufactured on the day of the study in the Cyclotron Facility of the University of Pennsylvania, and used at a dose of 0.08–0.16 mCi/kg (slow intravenous infusion) within 2–3 h of its preparation. All glycemic medications must be stopped prior to the study. The study is done under general anesthesia in a hybrid scanner that initially captures the nuclear signal (γ-radiation) and then generates low-dose (x-radiation) CT scan of the abdomen without changing the patient's position. The nuclear signal is captured at 10-min intervals during only the first 50 min post injection because after that time the tracer accumulates in the liver, gallbladder, biliary tree and duodenal lumen, which can lead to false positive images. Focal lesions are seen as bright spots over a darker background, whereas in cases of diffuse disease the tracer is homogeneously distributed throughout the organ (Fig. 45.3). In our experience with more than 160 studies, the sensitivity of the ^{18}FPET/CT to detect a focal lesion has been 84%. In the 16% that were erroneously diagnosed as diffuse disease, the focal lesions were particularly

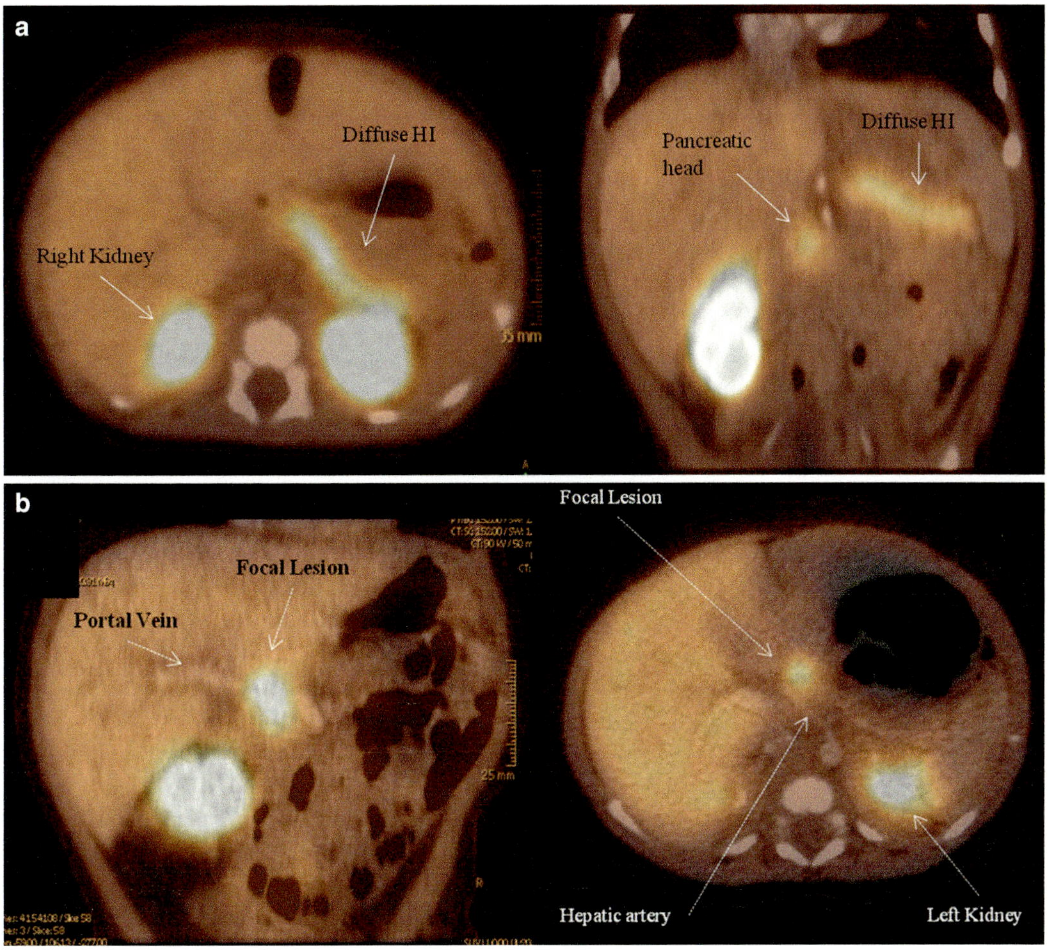

Fig. 45.3 [18]Fluoro-L-3–4 dihydroxyphenylalanine positron emission tomography merged with a low-dose radiation computerized tomography (^{18}F-PET/CT). (**a**) Diffuse disease: the entire pancreas uptakes the tracer homogeneously. Coronal and axial views. (**b**) Focal disease: the lesion is a discrete bright spot in the pancreatic head over a darker background. Merging the PET images to the CT images helps to determine the exact location of the focal lesion and its relation to surrounding structures

small (although the size of the lesion does not always correlates with the intensity of the signal), had an unusual shape, or were an atypical case in which the focal lesion occupied most of the pancreas [41]. The [18]FPET/CT is also sensitive in the detection of the very rare ectopic focal lesions [14, 42]. When a focal lesion is identified on the [18]FPET/CT, the correlation with the actual location determined during the surgery is nearly 100%. In cases with subtle differences in the signal intensity throughout the organ, we do a quantitative activity analysis using the ratio between the peak intensity at the point of interest to the intensity at the background. A ratio ≥ 1.5 is considered diagnostic of focal disease.

45.11 Surgical Management

All open operations are approached using a transverse supraumbilical laparotomy. The pancreas is completely exposed by an extended Kocher maneuver, entry into the lesser sac, and mobilization of the inferior border. It is not necessary to mobilize the spleen. The pancreas is inspected under 3.5X loupe magnification in an attempt to visualize a focal lesion, and it is also thoroughly palpated. If no focal lesion is identified, then 2-3 mm biopsies are taken from the pancreatic head, body, and tail. Patients with diffuse HI confirmed by intraoperative frozen analysis undergo near-total pancreatectomy. Near-total pancreatectomy (95–98%) involves the resection of the entire pancreas with the exception of a tiny residual piece of pancreatic tissue between the common bile duct and the duodenal wall. The intrapancreatic segment of the common bile duct (CBD) must be completely dissected to perform an for an adequate near-total pancreatectomy. To help with the dissection of the CBD, we place a vessel loop around the extrapancreatic distal CBD and then swing it within the duodenal C-loop to trace the CBD through the head of the pancreas until it enters the duodenum. This maneuver is not needed if the CBD follows a course posterior to the pancreatic head. In children with diffuse disease treated by near-total pancreatectomy, a gastrostomy tube is also placed to provide enteral access for glucose or overnight feeds if needed. When the intraoperative biopsies demonstrate normal pancreatic histology, a further search for the focal lesion using the preoperative localization data is conducted. Intraoperative high-resolution ultrasound has been reported to provide some help in localization because focal lesions may be hypoechoic, but we have been unable to confirm the utility of this radiologic modality [43]. Additional biopsies of suspicious areas are obtained until the focal lesion is identified by frozen section. Expert pediatric pathologic interpretation is vitally important.

Focal lesions tend to be less than 10 mm in diameter (although they can be much larger) and frequently are irregularly shaped. Some lesions have octopus-like extensions that make imperative the intraoperative confirmation of clear margins by frozen section analysis. Focal lesions often have subtle differences in their appearance compared to normal tissue, or may feel firmer than the surrounding normal pancreas. The preoperative PET/CT study greatly facilitates the search. We have been able to identify by visualization and/or palpation approximately two-thirds of all focal lesions. Focal lesions, however, can be buried within the pancreas and be impossible to see or feel. Once the focal lesion is identified, a partial pancreatectomy is performed using frozen sections of margins to ensure a complete resection. Small and superficial lesions in the body or tail can be treated by simple resection. Deep periductal lesions in the body and tail usually are treated by distal pancreatectomy. Superficial and small lesions in the head of the pancreas can also be treated by simple resection. On the other hand, deep pancreatic head lesions close to the common bile duct and pancreatic duct can be tricky to excise completely, particularly if there are tentacles of diseased tissue that emanate from the lesion. To ensure complete lesion resection in these challenging cases, we remove most or all of the pancreatic head, and follow with a Roux-en-Y pancreaticojejunostomy to drain the pancreatic body and tail. By doing this, the endocrine and exocrine functions of the remaining normal pancreas are preserved. In our experience, this approach has been needed in about 40% of focal lesions within the pancreatic head. The end of a retrocolic, 25 cm-long Roux-en-Y jejunal limb is meticulously anastomosed to the capsule of the pancreatic body (just *beyond* the cut surface of the pancreas) with fine interrupted 5-O monofilament suture to effectively tuck the cut end of the pancreas into the jejunal lumen (Fig. 45.4). The posterior aspect of the anastomosis is performed first, with all sutures placed first and then tied serially leaving the knots on the inside of the anastomosis, and the anterior aspect is performed last, in the same manner, but leaving the knots on the outside. The omentum is then freed from the transverse colon, wrapped around the anastomosis and sutured into place for additional security. Rarely, a focal lesion in the head will extend into the duodenal wall in which case a Whipple procedure may be needed. In cases of near-total or pancreatic head resections it is important to preserve the gastroduodenal artery as well as the vessels supplying the third and fourth portion of the duodenum (superior and inferior pancreaticoduodenal arteries) to avoid duodenal ischemia [16]. We do not use drains after any pancreatic resection for HI.

We have used laparoscopic surgery in patients with HI. In cases of focal disease of the body or

a b

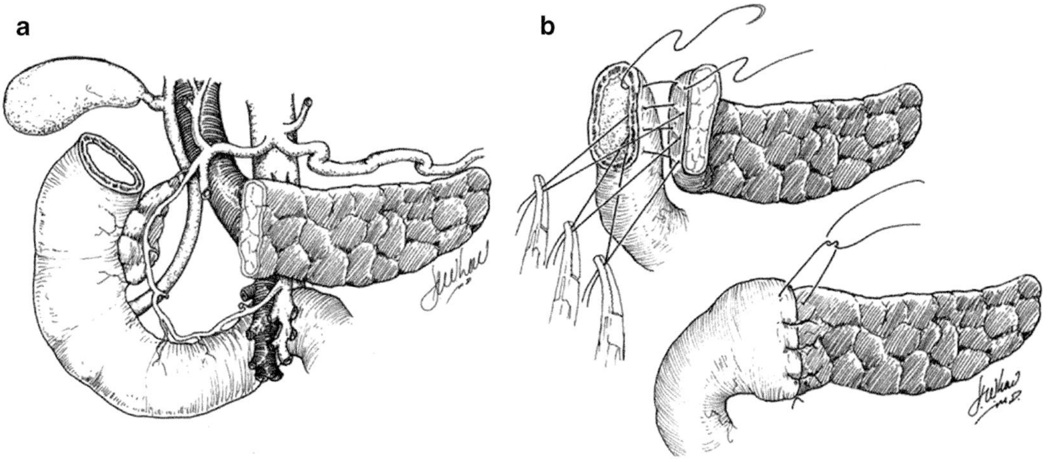

Fig. 45.4 To ensure complete lesion resection of deep pancreatic head lesions close to the common bile duct and pancreatic duct, we remove most or all of the pancreatic head followed by Roux-en-Y pancreaticojejunostomy to drain the remaining pancreatic body and tail to preserve the endocrine and exocrine functions of the remaining normal pancreas. The end of a retrocolic, 25 cm-long Roux-en-Y jejunal limb is meticulously anastomosed to the capsule of the pancreatic body (just *beyond* the cut surface of the pancreas) to effectively tuck the cut end of the pancreas into the jejunal lumen. The posterior aspect of the anastomosis is performed first, with all sutures placed first and then tied serially leaving the knots on the inside of the anastomosis, and the anterior aspect is performed last, in the same manner, but leaving the knots on the outside. From Laje P, Stanley CA, Palladino AA, et al. Pancreatic head resection and Roux-en-Y pancreaticojejunostomy for the treatment of the focal form of congenital hyperinsulinism. J Pediatr Surg, 2012;47 [1]:131–135; used with permission

tail, the approach is straightforward. To facilitate pancreatic body and tail exposure during laparoscopy, it is useful to sew the stomach up to the anterior abdominal wall using 2–3 transabdominal sutures to the anterior gastric wall close to the greater curvature (Fig. 45.5). The carbon dioxide pneumoperitoneum further suspends the stomach anteriorly and also helps to expose the pancreatic body and tail. The laparoscopic procedure is performed via four 3–5 mm ports, and this permits biopsies, complete resection of a visible peripherally located focal lesion, or a distal pancreatectomy if needed. The major drawback to the laparoscopic approach is that there is little tactile feedback to help locate a non-visible focal lesion. Near-total pancreatectomies and pancreatic head resections are significantly more demanding by laparoscopy than by open surgery, and while they are technically feasible, their complication rate such as bleeding and common bile duct injury is higher. The effectiveness of this approach is currently not as good as the open approach given that most reported cases are actually 75—90% pancreatectomies because the CBD is not dissected [44–46]. Perhaps an intraoperative laparoscopic ultrasound probe could facilitate visualization of the CBD to allow precise dissection of this structure.

45.12 Postoperative Management

Postoperative pain is managed by an epidural infusion of bupivacaine, which is kept for 3–4 days, and intravenous narcotics if needed as a continuous infusion or rescue boluses. Patients are kept NPO until bowel function resumes. The intravenous GIR is re-started at a low dose (2 mg/kg/min) because the stress of the surgery induces hepatic glycogenolysis. The GIR is advanced to 5 mg/kg/min 12–18 h after the surgery and to 8 mg/kg/min (equivalent to the physiological hepatic glucose release during fasting periods) 24—36 h after the surgery. Plasma glucose levels are measured hourly in the beginning and spaced out as they become stable. If the plasma glucose levels are excessively high (>400 mg/dL) we assess the presence of ketonic bodies in the urine, and if they are present, an intravenous insulin

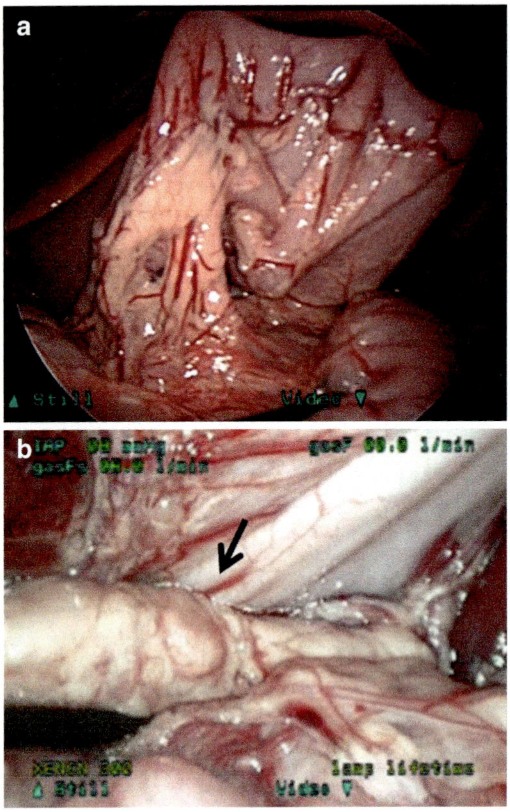

Fig. 45.5 Laparoscopic pancreatectomy. (**a**) To facilitate pancreatic exposure, the stomach is tacked up to the anterior abdominal wall using transabdominal sutures to the anterior gastric wall close to the greater curvature. (**b**) A focal lesion is clearly seen on the anterior-inferior aspect of the pancreatic body. Notice the difference in color between the lesion and the adjacent normal pancreas

infusion is started. The immediate postoperative oscillations in the plasma glucose levels are not reflective of the eventual long-term outcome, because factors like surgical stress and pain can alter glucose homeostasis. When bowel function is evident, enteral feeds are restarted. We start with 1/3 of the goal volume and advance daily by thirds. Simultaneously, the GIR is gradually weaned as the feeding volume increases. When patients are exclusively on enteral feeds, a "cure" fasting test is performed. If patients are able to maintain euglycemia for 18 h, they are considered completely cured. If the time to hypoglycemia is less than 18 h the next step is to determine a regimen of frequent feeds and short fasting periods that will allow the patient to be managed safely at home. Patients that are unable to be weaned from the intravenous glucose infusion rate are obviously not cured and will need further assessment.

45.13 Postoperative Complications

Our overall surgical complication rate after pancreatic surgery for HI is low. General potential complications are bowel obstruction due to adhesions and small intestine to small intestine intussusception (which occurs within the first 2 postoperative weeks) [47]. Specific complications include chyle leaks, pancreatic leaks, and CBD injuries, all of which are very rare in our experience.

45.14 Long-Term Outcomes After Surgery

In our experience with more than 300 pancreatectomies, about 95% of patients with focal disease are cured after surgery. The remaining 5% require some degree of support that is usually consists of a strict feeding regimen, and these cases are presumed to be secondary to microscopic residual disease. In cases of diffuse HI, approximately 50% of cases continue to have hypoglycemia after surgery and may require supportive management with octreotide and frequent feeds, and 25% develop diabetes requiring insulin. These patients, despite not being cured, are much easier to manage than before the surgery. Finally, approximately 25% of diffuse HI cases are well controlled with no medications. Long term follow-up is mandatory since insulin-dependent diabetes can develop even a decade, or more, later.

References

1. Stanley CA. Hyperinsulinism in infants and children. Pediatr Clin North Am. 1997;44:363–74.
2. Arnoux JB, de Lonlay P, Ribeiro MJ, et al. Congenital hyperinsulinism. Early Hum Dev. 2010;86(5):287–94.
3. McQuarrie I. Idiopathic spontaneously occurring hypoglycemia in infants; clinical significance of problem and treatment. Am J Dis Child. 1954;87(4):399–428.

4. Graham EA, Hartmann AF. Subtotal resection of the pancreas for hypoglycaemia. Surg Gynecol Obstet. 1934;59:474–9.
5. Yalow RS, Berson SA. Immunoassay of endogenous plasma insulin in man. J Clin Invest. 1960;39:1157–75.
6. Yakovac WC, Baker L, Hummeler K. Beta Cell nesidioblastosis in idiopathic hypoglycemia of infancy. J Pediatr. 1971;79(2):226–31.
7. Rahier J, Fält K, Müntefering H, et al. The basic structural lesion of persistent neonatal hypoglycaemia with hyperinsulinism: deficiency of pancreatic D cells or hyperactivity of B-cells? Diabetologia. 1984;26:282–9.
8. Palladino AA, Stanley CA. The hyperinsulinism/hyperammonemia syndrome. Rev Endocr Metab Disord. 2010;11(3):171–8.
9. Stanley CA. Two genetic forms of hyperinsulinemic hypoglycemia caused by dysregulation of glutamate dehydrogenase. Neurochem Int 2010 2. 2011;59(4):465–72.
10. Kassem S, Bhandari S, Rodríguez-Bada P, et al. Large islets, beta-cell proliferation, and a glucokinase mutation. N Engl J Med. 2010;362(14):1348–50.
11. Glaser B, Kesavan P, Heyman M, et al. Familial hyperinsulinism caused by an activating glucokinase mutation. N Engl J Med. 1998;338(4):226–30.
12. Li C, Chen P, Palladino A, et al. Mechanism of hyperinsulinism in short-chain 3-hydroxyacyl-CoA dehydrogenase deficiency involves activation of glutamate dehydrogenase. J Biol Chem. 2010;285(41): 31806–18.
13. Rahier J, Guiot Y, Sempoux C. Morphologic analysis of focal and diffuse forms of congenital hyperinsulinism. Semin Pediatr Surg. 2011;20(1):3–12.
14. Peranteau WH, Bathaii SM, Pawel B, et al. Multiple ectopic lesions of focal islet adenomatosis identified by positron emission tomography scan in an infant with congenital hyperinsulinism. J Pediatr Surg. 2007;42(1):188–92.
15. Suchi M, MacMullen C, Thornton PS, et al. Histopathology of congenital hyperinsulinism: retrospective study with genotype correlations. Pediatr Dev Pathol. 2003;6(4):322–33.
16. Laje P, Stanley CA, Palladino AA, et al. Pancreatic head resection and Roux-en-Y pancreaticojejunostomy for the treatment of the focal form of congenital hyperinsulinism. J Pediatr Surg. 2012;47(1):131–5.
17. Bellanné-Chantelot C, Saint-Martin C, Ribeiro MJ, et al. ABCC8 and KCNJ11 molecular spectrum of 109 patients with diazoxide-unresponsive congenital hyperinsulinism. J Med Genet. 2010;47(11):752–9.
18. Flanagan SE, Clauin S, Bellanné-Chantelot C, et al. Update of mutations in the genes encoding the pancreatic beta-cell K(ATP) channel subunits Kir6.2 (KCNJ11) and sulfonylurea receptor 1 (ABCC8) in diabetes mellitus and hyperinsulinism. Hum Mutat. 2009;30:170–80.
19. Huopio H, Reimann F, Ashfield R, et al. Dominantly inherited hyperinsulinism caused by a mutation in the sulfonylurea receptor type 1. J Clin Invest. 2000;106(7):897–906.
20. Pinney SE, MacMullen C, Becker S, et al. Clinical characteristics and biochemical mechanisms of congenital hyperinsulinism associated with dominant KATP channel mutations. J Clin Invest. 2008;118:2877–86.
21. Dekel B, Lubin D, Modan-Moses D, et al. Compound heterozygosity for the common sulfonylurea receptor mutations can cause mild diazoxide-sensitive hyperinsulinism. Clin Pediatr. 2002;41:183–6.
22. Dullaart RP, Hoogenberg K, Rouwe CW, et al. Family with autosomal dominant hyperinsulinism associated with A456V mutation in the glucokinase gene. J Intern Med. 2004;255:143–5.
23. Christesen HB, Tribble ND, Molven A, et al. Activating glucokinase (GCK) mutations as a cause of medically responsive congenital hyperinsulinism: prevalence in children and characterisation of a novel GCK mutation. Eur J Endocrinol. 2008;159:27–34.
24. Molven A, Matre GE, Duran M, et al. Familial hyperinsulinemic hypoglycemia caused by a defect in the SCHAD enzyme of mitochondrial fatty acid oxidation. Diabetes. 2004;53(1):221–7.
25. González-Barroso MM, Giurgea I, Bouillaud F, et al. Mutations in UCP2 in congenital hyperinsulinism reveal a role for regulation of insulin secretion. PLoS One. 2008;3(12):e3850.
26. Otonkoski T, Jiao H, Kaminen-Ahola N, et al. Physical exercise-induced hypoglycemia caused by failed silencing of monocarboxylate transporter 1 in pancreatic beta cells. Am J Hum Genet. 2007;81:467–74.
27. Flanagan S, Kapoor R, Mali G, et al. Diazoxide-responsive hyperinsulinemic hypoglycemia caused by HNF4A gene mutations. Eur J Endocrinol. 2010;162:987–92.
28. Marquard J, Palladino AA, Stanley CA, et al. Rare forms of congenital hyperinsulinism. Semin Pediatr Surg. 2011;20(1):38–44.
29. Suchi M, MacMullen CM, Thornton PS, et al. Molecular and immunohistochemical analyses of the focal form of congenital hyperinsulinism. Mod Pathol. 2006;19(1):122–9.
30. Peranteau WH, Ganguly A, Steinmuller L, et al. Prenatal diagnosis and postnatal management of diffuse congenital hyperinsulinism: a case report. Fetal Diagn Ther. 2006;21(6):515–8.
31. Ismail D, Smith VV, de Lonlay P, et al. Familial focal congenital hyperinsulinism. J Clin Endocrinol Metab. 2011;96(1):24–8.
32. Laje P, Halaby L, Adzick NS, et al. Necrotizing enterocolitis in neonates receiving octreotide for the management of congenital hyperinsulinism. Pediatr Diabetes. 2010;11:142–7.
33. Palladino AA, Stanley CA. A specialized team approach to diagnosis and medical versus surgical treatment of infants with congenital hyperinsulinism. Semin Pediatr Surg. 2011;20(1):32–7.
34. Lovvorn HN 3rd, Nance ML, Ferry RJ Jr, et al. Congenital hyperinsulinism and the surgeon: lessons learned over 35 years. J Pediatr Surg. 1999;34(5):786–92.

35. Doppman JL, Miller DL, Chang R, et al. Insulinomas: localization with selective intraarterial injection of calcium. Radiology. 1991;178(1):237–41.
36. Brunelle F, Negre V, Barth MO, et al. Pancreatic venous samplings in infants and children with primary hyperinsulinism. Pediatr Radiol. 1989;19(2):100–3.
37. Adzick NS, Thornton PS, Stanley CA, et al. A multidisciplinary approach to the focal form of congenital hyperinsulinism leads to successful treatment by partial pancreatectomy. J Pediatr Surg. 2004;39(3):270–5.
38. Hoegerle S, Schneider B, Kraft A, et al. Imaging of a metastatic gastrointestinal carcinoid by F-18-DOPA positron emission tomography. Nuklearmedizin. 1999;38(4):127–30.
39. Ribeiro MJ, De Lonlay P, Delzescaux T, et al. Characterization of hyperinsulinism in infancy assessed with PET and 18F-fluoro-L-DOPA. J Nucl Med. 2005;46(4):560–6.
40. Otonkoski T, Näntö-Salonen K, Seppänen M, et al. Noninvasive diagnosis of focal hyperinsulinism of infancy with [18F]-DOPA positron emission tomography. Diabetes. 2006;55(1):13–8.
41. Hardy OT, Hernandez-Pampaloni M, Saffer JR, et al. Accuracy of [18F]fluorodopa positron emission tomography for diagnosing and localizing focal congenital hyperinsulinism. J Clin Endocrinol Metab. 2007;92(12):4706–11.
42. Hussain K, Seppänen M, Näntö-Salonen K, et al. The diagnosis of ectopic focal hyperinsulinism of infancy with [18F]-dopa positron emission tomography. J Clin Endocrinol Metab. 2006;91(8):2839–42.
43. von Rohden L, Mohnike K, Mau H, et al. Visualization of the focus in congenital hyperinsulinism by intraoperative sonography. Semin Pediatr Surg. 2011;20(1):28–31.
44. Bax NM, van der Zee DC, de Vroede M, et al. Laparoscopic identification and removal of focal lesions in persistent hyperinsulinemic hypoglycemia of infancy. Surg Endosc. 2003;17(5):833.
45. Al-Shanafey S. Laparoscopic vs open pancreatectomy for persistent hyperinsulinemic hypoglycemia of infancy. J Pediatr Surg. 2009;44(5):957–61.
46. Pierro A, Nah SA, et al. Surgical management of congenital hyperinsulinism of infancy. Semin Pediatr Surg. 2011;20(1):50–3.
47. Laje P, Stanley CA, Adzick NS. Intussusception after pancreatic surgery in children: a case series. J Pediatr Surg. 2010;45(7):1496–9.

Part VI

Abdominal Wall Defects

Gastroschisis and Exomphalos

46

Basem A. Khalil and Paul D. Losty

Abstract

The earliest description(s) of exomphalos date from antiquity though credit is linked with the French surgeon Ambrose Pare for providing the first accurate account of the malformation and its grave prognosis in the sixteenth century. Exomphalos was considered universally fatal until success with surgical treatment was published in the early 1800s. Scarpa (1814) later emphasized a spectrum of malformation severity. In 1899 Ahfield introduced the concept of conservative management by applying alcohol dressings to the exposed sac. This method was modified by Grob some 60 years later with the introduction of mercurochrome. Creation of a 'skin silo' by mobilising abdominal wall skin to cover the intact sac in large exomphalos lesions was advocated by Olshausen (1877), Williams (1930) and later Robert Gross at Children's Hospital Boston in 1948.

Keywords

Exomphalos • Omphalocoele • Gastroschisis • Human embryology Surgical management • Silo • Staged closure • Outcomes

46.1 History

The earliest description(s) of exomphalos date from antiquity though credit is linked with the French surgeon Ambrose Pare for providing the first accurate account of the malformation and its grave prognosis in the sixteenth century. Exomphalos was considered universally fatal until success with surgical treatment was published in the early 1800s. Scarpa (1814) later emphasized a spectrum of malformation severity. In 1899 Ahfield introduced the concept of conservative management by applying alcohol dressings to the exposed sac [1]. This method was

B.A. Khalil, MPH, PhD, FRCS(Paed)
Department of Pediatric Surgery, SIDRA, Doha, Qatar

P.D. Losty, MD, FRCS(Paed), FEBPS (✉)
Department of Paediatric Surgery, Institute of Translational Medicine, Alder Hey Children's Hospital NHS Foundation Trust, University of Liverpool, Liverpool, UK
e-mail: paul.losty@liverpool.ac.uk

P.D. Losty et al. (eds.), *Rickham's Neonatal Surgery*, https://doi.org/10.1007/978-1-4471-4721-3_46

modified by Grob some 60 years later with the introduction of mercurochrome [1, 2]. Creation of a 'skin silo' by mobilising abdominal wall skin to cover the intact sac in large exomphalos lesions was advocated by Olshausen (1877), Williams (1930) and later Robert Gross at Children's Hospital Boston in 1948 [1–4].

Early descriptions of gastroschisis ('belly cleft') by teratologists in the nineteenth and early twentieth century had links with exomphalos (or ruptured sacs) [1]. Moore and Stokes (1953) later suggested the term gastroschisis should be strictly reserved for index cases in which the exposed viscera without a sac covering and abdominal wall defect lay adjacent to a normally inserted umbilical cord. Watkins in 1943 was the first to report surgical success [5, 6].

Staged abdominal wall closure with prosthetic materials was popularised by Schuster (1967) for management of exomphalos [7]. Intravenous nutrition heralded significant advances in survival of newborns with abdominal wall defects and gut related dysmotility notably in babies with gastroschisis [8]. Fetal medicine with prenatal imaging has now permitted accurate diagnosis, in utero monitoring, delivery planning and early surgery [9, 10]. Today many strategies are available for the paediatric surgeon to manage even the most challenging cases with the availability of preformed silos, tissue expander devices and artificial biomatrix materials to support skin grafting/abdominal wall closure [11–15]. In the modern era of care 95% survival is achievable in newborns with gastroschisis [16]. Exomphalos has also witnessed modest improvements in outcome(s) with 60–80% survival possible in selected cases (even with congenital heart disease) and those without major chromosomal anomalies.

46.2 Epidemiology

Exomphalos is estimated to occur in 1:3000–4000 births in Western countries [16]. In Japan the prevalence reported by the Japan Association of Obstetricians and Gynecologists Birth Defects Registry was 1:2500 births [17]. Gastroschisis has an incidence of 3–4.5 cases per 10,000 live births [18]. For reasons not fully understood abdominal wall defects have been observed to be increasing steadily in prevalence in the UK, Europe and North America [19, 20]. A 2011 EUROCAT report showed a rising prevalence particularly of gastroschisis [20]. Young maternal age with teenage pregnancy appears to be a risk factor. Low socioeconomic group status, poor nutrition, smoking and illicit substance abuse have also been cited [21, 22]. Clustering of index cases of gastroschisis within defined geographic regions suggests potential role(s) for environmental teratogens and pollutants [23]. Only 1%–2% infants with gastroschisis will have chromosome abnormalities [24]. By contrast exomphalos carries a significant risk, up to 30–40%, for presence of chromosomal lesions—trisomy 13, 18 or 21 [24, 25].

46.3 Embryology

During the 6th week of early human development the intestines with rapid growth herniate through the umbilical ring contributing to the 'physiological umbilical hernia'. By the 10th week the midgut then begins the process of returning to the abdominal cavity undergoing a 270° counterclockwise rotation fixing the gut in a normal axis of rotation [26, 27]. Exomphalos results from failure of the physiological hernia/gut loops to return to the abdominal cavity through an insult likely occurring to the lateral embryonic folds that fail to fuse in the midline. The lesion occupies a central location on the abdominal wall and can vary greatly in size from a small minor defect—2 cm diameter to a major malformation 5 cm or greater with liver and bowel loops herniated from the abdominal cavity and contained in a membranous covering sac composed of peritoneum, Wharton's jelly and amnion—(Fig. 46.1) The thoracic cavity may be maldeveloped also leading to significant restriction(s) on lung, airway growth, and diaphragm function contributing to pulmonary hypoplasia and bronchomalacia [28, 29]. Defects of the lower sternum and adjacent diaphragm may moreover contribute to co-existent anterior diaphragmatic hernia defects with pericardial

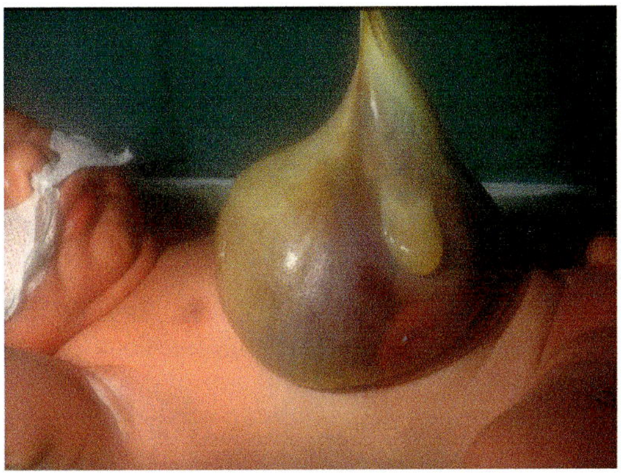

Fig. 46.1 Exomphalos—a major defect. A large sac can be seen covering the liver and intestines. The cord structures are evident at the apex of the sac

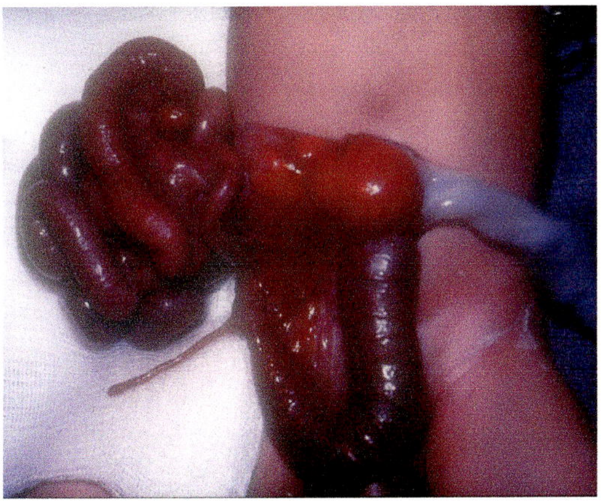

Fig. 46.2 Newborn with gastroschisis. The gut can be clearly seen herniated through an abdominal wall defect to the right side of the umbilical cord. In this case the bowel is in a healthy condition without any evidence of matting or peel formation

sac and cardiac anomalies as seen in infants with 'Pentalogy of Cantrell' syndrome [30].

Gastroschisis is characterized by the herniation of intestinal loops through an abdominal wall defect to the right side of a normally sited umbilical cord—(Fig. 46.2). Various theories regarding pathogenesis are proposed. These have included in utero rupture of the 'physiological hernia' from weakness occurring on the right side of the umbilical cord (Devries 1980) [31]. Stevenson (2009) also recently hypothesized gastroschisis may result from failure of the yolk sac and vitelline structures to be incorporated into the umbilical stalk leading to gut herniation [32]. Alongside visceral herniation testes and ovaries, fallopian tubes and bladder may also be visibly extruded through the defect.

46.4 Prenatal Diagnosis

Exomphalos and gastroschisis are readily diagnosed in over 90% cases from antenatal ultrasound imaging performed in the late first and second trimester periods of pregnancy [9, 24]. Maternal serum alphafetoprotein levels may also be raised [33]. First trimester prenatal diagnosis of exomphalos is associated with a greater than 50% risk of chromosomal abnormalities in addition to other major anomalies notably involving the cardiac and central nervous system(s). Distinguishing the abdominal wall defects is crucially important as fetal karyotyping should be routinely offered to pregnant women with a suspected diagnosis of exomphalos [24]. Fetal echocardiography and screening for other structural anomalies is additionally indicated as these greatly influence prognosis. Gastroschisis is not considered to have associations with chromosomal disorders though some 10–15% babies may have other anomalies notably co-existent intestinal atresia(s) [24]. A major focus of prenatal diagnosis in the current era has been the accurate identification of predictors of postnatal outcome that may influence parental counselling, timing of delivery and surgical management. Ultrasound and/or MRI may provide valuable information on risks of pulmonary hypoplasia developing in fetuses with giant exomphalos lesions by measuring the lung/thorax transverse area ratios (L/T) [28]. Some authors have also cited the value of measurement of largest exomphalos diameter compared to abdominal circumference in an effort to predict the need for primary versus staged closure, risk(s) of respiratory insufficiency and survival [29]. For many infants with exomphalos timing of delivery is scheduled near term with vaginal birth permissible for small lesions not containing liver. By contrast caesarean section is advised in those fetuses with the larger size defects containing herniated liver to avert hepatic injury occurring exiting the birth canal. In fetuses with gastroschisis much attention has focused on prenatal risk factors such as bowel dilatation and the potential risk(s) of intestinal damage to exposed bowel loops from amniotic fluid exposure [34, 35]. Several authors proposed amnioexchange based on experimental work on animal models. The rationale for amniotic fluid volume exchange derived from evidence linking inflammatory mediators in the liquor fluid to bowel injury. However, Midrio and colleagues carefully evaluated the role of amnioinfusion in a series of human fetuses with gastroschisis which then showed no benefit from amnioexchange in terms of reduction of intestinal injury and postnatal outcome [35]. Amnioinfusion though would still appear to have a potential valuable role as prenatal therapy in restoring liquor volume in those maternal cases complicated by severe oligohydramnios [35]. Bowel dilatation in utero has been cited as an adverse risk factor in fetuses with gastroschisis [36–38]. Specifically of concern is reference to progressive dilatation of the contained intra-abdominal loops which may indicate the existence of intestinal atresia and worse postnatal outcomes. These sonographic findings have led fetal medicine specialists to advocate more frequent surveillance ultrasound imaging to assure wellbeing.

More recent studies including a comprehensive systematic review have now challenged these observations by failing to show convincing evidence to indicate an increased risk of adverse postnatal events in fetuses with the presence of prenatal bowel dilatation [36]. Timing and mode of delivery has been widely debated in the fetus with gastroschisis [39]. Among many published studies (including a Cochrane review), none have convincingly shown outcome benefits for—(1) early preterm delivery <36 weeks, (2) caesarean section versus vaginal delivery unless specific obstetrical factors (fetal and/or maternal distress) prevail [39, 40]. Current evidence therefore strongly supports spontaneous or induced vaginal delivery of prenatally diagnosed gastroschisis fetuses after 36 weeks [40, 41]. It is self evident that all fetuses with a prenatally diagnosed abdominal wall defect should be delivered in obstetrical centres with appropriate expertise and access to a multidisciplinary team of NICU specialists and surgeons.

46.5 Newborn Management

Immediate management of a newborn with exomphalos or gastroschisis requires fluid replacement, gut decompression via passage of an NG tube, avoidance of hypothermia and local care to the exomphalos sac or herniated viscera—(Fig. 46.3). Cardio-respiratory support may also be indicated in babies with giant exomphalos lesions due to associated lung hypoplasia and/or congenital heart lesions. In infants with gastroschisis the bowel should be carefully inspected to ensure the gut is not injured/perforated, twisted or constricted by a narrow ring or band at the base of the abdominal wall defect. Testes, ovaries, fallopian tubes and bladder may be sometimes herniated through the defect also. The exposed viscera should be protected by wrapping a layer of transparent cling-film/cellophane bag over the gut and torso. Alternatively the gut may be placed in large medical grade plastic bag with drawstrings. The bowel should be always visible to the primary care team and the infant positioned with the exposed gut supported to avoid kinking the mesentery or strangulating the lesion at the base of the defect. It is often therefore best to advise that newborns are nursed on their right side (protecting gut perfusion/no mesentery kinking) whilst being transported by a retrieval team to a surgical facility. In infants with exomphalos inspection of the quality of the

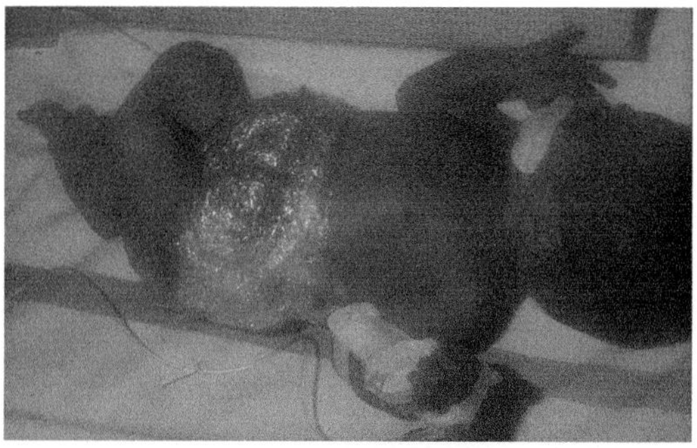

Fig. 46.3 Newborn with gastroschisis on arrival to the surgical unit following transport. Note the exposed viscera covered with a cling-film torso wrap to protect the gut and reduce heat loss. A nasogastric tube in situ facilitates gut decompression and reduces the risks of aspiration. An intravenous line allows delivery of crystalloid fluids and administration of antibiotics

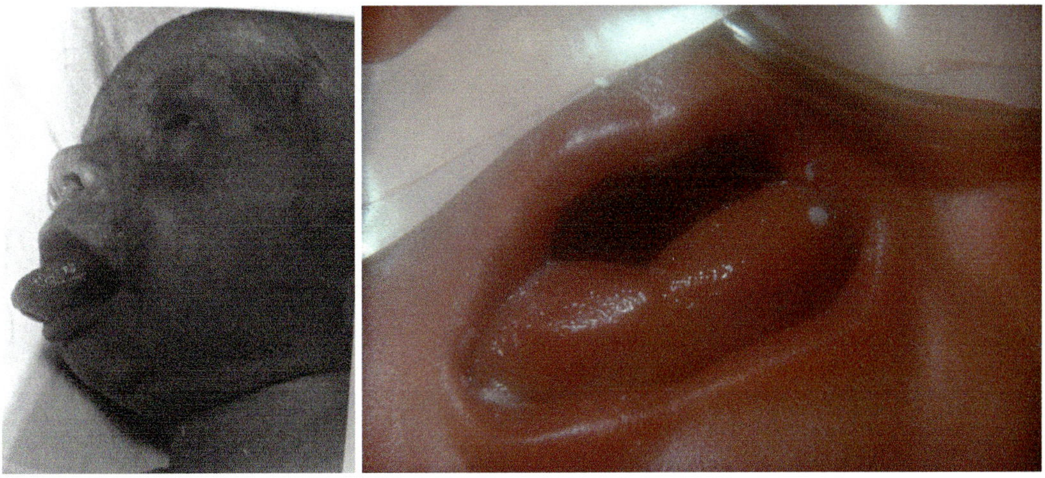

Fig. 46.4 Beckwith-Wiedemann syndrome in newborn with exomphalos. Note the coarse facial features and large tongue—'macroglossia'

exposed sac is important looking for tears or rupture that may greatly influence subsequent management. Contents may be clearly visible notably liver and/or gut defining the complexity of the lesion as a 'major' or 'minor' defect. All infants should be fully examined to exclude syndromic associations particularly in those with exomphalos where for example the presence of a large protruding tongue 'macroglossia' may indicate Beckwith-Wiedemann syndrome—(Fig. 46.4) [42]. Such infants are prone to neonatal hypoglycaemia and require glucose supplementation. Vascular access via a peripheral vein is secured with isotonic crystalloid fluids containing 10% dextrose and sodium chloride delivered to ensure adequate tissue perfusion and urine output. Nasogastric losses should be replaced with 0.9% normal saline. Fluid boluses are administered as indicated by low urine output. As heat is rapidly lost with exposed viscera newborns with abdominal wall defects should be nursed in a thermoregulated controlled environment to avert hypothermia.

46.6 Surgical Management

Surgical management of exomphalos is largely dictated by the size and complexity of the lesion and patient status [24]. An intact sac is protective to the underlying viscera and liver. Operation should not be delayed beyond 24 h for small defects <5 cm in size containing intestine with minimal liver herniation as primary fascial closure with or without prosthetic abdominal wall patch insertion can be accomplished. Commencing with sac excision care should be taken as the membrane covering is dissected from the bowel loops and liver. In the vicinity of the liver, sac may be adherent and should be left in place. Additionally the liver often encroaches occupying the midline plane such that the hepatic veins may be superficially located and injured if appropriate care is not taken. At the time of primary exomphalos operation where possible the surgeon should inspect the diaphragm for an anterior defect (Pentalogy of Cantrell) as this will additionally require repair or a prosthetic patch [30]. We have managed several cases where diaphragm defects have been undetected at exomphalos repair with chest film radiology weeks or months later revealing a defect. Stretching of the abdominal wall will facilitate viscera reduction and primary fascial closure. Likewise lateral flank relieving incisions can aid skin closure. Management of newborns and premature babies with large lesions (>5 cm) /giant exomphalos defects poses considerable challenges because of (1) lack of abdominal domain and/or (2) associated pulmonary hypoplasia with ventila-

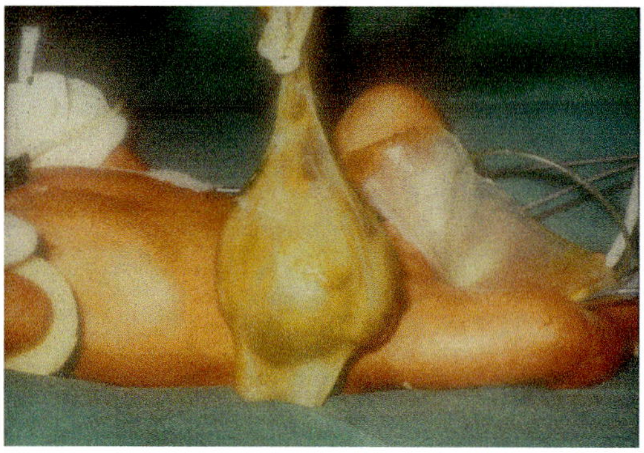

Fig. 46.5 Conservative management exomphalos major. The sac was treated with a topical agent silver sulfadiazine to promote healing

tor dependency. Conservative therapy is advocated here allowing the exposed sac to epithelialize. Several agents may accelerate and promote this process. This was successfully accomplished in the past using mercurochrome based compounds or povidone iodine solutions with toxicity problems later apparent which also included thyroid metabolic dysfunction [43–45]. Experience with burn wound care promoted the wider use of topical silver sulphadiazine which achieves excellent results with eschar formation aiding new skin cover and creating a ventral hernia defect—(Fig. 46.5) [46]. Staged ventral hernia repair can be scheduled in later years when the patient's medical status is improved. Conservative management may involve a lengthy hospital stay requiring dedicated nursing care to prevent sac infection. Trauma to the sac including tears and rupture can also occur. Sepsis if it develops can be difficult to eradicate despite antibiotic therapy which may then require emergent sac excision. In these challenging cases where primary closure or prosthetics cannot be deployed we have successfully utilised skin substitutes i.e. Integra artificial skin, which provides a collagen matrix as a temporary scaffold for subsequent native mesh skin grafting—(Fig. 46.6) [15]. Finally, tissue expanders are also a novel option to consider when confronted with giant exomphalos lesions to facilitate staged defect closure [13].

In newborns with gastroschisis primary closure of the defect can be achieved in some 75% cases with timely emergent operation [24, 41, 47]. To achieve these goals it is crucial cases are transported with some urgency after maternal delivery to the surgical team. Undue delay results in the infant's herniated bowel becoming matted and oedematous making silo placement and staged repair more likely.

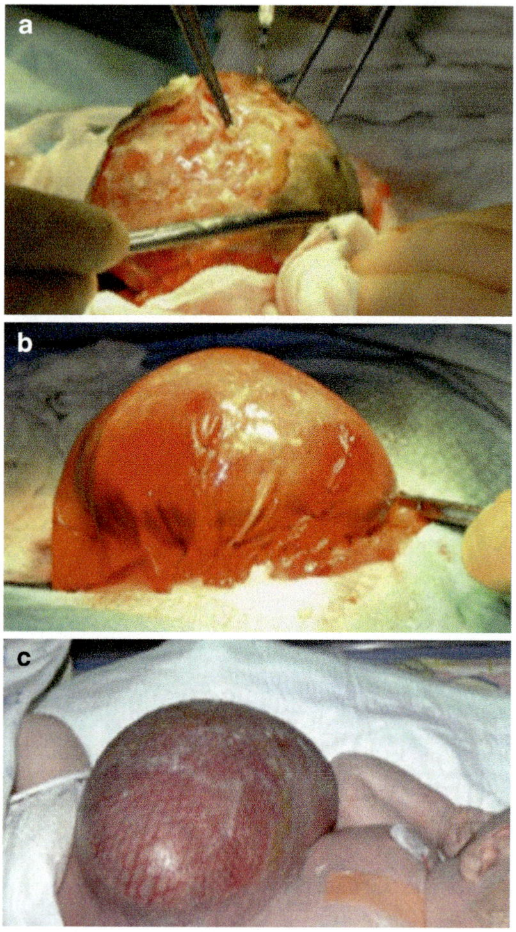

Fig. 46.6 Use of Integra artificial skin substitute as a rescue therapy to facilitate subsequent skin grafting in a 38 week gestation 2.8 kg newborn with giant exomphalos and cardiac anomaly. In this case primary conservative management was complicated with sac infection and systemic sepsis. Integra provided and created a scaffolding platform for native mesh skin graft placement after several days. The patient now a healthy teenager underwent uncomplicated staged ventral hernia repair as a toddler. Panels show (**a**) excision of infected sac day 15 after birth (**b**) Integra artificial skin substitute in place day 19—the composite material consists of a bovine porous collagen matrix covered by a thin sheet of silastic (**c**) Appearance after mesh skin grafting on week 11 after birth

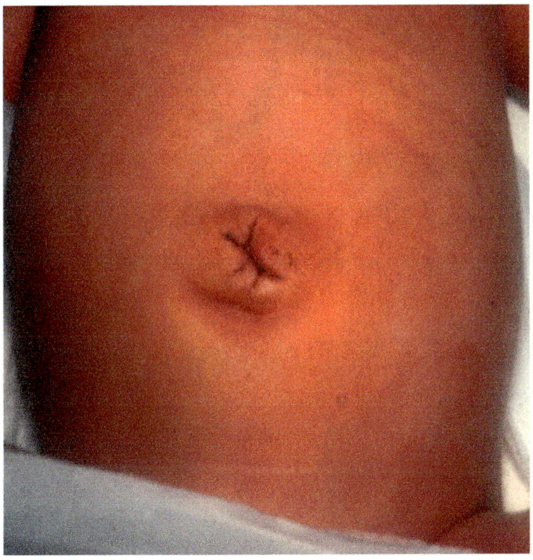

Fig. 46.7 Newborn with gastroschisis following primary repair with umbilicoplasty

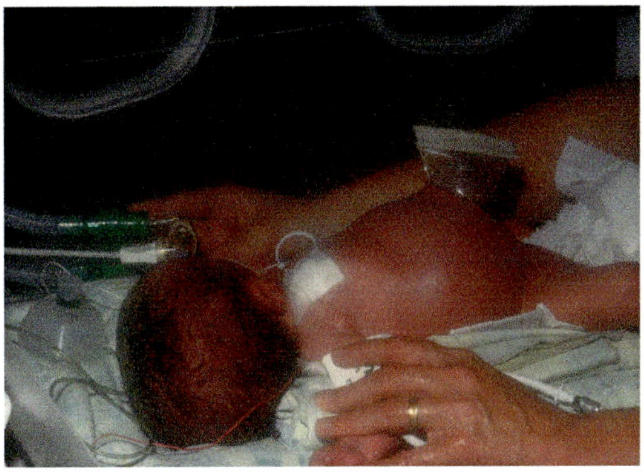

Fig. 46.8 Silo (reinforced silastic) creation in a newborn with gastroschisis and associated viscero-abdominal disproportion. The silo pouch was placed in this case to avert development of abdominal compartment syndrome. The silo is sutured to the fascial layers of the abdominal wall with interrupted monofilament sutures. Staged closure was later accomplished in 10 days

At operation the surgeon should carefully inspect the quality and integrity of the bowel particularly looking for intestinal atresia(s) seen in 10–15% cases. Where the gut appears healthy, stretching of the defect ring with retractors and/or a cephalad fascial incision will facilitate gentle bowel reduction. Primary fascial closure with preservation of the native umbilical cord or purse string creation of an umbilicus with cord excision 'umbilicoplasty' is desirable—(Fig. 46.7). Close co-operation between surgical and the anaesthetic teams is vital to ensure physiological safety of primary closure and avoidance of abdominal compartment syndrome characterized by ventilatory compromise, intestinal and renal ischaemia and impaired lower limb perfusion. The authors routinely assay arterial blood lactate levels during the procedure therefore to guide surgical management. Increased requirements for ventilation notably raised ventilator pressure(s) indicating impaired lung compliance may indicate the safer option of placing a silo and scheduling staged repair. In circumstances where bowel is extensively matted and oedematous and in premature babies with little abdominal domain, a silo should be fashioned by the surgeon permitting gradual staged visceral reduction with delayed repair. Debate exists with regard management of intestinal atresia at primary operation [48, 49]. Where the bowel appears very healthy some surgeons would elect to perform resection and primary anastomosis. In circumstances when bowel is inflamed, matted and oedematous a stoma may be created or the abdominal wall defect repaired with the aim to undertake atresia resection several weeks later. Silo placement likewise with delayed defect repair may be indicated with or without creation of a stoma. Several techniques may be deployed when electing to create a silo and plan staged repair. Traditionally reinforced silastic sheeting or prolene mesh may be sutured to the abdominal wall fascial layer at operation to create a 'silo pouch' protecting the gut—(Fig. 46.8). Some authors have also promoted the use of bedside spring-loaded silos in primary management of gastroschisis [11, 12]. At presentation to the newborn surgical unit the silo is placed over the exposed bowel without anaesthesia with the aim to undertake delayed staged repair some days later. Opinion is widely divided on the merits of this approach. Perhaps the real advantage here may be the 'out of hours' emergent care surgical residents can deploy to protect the infant's exposed bowel on the ward with the opportunity to undertake primary defect closure in normal working hours. Sutureless gastroschisis closure i.e. 'awake reduction' with umbilical capping in newborns without anaesthesia or silo placement was first proposed by Bianchi and Dickson [50]. Early reports steered some enthusiasm for this technique which was largely applicable in a select group of newborns with healthy bowel that could be easily reduced into the abdominal cavity. Whilst feasible great care is needed in decision making as the procedure is not without risk(s) indeed some authors have cited poor outcomes [51]. A meta-analysis concluded that infants managed by primary defect closure have much improved outcomes [52]. In the postoperative period infants with gastroschisis require ventilation for a number of days (primary closure vs. silo), antibiotics and total parenteral nutrition (TPN) delivered via a Broviac central venous line (or peripheral long line) until gut function normalises. Trophic enteral feeding (breast milk or formula) is commenced when NG bile aspirates diminish in volume to minimise TPN associated liver disease. The severity of the gastroschisis lesion will greatly influence hospital stay (4 weeks average—many months) as factors here to consider include intestinal dysmotility, risk(s) of development of necrotising enterocolitis, short gut syndrome, presence or absence of intestinal atresia(s) in 'complex' cases and staged repair [24, 51–56]. Feed intolerance should alert the surgeon to consider 'missed' atresia lesion, adhesive obstruction or a dysmotility syndrome which may require upper and lower GI contrast imaging to facilitate diagnosis.

46.7 Long Term Outcome(s)

Overall survival for newborns with gastroschisis in the current era is now well over 90–95% cases [24, 41, 47]. Factors determining survival here include 'simple' or 'complex' gastroschisis defects, 'vanishing lesions' with risks of non viable gut/extreme short gut, morbidity from TPN dependency and dysmotility, staged repair, adjunct procedures i.e. tapering, intestinal lengthening and 're-do' operations for necrotising enterocolitis, adhesive obstruction or volvulus [54–56]. The need for surgery beyond the neonatal period may be significant with a study showing that 25% of patients required operation for a gastroschisis related complication most commonly bowel obstruction in the first year of life [55]. The most severely affected patients with gut failure may ultimately require intestinal transplantation [24, 54]. Growth in early years may be suboptimal but many children 'catch up' milestones [57]. Neurodevelopmental outcomes are generally good with equivalence to aged match cohorts [58]. In boys with gastroschisis one-third may be noted to have undescended testes on office follow up visits. Spontaneous descent is observed to occur in almost half with orchidopexy required in a minority [59]. Dissatisfaction with abdominal wall scarring and absence of a 'normal umbilicus' is a significant aesthetic issue for many young people and older patients [60, 61]. Quality of life and physical functioning as adult survivors is perceived as equal to the general population [60, 62].

Outcomes of exomphalos survivors show a spectrum of illness severity linked with associated anomalies [24, 62, 63]. Respiratory and feeding problems are prevalent including ventilator dependency in the first year of life secondary to pulmonary hypoplasia, bronchomalacia and diaphragm malfunction [63, 64]. Studies have shown survivors can also develop reactive airway disease, pulmonary and systemic hypertension [24, 64, 65–67]. Neurodevelopmental outcomes are impaired in those requiring a high burden of intensive care in early life i.e. ventilation, tracheostomy, supplemental feeding [24, 68]. Further operations in early years may be required to manage adhesive bowel obstruction, staged ventral hernia repair, groin hernia(s), undescended testes, including surgery for gastroesophageal reflux [24, 59, 61, 68–70]. Quality of life for many adult survivors is perceived as equivalent to the healthy population [62, 63].

References

1. Irving IM. Umbilical abnormalities. In: Lister J, Irving IM, editors. Neonatal Surgery 3rd edn. London: Butterworths; 1990. p. 376–402.
2. Grob M. Conservative treatment of exomphalos. Arch Dis Child. 1963;54:441–4.
3. Williams C. Congenital defects of the anterior abdominal wall. Surg Clin North Am. 1930;10:805–9.

4. Gross RE. A new method for surgical treatment of large omphalocoeles. Surgery. 1948;24:277–92.
5. Moore TC, Stokes GE. Gastroschisis. Surgery. 1953;33:112–20.
6. Watkins DE. Gastroschisis. Virginia Med Mon. 1943;70:42–4.
7. Schuster SR. A new method for the staged repair of large omphalocoeles. Surg Gynecol Obstet. 1967;125:837–50.
8. Dudrick SJ, Wilmore DW, Vars HM, et al. Can intravenous feeding as the sole means of nutrition support growth in the child and restore weight loss in the adult ? Ann Surg. 1969;169:974–84.
9. Redford DH, McNay MB, Whittle MJ. Gastroschisis and exomphalos: precise diagnosis by mid-pregnancy ultrasound. Br J Obstet Gynaecol. 1985;92:54–9.
10. Nakayama DK, Harrison MR, Gross BH, et al. Management of the fetus with an abdominal wall defect. J Pediatr Surg. 1984;19:408–13.
11. Shermeta DW, Haller JA Jr. A new preformed transparent silo for the management of gastroschisis. J Pediatr Surg. 1975;10:973–5.
12. Minkes RK, Langer JC, Mazziota MV, et al. Routine insertion of a silastic spring loaded silo for infants with gastroschisis. J Pediatr Surg. 2000;35:843–6.
13. Bax NM, van der Zee D, Pull ter Gunne AJ, et al. Treatment of giant omphalocoele by enlargement of the abdominal cavity with a tissue expander. J Pediatr Surg. 1993;28:1181–4.
14. Clifton MS, Heiss KF, Keating JJ, et al. Use of tissue expanders in the repair of complex abdominal wall defects. J Pediatr Surg. 2011;46:372–7.
15. Almond SL, Goyal A, Jesudason EC, et al. Novel use of skin substitute as rescue therapy in complicated giant exomphalos. J Pediatr Surg. 2006;41:e1–2.
16. Wilson RD, Johnson MP. Congenital abdominal wall defects: an update. Fetal Diagn Ther. 2004;19:385–98.
17. Japan Association of Obstetricians and Gynecologists. Annual reports of congenital malformations. 1997–2006.
18. Kilby MD. The incidence of gastroschisis. BMJ. 2006;332:250–1.
19. Loanne M, Dolk H, Bradbury I. EUROCAT Working Group. Increasing prevalence of gastroschisis in Europe 1980–2002: a phenomenon restricted to younger mothers ? Paediatr Perinat Epidemiol. 2007;143A:660–71.
20. Loanne M, Dolk H, Kelly A, et al. Paper 4: EUROCAT statistical monitoring: identification and investigation of ten year trends of congenital anomalies in Europe. Birth Defects Res A Clin Mol Teratol. 2011;91:S31–43.
21. Torfs CP, Katz EA, Bateson TF, et al. Maternal medications and environmental exposures as risk factors for gastroschisis. Teratology. 1996;54:84–92.
22. Draper ES, Rankin J, Tonks AM, et al. Recreational drug use: a major risk factor for gastroschisis ? Am J Epidemiol. 2008;167:485–91.
23. Root ED, Meyer RE, Emch ME. Evidence of localized clustering of gastroschisis. Births in North Carolina 1999–2004. Soc Sci Med. 2009;68:1361–7.
24. Gamba P, Midrio P. Abdominal wall defects: prenatal diagnosis, newborn management and long-term outcomes. Semin Pediatr Surg. 2014;23:283–90.
25. Mastroiacovo P, Lisi A, Castilla EE, et al. Gastroschisis and associated defects: an international study. Am J Med Genet A. 2007;143A:660–71.
26. Gray SW, Skandalakis JE. Embryology for surgeons. Philadelphia: Saunders; 1972.
27. Kluth D, Jaeschke-Melli S, Fiegel H. The embryology of gut rotation. Semin Pediatr Surg. 2003;12:275–9.
28. Kamata S, Usui N, Sawai T, et al. Prenatal detection of pulmonary hypoplasia in giant omphalocoele. Pediatr Surg Int. 2008;24:107–11.
29. Danzer E, Victoria T, Bebbington MW, et al. Fetal MRI-calculated total lung volumes in the prediction of short-term outcome in giant omphalocoele: preliminary findings. Fetal Diagn Ther. 2012;31:248–53.
30. Cantrell JR, Haller JA, Ravitch MM. A syndrome of congenital defects involving the abdominal wall, sternum, diaphragm, pericardium and heart. Surg Gynecol Obstet. 1958;107:602–14.
31. Devries PA. The pathogenesis of gastroschisis and omphalocoele. J Pediatr Surg. 1980;15:245–51.
32. Stevenson RE, Rogers RC, Chandler JC, et al. Escape of the yolk sac: a hypothesis to explain the embryogenesis of gastroschisis. Clin Genet. 2009;75:326–33.
33. Palomaki GE, Hill LE, Knight GJ, et al. Second trimester maternal serum alpha-fetoprotein levels in pregnancies associated with gastroschisis and omphalocoele. Obstet Gynecol. 1988;71:906–9.
34. Bond SJ, Harrison MR, Filly RA, et al. Severity of intestinal damage in gastroschisis: correlation with prenatal sonographic findings. J Pediatr Surg. 1988;23:520–5.
35. Midrio P, Stefanutti G, Mussap M, et al. Amnioexchange for fetuses with gastroschisis: is it effective? J Pediatr Surg. 2007;42:777–82.
36. Tower C, Ong SSC, Ewer AK, et al. Prognosis in isolated gastroschisis with bowel dilation: a systematic review. Arch Dis Child Fetal Neonatal Ed. 2009;94:F268–74.
37. Kuleva M, Khen-Dunlop N, Dumez Y, et al. Is complex gastroschisis predictable by prenatal ultrasound? BJOG. 2012;119:102–9.
38. Lato K, Poellmann M, Knippel AJ, et al. Fetal gastroschisis: a comparison of second vs. third-trimester bowel dilatation for predicting bowel atresia and neonatal outcome. Ultraschall Med. 2013;34:157–61.
39. Segal SY, Marder SJ, Parry S, et al. Fetal abdominal wall defects and mode of delivery: a systematic review. Obstet Gynecol. 2001;98:867–73.
40. Grant NH, Dolring J, Thornton JG. Elective preterm birth for fetal gastroschisis. Cochrane Database Syst Rev. 2013;6:CD009394.
41. Skarsgard ED. Management of gastroschisis. Curr Opin Pediatr. 2016;28:363–9.
42. Beckwith JB, Wang CL, Donnell GN, et al. Hyperplastic fetal visceromegaly with macroglossia, omphalocoele, cytomegaly of adrenal fetal cortex, postnatal somatic gigantism and other abnormalities:

newly recognized syndrome. Proc Am Pediat Soc, Seattle, WA, June 16–18, 1964 (Abstr 41).
43. Beasley SW, Jones PG. Use of mercurochrome in the management of the large exomphalos. Aust Paediatr J. 1986;22:61–3.
44. Mullins ME, Horowitz BZ. Iatrogenic neonatal mercury poisoning from mercurochrome treatment of a large omphalocoele. Clin Pediatr (Phila). 1999;38:111–2.
45. Whitehouse JS, Gourlay DM, Masonbrink AR, et al. Non operative management of giant omphalocoele with topical povidone-iodine and its effects on thyroid function. J Pediatr Surg. 2010;45:1192–7.
46. Ein SH, Langer JC. Delayed management of giant omphalocoele using silver sulfadiazine cream: an 18 year experience. J Pediatr Surg. 2012;47:494–500.
47. Khalil BA, Baath ME, Baillie CT, et al. Infections in gastroschisis; organisms and factors. Pediatr Surg Int. 2008;24:1031–5.
48. Hoehner JC, Ein SH, Kim PC. Management of gastroschisis with concomitant jejuno-ileal atresia. J Pediatr Surg. 1998;33:885–8.
49. Fleet MS, de la Hunt MN. Intestinal atresia with gastroschisis: a selective approach to management. J Pediatr Surg. 2000;35:1323–5.
50. Bianchi A, Dickson AP. Elective delayed reduction and no anesthesia: 'minimal intervention management' for gastroschisis. J Pediatr Surg. 1998;33:1338–40.
51. Dolgin SE, Midulla P, Shlasko E. Unsatisfactory experience with 'minimal intervention management' for gastroschisis. J Pediatr Surg. 2000;35:1437–9.
52. Kunz SN, Tieder JS, Whitlock K, et al. Primary fascial closure versus staged closure with silo in patients with gastroschisis; a meta-analysis. J Pediatr Surg. 2013;48:845–57.
53. Shetty S, Kennea N, Desai P, et al. Length of stay and cost analysis of neonates undergoing surgery at a tertiary neonatal unit in England. Ann R Coll Surg Engl. 2016;98:56–60.
54. Coletta R, Khalil BA, Morabito A. Short bowel syndrome in children: surgical and medical perspectives. Semin Pediatr Surg. 2014;23:291–7.
55. Friedmacher F, Hock A, Castellani C, et al. Gastroschisis-related complications requiring further surgical interventions. Pediatr Surg Int. 2014;30:615–20.
56. Bergholz R, Boettcher M, Reinshagen K, et al. Complex gastroschisis is a different entity to simple gastroschisis affecting morbidity and mortality—a systematic review and meta-analysis. J Pediatr Surg. 2014;49:1527–32.
57. van Manen M, Hendson L, Wiley M, et al. Early childhood outcomes of infants born with gastroschisis. J Pediatr Surg. 2013;48:1682–7.
58. Gorra AS, Needelman H, Azarow KS, et al. Long-term neurodevelopmental outcomes in children born with gastroschisis; the tiebreaker. J Pediatr Surg. 2012;47:125–9.
59. Yardley IE, Bostock E, Jones MO, et al. Congenital abdominal wall defects and testicular maldescent: a 10 year single-center experience. J Pediatr Surg. 2012;47:118–22.
60. Harris EL, Minutillo C, Hart S, et al. The long-term physical consequences of gastroschisis. J Pediatr Surg. 2014;49:1466–70.
61. Davis BW, Stringer MD. The survivors of gastroschisis. Arch Dis Child. 1997;77:158–60.
62. Koivusalo A, Lindahl H, Rintala RJ. Morbidity and quality of life in adult patients with a congenital abdominal wall defect: a questionnaire survey. J Pediatr Surg. 2002;37:1594–601.
63. Van Eijick FC, Hoogeveen YL, van Weel C, et al. Minor and giant omphalocoele: long-term outcomes and quality of life. J Pediatr Surg. 2009;44:1355–9.
64. Danzer E, Hedrick HL, Rintoul NE, et al. Assessment of early pulmonary function 65. Abnormalities in giant omphalocoele survivors. J Pediatr Surg. 2012;47:1811–20.
65. Danzer E, Gerdes M, D'Agostino JA, et al. Prospective interdisciplinary follow up of children with prenatally diagnosed giant omphalocoele: short-term neurodevelopmental outcome. J Pediatr Surg. 2010;45:718–23.
66. Partridge EA, Hanna BD, Panitch HB, et al. Pulmonary hypertension in giant omphalocoele infants. J Pediatr Surg. 2014;49:1767–70.
67. Pernanteau WH, Tharakan SJ, Partridge E, et al. Systemic hypertension in giant omphalocoele: an underappreciated association. J Pediatr Surg. 2015;50:1477–80.
68. Danzer E, Gerdes M, D'Agostino JA, et al. Patient characteristics are important determinants of neurodevelopmental outcome during infancy in giant omphalocoele. Early Hum Dev. 2015;91:187–93.
69. Partridge EA, Peranteau WH, Flake A, et al. Frequency and complications of inguinal hernia repair in giant omphalocoele. J Pediatr Surg. 2015;50:1673–5.
70. Beaudoin S, Kieffer G, Sapin E, et al. Gastroesophageal reflux in neonates with congenital abdominal wall defect. Eur J Pediatr Surg. 1995;5:323–6.

Omphalomesenteric Duct and Urachal Remnants

47

Nada Sudhakaran and Bruce Okoye

Abstract

The umbilical cord remnant usually separates in the neonatal period and its persistence beyond the first couple of months is considered abnormal.

Umbilical abnormalities may present with failure of the umbilical cord to separate, omphalitis, mass lesions, or discharge. The commonest umbilical lesion in the neonate is an umbilical granuloma. Other abnormalities are umbilical polyps, omphalomesenteric duct and urachal remnants. It is essential to distinguish between these conditions in order to initiate appropriate treatment.

Keywords

Human embryology • Umbilical disorders • Meckel's diverticulum Urachal abnormalities

47.1 Introduction

The umbilical cord remnant usually separates in the neonatal period and its persistence beyond the first couple of months is considered abnormal [1].

Umbilical abnormalities may present with failure of the umbilical cord to separate, omphalitis, mass lesions, or discharge. The commonest umbilical lesion in the neonate is an umbilical granuloma [1, 2] Other abnormalities are umbilical polyps, omphalomesenteric duct and urachal remnants. It is essential to distinguish between these conditions in order to initiate appropriate treatment.

47.2 Omphalomesenteric Duct Remnant

47.2.1 History

Fabricius Hildanus was the first to report this congenital anomaly in 1598 [3, 4]. Morgagni further defined the anatomy and clinical presentation of Meckel's diverticulum [5–7].

N. Sudhakaran, MBBS, MRCS, FRCS(Paeds)
Department of Paediatric Surgery, Gold Coast University Hospital, Gold Coast, QLD, Australia

B. Okoye, MBBS, MD, FRCS(Paeds) (✉)
St. Georges University Hospital NHS Trust, London, UK
e-mail: bruce.okoye@nhs.net

P.D. Losty et al. (eds.), *Rickham's Neonatal Surgery*, https://doi.org/10.1007/978-1-4471-4721-3_47

In 1809 Johann Friedrich Meckel, described the embryology and the clinical features of this condition. His study of 22 paediatric cadavers gave rise to his description of the various forms of omphalomesenteric duct remnants namely, omphalomesenteric fistulas, omphalomesenteric cysts, umbilical sinuses and mesodiverticular bands. Meckel deduced that these malformations arose from the incomplete obliteration of the omphalomesenteric duct [4, 8, 9].

47.2.2 Epidemiology

The commonest Omphalomesenteric duct (OMD) remnant is the Meckel's diverticulum (MD). MD is also the commonest congenital abnormality of the gastrointestinal tract. It is referred to as the disease of "2s": It occurs in 2% of the population, arises 2 feet from the ileocoecal valve (adults), is about 2 in. long, about 2 cm in diameter, symptoms are often seen before the age of 2 and males are reported to be twice more likely to present with clinical symptoms [10, 11].

Meckels diverticulum is sporadic, but its presence is reportedly increased in children with Hirschsprung's disease, Down syndrome, esophageal atresia, duodenal atresia, malrotation, and congenital cardiac abnormalities [1].

47.2.3 Embryology

The yolk sac, is an extra embryonic extension from the primitive mid gut. This is formed by the 4th week of gestation. As the cranial and caudal body of the embryo folds, the neck of the yolk sac narrows. The lateral edges of the embryonic disk then start to fuse in the midline. The ectoderm covers the entire embryo, except where the yolk sac and connecting stalk emerge.

By the 6th week of gestation, the yolk sac is narrowed to a slim stalk now, known as the vitelline duct, omphalomesenteric duct or the yolk stalk [12] (Fig. 47.1).

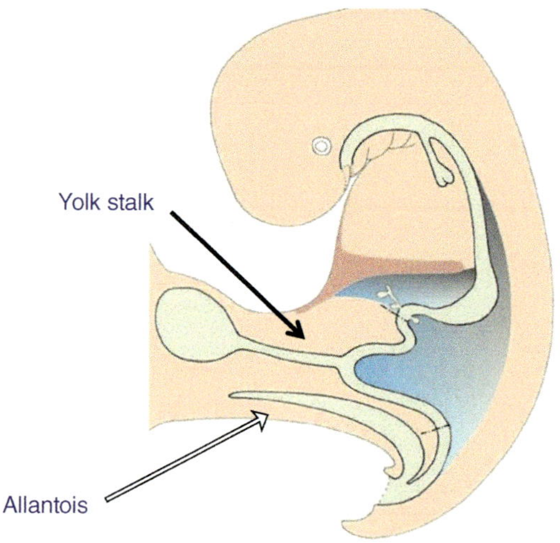

Fig. 47.1 Diagram of a fetus. *Black arrow*: Yolk stalk attached to the yolk sac on the left and the developing midgut on the right. *White arrow*: The allantois, which later becomes the urachus

The yolk stalk is thought to provide nutrients from the yolk sac to the developing embryo [13] After the 6th week, the yolk sac and yolk stalk disappear, along with the vitelline arteries [14]. Failure of this regression, creates the various forms of omphalomesenteric remnants. Although a number of other OMD anomalies can occur, MD is by far the most common.

As the yolk sac is continuous with the developing intestine, it contains all the layers of the intestinal wall as does a MD. Approximately 55–70% of MD contain ectopic tissue, usually either heterotopic gastric or pancreatic mucosa [15, 16]. The exact cause for this ectopic tissue in the diverticulum is unknown [17–19]. There have been suggestions that small buds of the pancreas are left on the foregut prior to its fusion, which then moves with the elongation of the gut onto the MD [20, 21]. There have been case reports of other ectopic tissues such as, colonic, duodenal, jejunal, hepatic, and endometrial, however these cases are rare and are isolated findings [22–25].

47.2.4 Anatomy

Meckels diverticulum is usually located on the antemesenteric border of the ileum [26]. It contains all five layers of the small intestine and is supplied by the vitelline artery (Fig. 47.2). This feature distinguishes it from a duplication cyst. The vitelline artery arises directly off the aorta [13, 27–30]. In addition to the mesenteric location of the ileum, MD has also been reported involving the proximal jejunum and the rectum [31]. The MD may be free (74%) or attached (26%) by fibrous bands to the umbilicus [32].

47.2.5 Clinical Presentation

Omphalomesenteric duct (OMD) remnants present clinically with a complication at an incidence of 4—6% [26, 33]. It has been noted that this incidence decreases with age. Clinical presentation is very varied and is related to the degree and pattern of patency or obliteration of the OMD. This may range from a completely patent omphalomesenteric duct at the umbilicus communicating with the bowel to a variety of lesser remnants, including the MD.

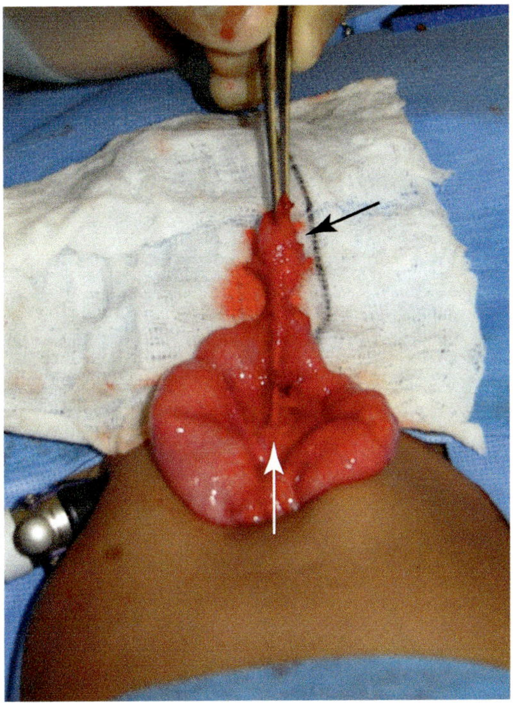

Fig. 47.2 *Black arrow*: Meckel's diverticulum; *White arrow*: vitelline artery arising from the mesentery, supplying the MD

Omphalomesenteric duct remnants may present with the persistent discharge of bowel content or mucus from the umbilicus, intussusception, prolapse of ileum at the umbilicus, intestinal obstruction, melena, anaemia and peritonitis [2].

Symptoms occur most frequently during childhood years (especially in the first 2 years of life) [34] The commonest modes of presentation are obstruction (30%), bleeding (27%), intussusception (19%), omphalitis (1%), and others (23%) [11, 35]. In the neonatal period MD may present with perforation, intussusception, ileal volvulus and less commonly, bleeding [2, 11].

Bowel obstruction is usually due to a mesodiverticular band, which is a fibrous remnant of the vitelline artery. This band, extending from the mesentery into the diverticulum, may trap a portion of the bowel [4, 36, 37]. In addition, volvulus of the bowel may occur around a persistent vitelline duct or band which connects the diverticulum to the umbilicus [16]. This may lead to bowel obstruction, perforation and peritonitis. Less commonly, an axial torsion of the MD may also occur. This occurs around its base when it is attached to either the umbilicus or ileal mesentery [26, 38]. Perforation of the MD may occur due to distal intestinal obstruction such as with Hirschsprungs disease or distal atresia [39].

Gastrointestinal bleeding is an important clinical presentation of MD. The incidence of bleeding in childhood has been recorded as high as 70% [4]. Bleeding occurs due to the presence of gastric or pancreatic tissue within the MD. Gastric tissue tends to be the more prevalent of the two, seen in 60–65% of cases, with pancreatic tissue seen in 5% of cases [15, 16]. The acidic secretions of the gastric tissues and alkaline secretions from the pancreatic tissues cause ulcerations to the adjacent normal ileal mucosa at the base of the MD, often upstream. This ultimately leads to the early detection of the diverticulum and may explain why it is most commonly found in children [22, 25]. The bleeding is often bright red fresh bleeding if large in volume or may be darker in colour. Melaena is unusual. The painless bleeding can be catastrophic, sometimes requiring urgent blood transfusion [4].

Ileo-ileal intussusception results when the MD, an aperistaltic segment of ileum, is pushed into the adjacent ileum or when the MD falls into the bowel lumen becoming a lead point for the intussusception. The intussusception may progress into the colon becoming ileo-colic [4].

MD have also been reported within inguinal or umbilical herniae (Littres hernia) [36, 40].

A small proportion of OMD may present with omphalitis, often, due to an infected OMD cyst. These cysts are what remains when the umbilical and bowel margins of the OMD obliterates but the central portion remains patent. Inflammation within an MD may occur but is unusual in the neonatal period. In addition, OMDs may present as an umbilical sinus, an unconnected collection of ectopic mucosa of ileal or gastric origin or pancreatic tissue at the umbilicus [10].

47.2.6 Management

Management varies with clinical presentation. Most importantly, following acute presentation such as bleeding, bowel obstruction, intusscusception or peritonitis, adequate rescusitation is the key priority. Crystalloid, blood products and antibiotics should be administered as needed with insertion of a naso gastric tube to aid bowel decompression and prevent pulmonary aspiration.

In some cases, such as with bowel volvulus, obstruction or peritonitis, the diagnosis will only be made following emergency laparotomy or laparoscopy. Surgery in cases of peritonitis or suspected bowel ischaemia must not be delayed in an attempt to obtain a precise diagnosis. Differential diagnoses in such cases will include the full spectrum of possible causes of acute abdomen or obstruction in the neonate such as malrotation, intussusception or bowel atresia.

In a stable child with an uncertain diagnosis further investigation may include plain radiography, ultrasonography, or imaging of the small and large bowel through contrast follow through or enema.

Obvious umbilical lesions with prolapsed intestinal mucosa would require surgical resection. If the baby presents with omphalitis or a mass under the umbilicus, then an ultrasound scan can be done prior to surgery. If the diagnosis is still unclear following radiological investigations in a stable child, diagnostic laparoscopy may be useful. Laparoscopy is increasingly used in both the diagnosis and treatment of MD. The diverticulum can be exteriorized via a periumbilical incision allowing either diverticulectomy or segmental resection and reanastomosis [41–45].

A "well" baby presenting with significant rectal bleeding will require a Meckel's scan. This scan utilizes Tc99 sodium pertechnetate given intravenously. The presence of ectopic gastric mucosa is highlighted by scintigraphy (Fig. 47.3).

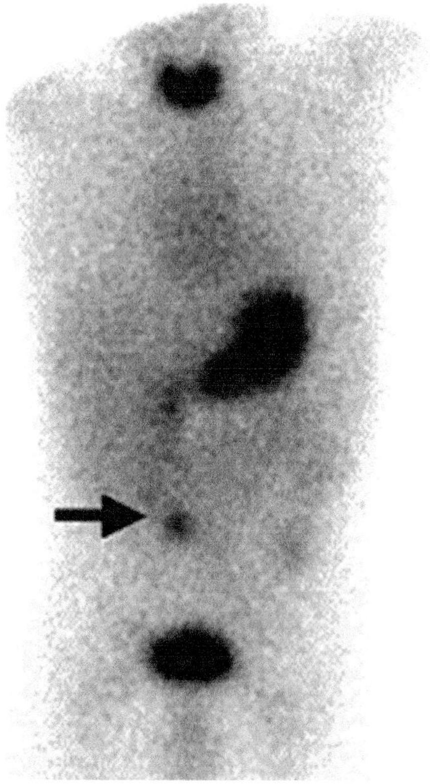

Fig. 47.3 Meckels Scan using Tc99 sodium pertechnetate, the arrow showing an area of ectopic gastric mucosa. Also highlighted are the thyroid gland, stomach and the urinary bladder

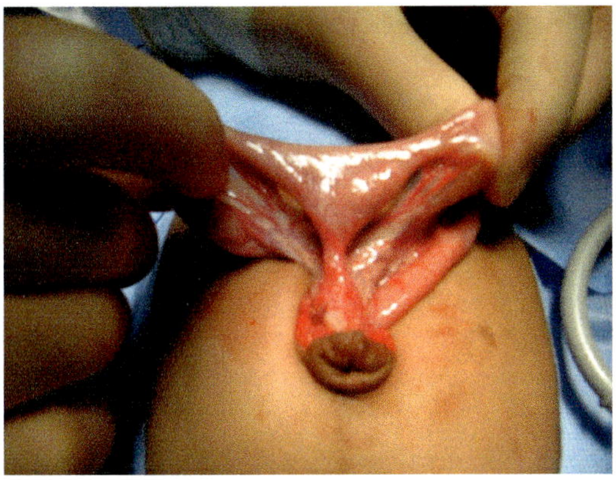

Fig. 47.4 Meckel's diverticulum attached to the umbilicus

The isotope has a high affinity for parietal cells of gastric mucosa. The residual isotope is concentrated in the urinary bladder. A positive scan shows abnormal uptake of the isotope outside the stomach and urinary bladder. The Meckel's scan has a reported sensitivity of 25–92% [41, 46–50]. Prescribing pentagastrin, histamine-2 (H-2) blockers and glucagon, have been reported to increase the diagnostic yield of the Meckel's study [33, 51]. In view of the wide variation in the sensitivity of the meckles scan, consideration should be given to early laparoscopy or laparotomy in children with suspicious clinical presentation (Fig. 47.4).

MD presenting with intestinal bleeding should have a segmental ileal resection along with the MD as the bleeding is often form ulcerated ileal mucosa adjacent to the MD. In addition, the heterotropic tissues may be found at the base of the MD. Hence a simple diverticulectomy is insufficient. A wedge excision or a segmental ileal resection would ensure complete resection of abnormal tissue [33].

47.2.7 Incidental Finding of Meckel's Diverticulum

Meckels diverticulum may be found incidentally during laparotomy or laparoscopy. There is varying opinion regarding the need to resect the MD in this situation. It has been suggested that diverticuli less than 2 cm in length, with no heterotopic palpable mucosa, constitute a lower risk group [52]. There are concerns that resecting an MD in a "clean" operation potentially converts it into a "dirty" or contaminated one. In addition, it is argued that the risk of the MD becoming symptomatic is small and that resection could result in a longer hospital stay with a risk of anastamotic leaks bowel obstruction, or infection [17, 53].

Proponents of resection suggest that the morbidity or mortality of the primary procedure may not be increased and that the palpable characteristics of the diverticulum may be unreliable [54, 55]. Tumors have rarely been reported within MD. These may be benign, such as lipoma, neuromuscular and vascular hamartomas, or malignant with carcinoids making up the majority of such cases [4, 56].

Two large studies looking at 50 years of data have shown an approximately 6% risk of complications arising from MD. Diverticulectomy performed in the presence of complications carries an operative mortality and morbidity of approximately 2% and 12% respectively [51, 57]. However, this risk must be weighed against the risks of complications from an incidental resection, a morbidity figure of around 1—2% [51, 57].

47.3 Urachal Abnormalities

The urachus is a fibrous, midline, tubular structure that extends from the dome of the bladder to the umbilicus. It represents an incomplete regression of the allantois. Urachal remnants may be completely asymptomatic but can also cause significant morbidity.

47.3.1 Epidemiology

Urachal remnants are considered rare. In pediatric autopsy studies, an incidence of 1 in 7610 cases for patent urachus and 1 in 5000 cases for urachal cysts has been documented [58]. However the incidence of symptomatic presentation with a urachal remnant is significantly smaller with the most common abnormality being urachal cysts [59].

In one review of 56 children with urachal abnormalities, about half were identified incidentally [60]. Babies with umbilical discharge and a patent urachus usually present at birth while non discharging anomalies usually present before 5 years of age [61, 62].

47.3.2 Embryology

The allantois is a finger like projection, connected to the cloaca of the primitive hindgut. The cloaca separates to form the urogenital sinus anteriorly and the rectum posteriorly [63–66] (Fig. 47.1).

The fetal bladder descends from the umbilicus into the pelvis around the fourth or fifth month of gestation. The allantois, which is attached to the dome of the bladder, stretches and progressively narrows down. It forms an epithelialized fibromuscular tube, the urachus. The urachus obliterates by fibrosis and forms the median umbilical ligament by about the 4th or 5th month of gestation [66, 67]. The precise aetiology of urachal anomalies remains undefined, however its presence has historically been attributed to bladder outlet obstruction. This "pop-off" anatomic theory is not well supported in the literature. One study reports up to 14% of patients with urachal abnormalities had evidence of bladder outlet obstruction, this finding is disputed in larger series [68, 69]. Urachal remnants can present as Umbilicourachal sinus (an incomplete tract from the umbilicus) or a complete one (patent urachus), urachal cysts or a vesicourachal diverticulum (Fig. 47.5). The most common abnormality, urachal cyst, can occur anywhere between the bladder and umbilicus and mostly occur in the distal third of the urachus. Vesicourachal diverticuli are rare, consisting of outpouchings of the bladder at the insertion of the urachus [69]. Other genitourinary conditions such as vesico-ureteric reflux, hypospadias and crossed renal ectopia are associated with urachal anomalies [70, 71].

47.3.3 Anatomy

The urachal remnant remains as a fibrous band lying in the retropubic, preperitoneal, perivesical space between the transversalis fascia and the parietal peritoneum, extending from the dome of the bladder to the umbilicus [65, 67] (Fig. 47.6). Its length varies from 3 to 10 cm and from 8 to

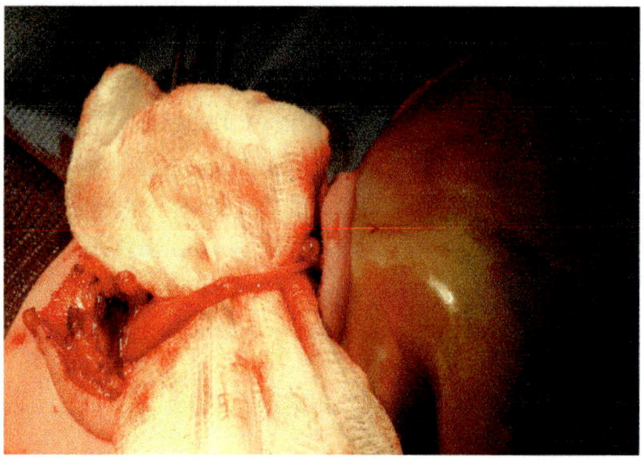

Fig. 47.6 Patent urachus attached to the bladder on the left, extending into an omphalocoele sac

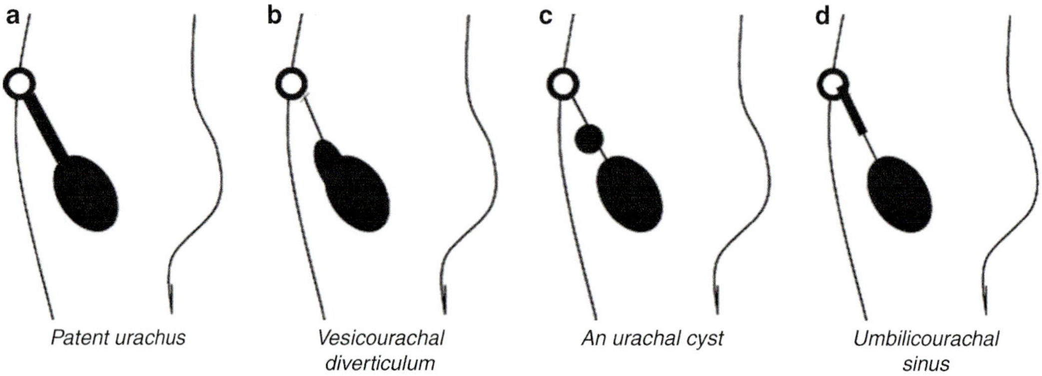

Fig. 47.5 Different forms of urachal remnants

10 mm in diameter [72, 73] Coexistence of a vitelline and urachal remnant is also uncommon, although reported [74].

47.3.4 Clinical Presentation

A patency of the embryologic urachal remnant after birth may give rise to various clinical problems. These include umbilical discharge, local infection, lower abdominal pain, and urinary tract infection. They may also be asymptomatic and be discovered incidentally [61, 62]. In a recent series, with 56 patients, the presentation was as follows: umbilical discharge (43%), umbilical infection (43%), and palpable cysts or masses associated with pain (14%). In this same group of patients, further investigations revealed that 14% had an associated genitourinary abnormality including vesico-ureteric reflux, a duplicated collecting system, hypospadias, meatal stenosis, bladder diverticulum, periurethral polyp, and renal dysplasia [69]. A patent urachus is estimated to account for about 10–15% of urachal anomalies [75]. These may sometimes present as a pseudocyst of the cord in the antenatal/fetal period [76].

As urachal remnants are rare, the literature on presentation in the neonatal period consists largely of case reports. These include prolapse of the urinary bladder, giant umbilical cord or with an omphalocoele [77–80]. There is a report of urinary ascites following trauma to a urachal remnant during umbilical artery catheterisation [81]. A subtle clinical sign of the presence of urachal remnant is the retraction of the umbilicus during voiding. This is often associated with pain [82]. Some urachal cysts are identified on ultrasound scan for another indication [83].

In an older child or young adult, infected urachal cysts can present with signs mimicking appendicitis, this is often an unsuspected finding at operation [84, 85].

47.3.5 Management

Clinical management depends on the mode of presentation. If the baby presents with an infected urachal cyst or urinary tract infection, it is important to treat the acute condition, with antibiotics, and appropriate fluid resuscitation. Ultrasound scan will assist with confirming the diagnosis and planning definitive treatment [86]. The presence of an abscess is traditionally managed in two stages: initially with antibiotics and drainage (either surgical or via interventional radiology), followed by delayed resection once the infection has resolved [86–89].

A micturating cysto-urethrogram (MCUG) may not always provide the diagnosis of a urachal remnant, especially if there is no connection with the bladder. However it may be informative in patients with a patent urachus and in whom a posterior urethral valves are a consideration [61, 69, 90]. A recent large study of 66 children with urachal remnant, from the Mayo clinic showed that of those who had a MCUG, 71% had grade 3 or less of vesico ureteric reflux and 12% had grade 4/5 reflux [91].

There have been reports of a patent urachus closing in the early newborn period. Some centres would advocate following some of these asymptomatic urachal remnants with serial ultrasound scans and conservative management [60, 75, 92]. However the long term risks of leaving these urachal remnants are stone formation and malignancy. The risk of future cancer in urachal remnants is well recognized. Urachal cancers account for 1–10% of adult bladder cancers, with a 10-year disease-free survival of about 50% [93, 94]. There have also been reports of cancers arising from urachal remnants in adolescence [95]. Urachal cancers are usually adenocarcinomas, although transitional cell, squamous cell and sarcomas have been reported [96–98].

For these reasons, the treatment of choice should be surgical resection. The tract along with the cyst and a small cuff of bladder at the insertion are removed. Mucosa should not be left at the umbilicus because of the concern that the urachal remnant may harbour a future carcinoma. This procedure can be performed by either open techniques or via laparoscopy. An open procedure may be performed via a curvilinear umbilical incision in infants. A transverse incision midway between the umbilicus and the pubis provides better exposure in older children [43–45, 99–101].

References

1. Ente G, Penzer PH. The umbilical cord: normal parameters. J R Soc Health. 1991;111(4):138–40.
2. Snyder CL. Current management of umbilical abnormalities and related anomalies. Semin Pediatr Surg. 2007;16:41–9.
3. Pollak R. Adjunctive procedure in intestinal surgery. In: Fischer JE, editor. Mastery of surgery. 5th ed. Philadelphia: Lippincott Williams & Wilkins; 2007. p. 1392–3.
4. Sharma R, Jain V. Emergency surgery for Meckel's diverticulum. World J Emerg Surg. 2008;3:27.
5. Morgagni GB. The seats and causes of disease investigated by anatomy (Translated from the Latin by Benjamin Alexander). London: A Millar and T Cadell; 1769. p. 141.
6. Amos C. Meckel's diverticulum: a pathological study of 63 cases. Am J Dis Child. 1931;42:544–53.
7. Hadley MN, Cogswell HD. Unusual origin of a Meckel's diverticulum from the base of the appendix. JAMA. 1936;106:537–8.
8. Meckel JF. Uber die divertikel am darmkanal. Arch Physiol. 1809;9:421–53.
9. Gokhan Y, Sadettin C, Turgut T. Perforation of Meckel's diverticulumby a chicken bone, a rare complication: report of a case. Surg Today. 2004;34:606–8.
10. Uppal K, Tubbs RS, Matusz P, Shaffer K, Loukas M. Meckel's diverticulum: a review. Clin Anat. 2011;24:416–22.
11. Ruscher KA, Fisher JN, Hughes CD, Neff S, Lerer TJ, Hight DW, Bourque MD, Campbell BT. National trends in the surgical management of Meckel's diverticulum. J Pediatr Surg. 2011;46:893–896.
12. Schoenwolf GC, Bleyl SB, Brauer PR, Francis-West PH. 2009. Larsen's human embryology. 4th edn. Philadelphia: Churchill Livingstone. p. 15, 106, 128–162.
13. Malik AA, Shams-ul-Bari WKA, Khaja AR. Meckel's diverticulum- revisited. Saudi J Gastroenterol. 2010;16:3–7.
14. Manning VR, McLaughlin EF. Persistent omphalomesenteric (vitelline) artery causing intestinal obstruction and gangrene of Meckel's diverticulum. Ann Surg. 1947;126:358–65.
15. Haubrich WS, Schaffner F, Berk JE, editors. Gastroenterology. Philadelphia: Saunders; 1995. p. 12–4.
16. Giusti S, Iacconi C, Giusti P, Minuto M, Caramella D, Bartolozzi C. Ileal invaginated Meckel's diverticulum: imaging diagnosis (2004:9b). Eur Radiol. 2004;14:2368–71.
17. Artigas V, Calabuig R, Badia F, Ruis X, Allende L, Jover J. Meckel's diverticulum: value of ectopic tissue. Am J Surg. 1986;151:631–4.
18. Turgeon DK, Barnett JL. Meckel's diverticulum. Am J Gastroenterol. 1990;85:777–81.
19. Madhyastha S, Prabhu VL, Saralaya V, Prakash. Meckel's diverticulum: A case report. Int J Morphol. 2007;25:519–22.
20. Horgan EJ. Accessory pancreatic tissue. Arch Surg. 1921;2:521–34.
21. Ogata H, Takehito O, Hiroki I, Shuichi T, Minoru Y. Heterotopic pancreas in children: review of the literature and report of 12 cases. Pediatr Surg Int. 2008;24:271–5.
22. Williams RS. Management of Meckel's diverticulum. Br J Surg. 1981;68:477–80.
23. Garretson DC, Frederich ME. Meckel's diverticulum. Am Fam Physician. 1990;42:115–9.
24. DiGiacomo JC, Cottone FJ. Surgical treatment of Meckel's diverticulum. South Med J. 1993;86:671–5.
25. Martin JP, Pamela DC, Kerri C. Meckel's diverticulum. Am Fam Physician. 2000;61:1037–42.
26. Limas C, Konstantinos S, Anagnostoulis S. Axial torsion and gangrene of a giant Meckel's diverticulum. J Gastrointest Liver Dis. 2006;15:67–8.
27. Segal SD, Albrecht DS, Belland KM, Elster EA. Rare mesenteric location of Meckel's diverticulum, a forgotten entity: a case study aboard USS Kitty Hawk. Am Surg. 2004;70:985–8.
28. Jay GD III, Margulis RR, McGraw AB, Northrip RR. Meckel's diverticulum; a survey of one hundred and three cases. Arch Surg. 1950;61:158–69.
29. Hollinshead WH. The jejunum, ileum and colon. In: Hollinshead WH, editor. Anatomy for surgeons, vol. 2. New York: Harper & Row; 1971. p. 478–86.
30. Manukyan MN, Kebudi A, Midi A. Mesenteric Meckel's diverticulum: A case report. Acta Chir Belg. 2009;109:510–2.
31. De Boer NK, Kuyvenhoven JP. Rectal Meckel's diverticulum. Endoscopy. 2009;41:E258.
32. Moore GP, Burkle FM. Isolated axial volvulus of a Meckel's diverticulum. Am J Emerg Med. 1988;6:137–42.
33. Menezes M, Tareen F, Saeed A, Khan N, Puri P. Symptomatic Meckel's diverticulum in children: a 16-year review. Pediatr Surg Int. 2008;24:575–7.
34. Hajivassiliou CA. Intestinal obstruction in neonatal/pediatric surgery. Semin Pediatr Surg. 2003;12(4):241–53.
35. Moore TC. Omphalomesenteric duct malformations. Semin Pediatr Surg. 1996;5:116–23.
36. Perlman JA, Hoover HC, Safer PK. Femoral hernia with strangulated Meckel's diverticulum (Littre's hernia). Am J Surg. 1980;139:286–9.
37. Brunicardi FC. 2005. Schwartz's Principles of Surgery. 8th Ed. New York: McGraw-Hill. p 1043–1044. Stewart IC. 1985. Neurovascular hamartoma in a Meckel's diverticulum. Br J Clin Pract 39:411–412.
38. Malhotra S, Roth DA, Gouge TH, Hofstetter SR, Sidhu G, Newman E. Gangrene of Meckel's diverticulum secondary to axial torsion: a rare complication. Am J Gastroenterol. 1998;93:1373–5.

39. Sy ED, Shan YS, Yang YR, et al. Hirschsprung's disease, a rare precipitating factor in neonatal perforated Meckel's diverticulum. J Pediatr Surg. 2006;41:1319–21.
40. Mishalany HG, Pereyra R, Longerbeam JK. Littres hernia in infancy presenting as undescended testis. J Pediatr Surg. 1982;17(1):67–9.
41. Lee KH, Yeung CK, Tam YH, Ng WT, Yip KF. Laparoscopy for definitive diagnosis and treatment of gastrointestinal bleeding of obscure origin in children. J Pediatr Surg. 2000;35(9):1291–3.
42. Yau KK, Siu WT, Law BK, et al. Laparoscopy-assisted surgical management of obscure gastrointestinal bleeding secondary to Meckel's diverticulum in a pediatric patient: case report and review of literature. Surg Laparosc Endosc Percutan Tech. 2005;15(6):374–7.
43. Murphy FJ, Mohee A, Khalil B, et al. Versatility of the circumumbilical incision in neonatal surgery. Pediatr Surg Int. 2009;25:145–7.
44. Scoutter AD, Askew AA. Transumbilical laparotomy in infants: a novel approach for a wide variety of surgical disease. J Pediatr Surg. 2003;38:950–2.
45. Suri M, Langer JC. A comparison of circumumbilical and transverse abdominal incisions for neonatal abdominal surgery. J Pediatr Surg. 2011;46:1076–80.
46. St-Vil D, Brandt ML, Panic S, Bensoussan AL, Blanchard H. Meckel's diverticulum in children: a 20-year review. J Pediatr Surg. 1991;26(11):1289–92.
47. Yahchouchy EK, Marano AF, Etienne JF, Fingerhut AL. Meckel's diverticulum. J Am Coll Surg. 2001;192(5):658–61.
48. Cooney DR, Duszynski DO, Camboa E, Karp MP, Jewett TC Jr. The abdominal technetium scan (a decade of experience). J Pediatr Surg. 1982;17(5):611–9.
49. Swaniker F, Soldes O, Hirschl RB. The utility of technetium 99 m pertechnetate scintigraphy in the evaluation of patients with Meckel's diverticulum. J Pediatr Surg. 1999;34(5):760–5.
50. Poulsen KA, Qvist N. Sodium pertechnetate scintigraphy in detection of Meckel's diverticulum: is it usable? Eur J Pediatr Surg. 2000;10:228–31.
51. Rerksuppaphol S, Hutson JM, Oliver MR. Ranitidine enhanced 99 m technetium pertechnetate imaging in children improves the sensitivity of identifying heterotopic gastric mucosa in Meckel's diverticulum. Pediatr Surg Int. 2004;20:323–5.
52. Mackey WC, Dineen P. A fifty year experience with Meckel's diverticulum. Surg Gynecol Obstet. 1983;156(1):56–64.
53. Peoples JB, Lichtenberger EJ, Dunn MM. Incidental Meckel's diverticulectomy in adults. Surgery. 1995;118(4):649–52.
54. Michas CA, Cohen SE, Wolfman EF Jr. Meckel's diverticulum: should it be excised incidentally at operation. Am J Surg. 1975;129(6):682–685.
55. Mukai M, Takamatsu H, Noguchi H, et al. Does the external appearance of a Meckel's diverticulum assist in choice of the laparoscopic procedure? Pediatr Surg Int. 2002;18(4):231–3.
56. Kittle SF, Jenkins HP, Dragstedt LR. Patent omphalomesenteric duct and its relation to the diverticulum of Meckel. Arch Surg. 1947;54:10–36.
57. Cullen JJ, Keith K, Moir C, Hodge D, Zinsmeister A, Melton J. Surgical management of Meckel's diverticulum. Ann Surg. 1994;220:564–9.
58. Rubin A. A handbook of congenital malformations. Philadelphia (Pa): Saunders; 2009.
59. Patel PJ, Kolawole TM, Izzidien Al-Samarrai AY. Vesicourachal diverticulum in association with other urological anomalies. Eur Urol. 1987; 13(6):417–8.
60. Ueno T, Hashimoto H, Yokoyama H, Ito M, Kouda K, Kanamaru H. Urachal anomalies: ultrasonography and management. J Pediat Surg. 2003;38(8):1203–7.
61. McCollum MO, MacNeily AE, Blair GK. Surgical implications of urachal remnants: presentation and management. J Pediatr Surg. 2003;38:798–803.
62. Mesrobian HG, Zacharias A, Balcom AH, et al. Ten years of experience with isolated urachal anomalies in children. J Urol. 1997;158:1316–8.
63. Begg RC. The urachus: its anatomy, histology and development. J Anat. 1930;64:170–83.
64. Kluth D, Hillen M, Lambrecht W. The principles of normal and abnormal hindgut development. J Pediatr Surg. 1995;30:1143–7.
65. Parrot TS, Gray SW, Skandalakis JE. The bladder and urethra. In: Skandalakis JE, Gray SW, editors. Embryology for surgeons. 2nd ed. Philadelphia: Saunders.
66. Moore KL. The urogenital system. In: Moore KL, editor. The developing human. 3rd ed. Philadelphia: Saunders; 1982. p. 255–97.
67. Blichert-Toft M, Nielsen OV. Congenital patient urachus and acquired variants. Diagnosis and treatment. Review of the literature and report of five cases. Acta Chir Scand. 1971;137:807–14.
68. Gearhart JP, Jeffs RD. Urachal abnormalities. In: Walsh PC, Retik AB, Vaughan ED, et al., editors. Campbell's urology, 7th ed. Philadelphia WB Saunders; 1998. p. 1984-1987.
69. Little DC, Shah SR, St. Peter SD, et al. Urachal anomalies in children: the vanishing relevance of the preoperative voiding cystourethrogram. J Pediatr Surg. 2005;40(12):1874–6.
70. Lane V. Congenital patent urachus associated with complete (hypospadiac) duplication of the urethra and solitary crossed renal ectopia. J Urol. 1982;127:990–2.
71. Rich RH, Hardy BE, Filler RM. Surgery for anomalies of the urachus. J Pediatr Surg. 1983;18:370–3.
72. Berman SM, Tolia BM, Laor E, et al. Urachal remnants in adults. Urology. 1988;31:17–21.
73. Schubert GE, Pavkovic MB, Bethke-Bedurftig BA. Tubular urachal remnants in adult bladders. J Urol. 1982;127:40–2.

74. Ozel LZ, Talu M, User Y, et al. Coexistence of a Meckel's diverticulum and a urachal remnant. Clin Anat. 2005;18(8):609–12.
75. Cuda SP, Vanasupa BP, Sutherland RS. Nonoperative management of a patent urachus. Urology. 2005;66(6):1320.
76. Osawa K, Ito M, Sugiyama M, et al. A case of fetal vesicoallantoic cyst in the umbilical cord. Fetal Diagn Ther. 2003;18(2):87–90.
77. Yeats M, Pinch L. Patent urachus with bladder eversion. J Pediatr Surg. 2003;38:E56.
78. Dorai CRT. Umbilical evagination of the bladder with omphalocele minor. Pediatr Surg Int. 2000;16:128–9.
79. Lugo B, McNulty J, Emil S. Bladder prolapse through a patent urachus: fetal andneonatal features. J Pediatr Surg. 2006;41:E5–7.
80. Nobuhara KK, Lukish JR, Hartman GE, et al. The giant umbilical cord: an unusual presentation of a patent urachus. J Pediatr Surg. 2004;39(1):128–9.
81. Mata JA, Livne PM, Gibbons MD. Urinary ascites: complication of umbilical artery catheterization. Urology. 1987;30(4):375–7.
82. Rowe PC, Gearhart JP. Retraction of the umbilicus during voiding as an initial sign of a urachal anomaly. Pediatrics. 1993;91(1):153–4.
83. Ozbek SS, Pourbagher MA, Pourbagher A. Urachal remnants in asymptomatic children: gray-scale and color Doppler sonographic findings. J Clin Ultrasound. 2001;29(4):218–22.
84. Yu JS, Kim KW, Lee HJ, et al. Urachal remnant diseases: spectrum of CT and US findings. Radiographics. 2001;21(2):451–61.
85. Risher WH, Sardi A, Bolton J. Urachal abnormalities in adults: the Ochsner experience. South Med J. 1990;83(9):1036–9.
86. Avni EF, Matos C, Diard F, et al. Midline omphalovesical anomalies in children: contribution of ultrasound imaging. Urol Radiol. 1988;10(4):189–94.
87. MacNeily AE, Koleilat N, Kiruluta HG, et al. Urachal abscesses: protean manifestations, their recognition, and management. Urology. 1992;40(6):530–535.
88. Masuko T, Nakayama H, Aoki N, et al. Staged approach to the urachal cyst with infected omphalitis. Int Surg. 2006;91(1):52–6.
89. Minevich E, Wacksman J, Lewis AG, et al. The infected urachal cyst: primary excision versus a staged approach. J Urol. 1997;157(5):1869–72.
90. Cilento BG Jr, Bauer SB, Retik AB, et al. Urachal anomalies: defining the best diagnostic modality. Urology. 1998;52(1):120–2.
91. Fox JA, McGee SM, Routh JC, Granberg CF, Ashley RA, Hutcheson JC, Vandersteen DR, Reinberg YE, Kramer SA. Vesicoureteral reflux in children with urachal anomalies. J Pediatr Urol. 2011;7(6):632–5.
92. Cappele O, Sibert L, Descargues J, et al. A study of the anatomic features of the duct of the urachus. Surg Radiol Anat. 2001;23(4):229–35.
93. Pinthus JH, Haddad R, Trachtenberg J, et al. Population based survival data on urachal tumors. J Urol. 2006;175(6):2042–7. discussion 2047
94. Wright JL, Porter MP, Li CI, et al. Differences in survival among patients with urachal and non-urachal adenocarcinomas of the bladder. Cancer. 2006;107(4):721–8.
95. Rankin LF, Allen GD, Yuppa FR, et al. Carcinoma of the urachus in an adolescent: a case report. J Urol. 1993;150(5 Pt 1):1472–3.
96. Brick SH, Friedman AC, Pollack HM, et al. Urachal carcinoma. Radiology. 1988;169:377–81.
97. Beck AD, Gaudin JH, Bonhan GD. Carcinoma of the urachus. Br J Urol. 1970;42:555–62.
98. Mostofi FK. Potentialities of bladder epithelium. J Urol. 1954;71:705–14.
99. Cutting CW, Hindley RG, Poulsen J. Laparoscopic management of complicated urachal remnants. BJU Int. 2005;96(9):1417–21.
100. Peters CA. Laparoscopic and robotic approach to genitourinary anomalies in children. Urol Clin North Am. 2004;31(3):595–605.
101. Khurana S, Borzi PA. Laparoscopic management of complicated urachal disease in children. J Urol. 2002;168(4 Pt 1):1526–8.

The Exstrophy Complex: Bladder and Cloacal Exstrophy

48

Peter P. Stuhldreher and John P. Gearhart

Abstract

The care of a newborn with the exstrophy-epispadias complex presents a formidable challenge to the pediatric surgical community. The approach to these children is a multi-disciplinary effort involving multiple subspecialties including urologists, surgeons, orthopedists, pediatric anesthesiologists and specialty nurses. Advances in the basic and clinical sciences in the past two decades have yielded insight into the embryologic, genetic, and the physiology of exstrophy. Despite multiple approaches to the surgical management of the exstrophic patients are used throughout the world, the critically important part of the surgical care is a successful primary closure. The best long-term outcomes can only be achieved with a successful primary closure, and each failure decreases a patient's chance at voided continence. This chapter aims to examine all aspects of the exstrophy patient including the surgical management and long term prognosis.

Keywords

Bladder exstrophy • Cloacal exstrophy • Embryology • Surgical management • Outcomes

48.1 Introduction

The care of a newborn with the exstrophy-epispadias complex presents a formidable challenge to the pediatric surgical community. The approach to these children is a multi-disciplinary effort involving multiple subspecialties including urologists, surgeons, orthopedists, pediatric anesthesiologists and specialty nurses. Advances in the basic and clinical sciences in the past two decades have yielded insight into

P.P. Stuhldreher, MD
Johns Hopkins Hospital, James Buchanan Brady Urological Institute, Baltimore, MD, USA

J.P. Gearhart, MD, FACS, FRCS(Hon) (Ed) (✉)
James Buchanan Brady Urological Institute, Johns Hopkins Hospital,
600 N. Wolfe St, Marburg 135, Baltimore, MD 21287, USA
e-mail: jgearha2@jhmi.edu

P.D. Losty et al. (eds.), *Rickham's Neonatal Surgery*, https://doi.org/10.1007/978-1-4471-4721-3_48

the embryologic, genetic, and the physiology of exstrophy. Despite multiple approaches to the surgical management of the exstrophic patients are used throughout the world, the critically important part of the surgical care is a successful primary closure. The best long-term outcomes can only be achieved with a successful primary closure, and each failure decreases a patient's chance at voided continence. This chapter aims to examine all aspects of the exstrophy patient including the surgical management and long term prognosis.

48.2 History

Interestingly, the first description of exstrophy dates back to 2000 BC, and is documented in the British Museum archives on an ancient Assyrian tablet [1]. The first recorded us of ureterosigmoidostomy in an exstrophy patient was by Syme in 1852 [2]. Followed in 1871 by Maury who successfully used abdominal and scrotal skin flaps to cover the exstrophy bladder and in 1885 by Wyman who is credited with the first successful neonatal primary bladder closure [3]. The use of osteotomy was introduced by Trendelenburg in 1892 starting with bilateral sacroiliac osteotomy to close the pelvis and fix the bladder, leading to subsequent operative refinement and its eventual integration as a mainstay in exstrophy closure [4]. Hugh Hampton Young was the first surgeon to perform a successful bladder exstrophy closure that resulted in a continent patient in 1942 [5]. The patients with the most severe end of the spectrum, cloacal exstrophy, frequently died in infancy or childhood, and it was not until 1960 that Rickham and Johnston in Liverpool reported the first long-term surviving case of cloacal exstrophy [6]. This successful management of the exstrophy and cloacal exstrophy patient led to significant advancements in the 1970s and 1980s in improved surgical techniques and strategies, including the advent of the modern staged repair by Jeffs, that led to the continence rates in exstrophy patients improving four-fold to 70–80% [7–9].

48.3 Classification

The exstrophy-epispadias complex (EEC) presents as a spectrum of disorders from epispadias to bladder exstrophy (BE) to cloacal exstrophy (CE). Depending on the point where embryologic development is disrupted, exstrophy can present from its milder forms to its more severe variant, the omphalocele-exstrophy-imperforate anus-spinal defect (OEIS) complex, otherwise known as CE [10].

Epispadias, the mildest variant in the EEC, typically presents with a urethra that is open on its dorsal aspect, and depending on the degree of severity, mildly separated pubic rami and rectus muscles. In more severe variants, the external urinary sphincter may be involved resulting in incontinence. This defect can be only glanular or extend to the bladder neck. Classic BE is the most common form of the defect and is characterized by an exstrophic bladder with the bladder mucosa exposed on the abdominal wall, a widened pubic diastasis, laterally rotated bony pelvic halves, divergent rectus muscle and fascia and an epispadiac phallus or bifid clitoris. Figures 48.1 and 48.2 illustrate these findings in both a male and female infant respectively. Cloacal exstrophy, now commonly referred to as the OEIS complex is the severest variant in the EEC. In addition to an exstrophied bladder template, the bladder halves are often separated, and a hindgut remnant is herniated in the midline. Spinal defects, omphalocele, extreme pubic diastasis, amorphic

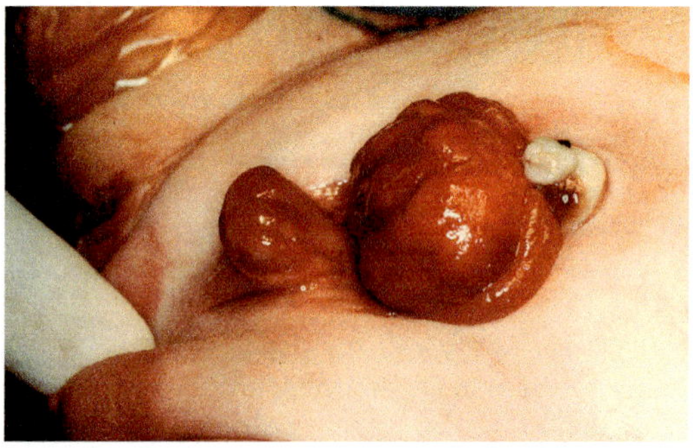

Fig. 48.1 Newborn male infant with classic bladder exstrophy

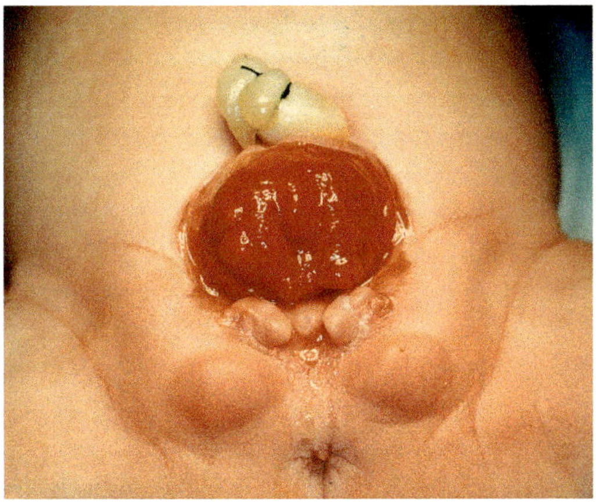

Fig. 48.2 Newborn female infant with classic bladder exstrophy

bony pelvic and hip anomalies, imperforate anus, and renal anomalies also accompany this variant of the EEC [11].

48.4 Prognosis

The published exstrophy literature is rife with different measures of success, and different prognostic factors that either lead or contribute to these outcomes. The universal tenets of successful neonatal repair of bladder exstrophy are: (1) a secure abdominal wall and bladder closure; (2) functional and cosmetic genital reconstruction; (3) achievement of urinary continence; and (4) preservation of renal function [12]. The principles for cloacal exstrophy closure are similar with the addition of: (5) neurosurgical stabilization of any spinal defects; (6) prevention of short bowel syndrome; and (7) achievement of fecal continence [13]. The literature on the exstrophy complex primarily consists of retrospective reviews, which is complicated as exstrophy is historically treated with several different techniques in multiple centers, injecting modest amounts of bias into the outcomes. Overall, the prognosis and outcome of the surgical reconstruction of the EEC can be evaluated in three major subcategories: physiological function, cosmetic appearance and psychological health [14].

48.5 Epidemiology

The incidence of bladder exstrophy in the general population is estimated in the literature to be 1 in 10,000 to 1 in 50,000 live births [15]. This is supported from data from the International Clearinghouse for Birth Defects monitoring system which quotes the incidence to be 3.3 in 100,000 live births [16]. There is a male preponderance noted in the exstrophy population in most contemporary series; the ratio is reported at 5:1–6:1 male-to-female exstrophy births [15, 16]. However, a recent epidemiological study based off of a national inpatient databank in the United States estimates that the male to female ratio may be equivalent [17]. The risk of recurrence of bladder exstrophy in a family with a child born with BE is approximately one in 100 [16]. Offspring of individuals with bladder exstrophy and epispadias having a recurrence of exstrophy recurrent is one in 70 live births, a 500-fold greater incidence than that in the general population [18]. Three isolated trends are noted that lead to increasing the incidence of bladder exstrophy: (1) decreasing maternal age; (2) high-parity pregnancies; and (3) in-vitro fertilization assisted pregnancy [16, 19].

The OEIS complex is found to occur in one in 200,000 to one in 400,000 live births according to published reports [20]. However, the incidence increases to 1:10,000 to 1:50,000 when stillborn infants are included in the analysis [21]. Similar to what is historically noted in BE, there is an increased incidence in the male population with a twofold higher incidence over the female population [22]. The only predilection data comes from an epidemiological study from New York where the incidence of OEIS was highest in Hispanic mothers and lowest in black, non-Hispanic mothers [23].

48.6 Genetics

Due to the rarity of the condition, genetic studies have been carried out on small populations of patients and no strong studies exist. One study looking for chromosomal anomalies revealed several abnormalities such as 47,XXX; 47XXY; 47XYY; and 45, XO/46,XX mosaicism in a group of 20 patients. The ultimate conclusion is that none of these chromosomal aberrations were causative of the EEC, although interestingly six of these patients also had Down's syndrome [24].

Insufficient folic acid intake during the antenatal period and deficient folate metabolism in pregnant mothers is a known risk factor for several midline birth defects [25]. The effects of folate on the development of the EEC have mixed results in the literature. In 2005, Mills et al. suggested that one polymorphism of metabolism in a DNA synthesis pathway resulted in an unstable protein that showed an increased risk ($p = 0.035$) for the development of omphalocele [26]. However, a family-based association study of that specific genetic polymorphism in the EEC showed no significant deviation in the exstrophy population from random transmission [27]. This was further supported in a study of 214 cases of EEC where folate supplementation showed no protective effect in preventing formation or decreasing the severity of the variant of EEC [28].

Recent advances in DNA technologies have allowed for significant discoveries in the alterations that may lead to the EEC. Genome wide association studies (GWAS) have shown strong evidence for variations in the *ISL1* gene being the candidate gene for bladder exstrophy, with the most significant SNP marker found to date being rs9291768 [29]. This has been supported by follow up studies showing rs9291768 as a strong candidate susceptibility locus for CBE [30]. Murine models support these findings as ISL1 is expressed in the critical time frame for CBE development, and expressed in the peri-cloacal mesenchyme and urorectal septum [31]. Continued study of the *ISL1* gene in the bladder exstrophy population is ongoing, and may lead to a better understanding of the pathogenesis of the EEC.

48.7 Animal Models

Animal models of the EEC are primarily mechanically induced and not transgenic or spontaneous animal models [11]. Naturally occurring cases of the EEC complex in animals are rare and are scantly described in the literature, with only isolated references to a feline occurrence in 1832 and a rhesus monkey with CBE in 2002 [32, 33]. Muecke was the first to report cloacal membrane maldevelopment in chicks resulting in exstrophy [34]. Subsequent studies on pig and chick embryos have demonstrated that disruption of the cloacal membrane leads to anorectal malformations and even cloacal exstrophy [35, 36]. Several other animal studies have been performed including embryological studies of the EEC on a rat model, a lamb model, and a female dog model [37–39]. However, all of these models share the same limitation as they are all mechanically and not genetically induced.

48.8 Embryology

The embryology of the EEC has been attributed by Muecke to the failure of the cloacal membrane to be reinforced by in-growth of mesoderm [34]. The cloacal membrane is situated caudally in the embryo, and is a double layer of tissue the makes up the infra-umbilical abdominal wall. Mesenchymal ingrowth between the ectodermal and endodermal layers of the cloacal membrane normally forms the bony pelvis and muscles of the lower abdominal wall. Once the mesenchymal grows inward, the urorectal septum grows downward and splits the cloacal cavity into anterior (bladder) and posterior (rectum) cavities. Paired genital tubercles will then migrate in a medial fashion to fuse in the midline cephalad to the dorsal membrane before spontaneous perforation of the cloacal membrane occurs. If the cloacal membrane is subject to premature rupture or is impeded from migration during development, the EEC may result. Depending on how far along during development the embryo is when membrane rupture occurs determines if epispadias, BE, or CE will result [40].

Multiple theories have been proposed, but Marshall and Muecke maintain that the primary etiology of the defect is an abnormal overdevelopment of the cloacal membrane. This subsequently, prevents medial migration of the mesenchyme and inhibits proper lower abdominal wall and pelvic development [41].

48.9 Associated Anomalies

Exstrophy is part of a spectrum of anomalies involving the urinary tract, genital tract, musculoskeletal system, the gastrointestinal tract, and the neurologic system.

48.9.1 Bladder Exstrophy

The musculoskeletal system in patients with bladder exstrophy is characterized by a widening of the pubic symphysis caused by malrotation of the innominate bones of the pelvis. Bony pelvic findings include a mean external rotation of the posterior aspect of the pelvis of 12° bilaterally; the acetabula of the hip are retroverted, the anterior pelvis is outwardly rotated by a mean of 18° and the pubic rami are 30% foreshortened [42]. These rotational deformities of the pelvic skeletal structures contribute to the short, pendular penis seen in bladder exstrophy. Additionally, this rotation also accounts for the increased distance between the hips, waddling gait, and the outward rotation of the lower limbs in these children. The sacroiliac joints are also externally rotated, the pelvis is rotated inferiorly, and the pelvic volume in exstrophy patients is larger than normal controls [43]. However, reports by Stec et al. have shown that fetal bony histology in the exstrophy child is identical to controls and bone development occurs at an equivalent rate [44].

In addition to the bony structures of the pelvis being laterally rotated, the large muscle groups constituting the pelvic floor are also flattened and laterally splayed. The pelvic floor covers a two-fold greater surface area in the exstrophy complex and each levator ani half is outwardly rotated 38° from midline. The levator ani complex is more flattened and only 32% of the puborectal sling is located anterior to the rectum for pelvic support as compared to 50% in controls [45]. MRI studies on the pelvic floor musculature have demonstrated one additional caveat: the degree of pubic and bony diastasis does not solely account for all of the derangements in the pelvic floor anatomy [46].

The abdominal wall is characterized by a fascial defect that is limited inferiorly by the intrasymphyseal band, representing the divergent urogenital diaphragm. This band connects the bladder neck and posterior urethra to the pubic ramus on while the anterior sheath of the rectus muscles fans out behind the urethra and bladder neck to inserts into the intrasymphyseal band. In exstrophy, the distance between the umbilicus and the anus is foreshortened, an umbilical hernia is usually present, and the incidence of inguinal hernia is high, occurring in 81.8% of boys and 10.5% of girls [47].

Anorectal defects are common as the perineum is short and broad, with the anus situated directly behind the urogenital diaphragm, displaced anteriorly. The divergent pelvic floor musculature may distort the anatomy around the external sphincter and contribute to varying degrees of anal incontinence and rectal prolapse.

The male genital defect may be severe with wide separation of the crural attachments, prominent dorsal chordee, and a shortened urethral groove. Magnetic resonance imaging (MRI) has demonstrated that the anterior corporal length in male patients with bladder exstrophy is almost 50% shorter than that of normal controls [48]. Female genital defects include a vagina that is shorter than normal, hardly greater than 6 cm in depth but of normal caliber. The vaginal orifice is frequently stenotic and displaced anteriorly; the clitoris is bifid. The labia, mons pubis, and clitoris are divergent depending on the severity of the phenotype. Typically, the uterus enters the vagina superiorly so that the cervix is in the anterior vaginal wall and the fallopian tubes and ovaries are normal.

The urinary tract is abnormal, with the bladder mucosa exstrophied on the abdominal wall. The bladder mucosa may appear to be normal, however hamartomatous polyps may be present on the bladder surface [49]. The upper urinary tract is usually normal, but anomalous development does occur. Horseshoe kidney, pelvic kidney, hypoplastic kidney, solitary kidney, and dysplasia with megaureter are all encountered in these patients. The ureters run through an abnormal course in their termination; the peritoneal pouch of Douglas between the bladder and the rectum is unusually deep, forcing the ureter down laterally in its course across the true pelvis. The distal segment of ureter approaches the bladder inferiorly and laterally, enters the bladder with little obliquity and therefore vesicoureteral reflux in the closed exstrophy bladder occurs in 100% of cases [50].

48.9.2 Cloacal Exstrophy

The above noted defects seen in the bladder exstrophy complex are all generally present in the OEIS complex, however they usually present as much more severe variants (Fig. 48.3). The gastrointestinal issues are usually the most profound addition to the spectrum with an ileocecal exstrophy, omphalocele, hindgut remnant and imperforate anus being the most common [51]. Omphaloceles are present in 88—100% of cases and may contain portions of small bowel or even liver depending on their size [52]. Short bowel syndrome and absorptive defects are commonly observed while other defects such as duplication anomalies, gastroschisis, anal ectopia, malrotation and exstrophied colonic segments may also be present [53].

The central nervous system typically is abnormal with spinal anomalies such as myelomeningocele, or tethered cords presenting in 64–100% of cases [21, 54]. Routine screening of neonates with OEIS is recommended. The innervation of the hemi-bladders arise from a pelvic plexus around the rectum, travelling along the postero-inferior surface of the rectum and extending out

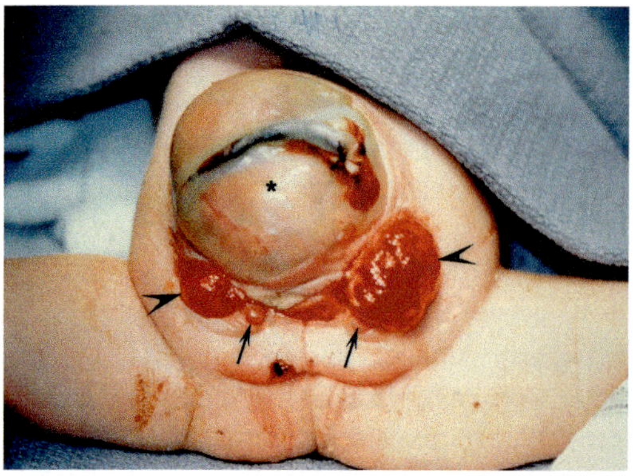

Fig. 48.3 Newborn infant with cloacal exstrophy

laterally to the bladder halves, placing them at risk for iatrogenic injuries at time of closure [55].

The OEIS complex is characterized by more profound bony abnormalities than bladder exstrophy. Spinal issues such as kyphosis, scoliosis, and abnormal vertebrae are present in 22–60% of the reported series [51, 53]. The pelvis is deformed with widely separated iliac wings, an extreme pubic diastasis, and vastly asymmetric pelvic halves [42]. Lower extremity malformations are also commonly seen in cloacal exstrophy. Club foot, equinovarus deformities, limb hypoplasia, absence, split foot, and additional digits are all noted within the complex at a rate of 17–26% [56].

Again, genitourinary aberrations are much more commonly seen in cloacal exstrophy. Upper urinary tract malformations such as renal agenesis, pelvic kidney and hydronephrosis may be observed in 1/3 of patients. Additionally, fusion anomalies, horseshoe kidney and ureteral abnormalities may also be found [52]. Testes in the male are frequently undescended with scrotal and labial halves widely separated. The phallus or clitoris is almost always bifid, underdeveloped or potentially absent. Inguinal hernias are common. In females, uterine duplication, vaginal duplication and vaginal agenesis are also reported in 25–95% of cases [21, 52].

48.10 Antenatal Presentation

48.10.1 Bladder Exstrophy

With modern prenatal ultrasound, it is possible to diagnose classic bladder exstrophy in the antenatal period [57, 58]. Two major criteria exist on prenatal ultrasound to suggest the diagnosis of bladder exstrophy: (1) the absence of a normal fluid-filled bladder on repeat examinations; and (2) a mass of echogenic tissue on the lower abdominal wall [58]. Furthermore, in a retrospective review of 25 prenatal ultrasound examinations resulting with the birth of classic bladder exstrophy, several observational findings were made: (1) absence of bladder filling; (2) a low-set umbilicus; (3) widening of the pubic ramus; (4) diminutive genitalia; and (5) a lower abdominal mass which increased in size as the pregnancy progressed [59].

48.10.2 Cloacal Exstrophy

Ultrasound is also the mainstay in the prenatal diagnosis of cloacal exstrophy, although it still is not 100% accurate. First described in 1985, major findings on prenatal ultrasonography include inability to visualize a full bladder, a large midline lower abdominal mass, and possible myelomeningocele [60]. An identifier that differentiates cloacal and bladder exstrophy is the trunk-like appearance of the exstrophied ileocecal segment that can be detected on ultrasound [61]. Further characterization of this issue has led to major criteria (occurring in >50% of cases) for prenatal diagnosis: non-visualization of the bladder, large anterior midline abdominal wall defect, cystic midline structure, omphalocele, and myelomeningocele; minor criteria (occurring in <50% of cases) include: lower extremity defects, renal anomalies, ascites, widened pubic rami, hydrocephalus, a single umbilical artery, and a narrow thorax [62]. When the prenatal diagnosis of the OEIS complex is obtained, consideration for termination of the pregnancy is an option for discussion with the parents [63].

48.11 Clinical Presentation, Diagnosis, and Postnatal Care

In the absence of prenatal diagnosis, the exstrophy complex can be diagnosed by physical examination at the time of birth. Typically children with exstrophy are most often born at term and in no particular distress. In BE, the exstrophic bladder template is visible as a circular patch of reddened mucosa from which the ureteral orifices will actively drain urine. Hamartomatous polyps may be present, the pubic symphysis is open and the diastasis between the two sides is palpable. The appearance of the genitalia is variable, with the urethra in males lying open on the dorsal surface of the corporal bodies with the penis splayed open dorsally. In females, the pubic diastasis results in an absence of a mons pubis with a bifid clitoris and lateral displacement of the labia. In CE, the above mentioned findings are present, however the bladder halves may be separated with a hindgut remnant located in the midline; the pubic diastasis may be extreme, and an omphalocele and/or myelomeningocele may be visible. Typically the abnormal vertebral defects and lower limb defects are visibly apparent in the newborn.

No immediate laboratory information is required, except in children who will undergo immediate surgery where a type and screen with baseline CBC, serum electrolytes and coagulation studies will assist preoperatively. Additionally, karyotyping should be performed in cases of the OEIS complex to better delineate chromosomal sexual determination. Imaging should be performed in the immediate postnatal period including a plain abdominal radiograph for precise measurement of the pubic diastasis, and characterization of the pelvic and vertebral defects. A renal ultrasound and spinal ultrasound allow for identity of baseline renal characteristics and to rule out spinal anomalies and tethered chord. The use of CT or MRI in the newborn is currently for academic and investigational purposes and is considered optional.

Postnatal care is similar for both BE and CE; starting in the delivery room, the umbilical cord should be tied with 2-0 silk sutures close to the abdominal wall so that the umbilical clamp does not traumatize the exposed mucosa. The bladder may be covered with a non-adherent film of plastic wrap (i.e. Saran Wrap) to prevent the mucosa from sticking to clothes or diapers. In addition, each time the diaper is changed the plastic wrap should be removed, the bladder surface irrigated with sterile saline, and a new square of plastic wrap placed. Consultation of surgical teams with expertise in the exstrophy complex should be obtained including a pediatric urologist or pediatric surgeon, an orthopedist, and in cases of OEIS a pediatric surgeon and a neurosurgeon when necessary. Cardiopulmonary and general physical assessment can be carried out in the first few hours of life. A thorough neonatal and subspecialist assessment may have to be deferred until transportation to a major children's medical or exstrophy center can be arranged.

48.12 Surgical Management of Bladder Exstrophy

48.12.1 Primary Bladder Closure

Over the past three decades, improved techniques in the functional bladder closure have contributed to higher success rates and improved long term outcomes in the exstrophy population. The objective of primary closure, whether as an infant or older, is to convert a patient with an exstrophic bladder into one with complete epispadias with incontinence. This allows for a low posterior urethral outlet resistance and ensures preservation of renal function. Typically epispadias repair is now performed between 6 and 10 months of age. In some very select cases, surgeons may elect to combine the bladder closure and epispadias repair into one procedure in the newborn. Initial repair is of paramount importance as it has been demonstrated that a successful closure of a good quality bladder template in a newborn is the single most important predictor of eventual voided continence [64].

Preoperatively it may be evident that a bladder template may be small and fibrotic and is not elastic or contractile enough for the usual closure procedure (Fig. 48.4). Examination with the patient under anesthesia may be required to assess the bladder adequately, particularly if edema, excoriation, and polyps are present on the mucosal surface (Fig. 48.5). The suitability of a bladder for closure or the need to perform a delayed closure should only be made by experienced surgeons as a failed closure may be catastrophic in the long term, while it has been shown in small series that delayed closure can have comparable continence outcomes long term to immediate primary bladder closure [65].

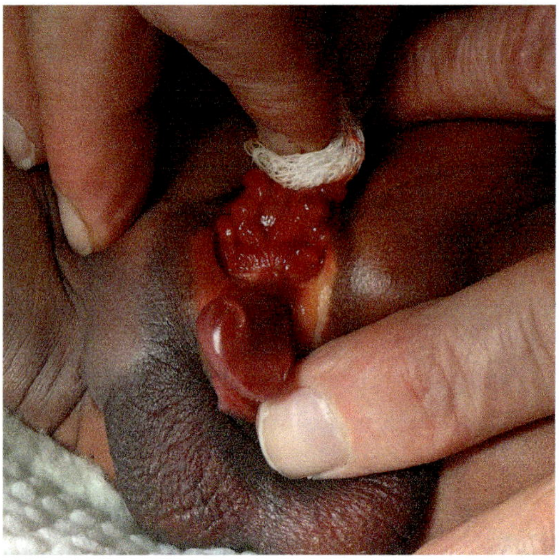

Fig. 48.4 Bladder template on a newborn with classic bladder exstrophy deemed too small for primary closure during the newborn period

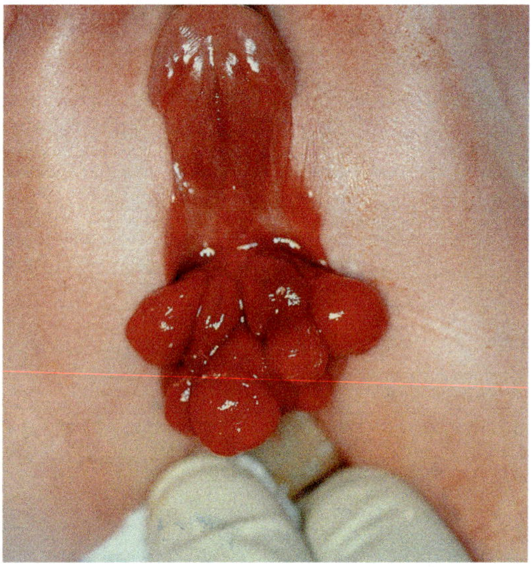

Fig. 48.5 Fibrotic bladder filled with hamartomatous polyps deemed unsuitable for primary closure during the newborn period

48.12.2 Pelvic Osteotomy

If primary closure is undertaken within 72 h of birth, majority of times the pelvic bones are not completely calcified and are malleable. At the beginning of the closure procedure, if the pelvis can be manually manipulated and closed without significant tension, then one may choose to forgo a formal pelvic osteotomy. In this case the pubis is re-approximated later in the procedure and the child is immobilized post-operatively with traction. If the closure is being performed after 72 h of life, if the pelvis is not malleable, or if the pubic diastasis is over 4 cm, then osteotomies should be performed at the time of primary bladder closure. If osteotomy is not utilized in the primary closure, postoperatively the infant is immobilized in modified Bryant's traction in a position in which the hips have 90° flexion for 4 weeks [66].

A pelvic osteotomy provides security to the closure as it brings the pubic symphysis together, diminishes tension on the abdominal wall closure, facilitates placement of the vesicourethral junction deep within the pelvis, and brings the pelvic floor musculature more anterior in the pelvis. A well performed osteotomy will add extra time under anesthesia for the infant; however security of the closure is paramount to prevent the procedure from failing.

Multiple techniques and approaches exist for performing pelvic osteotomy; however the technique that enjoys the most published results is the bilateral transverse innominate and vertical iliac osteotomy. Osteotomy should be performed as the initial step prior to attempting bladder closure [67]. The osteotomy may be performed with the infant in the same position required for bladder closure with the same whole body surgical prep. The pelvis is approached from the anterior body wall and exposure is gained from the iliac wings inferiorly to the pectineal tubercle and posteriorly to the sacroiliac joints. Both the transverse innominate osteotomy and the posterior iliac osteotomy may be performed through this anterior approach. Two fixator pins are placed in the inferior osteotomized segment and a single pin is placed in the wing of ileum superiorly. Radiographs are obtained to confirm pin placement, the soft tissues are closed, and the urologic portion of the procedure may then be performed. At the end of the procedure, an external fixator is applied and the patient is placed in Buck's traction for 4 weeks to prevent dislodgement of tubes and destabilization of the pelvis. Postoperatively, in newborns that undergo closure with-out osteotomy in the first 48–72 h of life, the baby is immobilized in modified Bryant's traction in a position in which the hips have 90° flexion. When modified Bryant's traction is used, the traction is employed for 4 weeks.

48.12.3 Bladder, Posterior Urethral, and Abdominal Wall Closure

The patient is given broad-spectrum antibiotics in an attempt to convert a contaminated field into a clean surgical wound. The various steps in primary bladder closure are illustrated in Figs. 48.6 and 48.7. The initial incision is created from just above the umbilicus and carried down around the bladder and paraexstrophy skin to approximately the level of the urethral plate. To ensure later posterior urethral and prostatic closure, a mucosal strip 2 cm wide is marked out from the trigone to just below the verumontanum in the male and the vaginal orifice in the female patient as seen in Fig. 48.6a, b. Male urethral length is typically sufficient and no longer are urethral transection and paraexstrophy skin flaps recommended in the modern repair.

The posterior plane behind the bladder template is entered just above the umbilicus and is established between the rectus fascia and the bladder. Each umbilical vessel is doubly ligated and incised allowing the peritoneum to be peeled off the dome of the bladder (Fig. 48.6c). The peritoneum should be separated from at least 50% of the bladder at this point allowing the bladder to be placed deeply into the pelvis at the time of closure. This plane of dissection is continued laterally in a caudal direction between the bladder and the rectus fascia until the urogenital diaphragm fibers are encountered (Fig. 48.6d). The pubis will also be encountered at this juncture and it should be retracted laterally allowing for the incision of the urogenital diaphragm fibers. This step facilitates the radical mobilization of the bladder neck and posterior urethra from the pubic bone (Fig. 48.7a).

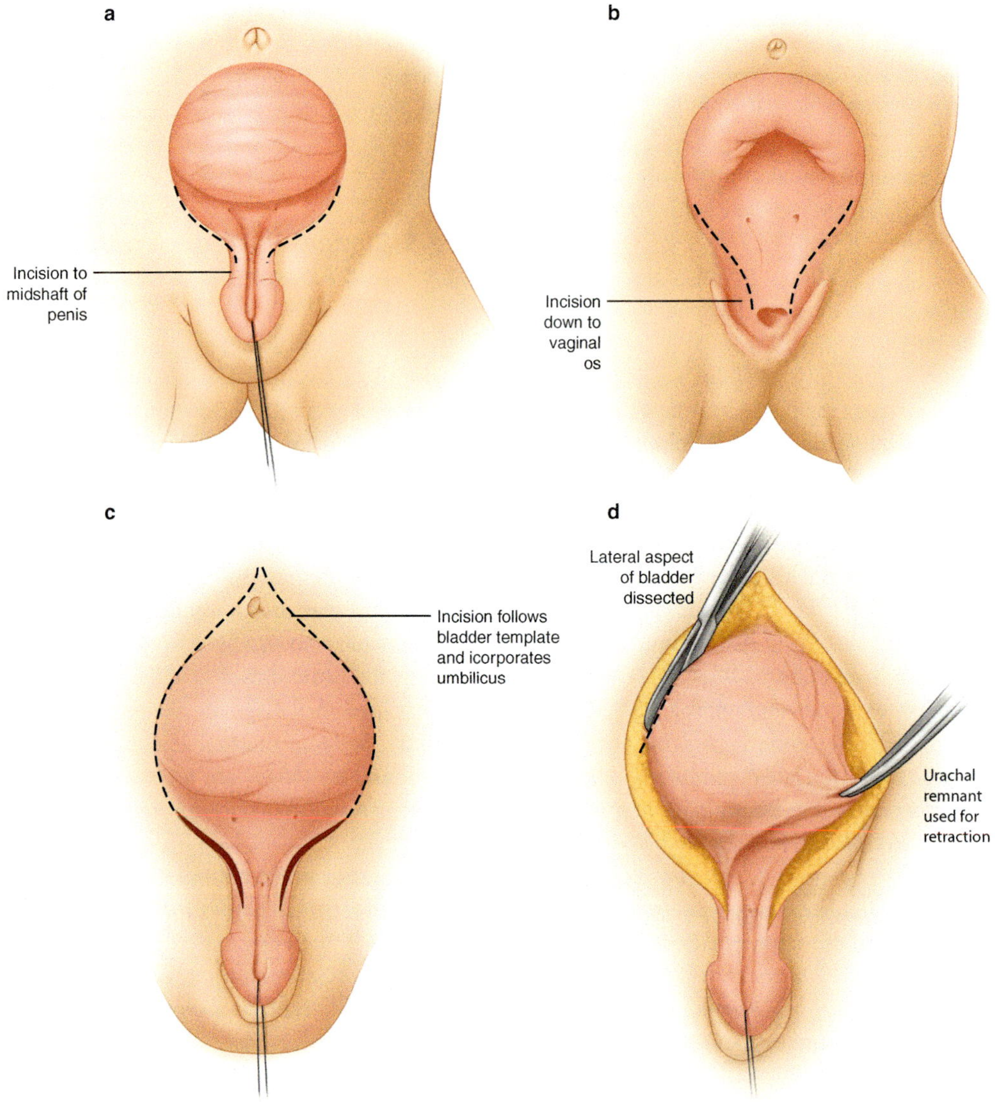

Fig. 48.6 Initial steps in primary bladder exstrophy closure. (**a**) Outline of initial incisions in a male exstrophy patient, (**b**) Outline of initial incisions in a female exstrophy patient, (**c**) Periumbilical incision and initial bladder dissection, (**d**) Further bladder dissection into the retropubic space and division of lateral bladder attachments

Gentle traction on the glans of the penis at this point will show the insertion of the corporal body on the lateral inferior aspect of the pubis. Care should be taken to avoid radical mobilization of the corpora as their blood supply may be aberrant in the exstrophy complex. The corporal bodies are not brought together at this juncture, as the epispadias repair will be performed as a second stage procedure around 6 months of age. The urogenital fibers are then incised with electrocau-

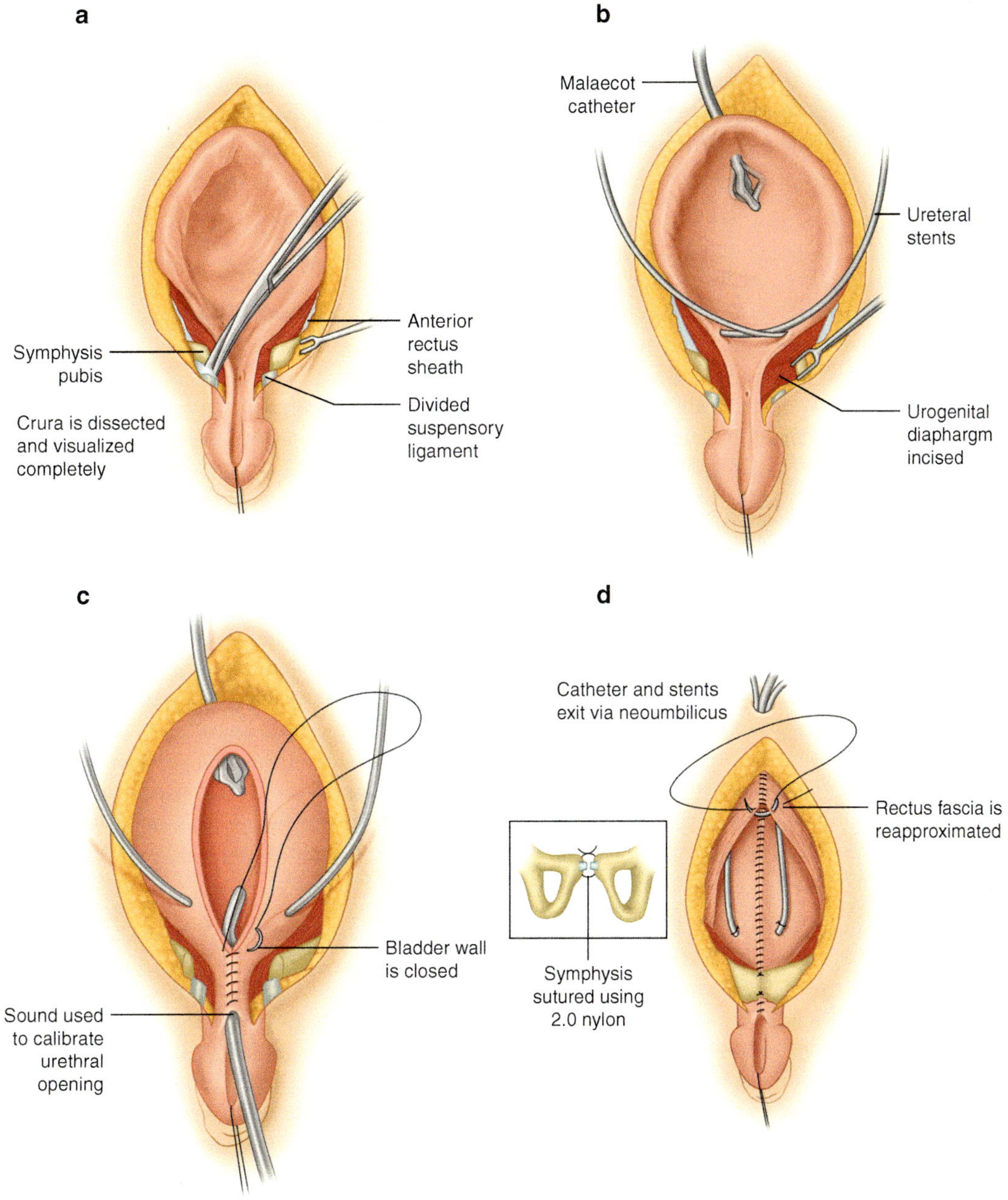

Fig. 48.7 Continued steps in primary bladder exstrophy closure. (**a**) Freeing of the urogenital diaphragm from the pubis, (**b**) Incision of the urogenital diaphragm fibers and placement of a suprapubic tube, (**c**) placement of ureteral catheters and bladder wall closure, (**d**) Fascial closure following reapproximation of the pubic symphysis

tery down to the pelvic floor in their entirety. This step is crucial in allowing the vesicourethral junction to be placed as deeply in the pelvis as possible. If the urogenital fibers are left intact, when the pubic bones are re-approximated, the posterior vesicourethral unit will be brought anteriorly in an unsatisfactory position.

After their incision, the wide band of fibrous and muscular tissue representing the urogenital diaphragm is detached subperiostally from the pubis bilaterally (Fig. 48.7b). At this stage the bladder should be freely mobile from surrounding structures while its postero-lateral blood supply is preserved. Paraexstrophy skin may then be discarded if not required during the repair. The mucosa and muscle of the bladder, and the posterior urethra are then closed in the midline anteriorly. This urethral orifice should calibrate to 12–14 French allowing enough resistance to aid in the bladder adaptation while avoiding increased outlet resistance and potential upper tract damage. This sized urethral opening will also primarily preventing prolapse through the urethra. If possible, a second layer closure with local tissue should be performed over the posterior urethra and bladder neck (Fig. 48.7c).

A suprapubic non-latex Malecot catheter is left in the bladder and ureteral stents are left in the ureters for 4 weeks to promote maximal urinary drainage. Ureteral stents allow for free renal drainage as swelling in the bladder floor may induce temporary ureteral obstruction. Urethral stents are avoided to prevent necrosis and accumulation of secretions in the neourethra.

Following bladder closure and drainage tube placement, the pubis is then re-approximated. If osteotomies have been performed, the fixator pins may be used to manipulate the pelvis closed, otherwise pressure over the greater trochanters bilaterally allows the pubic bones re-approximated in the midline. Horizontal No. 2 nylon mattress sutures are placed in the pubis and tied with a knot away from the neourethra (Fig. 48.7d).

An umbilicoplasty is then performed and the ureteral stents and suprapubic tube are brought out through the neoumbilicus. The author's primarily use a V-shaped flap of abdominal skin at the orthotopic umbilical location tacked down to the abdominal fascia in the method described by Hanna [68]. The abdominal fascia is closed with interrupted sutures. Care should be taken so that the drainage tubes exit the abdominal fascia superiorly with minimal tunneling under the skin to prevent erosion of the skin. The subcutaneous tissue and skin are then closed. The infant is then placed in traction, extubation is attempted is possible and the patient is transported to the intensive care unit for monitoring.

48.12.4 Combined Bladder Closure and Epispadias Repair

This surgical technique for complete primary exstrophy closure (CPRE) combines both the bladder closure and epispadias reconstruction into one procedure on the newborn. This technique was first described by Lattimer and Smith for primary closures and in 1991 for failed exstrophy closures [15, 69]. Today, renewed international interest exists in using a combined procedure on newborn patients, and the critical steps of the procedure have been outlined by Grady and Mitchell [70]. Initially, a similar dissection is performed to isolate the bladder, beginning superiorly and carried out inferiorly. Once the bladder template is dissected free, the penile dissection begins ventrally. Dissection of the corpora progresses medially and the penis is completely disassembled with care being taken to ensure the urethral plate preservation [71]. Deep proximal dissection frees the vesicourethral unit from the intrasymphyseal ligaments. The bladder is then closed, the penis is reassembled anatomically with a hypospadiac urethral opening (in 70% of patients) and the abdominal wall and skin closure is completed [70]. However, with this approach there have been several reports of significant soft tissue (glans and corporal) loss with this technique [72].

48.12.5 Radical Soft Tissue Mobilization (The Kelly Repair)

Another surgical option for a staged repair of exstrophy is the Kelly repair, or radical soft tissue mobilization. Briefly, this is a multi-staged technique that closes the bladder and abdominal wall without osteotomy after birth. Several months later a radical soft tissue surgical mobilization of the urogenital diaphragm from its periosteal attachments is performed to allow closure of the pelvis and pelvic floor. The penis is made hypospadiac and later penile repair is performed. Osteotomy is not routinely used in this repair [73].

48.13 Surgical Management of Cloacal Exstrophy

Cloacal exstrophy presents a much more complex treatment plan than bladder exstrophy. In the OEIS complex, spinal anomalies and myelomeningocele frequently occur. In the situation with a concomitant neurological issue, neurosurgical consultation and closure of the defect should be performed as soon as the infant is medically stable to undergo the procedure. The remainder of the surgical closure requires a coordinated effort by both a pediatric urologist and a pediatric surgeon. As both bowel and bladder are exstrophic and intertwined and the degree of severity is varied, individualized treatment strategies for each patient result in the best long-term results [74]. Most importantly, the pediatric surgeon and pediatric urologist should have a unified management plan regarding initial closure of both bowel and bladder with a long-term treatment plan for subsequent surgical reconstruction as the child ages [75].

A newborn cloacal exstrophy is typically brought to the operating room within 48–72 h of life for a closure procedure and abdominal exploration from the multi-disciplinary team. Various algorithms have been proposed as to single stage versus multi-stage procedures for initial repair, however all approaches emphasize several basic tenets: (1) omphalocele repair; (2) separation of the cecal plate from the bladder halves; and (3) hindgut preservation [13, 76]. The goal of urologic repair is to preserve and possibly close the two bladder halves while providing minimal opportunity for renal compromise [77]. The gastrointestinal objectives are to identify and quantify all available intestinal components, assess their continuity and ensure preservation of all intestinal length [78]. Individual steps of each procedure will not be detailed, but the guiding tenets of each portion of the repair and the optional treatment steps will be outlined in further detail.

The omphalocele defect in cloacal exstrophy ranges in size and may contain small bowel and even other solid abdominal viscera depending on its size. In almost all circumstances, attempts should be made to close the omphalocele at the time of the initial closure procedure as this facilitates successful closure of the abdominal wall. In most series this can be performed successfully after the abdominal exploration, bladder realignment and fecal diversion are performed. In cases of extremely large defects, alternatives are occasionally required instead of primary closure [54]. If the omphalocele cannot initially be reduced, a silo device may be employed with slow gradual reduction of the defect until it is small enough for closure. Alternatively, the omphalocele may be allowed to epithelialize creating a controlled ventral hernia for which repair may be deferred until the child has undergone some longitudinal growth [79]. Despite the availability of alternatives, most exstrophy experts attempt to close the omphalocele primarily in the initial surgical foray.

The cecal plate must be separated from the bladder halves. Once the entire hindgut remnant is free from the urinary tract, an attempt at bladder closure may be made if deemed appropriate. If performed, the bladder halves may be joined back in the midline with care to identify the ureteral orifices at the time of realignment. The bladder closure technique described above for bladder exstrophy may be used as the guiding principle for repair. If a complete closure is performed, then osteotomy may be employed in these patients at the same time however in the malformed pelvis of these infants, the task is difficult. At the author's institution, it is preferred to rejoin the bladder halves on the anterior abdominal wall and leave the bladder exstrophied. Subsequently in a delayed fashion around 1 year of age, the bladder may be closed with a staged osteotomy to close the pelvis if there is an extreme diastasis (>6 cm) [80, 81]. Additionally, the staged approach to bladder closure is supported by the increased incidence of tethered cord as well as the extensive dissection to close the bladder and pelvis through areas that innervates the bladder potentially placing the upper urinary tracts at unnecessary risk to justify one stage procedures [82]. However, in rare cases with a small omphalocele, good sized bladder template, and narrow pubic diastasis, a single staged closure can be safely performed.

The goal of gastrointestinal (GI) reconstruction at the time of primary closure is to characterize existing bowel, free it from the urinary bladder, divert the fecal stream and preserve all available bowel length. The typical anatomic presentation of the GI tract is to have the ileocecal segment of the gut exstrophied on the abdominal wall with the herniated ileum protruding out like an elephant trunk. In addition there may be hindgut a hindgut remnant or other detached colonic segments distally not in continuity with the intestinal stream [78]. Majority of patients (96%) in a large series have been found to have between 2 and 20 cm of total colonic length with the remainder having greater than 20 cm. Typically small bowel length is preserved and is close to normal in these infants [83]. The initial step is to mobilize the cecal plate from the bladder halves. This cecal plate must be tubularized so care needs to be taken to ensure adequate width to allow for tubularization. This step must be followed by careful inspection of the abdomen to identify any remaining segments of large intestine that are distal to or attached to the cecal plate. If any segments are discontinuous, continuity of the bowel should be reestablished by re-anastomosing the segments. The distal end of the large bowel segment is then brought out to the skin as a colostomy to divert the fecal stream. Careful attention to the GI reconstruction at this initial surgical closure procedure attempts to minimize short gut syndrome and maximize intestinal length for the consideration of future reconstruction [84].

48.14 Complications and Special Considerations

48.14.1 Primary Bladder Closure Failure

Regardless of the technique chosen to close the exstrophic bladder, the goals are the same: successful closure of the abdominal wall, pelvis and bladder; preservation of the urogenital soft tissues, and protection of the upper tracts from outlet obstruction and pyelonephritis. Primary bladder closure can fail in three primary ways in the postoperative period, either through dehiscence of the abdominal wall and bladder, prolapse of the bladder through the urethral opening, or the development of outlet obstruction [85].

Dehiscence of the abdominal wall and bladder is one of the primary reasons for failure of a closure procedure in the immediate postoperative setting. Dehiscence presents as opening of the abdominal wall and fascia and re-exposure of the exstrophic bladder mucosa on the abdominal wall; dehiscence is handily diagnosed on physical examination of the surgical wound. Dehiscence is mainly attributed to tension on the abdominal wall, bladder and pelvic closure. Tension must be minimized by good closure of the bony pelvis, deep placement of the bladder within the pelvis, and proper post-operative care including immobilization, sedation, proper urinary drainage, and avoidance of abdominal distension.

Bladder prolapse and outlet obstruction are problems that occur at the vesicourethral junction or the urethral opening following a primary closure procedure. Bladder prolapse can be partial or complete and is identified by the reddish bladder mucosa protruding through the urethral orifice. Incomplete closure of the pelvis or pelvic floor or creation of a neourethral segment that is considerably wider than 12 French can result in lack of support leading to prolapse through a capacious orifice. Additionally, avoidance of increased abdominal pressure or distension should be protective [86]. This can be accomplished through pain control measures to minimize unnecessary or abrupt movement of the infant, urinary drainage to keep the bladder decompressed, and avoidance of early post-operative abdominal distension from early feeding and avoidance of ileus.

Outlet obstruction, that can lead to upper tract deterioration stems from stricture of the neourethra, either from over-tightening of the neourethra or from erosion of the pubic stitch into the urethral channel [87]. This predisposes both the bladder and the upper urinary tracts to stress, dilatation and renal damage. This ultimately may result in recurrent pyelonephritis, renal insufficiency and detrusor muscle fatigue [88]. Both prolapse and outlet obstruction obviates the surgeon to perform a re-closure procedure or reconstructive procedure to open the bladder for urinary drainage.

Wound infections in the post-operative period are the enemy of any reconstructive surgery. Prophylactic antimicrobials are recommended for the postoperative period to prevent surgical site wound infections, which have been attributed as causative factors in wound dehiscence and scar tissue formation. Additionally, antimicrobial prophylaxis prevents urinary tract infections while drainage tubes are indwelling in the ureters and bladder [89]. During the post-operative period when the suprapubic tube and ureteral stents are in place, keeping them secure is of significant importance as early dislodgement of urinary drainage tubes has also been implicated as reasons for early surgical failures [90].

48.14.2 Genitourinary Soft Tissue Loss

The complete primary repair of exstrophy (CPRE), where epispadias repair is performed on the infant in the same surgical setting as primary bladder closure, has a unique series of complications reported with the loss of urethral, penile and glanular soft tissues [72]. The mechanism of injury is hypothesized to be ischemic in nature, with either compression of the pudendal blood vessels at time of pelvic closure or direct injury to the blood supply due to aggressive dissection compromising the already tenuous blood supply to the lower GU tract [91]. In capable hands at major exstrophy centers this complication can be avoided, however large referral centers internationally are reporting this complication with greater frequency [92, 93]. Unfortunately at this time, loss of glanular and corporal tissues are not replaceable and pose grave risks to future genital reconstructive efforts.

48.14.3 Bowel Complications in Cloacal Exstrophy Reconstruction

Primary bowel complications in the immediate post-operative period are rare, but the long term developmental issues and reconstructive issues are directly related to the primary procedure. Careful preservation of all intestinal length is of paramount importance as in 25% of the cases of children born with the OEIS complex, short bowel syndrome has been reported [20, 22]. If proper handling of the bowel is performed in infancy, potential exists for these children to have their colostomy reversed later on during childhood. Candidacy for an intestinal pull through procedure depends on both the ability to form solid stool and development of adequate perineal musculature and function. Careful dissection around the pelvic floor and preservation of bowel length at initial and subsequent reconstructive procedures maximizes the potential for anatomic reconstruction of the cloacal exstrophy child's distal GI tract later in life [94].

48.15 Quality of Life and Long-Term Outcomes

Urinary continence is a primary measure of long term outcome in both bladder and cloacal exstrophy reconstruction. In the bladder exstrophy patient population, volitional voided continence is achievable and well reported in the literature following surgical reconstruction. Rates of continence following reconstruction are reported as ranging from 18 to 83% [14]. The single most agreed-upon determinant of potential volitional voided continence is the success of the primary surgical bladder closure procedure [64]. Some reports of continence being achieve by primary closure or complete primary repair alone do exist, but most series acknowledge that the exstrophy child will eventually require a bladder neck reconstruction or outlet procedure [95]. Following bladder neck reconstruction, in patients who had a successful primary repair, continence rates have been reported as high as 83% in large series [96]. In infants that have had a failed re-closure procedure, the volitional continence rates only approach the 50% range. Many of these children ultimately have to go augmentation cystoplasty and continent catheterizable channels to become dry of urine [97]. In cloacal exstrophy, the reports of volitional voided continence are rare although some reports utilizing a complete primary repair at birth or through bladder neck reconstruction are reported [54, 98]. It is generally accepted that majority of patients with the OEIS complex will undergo a continent urinary diversion at some point during reconstruction to achieve urinary dryness [99].

Fecal continence is expected in the bladder exstrophy population. Several reports exist of exstrophy patients having long-term pelvic floor compromise and issues with partial fecal incontinence [100, 101]. Hypothesized theories for these issues are compromised pelvic floor muscular anatomy in the exstrophy complex and long term fatigue or stress on the pelvic floor manifesting earlier in life than in the healthy adult population. In cloacal exstrophy fecal continence is directly correlated to the ability of the remaining large intestine to form solid stool and the development of the perineal musculature in the children as they age. Decisions for eventual intestinal pull through procedures are made by a pediatric surgeon after longitudinal assessment of these two variables during infancy and childhood.

The psychological impact on children and adolescents with the exstrophy complex are a significant and chronic health condition that is similar to that seen in other major congenital birth defects [102]. Exstrophy patients are challenged in life and relationships and must cope with anxiety stemming from their physical differences potentially numerous operative procedures [103]. The quality of life of children with exstrophy is in many ways determined by their ability to develop essential coping mechanisms; however reports of increased post-traumatic stress and suicidal ideations are a cause for significant concern. Active surveillance of these children's' mental health by their pediatric surgeon and urologist is essential as in many cases these physicians serve in a primary care capacity for this patient population. When recognized, psychological or psychiatric referral should be obtained for those felt to be in need [104].

Long-term sexual outcomes of both male and female health are the source of ongoing studies. The male phallus is typically functional and suitable for intercourse; anatomically the penis will be shorter but wider than average with some degree of dorsal chordee or upward deflection [48]. Female patients with the exstrophy complex are the best characterized to date. The exstrophic female vaginal canal and internal genitalia are reasonably normal. The vaginal orifice may be stenotic, but vaginal depth is sufficient for intercourse and internal vaginal caliber is typically normal. The appearance of the external genitalia is dependent upon the surgical reconstruction. A series of 42 women with the exstrophy complex demonstrated that 34 engaged in vaginal intercourse; however 30 required either modified episiotomy or vaginoplasty to obviate the stenosis frequently encountered at the vaginal introitus [105]. Sexual desire has also been found to be appropriate and consistent with the unaffected population, at least in the bladder exstrophy population [106].

The fertility of patients in bladder exstrophy is primarily based on retrospective studies and observations. Males with bladder exstrophy are thought to have difficulty with antegrade ejaculation however a recent series of adult male exstrophy patients who underwent a single stage repair have shown achievable antegrade ejaculation in 94%. In these patients however, sperm quality was severely diminished [107]. The advancements in modern infertility treatments, such as intracytoplasmic sperm injection and IVF have made reproduction a viable possibility for the exstrophy male [108]. Several series have documented adult females with exstrophy who have become pregnant via vaginal insemination, who then carried and successfully delivered children [105]. Females however due to the widened pubic diastasis and weakened pelvic floor are particularly prone to vaginal and rectal prolapse; for this reason, delivery by Caesarian section is typically recommended in the exstrophy female population [106].

References

1. Buyukunal CS, Gearhart JP. A short history of bladder exstrophy. Semin Pediatr Surg. 2011;20(2):62–5.
2. Syme J. Ectopia vesicae. Lancet. 1852;2.
3. Murphy L. The history of urology. Springfield: Charles C. Thomas; 1972.
4. Trendelenburg F. De la cure operatoire de l'exstrophie vesicale et de l'epispadias. Arch Klin Chir. 1892;43:394.
5. Young, H., Exstrophy of the bladder: the first case in which a normal bladder and urinary control have been obtained by plastic operation. Surg Gynecol Obstet. 1942;74:729–37.
6. Rickham PP. Vesico-intestinal Fissure. Arch Dis Child. 1960;35(179):97–102.
7. Hollowell JG, Ransley PG. Surgical management of incontinence in bladder exstrophy. Br J Urol. 1991;68(5):543–8.
8. Lepor H, Jeffs RD. Primary bladder closure and bladder neck reconstruction in classical bladder exstrophy. J Urol. 1983;130(6):1142–5.
9. Mesrobian HG, Kelalis PP, Kramer SA. Long-term followup of 103 patients with bladder exstrophy. J Urol. 1988;139(4):719–22.
10. Stec AA. Embryology and bony and pelvic floor anatomy in the bladder exstrophy-epispadias complex. Semin Pediatr Surg. 2011;20(2):66–70.
11. Ludwig M, et al. Bladder exstrophy-epispadias complex. Birth Defects Res A Clin Mol Teratol. 2009;85(6):509–22.
12. Woodhouse CR, North AC, Gearhart JP. Standing the test of time: long-term outcome of reconstruction of the exstrophy bladder. World J Urol. 2006;24(3):244–9.
13. Ricketts RR, et al. Modern treatment of cloacal exstrophy. J Pediatr Surg. 1991;26(4):444–8; discussion 448–50
14. Gargollo PC, Borer JG. Contemporary outcomes in bladder exstrophy. Curr Opin Urol. 2007;17(4): 272–80.
15. Lattimer JK, Smith MJ. Exstrophy closure: a followup on 70 cases. J Urol. 1966;95(3):356–9.
16. Epidemiology of bladder exstrophy and epispadias: a communication from the International Clearinghouse for Birth Defects Monitoring Systems. Teratology. 1987;36(2): 221–7.
17. Nelson CP, Dunn RL, Wei JT. Contemporary epidemiology of bladder exstrophy in the United States. J Urol. 2005;173(5):1728–31.
18. Shapiro E, Lepor H, Jeffs RD. The inheritance of the exstrophy-epispadias complex. J Urol. 1984;132(2): 308–10.
19. Wood HM, Trock BJ, Gearhart JP. In vitro fertilization and the cloacal-bladder exstrophy-epispadias complex: is there an association? J Urol. 2003;169(4): 1512–5.
20. Hurwitz RS, et al. Cloacal exstrophy: a report of 34 cases. J Urol. 1987;138(4 Pt 2):1060–4.
21. Keppler-Noreuil KM. OEIS complex (omphalocele-exstrophy-imperforate anus-spinal defects): a review of 14 cases. Am J Med Genet. 2001;99(4):271–9.
22. Diamond DA, Jeffs RD. Cloacal exstrophy: a 22-year experience. J Urol. 1985;133(5):779–82.
23. Caton AR, et al. Epidemiology of bladder and cloacal exstrophies in New York State, 1983–1999. Birth Defects Res A Clin Mol Teratol. 2007;79(11): 781–7.
24. Smith NM, et al. The OEIS complex (omphalocele-exstrophy-imperforate anus-spinal defects): recurrence in sibs. J Med Genet. 1992;29(10):730–2.
25. Botto LD, Mulinare J, Erickson JD. Occurrence of omphalocele in relation to maternal multivitamin use: a population-based study. Pediatrics. 2002;109(5): 904–8.
26. Mills JL, et al. Folate and vitamin B12-related genes and risk for omphalocele. Hum Genet. 2012;131(5):739–46.
27. Reutter H, et al. Family-based association study of the MTHFR polymorphism C677T in the bladder-exstrophy-epispadias-complex. Am J Med Genet A. 2006;140(22):2506–9.
28. Gambhir L, et al. Epidemiological survey of 214 families with bladder exstrophy-epispadias complex. J Urol. 2008;179(4):1539–43.
29. Draaken M, et al. Genome-wide association study and meta-analysis identify ISL1 as genome-wide significant susceptibility gene for bladder exstrophy. PLoS Genet. 2015;11(3):e1005024.
30. Joan Ko KL, Yan G, Di Carlo H, Isaacs W, Gearhart J. Rs9291768 risk allele frequency in patients with bladder exstrophy-epispadias complex, in The Society for Pediatric Urology Annual Meeting, 2016, San Diego, CA.
31. Reutter H, et al. Genetics of bladder-exstrophy-epispadias complex (BEEC): systematic elucidation of Mendelian and multifactorial phenotypes. Curr Genomics. 2016;17(1):4–13.
32. Geoffroy-Saint-Hilaire I. Historie generale et particulaire des anomalies de lorganisation chez l'homme et les animaux, ouvrage comprenant des recherches sur les caracteres, la classification, linfluence physiologique et pathologique, les rapports generaux, les lois et les causes des monstruosities, des varietes et vices de conformation. Traite de teratologie. Paris: JP Bailliere; 1832.
33. Stec AA, et al. Classic bladder exstrophy in a non-human primate: a comparative analysis. Urology. 2002;59(2):180–3.
34. Muecke EC. The role of the Cloacal membrane in exstrophy: the first successful experimental study. J Urol. 1964;92:659–67.
35. van der Putte SC. Normal and abnormal development of the anorectum. J Pediatr Surg. 1986;21(5): 434–40.
36. Thomalla JV, et al. Induction of cloacal exstrophy in the chick embryo using the CO_2 laser. J Urol. 1985;134(5):991–5.

37. Slaughenhoupt BL, Chen CJ, Gearhart JP. Creation of a model of bladder exstrophy in the fetal lamb. J Urol. 1996;156(2 Pt 2):816–8.
38. Mildenberger H, Kluth D, Dziuba M. Embryology of bladder exstrophy. J Pediatr Surg. 1988;23(2): 166–70.
39. Fein RL. Artificial exstrophy in the dog for separated renal function studies. J Surg Res. 1969;9(4):235–9.
40. Ambrose SS, O'Brien DP 3rd. Surgical embryology of the exstrophy-epispadias complex. Surg Clin North Am. 1974;54(6):1379–90.
41. Marshall VF, Muecke EC. Handbuch de Urologie. New York: Springer-Verlag; 1968.
42. Sponseller PD, et al. The anatomy of the pelvis in the exstrophy complex. J Bone Joint Surg Am. 1995;77(2):177–89.
43. Stec AA, et al. Evaluation of the bony pelvis in classic bladder exstrophy by using 3D-CT: further insights. Urology. 2001;58(6):1030–5.
44. Stec AA, et al. Fetal bony pelvis in the bladder exstrophy complex: normal potential for growth? Urology. 2003;62(2):337–41.
45. Stec AA, et al. Pelvic floor anatomy in classic bladder exstrophy using 3-dimensional computerized tomography: initial insights. J Urol. 2001;166(4): 1444–9.
46. Williams AM, et al. 3-dimensional magnetic resonance imaging modeling of the pelvic floor musculature in classic bladder exstrophy before pelvic osteotomy. J Urol. 2004;172(4 Pt 2):1702–5.
47. Connolly JA, et al. Prevalence and repair of inguinal hernias in children with bladder exstrophy. J Urol. 1995;154(5):1900–1.
48. Silver RI, et al. Penile length in adulthood after exstrophy reconstruction. J Urol. 1997;157(3):999–1003.
49. Novak TE, et al. Polyps in the exstrophic bladder. A cause for concern? J Urol. 2005;174(4 Pt 2):1522–6; discussion 1526
50. Canning DA, et al. The cephalotrigonal reimplant in bladder neck reconstruction for patients with exstrophy or epispadias. J Urol. 1993;150(1):156–8.
51. Mathews R, et al. Cloacal exstrophy—improving the quality of life: the Johns Hopkins experience. J Urol. 1998;160(6 Pt 2):2452–6.
52. Diamond DA. Management of cloacal exstrophy. Dial Pediatr Urol. 1990;13:2.
53. McHoney M, et al. Cloacal exstrophy: morbidity associated with abnormalities of the gastrointestinal tract and spine. J Pediatr Surg. 2004;39(8):1209–13.
54. Lund DP, Hendren WH. Cloacal exstrophy: a 25-year experience with 50 cases. J Pediatr Surg. 2001;36(1):68–75.
55. Schlegel PN, Gearhart JP. Neuroanatomy of the pelvis in an infant with cloacal exstrophy: a detailed microdissection with histology. J Urol. 1989;141(3):583–5.
56. Jain M, Weaver DD. Severe lower limb defects in exstrophy of the cloaca. Am J Med Genet A. 2004;128A(3):320–4.
57. Gearhart JP, et al. Criteria for the prenatal diagnosis of classic bladder exstrophy. Obstet Gynecol. 1995;85(6):961–4.
58. Mirk P, Calisti A, Fileni A. Prenatal sonographic diagnosis of bladder exstrophy. J Ultrasound Med. 1986;5:291–3.
59. Verco PW, et al. Ectopia vesicae in utero. Australas Radiol. 1986;30(2):117–20.
60. Meizner I, Bar-Ziv J. Prenatal ultrasonic diagnosis of cloacal exstrophy. Am J Obstet Gynecol. 1985;153(7):802–3.
61. Hamada H, et al. New ultrasonographic criterion for the prenatal diagnosis of cloacal exstrophy: elephant trunk-like image. J Urol. 1999;162(6):2123–4.
62. Austin PF, et al. The prenatal diagnosis of cloacal exstrophy. J Urol. 1998;160(3 Pt 2):1179–81.
63. Arnaoutoglou C, et al. Outcome of antenatally diagnosed fetal anterior abdominal wall defects from a single tertiary centre. Fetal Diagn Ther. 2008;24(4):416–9.
64. Chan DY, Jeffs RD, Gearhart JP. Determinants of continence in the bladder exstrophy population: predictors of success? Urology. 2001;57(4):774–7.
65. Dodson JL, et al. The newborn exstrophy bladder inadequate for primary closure: evaluation, management and outcome. J Urol. 2001;165(5):1656–9.
66. Gearhart JP, et al. A combined vertical and horizontal pelvic osteotomy approach for primary and secondary repair of bladder exstrophy. J Urol. 1996;155(2):689–93.
67. Wild AT, et al. The role of osteotomy in surgical repair of bladder exstrophy. Semin Pediatr Surg. 2011;20(2):71–8.
68. Hanna MK. Reconstruction of umbilicus during functional closure of bladder exstrophy. Urology. 1986;27(4):340–2.
69. Gearhart JP, Jeffs RD. Management of the failed exstrophy closure. J Urol. 1991;146(2 Pt 2): 610–2.
70. Grady RW, Mitchell ME. Complete primary repair of exstrophy. J Urol. 1999;162(4):1415–20.
71. Mitchell ME, Bagli DJ. Complete penile disassembly for epispadias repair: the Mitchell technique. J Urol. 1996;155(1):300–4.
72. Husmann DA, Gearhart JP. Loss of the penile glans and/or corpora following primary repair of bladder exstrophy using the complete penile disassembly technique. J Urol. 2004;172(4 Pt 2):1696–700; discussion 1700–1
73. Jarzebowski AC, et al. The Kelly technique of bladder exstrophy repair: continence, cosmesis and pelvic organ prolapse outcomes. J Urol. 2009;182(4 Suppl):1802–6.
74. Stolar CH, Randolph JG, Flanigan LP. Cloacal exstrophy: individualized management through a staged surgical approach. J Pediatr Surg. 1990;25(5):505–7.
75. Soffer SZ, et al. Cloacal exstrophy: a unified management plan. J Pediatr Surg. 2000;35(6):932–7.

76. Howell C, et al. Optimal management of cloacal exstrophy. J Pediatr Surg. 1983;18(4):365–9.
77. Phillips TM. Spectrum of cloacal exstrophy. Semin Pediatr Surg. 2011;20(2):113–8.
78. Sawaya D, Gearhart JP. Gastrointestinal reconstruction and outcomes for patients with the OEIS complex. Semin Pediatr Surg. 2011;20(2):123–5.
79. Gearhart JP, Jeffs RD. Techniques to create urinary continence in the cloacal exstrophy patient. J Urol. 1991;146(2 Pt 2):616–8.
80. Silver RI, Sponseller PD, Gearhart JP. Staged closure of the pelvis in cloacal exstrophy: first description of a new approach. J Urol. 1999;161(1):263–6.
81. Mathews R, et al. Staged pelvic closure of extreme pubic diastasis in the exstrophy-epispadias complex. J Urol. 2006;176(5):2196–8.
82. Thomas JC, et al. First stage approximation of the exstrophic bladder in patients with cloacal exstrophy—should this be the initial surgical approach in all patients? J Urol. 2007;178(4 Pt 2):1632–5; discussion 1635–6
83. Sawaya D, et al. Gastrointestinal ramifications of the cloacal exstrophy complex: a 44-year experience. J Pediatr Surg. 2010;45(1):171–5; discussion 175–6
84. Mitchell ME, Plaire C. Management of cloacal exstrophy. Adv Exp Med Biol. 2002;511:267–70; discussion 270–3.
85. Novak TE, et al. Failed exstrophy closure: management and outcome. J Pediatr Urol. 2010;6(4):381–4.
86. Meldrum KK, Baird AD, Gearhart JP. Pelvic and extremity immobilization after bladder exstrophy closure: complications and impact on success. Urology. 2003;62(6):1109–13.
87. Baker LA, Jeffs RD, Gearhart JP. Urethral obstruction after primary exstrophy closure: what is the fate of the genitourinary tract? J Urol. 1999;161(2):618–21.
88. Husmann DA. Surgery insight: advantages and pitfalls of surgical techniques for the correction of bladder exstrophy. Nat Clin Pract Urol. 2006;3(2): 95–100.
89. Schaeffer AJ, et al. Complications of primary closure of classic bladder exstrophy. J Urol. 2008;180(4 Suppl):1671–4; discussion 1674
90. Husmann DA, McLorie GA, Churchill BM. Closure of the exstrophic bladder: an evaluation of the factors leading to its success and its importance on urinary continence. J Urol. 1989;142(2 Pt 2):522–4; discussion 542–3
91. Cervellione RM, et al. Penile ischemic injury in the exstrophy/epispadias spectrum: new insights and possible mechanisms. J Pediatr Urol. 2010;6(5):450–6.
92. Schaeffer AJ, et al. Complete primary repair of bladder exstrophy: a single institution referral experience. J Urol. 2011;186(3):1041–6.
93. Lazarus J. Penile loss following complete primary repair of bladder exstrophy. J Pediatr Urol. 2009;5(6):519–20.
94. Levitt MA, et al. Cloacal exstrophy—pull-through or permanent stoma? A review of 53 patients. J Pediatr Surg. 2008;43(1):164–8; discussion 168–70
95. Shnorhavorian M, et al. Long-term followup of complete primary repair of exstrophy: the Seattle experience. J Urol. 2008;180(4 Suppl):1615–9; discussion 1619–20
96. Surer I, et al. Combined bladder neck reconstruction and epispadias repair for exstrophy-epispadias complex. J Urol. 2001;165(6 Pt 2):2425–7.
97. Gearhart JP, et al. The multiple reoperative bladder exstrophy closure: what affects the potential of the bladder? Urology. 1996;47(2):240–3.
98. Lee RS, et al. Can a complete primary repair approach be applied to cloacal exstrophy? J Urol. 2006;176(6 Pt 1):2643–8.
99. Mathews R. Achieving urinary continence in cloacal exstrophy. Semin Pediatr Surg. 2011;20(2):126–9.
100. Miles-Thomas J, Gearhart JP, Gearhart SL. An initial evaluation of pelvic floor function and quality of life of bladder exstrophy patients after ureterosigmoidostomy. J Gastrointest Surg. 2006;10(4): 473–7.
101. El-Hout Y, et al. Do patients with classic bladder exstrophy have fecal incontinence? A web-based study. Urology. 2010;75(5):1166–8.
102. Wilson CJ, et al. The psychosocial impact of bladder exstrophy in adolescence. J Adolesc Health. 2007;41(5):504–8.
103. Reiner WG. A brief primer for pediatric urologists and surgeons on developmental psychopathology in the exstrophy-epispadias complex. Semin Pediatr Surg. 2011;20(2):130–4.
104. Reiner WG, Gearhart JP, Jeffs R. Psychosexual dysfunction in males with genital anomalies: late adolescence, Tanner stages IV to VI. J Am Acad Child Adolesc Psychiatry. 1999;38(7):865–72.
105. Woodhouse CR, Hinsch R. The anatomy and reconstruction of the adult female genitalia in classical exstrophy. Br J Urol. 1997;79(4):618–22.
106. Mathews RI, Gan M, Gearhart JP. Urogynaecological and obstetric issues in women with the exstrophy-epispadias complex. BJU Int. 2003;91(9):845–9.
107. Ebert AK, et al. Genital and reproductive function in males after functional reconstruction of the exstrophy-epispadias complex—long-term results. Urology. 2008;72(3):566–9; discussion 569–70
108. D'Hauwers KW, Feitz WF, Kremer JA. Bladder exstrophy and male fertility: pregnancies after ICSI with ejaculated or epididymal sperm. Fertil Steril. 2008;89(2):387–9.

Part VII

Nervous System

Hydrocephalus

49

Jawad Yousaf, Stephano R. Parlato,
and Conor L. Mallucci

Abstract

The term Hydrocephalus relates to the presence of an excessive amount of cerebrospinal fluid (CSF), which may cause an increase in intracranial pressure with or without associated abnormal enlargement of the cerebral ventricles. Hydrocephalus is not a single pathological disease entity rather it is secondary to a variety of pathological processes or insults that cause an imbalance between the production and absorption of CSF.

Keywords

Hydrocephalus • Pathophysiology • Classification • Venticulo-peritoneal shunt • Ventriculostomy

49.1 Introduction

The term Hydrocephalus relates to the presence of an excessive amount of cerebrospinal fluid (CSF), which may cause an increase in intracranial pressure with or without associated abnormal enlargement of the cerebral ventricles. Hydrocephalus is not a single pathological disease entity rather it is secondary to a variety of pathological processes or insults that cause an imbalance between the production and absorption of CSF. The estimated prevalence of congenital and infantile hydrocephalus is between 0.5 and 0.8 per 1000 births (live and still) [1–3].

The treatment of hydrocephalus has been revolutionized since the advent of shunts in 1950s. This transformed a usually fatal condition into a manageable disease. While CSF shunting remains the mainstay of treatment for neonatal hydrocephalus, endoscopic third ventriculostomy is an important surgical treatment option in certain disease entities. Better understanding of CSF dynamics and pathophysiology and technological advances in neuro-imaging, neuro-navigation and shunt hardware have allowed for a patient specific approach in management of this complex pathological entity. Early diagnosis and treatment is warranted to limit pathological damage, maximise neurological development and improve patient outcome.

J. Yousaf, MBBS, MRCS • S.R. Parlato, MD
Alder Hey Children's NHS Foundation Trust,
Liverpool, UK

C.L. Mallucci, MBBS, FRCS(Surgical Neurology) (✉)
Department of Neurosurgery, Alder Hey Children's
NHS Foundation Trust, Liverpool, UK
e-mail: conor.mallucci@alderhey.nhs.uk

P.D. Losty et al. (eds.), *Rickham's Neonatal Surgery*, https://doi.org/10.1007/978-1-4471-4721-3_49

49.1.1 CSF Physiology

The total CSF volume, on average, is 140 mL and this is divided between the ventricular system (25% or 35 mL), spinal canal (30—70 mL) and the cranial subarachnoid space [4–9]. In young children the total amount of CSF is smaller, around 70 ml, divided between the various compartments in a way similar to adults. The three components influencing CSF dynamics are production, circulation and drainage. Most CSF is produced by a highly vascular ingrowth through the ependymal lining of the ventricles known as the choroid plexus (Fig. 49.1). CSF is derived by adenosine triphosphate (ATP) dependant active secretion from cerebral arterial blood across epithelial walls. Mean CSF production in humans is 0.36 mL/min (approximately 20 mL/h, or 500 mL/day) although in young children the total daily production is smaller than in adults, possibly half [5–8, 10–14]. The choroid plexus has a blood supply ten times that of the cortex, and can produce CSF at a rate up to 0.21 mL/min/g tissue, a rate higher than any other secretory epithelium. The current widely accepted view is that CSF circulation is via bulk flow [15]. CSF is produced mainly within the lateral, third and fourth ventricles. Net bulk flow occurs from the lateral to the third ventricle via the foramen of Monro, on into the fourth ventricle via the aqueduct of Sylvius, and then out of the fourth ventricle via the midline foramen of Magendie, and the lateral foramina of Lushka into the subarachnoid space [16] (Fig. 49.2). Once produced, CSF circulation is limited by the cells, membranes, and junctional barriers lining the ventricular and subarachnoid spaces. The dynamics of CSF flow are in part governed by these anatomical configurations, and hence abnormalities within the system can affect CSF flow. The subarachnoid space comprises of an interconnecting network of basal CSF cisterns. CSF rapidly moves around the basal cisterns, and then moves more slowly into the subarachnoid space on the cortical convexity and to a lesser extent the spinal subarachnoid space, until reabsorption into the systemic circulation occurs via the venous system at the arachnoid

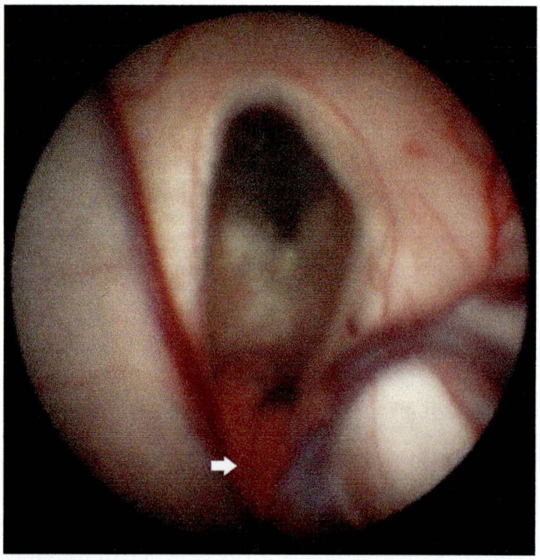

Fig. 49.1 Endoscopic view of the right foramen of Monro showing the choroid plexus (*white arrow*)

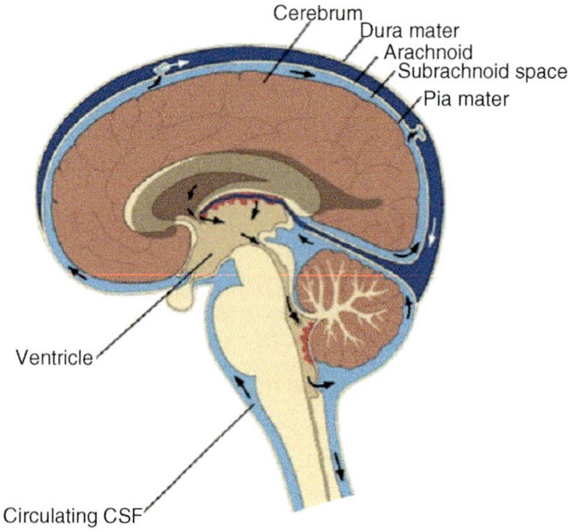

Fig. 49.2 CSF drainage pathways. A schematic section through the brain and spinal cord showing the drainage pathways for CSF. The CSF is formed by the choroid plexuses of the lateral ventricles with a small portion derived from fluid exudate from the cerebral parenchyma. Once formed the CSF passes through the foramina of Monro into the third ventricle. CSF then flows through the cerebral aqueduct of Sylvius into the fourth ventricle, which has a single-sided sheet-like plexus. From there fluid exits into the various basal cisterns and then into the subarachnoid space through paired foramina of Luschka and the single foramen of Magendie. CSF flows through SAS over the surface of the cortex. Some fluid drains back into the blood via the arachnoid granulations into the superior sagittal sinus, some via the spinal nerve roots and the remainder via the olfactory tracts

granulations in the superior sagittal sinus, the lymphatics across the cribiform plate, and the nerve root subarachnoid angles [17].

49.1.2 Classification

The classification of hydrocephalus remains a source of continued discussion due to our evolving understanding of pathogenesis and treatment of hydrocephalus. Hydrocephalus can be classified as Obstructive (block proximal to arachnoid granulations) and Communicating (block at arachnoid granulations) or Congenital and Acquired (see Box 49.1).

49.1.3 New Concepts

Recently Rekate [18] has defined hydrocephalus as "an active distention of ventricular system of the brain resulting from inadequate passage of cerebrospinal fluid and its point of production within the cerebral ventricles to its point of absorption into the systemic circulation". This concept assumes all hydrocephalus to be obstructive and defines hydrocephalus as an active process with a mismatch between CSF production and absorption. Rekate classification is based on point of obstruction and developed on a mathematical model. Figure 49.3 shows different points of obstruction along the CSF pathway.

Box 49.1 Common causes of hydrocephalus

Congenital causes

- Chiari malformation or spina bifida
- Danday-Walker complex
- Atresia of foramen of Munroe
- Aqueduct stenosis (X-linked)
- Congenital arachnoid cysts

Acquired causes

- Haemorrhage
- Infection
- Traumatic head injury
- Tumour

49.2 Causes of Hydrocephalus

49.2.1 Post-haemorrhagic

Intraventricular haemorrhage (IVH) is one of the most serious complications in premature infants and an important cause of mortality and long-term neurological sequelae in this group.

When infants are born prematurely, they are essentially arrested at a gestational stage during which the development of the highly vascularized germinal matrix in the brain is ongoing. Because the capillary network of this structure is still anatomically immature in these infants, the vessels are especially fragile and susceptible to rupture in the face of fluctuating cerebral blood flow or cerebral venous pressure, both common in premature babies, especially during periods of respiratory distress. If these vessels rupture, it can result in bleeding into the germinal matrix and subsequently into the ventricles of the brain [19]. The subsequent development of hydrocephalus is usually ascribed to fibrosing arachnoiditis, meningeal fibrosis and subependymal gliosis, which impair flow and resorption of cerebrospinal fluid (CSF).

IVH is characterized by a spectrum of lesions amenable to classification by grade of severity. The first classification scheme, proposed by Papile et al. [20] was based on computerized tomography (CT) scan findings of the extent of bleeding and recognizes four grades of IVH that are cumulative and numbered from mild to severe:

- Grade I: germinal matrix hemorrhage (GMH) only
- Grade II: GMH + IVH with no ventricular distension
- Grade III: GMH + IVH + ventricular distension
- Grade IV: GMH + IVH + intraparenchymal hemorrhage

Mild IVH (grades I and II) is generally benign [21], while grade III and particularly grade IV may be related to early complications, such as posthemorrhagic hydrocephalus (PHH) with

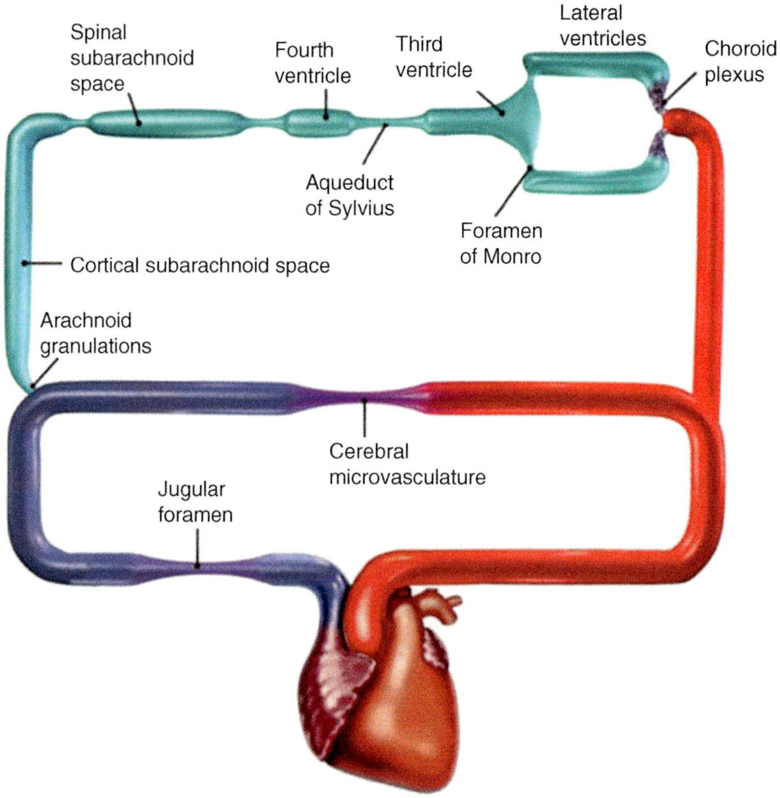

Fig. 49.3 Intracranial hydrodynamics represented as a circuit diagram with a parallel pathway of CSF flow and cerebral blood flow [18]

concomitant neurodevelopmental disabilities and high mortality. Grades II and III include intraventricular hemorrhages of variable severity as judged by the percentage of ventricle that contains blood or by the presence or absence of ventricular enlargement. IVH occurs in approximately 80% of cases with germinal matrix bleeding [22]. If the hemorrhage is large, it may even extend into adjacent parenchymal tissue [20], where the degree of injury dramatically impacts the neurological outcome. The correlation between the development of IVH and the actual gestational age at birth is thus dependent upon the stage of anatomical development of the germinal matrix, with the occurrence of IVH relatively uncommon after week 32. Estimated frequencies of germinal matrix bleeding and IVH range from 50 to 75% for infants born at less than 26 weeks, decline sharply after the 30th week of gestation, and decrease to less than 5% among unselected full-term infants [23].

The term post-hemorrhagic hydrocephalus (PHH) is generally applied when there is progressive accumulation of cerebral spinal fluid (CSF) under pressure with ventricular ballooning (ventriculomegaly or VM) and accompanying enlargement of the head [19, 24] (Figs. 49.4 and 49.5). VM typically develops 1–3 weeks following the initial intraventricular bleed [25, 26] in 55–80% of the IVH population, with 26–85% of these cases progressing to PHH. PHH should be suspected whenever IVH of grade II or higher is diagnosed.

PHH typically presents with symptoms of rising ICP, including apnea, vomiting, and abnormal posture, as well as rapidly increasing head circumference that crosses over the initial percentile or enlarges over 1.5 cm per week, a bulging anterior fontanel, and separation of the cranial sutures. However, the measurement of an enlarged head circumference is not sufficiently sensitive to aid in the diagnosis of hydrocephalus in the premature infant because ventricular dilatation can occur days to weeks prior to a detectable increase in the rate of head growth [27]. For the majority (65%) of newborns with PHH, the

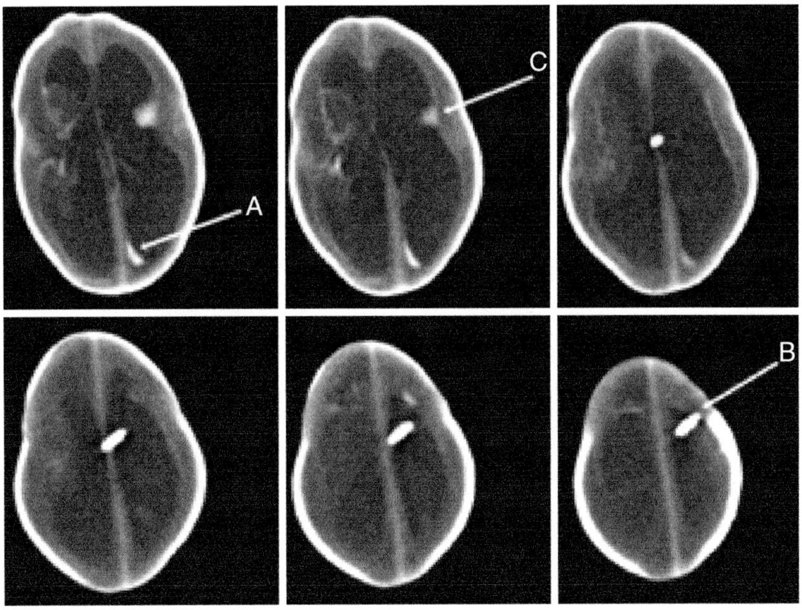

Fig. 49.4 Non-contrast axial CT (corrected age 29 weeks) images demonstrating the presence of a small amount of intraventricular hemorrhage (layering posteriorly within the occipital horn of the left lateral ventricle) (*A*), ventriculomegaly and the left frontal ventricular catheter portion of a ventricular catheter-reservoir (*B*). Small regions of thrombus are present within the lateral ventricles (*C*)

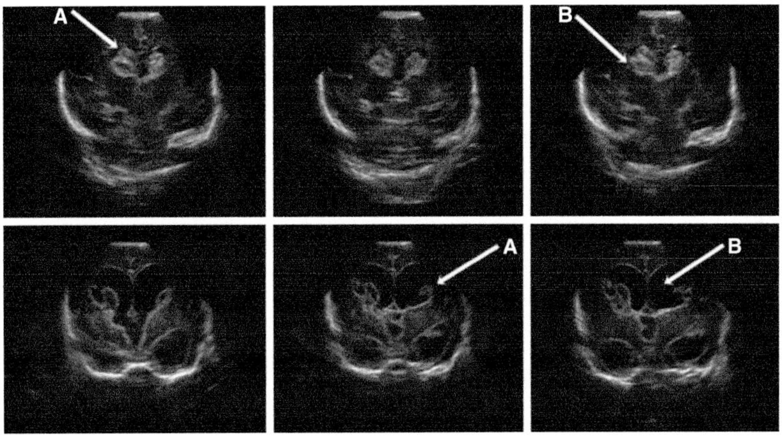

Fig. 49.5 *Upper panel*: Coronal cranial ultrasound images (corrected age 27 weeks) demonstrating the presence of bilateral IVH (*A*), right caudate nucleus hemorrhage (*B*) and ventriculomegaly. *Lower panel*: Subsequent cranial ultrasound images (corrected age 29 weeks) show evolving IVH (*A*) and progressive ventriculomegaly (*B*)

condition resolves spontaneously within a month, either regressing or stabilizing at an acceptable ICP (<approximately 80–110 mmH_2O), and these patients never require medical or surgical intervention [22]. Therefore, if the monitored progression continues at a slow rate, surveillance alone is the most appropriate management program. However, if close monitoring reveals rapid progression (increase in serial head circumference measurements of 2 cm/week with a full fontanel and split sutures) or if the slow progression persists beyond 2–4 weeks, interventions are indicated [28, 29].

The risk of IVH in the pre-term infant has been significantly reduced by measures that may indirectly ameliorate fluctuations in cerebral blood flow such as surfactant to reduce pulmonary hypertension and antenatal steroid administration [30, 31]. Some also advocate that premature infants should be maintained on paralytics and sedation for the first 72 h following birth to reduce the risk of IVH [31]. Once PHH has been diagnosed radiologically, temporising interventional methods may be employed as some patients may either be too unstable for surgery or their hydrocephalus resolves with degradation of the IVH without obvious lasting imbalance to the CSF dynamics. Most cases of PHH occurs 3–4 weeks after IVH but it is important to note that many of these cases are clinically silent and early detection requires a high index of suspicion and serial radiological monitoring. Of those that develop PHH, over 50% become shunt dependant with a high rate of neurodevelopmental disabilities.

More recently, the DRIFT trial has suggested reduction in cognitive disability at 2 years in premature neonates with PHH treated with continuous ventricle washout and intraventricular infusion of Tissue Plasminogen Activator [32]. The treatment did not have any impact on the incidence of shunt dependence. Medical and surgical management options for PHH are discussed in the proceeding sections of this chapter.

49.2.2 Post-infectious

Post infectious hydrocephalus (PIH) is an important cause of hydrocephalus is the developed world and is most common cause of hydrocephalus in the developing world. Intrauterine infection can cause hydrocephalus when they involve the central nervous system. Infection not only impairs CSF flow and absorption but also compromise parenchymal development. These infections include Toxoplasmosis, cytomegalovirus, mumps and syphilis. Postnatal meningitis may result from amniotic infection where the membranes have been ruptured for a prolonged period. In the first 2 weeks of life, the organism is usually Escherichia coli and other Gram-negative enteric bacilli. In the second 2-week period, the pathogens are more likely to be Gram-positive cocci, Listeria and Pseudomonas [33–35]. In low birth weight neonates, pathogenic organisms include coagulase negative staphalococci, gram positive cocci and Candida species. In the developing world B-haemolytic streptococci and tuberculosis remain important causes of neonatal hydrocephalus. PIH typically occurs 2–3 weeks following diagnosis of bacterial meningitis and studies have shown that associated complications include abscess formation, ventriculitis and subsequent CSF loculations and intraventricular septations [35, 36]. The management is difficult and frequently requires multiple shunt placements and revisions with associated poor developmental outcome and high morbidity and mortality rates.

49.2.3 Chiari Malformation and Spina Bifida

Chiari malformations are a group of conditions with different etiologies which involve abnormalities in the posterior fossa and craniovertebral junction. These abnormalities are often associated with the presence of hydrocephalus due to changes they cause in cerebrospinal fluid (CSF) flow at the level of the craniovertebral junction. The Chiari I malformation (CM I), or hindbrain herniation syndrome, consists of downward herniation of the cerebellar tonsils through the foramen magnum into the cervical spinal canal [37, 38]. The degree of displacement is typically greater than 5 mm below the plane of the foramen magnum on sagittal magnetic resonance image (MRI) [38–42]. The vermis, fourth ventricle and brainstem are relatively normal. Syringomyelia occurs in 45–68% of cases [41, 43, 44]. It is associated with scoliosis in 42%, abnormal retroflexed odontoid process in 26%, and basilar invagination in 12% [39, 40, 42, 45–47]. The average age of onset is in the mid 30s, but it can occur in those as young as 3 months [45].

Chronic tonsillar herniation in CM I is most likely secondary to underdevelopment of the occipital bone and overcrowding of the cerebellum in a small posterior fossa. The fundamental defect is thought to involve underdevelopment of the occipital somites originating from the paraaxial mesoderm.

The most common symptom, occurring in up to 81% of patients, is suboccipital headache that is worsened with head dependency and valsalva-type maneuvers such as coughing, straining and exertion [48–50]. Over 70% of patients present with either ocular disturbances (such as diplopia, blurred vision or retro-orbital pain), or otoneurological disturbances (such as dizziness, disequilibrium, tinnitus or ear pressure). Lower cranial nerve, brainstem and cerebellar findings include dysphagia, sleep apnea, dysarthria, tremors, impaired gag reflex and poor coordination. Permanent nocturnal central hypoventilation requiring ventilation has been reported [51]. Sensory and motor findings due to spinal cord dysfunction are common, especially when associated with syringomyelia. Over 90% of patients with syringomyelia present with spinal cord disturbances such as paresthesias, pain, burning dysesthesias or anesthesia, weakness, spasticity, atrophy, incontinence, trophic phenomena, impaired position sense, or hyperreflexia [52]. Scoliosis, which can occur in children with Chiari I—related syringomyelia, has been shown to improve following craniovertebral decompression.

The Chiari II malformation (CM II) is intimately associated with myelomeningocele, and involves vermian herniation with descent of the brainstem and fourth ventricle through a widened foramen magnum (see Fig. 49.6). The vermian "peg" may descend as low as the upper thoracic level [52–54]. Other findings include cerebellar inversion with absent cisterna magna ("banana sign" on ultrasonography), hypoplastic tentorium that inserts very low placing the torcular herophili just above the foramen magnum, and a medullary "kink" in two thirds of patients due to posterior displacement of a relatively mobile medulla along with a fixed spinal cord [52–54]. CM II is associated with many brain anomalies. Skull findings include enlarged foramen magnum, craniolacunia, scalloping of the petrous bones, jugular tubercles and frontal bone (known as the lemon sign on ultrasound), increased concavity of the basioccipital clivus, low inion and sometimes basilar impression and assimilation of the atlas [52, 55, 56]. Cerebral findings include enlarged massa intermedia, polygyria, and agenesis of the corpus callosum. Below-average intelligence occurs in over half of patients [57]. Other findings include prominent anterior commissure, absence of the falx with interdigitation of the occipital and parietal lobes, agenesis of the olfactory tract, absence of the cingulate gyrus, heterotopic gray matter, fusion of the colliculi (tectal beaking), cranial nerve nuclei malformation, and decreased cerebellar volume with dysplastic or absent folia. In CM II, cranial and upper cervical nerves display an upward course [52].

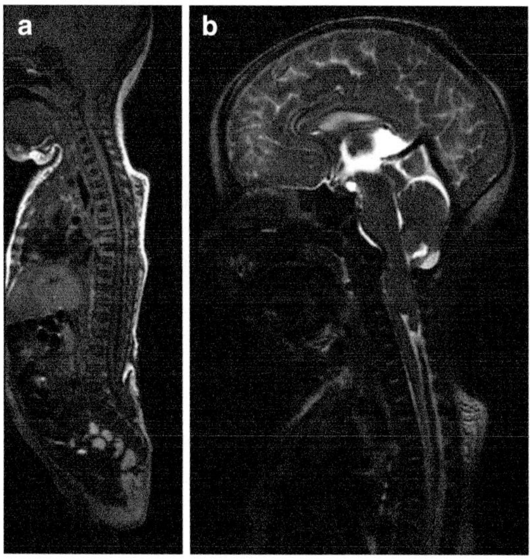

Fig. 49.6 Sagittal T1 (**a**) and T2 (**b**) weighted MRI images obtained following closure of lumbosacral myelomeningocoele demonstrating Chiari II malformation

CSF flow abnormalities are abundant in CM II. Hydrocephalus is seen in approximately 90% [52] (see Fig. 49.7). Other common ventricular abnormalities include a small, elongated low lying fourth ventricle that can be displaced into the cervical canal, with outwardly projecting choroid plexus (embryological location), small aqueduct, "shark tooth deformity" of the third ventricle (anterior diverticulum), colpocephalic lateral ventricles, "beaking" of the frontal horns, occasionally absent inferior medullary velum and occasionally absent foramen of Magendie [52]. Development of the CM II is likely associated with the open neural tube defect and drainage of CSF through the central canal during development [58]. Without ventricular distention, the posterior fossa does not develop normally. This theory also explains the development of hydrocephalus, due to blocked CSF outflow at the foramina of Lushka and Magendie [58]. Nearly every patient with CM II presents initially with an open neural tube defect. Frequently, the diagnosis is made in utero.

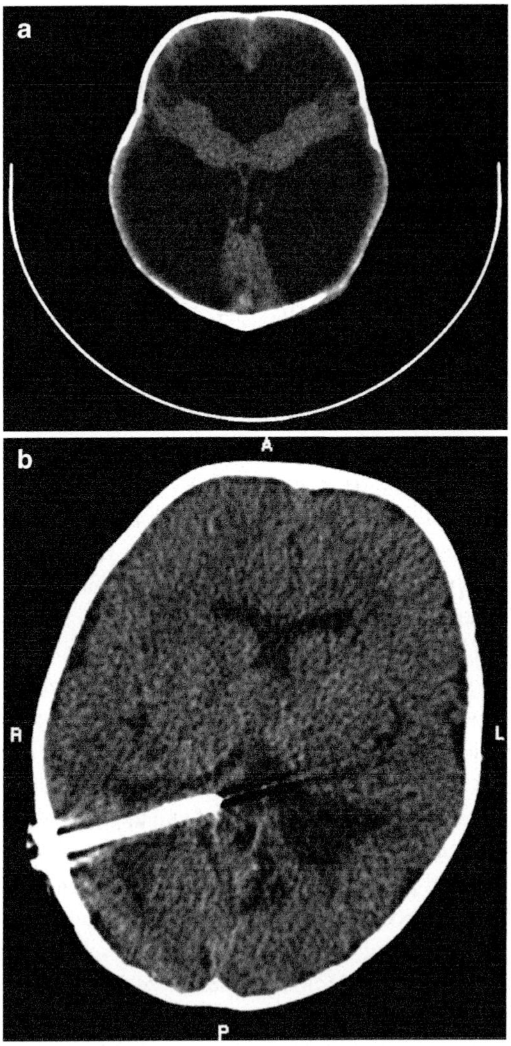

Fig. 49.7 Axial CT images demonstrating ventriculomegaly (**a**). The hydrocephalus was treated with insertion of ventriculoperitoneal shunt with resolution of ventriculomegaly as demonstrated on the CT scan obtained 1 year after shunt insertion (**b**)

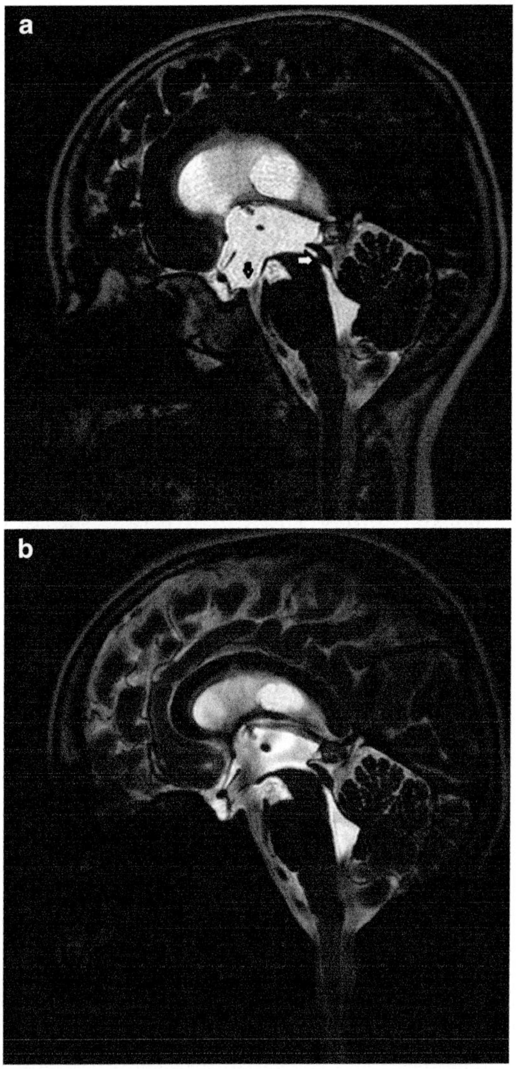

Fig. 49.8 CINE sequence sagittal MRI images demonstrating membranous occlusion of the aqueduct with dilatation of the proximal part of the aqueduct (*white arrow*) and depressed floor of the third ventricle (*black arrow*) indicating hydrocephalus (**a**). This was treated with endoscopic third ventriculostomy. Post operative CINE sequence MRI image demonstrates restoration of the normal architecture of the third ventricular floor and a flow void in the prepontine CSF cistern demonstrating patent third ventriculostomy (**b**)

Symptoms attributable to CM II vary with age. In all age groups, symptoms are worsened with the presence of hydrocephalus.

49.2.4 Aqueduct Stenosis

Aqueductal stenosis is responsible of 6–66% of cases of hydrocephalus in children (more than 50% presenting in the first year of life) [59–61] (Fig. 49.8). Ceddia and co-workers reported an incidence of congenital hydrocephalus of 0.3–2.5/thousand born alive, 20% associated to aqueduct stenosis [62]. There is a mild male prevalence and there are two peaks of distribution for age including one in the first year of life [59]. In about three quarters of patients with aqueduct

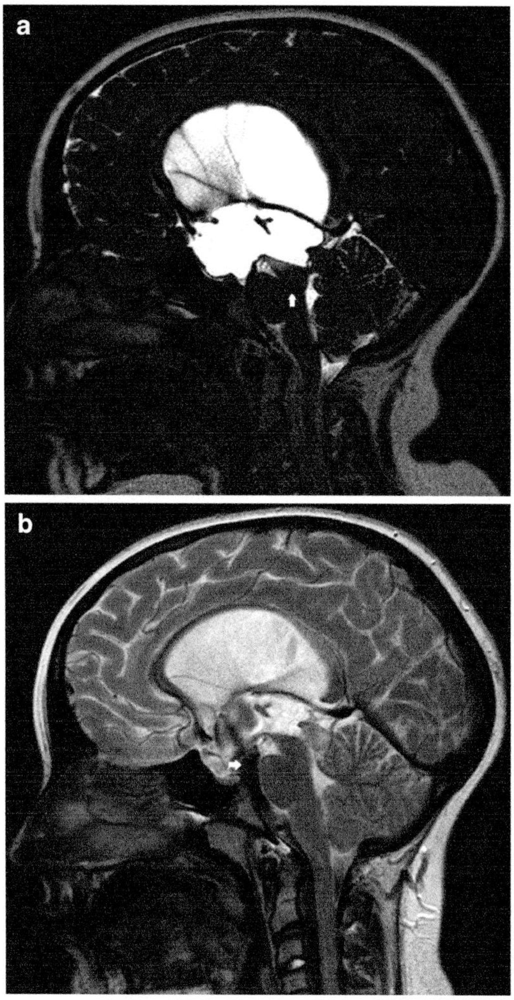

Fig. 49.9 Pre-operative (**a**) and postoperative (**b**) CINE sequence sagittal MRI images demonstrating hydrocephalus secondary to a tectal plate tumour (*white arrow*) causing aqueduct stenosis. Again note the depressed floor of the third ventricle in (**a**). This was treated with Endoscopic third ventriculostomy. Note the flow void through the ventriculostomy (*white arrow*) in (**b**)

stenosis the etiology of the disorder is not known [60]. In remaining cases it can be attributed to different causes including rare X-linked syndromic cases, infectious, haemorrhagic, neoplastic (e.g. tectal tumours) (Fig. 49.9), and vascular (Vein of galen aneurysms). Aqueductal stenosis has also been reported in association with different CNS malformations, such as Spina Bifida, Dandy-Walker complex, retrocerebellar and supracollicular cysts [60, 63, 64].

49.2.5 Dandy Walker Complex

The classic Dandy Walker Malformation (DWM) is defined by the presence of a large median posterior fossa cyst (diverticulum) widely communicating with the fourth ventricle, associated with a rotated, elevated and hypoplastic or aplastic cerebellar vermis contacting an upwardly displaced tentorium and similarly displaced transverse sinuses. There is in addition posterior bossing of the posterior fossa contributing to its enlargement and antero-lateral displacement of normal or hypoplastic cerebellar hemispheres [65]. The cystic dilatation of the fourth ventricle fills the posterior fossa and extends into the cisterna magna, which is compressed between the dilated fourth ventricle and the posterior fossa dura. The cystic CSF collection in the posterior fossa does not communicate freely with the basal cisterns (Fig. 49.10).

Dandy Walker Complex (DWC) was described by Berkovich et al. to denote a spectrum of disorders including classic DWM at one extreme all of which include a cyst communicating with the fourth ventricle [66]. The crucial point according to Barkovich et al. is to assess the axial images at the mid-fourth ventricle level; no vermian tissue interposed between the fourth ventricle and the cyst indicates a Type A DWC which is either a classic DWM or a 'Dandy Walker Variant' (DWV). The Dandy Walker Variant being, effectively, the same widely communicating cyst without all of the features of a classic DWM, particularly the enlargement of the posterior fossa. If vermis is interposed between the cyst and the fourth ventricle at the level of the mid-fourth ventricle then this is referred to as a type B DWC lesion, the equivalent, traditional term being mega cisterna magna (MCM).

Dandy walker complex accounts for around 4% of all cases of hydrocephalus with the incidence of the order of 1:25,000–1:30,000 live births [67–69]. The majority of foetuses with prenatally diagnosed DWM or DWV will not survive to term [70].

The Dandy Walker Complex can arise in the context of mendelian disorders, chromosomal disorders (trisomies, deletions and duplications)

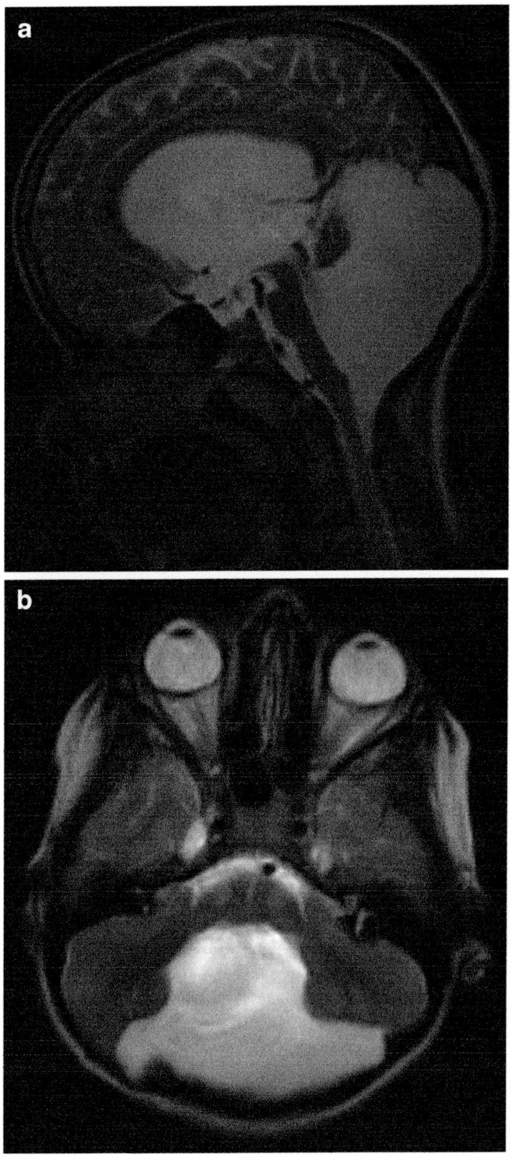

Fig. 49.10 Dandy Walker Malformation (DWM). T2 W MR images in the midsagittal (**a**) and mid-fourth ventricle axial (**b**) plains show the salient features of the classic DWM namely the rotated and partially agenetic vermis, the high insertion of the torcular, the enlarged posterior fossa and the wide communication between the fourth ventricle proper and the 'cyst'. Note the widely patent aqueduct with flow void

and with teratogen exposure (alcohol, viral infection, drugs). In addition the DWC may be associated with other brain malformations in 68% of cases [71] including aqueduct stenosis, callosal agenesis and neural tube defects. In addition significant extracerebral malformations; particularly of the heart, the kidneys, the palate, the perineum and the vertebrae, are present in about 45% [67, 68]. For these reasons it is imperative that every new case of the DWC is assessed by a clinical geneticist and other abnormalities identified.

49.2.6 Craniosynostosis

Craniosynostosis is an uncommon cause of neonatal hydrocephalus. The pathogenesis of hydrocephalus in craniosynostosis involves mechanical obstruction of CSF outflow due to crowding of the posterior fossa [72] and impaired CSF absorption resulting from venous outlet obstruction [72].

49.2.7 Uncommon Congenital Malformations

49.2.7.1 Encephalocoele

The term encephalocoele is used to describe all congenital cranial herniations. Traditionally encephalocoeles are divisible into posterior and anterior encephalocoeles. Posterior lesions are commoner and classified into parietal and occipital lesions with the occipital lesions including supra and infratorcular subtypes. These are cystic swellings with variable skin coverage. A significant subgroup of these includes the atretic encephalocoele, which is usually flat and non-cystic. The rarer anterior encephalocoeles are herniations through the anterior skull base and they are classified as, sincipital, where the herniation is through the foramen cecum anterior to the cribriform plate or basal where the herniation is through the sphenoid bone and sinus.

Posterior encephalocoeles are associated with very significant brain abnormalities including hydrocephalus, agenesis of the corpus callosum, DWC, grey matter heterotopias and venous drainage anomalies (Fig. 49.11). Parietal lesions are

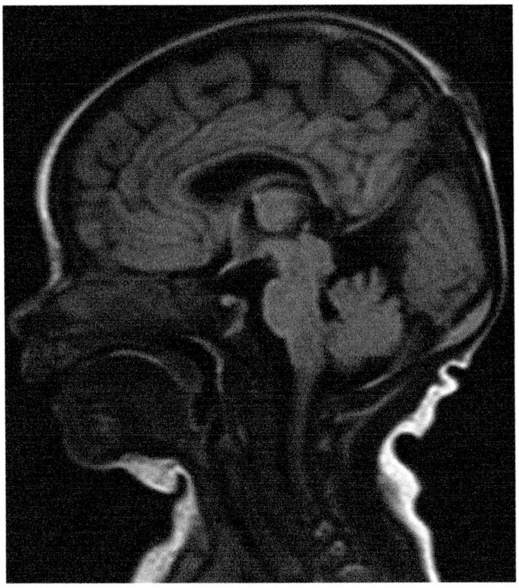

Fig. 49.11 Sagittal T1-weighted MRI scan of a new born with a midline occipital lump covered with tuft of hair. The lesion was resected and histology confirmed it to be an encephalocoele. Note the aberrant straight sinus

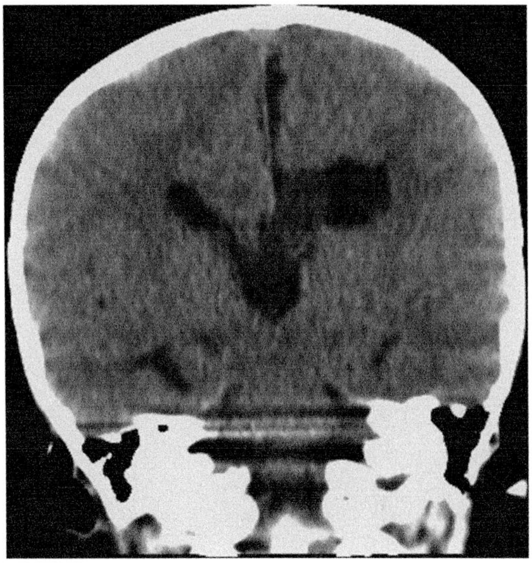

Fig. 49.12 Coronal CT image showing partial agenesis of the corpus callosum and an associated cyst

particularly associated with dorsal interhemispheric cysts which may communicate directly with the ventricular system, in extreme cases they may be associated with holoprosencephaly. MRI is mandatory before exploring these lesions to delineate other abnormalities and MRV may help delineate venous anatomy which is frequently abnormal. The incidence of hydrocephalus in encephalocoeles is variably reported with the association reportedly higher with posterior encephalocoeles.

49.2.7.2 Agenesis of Corpus Callosum

The corpus callosum is the major commissural structure and its complete or partial agenesis is a common brain malformation with a prevalence of 0.5–70 per 10,000 in children with developmental delay. It is rarely isolated and is often associated with other serious brain malformations i.e., DWC, Chiari malformations, holoprosencephaly and interhemispheric cysts [73] (Fig. 49.12).

A large survey of the aetiology of congenital hydrocephalus indicated that agenesis of the corpus callosum was a relatively common cause of foetal and to a lesser extent infantile hydrocephalus [74]. In a large literature review encompassing 705 cases of agenesis of the corpus callosum (ACC) hydrocephalus was present in some 23%, often associated with distinct syndromic states (Aicardi, Acrocallosal, Andermann and Shapiro syndromes) [75]. More recently it has been realised that X-linked hydrocephalus overlaps with X-linked agenesis of the corpus callosum and a number of other conditions resulting in a spectrum of disorders which include all or some of: corpus callosum hypolpasia, mental retardation, adducted thumbs, spastic paraplegia and hydrocephalus. It has gained the acronym CRASH syndrome and they are related to mutation in the L1 cellular adhesion molecule gene [76]. ACC can be associated with the finding of interhemispheric arachnoid cysts which again may be related to hydrocephalus.

49.2.7.3 Hydrancephaly

Hydranencephaly describes a severe brain malformation in which, although remnants of nonfunctional cortex may be present, there is an extensive reduction in brain parenchyma that has

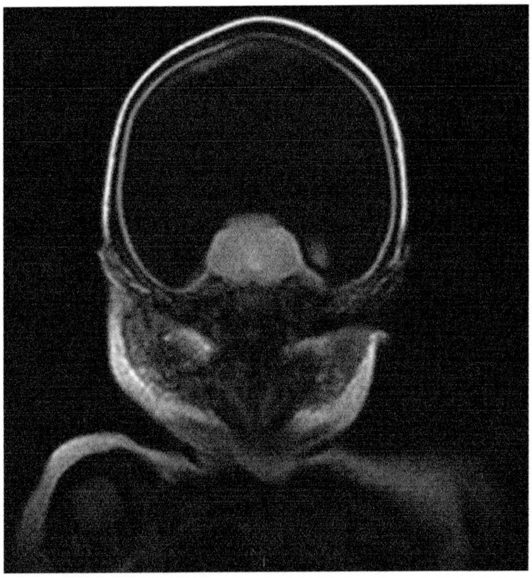

Fig. 49.13 Coronal T1-weighted MRI scan demonstrating hydrancephaly

been replaced with CSF (Fig. 49.13). The aetiology is variable and infants have a limited lifespan. Ventriculoperitoneal shunts have been inserted to control head size in infants and although the literature is sparse there are reports of relatively prolonged survival [77]. Children with hydranencephaly never gain consciousness or awareness regardless of shunt insertion but with aggressive nursing care can have prolonged survival and control of head size reduces the incidence of cranial pressure sores [78].

49.2.7.4 Holoprosencephaly

Holoprosencephaly (HPE) is a complex, congenital brain malformation the essence of which is the failure of the forebrain to split into two hemispheres; it is associated with facial anomalies. It occurs in 1:250 pregnancies approximately but only 3% of foetuses will survive to term so the live birth prevalence is of the order of 1 in 10,000 [79–81].

The incidence of hydrocephalus increases in the more severe forms of the malformation and an important guide is that the majority of children with HPE have microcephaly, when it is not present the child should be investigated for potential hydrocephalus [82]. Although the functional status achieved by children with severe forms of HPE is very limited insertion of a ventriculoperitoneal shunt can make nursing care easier [83].

49.2.8 Neoplasms

Neoplasms are uncommon but important cause of hydrocephalus in neonates. Hydrocephalus can arise from obstruction at various points of CSF pathway. Neoplasm associated hydrocephalus can be further subdivided according to tumour location into three types, supratentorial, infratentorial and spinal. The commonest types in newborns are often of neuroectodermal origin and are more commonly supratentorial.

49.2.9 External Hydrocephalus

This controversial pathological entity is also linked to or referred to as 'pseudohydrocephalus', 'benign subdural effusion', benign enlargement of the subarachnoid spaces' and 'benign pericerbral effusion'. Its etiology and pathophysiology in relation to CSF dynamics is uncertain but include abnormal collections of fluid in the subarachnoid or subdural space overlying the cerebral convexity. The condition occurs while the cranial sutures are open. Although most cases do not require intervention and maintain a benign course some patients present with features related to mass effect and raised intracranial pressure and in rare cases may require management with a subdural-peritoneal shunt.

49.2.10 Overproduction

Choroid plexus papillomas are rare intraventricular tumours that may cause overproduction of CSF resulting in massive ventricular enlargement. They are most often found in the lateral ventricle and appear as homogenously enhancing lesions on MRI. They are vascular lesions and resection of the tumour may be curative if the tumour is benign.

49.3 Clinical Presentation of Hydrocephalus in Neonates

The clinical presentation of hydrocephalus is remarkably similar despite the varied etiology and is related to signs and symptoms of localised or generalised raised intra-cranial pressure (see Box 49.2).

An increase in head size is the major feature of hydrocephalus in the neonate, with an increasing deviation of head circumference from the normal centiles for age. Incremental plotting of head circumference is essential in this regard, using a centile chart such as that produced by Gairdner and Pearson, allowing for gestational age at birth [84]. It should be noted that there are causes for head enlargement other than hydrocephalus (e.g. a familial tendency for a large head, osteofibromatosis, macrocephaly or intracranial cysts). The head-shape may also be abnormal.

Box 49.2 Symptoms and signs of raised intracranial pressure in newly diagnosed hydrocephalus or shunt malfunction in the infant and young child

- Irritability
- Impaired level of consciousness
- Vomiting
- Failure to thrive
- Poor feeding
- Developmental delay
- Increasing head circumference crossing centiles
- Poor head control
- Tense anterior fontanelle
- Dilated scalp veins
- "Setting sun" sign (combination of upper eyelid retraction and failure of upgaze)
- Bradycardia
- Apnoeic spells
- Seizures

Bulging of the anterior fontanelle with a variably open posterior fontanelle, separation of the suture lines and dilatation of superficial scalp veins (due to venous reflux from cerebral sinuses) are classical feature of raised intracranial pressure in hydrocephalus. "Setting sun sign", an upward gaze palsy may be seen with the superior sclera visible. The component parts of this phenomenon consist of downward rotation of the eyeballs and retraction of the upper eyelids and may be accompanied by brow raising. It may be intermittent, disappearing when ICP is reduced. However, this sign can also be seen and elicited though rarely in normal infants. Sixth nerve palsy can be seen as this nerve is most sensitive to pressure due to is long intracranial course. Papilloedema, decreased level of consciousness and other focal neurological deficit can be presenting signs too. Opisthotonic posturing, bradycardic and apnoeic episodes are critical signs of raised intracranial pressure suggesting brainstem compromise and requires emergent neurosurgical assessment and treatment.

Other important presenting symptoms of hydrocephalus in the infant are related to raised intracranial pressure such as irritability, lethargy, poor feeding, vomiting, failure to thrive, and delayed motor development. The clinical presentation may also include features specifically related to the associated causative pathology.

49.4 Imaging and Investigations

Skull X-rays may shows signs of raised intracranial pressure however they are largely obsolete and are not used as part of the standard diagnostic workup and management of hydrocephalus in the newborn. Historically, widening of the sutures beyond 3 mm can be seen with associated *lacunar* skull defects ("copper beating") and erosion of posterior clinoids at the dorsum sella.

Ultrasonography is exceptionally useful as a non-invasive technique [85–87] (Fig. 49.5) Antenatal sonography can detect hydrocephalus in utero and is the screening procedure of choice in patients under the age of 18 months.

Measurements of both the ventricle size and the cortical mantle are possible. Serial ultrasonography has not only improved the ability to detect hydrocephalus, but has also resulted in more prompt treatment of this condition and has proved extremely useful in detecting IVH and hydrocephalus in premature infants. It is considered the initial investigation of choice for neonates with hydrocephalus and can be performed at the bedside. It is worth noting that although ultrasound is sensitive and specific for the diagnosis of hydrocephalus, clarification of its aetiology usually necessitates subsequent CT or MR imaging.

Computed topography (CT) is widespread, rapid and easy to interpret tool. CT diagnosis of hydrocephalus is based on ventriculomegaly including ballooning of frontal horns of lateral ventricles and periventricular low density suggesting trans-ependymal absorption of CSF secondary to raised pressure (see Fig. 49.7). CT however is less efficient in defining the pathoanatomical substrate as compared to Magnestic resonance imaging. In addition it exposes the child to radiation the cumulative doses of which can be significant through the lifetime of treatment.

Magnetic resonance imaging (MRI) is the gold standard for diagnosing hydrocephalus related causative pathology and demonstrates the ventricular and CSF anatomy in exquisite detail. Pathological entities such as aqueduct stenosis, Chiari malformations and neoplastic lesions are readily identifiable. MRI also allows for detailed surgical planning when considering the options of endoscopic third ventriculostomy, shunting, posterior fossa surgery and so forth. MRI T1 and T2 weighted dynamic flow sequences can highlight the relevant ventricular, periventricular and CSF flow with remarkable clarity [88]. This is particularly useful when assessing the anatomy of the third ventricle and aqueduct in relation to determining the surgical procedure of choice. Volume data-sets for both CT and MRI are now readily obtainable which are compatible to bespoke three-dimensional neuronavigation workstations for shunting and neuroendoscopic procedures. MRI is increasingly used for antenatal investigation and is valuable in both outlining congenital malformations and haemorrhage [89].

Postoperative imaging to assess ventricular size after shunting or neuroendoscopy can be performed with both CT and MRI. However after a third ventriculostomy, phase contrast dynamic MRI sequences are required to identify CSF flow through the ventriculostomy and is best visualised on sagittal images [88, 90]. Invasive pressure measurements such as fontonometry are less often justified as they are unreliable when compared with modern methods of imaging.

An antibody screen should be carried out if an intrauterine infection is considered. CSF analysis is indicated where infection or haemorrhage is suspected, as these factors may influence the subsequent clinical management. A raised protein level, or indeed bloodstained CSF, is not necessarily a contraindication to shunting but is taken into consideration when determining the timing of shunt placement. It may be appropriate to delay surgery until the protein count and/or the blood in the CSF clears to an acceptable degree. If active infection is suspected then a temporising external ventricular drain would be preferred before a permanent shunt can be implanted once the infection has been treated and confirmed with sterile CSF samples.

49.5 Management Options

The complications associated with surgery in the low-birth weight neonate or neonates with co-existing unstable medical conditions raises the need to explore non-surgical means of managing hydrocephalus. The additional possibility of occasionally self-limiting conditions such as PHH may only require temporising management options. However, pharmacotherapeutic agents such as acetozolomide, frusemide and steroids have not been shown to be effective in reducing the rate of shunting and cannot be recommended [91, 92]. Although historically a common practice, serial lumbar punctures should probably no longer be used. A published meta-analysis concluded that no evidence of benefit was demonstrated with a significant risk of secondary infection [93]. Similarly serial multiple percutaneous ventricular taps have been abandoned by most large tertiary neurosurgical centres due to the numerous associated complications such 'puncture porencephaly', infection and encephalomalacia [94, 95].

Surgery remains the overwhelming mainstay of treatment for hydrocephalus in the newborn. CSF Shunting has converted hydrocephalus from an almost exclusively fatal disease to a frequently curable condition. The first permanent CSF diversion for hydrocephalus was performed by Mikulicz in 1893 in the form of a ventriculo-subarachnoid-subgaleal shunt [96]. This procedure was also simultaneously the first intrathecal ventriculostomy. Since then virtually every anatomical cavity has been utilised as a potential reservoir or conduit for CSF drainage with varying degrees of success. These include subcutaneous tissues of the scalp, atria, pleura, ureters, gallbladder and thoracic duct. Most of these are no longer considered in standard 'first line' practice in newborn hydrocephalus. This section outlines the most common surgical techniques in newborn hydrocephalus surgery.

49.5.1 External Ventricular Drainage

EVD has been widely used in the temporary treatment of hydrocephalus for several decades. The frontal and occipital horns of the lateral ventricles are the site of choice via a single burr-hole and the CSF is drained into a sterile closed circuit system which can be continuously controlled by a simple gravity based outflow valve. In situations of acute symptomatic hydrocephalus secondary to operable or potentially operable lesion, EVD can be employed to provide necessary control until such time as to allow further assessment and definitive treatment of hydrocephalus. It is of particular use in the presence of active infection whereby a permanent shunt system cannot be placed until the infection has been successfully treated and also until a high related CSF protein level (as seen in some peri and post infectious settings) normalises to allow shunt placement. It also allows for the direct administration of intrathecal antibiotics into the infected CSF space. EVD is also potentially useful in IVH or PHH as a temporising measure before either persistent hydrocephalus has been confirmed or the blood load has reduced. In PHH, EVDs have also been used in several studies for administration of intraventricular fibrinolytic therapies and CSF irrigation however these have not translated to proven clinical practice and remain experimental [95, 97].

Potential complications associated with EVDs include infection and catheter dislodgement. Recent introduction of antibiotic impregnated EVD systems have reduced the risk of infection however it remains the major source of EVD related patient morbidity.

49.5.2 Subcutaneous Reservoir Ventricular Catheter Placement

This device comprises of a frontal subcutaneous reservoir with a catheter entering the ventricle (Figs. 49.14, 49.15, and 49.16). It is

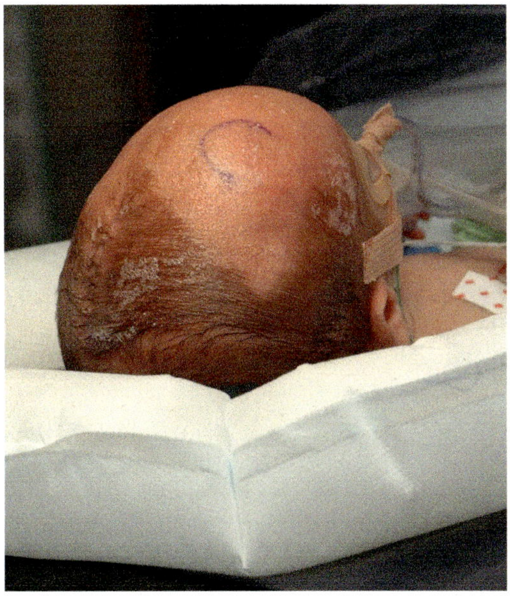

Fig. 49.14 Preoperative skin marking for insertion of a right frontal subcutaneous CSF reservoir

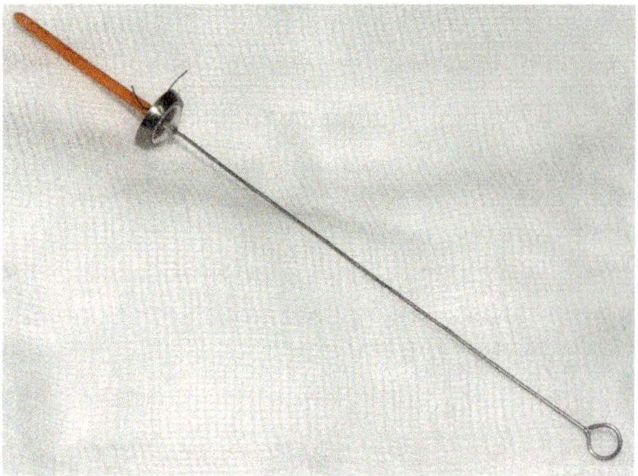

Fig. 49.15 Intraoperative image of ventricular catheter connected to subcutaneous reservoir. (A stylet has been inserted through the reservoir and the catheter to aid insertion)

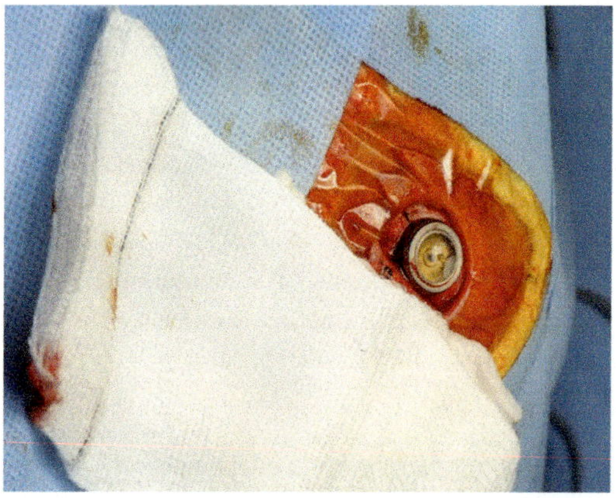

Fig. 49.16 Intraoperative image following insertion of subcutaneous CSF reservoir. The stylet shown in Fig. 49.15 has been removed. Note the xanthochromic fluid in the reservoir typical of post haemorrhagic hydrocephalus

mainly used in neonates with symptomatic hydrocephalus whose low birth weight and/or the potential for spontaneous arrest of the hydrocephalus preclude the immediate need for a permanent shunt. It is a viable option in PHH. The reservoir allows repeated bedside aspiration of CSF, has lower infection rates compared to EVD and also allows access for administration of intraventricular antibiotics. Complications and limitations include skin erosion and only intermittent intracranial pressure control.

49.5.3 Ventriculoperitoneal Shunt

49.5.3.1 Overview

Ventriculoperitoneal shunt is the most common form of implantable CSF shunts. The method was first described in 1908 and was initially less favoured than the ventriculo-atrial (VA) or ventriculopleural shunt [96]. The peritoneum has since become the drainage site of choice due to complications with VA shunts such as sudden death from pulmonary embolism, endocarditis and nephritis were noted. Another recognised problem in many VA shunts in the neonate is the need to lengthen the lower end as the child grows and the catheter pulls up out of the atrium. This can be obviated with VPS in the neonate with a longer intraperitoneal catheter. VPS hardware includes a ventricular catheter, CSF reservoir, a one way shunt valve and distal peritoneal catheter.

The choice of valve type remains a personal choice and a regular source of debate within the neurosurgical community as there is no high quality evidence favouring one type over another. Valve types include differential-pressure, flow-regulating, gravity-actuated and programmable valves. All the valve types only allow unidirectional flow of the CSF. An anti-siphon device may be included in the system to prevent over-drainage. In practice some factors that may influence decision making include valve size and profile in relation to newborn/premature neonate scalp skin, cortical mantle thickness, cost and individual surgeon experience. Some authors advocate a flow control valve for shunts in the newborn to avoid the later complication of slit ventricle syndrome. This is related to chronic over-drainage and is seen most commonly in patients who have a shunt implanted in the first 2 years of life [98]. Over-drainage and development of subdural haematomas in newborns with large ventricles and thin cortical mantle may be avoided with high-resistance valves [99].

The catheters are usually made from synthetic silicone rubber. The use of antibiotic impregnated and silver coated shunt tubing with in-vivo antibacterial activity is gaining popularity and may confer a protective benefit against infection, particularly in the neonatal setting [100]. Further randomised studies are required to confirm this.

Both frameless, and frame-based neuronavigation systems have been utilised to reduce the incidence of poorly sited ventricular catheters and recent studies have shown benefit in catheter placement accuracy but it remains to be seen if this relates to a significant reduction in shunt revision rates in the long-term [101]. With the bespoke electromagnetic (EM) frameless neuronavigation system no rigid head fixation, pins or screws is required and this confers a significant advantage for neonatal shunt surgery. Previous studies on endoscopic versus non-endoscopic catheter placement have not demonstrate any difference in shunt revision rates [102].

49.5.3.2 Surgical Technique

Routine preoperative preparations such as blood parameters are a necessity. The patient is positioned whilst under general endotracheal anaesthesia. Antibiotic prophylaxis is recommended such as a cephalosporin e.g. Cefotaxime at the time of induction. The head is rotated to the opposite side to the shunt with the neck extended to create a straight line between the scalp and abdominal incision. The site of the burr-hole and abdominal incision should be marked prior to skin preparation and draping. (Fig. 49.17) Occipital burrholes are usually 3–4 cm from the midline along the lambdoid suture. Frontal burrholes are 2–3 cm along the coronal suture from midline. It is vital to tailor the burr-hole to the ventricular morphology on imaging so as to ensure optimal ventricular catheter placement. In infants with splayed sutures, access can be achieved via an opening of the sutures. The site of burrhole is of surgeon's preference as there is little evidence showing advantages of one over the other. Occipital burrholes are traditionally used as they are more cosmetically acceptable. Durotomy is made and the brain pia is cauterised. Dural opening should be kept minimal to reduce the risk of CSF escape around the ventricular catheter and hence promoting CSF leak.

The abdominal incision is usually performed on the same side either upper midline or paraumbilical site, however the site is unimportant. The most prudent part is to be sure the peritoneum space is opened. Open technique, use of trocar [103] and more recently laparoscopic assistance have been described [104]. The distal catheter is tunnelled subcutaneously from the burrhole site to the abdominal opening, or vice versa (Fig. 49.18). If a frontal burrhole is used, an intervening incision is made at the occiput.

The ventricular catheter is introduced mounted on a stylet. The trajectory is determined according to external landmarks. From the occipital burrhole, a target at the midpoint of the forehead at the hairline so that the lateral frontal horn will be entered. From a frontal burrhloe, aim for a target of the intersecting planes midpupillary line and the external auditory meatus. Intraoperative ultrasonography or image guided stereotaxy (for example EM guidance) [101] can be used for

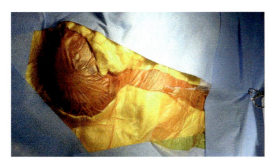

Fig. 49.17 Intraoperative image during insertion of right parietal ventriculoperitoneal shunt after skin preparation and draping

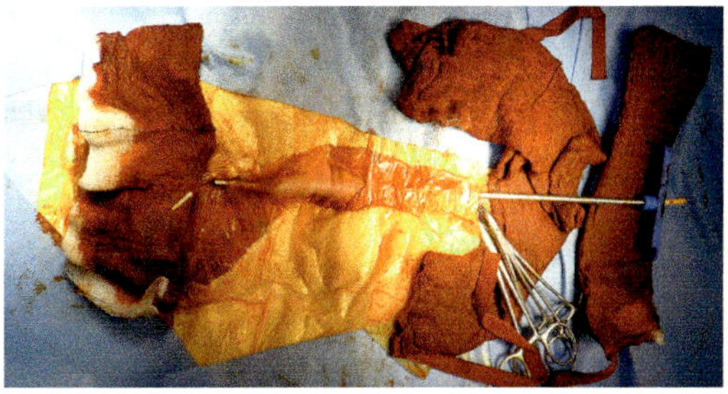

Fig. 49.18 Intraoperative image during insertion of ventriculoperitneal shunt. The tunneller has been passed from the abdomen to the right parietal incision

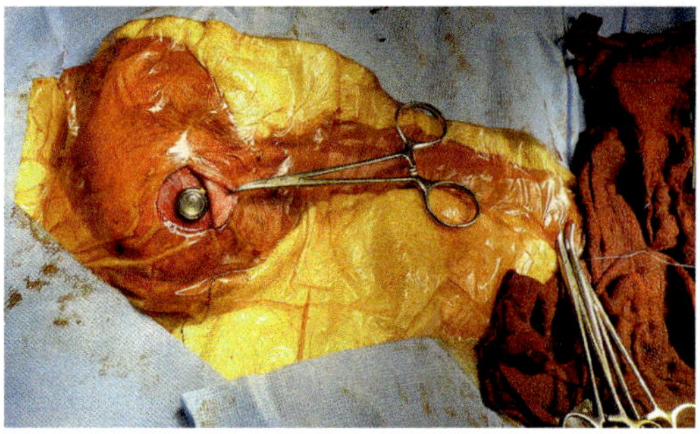

Fig. 49.19 Intraoperative image during insertion of ventriculoperitoneal shunt. The right parietal burrhole seated reservoir is visible with the attached distal catheter

more accurate positioning of the catheter. CSF Pressure may be measured at this point and a sample of CSF taken for biochemical and microbiological examinations. The proximal catheter is connected to the distal catheter via a reservoir (Fig. 49.19) and a valve system, depending on what type is being used.

The distal end is examined to ensure that there is free flowing CSF. The distal catheter is placed within the peritoneum. The peritoneum is closed using absorbable sutures, the muscle layers and skin are then closed.

49.5.3.3 Image Guided Placement of Ventricular Catheter

Both frameless and frame-based neuronavigation systems have been utilised to reduce the incidence of poorly sited ventricular catheters and recent studies have shown benefit in catheter placement accuracy but it remains to be seen if this relates to a significant reduction in shunt revision rates in the long-term [101]. With the bespoke electromagnetic (EM) frameless neuronavigation system no rigid head fixation, pins or screws is required and this confers a significant advantage for neonatal shunt surgery. Previous studies on endoscopic versus non-endoscopic catheter placement did not demonstrate any difference in shunt revision rates [102].

49.5.3.4 Complications

Complications of VPS most commonly includes infection, malposition of the ventricular catheter, mechanical failure leading to suboptimal drainage or blockage, overdrainage, shunt migration/disconnection and less commonly intra-abdominal sequelae such as bowel perforation, hernias, hydrocoeles, appendicitis and peritonitis. Shunt complication rates are significantly higher in the newborn and studies have shown low-birth weight to be linked to a higher incidence of shunt infection and revision rates [105]. If the CSF is sterile on insertion, the usual organisms causing postoperative shunt infection are skin commensals such as Staphylococcus epidermidis (Coagulase negative Staphalococcus). Where infection has been proven, the removal of the entire system and temporary CSF diversion via an EVD and concomitant intrathecal antibiotic administration is usually necessary. The treatment of shunt infections has been reviewed extensively by Bayston et al. [106].

Unfortunately despite advances in neuronavigation and shunt tubing material, shunt failure remains a considerable source of morbidity for hydrocephalus patients with up to 40% of shunts failing in the first year [107]. Indeed, shunt failure remains an almost inevitable consequence during a patient's life up to 80% of shunts requiring revision after 12 years [108].

49.5.4 Ventriculoatrial Shunt

Ventriculo-atrial shunts are indicated in patients with intraabdominal pathologies precluding the use of peritoneum as a drainage site. These include necrotising enterocilitis, peritonistis and adhesions secondary to extensive abdominal surgery.

These may be performed in a similar fashion to ventriculo-peritoneal shunts except for the lower incision which is over the right side of the neck. The objective is for the shunt tip to lie in the superior vena cava just rostral to the tricuspid valve. The two most common methods are open versus percutaneous insertion. Access to the jugular vein can be achieved by exposing the common facial vein, which is tied proximally and held with a stay suture at the venotomy site, the distal catheter is fed into the superior vena cava. Intra-operative fluoroscopy or X-rays are helpful in achieving the ideal position. Throughout the procedure, the anesthiologist should inform you of any cardiac alterations or rhythm changes. A purse-string suture is closed around the catheter sufficiently to prevent hemorrhage, but not so tight as to cause obstruction to the catheter. Percutaneous methods into the jugular or subclavian veins can be achieved with the aid of ultrasound guidance and fluoroscopy [109–111].

Complications include the need to repeatedly lengthen the distal catheter as the child grows, higher risk of bacteremia and sepsis and specific vascular complications including thrombosis, micro-emboli with secondary pulmonary hypertension and corpulmonale, macroemboli with pulmonary embolism and vascular perforation.

49.5.5 Ventriculopleural Shunt

Ventriculo-pleaural shunts are only used in cases where peritoneum and right atrium cannot be used as sites for CSF diversion. It is rarely performed in neonates or indeed infants and not recommended in this age group as the pleural cavity cannot cope with the benign pleural effusion that results from CSF drainage.

The proximal approach is identical to the ventriculo-peritoneal shunt placement. The pleural space can be entered at a variety of sites however along the anterior axillary line in the fifth intercostal space is both convenient and safe. Intercostal muscle layers are split on the upper border of the rib to avoid the neurovascular bundle to reveal the pleura. It is then opened, the distal catheter is then introduced into the space gently to avoid entering the lung parenchyma. The muscle is closed to avoid further air entry into the pleural space. Distal catheter placement may be aided by thoracoscopy [104]. Contraindications for this technique include previous thoracic surgery, acute or chronic pulmonary disease and poor pulmonary function. CSF will usually accumulate as benign pleural effusion, however if this is progressive it may lead to respiratory distress and therefore vigilance for this complication is important. This technique however is rarely applicable in newborns or indeed infants as the pleural cavity cannot cope with the CSF load at this age. The technique is thus usually reserved for very rare cases where few options for the distal catheter remain in older children.

Other contraindications include previous thoracic surgery, acute or chronic pulmonary disease and poor pulmonary function.

49.5.6 Post Operative Care of Shunted Patients

Post operative scans are obtained and act as a reference to future surgery and shunt positioning. Continual monitoring of head circumference is required.

49.5.7 Endoscopic Third Ventriculostomy

Endoscopic third ventriculostomy has re-emerged in the past 30 years and introduced a new dimension to management of hydrocephalus. Open third ventriculostomy was first performed by Dandy in 1922 [112] and later as an endoscopic procedure by Mixter in 1923. Advances in fiberoptic camera technology combined with high resolution MRI have been chiefly responsible for emergence of ETV as a therapeutic option for hydrocephalus.

The aim of ETV is to re-direct CSF through a "short-cut" from the third ventricle into the subarachnoid space to allow circulation and natural absorption of CSF. This re-route allows for natural absorption of CSF as opposed to external re-routing via a shunt.

49.5.7.1 Indications

The obvious advantages of shunt independence have made this an attractive surgical option however current evidence suggests that patient selection is crucial to outcome success rates. ETV in obstructive hydrocephalus with maintained CSF absorption such as in congenital aqueduct stenosis is associated with the highest success rates. ETV is seldom successful in hydrocephalus secondary to IVH and meningitis which account for the majority of cases of neonatal hydrocephalus. This is due to a difference in aetiology with the obstruction being at the level of the subarachnoid space secondary to scarring and inflammation and possibly also involving failure of CSF absorption. While in older children, the indications for endoscopic treatment have been relatively well defined, much debate continues on the value of this treatment in the first few months of life [113–115]. While various studies have reported differing success rates there remains a lack of consensus on the value of third ventriculostomy in infants and neonates.

The role of ETV as a secondary treatment option after initial or multiple shunt failures is gaining popularity with encouraging success rates [116]. This is relevant to the newborn with PHH or PIH who may benefit from a primary shunt (where primary ETV is ineffective) and then be considered for a secondary ETV when presenting with a future shunt failure.

ETV may also have an important role in the treatment of hydrocephalus in developing countries [117]. The lack of a follow-up service for children in developing countries having permanent shunt implants re-inforces the obvious advantage of a shunt-free therapeutic option—ETV. PIH accounts for up to 60% of hydrocephalus cases in certain developing countries [117]. In keeping with results published for developed country ETV success rates in infants, success rates in a relatively large series of patients treated in a developing country in the under 1 year group was lower than in the older child. Nevertheless, up to a 60% shunt avoidance rate has been reported in developing country infants presenting with PIH aqeuduct stenosis undergoing ETV [117]. The challenge posed by the lack of a shunt follow-up service in developing countries and the consequent impetus for ETV as a treatment modality had also potentially leads to a clinical situation in which ETV may be performed on a patient whose CSF absorption capability has not recovered sufficiently. Whereas these patients would probably have been treated with a shunt in a developed country. The combination of ETV and choroid plexus cauterization (CPC) may be a viable option in temporarily reducing the rate of CSF production until the absorptive function potentially returns. Results from a study employing this management technique on patients in the developing world reported a success rate of over 70% in infants under 1 year with PIH and an open aqueduct [118].

Other applications of neuroendoscopy include aqueduct stenting for isolated fourth ventricle enlargement, multiloculated hydrocephalus requiring communication of CSF spaces via septum pellucidotomies, cyst fenestrations and as an adjunct to shunt surgery by aiding shunt placement under direct endoscopic vision.

49.5.7.2 Surgical Technique

The technique involves a single paramedian coronal burrhole to gain access into the lateral ventricle. The ventricle is then cannulated using a 10 or 12 Fr cannula which then acts as a conduit for rigid or flexible endoscope. The endoscope is then introduced and navigated through the enlarged foramen of Munroe into the third ventricle (Fig. 49.1). The landmarks on the third ventricle floor are identified including the mammillary bodies and pituitary red spot. A midline fenestration is then made in the thinnest part of the third ventricle floor avoiding critical structures including the basilar artery (Fig. 49.20). The endoscope is then advanced through the fenestration to identify and fenestrate any further obstructive membranes thereby ensuring that an effective communication is achieved between the third ventricle and the inter-peduncular and prepontine subarachnoid CSF cisterns. Upon completion, the endoscope and the cannula are withdrawn and no hardware is left in situ.

Although a safe procedure in well trained and experienced hands the complications of neuroendoscopy can be devastating. Severe haemorrhage, cardiac arrest, cerebral infarction, diabetes insipidus and damage to the fornices resulting in memory deficit have all been reported [119]. In addition it is important to mention the rare but potential risk of sudden post ETV death due to closure of the ventriculostomy [119].

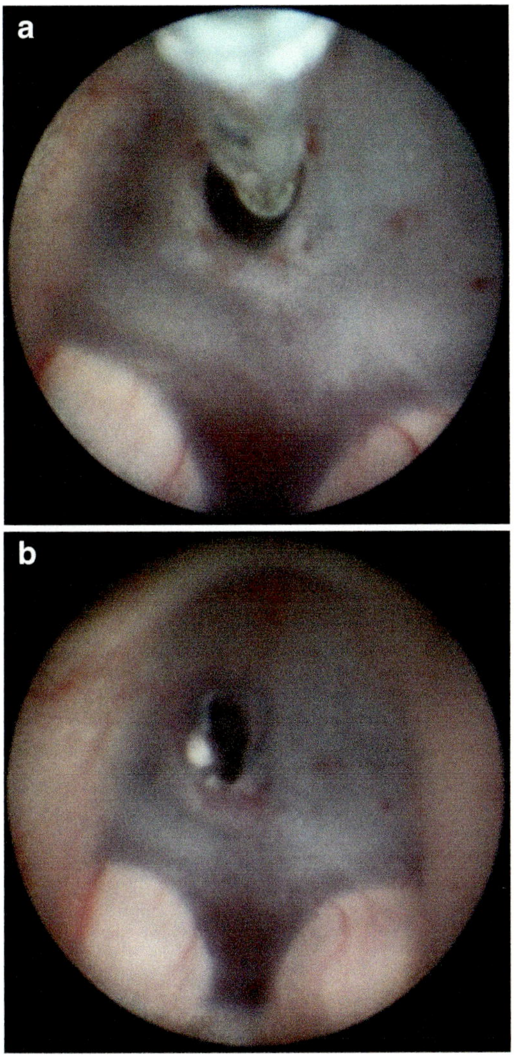

Fig. 49.20 Intraoperative images (obtained during endoscopic third ventriculostomy) demonstrating passage of the balloon through the floor of the third ventricle. Note the pituitary *red spot* is upper half and the mammillary bodies in the lower half of the picture (**a**) The balloon tip cab be seen across the stoma. (**b**) The stoma after the balloon has been withdrawn

49.5.8 Fetal Surgical Therapy

In utero diagnosis of hydrocephalus by fetal ultrasounds has raised the possibility of prenatal intervention and treatment of hydrocephalus. Extensive experimental work and certain human studies have been performed in countries where abortion is legally banned but thus far the results are poor and majority of patients who underwent fetal surgery for hydrocephalus required VPS insertion after birth. This method of management is therefore not currently recommended [120].

More recently the MOMS (Management of Myelomeningocoele study) trial [121] has shown that prenatal repair of myelomeningocoele reduced the need for shunting from 82 to 40% and improved motor outcomes at 30 months albeit at an increased risk of fetal and maternal complications. This is therefore a viable management option in countries where abortion is legally banned and expertise for prenatal intervention is available.

49.6 Outcome

The outcome of hydrocephalus is ultimately determined by the underlying causative pathological entity. Other factors influencing outcome include the treatment selected and avoidance of the treatment related complications. Historically, successful hydrocephalus treatment was defined as satisfactory ventricular catheter position on cranial imaging, absence of postoperative complications (such as infection or haemorrhage) requiring further surgery, and relief of symptoms of raised intracranial pressure. Such measures are however crude and an absence of shunt failure does not necessarily equate to success. In a cohort of UK patients with spina bifida followed from birth, patient reported outcomes indicated a poor prognosis for independent living into adulthood [122]. More recently small prospective case series have evaluated the role of neuropsychological testing in patients with spina bifida and showed that reading and writing function remain deficient into adulthood and that memory status is positively correlated with functional independence [123]. These tests are time consuming to administer and interpret but provide an indication of the potential for independent living for patients.

Several researchers have developed objective outcome measures that are primarily aimed at paediatric cohorts and patients with spina bifida living into adulthood. These tools range from prospective lifestyle and health assessment questionnaires (patient reported outcomes) to objective measures of physical, social-emotional, and cognitive function (the hydrocephalus outcome questionnaire). The hydrocephalus outcome questionnaire has been validated and can be administered to children older than 5 years who are shunt dependent to measure development and the effects of episodes of shunt malfunction on neurological development and social integration [124].

49.7 Ongoing Research

Research into the pathophysiology of hydrocephalus continues and is beyond the scope of this chapter. One such current research is the study by J. Miyan at the University of Manchester to investigate the role of CSF in developmental of cerebral cortex and developmental defect associated with fetal-onset hydrocephalus and neural tube defects. The study is based on the results of rat hydrocephalus model and aims to determine if the imbalance in a folate enzyme (10-formyltetrahydrofolate dehydrogenase), Transforming Growth Factor-beta, Brain Derived Neurotropic Factor and Basic Fibroblast Growth Factor concentrations that is present in rat model of hydrocephalus is also present in the CSF of human infant with hydrocephalus.

Ongoing surgical research trials aim to further improve the management of hydrocephalus. The International Infant Hydrocephalus Study (www.iihsstudy.org) is a multicentre trial randomising infants with defined aqueduct stenosis and triventricular hydrocephalus to receive either endoscopic third ventriculostomy or CSF shunting. This study was initiated under the aegis of the International Study Group for Neuro-endoscopy and the International Society for Paediatric Neurosurgery and aims to provide long term outcome analysis on shunt dependence and a more comprehensive analysis of treatment effect and patient outcome (including various aspects of quality of life such as hospitalisation or other sickness time and neurodevelopmental evaluations over the course of 5–7 years).

British Antibiotic and Silver Impregnated Catheters for ventriculoperitoneal Shunts is a multi-centre randomised controlled trial (BASICS trial) funded by the National Institute for Health Research. The trial is led by the departments of neurosurgery in Alder Hey Children's Hospital and the Walton Centre for Neurology and Neurosurgery in Liverpool and aims to compare standard silicone, antibiotic impregnated and silver impregnated catheters in the incidence of shunt infections.

References

1. Blackburn BL, Fineman RM. Epidemiology of congenital hydrocephalus in Utah, 1940–1979: report of an iatrogenically related "epidemic". Am J Med Genet. 1994;52:123–9.
2. Fernell E, Hagberg G, Hagberg B. Infantile hydrocephalus epidemiology: an indicator of enhanced survival. Arch Dis Child Fetal Neonatal Ed. 1994;70:F123–8.
3. Stein S, Feldman H, Kohl S, et al. The epidemiology of congenital hydrocephalus: a study in Brooklyn NY 1968–1976. Childs Brain. 1981;8:253–62.
4. Kohn MI, Tanna NK, et al. Analysis of brain and cerebrospinal fluid volumes with MR imaging. Part I. Methods, reliability, and validation. Radiology. 1991;178(1):115–22.
5. Davson H, Segal MB. Physiology of the CSF and blood brain barriers. Boca Raton: CRC Press; 1996.
6. Edsbagge M, Tisell M, et al. Spinal CSF absorption in healthy individuals. Am J Physiol Regul Integr Comp Physiol. 2004;287(6):R1450–5.
7. Kimelberg HK. Water homeostasis in the brain: basic concepts. Neuroscience. 2004;129(4):851–60.
8. Redzic ZB, Segal MB. The structure of the choroid plexus and the physiology of the choroid plexus epithelium. Adv Drug Deliv Rev. 2004;56(12):1695–716.
9. Xenos C, Sgouros S, Natarajan K. Ventricular volume change in childhood. J Neurosurg. 2002;97:584–90.
10. Cutler RW, Page L, et al. Formation and absorption of cerebrospinal fluid in man. Brain. 1968;91(4):707–20.
11. Milhorat TH, Kotzen RM, et al. Stenosis of central canal of spinal cord in man: incidence and pathological findings in 232 autopsy cases. J Neurosurg. 1994;80(4):716–22.
12. Shapiro K, Marmarou A, et al. Characterization of clinical CSF dynamics and neural axis compliance using the pressure-volume index: I. The normal pressure-volume index. Ann Neurol. 1980;7(6):508–14.
13. Rosenberg GA. Brain fluids and metabolism. Oxford: Oxford University Press; 1990.

14. Smith DE, Johanson CE, et al. Peptide and peptide analog transport systems at the blood-CSF barrier. Adv Drug Deliv Rev. 2004;56(12):1765–91.
15. Abbott NJ. Evidence for bulk flow of brain interstitial fluid: significance for physiology and pathology. Neurochem Int. 2004;45(4):545–52.
16. Williams PL, Warwick R, Dyson M, Bannister LH, editors. Gray's anatomy. 37th ed. Churchill Livingstone: London; 1989.
17. Netter FH. The nervous system. In: Netter FH, editor. The Ciba collection of medical illustrations, vol. 1. Summit: Ciba Pharmaceutical Products; 1953. p. 44.
18. Rekate HL. The definition and classification of hydrocephalus: a personal recommendation to stimulate debate. Cerebrospinal Fluid Res. 2008;5:2.
19. Cherian S, Whitelaw A, Thoresen M, Love S. The pathogenesis of neonatal post-hemorrhagic hydrocephalus. Brain Pathol. 2004;14:305–11. (Review article).
20. Papile LA, Burstein J, Burstein R, Koffler H. Incidence and evolution of subependymal and intraventricular haemorrhage: a study of infants with birth weight less than 1500 gm. J Pediatr. 1978;92:529–34.
21. de Vries LS, Dubowitz LM, Dubowitz V, Kaiser A, Lary S, Silverman M, Whitelaw A, Wigglesworth JS. Predictive value of cranial ultrasound in the newborn baby: a reappraisal. Lancet. 1985;326:137–40.
22. Volpe JJ. Intracranial hemorrhage: germinal matrix-intraventricular hemorrhage of the premature infant. In: Volpe JJ, editor. Neurology of the newborn. 4th ed. Philadelphia: WB Saunders; 2001. p. 428–93.
23. Ichord RN. Neurologic complications. In: Witter FR, Keith LG, editors. Textbook of prematurity. Boston: Little, Brown; 1993. p. 305–20.
24. Whitelaw A. Intraventricular haemorrhage and posthaemorrhagic hydrocephalus: pathogenesis, prevention and future interventions. Semin Neonatol. 2001;6:135–146. (Review article).
25. Korobkin R. The relationship between head circumference and the development of communicating hydrocephalus in infants following intraventricular hemorrhage. Pediatrics. 1975;56:74–7.
26. Volpe JJ. Neonatal intracranial hemorrhage. Pathophysiology, neuropathology, and clinical features. Clin Perinatol. 1977;4:77–102.
27. Holt PJ. Posthemorrhagic hydrocephalus. J Child Neurol. 1989;4 Suppl:S23–31. (Review article).
28. Hansen AR, Snyder EY. Medical management of neonatal posthemorrhagic hydrocephalus. Neurosurg Clin North Am. 1998;9:95–104. (Review article).
29. Roland EH, Hill A. Germinal matrix-intraventricular hemorrhage in the premature newborn: management and outcome. Neurol Clin. 2003;21:833–51, vi–vii. (Review article).
30. Fernall E, Hagberg G, Hagberg B. Infantile hydrocephalus—the impact of enhanced preterm survival. Acta Paediatr Scand. 1990;79:1080–6.
31. Perlman JM, McMenamin JB, Volpe JJ. Fluctuating cerebral blood-flow velocity in respiratory-distress syndrome. Relation to the development of intraventricular hemorrhage. N Engl J Med. 1983;309(4):204–9.
32. Whitelaw A, Jary S, Kmita G, Wroblewska J, Musialik-Swietlinska E, Mandera M, Hunt L, Carter M, Pople I. Randomized trial of drainage, irrigation andfibrinolytic therapy for premature infants with posthemorrhagic ventricular dilatation: developmental outcome at 2 years. Pediatrics. 2010;125(4):e852–8.
33. Sáez-Llorens X, McCracken GH Jr. Bacterial meningitis in children. Lancet. 2003;361(9375):2139–48. (Review).
34. Chang Chien HY, Chiu NC, Li WC, et al. Characterisitcs of neonatal bacterial meningitis in a teaching hospital in Taiwan from 1984–1997. J Microbiol Immunol Infect. 2000;33(2):100–4.
35. Klinger G, Chin CN, Beyene J, Perlman M. Predicting the outcome of neonatal bacterial meningitis. Pediatrics. 2000;106(3):477–82.
36. Prats JM, López-Heredia J, Gener B, Freijo MM, Garaizar C. Multilocular hydrocephalus: ultrasound studies of origin and development. Pediatr Neurol. 2001;24(2):149–51.
37. Chiari H. Uber Veranderungen des Kleinhiens, des pons und der medulla oblongate. Folge von congenitaler hydrocephalie des grossherns. Deskschr Akad Wiss Wien. 1895;63:71–116.
38. Cleland J. Contribution to the study of spina bifida, encephalocoele and anencephalys. J Anat Physiol. 1883;17:257–91.
39. Dyste GN, Menezes AH, Van Gilder JC. Sympromatic Chiari malformations: an analysis of presentation, management and long-term outcome. J Neurosurg. 1989;71:159–68.
40. Elster AD, Chen MY. Chiari I malformations: clinical and radiologic reappraisal. Radiology. 1992;183:347–53.
41. Mikulis DJ, Diaz O, Egglin TK, Sanchez R. Variance of the position of the cerebellar tonsils with age: preliminary report. Radiology. 1992;183:725–8.
42. Milhorat TH, Chou MW, Trinidad EM, Kula RW, Mandell M, Wolpert C, Speer MC. Chiari I malformation redefined: clinical and radiographic findings for 364 symptomatic patients. Neurosurgery. 1999;44:1005–17.
43. Park JK, Gleason PL, Madsen JR, Goumnerova LC, Scott RM. Presentation and management of Chiari malformation in children. Pediatr Neurosurg. 1997;26:190–6.
44. Greenlee JDW, Donovan KA, Hasan DM, Menezes AH. Chiari I malformation in the very young child: the spectrum of presentations and experience in 31 children under age 6 years of age. Pediatrics. 2002;110:1212–9.
45. Menezes AH, Greenlee JDW, Donovan KA. Honored guest presentation: lifetime experiences and where are we going: Chiari I with syringohydromyelia—controversies and development of decision trees. Clin Neurosurg. 2005;52:297–305.

46. Dyste GN, Menezes AH. Presentation and management of pediatric Chiari malformations without myelodysplasia. Neurosurgery. 1988;23:589.
47. Menezes AH. Comments: incidentally identified syringomyelia associated with Chiari I malformations: is early interventional surgery necessary. Neurosurgery. 2001;49:641.
48. Alzate JC, Kothbauer KF, Jallo GI, Epstein FJ. Treatment of Chiari type I malformation in patients with and without syringomyelia: a consecutive series of 66 cases. Neurosurg Focus. 2001;11:1–9.
49. Menezes AH. Chiari I malformations and hydromyelia—complications. Pediatr Neurosurg. 1991–1992;17:146–54.
50. Tubbs RS, McGirt MJ, Oaks WJ. Surgical experience in 130 pediatric patients with Chiari malformations. J Neurosurg. 2003;99:291–6.
51. Bhangoo R, Sgouros S, Walsh AR, Clarke JR. Hindbrain-hernia-related syringomyelia without syringobulbia, complicated by permanent nocturnal central hypoventilation requiring non-invasive ventilation. Childs Nerv Syst. 2006;22(2):113–6.
52. Oakes WJ, Tubbs RS. Chiari malformations. In: Winn HR, editor. Youman's neurological surgery. 5th ed; 2005. p. 3347–61.
53. el Gammal T, Mark EK, Brooks BS. MR imaging of Chiari II malformation. Am J Roentgenol. 1988;150:163–70.
54. McLone DG, Nakahara S, Knepper PA. Chiari II malformation: pathogenesis and dynamics. Concepts Pediatr Neurosurg. 1991;11:1–17.
55. Nicolaides KH, Campbell S, Gabbe SG, Guidetti R. Ultrasound screening for spina bifida: cranial and cerebellar signs. Lancet. 1986;2:72–4.
56. Naidich TP, Pudlowski RM, Naidich JB. Computed tomographic signs of Chiari KK malformation II: midbrain and cerebellum. Radiology. 1980;134:391–8.
57. Venes JL, Black KL, Latack JT. Preoperative evaluation and surgical management of the Arnold-Chiari II malformation. J Neurosurg. 1986;64:363–70.
58. McLone DG, Knepper PA. The cause of Chiari II malformation: a unified theory. Pediatr Neurosci. 1989;15:1–12.
59. Hirsch JF, Hirsch E, Sainte-Rose C, et al. Stenosis of the aqueduct of Sylvius (etiology and treatment). J Neurosurg Sci. 1986;30:29–39.
60. Jellinger G. Anatomopathology of nontumoral aqueduct stenosis. J Neurosurg Sci. 1986;30:1–16.
61. Robertson JA, Leggate JRS, Miller JD, et al. Aqueductal stenosis-presentation and prognosis. Br J Neurosurg. 1990;4:101–6.
62. Ceddia A, Di Rocco C, Iannelli A, et al. Idrocefalo neonatale ad eziologia non tumorale. Minerva Pediatr. 1992;44:445–50.
63. McFarlane A, Maloney AFJ. The appearance of aqueduct and its relationship with hydrocephalus in the Arnold-Chiari malformation. Brain. 1957;80:479–91.
64. Cinalli G, Spennato P, Del Basso De Caro ML, Buonocore MC. Hydrocephalus and Dandy Walker malformation. In: Cinalli C, Maixner WJ, Sainte-Rose C, editors. Pediatric hydrocephalus. Milan: Springer; 2004. p. 259–77.
65. Klein O, Pierre-Kahn A, Boddaert N, et al. Dandy-Walker malformation: prenatal diagnosis and prognosis. Childs Nerv Syst. 2003;19:484–9.
66. Barkovich AJ, Kjos BO, Norman D, et al. Revised classification of posterior fossa cysts and cyst-like malformations based on the results of multiplanar MR imaging. Am J Neuroradiol. 1989;153(6):1289–300.
67. Hirsch JF, Pierre-Kahn A, Renier D, et al. The Dandy-Walker malformation. A review of 40 cases. J Neurosurg. 1984;61:515–22.
68. Pascual-Castroviejo I, Velez A, Pascual-Pascual SI, et al. Dandy Walker malformation: analysis of 38 cases. Childs Nerv Syst. 1991;7:88–97.
69. Has R, Ermis H, Ibrahimoglu L, et al. Dandy-Walker malformation: a review of 78 cases diagnosed by prenatal songraphy. Fetal Diagn Ther. 2004;19(4):342–7.
70. Osenbach RK, Menezes AH. Diagnosis and management of the Dandy Walker malformation: 30 years experience. Pediatr Neurosurg. 1992;18:179–89.
71. Hart MN, Malamud N, Ellis WG. The Dandy-walker syndrome. A clinico-pathological study based on 28 cases. Neurology. 1972;22:771–80.
72. Cinalli G, Renier D, Sebag G, et al. Chronic tonsillar herniation in Crouzon's and Apert's syndromes: the role of premature synostosis of the lambdoid suture. J Neurosurg. 1995;83:575–82.
73. Moutard ML, Kieffer V, Feingold J, et al. Agenesis of the corpus callosum: prenatal diagnosis and prognosis. Childs Nerv Syst. 2003;19(7–8):471–6.
74. Moritake K, Nagai H, Miyazaki T, et al. Nationwide survey of the etiology and associated conditions of prenatally and postnatally diagnosed congenital hydrocephalus in Japan. Neurol Med Chir (Tokyo). 2007;47(10):448–52.
75. Jeret JS, Serur D, Wisniewski KE, et al. Clinicopathological findings associated with agenesis of the corpus callosum. Brain Dev. 1987;9(3):255–64.
76. Fransen E, Van Camp G, Vits L, et al. L1-associated diseases: clinical geneticists divide, molecular geneticists unite. Hum Mol Genet. 1997;6(10):1625–32.
77. McAbee GN, Chan A, Erde EL. Prolonged survival; with hydranencephaly: report of two patients and literature review. Pediatr Neurol. 2000;23(1):80–4.
78. Dieker T, Bruno RD. Sensory reinforcement of eyeblink rate in decorticate human. Am J Ment Defic. 1976;80(6):665–7.
79. Matsunaga E, Shiota K. Holoprosencephaly in human embryos: epidemioloc studies of 150 cases. Teratology. 1977;16(3):261–72.
80. Cohen MM Jr. Perspectives on holoprosencephaly: Part I. Epidemiology, genetics and syndromology. Teratology. 1989;40(3):211–35.
81. Bullen PJ, Rankin JM, Robson SC. Investigation of the epidemiology and prenatal diagnosis of

holoprosencephaly in the North of England. Am J Obstet Gynecol. 2001;184(6):1256–62.
82. Plawner LL, Delgado MR, Miller VS, et al. Neuroanatomy of holprosencephaly as a predictor of function: beyond the face predicting the brain. Neurology. 2002;59(7):1058–66.
83. Hahn JS, Plawner LL. Evaluation of management of children with holoprosencephaly. Pediatr Neurol. 2004;31(2):79–88.
84. Zahl SM, Wester K. Routine measurement of head circumference as a tool for detecting intracranial expansion in infants: what is the gain? A nationwide survey. Pediatrics. 2008 Mar;121(3):e416–20.
85. International Society of Ultrasound in Obstetrics and Gynecology. Sonographic examination of fetal central nervous system: guidelines for performing the 'basic examination' and the 'fetal neurosonogram'. Ultrasound Obstet Gynecol. 2007;29:109–16.
86. Quinn MW. The Doppler characteristics of hydrocephalus. MD thesis. Dublin: Trinity College, Dublin University; 1991.
87. Goh D, Minns RA, Pye SD. Transcranial Doppler ultrasound as a non-invasive means of monitoring cerebrohaemodynamic change in hydrocephalus. Eur J Paediatr Surg 1991;1(Suppl. I):14–17.
88. Mallucci Cl, Sgourous S Cerebrospinal fluid disorders. Informa Healthcare. 2010 Ch.3;71–5.
89. Papadias A, Miller C, Martin WL, Kilby MD, Sgouros S. Comparison of prenatal and postnatal MRI findings in the evaluation of intrauterine CNS anomalies requiring postnatal neurosurgical treatment. Childs Nerv Syst. 2008;24(2):185–92. Epub 2007 Aug 21
90. O'Brien DF, Seghedoni A, Collins DR, Hayhurst C. Mallucci CL is there an indication for ETV in young infants in aetiologies other than isolated aqueduct stenosis? Childs Nerv Syst. 2006;22(12):1565–72. Epub 2006 Sep 19. (Review)
91. Kennedy CR, Ayers S, Campbell MJ, Elbourne D, Hope P, Johnson A. Randomized, controlled trial of acetazolamide and furosemide in posthemorrhagic ventricular dilation in infancy: follow-up at 1 year. Pediatrics. 2001;108(3):597–607.
92. Whitelaw A, Kennedy CR, Brion LP. Diuretic therapy for newborn infants with posthemorrhagic ventricular dilatation. Cochrane Database Syst Rev. 2001;(2):CD002270. (Review).
93. Whitelaw A. Repeated lumbar or ventricular punctures in newborns with intraventricular hemorrhage. Cochrane Database Syst Rev. 2001;(1):CD000216. (Review). doi:https://doi.org/10.1002/14651858.CD000216.
94. Hudgins RJ. Posthemorrhagic hydrocephalus of infancy. Neurosurg Clin North Am. 2001;12(4):743–51, ix. (Review)
95. Shooman D, Portess H, Sparrow O. A review of the current treatments of posthaemorrhagic hydrocephalus of infants. Cerebrospinal Fluid Res. 2009;6:1.
96. Lifshutz JI, Johnson WD. History of hydrocephalus and its treatments. Neurosurg Focus. 2001;11(2):E1.
97. Cherian S, Whitelaw A, Thoresen M, Love S. The pathogenesis of neonatal post-hemorrhagic hydrocephalus. Brain Pathol. 2004;14(3):305–11. (Review)
98. Jain H, Sgouros S, Walsh AR, Hockley AD. The treatment of infantile hydrocephalus: "differential-pressure" or "flow-control" valves. A pilot study. Childs Nerv Syst. 2000;16(4):242–6.
99. Rekate HL. The slit ventricle syndrome: advances based on technology and understanding. Pediatr Neurosurg. 2004;40(6):259–63.
100. Hayhurst C, Cooke R, Williams D, Kandasamy J, O'Brien DF, Mallucci CL. The impact of antibiotic-impregnated catheters on shunt infection in children and neonates. Childs Nerv Syst. 2008;24(5):557–62. Epub 2007 Oct 26
101. Clark S, Sangra M, Hayhurst C, Kandasamy J, Jenkinson M, Lee M, Mallucci C. The use of noninvasive electromagnetic neuronavigation for slit ventricle syndrome and complex hydrocephalus in a pediatric population. J Neurosurg Pediatr. 2008;2(6):430–4.
102. Kestle JR, Drake JM, Cochrane DD, Milner R, Walker ML, Abbott R 3rd, Boop FA, Endoscopic Shunt Insertion Trial Participants. Lack of benefit of endoscopic ventriculoperitoneal shunt insertion: a multicenter randomized trial. J Neurosurg. 2003;98(2):284–90.
103. Goitein D, Papasavas P, Gagné D, Ferraro D, Wilder B, Caushaj PJ. Single trocar laparoscopically assisted placement of central nervous system-peritoneal shunts. Laparoendosc Adv Surg Tech A. 2006;16(1):1–4.
104. Kurschel S, Eder HG, Schleef J. CSF shunts in children: endoscopically-assisted placement of the distal catheter. Childs Nerv Syst. 2005;21(1):52–5. Epub 2004 Sep 8
105. Adams-Chapman I, Hansen NI, Stoll BJ, Higgins R, NICHD Research Network. Neurodevelopmental outcome of extremely low birth weight infants with posthemorrhagic hydrocephalus requiring shunt insertion. Pediatrics. 2008;121(5):e1167–77. Epub 2008 Apr 7
106. Bayston R. Epidemiology, diagnosis, treatment, and prevention of cerebrospinal fluid shunt infections. Neurosurg Clin N Am. 2001;12(4):703–8. viii
107. Drake JM, Sainte-Rose C. The shunt book. New York: Blackwell Scientific; 1995.
108. Sainte-Rose C, Piatt JH, Renier D, et al. Mechanical complications in shunts. Pediatr Neurosurg. 1991;17:2–9.
109. Decq P, Blanquet A, Yepes C. Percutaneous jugular placement of ventriculo-atrial shunts using a split sheath. Acta Neurochir (Wien). 1995;136(1–2):92–4. Technical note
110. Sheth SA, McGirt M, Woodworth G, Wang P, Rigamonti D. Ultrasound guidance for distal insertion of ventriculo-atrial shunt catheters: technical note. Neurol Res. 2009;31(3):280–2. Epub 2008 Nov 26
111. Ellegaard L, Mogensen S, Juhler M. Ultrasound-guided percutaneous placement of ventriculoatrial

shunts. Childs Nerv Syst. 2007;23(8):857–62. Epub 2007 Mar 21
112. Dandy W. An operative approach for hydrocephalus. Bull Johns Hopkins Hospital. 1922;33:189–90.
113. Wagner W, Koch D. Mechanisms of failure after endoscopic third ventriculostomy in young infants. J Neurosurg. 2005;103(1 Suppl):43–9.
114. Javadpour M, Mallucci C, Brodbelt A, Golash A, May P. The impact of endoscopic third ventriculostomy on the management of newly diagnosed hydrocephalus in infants. Pediatr Neurosurg. 2001;35(3):131–5.
115. Buxton N, Macarthur D, Mallucci C, Punt J, Vloeberghs M. Neuroendoscopy in the premature population. Childs Nerv Syst. 1998;14(11):649–52.
116. O'Brien DF, Javadpour M, Collins DR, Spennato P, Mallucci CL. Endoscopic third ventriculostomy: an outcome analysis of primary cases and procedures performed after ventriculoperitoneal shunt malfunction. J Neurosurg. 2005;103(5 Suppl):393–400.
117. Warf BC. Hydrocephalus in Uganda: the predominance of infectious origin and primary management with endoscopic third ventriculostomy. J Neurosurg. 2005;102(1 Suppl):1–15.
118. Warf BC. Comparison of endoscopic third ventriculostomy alone and combined with choroid plexus cauterization in infants younger than 1 year of age: a prospective study in 550 African children. J Neurosurg. 2005;103(6 Suppl):475–81.
119. Javadpour M, May P, Mallucci C. Sudden death secondary to delayed closure of endoscopic third ventriculostomy. Br J Neurosurg. 2003;17(3):266–9.
120. Von Koch CS, Gupta N, Sutton LN, Sun PP. In utero surgery for hydrocephalus. Childs Nerv Syst. 2003;19(7–8):574–86. Epub 2003 Jul 25. (Review)
121. Adzick NS, Thom EA, Spong CY, et al., for the MOMS Investigators. A randomized trial of prenatal versus postnatal repair of myelomeningocele. N Engl J Med. 2011;364:993–1004.
122. Hunt GM, Oakeshott P. Outcome in people with open spina bifida at age 35: prospective community based cohort study. BMJ. 2003;326:1365–6.
123. Dennis M, Jewell D, Drake J, Misakyan T, Spiegler B, Hetherington R, et al. Prospective, declarative, and nondeclarative memory in young adults with spina bifida. J Int Neuropsychol Soc. 2007;13:312–23.
124. Kulkarni AV, Shams I, Cochrane DD, McNeely PD. Quality of life after endoscopic third ventriculostomy and cerebrospinal fluid shunting: an adjusted multivariable analysis in a large cohort. J Neurosurg Pediatr. 2010;6:11–6.

50 Neural Tube Defects

Martin T. Corbally

Abstract

Neural Tube Defects (NTD) or Spina Bifida are disorders of neural tube development and closure and include a wide variety of abnormalities ranging from spina bifida occulta to anencephaly. Although the incidence of neural tube defects is less common today (0.5–1/1000 live births in some reports) and is falling, NTDs remain the most common congenital central neural system developmental disorder. The factors contributing to this decreasing incidence are in some part geographic and related to antenatal screening and termination of pregnancy but also relate to improved nutrition and folic acid supplementation. Improved standards of living and a falling birth rate have also impacted on a declining incidence. Despite this Spina Bifida is a cause of major morbidity with significant implications to the quality of life of the child but which also impacts significantly on the wellbeing of the family unit as a whole. Not surprisingly the management of these children involves a multi-disciplinary team approach with significant input from specialist paediatric surgeons, neurosurgeons, urologists, orthopaedic surgeons, paediatricians (especially rehabilitation) social workers, nursing, physiotherapy and child psychology.

Keywords

Neural tube defects • Spina bifida • Encephalocoele • Surgical management Outcomes

50.1 Introduction

Neural Tube Defects (NTD) or Spina Bifida are disorders of neural tube development and closure and include a wide variety of abnormalities ranging from spina bifida occulta to anencephaly. Although the incidence of neural tube defects is less common today (0.5–1/1000 live births in some reports) and is falling, NTDs remain the

M.T. Corbally, MB, BCh, BAO, MCh, FRCS(Ed)
Department of Surgery, RCSI Medical University, King Hamad University Hospital, Al Sayh, Bahrain
e-mail: martin.corbally@khuh.org.bh

P.D. Losty et al. (eds.), *Rickham's Neonatal Surgery*, https://doi.org/10.1007/978-1-4471-4721-3_50

most common congenital central neural system developmental disorder [1]. The factors contributing to this decreasing incidence are in some part geographic and related to antenatal screening and termination of pregnancy but also relate to improved nutrition and folic acid supplementation. Improved standards of living and a falling birth rate have also impacted on a declining incidence. Despite this Spina Bifida is a cause of major morbidity with significant implications to the quality of life of the child but which also impacts significantly on the wellbeing of the family unit as a whole. Not surprisingly the management of these children involves a multi-disciplinary team approach with significant input from specialist paediatric surgeons, neurosurgeons, urologists, orthopaedic surgeons, paediatricians (especially rehabilitation) social workers, nursing, physiotherapy and child psychology.

An unexpected diagnosis of NTD can have devastating consequences for the family and great support is necessary from birth onwards. The objective of management is to achieve early back closure, deal with hydrocephalus if required and to provide a meaningful structure for the child and family to allow as good a quality of life with normal or near normal integration into society as possible. There is no immediate cure for this often severe congenital deformity but modern techniques of back closure combined with precise hydrocephalus management enable the paediatric surgeon or paediatric neurosurgeon deliver not only life saving initial surgery but also provide a more holistic individualised management plan that improves not only the child's life quality but also that of the immediate family. This involves regular review at a dedicated Spina Bifida clinic which aims to minimise the disruption to family life by providing a multidisciplinary team presence (paediatric and orthopaedic surgery, social workers, specialist nurse and experts in paediatric rehabilitation) at each follow up.

It is important that each clinic visit focuses not only on identified problems e.g. posture control, mobility and hip issues with correction of talipes but also monitors potential problems such as the neuropathic bladder and its consequences especially long-term renal damage. A "one stop" properly structured clinic is a resource of great value to parents managing a child with a NTD and enables not only the medical and surgical aspects to be addressed but can focus on social and housing issues and on integration into mainstream education.

This chapter will focus briefly on the embryology of neural tube defects, the types commonly seen and their management including closure. For descriptive reasons most emphasis will be placed on the treatment of myelomeningocoele as this is the commonest type of NTD seen.

50.2 Embryology and Pathogenesis

Spina Bifida is a congenital abnormality affecting growth and development of the spine in which development and fusion of the vertebral arches and overlying skin and muscle has failed with or without protrusion and dysplasia of the spinal cord and its meninges.

The neural tube begins to form at around 14 days of age by the formation of the neural plate which is derived from the ectodermal tissue. Longitudinal in-folding of the plate (neurulation) (Fig. 50.1) proceeds from the mid portion (cervical) of the tube in a cephalad and caudal direction. The precise control of neurulation is not fully understood but the notochord which lies deep to the neural plate probably induces in-folding. The two ends of the neural tube are the last to close and these are called the anterior and posterior neuropores with the anterior or cranial neuropore closing at 24 days. Failure of closure of either neuropore can explain anencephaly or Myelomeningocoele. Alternatively the neuropores could close normally but failure of CSF drainage through the fourth ventricle causes hydrocephalus which ruptures the newly formed and delicate neural tube.

At this stage of development there are two layers of ectodermal tissue one more medially placed which on closure forms the neural tube and the more laterally placed ectoderm provides complete neural tube closure. By 21 days the neural tube has formed and the mesodermal elements begin to arrange into the vertebra and dura.

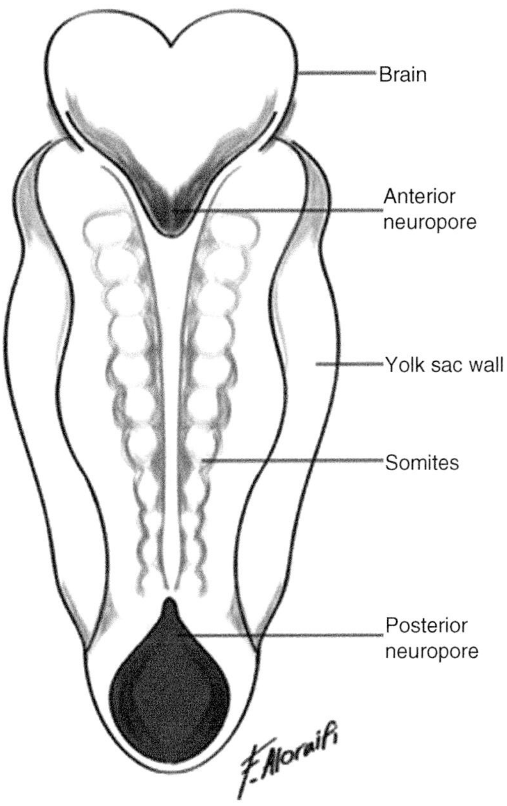

Fig. 50.1 Neurulation is proceeding and the anterior and posterior neuropores are visible

This occurs by migration of mesodermal elements into the notochord area to begin the formation of vertebra and intervertebral discs. Abnormalities of mesodermal arrangement or inclusion or persistence of some totipotent cells can result in other abnormalities such as diastematomyelia, lipo-myelomeningocoele abnormal vertebrae, sacro-coccygeal teratoma. If the notochord splits and the yolk sac herniates then the result can be the split notochord syndrome sinus or a fistula with ectopic bowel.

50.3 Aetiology

While we have significant insight into the development of the neural tube we do not know the precise aetiology of NTDs. A variety of factors have been suggested some of them genetic, some nutritional and some teratogenic.

50.3.1 Nutritional Factors

There is sufficient data to support a causal relationship between myelomeningocoele and folic acid metabolism. This may reflect environmental factors interacting with a genetic predisposition. Whatever the reason, there is substantial evidence now that peri-conceptual folic acid in a dose of 0.1–0.4 mg/day will reduce the incidence of NTDs in all pregnancies with or without added or existing risk. The Medical Research Council Vitamin study in1991 reported on the results of a randomised double blind trial in 33 centres in 7 countries in women at risk and demonstrated a significant reduction in the incidence of NTD in such pregnancies [1, 2]. Peri-conceptual folic acid is now recommended for all women whether or not there is a perceived genetic risk. In women at risk the dose of peri conceptual folic acid is 4–5 mg/kg per day. The incidence seems to be higher in women who have preconception obesity and diabetes with poor glucose control.

50.3.2 Genetics

The incidence of Spina Bifida continues to decline and its real incidence is hard to define especially when considered against the rates of termination for the condition. While the NIH list the condition as rare there are over 240 live births per year in the USA but over 4000 pregnancies with an antenatal diagnosis of NTD the majority of whom do not reach term. In the UK the overall incidence is about 5.7/10,000 births. While there are clear genetic associations the exact mode of inheritance is not known, and it is likely that there is a multifactorial hereditary predisposition. This is suggested by ethnic variation (more common in Caucasians and Hispanics), females more likely affected, familial tendency and increased incidence in parental consanguinity. If there has been a previous pregnancy affected by NTD the risk is of the order of 1 in 20–25 of a subsequent pregnancy being affected. This increases to 1 in 8 if there are two children with a NTD. The risk if one parent had an NTD is 1 in 200.

50.3.3 Teratogens

Foetal exposure to Sodium Valproate and Carpamazine carry a 1.2% risk of NTD while hyperthermia and certain viruses have also been associated with increased risk.

50.4 Historical

The earliest cited reference to an NTD abnormality may be that of Casper Bauhin (1605) from a work by Morgagni in1761 [3]. However the term spina bifida dorsi was introduced by Talpius in 1641 who also attempted to excise the sac with fatal results. Similar surgical efforts were invariably fatal as were attempts to aspirate the sac. Although there were some reports of successful surgery in the latter part of the nineteenth century it was not until techniques were developed to effectively deal with hydrocephalus in the late 1950s that real improvements in survival and outcome were seen. Earlier attempts had attempted to reduce CSF production by choroid plexus ablation. It was not until the introduction of the Spitz-Holter valve that the management of these children was revolutionised and a more aggressive approach to primary back closure acceptable [4]. Longterm survival of these children was now the norm and necessitated the progression of strategies to deal with neurogenic bladder and orthopaedic issues.

However survival of greater numbers of children who were severely incapacitated with a poor life quality prompted a re-appraisal of an aggressive attitude and sentinel works by Lorber and Schofield [5] and others suggested that in selected patients aggressive surgical management was not appropriate. Major ethical dilemmas were raised which called into question the decision to select infants in this way and to with hold primary back closure in those regarded as having poor outcomes. Patients born with thoracolumbar lesions, severe kyphosis, gross paraplagia, severe hydrocephalus (>90th centile by 2 cm) and other significant associated congenital lesions were considered to be incompatible with survival or good quality of life and primary operative closure was not advised. Conservative management of these infants with demand feeding and sedation was recommended after discussion with parents. While it achieved time for parents to consider the recommended treatment it also became apparent that many infants managed in this way survived and that their quality of life may have been adversely affected by the decision to manage them without primary back closure [6].

Today the majority of infants with Spina Bifida are managed operatively but this nevertheless accepts that treatment in all such infants should be individualized. Of course the widespread use of antenatal Ultrasound and prenatal counseling allows for early termination, if legislated and based on parental request, and is based on an assessment of severity of the lesion. Parents must be fully informed about the anticipated quality of life potential if they decide against termination. This clearly contributes to fewer children being born with severe lesions.

50.5 Classification and Types

NTD defects vary from anencephaly to spina bifida occulta but the most commonly seen is myelomeningocoele and for the most part it will form the basis of this chapter.

A. Brain
   1. Encephalocoele. is a herniation of brain (anterior or posterior) through a congenital defect of the skull which is covered by meninges and skin.
   2. Anencephaly is a uniformly fatal congenital NTD defect where the brain is very severely malformed with poor skull and soft tissue development
   3. Exencephaly is extremely rare with no skin or skull coverage

B. Brain and Spine

   Craniorachisis involves both the brain and the spine

C. Spine (Spina Bifida Cystica)
   1. Myelomeningocoele. (Fig. 50.2) is the commonest form of spina bifida and presents as a cord defect anywhere from the

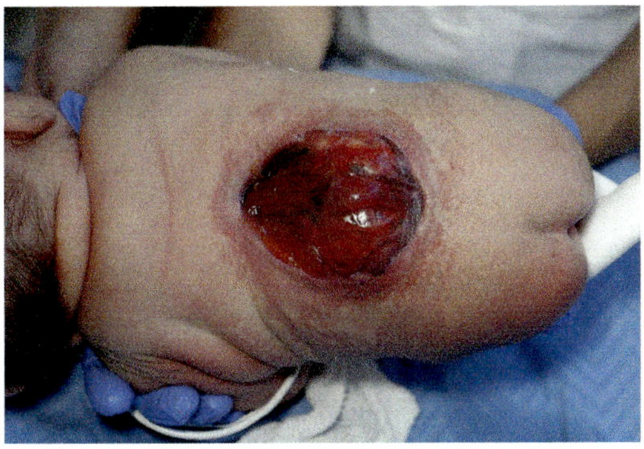

Fig. 50.2 Typical thoracic-lumbar myelomeningocoele showing exposed meninges and neural plaque

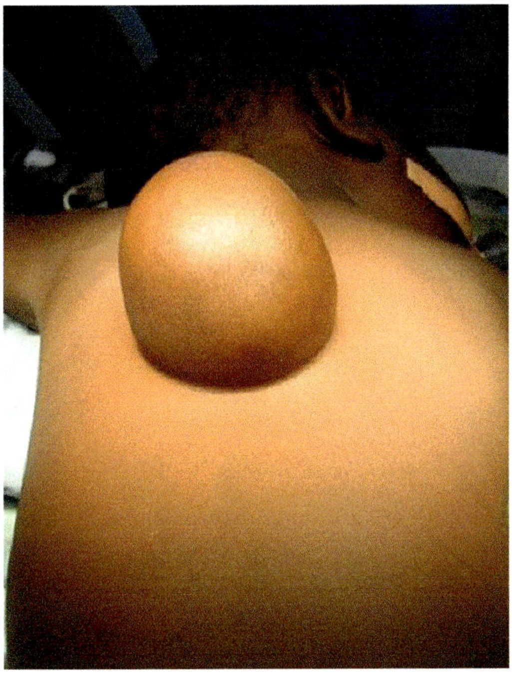

Fig. 50.3 Intact skin covering sac of investing meninges

cervical to sacral region. The defect may have a flimsy attenuated meninges and partial skin covering or partially covering a centrally placed neural plaque.

2. Meningocoele (Fig. 50.3) is a defect in the vertebra and muscle but the skin is intact. Generally the cord is covered by a meningeal sac.
3. Spina Bifida Occulta. The skin is intact but there are absent vertebral components (spinous processes) and there is usually a large tuft of hair or there may be an associated tethered cord, haemangioma or lipoma.

50.6 Antenatal Diagnosis

It is more likely today that antenatal scans will have detected a neural tube defect and termination is possible if that is both legal and in keeping with parental wishes. Maternal alpha feto-protein (AFP) can be used as a screening test in early pregnancy and will be raised with open NTDs as early as 16–18 weeks gestation. This should prompt more detailed investigation either by ultrasound and or MRI scan especially if persistently raised at this stage of pregnancy. 3-D ultrasonography is more sensitive than 2-D U/S and more widely available than foetal MRI scan with a reported sensitivity of 94% [7]. It does need significant training however and all abnormal scans should be the subject of detailed multidisciplinary discussion before any decision is reached on management.

Antenatal ultrasound allows appropriate discussion and planning of delivery if the parents decide not to terminate the pregnancy. Discussions should involve the Obstetrician, Paediatric Surgeon or Paediatric Neurosurgeon and should present as realistic a view as possible considering the level and size of the lesion. This discussion should highlight the main areas of concern which with any spinal NTD will include mobility, presence or absence of hydrocephalus and likelihood of a ventriculo-peritoneal shunt, intellectual ability or disability, long term bladder and bowel issues and the likelihood of multiple surgeries and morbidity. When the decision is made to carry to term a decision should be reached about the mode and place of delivery as most would advocate planned Caesarean section which may positively affect functional outcome as well as facilitating team readiness for the child's delivery. Ideally such infants are best delivered close to a paediatric surgical hospital or a paediatric neurosurgical unit. There is as yet no clear benefit of foetal in-utero surgery to allow lesional coverage.

50.7 Initial Management

Following delivery the infant is assessed as regards site of the lesion and whether it is covered or not. Skin covered lesions require no urgent intervention but open lesions should be covered with cling film and a rapid assessment made of associated problems. It is important that the medical team looking after the infant have a series of discussions with the parents and provide as much information as possible at this time. This should include a frank but empathetic discussion of the clinical severity of the lesion, the assessments needed and the likely clinical plan. It is clearly helpful if parents have had an opportunity to meet the surgeon prior to delivery and the news is not so catastrophic for them. A plan of management needs to be developed that includes a structured imaging protocol and a full sensorimotor evaluation. This often demonstrates a flaccid paralysis and is best quantified by an experienced physiotherapist and is most useful when subsequently compared to post-operative function [8].

In addition to the obvious spinal lesion, patients with NTDs can have many other associated problems and these must be documented. Talipes, congenital hip dislocation and other spinal abnormalities are common and need the input of a paediatric orthopaedic surgeon and paediatric physiotherapist.

Most patients with a myelomeningocoele will have a patulous anus and some may have neonatal rectal prolapse. The majority of patients with myelomeningocoele will have features of a neuropathic bladder (decreased bladder compliance and sphincter dysfunction) causing a high pressure bladder with consequential risk of urinary stasis and Vesico-Ureteric Reflux with renal scarring. However these are rarely seen at birth apart from bladder dribbling and can be monitored by regular screening and earlier introduction of clean intermittent catheterisation as indicated by recurrent infection or renal damage on radioisotope (DMSA) scan. A baseline renal Ultrasound is performed and is generally normal at this stage.

Head circumference and a cranial U/S are performed to assess the degree of Hydrocephalus. Approximately 90% of myelomeningocoele patients will require a Ventriculo-Peritoneal shunt for increasing Hydrocephalus within the first 4 weeks of birth [8].

It is advisable that all spinal NTD patients have a cranio-spinal MRI scan performed at some stage to rule out any associated cord abnormalities such as a tethered cord (Figs. 50.4 and 50.5), the ubiquitous Arnold Chiari malformation (Fig. 50.6) or a cord syrinx (Figs. 50.6 and 50.7). Approximately 70% of NTD patients will also

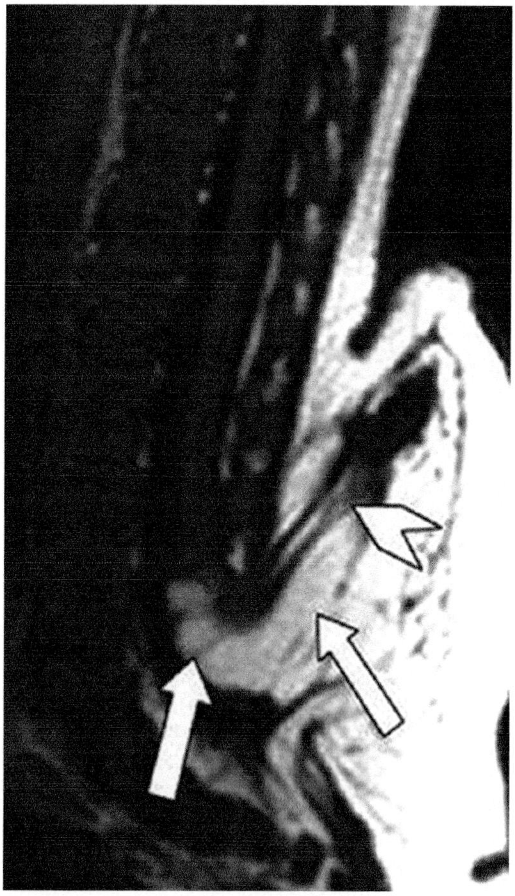

Fig. 50.4 Newborn male infant with a lipomyelomeningocoele. Sagittal T1 weighted image of the lower spine showing the low lying cord tethered by the filum (*white arrow head*) to the large lipomatous malformation (*white arrows*) that is contiguous with the subcutaneous fat through the posterior dysraphic elements

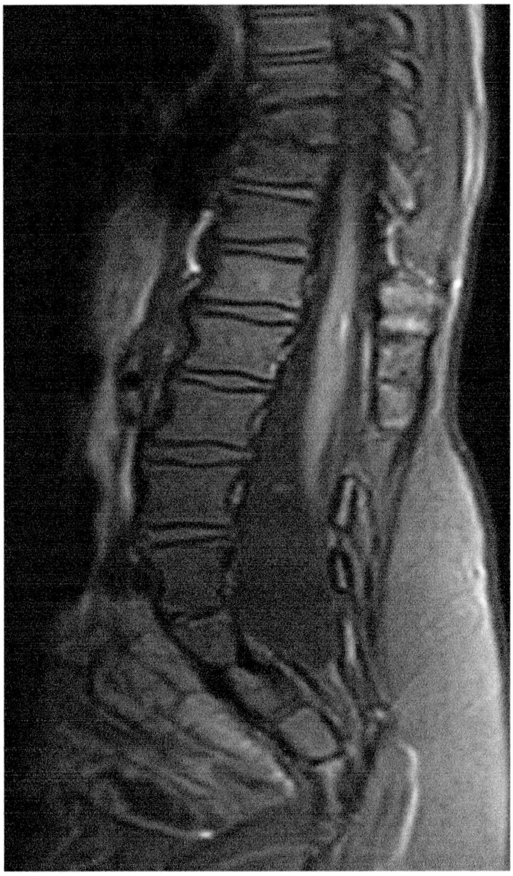

Fig. 50.5 Saggital T2 weighted image of the lower spine, showing the cord tethered at the level of L4 with a short syrinx above this

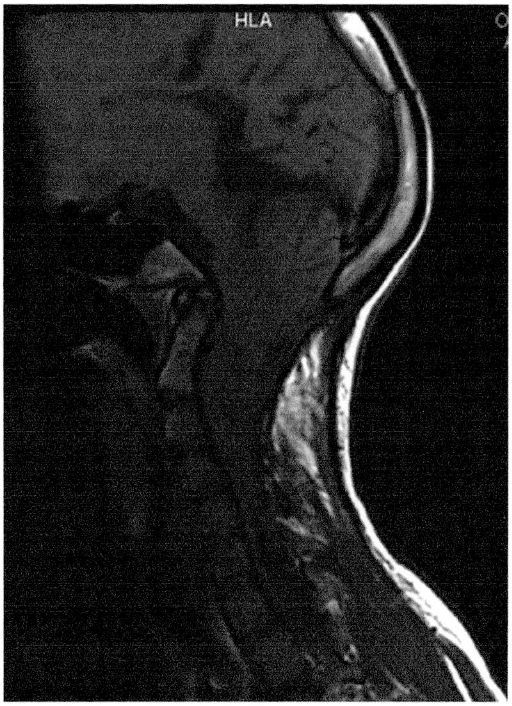

Fig. 50.6 Sagital T1 weighted image of the craniocervical junction showing a typical Arnold Chiari malformation, a small posterior fossa, large funnel shaped foramen magnum and herniation of cerebellar contents into the cervical canal behind the medulla. A large syrinx is also seen

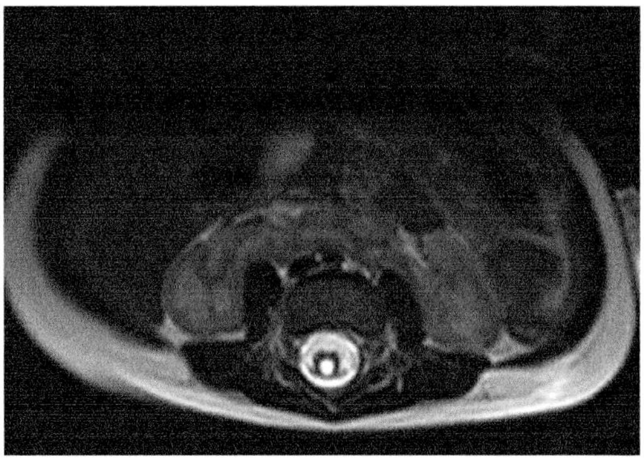

Fig. 50.7 Showing an axial T2 weighted image through the lower cord showing a central syrinx and a horseshoe kidney

have an abnormality of the corpus callosum. Spinal U/S is extremely sensitive to these abnormalities when performed from birth to 4/6 weeks postnatal.

Other investigations required are an X-ray of the spine to document the extent of the bony defect and also the degree of kyphosis (Fig. 50.8) which may require an osteotomy to facilitate closure. An orthopaedic opinion is obtained to assess and treat Talipes and dislocated hip if present. In general both of the latter abnormalities are managed conservatively.

It is important to provide support at all times to the parents, especially if there has not been an antenatal diagnosis, who can be and generally are shocked by the entire process. In general most infants undergo closure within 24–36 h unless there is a severe lesion or serious major associated abnormality. The objective of early closure is to prevent further neural deterioration from infection and prior to closure the lesion should be

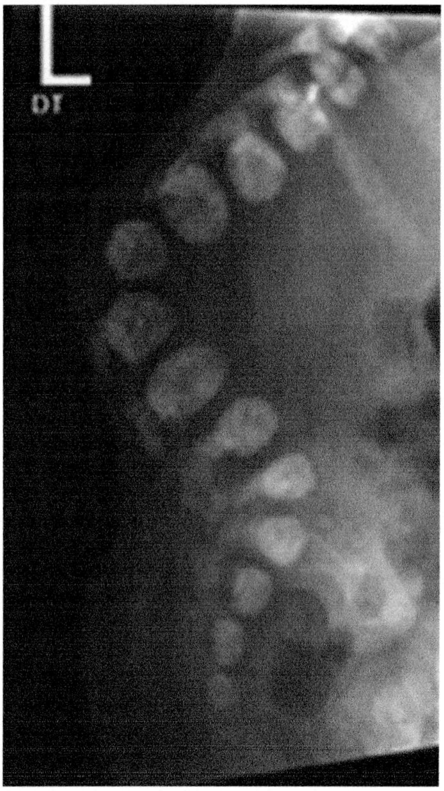

Fig. 50.8 Severe lumbar kyphosis associated with a myelomeningocoele. This lesion may require an osteotomy prior to complex soft tissue closure

protected with a Chorhexidine sponge and cling film over. Consideration should also be given to a broad spectrum antibiotic.

Most closures are well tolerated but occasionally closure can result in accelerated hydrocephalus which is generally compensated well with an open anterior fontanelle. Shunting will be required when the head circumference exceeds two standard deviations over the 90th centile or when there is rapid increase in hydrocephalus. It is also necessary if there is persistent CSF leakage from the closed back lesion.

50.8 Operative Details of Closure (As per Myelomeningocoele)

Following general anaesthesia and insertion of an endotracheal tube the patient is turned prone and cotton (Gamgee) supports placed under the pelvis and chest. It is important to place additional supports beneath each foot. It is not necessary to have blood available for this procedure but most would have a group and hold order with the laboratory. A neonatal diathermy pad is usually applied to the abdomen or chest. A warming bear hugger is routinely used. Bipolar diathermy should be used throughout. A swab for culture may be obtained at this point.

The skin is prepped with a povidone iodine solution and the lesion with chlorhexidene and draped with generous margins to facilitate additional skin dissection if required. An incision is made at the lowermost portion of the sac using a sharp scissors. This incision is carried cranially staying away from the neural plaque, which should not be handled where possible, and close to the sac-skin junction. Incision into the sac results in a release of CSF and some bleeding which is easily dealt with using bipolar diathermy. Nerve roots and blood vessels are now seen traversing the sac and disappearing anteriorly through the dural layer, and they should be preserved. The dural layer is clearly visible as a whitish fibrous layer. The sac is elevated taking care not to traumatise the neural plaque and the sac excised completely from the plaque. Bleeding from the neural edge is dealt with using biloar diathermy and with minimal handling of the plaque itself. At intervals chlorhexidene soaks may be applied to the area. Tubal reconstruction of the plaque is rarely indicated [8, 9].

The plaque will now be seen to lie on an easily recognisable dural layer. This fibrous layer is incised as far laterally as possible and the layer carefully dissected from the underlying fascia. This dissection is carried medially until the nerve roots come into view. Epidural veins may proof difficult at this point but these can be controlled by bipolar diathermy.

The mobilized dural layer is now tubularised over the exposed neural plaque using a running suture of 6/0 maxon on a 9 or 11 mm round bodied needle. A watertight closure is the expected aim. Occasionally it is not possible to complete the dural tube completely and a small portion of vertebral fascia is used to achieve closure. This

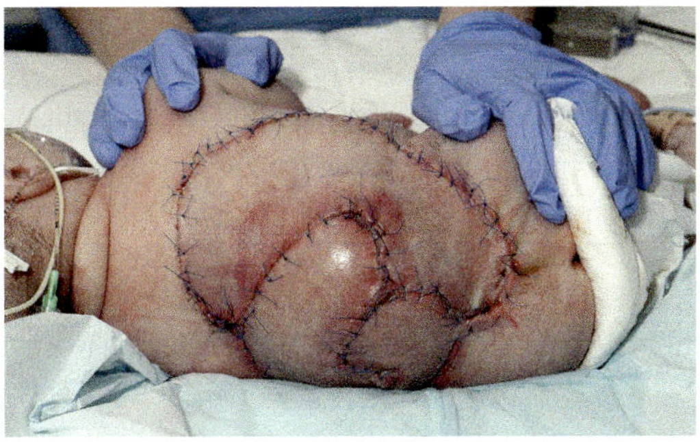

Fig. 50.9 Complex rotational flap repair in baby with severe kyphosis

is preferable to compromising the plaque. A small suction drain is placed to lie lateral to the dural lube and exited far laterally. This deals with any leakage of CSF which is usually short lived. Troublesome leakage usually responds to the insertion of a Ventriculo Peritoneal shunt. Where possible the dural tube is re-inforced using an additional fascial covering obtained by mobilising the fascia from the underlying muscle. It is usually impossible to cover the dural tube completely with fascia especially at the lower end.

The subcutaneous layer is approximated using a 3/0 absorbable suture. It is nearly always possible to close the skin layer using interrupted (4/0) sutures, but very rarely this requires considerable skin undermining or the use of lateral releasing skin incisions or complex flap repairs (Fig. 50.9). The skin closure is supported with wound strips and a dressing applied.

50.9 Post-Operatively

The baby is nursed prone or in a lateral position. Careful attention is paid to keeping the area clean. Feeds are not restricted. Weekly estimates of head circumference are performed and this is supplemented with cranial ultra-sound to monitor progress of the associated hydrocephalus. A Ventriculo-peritoneal shunt is inserted when the head circumference rises precipitously or when the Ventricular diameter increases beyond 50–60% of the diameter of the skull.

50.10 Other Considerations

Associated vertebral kyphosis may occasionally require an osteotomy to facilitate closure in the primary setting (Figs. 50.8 and 50.9). This is more likely with lesions treated conservatively initially and back closure performed as a secondary event

It is worth remembering that infants with NTDs may become sensitised to Latex rubber and that this should be avoided where possible even at the time of initial closure.

Encephalocoeles account for less than 10% of all neural tube defects and occur as a defect in the cranium through which the brain or part of the brain herniates. They are typically posterior and occipital but fronto-nasal may be more common in Asia. They may occur in other sites such as parietal. They are obvious at birth although fronto nasal lesions may be mistaken for dermoid cysts. Their size and complexity relate to the amount of brain tissue in the encephalocoele. The rest of the brain may abnormal also and there may be hydrocehalus. Imaging is with MRI and treatment is generally by excision unless there is a very significant amount of brain in the lesion in which case they may be, by necessity, managed conservatively.

50.11 Outcome

Patients with spina bifida pose serious problems to the family and the medical, nursing and allied professions. They need a multidisciplinary approach for their management with special emphasis on monitoring renal and bladder function, provision of physiotherapy services both in the community and hospital, proper evaluation of hearing and visual acuity, orthopaedic review and assistance with mobility either using calipers or a modified wheelchair. In addition the mobilisation of local paediatric and medical services with input from social services is vital to optimise their ultimate quality of life. Quality of life in these patients can be actively enhanced using clean intermittent catheterisation and bowel washout programmes.

The majority of meningomyelocoele patients have a neurogenic bladder and less than 10% are truly continent [8, 9]. Increased detrusor pressure is rarely a problem in the neonatal period and most infants empty with a dribbling stream. Over time urinary stasis and a high pressure system can be associated with vesico-ureteric reflux and be the cause of recurrent urinary tract infection and renal scarring. Consequently frequent renal tract imaging, cultures and urodynamics are required to determine whether or not there is a need for prophylactic antibiotics or early institution of bladder catheter drainage as in intermittent catheterisation (CIC). CIC may be introduced at a later time to confer social continence in the majority (>75%) and the remainder by a combination of pharmocology (anticholinergics) and surgery [10]. It is essential that the urinary tract is frequently monitored using Ultrasound and radionuclide imaging to ensure that silent renal damage does not occur or progress unnoticed.

The majority of myelomeningocoele patients have an active internal anal sphincter and tend to have a degree of constipation. This is considerably easier to manage with diet, fluids and laxatives as needed. Rectal retrograde washouts using systems like the Willis washout are largely effective although some degree of tolerance to the washout can occur over time. Antegrade washouts as in an antegrade colonic enema procedure may restore social faecal continence in these cases.

While virtually every NTD patient will have the Chiari malformation only a minority will have symptoms referable to brainstem compression such as cranial nerve palsies, headache. MRI scan is indicated to evaluate the need for foraminal decompression in selected symptomatic patients. A problem arises with regard to cord tethering which is a common finding in repaired myelomeningocoele. The issue is whether a tethered cord in itself warrants surgery since in all probability it will probably simply recur. A more rational approach is to monitor progress and reserve surgery for situations of neurological deterioration, change in ambulation (gait or toe clawing) or urinary function, the latter perhaps directed by deterioration on urodynamics. MRI is the investigation of choice to detect significant anatomical cord tethering (Figs. 50.4 and 50.5).

In general patients with lesions at L3 will be non-ambulatory while those at L5 will ambulate normally. Patients with lesions between these areas will require considerable support to walk and may spend intermittent periods in a wheelchair. However less than 1/3 patients are ambulatory in long term studies. Some of these may relate not to an inability to walk but to a personal choice as many find the wheelchair more acceptable and easier to use. Living circumstances must be reviewed constantly as the child grows older with interaction with social workers and occupational therapy.

Over 90% of myelo-meningocoele patients will require CSF shunting and these patients need constant review to ensure there is no shunt malfunction. Shunt series allow diagnosis of catheter fracture but a CT scan is needed to gain more useful information especially when the fontanelle has closed after 16 or 18 months of age.

NTD patients may have a variety of cognitive impairments especially if associated with shunt malfunction and episodes of infection. Shunt infection rates should be less than 3% using a no touch insertion technique. It is important that early remedial education is available and that these children are supported in mainstream schools as early and as far as possible.

50.12 Summary

Spina Bifida is a congenital disorder of neural tube closure that may occur anywhere from the cranium to the sacrum and vary from a life threatening condition to a mild and unnoticed defect. While the pattern of inheritance is not clear it is certain that there are both nutritional and genetic factors that weigh together to influence the occurrence of a neural tube defect. Antenatal diagnosis both by imaging and maternal Alpha Feto-protein (AFP) has changed the incidence of NTD dramatically in jurisdictions where medical terminations are legal. There has also been a real reduction in the overall population incidence however which appears to be independent of this and may relate to better overall nutrition. The addition of peri-conceptual folic acid has been shown to decrease incidence when given in doses of 0.1–0.4 mg/kg/day. Post natal management of NTD babies presents serious and complex ethical considerations if the lesion is severe and survival is questioned, especially if it is considered that a conservative approach is justified on the basis of quality of life. Most patients however are considered for early back closure and or Ventriculo Peritoneal Shunt insertion. Timing of surgical intervention may impact on variables such as mobilty and intellectual ability with early closure perhaps conferring a positive effect on these variables. Most patients will need Ventriculo-peritoneal shunting and all require lifelong surveillance to ensure preserved renal function. Issues surrounding bladder and renal function and continence with mobility, educational and psychosocial concerns are lifelong matters that require significant professional input. With modern interventional techniques and an all encompassing multidisciplinary approach, the majority can enjoy a good quality of life.

Acknowledgments Sincere thanks to Mr. John Caird, Consultant Paediatric Neurosurgeon and Dr. Claire Brenner, Consultant Paediatric Radiologist for permission to use their clinical photographs and Dr. Fatima AlOraifi, MRCSI, PhD for the art work.

References

1. Williams J, et al. Updated estimates of neural tube defects prevented by mandatory folic acid fortification—United States, 1995-2011. MMWR Morb Mortal Wkly Rep. 2015;64(1):1–5.
2. Medical Research Council Vitamin Study Group. Prevention of Neural Tube Defects. Lancet. 1991;338: 131–7.
3. Morgagni JB. Je Sedibus et causis morborum per indagatis. Typographia Simoniana: Naples; 1762.
4. Drake JM, et al. The shunt book. Cambridge: Blackwell; 1995.
5. Lorber J. Results of treatment of myelomeningocoele. An analysis of 524 unselected cases, with special reference to possible selection for treatment. Dev Med Child Neurol. 1971;13:279–303.
6. Surana RH, et al. Are the selection criteria for the conservative management in spina bifida still applicable? Eur J Pediatr Surg. 1991;1(Suppl. 1):35–7.
7. Romero R, et al. Accuracy of Ultrasound in the prenatal diagnosis of spinal anomalies. Am J Perinatol. 1989;6:320–3.
8. Corbally MT. Spina bifida and encephalocoele. In: Puri P, Höllwarth ME, editors. Pediatric surgery: diagnosis and management. Berlin: Springer; 2009. p. 765–74
9. Rudy DC, et al. The incontinent myelodysplastic patient. Urol Clin North Am. 1991;18:295–308.
10. Kasabian NB, et al. The prophylactic value of clean intermittent catheterization and anticholinergic medications in infants and newborns with myelodysplasia at risk of developing urinary tract deterioration. Am J Dis Child. 1992;146:840–3.

Neonatal Brain Tumours

51

Chris Barton, Jothy Kandasamy,
Benedetta Pettorini, Conor L. Mallucci,
and Barry Pizer

Abstract

Neonatal brain tumours (NBT) are a rare but important group of neoplasms within the field of paediatric neuro-oncology as they present particular technical and physiological challenges to the neuro-surgical team. Contemporary management requires the application of appropriate multimodal individualised therapeutic approaches.

Neonatal brain tumours (NBT) are a rare but important group of neoplasms within the field of paediatric neuro-oncology as they present particular technical and physiological challenges to the neuro-surgical team. Contemporary management requires the application of appropriate multimodal individualised therapeutic approaches.

Keywords

CNS tumours • Newborn brain tumours • Management • outcome

51.1 Epidemiology and Aetiology

Neonatal brain tumours represent a rare and heterogeneous group of neoplasms with an incidence of 1–3.5 per 100,000 newborns [1]. Central Nervous System (CNS) tumours diagnosed in the first year of life represent 7.2–10.9% of all perinatal tumours [2], but account for up to 20% of deaths from neoplastic disease within the neonatal age bracket [3]. The rarity and sporadic nature of many of these tumours means that case series tend to be small, with reporting over long periods during which investigations, diagnostic criteria and treatments may have changed, affecting epidemiological, clinical and survival data. Furthermore, it can be difficult to extract data

C. Barton, MB, ChB, BSc(Hons), MRCPCH
B. Pizer, MB, ChB, MRCP, FRCPCH, PhD (✉)
Department of Oncology, Alder Hey Children's Hospital, Liverpool, Merseyside, UK
e-mail: Barry.pizer@alderhey.nhs.uk

J. Kandasamy, FRCS(Neuro Surg)
Department of Neurosurgery, Royal Hospital for Sick Children, Edinburgh, Lothian, UK

B. Pettorini, MD
Department of Neurosurgery, Alder Key Children's Hospital, Liverpool, Merseyside, UK

C.L. Mallucci, MBBS, FRCS(Surgical Neurology)
Department of Neurosurgery, Alder Hey Children's NHS Foundation Trust, Liverpool, UK

P.D. Losty et al. (eds.), *Rickham's Neonatal Surgery*, https://doi.org/10.1007/978-1-4471-4721-3_51

regarding particular age ranges (e.g. <28 days or <1 year) from some reports, complicated further by the analysis of data within age ranges specific to the treatment strategy being considered (e.g. 0–3 years in protocols delaying radiotherapy).

51.2 Causative Factors

A higher incidence of infant brain tumours is seen with familial genetic conditions such as Gorlin Syndrome, Li-Fraumeni and Tuberose Sclerosis [1] (Fig. 51.1). Overall congenital abnormalities are seen in around 15% of neonatal tumours in general, suggesting an association with genetic defects [4].

Observational, biological, environmental and demographic studies have investigated potential relationships between causative factors and particular tumour subtypes or histotypes, with in utero exposure associations even more difficult to elucidate. Proposed factors include smoking, diet, racial characteristics, maternal age, maternal viral infections, pesticides and medications, with inconsistent, inconclusive and even contradictory findings from studies [1, 5].

51.3 Clinical Presentation

Obstetric complications of NBT include reduced foetal movements, polyhydramnios, enlarged uterine dimensions and premature labour, and tend to be vague, non-specific findings [3, 6]. While the widespread use of antenatal ultrasound as a routine tool in the monitoring of pregnancy has seen an increase in antenatal detection of intracranial lesions [6], in most cases this is as an incidental finding [2]. None the less, up to 18%

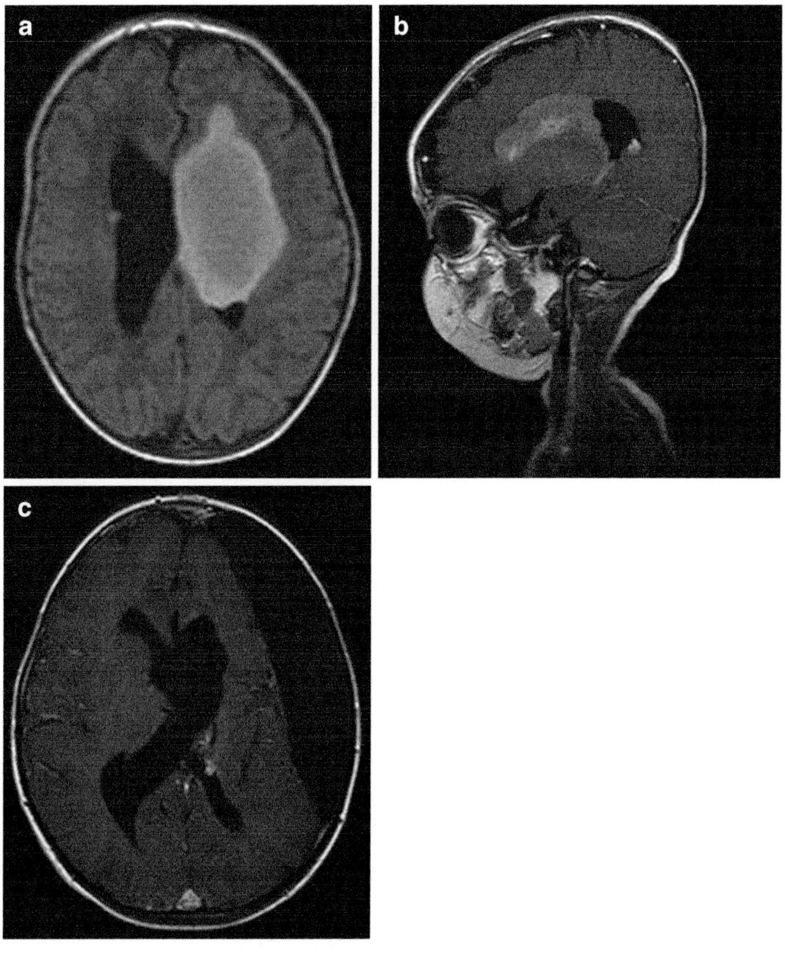

Fig. 51.1 (**a**) Axial and (**b**) sagittal T1 weighted MRI scans of a newborn child demonstrating a large intra-ventricular tumour. This tumour had been first diagnosed on the antenatal 22 week maternal ultra sound scan. A diagnosis of tuberose sclerosis was subsequently confirmed and the tumour was confirmed as a giant cell astrocytoma, which is pathognomic for tuberose sclerosis. The lesion slowly progressed on serial imaging leading to resection of the lesions at 6 months of age. (**c**) T1 weighted post-contrast study of the postoperative MRI scan showing complete resection of the lesion with associated asymptomatic subdural hygroma

of brain tumours presenting in the first year of life are diagnosed antenatally [2]. In utero magnetic resonance imaging (MRI) can help to elucidate further clinical information, and allow for better informed planning of delivery through the anticipation of peripartum problems such as dystocia.

The peripartum presentation of brain tumours includes dystocia, breech, stillbirth, and poor condition at birth [3]. Some of these correlate with neonatal presentations including macrocephaly, hydrops, hydrocephalus, seizures, nystagmus, apnoeas, cranial nerve lesions (e.g. hemifacial spasm) seizures and intracranial haemorrhage [3, 6, 7]. It must be appreciated that increased head circumference can manifest pre-, peri- or postpartum, and can significantly complicate the birthing process.

After birth, NBT can be insidious in their growth and presentation, and can reach a significant size before clinical manifestation. Subsequently, slowly progressive intracranial lesions can be obscured by normal growth, further complicated by the pliability of infant skull plates and potential to accommodate increasing intracranial pressure and masses. Common presentations include bulging fontanelles, rapidly increasing head circumference, separating sutures, prominent scalp veins, hydrocephalus [8], and optical manifestations such as sundowning [8] and nystagmus [7–9]. Other presentations include disordered growth e.g. failure-to-thrive (FTT), centile discrepancy (e.g. head/length/weight), lethargy, vomiting and seizures, with less commonly described presentations including irritability, head tilt, facial palsy, ptosis, hypotonia, incontinence and parapesis [7–9]. The association of particular symptoms with tumour types in infancy is also well established e.g. hypothalamic hamartoma and gelastic epilepsy (Fig. 51.2).

51.4 Neuroimaging

The anatomical locus of a tumour, apparent morphology (e.g. cystic, nodular, solid etc.), homogeneity and size, as identified from radiological findings can give an idea of a potential underlying diagnosis. As such, effective radiological input is key to the multidisciplinary management of NBT. Using non-ionising radiation, MRI is the modality of choice, posing less risk to the immature brain than computed tomography (CT), whilst offering clearer, higher resolution imaging of tumour morphology and anatomical relations. In the neonatal period, images can frequently be successfully acquired after infants have fed however MRI under general anaesthetic may be necessary to ensure imaging is of an adequate quality. Furthermore, the frequent presentation of some tumour types with leptomeningeal and subarachnoid spread means imaging of the entire CNS axis is required [6].

The higher water content and decreased myelination of the neonatal and infant brain decreases the differential appearance of white versus grey matter relative to the more mature brain of older children and adults. Subsequently, infant specific imaging protocols have been developed that not only address the time constraints of imaging, but also the specific technical challenges that arise [10].

CT does however haves a definite role in the further characterisation of some tumours, for example in determining the extent of calcification within tumours, and determining the extent of haemorrhage within lesions [1, 6]. Where surgical intervention has required the insertion of devices such as ventriculo-peritoneal (VP) shunts for the management of hydrocephalus, CT is the preferred modality for the investigation and monitoring of potential complications.

Newer advanced radiological techniques such as MRI spectroscopy are finding increasing application in clinical practice. The biochemical spectroscopic profiles of molecules such as choline, creatinine, amino acids and N-acetyl aspartate within normal brain tissues and lesions are measured relative to one another whilst nonspecific profiles are common, differences can help to distinguish between different disease processes (e.g. tumour vs. abscess) and suggest possible tumour grade and types [1].

Alongside the initial investigation and management of disease, radiological modalities are find-

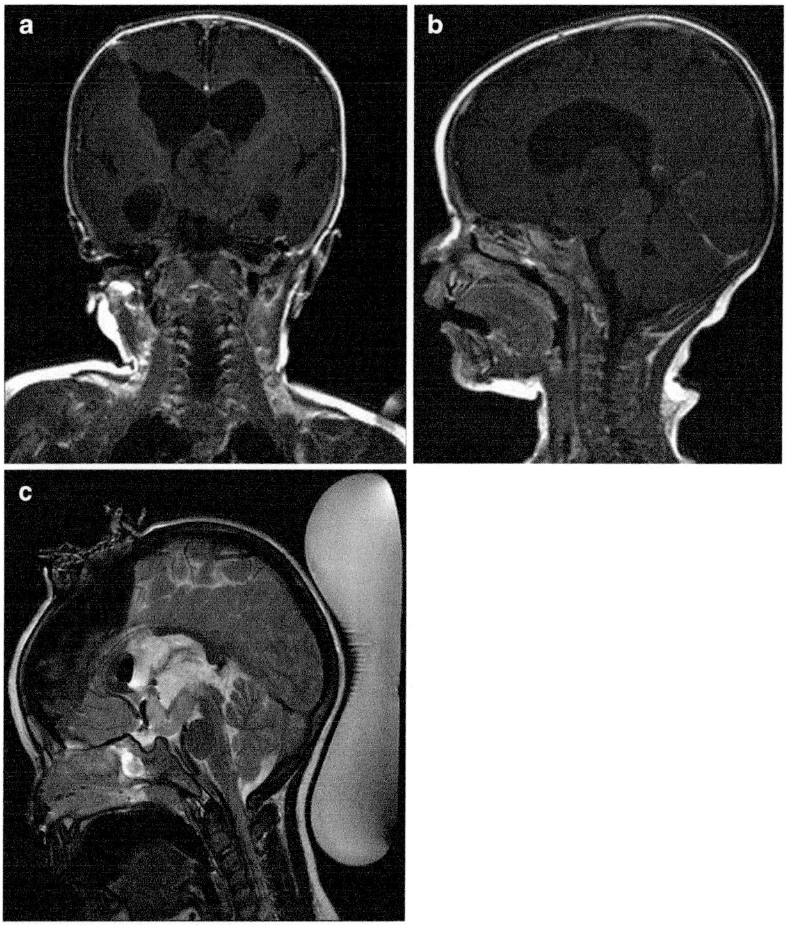

Fig. 51.2 (**a**) Coronal and (**b**) sagittal T1 weighted images demonstrating a large hypothalamic mass in a newborn child presenting with intractable gelastic epilepsy. The tumour had actually been diagnosed on antenatal ultrasound and MRI. Management initially consisted of observation only after an endoscopic biopsy confirmed a hypothalamic hamartoma. (**c**) The patient progressed to have medically intractable epilepsy, and at age 3 she had a subtotal resection of the hypothalamic hamartoma. The figure demonstrates the intra-operative MRI (sagittal T2) of the lesion during surgery

ing increased applications in preoperative and intraoperative planning. The anatomic relationship of a tumour and surrounding functional neurological and vascular structures can be mapped for preoperative planning, and imported into a surgical navigation system for intra-operative guidance.

51.5 Surgical Management

Despite an increasing incidence, NBT remain rare, and represent a highly heterogeneous group of diseases. Surgical management in specialised centres is essential to facilitate the frequent and cumulative exposure of clinicians to new cases in all age ranges and populations. With modern neurosurgical techniques, there is increasing evidence linking gross total tumour resection in various histological types to improved outcomes and progression free survival in older children. The data for neonatal surgery remains less well defined.

Surgical intervention usually incorporates the following objectives: (1) control of raised intracranial pressure due to hydrocephalus by diversion of CSF, (2) obtaining tissue for pathological diagnosis; (3) attempted curative resection of benign lesions and (4) improving survival for malignant tumours. Other important factors to consider are surgeon experience, expectations of the family with regard to treatment outcomes, and accessibility of the underlying lesion. Obtaining a histopathological diagnosis to guide the surgical objective and management strategy is vital to providing such patients with optimal care.

Relative to the size of the neonatal and infant brain, NBT can often occupy several cranial compartments, accounting for a significant portion of the intracranial vault [1]. Even with such extensive development, NBT may only manifest in the first instance as the result of an acute change or deterioration. Intratumoural haemorrhage, reflecting the increased vascularity of large tumours is common, and the sudden, spontaneous rapid growth of biologically "benign" tumours is well recognised. This increased vascularity of neonatal tumours also complicates surgery, greatly increasing the risk of intraoperative bleeding. The reduced circulating volume seen in neonates increases their susceptibility to hypovolaemia and associated problems such as haemocoagulative disorders [11, 12], complicated further by difficulties regulating metabolic homeostasis and temperature regulation in this population whilst under general anaesthetic.

The size constraints of the infant head impose highly restrictive dimensions on the operative field, and the fragility of the infant brain often limits the extent of surgery that can be planned. Alongside this, the anatomical site of an NBT is a determinant factor in the appropriateness and nature of planned surgery. Fundamental to this is whether the site is supratentorial (cerebral) or infratentorial (cerebellar), with approximately 60% of IBT supratentorial in nature, a figure seen in numerous case series (Serowka et al., 2010: n = 33, 63% supratentorial [8] and Young and Johnston, 2004: n = 16, 62.5% supratentorial [9]).

The location of NBT relative to the tentorium has significant practical implications, implicit in differential diagnoses, surgical accessibility (and hence potential complications and morbidity), and the long-term clinical implications of tumours resistant to treatment (i.e. continued growth and infiltration into surrounding structures). Neonatal tumours demonstrate a predilection for midline and periventricular loci, probably as result of the neoplastic transformation of physiologically proliferating primitive cell populations within these regions [1]. Midline locations such as the optic-hypothalamic region and brainstem make gross total resection impossible in certain cases, and the infiltration of normal brain structures in malignant tumour types contributes significantly to poor resectability.

Improvements in neurosurgical techniques, imaging (including intraoperative MRI) and importantly perioperative care in regional specialist centres have led to a more aggressive surgical strategy with radical or wide surgical resections sometimes the goal. Frameless and wireless neuronavigation as well as the use of intraoperative evoked potentials may further increase the safety and effectiveness of neurosurgical procedures even in these very young patients. Minimally invasive procedures such neuroendoscopic surgery (burr-hole transventricular approaches) can be used to obtain tumour samples, where present, simultaneously treat associated hydrocephalus via CSF diversion procedures such as an endoscopic third ventriculostomy [6].

Nevertheless, the rate of radical tumour excision remains relatively low compared to older children and adults [13]. The International Society for Pediatric Neurosurgery survey (1991) reported on 876 children with brain tumors of the first year of life with a gross total tumour resection rate of 44% [14]. A staged-surgery strategy is adopted in many centres to allow the surgeon to remove large neonatal brain tumours in two or more operating sessions. In theory this may reduce surgical risk by having multiple shorter operations, thereby allowing for easier maintenance and control of intraoperative metabolic and thermal homeostasis, reducing intraoperative blood loss, and reducing postoperative complications resulting from sudden intracranial decompression e.g. subdural fluid collections secondary to cranio-encephalic disproportion. Intraoperative bleeding which can cause physiological imbalances in the neonate can be further reduced by means of thrombin based haemostatic agents, intraoperative isovolemic haemodilution and intraoperative blood recovery to help in decreasing the risk of haemotransfusion [15].

Preoperative endovascular embolization of the tumors such as choroid plexus papilloma and carcinoma has been reported as a valid option to decrease the risk of severe intraoperative haemorrhage [16]. Furthermore, some authors have reported the successful use of neoadjuvant chemotherapy to allow for tumour shrinkage and reduction of vascularity before planning surgical resection. The use of preoperative chemotherapy has been reported for choroid plexus tumors, posterior fossa malignant glioma, optic-hypothalamic glioma and unresectable brainstem gliomas [1].

It is important to understand that all the published series on neonatal brain tumours report on a sizable group of infants who do not undergo any surgical resection. The reasons are not necessarily clearly outlined in the published literature but factors that are considered will include clinical and ethical considerations with regards to survival and prognosis, situations where there is agreement on the radiological diagnosis with no possibility of successful resection and/or adjuvant therapy. These decisions are best made in conjunction with a specialist paediatric neuro-oncology multidisciplinary team.

Nevertheless, new surgical techniques continue to develop, as do strategies to support surgical procedures and planning. Intraoperative MRI and ultrasound have improved the safety of operative techniques and helped to maximise the extent of resection through real time analysis of resected tumour relative to surrounding tissues. Distinct from this, the use of 5ALA, a dye that when applied to tumour cells, glows red under an ultraviolet light, potentially allows the intraoperative assessment of any residual tumour burden, also aiming to maximise the extent of resection [17]. Robot assisted neuroendoscopy systems continue to be refined, aiming to minimise the risk of damage to intracranial structures, as distinct from the development of techniques that allow optical imaging of brainstem nuclei and nerve tracts, that enable safer surgery in difficult regions such as the brain stem.

51.6 Adjuvant Therapies

Irradiation of the developing brain is associated with considerable long term morbidity, including learning difficulties, attention and concentration disorders, short term memory deficits, social adjustment and personality disorders, disorders of speech, language and communication, and physiological problems such as pituitary and hypothalamus related growth disturbance [18]. Subsequently, its avoidance until well beyond the infant period has become a standard in the design of most neonatal and infant brain tumour treatment protocols, ideally extending this period to the fourth year of life where possible.

51.7 Chemotherapy

As with all chemotherapy, therapeutic benefits have to be considered against the considerable toxicity profiles of chemotherapeutic agents, and long-term or late effects such as second malignancies. No chemotherapy protocols have been developed specifically for the management of neonatal brain tumours, although a number of so-called 'baby brain' protocols have been developed with the aim of using prolonged relatively low-intensity chemotherapy schedules to delay of avoid the use of radiation therapy [19–21].

With regard to designing such protocols, a number of fundamental pharmacokinetic differences between infants and older children/adults need to be considered [22]. These include significant differences in drug transport, drug metabolism and increased half-life arising from altered renal function, immature gastrointestinal systems and decreased glomerular filtration rate, with a greater body water composition and decreased plasma concentrating ability, as well as altered end organ differences such as decreased myelination [22, 23].

51.8 Multidisciplinary Management

The rarity and heterogeneity of NBT, alongside difficulty in their accurately classification and diagnosis demands multidisciplinary case review and management, involving histopathology, neurosurgery, neurooncology, radiology, endocrine, clinical oncology and neurology amongst others. With the significant morbidity associated with neurosurgical procedures, and long terms problems associated with chemotherapy, an extended MDT including dietetics, social workers, clinical psychology and physiotherapy is often required. In the case of NBT, primary health services, and in particular health visitation is fundament with the potential for deranged growth and development, and significant long-term disability.

51.9 Genetic and Biological Characterisation of Tumours and Risk Stratification

Putative biological, genetic and molecular markers of tumour biology and behaviour are increasingly finding clinical application, in the staging and classification of tumours, in some instances determining treatment courses. The presence of certain phenotypic or genotypic markers has been validated as determinants of whether specific tumours need more or less intensive surgical intervention or chemotherapy. For example, a tumour with more aggressive profiles, with metastasis on investigation may warrant more radical surgery, or more intense chemotherapy, whereas lower risk lesions demand less intensive therapy, if long term health risks can be reduced without compromising survival.

The prime example of this new knowledge is in medulloblastoma, which is now sub-categorised into four molecularly distinct sub-groups [24]. Further research has demonstrated that probing alterations in tumour DNA is able to define a so-called CIMP-positive subtype of posterior fossa ependymoma that clearly has a poorer outcome than CIMP-negative tumours [25]. Similar genetic sub-typing is being demonstrated in high grade glioma, atypical teratoid/rhabdoid tumour and others.

51.10 Prognosis/Survival/ Outcomes

Due to the rarity of NBT, published literature tends towards being small cases series, limited to considering a heterogeneous group of tumours with distinct individual anatomical characteristics [9]. The small numbers can also mean that series can be from an extended periods, during which diagnostic methods, surgical techniques and treatment protocols may have changed [9]. This impacts greatly on the already difficult task of trying to generate survival data, and when counselling parents about the prognosis of diagnosed conditions.

The outcomes measured when considering survival following infant brain tumours, as with tumours at other loci include 5-year survival and 5 year progression free survival. The considerable anatomical and functional development of the brain, including skill acquisition and cognitive development, that occurs during infancy has resulted in an increased significance being given to long-term neurological, physical, behavioural and psychological sequelae. This involves monitoring for aberrant or delayed development in social, gross and fine motor and speech and language, including physical and sensory deficits, and the impact that these can have on the quality of life (QoL) of the child. It is essential to consider that long term morbidity dose not arise solely from the initial disease process and oncogenesis, but to a significant degree from treatment, whether surgical, chemotherapy or radiotherapy, as discussed. Increasingly, measures are being developed to consider long term outcomes, not only to identify the health needs of NBT survivors, but as part of the ongoing risk-benefit considerations that are part of all medical/surgical interventions, but also in comparing the efficacy of different treatment modalities in terms of long-term outcomes.

51.11 Low Grade Glioma (LGG) and High Grade Glioma (HGG)

Low Grade Gliomas include pilocytic, pilomyxoid, diffuse and pleomorphic astrocytoma (of which pilocytic astrocytoma is the most common). Individually, astrocytomas and are the most commonly identified group of tumours in infancy accounting for approximately 30% brain tumours, and are a significant in the neonatal period [26]. LGG can arise anywhere in the neuronal axis, but are most commonly supratentorial and midline tumours, involving the hypothalamic area and optic pathway [26]. In the neonatal period the mesencephalon and pons are also common primary sites [3]. While low-grade tumours classically demonstrate a more benign, indolent course in comparison to more aggressive, malignant high-grade tumours, infant astrocytomas represent a highly heterogeneous population of tumours in terms of their gross anatomy, histology and clinical behaviour [3]. Some display more aggressive pathological characteristics, with poorer outcomes and significantly reduced treatment responses than might be expected [26].

The treatment of choice is gross total resection for most low grade gliomas that are readily accessible, e.g. hemispheric, cerebellar, focal and dorsal exophytic brainstem and cervico-medullary tumors with the extent of resection has been reported as an important predictor of clinical outcome. Thus the usual post-operative recommendation for many patients with low grade glioma is serial imaging and clinical follow-up to detect disease progression. Repeat surgeries can be performed in the event of detected tumour progression or recurrence before the addition of adjuvant therapy.

The proximity of the common anatomical sites in which astrocytomas develop to fundamental structures such the optic pathway and the hypothalamus increases the risk of significant post-surgical complications and morbidity, and almost precludes gross total resection as a viable surgical strategy [26].

51.12 High Grade Glioma (HGG)

High Grade Gliomas are either anaplastic astrocytoma or glioblastoma multiforme, both rare in the neonatal age bracket. Infants with chemosensitive, histologically confirmed HGG in infancy have been described [26] with evidence to suggest that infants diagnosed below 6 months may have the best prognosis of all [26]. Figure 51.3 shows pre and post-operative images a high grade glioma in a 2 weeks old child who remains well at 2 years of age, following surgery and chemotherapy, with residual but static disease.

This is reflected in the results from baby brain protocols that suggest a much better prognosis for very young children with HGG than those in older children and adults, despite the avoidance of radiotherapy pointing to fundamental difference in the biology of these tumours at different ages. Of the patients with HGG, SEER data suggested that patients who underwent GTR had increased survival in patients <12 months [27], though previous studies have identified no such relationship between extent of surgery and survival [28].

51.13 Medulloblastoma

Medulloblastoma represent a group of highly malignant embryonal tumours [18]. On radiological imaging, medulloblastoma appear as solidly enhancing, homogenous masses, with or without cystic changes or calcification [18]. Presentation with obstructive hydrocephalus is common and leptomeningeal and cerebrospinal seeding occurs in a significant proportion of cases [3].

Neonatal medulloblastoma is associated with increased difficulty in performing gross total excision. Risk stratification considers tumours characteristics such as the degree of surgical excision, presence of disseminated/metastatic disease and histological subtype. A variety of chemotherapeutic options are used. Prognosis is generally very poor, although patients with desmosplastic histology have a better outcome.

51.14 Central Nervous System Primitive Neuroectodermal Tumours (CNS-PNET)

CNS-PNETs are embryonal tumours composed of poorly undifferentiated neuroepithelial cells, and represent a rare but highly malignant group of small cell tumours [3] and represent around 7.7% of IBT [29].

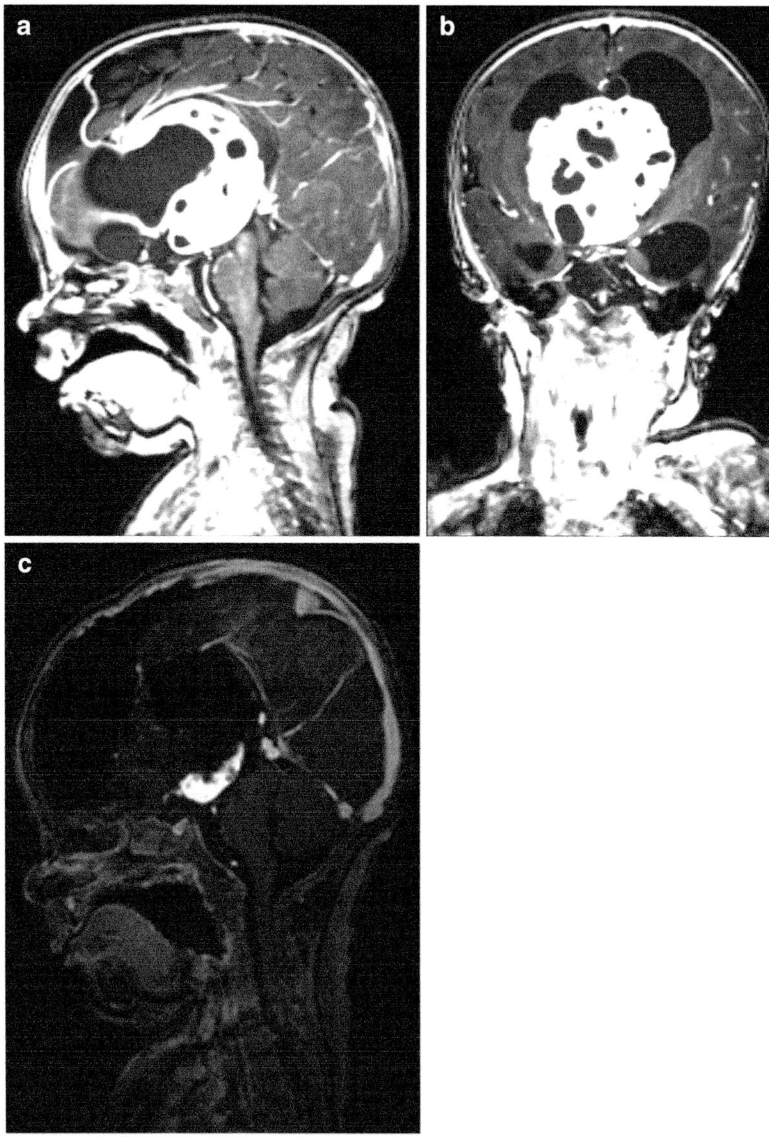

Fig. 51.3 (**a**) Sagittal and (**b**) coronal T1 images (with gadolinium) showing a large tumour in a 2 week old baby. The infant presented with a rapidly enlarging head circumference typical of acute hydrocephalus, but was clinically well otherwise. The tumour was diagnosed as a glioblastoma multiforme (WHO Grade 4) after biopsy. (**c**) Sagittal T weighted imaging (with gadolinium) following major resection, with a small amount of residual tumour left in the hypothalamic area. The child experienced no neurological deficits post operatively, but developed diabetes iInsipidus and required a ventriculoperitoneal shunt 2 weeks later

As a group of tumours, CNS-PNET can occur at several sites within the supratentorial brain including the pineal gland (pineoblastoma) [3]. Like medulloblastoma they demonstrate a propensity for dissemination through the CSF [3].

Prognosis in the neonatal and infant period is poor, with recommended treatment being maximal tumour resection and intensive chemotherapy [29]. Neonatally presenting StPNET tends to be more advanced, with larger tumours and more progressed disease, often meaning surgery is more complicated, if possible at all [3].

51.15 Atypical Teratoid/Rhabdoid Tumour (AT/RT)

Atypical teratoid/rhabdoid tumours (AT/RT) represent a group of tumours that have previously been misclassified as malignant entities such as medulloblastoma or choroid plexus teratomas. They are foremost a tumour of infants and young children and arise predominantly within the posterior fossa, but with the potential to manifest anywhere in the CNS often with disseminated disease [30]. ATRT is associated with the tumour suppressor gene hSNF5/INI1 and diagnosed is aided by the absence of the immunohistochemical expression of INI1 expression.

Response to chemotherapy alone is generally poor, with Rorke reporting only 14% showing chemosensitivity [29]. Gross total resection is probably beneficial [30] but the prognosis in infancy is very poor, especially in the presence of disseminated disease, and in early infancy treatment is usually palliative [26].

51.16 Teratoma

Teratomas account for approximately 25–55% of NBT, [1]. Larouche describes significant variation in the prevalence of teratomas between case series, attributing this in part to the increasing accuracy that with which other tumours, such as Desmoplastic Infantile Gliomas, are now being correctly identified [26]. Teratomas characteristically demonstrate endodermal, ectodermal and mesodermal elements, commonly with immature neuroglial cells. Tumours can erode though bony and cartilaginous anatomic relations, and often directly replacing brain tissue. Isaacs reports the difficulty that lies in identifying the anatomic origin of teratomas in approximately one third of patients, though common sites include the pineal gland, the hypothalamus, suprasellar region and cerebral hemispheres [3].

51.17 Ependymoma

Ependymoma represents 11% of NBT [3] and develop from ependymal cells; cliliated epithelial cells lining the ventricles involved with the production and circulation of CSF. Presentation is often with large tumours, with a higher risk of dissemination through the CSF in infancy [26]. In infancy most arise within the fourth ventricle.

The difficulty of treating ependymoma without radiation is well acknowledged [26]. The degree of resection is the major prognostic factor [26].

Accordingly, infratentorial tumours, especially those in the posterior fossa with involvement of the lateral recess, are traditionally accepted as having a poorer outcome. Surgery is complicated by the proximity of the brain stem, cranial nerves and the great vessels. Post-operative chemotherapy is usually administering following one of the so-called prolonged baby brain chemotherapy regimens mentioned previously.

51.18 Choroid Plexus Tumours (CPT)

Choroid plexus tumours include a spectrum of neoplasms including Choroid Plexus Papillomas (CPP) accounting for approximately 5% of NBT [31], so-called 'atypical' CPPs and the highly malignant Choroid Plexus Carcinomas (CPC). As a group they are highly vascular tumours that display significantly increased secretion of cerebrospinal fluid. Inadequate compensatory drainage results in ventricular dilation and rapidly progressive hydrocephalus, with associated manifestations such as increasing head circumference [31]. Choroid plexus tumours predominately present in the lateral ventricle, but can also develop in the third or fourth ventricles [31]. CPC can also disseminate through the cerebrospinal fluid [31].

Complete surgical resection when possible should be performed and is usually curative for CPP and is prognostically significant for CPC. Surgery may be complicated by the risk of significant haemorrhage from tumours that commonly have well-established vascular beds [31]. Adjuvant chemotherapy is given for CPC but despite this, the prognosis remains very poor [31].

51.19 Desmoplastic Infantile Astroglial Tumours

Desmoplastic Astrocytoma (DAI) and Ganglioma of Infancy (DIG) present as exclusively supratentorial tumours, and are frequently cystic on imaging [26, 32]. Complete resection may be limited because of large tumour size at presentation, widespread intracranial infiltration, a high degree of vascularity and commonly, multilobar involvement [26]. Staged operations and pre-operative angiography/embolisation have been advocated. The differentiation between the DAI and DIG is the presence of neuronal cells histologically in DIG, but otherwise they are morphologically and radiologically very similar. The main area for discussion with these tumours is the sometimes aggressive appearance on histology suggesting a more malignant tumour. However, the tumour is generally felt to be curable with surgery alone and adjuvant therapy is not usually recommended if complete resection can be effected, with a good prognosis if this can be achieved [32].

51.20 Discussion

Future work will continue to find the balance between aggressive tumour treatment and management and the long-term morbidity that survivors face. Advances continue to be made in our understanding of tumour biology and molecular biology, with risk stratification allowing the identification of those tumour types that demand more aggressive management compared with those in which less intensive therapy will not compromise cure or survival. Alongside this, biological and clinical work must continue to develop novel therapeutic approaches such as anti-angiogenesis and pro-apoptosis agents, and differentiation-promoting agents, all of which may improve the survival and quality of life of future paediatric brain tumour patients. Fundamental to this will be continued collaboration between multi-institutional groups, to develop and validate future therapeutic approaches in clinical trials.

References

1. Massimi L, Pettorini B, Tamburrini G, Caldarelli M, Di Rocco C. Advances in the management of brain tumours in infants. Curr Cancer Ther Rev. 2011;7(3):184–200.
2. Manoranjan B, Provias JP. Congenital brain tumours: diagnostic pitfalls and therapeutic interventions. J Child Neurol. 2010;26(5):599–614.
3. Isaacs H Jr. I. Perinatal brain tumours: a review of 250 cases. Pediatr Neurol. 2002;27(4):249–61.
4. Moore SW, Satge D, Sasco AJ, Zimmerman A, Plaschkes J. The epidemiology of neonatal tumours. Report of an international working group. Pediatr Surg Int. 2003;19(7):509–19.
5. Cordier S, Monfort C, Filipinni G, Preston-Martin S, Lubin F, Mueller BA, Holly EA, Peris-Bonet R, McRedie M, Choi W, Little J, Arslan A. Parental exposure to polycyclic aromatic hydrocarbons and the risk of childhood brain tumours: the SEARCH international childhood brain tumours study. Am J Epidemiol. 2004;159(12):1109–16.
6. Magdum SA. Neonatal brain tumours - a review. Early Hum Dev. 2010;86(10):627–31.
7. Shamji MF, Vassilyadi M, Lam CH, Montes JL, Farmer JP. Congenital tumours of the central nervous system: the MCH experience. Pediatr Neurosurg. 2009;45(5):368–74.
8. Serowka K, Chiu Y, Gonzalez I, Gilles F, McComb G, Krieger M, Dhall G, Britt LJ, Sposto R, Finlay JL. Central nervous system (CNS) tumours in the first six months of life: the Children's Hospital Los Angeles Experience, 1979-2005. Paediatr Haematol Oncol. 2010;27(2):90–102.
9. Young HK, Johnston H. Intracranial tumours in infants. J Child Neurol. 2004;19(6):424–30.
10. Saunders DE, Thompson C, Gunny R, Jones R, Cox T, Chong WK. Magnetic resonance imaging protocols for paediatric neurology. Pediatr Radiol. 2007;37:789–97.
11. Piastra M, Di Rocco C, Caresta E, Zorzi G, De Luca D, Caldarelli M, La Torre G, Conti G, Antonelli M, Eaton S, Pietrini D. Blood loss and short-term outcome of infants undergoing brain tumour removal. J Neurooncol. 2008;90(2):191–200.
12. Kane PJ, Phipps KP, Harkness WF, Hayward RD. Intracranial neoplasms in the first year of life: results of a second cohort of patients from a single institution. Br J Neurosurg. 1999;13(3):294–8.
13. Rutka JT, Kuo JS. Pediatric surgical neuro-oncology: current best care practices and strategies. J Neurooncol. 2004;69(1-3):139–50.
14. Di Rocco C, Iannelli A, Ceddia A. Intracranial tumors of the first year of life. Childs Nerv Syst. 1991;7:150–3.
15. Murto KTT, Splinter WM. Perioperative autologous blood donation in children. Transfus Sci. 1999;21(1):41–62.

16. Otten ML, Riina HA, Gobin YP, Souweidane MM. Preoperative embolization in the treatment of choroid plexus papilloma in an infant. Case report. J Neurosurg. 2006;104(6 Suppl):419–21.
17. Stummer W, Pichlmeier U, Meinel T, Wiestler OD, Zanella F, Reulen HJ, ALA-Glioma Study Group. Fluorescence-guided surgery with 5-aminolevulinic acid for resection of malignant glioma: a randomised controlled multicentre phase III trial. Lancet Oncol. 2006;7(5):392–401.
18. Dhall G. Medulloblastoma. J Child Neurol. 2009;24(11):1418–30.
19. Duffner PK, Horowitz ME, Krischer JP, Burger PC, Cohen ME, Sanford RA, Friedman HS, Kun LE. The treatment of malignant brain tumors in infants and very young children: an update of the Pediatric oncology group experience. Neuro Oncol. 1999;1(2):152–61.
20. Grundy RG, Wilne SH, Robinson KJ, Ironside JW, Cox T, Chong WK, Michalski A, Campbell RH, Bailey CC, Thorp N, Pizer B, Punt J, Walker DA, Ellison DW. Machin D; Children's cancer and leukaemia group (formerly UKCCSG) brain tumour committee. Primary postoperative chemotherapy without radiotherapy for treatment of brain tumours other than ependymoma in children under 3 years: results of the first UKCCSG/SIOP CNS 9204 trial. Eur J Cancer. 2010;46(1):120–33.
21. Grill J, Sainte-Rose C, Jouvet A, Gentet JC, Lejars O, Frappaz D, Doz F, Rialland X, Pichon F, Bertozzi AI, Chastagner P, Couanet D, Habrand JL, Raquin MA, Le Deley MC, Kalifa C. Treatment of medulloblastoma with postoperative chemotherapy alone: an SFOP prospective trial. Lancet Oncol. 2005;6(8):573–80.
22. Vasilatou-Kosmidis H. Cancer in neonates and infants. Med Pediatr Oncol. 2003;41(1):7–9.
23. Bleyer WA. Clinical pharmacology of intrathecal methotrexate. II. An improved dosage regimen derived from age related pharmacokinetics. Cancer Treat Rep. 1977;61:1419–25.
24. Taylor MD, Northcott PA, Korshunov A, Remke M, Cho YJ, Clifford SC, Eberhart CG, Parsons DW, Rutkowski S, Gajjar A, Ellison DW, Lichter P, Gilbertson RJ, Pomeroy SL, Kool M, Pfister SM. Molecular subgroups of medulloblastoma: the current consensus. Acta Neuropathol. 2012;123(4):465–72.
25. Mack SC, Witt H, Piro RM, Gu L, Zuyderduyn S, Stütz AM, Wang X, Gallo M, Garzia L, Zayne K, Zhang X, Ramaswamy V, Jäger N, Jones DT, Sill M, Pugh TJ, Ryzhova M, Wani KM, Shih DJ, Head R, Remke M, Bailey SD, Zichner T, Faria CC, Barszczyk M, Stark S, Seker-Cin H, Hutter S, Johann P, Bender S, Hovestadt V, Tzaridis T, Dubuc AM, Northcott PA, Peacock J, Bertrand KC, Agnihotri S, Cavalli FM, Clarke I, Nethery-Brokx K, Creasy CL, Verma SK, Koster J, Wu X, Yao Y, Milde T, Sin-Chan P, Zuccaro J, Lau L, Pereira S, Castelo-Branco P, Hirst M, Marra MA, Roberts SS, Fults D, Massimi L, Cho YJ, Van Meter T, Grajkowska W, Lach B, Kulozik AE, von Deimling A, Witt O, Scherer SW, Fan X, Muraszko KM, Kool M, Pomeroy SL, Gupta N, Phillips J, Huang A, Tabori U, Hawkins C, Malkin D, Kongkham PN, Weiss WA, Jabado N, Rutka JT, Bouffet E, Korbel JO, Lupien M, Aldape KD, Bader GD, Eils R, Lichter P, Dirks PB, Pfister SM, Korshunov A, Taylor MD. Epigenomic alterations define lethal CIMP-positive ependymomas of infancy. Nature. 2014;506(7489):445–50.
26. Larouche V, Huang A, Bartels U, Bouffet E. Tumours of the central nervous system in the first year of life. Pediatr Blood Cancer. 2007;49(7):1074–82.
27. Qaddoumi I, Sultan I, Gajjar A. Outcome and prognostic features in Pediatric Gliomas. Cancer. 2009;115(24):5761–70.
28. Duffner PK, Krischer JP, Burger PC, Cohen ME, Backstrom JW, Horowitz ME, Sanford RA, Friedman HS, Kun LE. Treatment of infants with malignant gliomas: the paediatric oncology group experience. J Neurooncol. 1996;28(2-3):245–56.
29. Rorke LB, Hart MN, McLendon RE. 2000. Supratentorial primitive neuroectodermal tumour (PNET). In: Kleihues P, Cavenee WK Pathology and genetics of tumours of the nervous system. Lyon: International Agency for Research on Cancer. 141-144.
30. Reddy TR. Atypical teratoid/rhabdoid tumours of the central nervous system. J Neurooncol. 2005;75: 309–13.
31. Lafay-Cousin L, Keene D, Carret AS, Fryer C, Brossard J, Crooks B, Eisenstat D, Johnston D, Larouche V, Silva M, Wilson B, Zelcer S, Bartels U, Bouffet E. Choroid plexus tumors in children less than 36 months: the Canadian Pediatric brain tumor consortium (CPBTC) experience. Childs Nerv Syst. 2011;27(2):259–64.
32. Mallucci C, Lellouch-Tubiana A, Salazar C, Cinalli G, Renier D, Sainte-Rose C, Pierre-Kahn A, Zerah M. The management of desmoplastic neuroepithelial tumours in childhood. Childs Nerv Syst. 2000;16(1):8–14.

Part VIII

Oncology

Epidemiology and Genetics of Neonatal Tumours

52

Charles Stiller

Abstract

Neoplasms are rare in neonates, although somewhat more frequent than in older children. In Great Britain, for birth years 1988–2007, the National Registry of Childhood Tumours recorded 394 cases of cancer (including non-malignant CNS tumours) in live-born infants less than 28 days of age. The risk of neonatal cancer was 27.6 per million live births or 1 in 36,170, equivalent to an incidence of 361 per million person-years and double the rate over the remainder of the first year of life. The most frequent cancers were germ-cell tumours (24%), neuroblastoma (23%), leukaemia (18%) and CNS tumours (13%). Cancers probably account for a minority of neonatal neoplasms, so that the total risk of benign and malignant tumours exceeds 1 in 18,000. While the short-term prognosis of neonatal cancer is rather poor, the probability of survival conditional on surviving one year from diagnosis is much higher than in older children. Survival from leukaemia, embryonal CNS tumours and rhabdomyosarcoma is especially poor for neonates, whereas neonates with neuroblastoma have much higher survival than children aged 1 year and over. The proportion of neonatal cancers associated with pathogenic germline mutations seems unlikely to be much lower than 10%; in addition, a substantial proportion are associated with chromosomal abnormalities. Exogenous risk factors are probably only relevant if exposure is prenatal. The most plausible from among the many that have been investigated are exposure to ionizing radiation and some pollutants during pregnancy and some dietary factors.

Keywords

Neonatal cancer • Epidemiology • Survival statistics • Outcomes

52.1 Incidence

Neoplasms are rare in neonates, although they occur somewhat more frequently than in older children. The most reliable incidence data are for

C. Stiller, MSc
National Cancer Registration and Analysis Service, Public Health England,
4150 Chancellor Court, Oxford Business Park South, Oxford OX4 2GX, UK
e-mail: charles.stiller@new.ox.ac.uk; charles.stiller@phe.gov.uk

P.D. Losty et al. (eds.), *Rickham's Neonatal Surgery*, https://doi.org/10.1007/978-1-4471-4721-3_52

cancers, defined according to the International Classification of Childhood Cancer, Third Edition (ICCC-3) [1] as malignant neoplasms together with non-malignant intracranial and intraspinal tumours, since these diseases are ascertained by population-based cancer registries. In Great Britain, for birth years 1988–2007, the National Registry of Childhood Tumours recorded 394 cases of cancer in live-born infants less than 28 days of age. There were 183 boys and 211 girls affected, a male:female ratio of 0.9:1. The risk of neonatal malignancy was 27.6 per million live births or 1 in 36,170. This is equivalent to an incidence of 361 per million person-years, double the rate of 177 per million person-years over the remainder of the first year of life. A similarly raised incidence in the first month has been observed in the United States [2]. As will be described below, the risk of cancer in the neonate would be considerably lower if a more restrictive definition of malignancy were applied. But even with the relatively inclusive definition in the International Classification of Diseases for Oncology (ICD-O-3), on which ICCC-3 is based, it seems likely that cancers account for a minority of neonatal neoplasms and that the total risk of benign and malignant tumours in the first 28 days of life exceeds 1 in 18,000.

Childhood cancer is a diverse collection of diseases. The distribution of tumour types varies markedly with age, not only through the years of childhood but even between the neonatal period and the rest of the first year. Table 52.1 gives details of the 394 neonatal cancers registered among neonates born in Britain in 1988–2007, together with those among older infants for comparison. Figure 52.1 shows the relative frequencies of the 12 main diagnostic groups of ICCC-3 in neonates, older infants, and children aged 1–4 years at diagnosis. Among neonates, the most frequent categories were germ-cell tumours (24%), neuroblastoma (23%), leukaemia (18%) and intracranial and intraspinal (central nervous system:CNS) tumours (13%). By contrast, while leukaemia, neuroblastoma and CNS tumours had fairly similar relative frequencies among older infants, germ cell and gonadal tumours accounted for only 4% and were outnumbered by retinoblastoma, renal tumours and soft-tissue tumours. As can been seen from Table 52.1, however, the higher total incidence among neonates meant that only lymphomas and renal cancers had a markedly higher incidence after the first 4 weeks.

Of the 71 cases of neonatal leukaemia, 36 (50%) were acute myeloid, 15 (21%) were acute lymphoblastic, 5 (7%) were JMML/CMML, 1 (1%) was myelodysplasia and 14 (20%) were of unspecified type. No lymphomas were registered in this age group.

Among the 50 CNS tumours, unspecified tumours accounted for 38%, reflecting the low biopsy rate for neonatal brain tumours. Of the 11 astrocytomas, 1 was pilocytic, 5 were high-grade and 5 were of unspecified grade. The 10 embryonal tumours comprised 3 medulloblastomas, 4 primitive neuroectodermal tumours and 3 atypical teratoid/rhabdoid tumours (ATRT). Of the 5 choroid plexus tumours, 4 were papillomas and 1 was a carcinoma. No ependymomas were registered. The "other glioma" category comprised one astroblastoma and three unspecified gliomas. The single mixed glial-neuronal tumour was a desmoplastic infantile ganglioglioma.

Neuroblastoma was the second most frequent malignant solid tumour of neonates. The similar numbers of boys and girls contrast with the male excess among older children [3]. In the present series, 38 cases (42%) had Stage 4S disease according to the International Neuroblastoma Staging system [4], 11 (12%) were Stage 4, 34 (37%) had localised disease and there was no record of tumour stage for the remaining 8 (9%). A series of 134 cases of neonatal neuroblastoma in the Italian Neuroblastoma Registry contained a similarly high proportion of Stage 4S but only a single case of Stage 4 [5]. Among the tumours tested, only 2% had amplification of the MYCN oncogene which is more frequent in older children and is associated with poor prognosis [5]. In the Quebec Neuroblastoma Screening Project, nearly all cases diagnosed by screening at age 3 weeks or detected clinically before then had favourable biological features and none had MYCN amplification [6]. Neuroblastoma may

Table 52.1 Incidence of cancer among live-born neonates born 1988–2007 in Great Britain

	Neonates aged 0–27 days				Infants aged 28–364 days		
ICCC-3	*N*	Risk/10^6 live births	Rate/10^6 py	M/F	*N*	Risk/10^6 live births	Rate/10^6 py
I. Leukaemias	71	5.0	65.0	0.9	498	34.9	37.8
(a) ALL	15	1.1					
(b) AML	36	2.5					
(d) JMML/CMML and MDS	6	0.4					
(e) Other and unspecified	14	1.0					
II. Lymphomas	0	0.0	0.0	—	11	0.8	0.8
III. CNS tumours	50	3.5	45.8	1.3	448	31.4	34.0
(a) (2) Choroid plexus tumours	5	0.4					
(b) Astrocytoma	11	0.8					
(c) Embryonal	10	0.7					
(d) Other gliomas	4	0.3					
(e) (4) Mixed glial neuromal	1	0.1					
(f) Unspecified	19	1.3					
IV. Neuroblastoma etc.	91	6.4	83.3	1.0	474	33.3	36.0
(a) Neuroblastoma	91	6.4					
V. Retinoblastoma	32	2.2	29.3	1.0	306	21.5	23.3
VI. Renal tumours	5	0.4	4.6	1.5	218	15.3	16.6
(a) (1) Wilms tumour	4	0.3					
(4) pPNET	1	0.1					
VII. Hepatic tumours	7	0.5	6.4	2.5	91	6.4	6.9
(a) Hepatoblastoma	7	0.5					
VIII. Bone tumours	1	0.1	0.9	0.0	5	0.4	0.4
(d) (2) Chordoma	1	0.1					
IX. Soft tissue sarcoma	38	2.7	34.8	1.1	150	10.5	11.4
(a) Rhabdomyosarcoma	13	0.9					
(b) (1) Fibrosarcoma	10	0.7					
(3) Mal haemangiopericytoma	1	0.1					
(d) (2) pPNET	2	0.1					
(3) Extra renal rhabdoid	5	0.4					
(6) Leiomyosaroma	1	0.1					
(8) Blood vessel tumours	1	0.1					
(9) Extra osseous osteosarcoma and chondrosarcoma	1	0.1					
(e) Unspecified	4	0.3					
X. Germ-cell and gonadal	93	6.5	85.1	0.5	97	6.8	7.4
(a) CNS germ cell tumours	13	0.9					
(b) Other non-gonadal germ-cell	78	5.5					
(c) Gonadal germ cell	2	0.1					
XI. Melanoma and carcinoma	3	0.2	2.7	0.0	9	0.6	0.7
(d) Malignant melanoma	3	0.2					

(continued)

Table 52.1 (continued)

ICCC-3	Neonates aged 0–27 days N	Risk/10⁶ live births	Rate/10⁶ py	M/F	Infants aged 28–364 days N	Risk/10⁶ live births	Rate/10⁶ py
XII. Other and unspecified	3	0.2	2.7	2.0	16	1.1	1.2
(a) Gastrointestinal stromal tumour	1	0.1					
(b) Unspecified	2	0.1					
Total	394	27.6	360.6	0.9	2325	163.1	176.7

Numbers of cases (*N*), risk per million live births, incidence per million person-years (py) and male/female ratio (M/F). Incidence rates ignore mortality from other causes and assume zero international migration. Numbers and rates among older infants given for comparison
Source: National Registry of Childhood Tumours

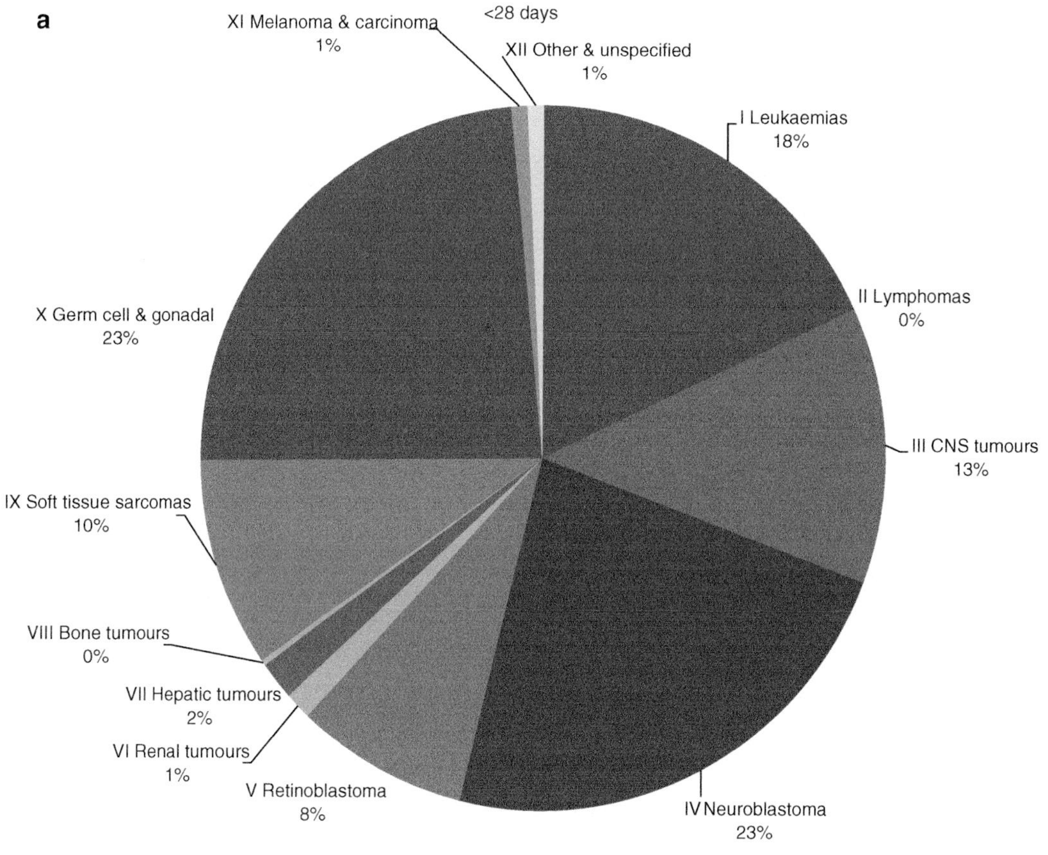

Fig. 52.1 Relative contributions of the 12 IICC-3 diagnostic groups to cancer incidence among young children in Britain by age group: (**a**) neonates aged 0–27 days, (**b**) infants aged 28–364 days, (**c**) children aged 1–4 years. *Source*: (**a**, **b**), Table 52.1; (**c**) National Registry of Childhood Tumours, unpublished data, 1988–2007

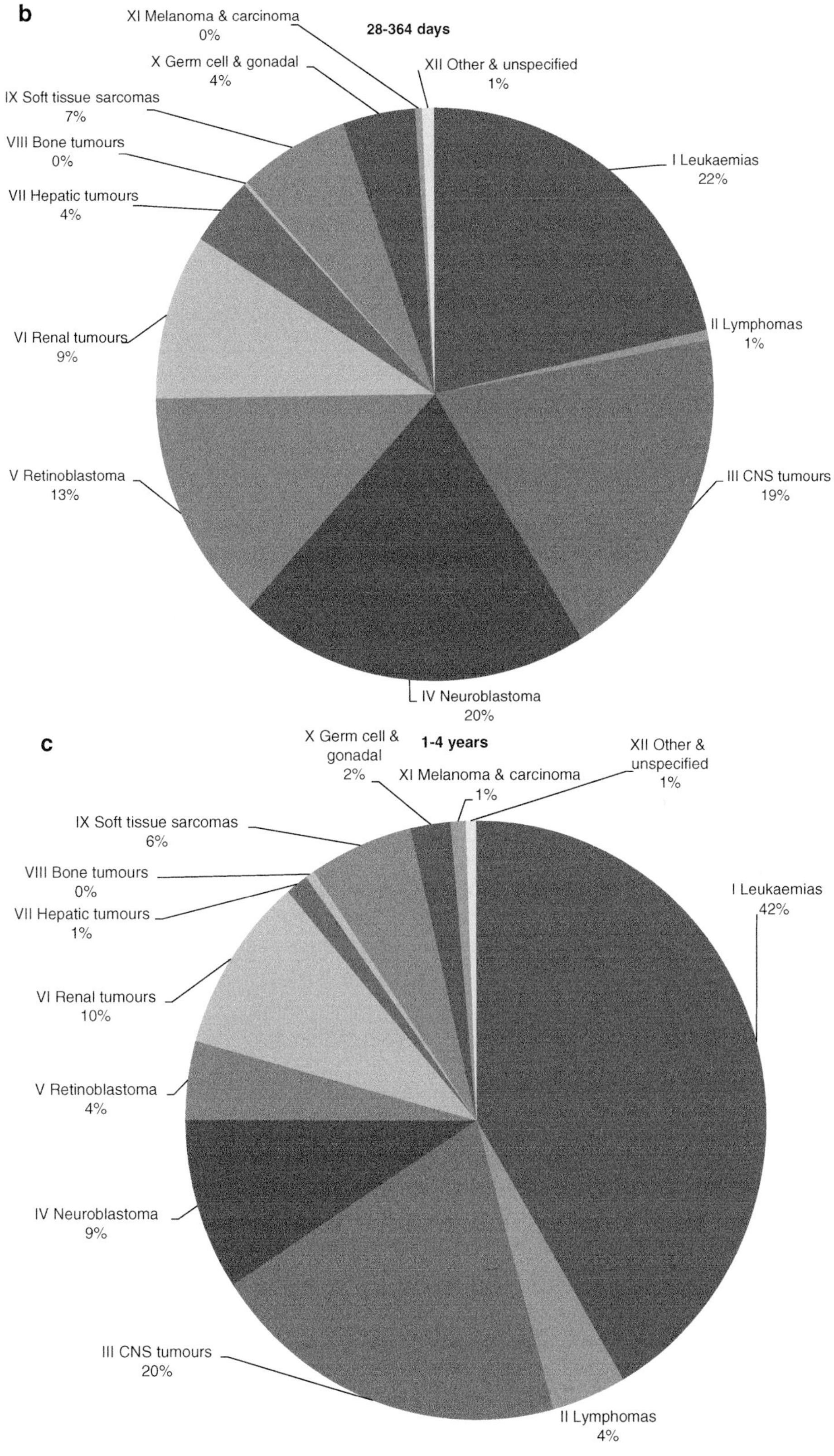

Fig. 52.1 (continued)

be detected prenatally by ultrasonography. Among 32 live-born cases of neonatal neuroblastoma diagnosed at paediatric oncology centres in Britain during 1986–94, 5 (16%) had a prenatal maternal ultrasound scan suggestive of neuroblastoma and another two had abnormal scans which could, with hindsight, be attributed to the tumour [7]. In the Italian Neuroblastoma Registry, 20% of neonatal cases diagnosed in 1980–2006 were detected prenatally, with little variation in the prenatal detection rate over the 27 year study period [5].

Of the 32 patients with retinoblastoma, 6 (19%) had unilateral and 25 (78%) had bilateral tumours.

Of the four cases of Wilms tumour, three were unilateral and one was bilateral. Although rhabdoid tumour of the kidney has its highest incidence in the first year of life, no cases were recorded among neonates. Hepatic cancer was more frequent than renal cancer; all seven cases were hepatoblastomas. A single case of chordoma was the only neonatal malignant bone tumour.

The 13 rhabdomyosarcomas were evenly divided between embryonal and alveolar subtypes, with six cases of each; the remaining case was of unknown subtype. An unusually high proportion of neonatal alveolar rhabdomyosarcoma may be of the fusion-negative variant which accounts for only 20% of cases in older patients [8, 9]. The primary sites were head and neck (3 cases), upper limb (1), lower limb (2), connective tissue of trunk (5) and bladder/prostate (2). All ten fibrosarcomas were of the infantile subtype. Primary site was known in nine cases: head and neck (2), upper limb (3), lower limb (2), and connective tissue of trunk (2). The single case of leiomyosarcoma was in the small bowel and might well be reclassified as gastro-intestinal stromal tumour if it were diagnosed today.

Germ-cell tumours were the most frequent group of tumours observed in this series. They were twice as frequent among girls as among boys. The 13 CNS tumours in this group were all teratomas, of which three were specified as malignant and three as benign. The 78 other non-gonadal germ cell tumours comprised 64 teratomas, 9 yolk-sac tumours, 4 mixed germ cell tumours, and 1 choriocarcinoma. The incidence of non-gonadal, non-CNS malignant germ cell tumours calculated here will be an over-estimate according to some definitions of malignancy. This is because immature teratoma is regarded as malignant in ICD-O-3. The present series included 38 cases described as immature teratoma with no malignant features, and if they were to be excluded, the incidence would fall from 5.5 per million live births to 2.8 per million. In a thirty-year population-based study with pathology review in the West Midlands region of England, all 49 extracranial germ cell tumours diagnosed in the first 4 months of life were classified as benign mature teratoma, although four recurred as malignant tumours [10]. The majority of the non-gonadal, non-CNS germ cell tumours in the present series (50/78, 64%)were in the sacrococcygeal region. Other primary sites were head and neck (12, 15%), mediastinum (6, 8%), intraabdominal (6, 8%) and unknown (4, 5%). The two gonadal germ-cell tumours were a testicular yolk-sac tumour and an ovarian teratoma.

It should be emphasised that the series described here does not provide an exhaustive catalogue of malignancies that can arise in neonates. For example, in the years before or after the study period, the NRCT has included neonatal cases of ocular medulloepithelioma, pancreatoblastoma [11] and pleuropulmonary blastoma. There are numerous reports of other very rare neonatal cancers in the literature.

The NRCT, like nearly all cancer registries, did not aim for complete ascertainment of benign tumours. It nevertheless contained a sizeable number of registrations for non-malignant tumours diagnosed in neonates over the same period as the malignant neoplasms discussed above. These registrations are enumerated in Table 52.2. Ascertainment was undoubtedly incomplete and biased towards (1) diagnoses most often referred to paediatric oncologists and (2) fatal tumours. The data can nevertheless provide minimum estimates of incidence for certain non-malignant neonatal tumours, also given in Table 52.2, and the proportion of tumours that are benign in some diagnostic groups.

Table 52.2 Incidence of non-malignant neoplasms among live-born neonates born 1988–2007 in Great Britain

Diagnostic group	*N*	Minimum risk/10⁶ live births	M/F
Langerhans cell histiocytosis	5	0.4	0.7
Renal tumours	45	3.2	1.0
Mesoblastic nephroma	41	2.9	
Cystic nephroma	1	0.1	
Unspecified	3	0.2	
Hepatic tumours	12	0.8	0.7
Haemangioendothelioma/haemangioma	10	0.7	
Unspecified	2	0.1	
Fibromatous tumours	13	0.8	1.4
Fibromatosis	5	0.4	
Myofibromatosis	3	0.2	
Haemangiopericytoma	4	0.3	
Fibroma	1	0.1	
Extrahepatic blood vessel tumours	30	2.1	1.3
Haemangioma	14	1.0	
Lymphangioma	16	1.1	
Other soft tissue tumours	5	0.4	0.5
Rhabdomyoma	3	0.2	
Leiomyoma	2	0.1	
Germ-cell tumours	203	14.2	0.4
Extragonadal teratoma	201	14.1	
Gonadal germ-cell tumours	2	0.1	
Other gonadal tumours	8	0.6	7.0
Juvenile granulosa cell tumour	6	0.4	
Leydig cell tumour	1	0.1	
Unspecified	1	0.1	
Melanoma	4	0.3	3.0
Other and unspecified	33	2.3	0.6
Gastrointestinal stromal tumour	1	0.1	
Sialoblastoma	1	0.1	
Unspecified	31	2.2	
Total	358	25.1	0.7

Numbers of registered cases (*N*), minimum estimate of risk per million live births, and male/female ratio (M/F). Note that ascertainment is incomplete and varies between diagnostic groups
Source: National Registry of Childhood Tumours

The risk of 0.4 per million live births for Langerhans cell histiocytosis (LCH) is almost certainly too low. In the German Childhood Cancer Registry the estimated incidence in the first month of life was between 1 and 2 per million live births [12]. In a series of over 1000 children from the Austrian/German/Swiss/Netherlands subcentre of the international LCH clinical trials, the disease manifested in the neonatal period in 61 cases but was only diagnosed within the first 4 weeks in 20 of them [12], which suggests that LCH may be present in 3–6 per million neonates.

Mesoblastic nephroma seems likely to be more completely registered than most benign neoplasms of infancy because of its eligibility for clinical trials of treatment for childhood renal tumours. The minimum risk estimate of 2.9 per million live births is very close to the 3.0 per million, based on 7 cases, in the West Midlands study where ascertainment was thought to be virtually complete [10]. The presence of 41 cases in the present series compared with four cases of Wilms tumour indicates that mesoblastic nephroma is at least ten times as frequent as Wilms tumour among neonates. By the age of 3 months, however, Wilms tumour is much more frequent than mesoblastic nephroma [13]. Among 47 cases of mesoblastic nephroma included in UK Wilms tumour trials, the median age at diagnosis was 1 month, an antenatal diagnosis of renal mass was made in 14 (30%) and a further 8 (17%) presented with an abdominal mass on routine postnatal examination [13]. This suggests that the great majority of neonatal mesoblastic nephromas are detected prenatally or diagnosed incidentally.

There are no population data on hepatic haemangioendothelioma and haemangioma but the fact that the NRCT series included ten cases, as against seven cases of hepatoblastoma, suggests that this is the most common neonatal liver tumour.

Because of its interest to oncologists, it seems likely that ascertainment of fibromatosis, including myofibromatosis, was relatively high. The data presented here suggest that these conditions are diagnosed in the neonatal period with a frequency similar to infantile fibrosarcoma.

By far the largest group of non-malignant tumours was the extragonadal teratomas which, even if ascertainment were complete, were almost three times as frequent as malignant germ-cell tumours. The excess of girls over boys was similar to that for malignant germ-cell tumours. The most frequent site was the sacrococcygeal region (144/201, 72%), followed by head and neck (33/201, 16%), intraabdominal (6/201, 3%) and intrathoracic (3/201, 1%); site was not specified in 15 cases (7%). Combining the numbers of malignant and non-malignant cases, the recorded incidence of neonatally diagnosed sacrococcygeal teratoma was 12.8 per million live births, or 1 in 78,000. This is somewhat lower that the rate of 1 in 58,700 live births for sacrococcygeal, sacral and pre-sacral teratomas in the West Midlands study, the great majority of which were diagnosed neonatally [10]. In a more recent population-based study in northern England the birth prevalence was 1 in 27,000 live births overall and 1 in 37,700 for tumours diagnosed neonatally [14]. This suggests that nationally only half of all sacrococcygeal teratomas, and 40% of non-malignant cases, were registered. In the northern England study, 50% of live born neonatal cases had been detected on prenatal ultrasound.

52.2 Genetic and Familial Associations

A substantial proportion of childhood cancers occur in association with genetic syndromes. In a large series of children and adolescents with cancer, 8.5% had germline mutations that were deemed to be definitely or probably pathogenic [15]. It seems very unlikely that the percentage is lower among neonates with cancer. In addition, a substantial proportion are associated with chromosomal abnormalities. Among young children with Down syndrome, the relative risk of leukaemia is about 50 and it is especially high for AML [16]. In the present series, 15/71 (21%) neonates with leukaemia had Down syndrome. These included 9 of the 36 with AML, 5 of the 14 with unspecified leukaemia and the single case of myelodysplasia; there were no cases of Down syndrome with ALL. These data do not include cases of transient abnormal myelopoiesis (TAM), a benign condition found in 10% of Down syndrome babies [17]. AML later develops in 20–30% of infants with Down syndrome and TAM, but virtually always beyond the neonatal period [18].

In the majority of acute leukaemia in infants, both ALL and AML, the malignant clone has a rearrangement involving the MLL gene on chromosome 11q23 [19]. Studies of neonatal blood spots have confirmed that the MLL rearrangement originates *in utero* [20]. A large number of studies has found associations between polymorphisms of several genes and the risk of childhood leukaemia but they have mostly related to types of leukaemia more often found in older children. There is some evidence that carriers of the inactivating polymorphism C609T in the NAD(P)H:quinine oxidoreductase 1 gene (NQ01) have an increased risk of ALL or of MLL+ leukaemia [21–23]. One recent study found that slow-acetylation phenotypes of N-Acetyl transferase 2 (NAT2) were associated with MLL+ and MLL- infant leukaemia [24]. The Brazilian Collaborative Study Group of Infant Acute Leukemia has found that polymorphisms of several other genes affect the risk of leukaemia in the first 2 years of life [25, 26]. In a cohort of 641 children with Noonan syndrome who were verified as carrying a germline PTPN11 mutation, 16 (2.5%) had JMML and 8 (1.2%) had other JMML-like myeloproliferative disorders (MPD) with onset in the neonatal period, and there were a further four cases of JMML and eight of MPD with onset later in childhood [27].

Genome-wide association studies have identified several genomic loci associated with predisposition to sporadic neuroblastoma [28]. Some of these are associated with high-risk disease [28], and thus of limited relevance to neonatal neuroblastoma which is predominantly low-risk. Four predisposition loci for low-risk neuroblastoma have also been identified [29], although with no proposed mechanism as yet [28]. Three further loci have been associated with predisposition to neuroblastoma of both high-risk and low-risk forms [28].

Only 1–2% of neuroblastoma is familial and the majority of pedigrees are associated with germline mutations of the anaplastic lymphoma kinase (ALK) gene [28]. Most of the remaining familial cases result from germline mutations of the paired-like homeobox 2B(PHOX2B) gene, and affected children also have a high risk of Hirschsprung disease and congenital central hypoventilation syndrome [28]. About 10% of familial neuroblastoma is not associated with either of these genes and their aetiology remains unknown. Genetic testing for germline ALK and PHOX2B mutations is recommended for infants with a family history of neuroblastoma [28].

Retinoblastoma is caused by mutation or, rarely, deletion of both copies of the tumour suppressor gene RB1on chromosome 13q14. In heritable cases the first mutation is in the germline, while in non-heritable cases both mutations are somatic [30]. The majority of children with heritable retinoblastoma have bilateral disease whereas non-heritable cases are invariably unilateral. Among the 32 cases of retinoblastoma in Table 52.1, there was a past family history of the disease in 24/25 bilateral and all six unilateral cases and this would undoubtedly have increased the likelihood of diagnosis during the neonatal period. Based on the criterion of having bilateral tumours or past family history, at least 31/32 (97%) of the cases of neonatal retinoblastoma were of the heritable form.

Germline mutations of the tumour suppressor gene TP53 confer increased risk of a wide range of childhood cancers including soft-tissue sarcomas and adrenocortical carcinoma, and are responsible for most occurrences of the Li-Fraumeni familial cancer syndrome [31]. In a study of children with sporadic rhabdomyosarcoma, 3/13 patients aged under 3 years at diagnosis harboured a constitutional TP53 mutation, compared with none of the 20 children over 3 years of age [32]. Two of the affected children had embryonal rhabdomyosarcoma and one had alveolar rhabdomyosarcoma. The youngest child with a TP53 mutation was diagnosed at 18 months and the youngest in the series was 5 months of age. Nevertheless, it is plausible that some cases of neonatal rhabdomyosarcoma are caused by germline TP53 mutations. A very high proportion of young children with adrenocortical carcinoma carry a germline mutation of TP53 [33, 34]. Adrenocortical carcinoma does occur in infancy, although there were no cases in the 20-year series of Table 52.1. In a study of mass screening of neonates in southern Brazil, where adrenocortical tumours are strongly associated with the germline TP53 mutation R337H, the mutation was carried by 0.27% of those were screened, and adrenocortical tumours were diagnosed in 2.4% of carriers compared with 0.0012% of non-carriers [35].

While nearly all sporadic chordomas occur in adults, 9 of the 11 published cases in patients with tuberous sclerosis complex (TSC) have been diagnosed in children under 5 years of age [36]. They include four cases arising in the sacrum, a rare site for sporadic chordoma, all of them diagnosed in the first week of life [37]. TSC is caused by inactivating germline mutations of either of the tumour suppressor genes TSC1 and TSC2, and chordoma has been found in both groups. Chordoma of the skull base, a much more frequent primary site for sporadic chordoma, has also been reported in association with TSC but the youngest infant so far recorded was diagnosed at 4 months of age [36]. Cardiac rhabdomyomas, usually diagnosed prenatally or in the neonatal period, are a major feature of TSC [38]. Subependymal giant cell astrocytoma, a low-grade glioma, occurs in 10% of patients with TSC [39] but is rarely diagnosed in neonates [38].

Rhabdoid tumour predisposition syndrome is associated with germline mutation or deletion of SMARCB1 (also known as INI1, hSNF5 or BAF47) on chromosome 22q and results in increased risk of rhabdoid tumour of the kidney, ATRT of the CNS, and extra-renal rhabdoid tumours of other sites [40].

Beckwith-Wiedemann syndrome is associated with increased risk of several childhood cancers including Wilms tumour, hepatoblastoma, adrenocortical carcinoma, rhabdomyosarcoma, neuroblastoma and pancreatoblastoma [41]. The cancers are nearly always diagnosed later than the first month of life but a few cases have been reported in neonates [11, 42, 43].

A wide range of other genetic syndromes is associated with increased risk of various childhood cancers but as they generally only manifest after the first month of life they are not discussed further here [44, 45].

There is little evidence that family members of children with germ cell tumours have a changed risk of cancer overall. In a North American case-control study of 274 children with malignant germ-cell tumours, family history of cancer before age 40 years or of ovarian or uterine cancers was associated with reduced risk of germ cell tumours in girls, whereas family history of cancer before age 40 or of melanoma was associated with increased risk in boys [46]. Nearly all neonatal germ cell tumours are extragonadal but results were not presented separately for extragonadal tumours, which accounted for less than half the cases in the study.

Several studies have found a higher relative risk of cancer in infancy than later in childhood among children with congenital abnormalities compared with children without abnormalities [47–50].

There is little evidence for any association between infant leukaemia and congenital abnormalities other than Down syndrome [51].

An excess risk of neuroblastoma in children with congenital abnormalities has been found repeatedly, but with limited consistency regarding the type of abnormality [52–55]. The association appears to be strongest for neuroblastoma diagnosed in infancy [54, 55], but it may also be more pronounced for tumours with MYCN amplification [54].

There have been numerous reports of associations between congenital abnormalities and childhood germ-cell tumours [48, 56–62]. In the largest case-control study the association was more pronounced for extragonadal tumours [63]. It also appeared to be limited to boys but this was largely accounted for by the highly significant association between cryptorchidism and testicular tumours [63]. There was little indication of association with any other specific abnormalities [63]. Sacrococcygeal teratomas are, however, frequent in infants with Currarino syndrome [64].

52.3 Other Birth Characteristics

High birth weight is associated with an increased risk of many childhood cancers. In parallel analyses of very large case-control data sets from the UK and USA, there were consistently raised risks of leukaemia, CNS tumours, renal tumours and soft-tissue sarcomas [65]. The results for leukaemia and CNS tumours were broadly similar to those in meta-analyses of previous studies [66, 67]. At least three studies have found an association with MLL+ leukaemia [68–70]. An increased risk of AML with low birth weight has also been found in some studies [65, 66], though this may be due to the fact that low birth weight is also associated with Down syndrome [65].

A meta-analysis of ten studies found that birth weight above 4000 g or below 2500 g was associated with increased risk of neuroblastoma [71], and a similarly U-shaped relationship was found in the recent UK/US study [65]. There is no consistent evidence for the increased risk being confined to a particular age group at diagnosis [52].

Low birth weight is an established risk factor for hepatoblastoma [65, 72], but it is nearly always diagnosed beyond the neonatal period and it is unclear how many cases are truly congenital [73].

There was a particularly marked trend towards higher risk of extragonadal, non-CNS germ-cell tumours with increasing birth weight in the UK/US study [65]. In the largest previous case-control study of children with malignant germ-cell tumours, there was a significantly increased risk with parentally reported birth weight above 3500 g but the increase was much smaller and non-significant in the subset of children whose medical records could be reviewed [74]. An earlier study which had also found an association with higher birth weight speculated that this might be due to higher levels of maternal oestrogen during pregnancy [75] but the more recent study failed to provide evidence that exposure to exogenous female hormones in pregnancy increased the risk of germ-cell tumours [74]. Results were not presented specifically for infants but some neonatal teratomas constitute an appreciable proportion of body weight and a high proportion of premature births among infants with sacrococcygeal teratoma is a consequence of the tumour [14, 76].

There appears to be no association of infant leukaemia with prior fetal loss, infertility or its treatment [68, 77]. There has been little consistency in findings for neuroblastoma in relation to reproductive history [52, 54, 55, 78–80], whether or not the data were subdivided according to age at diagnosis or MYCN status. One study of rhabdomyosarcoma found a highly significant association with neonatal prior history of stillbirth [81] but a more recent, larger study found no difference in history of fetal loss between case and control mothers [82].

The two largest cohort studies of cancer in children born following assisted reproduction technology found no significant overall increase in cancer risk [83, 84]. In the Netherlands an increased risk of retinoblastoma was reported among children born after in vitro fertilisation, based on five cases diagnosed during 2000–2002 [85]. Over the next five years, however, no significantly elevated risk was found [86]. There was also no evidence for increased risk of retinoblastoma in three other large cohort studies [83, 84, 87].

52.4 Exogenous Risk Factors

The very early age at diagnosis for neonatal cancer means that exogenous risk factors that have been investigated for childhood cancer in general are only at all likely to be relevant if exposure was prenatal.

While 15–20% of childhood leukaemia may be attributable to exposure to natural background ionising radiation, the proportion among neonates is negligible because of their low total exposure by that age [88, 89].

Therapy-related AML in patients who have received chemotherapy that inhibits DNA topisomerase II (topo-II) often has the same MLL abnormalities that are found in infant leukaemia, leading to the hypothesis that maternal exposure to topo-II inhibitors in diet or medications might result in MLL+ leukaemia in the infant [90]. The hypothesis gains limited support from associations of infant AML with maternal consumption of foods containing topo-II inhibitors [90, 91] but no effect has been found for other topo-II inhibitors or for MLL+ ALL. Maternal consumption of fresh fruit and vegetables during pregnancy has been associated with decreased risk of MLL+ infant leukaemia [91]. Exposure to petroleum products during pregnancy has been associated with MLL- infant leukaemia in one study [92]. In the Air Pollution and Childhood Cancers Study in California, there was a raised risk of neuroblastoma with prenatal exposure to several pollutants; the effect was more marked for infants under 6 months of age, but there was no information on stage or MYCN status [93]. In the same study, there was a raised risk of bilateral retinoblastoma with prenatal exposure to traffic-related pollution [94]. Maternal cigarette smoking during pregnancy is not associated with infant leukaemia but the evidence on alcohol and illicit drug use is inconsistent [95].

There are numerous case reports of various neonatal tumours in infants whose mother took a wide range of drugs during pregnancy but very few of these associations have been confirmed by epidemiological studies [96]. Following the appearance of reports of neuroblastoma associated with fetal alcohol syndrome, several case-control studies found increased risk of neuroblastoma with maternal alcohol consumption during pregnancy [52]. The proportion of case mothers who drank in pregnancy was generally low, however, and no consistent association was found in the study which was based on by far the largest number of cases [97]. Several studies reported an excess risk of neuroblastoma with intake of diuretics in pregnancy [52] but the numbers of exposed cases were very small. Excess risks associated with maternal use of analgesics and other nervous system drugs have also been reported but the results were not broken down by age at diagnosis [52, 98].

Two studies have found a reduction in risk of neuroblastoma with maternal vitamin intake in pregnancy, which did not vary with age at diagnosis [99, 100]. Only the more recent study analysed the data in relation to MYCN status, and the effect was more pronounced for MYCN non-amplified disease [100]. Incidence of neuroblastoma among infants in Ontario declined by 60% since the start of folic acid fortification of flour [101] but in Hungary the risk of neuroblastoma did not decrease during the first four years of a national policy of folic acid supplementation in pregnancy [102].

The largest case-control study of sporadic bilateral retinoblastoma arising from a new germline RB1 mutation found significant associations with gonadal radiation exposure to either parent before conception [103]. While the mutations may have been radiation-induced, the results could also be due to bias, confounding or chance.

Radiation exposure during pregnancy has been associated with rhabdomyosarcoma in the child, with the association being strongest for children diagnosed before 5 years of age and perhaps limited to embryonal rhabdomyosarcoma [82].

52.5 Survival

Table 52.3 shows survival rates for infants born in 1988–2007 who had cancer diagnosed in the neonatal period. Results are presented for all ICCC-3 groups, subgroups and divisions with at least five cases. Overall survival was 64% at 1 year from diagnosis and 62% at 3 years, considerably lower than the 88% 1-year and 78% 3-year survival rates for all childhood cancer diagnosed during 1991–2000 [13]. Thus, while the short-term prognosis of neonatal cancer is rather poor, the probability of survival conditional on surviving 1 year from diagnosis is very much higher than in older children. Survival from leukaemia, embryonal CNS tumours, renal tumours and rhabdomyosarcoma was especially poor for neonates compared with older children. By contrast, neonates with retinoblastoma had 100% 3-year survival. The 79% 3-year survival rate of neonates with neuroblastoma was slightly

Table 52.3 Survival from cancer among live-born neonates born 1988–2007 in Great Britain

ICCC-3	*N*	1-year survival	3-year survival
I. Leukaemias	71	34	30
(a) ALL	15	33	13
(b) AML	36	36	36
(d) JMML/CMML and MDS	6	67	67
(e) Other and unspecified	14	14	14
III. CNS tumours	50	42	42
(a) (2) Choroid plexus tumours	5	80	80
(b) Astrocytoma	11	64	64
(c) Embryonal	10	0	0
(f) Unspecified	19	37	37
IV. (a) Neuroblastoma	91	80	79
V. Retinoblastoma	32	100	100
VI. (a) Wilms tumour and renal pPNET	5	40	40
VII. (a) Hepatoblastoma	7	71	71
IX. Soft tissue sarcoma	38	45	37
(a) Rhabdomyosarcoma	13	54	38
(b) (1) Fibrosarcoma	10	70	70
(d) (3) Extra renal rhabdoid	5	20	0
X. Germ-cell and gonadal	93	76	76
(a) CNS germ cell tumours	13	31	31
(b) Other non-gonadal germ-cell	78	83	83
Total	395	64	62

Numbers of cases (*N*), 1-year and 3-year survival rates (%)

lower than the 84% 3-year survival of all infants under 1 year of age who were diagnosed with neuroblastoma in 1991–2000 but much higher than that for children aged 1 year and over at diagnosis [13].

Most survivors of childhood cancer go on to lead normal lives. They are, however, at increased risk of second cancers and a range of other late effects depending on the type of cancer and its treatment [104–108]. There is little information on these risks specifically as they relate to survivors of neonatal cancer. There is some evidence that the risk of second cancer following heritable retinoblastoma treated with radiotherapy is especially high when the retinoblastoma is diagnosed in the first month of life [109].

References

1. Steliarova-Foucher E, Stiller C, Lacour B, Kaatsch P. International Classification Of Childhood Cancer, Third Edition. Cancer. 2005;103:1457–67.
2. Gurney JG, Ross JA, Wall DA, Bleyer WA, Severson RK, Robison LL. Infant cancer In The U. S.: histology-specific incidence and trends, 1973 to 1992. J Pediatr Hematol Oncol. 1997;19:428–32.
3. Stiller C. Childhood cancer In Britain: incidence, survival, mortality. Oxford: Oxford University Press; 2007.
4. Brodeur GM, Pritchard J, Berthold F, NLT C, Castel V, Castleberry RP, et al. Revisions of the international criteria for neuroblastoma diagnosis, staging, and response to treatment. J Clin Oncol. 1993;11:1466–77.
5. Gigliotti AR, Di Cataldo A, Sorrentino S, Parodi S, Rizzo A, Buffa P, et al. Neuroblastoma in the newborn. A study of the Italian Neuroblastoma Registry. Eur J Cancer. 2009;45:3220–7.
6. Brodeur GM, Look AT, Shimada H, Hamilton VM, Maris JM, Hann HW, et al. Biological aspects of neuroblastomas identified by mass screening in Quebec. Med Pediatr Oncol. 2001;36:157–9.
7. Moppett J, Haddadin I, Foot AB. Neonatal neuroblastoma. Arch Dis Child Fetal Neonatal Ed. 1999;81:F134–7.
8. Grundy R, Anderson J, Gaze M, Gerrard M, Glaser A, Gordon A, et al. Congenital alveolar rhabdomyosarcoma: clinical and molecular distinction from alveolar rhabdomyosarcoma in older children. Cancer. 2001;91:606–12.
9. Slater O, Shipley J. Clinical relevance of molecular genetics to paediatric sarcomas. J Clin Pathol. 2007;60:1187–94.
10. Parkes SE, Muir KR, Southern L, Cameron AH, Darbyshire PJ, Stevens MC. Neonatal tumours: a thirty-year population-based study. Med Pediatr Oncol. 1994;22:309–17.
11. Koh TH, Cooper JE, Newman CL, Walker TM, Kiely EM, Hoffmann EB. Pancreatoblastoma in a neonate with Wiedemann-Beckwith syndrome. Eur J Pediatr. 1986;145:435–8.
12. Minkov M, Prosch H, Steiner M, Grois N, Pötschger U, Kaatsch P, et al. Langerhans cell histiocytosis in neonates. Pediatr Blood Cancer. 2005;45:802–7.
13. England RJ, Haider N, Vujanic GM, Kelsey A, Stiller CA, Pritchard-Jones K et al. Mesoblastic nephroma: a report of the United Kingdom Children's Cancer and Leukaemia Group (CCLG). Pediatr Blood Cancer. 2011; 56:744–8.
14. Swamy R, Embleton N, Hale J. Sacrococcygeal teratoma over two decades: birth prevalence, prenatal diagnosis and clinical outcomes. Prenat Diagn. 2008;28:1048–51.
15. Zhang J, Walsh MF, Wu G, Edmonson MN, Gruber TA, Easton J, et al. Germline mutations in predisposition genes in childhood cancer. N Engl J Med. 2015;373:2336–46.
16. Hasle H. Pattern of malignant disorders in individuals with Down's syndrome. Lancet Oncol. 2001;2:429–36.
17. Massey GV. Transient leukemia in newborns with Down syndrome. Pediatr Blood Cancer. 2005;44:29–32.
18. Crispino JD. *Gata1* mutations in down syndrome: implications for biology and diagnosis of children with transient myeloproliferative disorder and acute megakaryoblastic leukemia. Pediatr Blood Cancer. 2005;44:40–4.
19. Biondi A, Cimino G, Pieters R, Pui C-H. biological and therapeutic aspects of infant leukemia. Blood. 2000;96:24–33.
20. Greaves MF, Maia AT, Wiemels JL, Ford AM. Leukemia in twins: lessons in natural history. Blood. 2003;102:2321–33.
21. Guha N, Chang JS, Chokkalingam AP, Wiemels JL, Smith MT, Buffler PA. *Nq01* polymorphisms and de novo childhood leukaemia: a huge review and meta-analysis. Am J Epidemiol. 2008;168:1221–32.
22. Guha N, Chang JS, Chokkalingam AP, Wiemels JL, Smith MT, Buffler PA. Nq01 polymorphisms and de novo childhood leukaemia: a huge review and meta-analysis. Am J Epidemiol. 2009;169:1280.
23. Li C, Zhou Y. Association between NQO1 C609T polymorphism and acute lymphoblastic leukemia risk: evidence from an updated meta-analysis based on 17 case-control studies. J Cancer Res Clin Oncol. 2014;140:873–81.
24. Zanrosso CW, Emerenciano M, Gonçalves BA, Faro A, Koifman S, Pombo-de-Oliveira MS. *N*-Acetyltransferase 2 polymorphisms and susceptibility to infant leukemia with maternal exposure to dipyrone during pregnancy. Cancer Epidemiol Biomarkers Prev. 2010;19:3037–43.

25. Emerenciano M, Barbosa TC, Lopes BA, Blunck CB, Faro A, Andrade C, et al. ARID5B polymorphism confers an increased risk to acquire specific Mll rearrangements in early childhood leukemia. BMC Cancer. 2014;14:127.
26. Lopes BA, Emerenciano M, Gonçalves BAA, Vieira TM, Rossini A, Pombo-de-Oliveira MS. Polymorphisms in *CYP1B1*, *CYP3A5*, *GSTT1*, and *SULT1A1* are associated with early age acute leukemia. PLoS One. 2015;10:E0127308.
27. Strullu M, Caye A, Lachenaud J, Cassinat B, Gazal S, Fenneteau O, et al. Juvenile Myelomonocytic Leukaemia And Noonan Syndrome. J Med Genet. 2014;51:689–97.
28. Bosse KR, Maris JM. Advances in the translational genomics of neuroblastoma; from improving risk stratification and revealing novel biology to identifying actionable genomic alterations. Cancer. 2016;122:20–33.
29. Nguyen LB, Diskin SJ, Capasso M, Wang K, Diamond MA, Glessner J et al. Phenotype restricted genome-wide association study using a gene-centric approach identifies three low-risk neuroblastoma susceptibility loci. PLoS Genet. 2011;7:E1002026.
30. Lohmann DR, Gallie BL. Retinoblastoma: revisiting the model prototype of inherited cancer. Am J Med Genet C Semin Med Genet. 2004;129:23–8.
31. Varley JM. Germline Tp53 mutations and Li-Fraumeni syndrome. Hum Mutat. 2003;21:313–20.
32. Diller L, Sexsmith E, Gottlieb A, FP L, Malkin D. Germline P53 mutations are frequently detected in young children with rhabdomyosarcoma. J Clin Invest. 1995;95:1606–11.
33. Wagner J, Portwine C, Rabin K, Leclerc J-M, Narod SA, Malkin D. High frequency of germline P53 mutations in childhood adrenocortical cancer. J Natl Cancer Inst. 1994;86:1707–10.
34. Varley JM, Mcgown G, Thorncroft M, James LA, Margison GP, Forster G, et al. Are there low-penetrance Tp53 alleles? Evidence from childhood adrenocortical tumors. Am J Hum Genet. 1999;65:995–1006.
35. Custódio G, Ga P, Kiesel Filho N, Komechen H, Sabbaga CC, Rosati Ret AL. Impact of neonatal screening and surveillance for the TP53 R337H mutation on early detection of childhood adrenocortical tumors. J Clin Oncol. 2013;31:2619–26.
36. McMaster ML, Goldstein AM, Parry DM. Clinical features distinguish childhood chordoma associated with tuberous sclerosis complex (TSC) from chordoma in the general paediatric population. J Med Genet. 2011;48:444–9.
37. Lee-Jones L, Aligianis I, Davies PA, Puga A, Farndon PA, Stemmer-Rachamimov A, et al. Sacrococcygeal chordomas in patients with tuberous sclerosis complex show somatic loss of TSC1 or TSC2. Genes Chromosomes Cancer. 2004;41:80–5.
38. Yates JR, Maclean C, Higgins JN, Humphrey A, Le Maréchal K, Clifford M, et al. The tuberous sclerosis 2000 study: presentation, initial assessments and implications for diagnosis and management. Arch Dis Child. 2011;96:1020–5.
39. Crino PB, Nathanson KL, Henske EP. The tuberous sclerosis complex. N Engl J Med. 2006;355:1345–56.
40. Bourdeaut F, Lequin D, Brugières L, Reynaud S, Dufour C, Doz F, et al. Frequent hSNF5/INI1 germline mutations in patients with rhabdoid tumor. Clin Cancer Res. 2011;17:31–8.
41. Lapunzina P. Risk of tumorigenesis in overgrowth syndromes: a comprehensive review. Am J Med Genet C Semin Med Genet. 2005;137:53–71.
42. Kuroiwa M, Sakamoto J, Shimada A, Suzuki N, Hirato J, Park MJ, et al. Manifestation of alveolar rhabdomyosarcoma as primary cutaneous lesions in a neonate with Beckwith-Wiedemann syndrome. J Pediatr Surg. 2009;44:E31–5.
43. Worth LL, Slopis JM, Herzog CE. Congenital hepatoblastoma and schizencephaly in an infant with Beckwith-Wiedemann syndrome. Med Pediatr Oncol. 1999;33:591–3.
44. D'Orazio JA. Inherited cancer syndromes in children and young adults. J Pediatr Hematol Oncol. 2010;32:195–228.
45. Zimmerman R, Schimmenti L, Spector L. A catalog of genetic syndromes in childhood cancer. Pediatr Blood Cancer. 2015;62:2071–5.
46. Poynter JN, Radzom AH, Spector LG, Puumala S, Robison LL, Chen Z, et al. Family history of cancer and malignant germ cell tumors in children: a report from the Children's Oncology Group. Cancer Causes Control. 2010;21:181–9.
47. Agha MM, Williams JI, Marrett L, To T, Zipursky A, Dodds L. Congenital abnormalities and childhood cancer. Cancer. 2005;103:1939–48.
48. Bjørge T, Cnattingius S, Lie RT, Tretli S, Engeland A. Cancer risk in children with birth defects and in their families: a population based cohort study of 5.2 million children from Norway And Sweden. Cancer Epidemiol Biomarkers Prev. 2008;17:500–6.
49. Partap S, Maclean J, Von Behren J, Reynolds P, Fisher PG. Birth anomalies and obstetric history as risks for childhood tumors of the central nervous system. Pediatrics. 2011;128:E652–7.
50. Dawson S, Charles AK, Bower C, de Klerk NH, Milne E. Risk of cancer among children with birth defects: a novel approach. Birth Defects Res A Clin Mol Teratol. 2015;103:284–91.
51. Johnson KJ, Roesler MA, Linabery AM, Hilden JM, Davies SM, Ross JA. Infant leukemia and congenital abnormalities: a Children's Oncology Group Study. Pediatr Blood Cancer. 2010;55:95–9.
52. Heck JE, Ritz B, Hung RJ, Hashibe M, Boffetta P. The epidemiology of neuroblastoma: a review. Paediatr Perinat Epidemiol. 2009;23:125–43.
53. Menegaux F, Olshan AF, Reitnauer PJ, Blatt J, Cohn SL. Positive association between congenital anomalies and risk of neuroblastoma. Pediatr Blood Cancer. 2005;45:649–55.
54. Munzer C, Menegaux F, Lacour B, Valteau-Couanet D, Michon J, Coze C, et al. Birth-related characteristics, congenital malformation, maternal reproduc-

tive history and neuroblastoma: the ESCALE study (SFCE). Int J Cancer. 2008;122:2315–21.
55. Bjørge T, Engeland A, Tretli S, Heuch I. Birth and parental characteristics and risk of neuroblastoma in a population-based Norwegian cohort study. Br J Cancer. 2008;99:1165–9.
56. Johnston HE, Mann JR, Williams J, Waterhouse JA, Birch JM, Cartwright RA, et al. The Inter-Regional, Epidemiological Study of Childhood Cancer (IRESCC): case-control study in children with germ cell tumours. Carcinogenesis. 1986;7:717–22.
57. Fraumeni JF Jr, Li FP, Dalager N. Teratomas in children: epidemiologic features. J Natl Cancer Inst. 1973;51:1425–30.
58. Narod SA, Hawkins MM, Robertson CM, Stiller CA. Congenital anomalies and childhood cancer in Great Britain. Am J Hum Genet. 1997;60:474–85.
59. Altmann AE, Halliday JL, Giles GG. Associations between congenital malformations and childhood cancer. A register-based case-control study. Br J Cancer. 1998;78:1244–9.
60. Nishi M, Miyake H, Takeda T, Hatae Y. Congenital malformations and childhood cancer. Med Pediatr Oncol. 2000;34:250–4.
61. Merks JHM, Caron HN, Hennekam RCM. High incidence of malformation syndromes in a series of 1,073 children with cancer. Am J Med Genet A. 2005;134:132–43.
62. Rankin J, Silf KA, Pearce MS, Parker L, Ward Platt M. Congenital anomaly and childhood cancer: a population-based, record linkage study. Pediatr Blood Cancer. 2008;51:608–12.
63. Johnson KJ, Ross JA, Poynter JN, Linabery AM, Robison LL, Shu XO. Paediatric germ cell tumours and congenital abnormalities: a Children's Oncology Group Study. Br J Cancer. 2009;101:518–21.
64. Lynch SA, Wang Y, Strachan T, Burn J, Lindsay S. Autosomal dominant sacral agenesis: Currarino syndrome. J Med Genet. 2000;37:561–6.
65. O'Neill KA, Murphy MF, Bunch KJ, Puumala SE, Carozza SE, Chow EJ, et al. Infant birthweight and risk of childhood cancer: international population-based case control studies of 40 000 cases. Int J Epidemiol. 2015;44:153–68.
66. Caughey RW, Michels KB. Birth weight and childhood leukemia: a meta-analysis and review of the current evidence. Int J Cancer. 2009;124:2658–70.
67. Harder T, Plagemann A, Harder A. Birth weight and subsequent risk of childhood primary brain tumors: a meta-analysis. Am J Epidemiol. 2008;168: 366–73.
68. Spector LG, Davies SM, Robison LL, Hilden JM, Roesler M, Ross JA. Birth characteristics, maternal reproductive history, and the risk of infant leukemia: a report from The Children's Oncology Group. Cancer Epidemiol Biomarkers Prev. 2007;16:128–34.
69. Koifman S, Pombo-de-Oliveira MS, And The Brazilian Collaborative Study Group Of Infant Acute Leukemia. High birth weight as an important risk factor for infant leukemia. Br J Cancer. 2008;98:664–7.
70. O'Neill KA, Bunch KJ, Vincent TJ, Spector LG, Moorman AV, MFG M. Immunophenotype and cytogenetic characteristics in the relationship between birth weight and childhood leukemia. Pediatr Blood Cancer. 2012;58:7–11.
71. Harder T, Plagemann A, Harder A. Birth weight and risk of neuroblastoma: a meta-analysis. Int J Epidemiol. 2010;39:746–56.
72. Spector LG, Birch J. The epidemiology of hepatoblastoma. Pediatr Blood Cancer. 2012;59:776–9.
73. Turcotte LM, Georgieff MK, Ross JA, Feusner JH, Tomlinson GE, Malogolowkin MH, et al. Neonatal medical exposures and characteristics of low birth weight hepatoblastoma cases: a report from the Children's Oncology Group. Pediatr Blood Cancer. 2014;61:2018–23.
74. Shankar S, Davies S, Giller R, Krailo M, Davis M, Gardner K, et al. In Utero Exposure To Female Hormones And Germ Cell Tumors In Children. Cancer. 2006;106:1169–77.
75. Shu XO, Nesbit ME, Buckley JD, Krailo MD, Robison LL. An exploratory analysis of risk factors for childhood malignant germ-cell tumors: report from the Children's Cancer Group (Canada, United States). Cancer Causes Control. 1995;6:187–98.
76. Brace V, Grant SR, Brackley KJ, Kilby MD, Whittle MJ. Prenatal diagnosis and outcome in sacrococcygeal teratomas: a review of cases between 1992 and 1998. Prenat Diagn. 2000;20:51–5.
77. Puumala SE, Spector LG, Wall MM, Robison LL, Heerema NA, Roesler MA, et al. Infant leukemia and parental infertility or its treatment: a Children's Oncology Group report. Hum Reprod. 2010;25:1561–8.
78. Johnson KJ, Puumala SE, Soler JT, Spector LG. Perinatal characteristics and risk of neuroblastoma. Int J Cancer. 2008;123:1166–72.
79. Bluhm E, McNeil DE, Cnattingius S, Gridley G, El Ghormli L, Fraumeni JF Jr. Prenatal and perinatal risk factors for neuroblastoma. Int J Cancer. 2008;123:2885–90.
80. McLaughlin CC, Baptiste MS, Schymura MJ, Zdeb MS, Nasca PC. Perinatal risk factors for neuroblastoma. Cancer Causes Control.2008;20:289–301.
81. Ghali MH, Yoo K-Y, Flannery JT, Dubrow R. Association between childhood rhabdomyosarcoma and maternal history of stillbirths. Int J Cancer. 1992;50:365–8.
82. Grufferman S, Ruymann F, Ognjanovic S, Erhardt EB, Maurer HM. Prenatal X-ray exposure and rhabdomyosarcoma in children: a report from the Children's Oncology Group. Cancer Epidemiol Biomarkers Prev. 2009;18:1271–6.
83. Williams CL, Bunch KJ, Stiller CA, Murphy MFG, Botting BJ, Wallace WH, et al. Cancer risk among children born after assisted conception. N Engl J Med. 2013;369:1819–27.
84. Sundh KJ, Henningsen AK, Källen K, Bergh C, Romundstad LB, Gissler M, et al. Cancer in chil-

dren and young adults born after assisted reproductive technology: A Nordic cohort study from the Committee Of Nordic Art And Safety (Conartas). Hum Reprod. 2014;29:2050–7.
85. Moll AC, Imhof SM, Cruysberg JR, Schouten-van Meeteren AY, Boers M, van Leeuwen FE. Incidence of retinoblastoma in children born after in-vitro fertilisation. Lancet. 2003;361:309–10.
86. Marees T, Dommering CJ, Imhof SM, Kors WA, Ringens PJ, van Leeuwen FE, et al. Incidence of retinoblastoma in Dutch children conceived by IVF: an expanded study. Hum Reprod. 2009;24: 3220–4.
87. Foix-L'Hélias L, Aerts I, Marchand L, Lumbroso-Le Rouic L, Gauthier-Villars M, Labrune P et al. Are children born after infertility treatment at increased risk of retinoblastoma? Hum Reprod. 2012;27:2186–92.
88. Wakeford R, Kendall GM, Little MP. The proportion of childhood leukaemia incidence in great britain that may be caused by natural background ionizing radiation. Leukemia. 2009;23:770–6.
89. Kendall GM, Little MP, Wakeford R. Numbers and proportions of leukemias in young people and adults induced by radiation of natural origin. Leuk Res. 2011;35:1039–43.
90. Ross JA, Potter JD, Reaman GH, Pendergrass TW, Robison LL. Maternal exposure to potential inhibitors of DNA topoisomerase ii and infant leukemia (United States): a report from the Children's Cancer Group. Cancer Causes Control. 1996;7:581–90.
91. Spector LG, Xie Y, Robison LL, Heerema NA, Hilden JM, Lange B, et al. Maternal diet and infant leukemia: the dna topoisomerase ii inhibitor hypothesis: a report from the Children's Oncology Group. Cancer Epidemiol Biomarkers Prev. 2005;14:651–5.
92. Slater ME, Linabery AM, Spector LG, Johnson KJ, Hilden JM, Heerema NA, et al. Maternal exposure to household chemicals and risk of infant leukemia: a report from the Children's Oncology Group. Cancer Causes Control. 2011;22:1197–204.
93. Heck JE, Park AS, Qiu J, Cockburn M, Ritz B. An exploratory study of anmbient air toxics exposure inn pregnancy and the risk of neuroblastoma in offspring. Environ Res. 2013;127:1–6.
94. Ghosh JK, Heck JE, Cockburn M, Su J, Jerrett M, Ritz B. Prenatal exposure to traffic-related air pollution and risk of early childhood cancers. Am J Epidemiol. 2013;178:1233–9.
95. Slater ME, Linabery AM, Blair CK, Spector LG, Heerema NA, Robison LL, et al. Maternal prenatal cigarette, alcohol and illicit drug use and risk of infant leukaemia: a report from the Children's Oncology Group. Paediatr Perinat Epidemiol. 2011;25:559–65.
96. Satgé D, Sasco AJ, Little J. Antenatal therapeutic drug exposure and fetal/neonatal tumours: review of 89 cases. Paediatr Perinat Epidemiol. 1998;12:84–117.
97. Yang Q, Olshan AF, Bondy ML, Shah NR, Pollock BH, Seeger RC, et al. Parental smoking and alcohol consumption and risk of neuroblastoma. Cancer Epidemiol Biomarkers Prev. 2000;9:967–72.
98. Bonaventure A, Simpson J, Ansell P, Roman E, Lightfoot T. prescription drug use during pregnancy and risk of childhood cancer—is there an association? Cancer Epidemiol. 2015;39:73–8.
99. Michalek AM, Buck GM, Nasca PC, Freedman AN, Baptiste MS, Mahoney MC. Gravid health status, medication use, and risk of neuroblastoma. Am J Epidemiol. 1996;143:996–1001.
100. Olshan AF, Smith JC, Bondy ML, Neglia JP, Pollock BH. Maternal vitamin use and reduced risk of neuroblastoma. Epidemiology. 2002;13:575–80.
101. French AE, Grant R, Weitzman S, Ray JG, Vermeulen MJ, Sung L, et al. Folic acid food fortification is associated with a decline in neuroblastoma. Clin Pharmacol Ther. 2003;74:288–94.
102. Bognár M, Ponyi A, Hauser P, Müller J, Constantin T, Jakab Z, et al. Improper supplementation habits of folic acid intake by Hungarian pregnant women: improper recommendations. J Am Coll Nutr. 2008;27:499–504.
103. Bunin GR, Felice MA, Davidson W, Friedman DL, Shields CL, Maidment A, et al. Medical radiation exposure and risk of retinoblastoma resulting from new germline RB1 mutation. Int J Cancer. 2011;128:2393–404.
104. Reulen RC, Winter DL, Frobisher C, Lancashire ER, Stiller CA, Jenney ME, et al. Long-term cause-specific mortality among survivors of childhood cancer. JAMA. 2010;304:172–9.
105. Reulen RC, Frobisher C, Winter DL, Kelly J, Lancashire ER, Stiller CA, et al. Long-term risks of subsequent primary neoplasms among survivors of childhood cancer. JAMA. 2011;305:2311–9.
106. Armstrong GT, Liu Q, Yasui Y, Neglia JP, Leisenring W, Robison LL, et al. Late mortality among 5-year survivors of childhood cancer: a summary from the Childhood Cancer Survivor Study. J Clin Oncol. 2009;27:2328–38.
107. Diller L, Chow EJ, Gurney JG, Hudson MM, Kadin-Lottick NS, Kawashima TI, et al. Chronic disease in the childhood cancer survivor study cohort: a review of published findings. J Clin Oncol. 2009;27:2339–55.
108. Meadows AT, Friedman DL, Neglia JP, Mertens AC, Donaldson SS, Stovall M, et al. Second neoplasms in survivors of childhood cancer: findings from the childhood cancer survivor study cohort. J Clin Oncol. 2009;27:2356–62.
109. Abramson DH, Du TT, Beaverson KL. Neonatal retinoblastoma in the first month of life. Arch Ophthalmol. 2002;120:738–42.

Vascular Anomalies

53

R. Dawn Fevurly and Steven J. Fishman

Abstract

Vascular anomalies have long confused patients and physicians alike. Historically, it was believed that a mother's emotions or diet could imprint upon her unborn child, resulting in a vascular birthmark. This use of the terms "cherry", "strawberry", or "port wine stain" reflect this doctrine of maternal impressions. Virchow was likely the first to attempt to categorize vascular anomalies based upon histological features. Despite his attempts, overlapping vernacular and histopathologic terms continued to contribute to confusion, resulting in misdiagnosis, inappropriate treatment, and misdirected research. In 1983, Mulliken and Glowacki presented a reliable classification system for vascular anomalies, dividing the field into two major categories: hemangiomas and malformations. Following modification to tumors and malformations, this system was formally accepted by the International Society for the Study of Vascular Anomalies in 1996 and remains in use today.

Keywords

Arteriovenous malformation • Hemangioma • Lymphatic malformation • Kaposiformhemangioendothelioma • Vascular anomaly • Vascular malformation • Venous malformation

53.1 Introduction

Vascular anomalies have long confused patients and physicians alike. Historically, it was believed that a mother's emotions or diet could imprint upon her unborn child, resulting in a vascular birthmark [1]. This use of the terms "cherry", "strawberry", or "port wine stain" reflect this doctrine of maternal impressions [2]. Virchow was likely the first to attempt to categorize vascular anomalies based upon histological features [3]. Despite his attempts, overlapping vernacular and histopathologic terms continued to contribute to confusion, resulting in misdiagnosis, inap-

R.D. Fevurly, MD • S.J. Fishman, MD
Department of Surgery, Children's Hospital Boston, 300 Longwood Ave., Boston, MA 02115, USA
e-mail: steven.fishman@childrens.harvard.edu

P.D. Losty et al. (eds.), *Rickham's Neonatal Surgery*, https://doi.org/10.1007/978-1-4471-4721-3_53

propriate treatment, and misdirected research. In 1983, Mulliken and Glowacki presented a reliable classification system for vascular anomalies, dividing the field into two major categories: hemangiomas and malformations [1]. Following modification to tumors and malformations, this system was formally accepted by the International Society for the Study of Vascular Anomalies in 1996 and remains in use today [4].

The division of vascular anomalies into tumors and malformation is based upon cellular and clinical behavior, as well as unique radiographic and immunohistochemical differences. Vascular tumors are characterized by endothelial hyperplasia and include both hemangiomas and less common pediatric vascular tumors. Vascular malformations arise by vascular dysmorphogenesis and exhibit normal endothelial cell turnover [5]. Use of this bipartite system provides the framework for diagnosis, prognosis and a guide for therapy. Familiarly with the field, its classification system, and the correct nomenclature will aid clinicians in diagnosis and treatment and improve outcomes for patients affect by these lesions.

53.2 Vascular Tumors

53.2.1 Infantile Hemangioma

Infantile hemangioma (IH) is a benign tumor of endothelial cells. As the most common tumor of infancy, it affects approximately 4% of all Caucasian infants [6]. In dark-skinned babies, the incidence is lower. There is a female-to-male preponderance of 3:1–5:1 [5]. Extremely low birth weight infants (<1000 g) bear an increased risk for hemangioma with an overall incidence of 23%, with every 500 g decrease in birth weight increasing the risk by 40% [7, 8]. Additional risk factors of advanced maternal age, placental abnormalities, and multiple gestations are observed [9].

IH most commonly presents as a focal cutaneous lesion (72%), displaying a predilection for the head or neck (60%) [10, 11]. They also occur on the trunk (25%) and extremities (15%) [11]. Multiple tumors occur in 20% of cases, signaling potential involvement of extracutaneous organs such as the gastrointestinal tract or liver [5]. In infants displaying more than five hemangiomas, the risk for hepatic hemangiomas is greatly increased [12]. Hemangiomas typically present around one to 2 weeks of life. Nearly half of infants display a promontory mark, such as a pale spot or faint macular stain [5]. The superficial form develops into a raised, bosselated, crimson lesion, while deeper hemangiomas may present as raised bluish lesions with indistinct borders.

The predictable life cycle of the IH is its hallmark (Fig. 53.1). The *proliferative phase* last until 10–12 months of age and is characterized by rapid growth. A second stage of growth in proportion to the child then occurs, followed by the *involuting phase*, which spans the next 1–7 years. During this final phase, the endothelial matrix is replaced by loose fibrous or fibro-fatty tissue. By

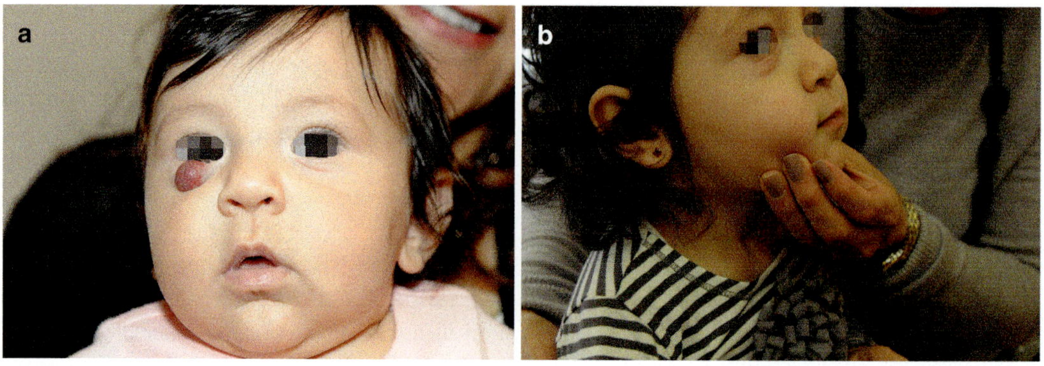

Fig. 53.1 Infantile hemangioma (IH). (**a**) Proliferating phase IH at 5 months of age. (**b**) Involuted IH at 4 years of age

age 5, 50% of tumors have completed involution. This increases to 70% by age 7, with the remainder involuted by ages 10–12 [13]. While half of patients display normal skin in the area of the hemangioma, larger tumors sometimes leave redundant skin and a fibrofatty residuum. In addition, ulcerated hemangiomas often leave scars or a yellowish discoloration [5].

While dangerous complications are rare, several situations are cause for added scrutiny [13]. Hemangiomas of the subglottis or cervicofacial region can lead to life-threatening airway obstruction [5]. Hoarseness and biphasic stridor beginning at 6–12 weeks of age provides clues to a subglottic IH. Ulcerating IH of the eyelid, nasal tip, lip, or ear can lead to disfigurement. IH located in the periorbital region can block the visual axis and lead to amblyopia. In such cases, a pediatric ophthalmologist should be involved. Through recognition of the anatomic distribution of IH, many complications may be averted with proper care and treatment. Intestinal hemangiomas can manifest as infantile bleeding and anemia, while hepatic hemangiomas can result in high-output cardiac failure, hypothyroidism, and abdominal compartment syndrome.

53.2.1.1 Etiology and Pathogenesis

Despite the prevalence of IH, insight into its etiology and pathogenesis remains limited. Several theories propose the endothelial stem/progenitor cell as the cellular source of hemangioma [14–16]. The source of these endothelial progenitors, however, remains elusive. Some studies suggest resident angioblasts, arrested in a stage of early development, give rise to these cells. A second theory proposes these cells are of placental origin, given their co-expression of several distinct markers: GLUT1, merosin, Lewis Y antigen, Fcγ-RIIb, indoleamine 2,3-deoxygenase, IGF-2 and type III iodothyronine deiodinase (DI03) [17–22]. Disruption of the maternal-fetal barrier may permit placental endothelial cells to reach fetal tissues, possibly accounting for the increased incidence of hemangioma observed with chorionic villus sampling due to local placental injury [23]. A third theory promotes IH formation stemming from angiogenesis dysregulation, as expression of vascular endothelial growth factor receptors (VEGFR) 1 and 2 are altered [24]. Activation of VEGFR2, which promotes endothelial cell proliferation, is upregulated in IH, while VEGFR1 levels, a decoy receptor that limits activation of VEGFR2 by binding ligands, are downregulated [25–28]. This may promote overgrowth of endothelial cells leading to disorganized blood vessels and studies in mice support this idea [27].

The clinical observation of growth and involution in IH are mirrored in the cellular activity of the tumor. During proliferation, overexpression of proangiogenic markers predominates with the presence of basic fibroblast growth factor, vascular endothelial growth factor, and matrix metalloproteinases [24, 29]. During involution, the majority of these markers are down regulated and angiogenesis decreases as endothelial cells undergo apoptosis [30]. Subsequently, angiogenesis inhibitors such as inteferon-β and tissue inhibitor of metalloproteinase are up regulated at this time, while proapoptotic markers mitochondrial cytochrome b and homer-2a also appear [30–32]. However, other key elements towards understanding hemangiomas, including triggers for involution, female proponderance, and trophism, remain unexplained.

53.2.1.2 Associated Structural Abnormalities

True hemangiomas are occasionally associated with other malformations.

A subgroup of patients typically with cervicofacial hemangioma exhibit associated structural anomalies of the brain (e.g. posterior fossa abnormality), cerebral vasculature (e.g. aneurysms, hypoplasia or absence of carotid or vertebral vessels), eye (e.g. cataracts, optic nerve hypoplasia), aorta (e.g. coarctation), and chest wall defects (e.g. sternal clefts) in the PHACES association [33–35]. Tumors overlying the lumbosacral region may signal spinal dysmorphism (e.g. lipomenigocele, tethered spinal cord) and affected infants less than 4 months of age should undergo screening ultrasound. Investigation at later ages generally requires MRI [36]. In addition, anorectal and genital anomalies may occur with IH of the pelvis or perineum.

53.2.1.3 Radiologic Features

Most hemangiomas can be readily diagnosed by history and physical examination. Radiographic imaging can play an important role in evaluating deep or atypical lesions. Under ultrasonographic evaluation, proliferating IH appear as fast-flow tissue masses with increased vessel density [37, 38]. MRI evaluation is reserved for cases of uncertainty and confirmation of tissue orientation. Like ultrasound, MRI of IH reveals a vascular solid mass with dilated feeding and draining vessels. Tissue is of indeterminate intensity on T1-weighted images and bright on T2-weighted images with flow voids present [38]. Involuted IH resembles an avascular fatty mass on MRI [39].

53.2.1.4 Treatment

Most IH regress without intervention, requiring only guidance, education, and support from a pediatrician or consultant. Care should be taken to recognize the emotional impact of the tumor, particularly in cases of disfiguring IH. In cases of equivocal diagnosis, dangerous location, large size, rapidity of growth, or potential for other complications, referral to a specialist is indicated.

Ulceration

Spontaneous epithelial breakdown, crusting, ulceration, and necrosis are the most common complications of IH, occurring in approximately 5% of cases. The most vulnerable areas include the lips, parotid, or perineum [40, 41]. Ulceration frequently takes place during the proliferation phase, perhaps due to overgrowth of the blood supply or growth in excess of the skin's elastic capabilities [42, 43]. Initial treatment involves cleansing of the wound, application of an antibiotic salve and use of viscous lidocaine for pain control. Superficial ulcerations heal within days to weeks, while deeper wounds may take several weeks [5]. Eschar should be sharply debrided, followed by wet-to-dry dressing changes in order to stimulate granulation tissue. Resection should be considered if the remaining scar would be similar to removal of the involuted area later.

Pharmacotherapy

For many years, corticosteroids were the mainstay of treatment for IH. Recently, a number of studies and reports have pointed to propranolol, a nonselective beta-blocker, as an effect pharmacologic agent in the treatment of IH [44–47]. Within 1–3 days of therapy, a softening and change in color of IH is noted, possibly due to inhibition of vasodilation [44, 47]. Blockage of proangiogenic signals VEGF, bFGF, and MMP 2/9 likely accounts for the halt of growth of the tumor [48]. Finally, the observation that beta-blockers can induce apoptosis in proliferating endothelial cells may account for the accelerated regression of the tumor [49, 50]. A prospective randomized trial is currently underway, the results of which will hopefully guide future therapy with this exciting treatment. Current treatment regimens recommend dosing of 0.5–0.7 mg/kg/dose tid (total daily dose of 2–3 mg/kg/day, divided tid), following a cardiology consultation [47, 51]. Potential side effects include bradycardia, hypotension, hypoglycemia, gastrointestinal complaints, and bronchospasm [46, 51–54]. A role for topical beta-blockers, such as timolol maleate, has also shown modest results [55].

Systemic corticosteroid therapy has been the most widely used treatment of endangering, ulcerating, problematic, or life-threatening IH. Oral prednisolone (2–3 mg/kg/day for 2–3 weeks) is generally favored, but in a life-threatening situation, such as airway constriction, an equivalent dose in intravenous form is recommended. Response is often evident in 1–2 weeks, which includes fading of color, a diminished rate of growth, and palpable softening. Upon stabilization, the dosage is tapered every 2–4 weeks to minimize steroid associated complications, with a goal of discontinuation by 10 months of age. Overall response rates are 80–90%. Potential side effects include Cushingoid facies (71%), growth delay (35%), personality changes (29%), gastric irritation (21%), hirsutism (13%), and hypertension [56–59]. The mechanism of action is thought to be secondary to corticosteroid suppression of vascular endothelial growth factor A, effectively limiting the vasculogenic potential of IH [60].

Intralesionalinjection of corticosteroid for small, well-localized cutaneous IH, particularly of the lip, cheek, nasal tip or eyelid, may be considered. Triamcinolone (25 mg/ml) is injected slowly at low pressure with a 3 mL syringe and 25 gauge needle, which minimizes the risk of embolization through draining veins. Dosage is typically 3–5 mg/kg per injection. This may be repeated at 6–8 weeks intervals, typically amounting to 3–5 sessions [61].

Recombinant interferon alpha (IFNα-2a or 2b) had previously been second-line therapy for IH, but has been avoided more recently due to reports of associated spastic diplegia [59]. This is a particular risk in infants less than 6 months age, occurring in 5–20% of treated patients [62]. Better second line therapy involves anti-angiogenic chemotherapy drugs, such as vincristine, which has been effective in some children unresponsive to corticosteroids [63, 64].

Embolic Therapy

Embolization is rarely indicated for instances of drug refractory IH causing severe congestive heart failure. The most common lesions necessitating embolization are hepatic hemangiomas. Arteriovenous collaterals and portohepatic shunts, not the proximal hepatic artery branches, in the tumor should be targeted. Pharmacologic therapy is continued even after successful embolization in these patients.

Laser Therapy

Flashlamp pulsed dye laser is ineffective in treating proliferating IH. Due to its superficial penetration of IH, it serves only to lighten the lesion, leaving proliferation unaffected. Small, flat lesions that do respond are typically those that would regress naturally with little to no scarring. Moreover, side effects of laser use include ulceration, partial-thickness skin loss, scarring, and hypopigmentation. Accepted indications for laser therapy include removal of persistenttelangiectasias in involuted IH or excision of a unilateral subglottic IH with continuous-wave carbon dioxide laser [65].

Surgical Therapy

Indications for surgical resection differ according to patient age and hemangioma state. Proliferating IH (during infancy) may be removed when exhibiting ulceration, obstruction, or recurrent bleeding. An upper eyelid IH unresponsive to medical management and causing visual obstruction is an example of this.

IH of the stomach, small intestine, or colon may cause recurrent GI bleeding. Endoscopy and/or laparoscopy may aid in localization of these lesions [66]. Supportive care with medical management and blood transfusions is all that is often necessary. Unresponsive tumors may benefit from endoscopic band ligation or segmental bowel or wedge resections. Unfortunately, most GI IH demonstrates patchy involvement, making surgical or endoscopic intervention difficult [67]. Surgical excision of hepatic hemangioma should almost never be necessary.

Removal of involuting IH may be beneficial in instances of large, protuberant IH. Indications for removal include inevitable excision, need for staged excision, ability to hide the scar, and desire to avoid an altered self-image [5]. Postponing resection until involution is best, as some IH involute without scarring and others leave behind excess skin and a fibrofatty residuum. In the latter instance, resection may minimize distortion and improve cosmetic appearance.

Minimizing the scar, regardless of the indication or timing of surgery, is of top priority [68]. The most common approach involves a lenticular excision with linear closure. The length of the excision must extend beyond the lesion in order to avoid permanent dog-ears. In convex areas, such as the face or forehead, central flattening often results with lenticular excision. Circular excision with intradermal purse-string closure is often more amenable to these cases. Radial folds resulting from this technique tend to smooth out within a few weeks of surgery [68].

53.2.2 Congenital Hemangioma

In contrast to IH, congenital hemangiomas evolve in utero and do not exhibit postnatal growth [69]. These tumors may be detected via prenatal screening as early as the 12th week of gestation [69–71]. Congenital hemangiomas are divided into two

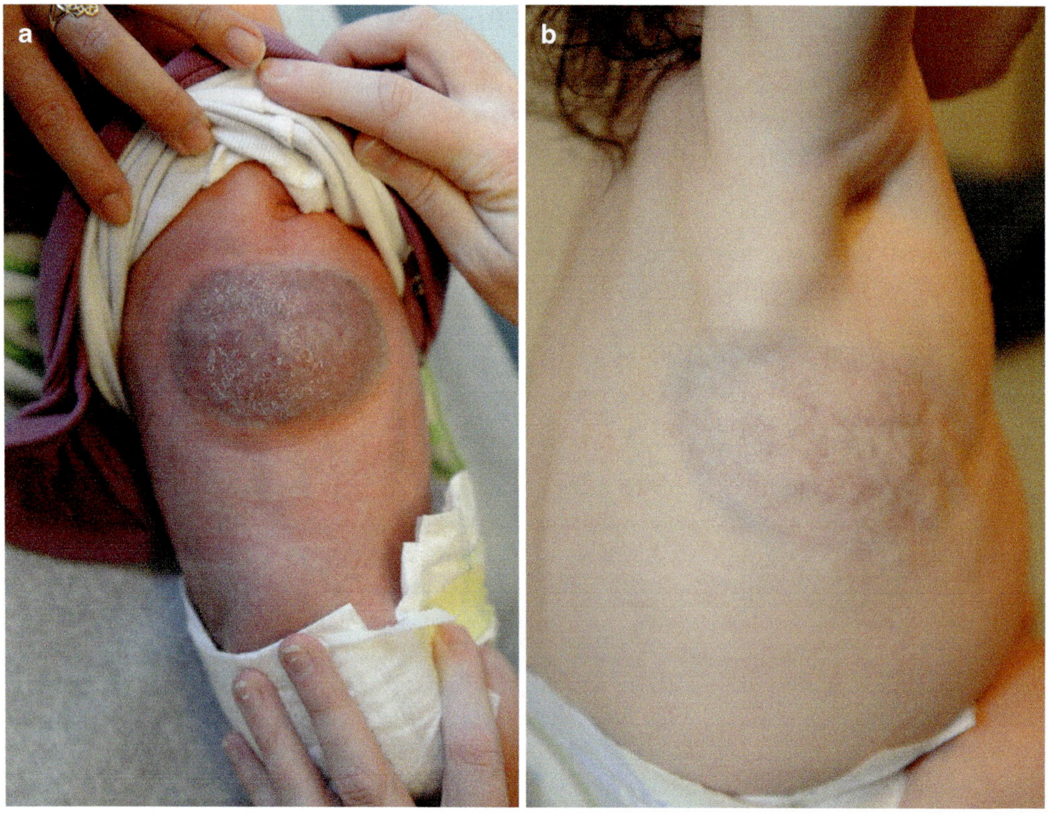

Fig. 53.2 Congenital hemangioma. (**a**) Rapidly Involuting Congenital Hemangioma (RICH) of chest at 10 days after birth. (**b**) Same child with involuting RICH at 1 year old

classes: rapidly involuting congenital hemangioma (RICH) and noninvoluting congenital hemangioma (NICH) (Fig. 53.2). Both lesions tend to be solitary and lack a gender bias. In addition, these lesions stain negatively for GLUT-1, unlike IH.

In RICH lesions, regression begins early and is complete by 9–14 months of age [69]. On examination, RICH lesions present as raised, grey to violaceous in color with a depression or central area of necrosis, often surrounded by a pale halo. Telangiectasias or ectatic veins may be present. They are commonly located on the head, neck or extremities [69, 72]. Following involution, the area appears flattened, lacking the usual fatty residuum of IH [72].

NICH lesions take on a more bossed, round-to-ovoid shape with shades of pink to purple. Like RICH, they may display coarse telangectasias. Commonly affected areas include the head/neck, followed by the limbs and trunk. NICH does not undergo involution and grows with the child [73].

Both RICH and NICH are fast-flow lesions under ultrasound evaluation. Large, superficial flow voids and areas of inhomogeneous contrast are characteristic of RICH lesions on MRI. Under angiography, arterial aneurysms and direct arteriovenous shunts are identified [72]. NICH resembles IH radiologically. Because infantile fibrosarcoma may appear similar to congenital hemangiomas, biopsy may be necessary in cases of uncertain diagnosis [74].

53.2.3 Hepatic Hemangioma

Hepatic hemangiomas (HH) in infants differ from so-called "hepatic hemangiomas" of adulthood. "Hepatic hemangiomas", also known as "cavernous hemangiomas", in adults are actually venous malformations. In contrast, HH of infancy are true vascular tumors. Three patterns are seen: focal, multifocal, and diffuse [75] (Fig. 53.3). Despite popular belief, the vast majority of these lesions are non-threatening.

Focal HH are akin to RICH lesions in that they stain negative for GLUT-1 and present fully formed at birth. In addition, involution tends to be more rapid than their IH counterparts. Infants with focal HH often possess no cutaneous hemangiomas and lesions demonstrate no gender bias. Antenatal detection is common with larger lesions [76]. Intralesional thrombosis occasionally causes transient thrombocytopenia and anemia. The vast majority of lesions require no treatment, however a small number of infants suffer from high-output cardiac failure secondary to macrovascular high-flow shunts (arteriovenous or portovenous). As the lesion involutes, these shunts typically close. While pharmacotherapy has been attempted, it is unclear what role it may play, as these lesions tend to undergo involution rapidly. Symptomatic shunts may be embolized by pediatric interventional radiologists, however, to improve heart failure. Rupture is very rare. Resection is rarely if ever indicated.

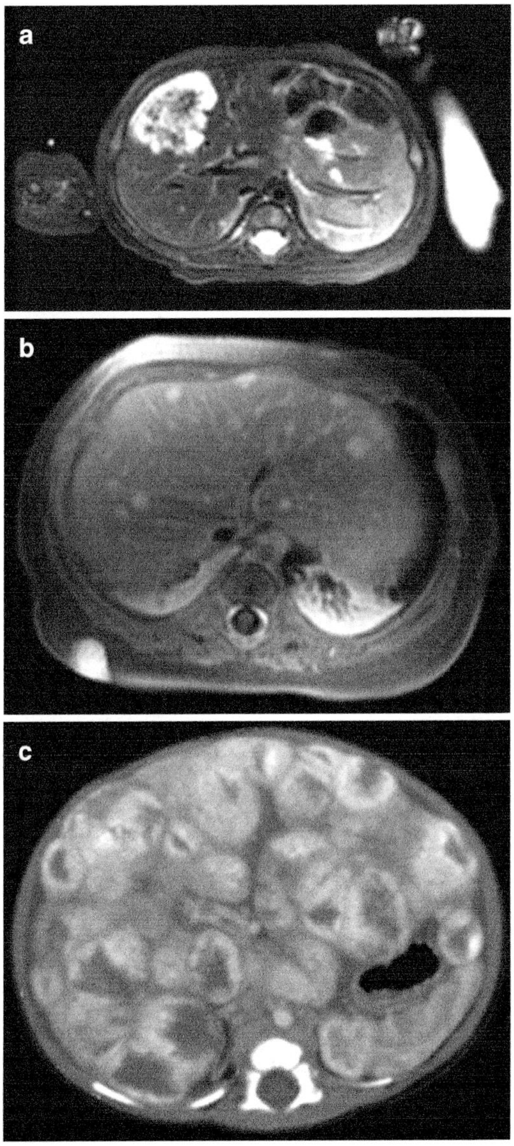

Fig. 53.3 Axial MRI images of hepatic hemangioma. (**a**) Focal hepatic hemangioma with typical heterogenous appearance. (**b**) Multifocal hepatic hemangiomas dispersed throughout liver. (**c**) Diffuse hepatic hemangioma with near complete replacement of liver parenchyma

Radiographic evaluation of focal HH reveals consistent patterns. On computed tomography (CT), focal HH are heterogeneous with centripetal enhancement. An area of central sparing is noted due to necrosis or thrombosis. Calcification is common, increasing as the lesion involutes [77]. MRI depicts focal HH as shows a well-defined, solitary, spherical tumor and appears hypointense on T1 and hyperintense on T2. Centripedal enhancement is seen on gadolinium sequences. Once again, central sparing is noted due to necrosis, thrombosis, or intralesional hemorrhage.

Multifocal HH are true infantile hemangiomas. They stain positive for GLUT-1 and possess a female preponderance. Discovery often occurs following a screening ultrasound due to multiple cutaneous lesions. Most multifocal HH are asymptomatic but a small subset may cause high-output cardiac failure due to macrovascular shunting. Traditionally, pharmacotherapy has centered around corticosteroids, but a role for propranolol is now emerging. Embolization of shunts can ameliorate the high-output state in medically unresponsive cases.

Diffuse HH warrant the greatest cause for concern. Once again, a female bias is noted. These lesions are typical IH but almost completely replace the liver parenchyma with innumerable, compact nodule tumors. The subsequent hepatomegaly can result in compression of the vena cava or thoracic cavity, effectively resulting in abdominal compartment syndrome, respiratory distress, or multiorgan failure. IH express type 3 iodothyronine deiodinase which converts thyroid hormone to its inactive forms [20]. Due to the sheer number of tumors in diffuse HH, there is an accelerated breakdown of thyroid hormone to its inactive form in these infants, resulting in sometimes dramatic acquired hypothyroidism. Levels of type 3 iodothyronine deiodinase correlate proportionally to tumor burden. In order to prevent mental retardation and cardiac failure, exogenous hormone replacement therapy, often in large quantities, is critical. All infants with diffuse and multifocal HH should undergo TSH screening. As the tumor involutes, hypothyroidism improves and hormone replacement therapy should be titrated. Additional pharmacotherapy may involve corticosteroids or propranolol. In extreme instances in which the detection and therapy are delayed, hepatic transplantation may be necessary [75].

Multifocal and diffuse HH appear similar on imaging. On CT, multiple well-defined, spherical lesions are evident. While multifocal HH demonstrates intervening normal liver parenchyma, diffuse HH often completely replaces this parenchyma. Contrast allows for centripedal enhancement of lesions. Shunting is indicated by enlarged vessels, often with flow voids in and around the lesion. On MRI, lesions enhance homogenously and are hypointense relative to liver on T1 and hyperintense on T2 [78].

Clinical and radiographic follow up is critical in infants with HH, as deterioration is possible. Differential diagnosis includes arteriovenous malformation, arterioportal fistula, mesenchymal hamartoma, hepatoblastoma, angiosarcoma, and metastatic neuroblastoma. Percutaneous biopsy is indicated in cases of uncertain diagnosis.

53.2.4 Pyogenic Granuloma

Pyogenic granuloma is a benign, acquired vascular lesion that is often confused with IH [79]. In contrast to IH, these lesions rarely present prior to 6 months of age (average age 6.7 years) and are associated with port wine stains. Growth is rapid, erupting through the skin on a pedicle or stalk. Common locations include the head and neck. Lesions tend to bleed easily [80]. Treatment includes curettage or full-thickness excision, shave excision with cautery, cautery alone, or laser phototherapy [81]. Failure of complete excision leads to a high recurrence rate (45%) [79].

53.2.5 Kaposiform Hemangioendothelioma and Kasabach-Merritt Phenomenon

Based upon the description of a child with profound thrombocytopenia, petechiae, and bleeding in the presence of a “giant hemangioma” in 1940, the Kasabach-Merritt phenomenon (KMP) was described [82]. Seventy years later, it is now clear that KMP is never associated with IH. Instead, KMP occurs with more invasive and aggressive vascular tumors known as *kaposiformhemangioendothelioma* (KHE) or *tufted angioma* (TA) [83–85]. Both tumors are generally present at birth, unifocal, and have a propensity for the trunk, shoulder, thigh, or retroperitoneum. On examination, TA resembles erythematous macules, while KHE is more extensive and can rapidly expand. The overlying skin in KHE appears deep red-purple in color with surrounding ecchymosis (Fig. 53.4). Generalized petechiae may accom-

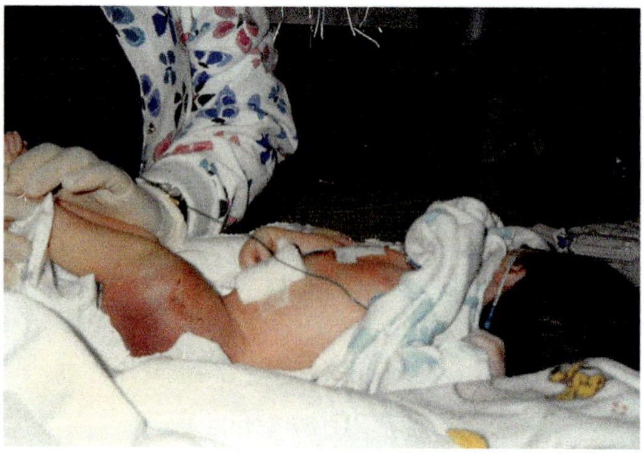

Fig. 53.4 KaposiformHemangioendothelioma (KHE) of thigh

pany the lesion in cases of profound thrombocytopenia (less than 10,000 cells/μL). Affected infants carry the additional risks of intracranial, pleural, pulmonary, peritoneal, and gastrointestinal hemorrhage with associated mortality hovering around 20–30% [86]. Thrombocytopenia results from intralesional trapping of platelets, and subsequent platelet transfusion leads to rapid expansion of the lesion [87–89]. Laboratory values reveal a normal to mildly elevated prothrombin time and activated partial thromboplastin time, an elevated D-dimer level, and a decreased fibrinogen value. Small areas of KHE (less than 8 cm in size) are less likely to suffer from KMP [90].

Histopathologic analysis of KHE reveals aggressive infiltration of normal tissues by sheets or nodules of slender epithelial cells and vascular spaces consisting of hemosiderin deposits and erythrocyte fragments [84]. TA consists of small tufts of capillaries (cannonballs) in the middle to lower dermis [85].

Radiographic evaluation of KHE and TA are similar. Both demonstrate poor tumor margin with extension into tissues across tissue planes. Like other vascular tumors, feeding and draining vessels are enlarged and enhanced signal on T2-weighted images is displayed. These vessels are small relative to tumor size, however. In addition, standing of the subcutaneous fat secondary to lymphatic invasion may occur [84].

Treatment of KHE or TA with KMP involves primarily medical care. Typical pharmacotherapeutic choices include corticosteroids, vincristine, or interferon. Vincristine has been associated with increased platelet counts and fibrinogen levels and may induce apoptosis in tumor endothelial cells, thus contributing to tumor necrosis [63, 91, 92]. Interferon-α possesses anti-angiogenic properties, but neurologic side effects such as spastic diplegia complicate its use [93, 94]. Recently, sirolimus had shown promising results for KHE with KMP and a clinical trial is now in progress [95, 96]. Heparin should be avoided as it may aggravate platelet trapping and stimulate tumor growth. In cases of KHE without KMP, treatment may be useful to diminish tumor size and long-term complications (such as joint contracture or myofascial pain syndromes) [90, 97].

53.3 Vascular Malformations

Vascular malformations are localized or diffuse errors of development affecting any segment of the vascular tree, including arterial, venous, capillary, and/or lymphatic vessels. They are typically divided in to two categories based upon channel type and flow characteristics. Slow flow anomalies include capillary malformations, lymphatic malformations, and venous malformations, while fast flow anomalies include arteriovenous malformations and arteriovenous fistulae. Complex, combined vascular malformations also exist. Congenital malformations have a prevalence of approximately 1.2–1.5% [98]. While most are sporadic, some inherited forms have been observed, often in an autosomal dominant pattern [99, 100]. Despite recent discoveries into the pathogenesis of such diseases, much still remains unclear.

53.3.1 Embryology and Development of the Vascular and Lymphatic Systems

The development of the vascular system during embryogenesis occurs by two separate but related processes: vasculogenesis and angiogenesis. Vasculogenesis involves the initial formation of blood vessels, while angiogenesis describes the formation of new vessels from existing vessels. Around the third week of development, mesodermally derived hemangioblasts congregate into blood islands. Cells in the center of these islands become hematopoietic stem cells, while those at the periphery differentiate into angioblasts, the precursors to blood vessels. These angioblasts subsequently proliferate into a capillary like network of tubes to establish a primary vascular bed. Reorganization of this plexus into a functional vascular system is achieved through angiogenesis, with the formation of new vessels and capillaries through sprouting [101].

The fate of endothelial precursors into their differentiated channel types is imprinted early in embryogenesis by distinct cell-surface markers

[102]. Arterial endothelial cells express ephrin-B2, while venous endothelial cells express its receptor, Eph-B4 [103]. Recruitment of periendothelial cells to the vessel wall promotes stabilization via inhibition of proliferation and migration. This effect is further aided by stimulation of the production of extracellular matrix and subsequent deposition of a basement membrane. This interaction is regulated by vascular endothelial growth factor, platelet derived growth factor-β, angiopoietins and their receptors, and transforming growth factor-β1 [104].

Development of the lymphatic system begins at the end of the sixth week of embryogenesis, only after the establishment of functional blood vessels [105]. Existing veins give rise to lymphatic sacs, which then reorganize to form the lymphatic vasculature [106, 107]. This process begins with the expression of lymphatic vessel endothelial hyaluronan receptor (LYVE-1) along the anterior cardinal vein [108]. Polarized expression of the transcription factor prospero-related homeobox 1 (PROX-1) then follows in a subpopulation of these cells. PROX-1 effectively serves as the master regulator of lymphatic endothelial cell development [109]. As lymphatic endothelial cells express the vascular endothelial growth factor receptor-3, they are drawn to its ligand, vascular endothelial growth factor-C, which directs budding and migration [110]. Lymphatic endothelial cells bud from the lymph sacs, undergo remodeling, and form the peripheral lymphatic system [105]. Malformations of the lymphatic system result in slow-flow anomalies and are described separately in this textbook.

53.3.2 Capillary Malformations

Capillary malformation (CM), more commonly known as port-wine stains, are dermal vascular anomalies occurring in around 0.3% of newborns [111]. They must be differentiated from the more common *nevus flammeusneonatorum* ("angel kiss" on the forehead or "stork bite" on the nuchal area), which are transient dilations of normal dermal vessels that fade over time. The latter are the most common vascular birthmark, affecting 50% of Caucasian neonates. CMs are present as birth and appear as flat, pink-red, cutaneous patches. Occurring anywhere on the body, they can be localized or extensive. CMs are composed of dilated, ectatic capillary-to-venule sized vessels in the superficial dermis. Histopathologic analysis reveals a paucity of surrounding nerves. Over time, these vessels tend to dilate due to lack of innervation, accounting for their observed darkening and nodular expansion [112]. Associated hypertrophy of the subcutaneous tissue, muscle, and bone underlying a CM is common. In cases of CM located on the extremity, leg length discrepancy may be observed. While the majority of CMs are sporadic, a familial pattern of autosomal dominant inheritance with incomplete penetration has been reported. Linkage analysis identified a locus on chromosome 5q13–15 termed CMC1, with the causative gene a negative regulator of ras termed RASA1 [113, 114].

CM may signal an underlying structural abnormality. A CM overlying the cervical or lumbar spine may be associated with an occult spinal dysraphism or tethered cord. An encephaloceleor ectopic meninges may underlie a midline occipital CM. Children with a CM along the ophthalmic and maxillary branches of the trigeminal nerve distribution should be evaluated for Sturge-Weber syndrome, an associated vascular anomaly of the ipsilateral choroid and leptomeninges. Clinical manifestations may include seizures, contralateral hemiplegia, and variable developmental motor and cognitive delay. CM may also be observed in complex-combined vascular malformations.

Treatment of CM is primarily aimed at cosmesis. Vascular-selective pulsed dye lasers are currently the treatment of choice, resulting in significant lightening in approximately 70% of patients. Early, thin CMs and those located on the face have the best outcomes [115]. The timing of therapy remains controversial, but beginning treatment by 6 months of age has shown promising early results [116, 117]. Surgical intervention may be required for associated soft tissue hypertrophy and limb length discrepancy.

53.3.2.1 Cutis Marmorata Telangiectasia Congenita

Cutis marmorata telangiectasia congenita (CMTC) is a rare congenital disorder in which affected newborns demonstrate a blue to deep purple discoloration with a characteristic reticular vascular pattern [118]. CMTC may occupy a localized, segmental, or generalized distribution, usually involving the trunk and extremities [119]. Histopathology reveals dilated capillaries in the papillary dermis and proliferation of blood vessels in the reticular dermis [120]. Occurrence is sporadic and without gender bias. Ulceration and bleeding of depressed areas or hypoplasia of the affected limb may occur. Associate stenosis of the common iliac and femoral arteries has also been observed [121]. Nearly all affected infants demonstrate steady improvement within the first year of life and into adolescence. Atrophy, pigmentation, and prominent veins often persist into adulthood.

53.3.2.2 Telangiectasia

Tiny acquired capillary vascular marks, commonly known as spider nevi or spider telangiectasias, can appear on preschool and school-aged children. No gender bias exists and epidemiological studies suggest they may be present in nearly half of children [98]. Spontaneous resolution is possible, but pulsed dye laser can remove the lesion.

Hereditary hemorrhagic telangiectasia (HHT; Osler-Weber-Rendu syndrome) is an autosomal dominant disorder affecting 1–2 per 100,000 of the Caucasian population (Fig. 53.5). HHT results from mutations in endoglin, activin receptor-like kinase 1, or Smad4. The genes encode proteins that control transforming growth factor-β signaling in vascular endothelial cells [122–124]. Diagnosis is made in the presence of at least three separate manifestations: mucocutaneous telangiectasia (such as on the fingertip, lips, oral mucosa, or tongue), spontaneous recurrent nosebleeds, visceral involvement (GI tract, pulmonary, hepatic, cerebral, or spinal AVM), and family history [125]. Spontaneous, recurrent nosebleeds often begin before school age. One third of affected individuals develop chronic anemia secondary to GI bleeding [125, 126].

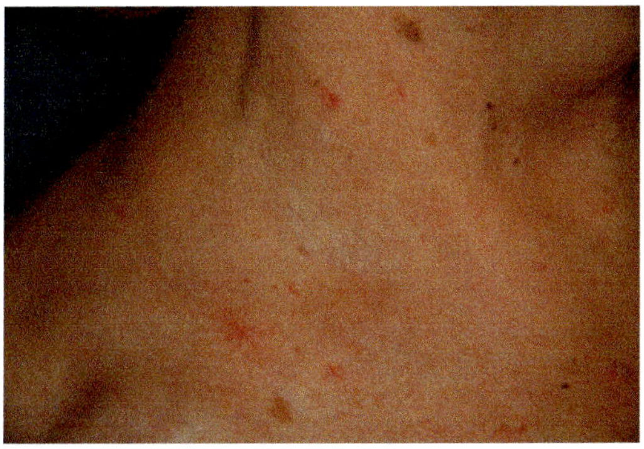

Fig. 53.5 Hereditary hemorrhagic telangiectasia (HHT)

Ataxia-telangiectasia (Louis-Bar syndrome) is an autosomal recessive neurovascular disorder appearing around 3–6 years of life. Affected children initially develop bright-red telangiectasias on the nasal and temporal area of the bulbar conjunctiva, which then progress to the face, neck, upper chest, and flexor surfaces of the forearms. Cerebellar ataxia develops synonymously, followed by progressive motor neuron dysfunction. Endocrine and immunologic deficiencies develop, with death usually occurring in the second decade of life from recurrent infections or malignancy. The defective gene, ATM, is believed to alter DNA repair mechanisms of double-stranded breaks [127].

53.3.3 Venous Malformation

Venous malformations (VMs), the most common of the vascular anomalies, are slow flow lesions often mislabeled as "cavernous hemangiomas." While present at birth, they are often not immediately evident. Common locations include the skin and soft tissues, but VMs may present anywhere in the body. Classically, a VM appears as a soft, blue, compressible, spongy mass, but presentation may range from simple varicosities to networks of channels within an organ (Fig. 53.6). VMs grow proportionally with a child and expand over time. Phlebothrombosis is common and may be painful. Histologically, VMs consist of thin-walled, dilated abnormal channels with surrounding smooth muscle deposited in clumps. This

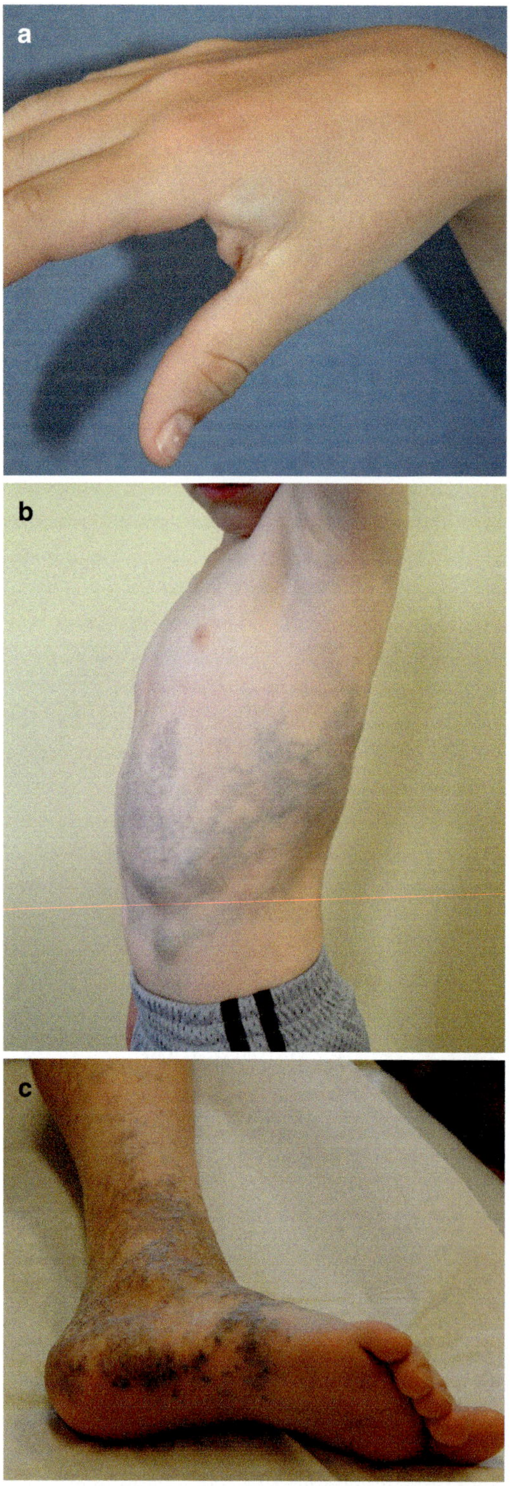

Fig. 53.6 Venous malformation (VM). (**a**) Localized VM involving thenar space of the hand. (*Middle*) Truncal VM. (**b**) Glomovenous malformation (GVM) of foot displaying cobblestone-like appearance

muscle abnormality attributes to the tendency of VMs to expand over time. There is often evidence of clot formation, fibrovascular ingrowth and phleboliths on microscopy.

Complications vary according to location of the VM. Head and neck VMs distort facial features and may cause exophthalmia, dental malalignment, and obstructive sleep apnea. Extremity VM can cause limb length discrepancies, painful hemarthrosis, and degenerative arthritis. Intraosseous VM may lead to structural weakening and pathologic fractures. GI tract lesions may be dispersed throughout the bowel, but are most commonly localized to the left colon, rectum, and surrounding pelvic and retroperitoneal structures [5, 67, 128]. Chronic bleeding and anemia may result [129]. Rectal VMs associated with ectasia of mesenteric veins are a risk factor for portomesenteric venous thrombosis [130].

The vast majority of VMs are sporadic. Half of sporadic lesions may be traced to mutations in Tie2, a receptor tyrosine kinase involved in vascular remodeling [131, 132]. Inherited VMs include *familial cutaneous mucosal VM*, an autosomal dominant condition occurring in 1–2% of the population. Affected individuals develop dome shaped lesions of the skin and GI mucosa ranging from tiny to several centimeters in size [100]. Deregulation of Tie2 is likely the cause [133, 134]. Histologically, lesions demonstrate a lack of an inner elastic membrane, possibly due to uncoupling of endothelial and smooth muscle cell signaling [135, 136]. *Glomovenous malformations* (GVMs) are another inherited condition that accounts for 5% of all lesions. GVMs appear as multiple blue nodular dermal lesions, giving a cobblestone-like appearance (Fig. 53.6). They localize on the extremities, are poorly compressible, and are often painful [137]. Histologically, dilated vessels are surrounded by epithelioid-like glomus cells expressing smooth muscle actin and vimentin [138]. A loss-of-function mutation in glomulin is to blame, resulting in defects in vascular smooth muscle differentiation [139].

Blue rubber bleb nevus syndrome (BRBNS) is a rare, sporadic disorder involving cutaneous and gastrointestinal VMs. Cutaneous lesions are generally blue to purple in color, often numerous, and have a predilection for the trunk, palms, and soles of the feet [140] (Fig. 53.7). A large, dominant VM is often present. Over time, lesions become progressively larger. Lesions of the GI tract are frequently situated in the small bowel, with chronic bleeding and anemia often the result. Lesions may also serve as a lead point for intussusception or volvulus. Capsule endoscopy is an effective tool in visualizing these lesions [141].

Imaging of VMs is best served by MRI. On T2 sequences, VMs demonstrate hyperintensity, an important contrast to that seen with lymphatic malformations, another slow flow lesion. Phleboliths are often seen as signal voids. High flow vessels are not seen within or around VMs. MRI is particularly helpful delineating deep venous anatomy of the extremity [39].

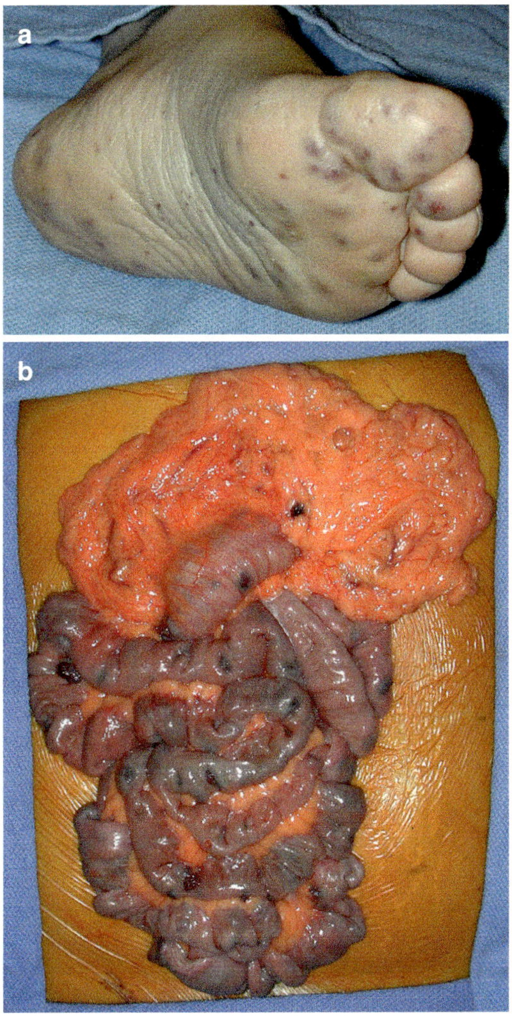

Fig. 53.7 Blue rubber bleb nevus syndrome (BRBNS). (**a**) Characteristic blue shaded cutaneous lesions of the foot. (**b**) Serosal lesions involving the bowel

53.3.3.1 Treatment

Indications for treatment of VMs include functional deficits, poor cosmetic appearance, bleeding and pain. Elastic compression stockings play an important role in management of extremity VMs. Low dose aspirin (81 mg per day) may also aid in prevention of phlebothromboses. The mainstay of treatment for VM, however, lies in sclerotherapy and surgical resection. Sclerosants act to induce endothelial damage, thrombosis, and, ultimately, scarring of the lumen. A multitude of agents have been introduced, with varying results [142]. Unfortunately, recannalization often occurs, requiring multiple treatments [143]. Local complications include blistering, full-thickness necrosis, and nerve injury, while systemic effects may include hemolysis, pulmonary hypertension, and cardiac and renal toxicities [144].

Surgical excision of a VM is often successful in instances of small, well-localized lesions. GVMs, in particular, benefit from excision due to their localized presentation and poor response to compression [137]. Larger lesions often undergo sclerotherapy in an attempt to shrink the VM prior to resection. Often, staged procedures may be required. Removal of bleeding GI lesions is indicated in cases of refractory anemia requiring frequent transfusion. Resection of GI lesions, particularly those of BRBNS, involves numerous wedge excisions and polypectomy by intussusception of successive lengths of intestine [66, 145]. Intraoperative enteroscopy aids with identification of lesions. Diffuse colorectal VMs causing significant bleeding may be treated with colectomy, anorectal mucosectomy, and coloanal pull-through [146].

53.3.4 Arteriovenous Malformations

Arteriovenous malformations (AVMs) are fast flow malformations consisting of disorganized arteries and veins that directly communicate

Table 53.1 Schobinger staging system of ateriovenous malformations (AVMs)

Stage	Clinical findings
I (Quiescence)	Pink-blue warm stain, shunting on Doppler examination
II (Expansion)	Enlargement, pulsation, thrill, bruit, tense veins
III (Destruction)	Dystrophic skin changes, ulceration, bleeding, pain, or tissue necrosis
IV (Decompensation)	Cardiac failure

(shunts), bypassing the high-resistance capillary bed. The shunts comprise the epicenter, or nidus, of the AVM. While AVMs may present at birth with life-threatening high-output cardiac failure, the majority are latent during infancy and childhood. During adolescence, they tend to expand, possibly as a result of hormonal changes [147]. Clinically, AVMs appear as a pink patch in the skin with an underlying thrill or bruit. Over time, ischemic changes, ulceration, pain, and intermittent bleeding may provide complications. A clinical staging system introduced by Schobinger helps document the natural history of the AVM Table 53.1.

The majority of AVMs are sporadic. Heritable forms have been identified, however. A capillary malformation-arteriovenous malformation (CM-AVM) is an autosomal disorder involving the presence of a randomly distributed CM along with a fast flow lesion. CM-AVM is caused by mutations in *RASA1*. Conditions that fall under this spectrum include intracranial or extracranial AVM, Parkes Weber Syndrome, and a vein of Galen aneurysmal malformation [148].

The fast flow of the AVM may be detected on ultrasonography and Doppler imaging. Dilated feeding arteries and draining veins appear as areas of contrast enhancement on CT, signal flow voids (black tubular structures) on MRI, and signal enhancement (white tubular structures) on MRA. The ability to discern the nidus may be complicated, but superselective angiography may improve detection [5] (Fig. 53.8). Muscle hypertrophy, bony changes, and increased fat may also be present on imaging.

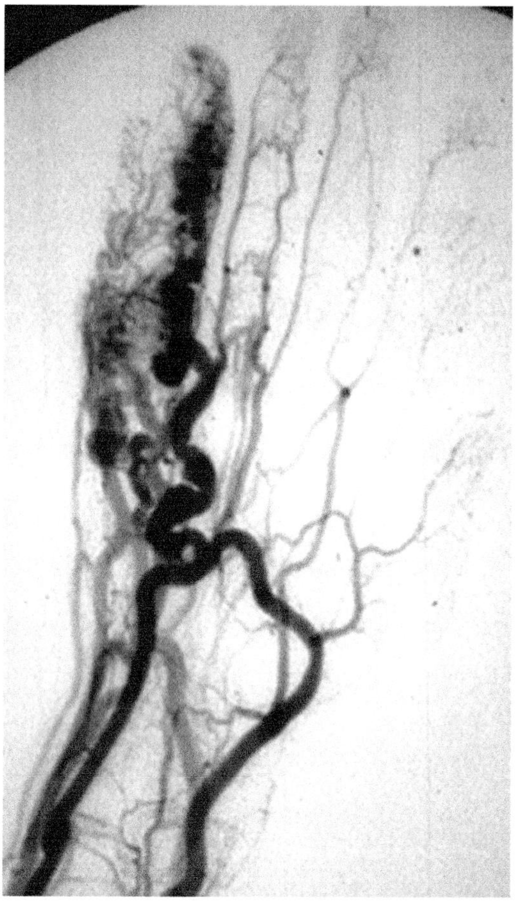

Fig. 53.8 Angiography of finger AVM displaying torturous vessels

53.3.4.1 Treatment

Due to their life-long expansion, many AVMs require treatment. The mainstay of treatment involves intravascular embolization with or without surgical excision. While infants suffering from AVM related postnatal congestive heart failure require early intervention, timing for therapy with the majority of patients is controversial. By convention, most therapy has been delayed until the presence of symptoms or endangering signs (e.g. persistent pain, bleeding, recurrent ulceration, or progression to Schobinger Stage III–IV). Attempted resection of early, poorly defined AVMs may result in incomplete resection, leading to recurrence and complicating future procedures. Alternatively, early AVMs may be more amenable to resection and complete removal. Children should undergo a complete diagnostic evaluation and be followed annually, taking care to evaluate for signs of limb length discrepancy or expansion. Often, Stage I and II AVMs are observed until progression to Stage III.

Regardless of stage, treatment should be directed towards the nidus. Ligation or embolization of proximal feeding arteries should be avoided, as this elicits rapid recruitment of flow from nearby arteries to supply the malformation and may preclude future embolization [143]. Instead, the preferred strategy involves arterial embolization of the nidus followed by surgical resection 2–3 days later. This often aids in decreasing intraoperative blood loss. Complete removal of the nidus and surrounding tissue is attempted in order to deter recurrence. The best results are seen with well-localized AVMs, while larger and more diffuse lesions may require staged procedures, skin grafting, or possible amputation. Unfortunately, many AVMs permeate deep into the soft tissue and skeletal system, allowing for only palliative embolization. Pharmacologic agents targeting angiogenesis and extracellular matrix remodeling are currently being explored for treatment in these dire situations [149].

53.3.5 Complex-Combined Vascular Malformations

Like single-channel-type malformation, complex-combined vascular malformations are divided into slow-flow and fast-flow categories. They are often associated with soft tissue hypertrophy and skeletal overgrowth.

53.3.5.1 Capillary-Lymphaticovenous Malformation

Capillary-lymphaticovenous malformation is commonly known as Klippel-Trenaunay syndrome. Affected individuals typically present at birth with an enlarged extremity, multiple capillary malformations arranged in a geographic pattern along the lateral side of the body, lymphatic vesicles, and visible varicosities [5] (Fig. 53.9). Newborns often display a macular CM, which

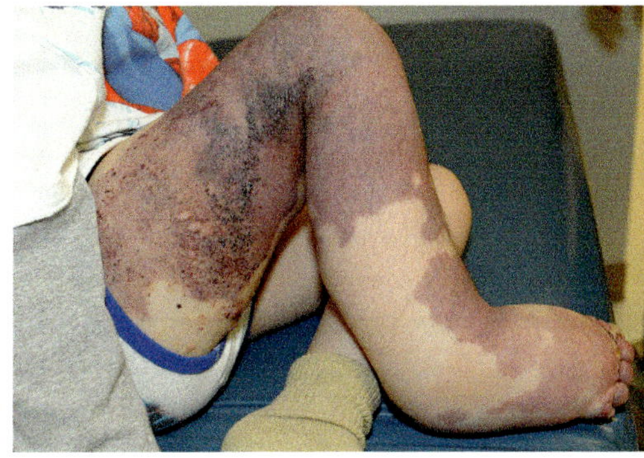

Fig. 53.9 Capillary-lymphaticovenous malformation (CLVM), also known as Klippel-Trenaunay Syndrome

undergoes progressive studding with lymphatic vesicles over time. CLVM most commonly involves the lower extremity (88%), but can involve the upper extremity (29%) and trunk (23%) [150]. Soft tissue and skeletal hypertrophy of the affected limb predominate. Lymphatic anomalies include lymphatic cysts (micro- or macro-), and lymphedema. Lymphatic vesicles often erupt through the CM, causing bleeding and/or lymphatic drainage. Lymphatic malformations (LM) are common and frequently involve the pelvis, perineum, and buttock. Pelvic masses may lead to constipation, recurrent infection, or bladder outlet obstruction. Venous abnormalities include the presence of persistent embryologic veins, most commonly the marginal vein of Servelle. Incompetent valves within these veins makes these more prominent, while a deep venous system may be entirely absent. VMs in the lower extremities may extend into the pelvis and connect with femoral veins, iliac veins, or the inferior vena cava. Pulmonary embolism results in 4–25% of cases [130].

MRI and MR venography (MRV) serve the most use in description of the vascular malformation of CLVM. MRV reliably maps the venous system, including the anomalous venous channels present. Often, a large lateral vein of Servelle is evident. Macrocystic, microcystic, or a combination of LM is typically present. Plain radiographs allow for identification and evaluation of leg-length discrepancies. Venography may also be utilized for planning of surgical intervention or sclerotherapy.

Treatment

Management of CLVM is typically conservative. Compression therapy, initiated following ambulation, is important to control swelling. Limb length discrepancies should be identified and followed by serial radiographs. Shoe-lifts are beneficial for discrepancies between 0.5–2 cm. For differences greater than 2 cm, epiphysiodesis of the distal femoral growth plate may be performed around 12 years of age. Grotesque enlargement of the foot may be treated with selective ablative procedures (i.e. ray, midfoot, or Syme amputation) [151]. Sclerotherapy targeting focal VMs, superficial veins, or lymphatic cysts may be of benefit. Leaking or bleeding lymphatic vesicles are also treated with sclerotherapy or laser ablation. Persistent embryonic veins are candidates for endovenous laser ablation or resection, particularly in instances of direct communication with femoral or iliac veins or the inferior vena cava in order to prevent pulmonary emboli.

Debulking procedures offer physical and psychological benefits to patients with CLVM. Evaluation of the location of soft tissue overgrowth is critical in preoperative planning. While extrafascial involvement is amenable to surgery, debulking of intrafascial overgrowth should be avoided due to risk of injury to major neurovascular structures or immobility. Staged repair may be necessary, particularly with thoracic or trunk involvement. Postoperative healing can be problematic due to involvement of abnormal tissue with poor lymphatic drainage and altered circulation. Prolonged suction drainage is used. Placement of an inferior vena cava filter and preoperative anticoagulation are used to decrease the risk of pulmonary embolism and deep venous thrombosis [151].

53.3.5.2 CLOVES Syndrome

CLOVES syndrome is characterized by congenital lipomatous overgrowth, vascular malformations, epidermal nevi, and skeletal anomalies [152, 153] (Fig. 53.10). Its key feature is a truncal lipomatous mass, typically present at birth. These masses are hypervascular and often infiltrative, extending into the retroperitoneum, mediastinum, and pleural cavity. Involvement of the spinal canal and epidural space may lead to compression of the cord, thecal sac, or nerve root. Slow-flow vascular lesions, CMs, and LMs have been identified. Large, phlebectatic VMs may pose a risk of pulmonary embolus. Parasapinal or intraspinal AVMs can result in paresis and spasticity. MRI with venous and arterial sequences aids in evaluation. Acral deformities include wide, delta-shaped hands and feet, macrodactyly, and a sandal gap appearance of the toes. Scoliosis is present in 50% of cases.

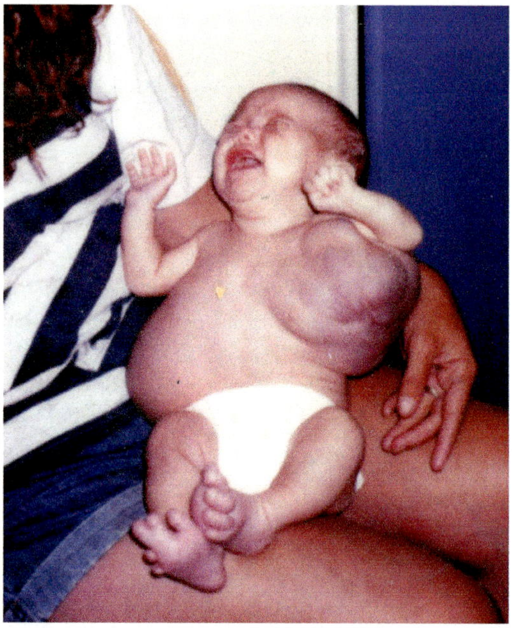

Fig. 53.10 CLOVES syndrome. Infant displaying truncal lipomatous mass, truncal capillary staining, macrodactyly, and wide, delta-shaped feet

53.3.5.3 Parkes Weber Syndrome

Parkes Weber syndrome is characterized by the presence of a patchy or confluent capillary malformation with underlying multiple micro arteriovenous fistulas (AVFs). These malformations are typically located in a lower extremity and associated with soft tissue and skeletal hypertrophy [154]. Lymphatic anomalies are often present as well. Length discrepancy can result. The stained areas are warm to palpation and thrill may be detected. Doppler examination often reveals increased flow. On imaging, the involved area displays subcutaneous, muscular, and bony overgrowth with diffuse microfistulae. Angiography and venography reveal generalized venous and arterial dilation with a soft tissue blush involving muscles and subcutaneous fat.

Treatment is reserved for symptomatic patients. While up to 30% of patients with Parkes Weber syndrome may exhibit signs of cardiac volume overload, this is typically well tolerated [154]. Rarely, cardiac failure due to shunting through the AVFs may develop. Children should be seen annually and monitored for axial overgrowth, signs of cardiac failure, and cutaneous problems related to ischemia. Repetitive superselective embolization may be employed to reduce flow and improve heart failure [5]. Limb amputation may be required for severe disease.

53.3.5.4 PTEN Hamartoma-Tumor Syndrome

PTEN hamartoma-tumor syndrome results from mutation of *PTEN* (phosphatase tensin homolog on chromosome 10), which encodes for a tumor suppressor protein involved in cell-cycle regulation. Two autosomal dominant disorders with a predisposition for cancer result: Bannayan-Riley-Ruvalcaba syndrome (BRRS) and Cowden syndrome (CS) [155]. BRRS is characterized by macrosomia at birth, macrocephaly, penile freckling, lipomas, hamartomatous intestinal polyposis, proximal myopathy, and variable degrees of developmental delay. CS consists of multiple hamartomas and neoplasias of ectodermal, mesodermal, and endodermal origin (particularly the breast, thyroid, and endometrium). Vascular anomalies are present in approximately 50% of patient with PTEN mutations and tend to be characterized as fast-flow radiographically [154]. Histopathologically, disordered growths of blood vessels, adipose, fibrous tissue is noted. Due to the increased risk for cancer, patients with fast-flows lesions should be evaluated for *PTEN* mutations.

Conclusions

The last three decades have witnessed remarkable advances into understanding the pathogenesis of vascular anomalies. An improved genetic-anatomic-histologic classification system has clarified the identification of vascular diseases and allowed for the development of multidisciplinary approaches toward disease management and treatment. Increased understanding of embryonic development has permitted novel therapeutic approaches. With continued strides and a combined management approach, those affected by vascular anomalies may benefit.

References

1. Mulliken JB, Glowacki J. Hemangiomas and vascular malformations in infants and children: a classification based on endothelial characteristics. Plast Reconstr Surg. 1982;69:412–22.
2. Mulliken JB, Young AE. Vascular birthmarks: hemangiomas and malformations. Philadelphia: Saunders; 1988.
3. Virchow R. Angioma in die krankhaften Geschwulste. Berlin: Hirschwald; 1863.
4. Enjolras O. Vascular tumors and vascular malformations: are we at the dawn of a better knowledge? Pediatr Dermatol. 1999;16:238–41.
5. Mulliken JB, Fishman SJ, Burrows PE. Vascular anomalies. Curr Probl Surg. 2000;37:517–84.
6. Holmdahl K. Cutaneous hemangiomas in premature and mature infants. Acta Paediatr. 1955;44:370–9.
7. Amir J, Metzker A, Krikler R, et al. Strawberry hemangioma in preterm infants. Pediatr Dermatol. 1986;3:331–2.
8. Drolet BA, Swanson EA, Frieden IJ. Infantile hemangiomas: an emerging health issue linked to an increased rate of low birth weight infants. J Pediatr. 2008;153:712–715. , 715.e711.
9. Haggstrom AN, Drolet BA, Baselga E, et al. Prospective study of infantile hemangiomas: demographic, prenatal, and perinatal characteristics. J Pediatr. 2007;150:291–4.
10. Chiller KG, Passaro D, Frieden IJ. Hemangiomas of infancy: clinical characteristics, morphologic subtypes, and their relationship to race, ethnicity, and sex. Arch Dermatol. 2002;138:1567–76.
11. Finn MC, Glowacki J, Mulliken JB. Congenital vascular lesions: clinical application of a new classification. J Pediatr Surg. 1983;18:894–900.
12. Horii KA, Drolet BA, Frieden IJ, et al. Prospective study of the frequency of hepatic hemangiomas in infants with multiple cutaneous infantile hemangiomas. Pediatr Dermatol. 2011;28:245–253. doi:2https://doi.org/10.1111/j.1525-1470.2011.01420.x. Epub 2011 Apr 26.
13. Bowers R, Graham E, Tomlinson K. The natural history of the strawberry birthmark. Arch Dermatol. 1960;82:667–80.

14. Boye E, Yu Y, Paranya G, et al. Clonality and altered behavior of endothelial cells from hemangiomas. J Clin Invest. 2001;107:745–52.
15. Bischoff J. Progenitor cells in infantile hemangioma. J Craniofac Surg. 2009;20:695–7.
16. Khan ZA, Boscolo E, Picard A, et al. Multipotential stem cells recapitulate human infantile hemangioma in immunodeficient mice. J Clin Invest. 2008;118:2592–9.
17. Marchuk DA. Pathogenesis of hemangioma. J Clin Invest. 2001;107:665–6.
18. North PE, Waner M, Mizeracki A, et al. A unique microvascular phenotype shared by juvenile hemangiomas and human placenta. Arch Dermatol. 2001;137:559–70.
19. Leon-Villapalos J, Wolfe K, Kangesu L. GLUT-1: an extra diagnostic tool to differentiate between haemangiomas and vascular malformations. Br J Plast Surg. 2005;58:348–52.
20. Huang SA, Tu HM, Harney JW, et al. Severe hypothyroidism caused by type 3 iodothyronine deiodinase in infantile hemangiomas. N Engl J Med. 2000;343:185–9.
21. Picard A, Boscolo E, Khan ZA, et al. IGF-2 and FLT-1/VEGF-R1 mRNA levels reveal distinctions and similarities between congenital and common infantile hemangioma. Pediatr Res. 2008;63:263–7.
22. Bree AF, Siegfried E, Sotelo-Avila C, et al. Infantile hemangiomas: speculation on placental trophoblastic origin. Arch Dermatol. 2001;137:573–7.
23. Kleinman ME, Tepper OM, Capla JM, et al. Increased circulating AC133+ CD34+ endothelial progenitor cells in children with hemangioma. Lymphat Res Biol. 2003;1:301–7.
24. Chang J, Most D, Bresnick S, et al. Proliferative hemangiomas: analysis of cytokine gene expression and angiogenesis. Plast Reconstr Surg. 1999;103:1–9; discussion 10.
25. Roberts DM, Kearney JB, Johnson JH, et al. The vascular endothelial growth factor (VEGF) receptor Flt-1 (VEGFR-1) modulates Flk-1 (VEGFR-2) signaling during blood vessel formation. Am J Pathol. 2004;164:1531–5.
26. Jinnin M, Medici D, Park L, et al. Suppressed NFAT-dependent VEGFR1 expression and constitutive VEGFR2 signaling in infantile hemangioma. Nat Med. 2008;14:1236–1246. Epub 2008 Oct 19.
27. Fong GH, Rossant J, Gertsenstein M, et al. Role of the Flt-1 receptor tyrosine kinase in regulating the assembly of vascular endothelium. Nature. 1995;376:66–70.
28. Jinnin M, Ishihara T, Boye E, et al. Recent progress in studies of infantile hemangioma. J Dermatol. 2010;37:939–55. doi:10.1111/j.1346--8138.2010.00927.x. Epub 2010 Aug 16.
29. Tille JC, Pepper MS. Hereditary vascular anomalies: new insights into their pathogenesis. Arterioscler Thromb Vasc Biol. 2004;24:1578–1590. Epub 2010 Jan 13.
30. Razon MJ, Kraling BM, Mulliken JB, et al. Increased apoptosis coincides with onset of involution in infantile hemangioma. Microcirculation. 1998;5:189–95.
31. Takahashi K, Mulliken JB, Kozakewich HP, et al. Cellular markers that distinguish the phases of hemangioma during infancy and childhood. J Clin Invest. 1994;93:2357–64.
32. Bielenberg DR, Bucana CD, Sanchez R, et al. Progressive growth of infantile cutaneous hemangiomas is directly correlated with hyperplasia and angiogenesis of adjacent epidermis and inversely correlated with expression of the endogenous angiogenesis inhibitor. IFN-beta Int J Oncol. 1999;14:401–8.
33. Goldberg NS, Hebert AA, Esterly NB. Sacral hemangiomas and multiple congenital abnormalities. Arch Dermatol. 1986;122:684–7.
34. Albright AL, Gartner JC, Wiener ES. Lumbar cutaneous hemangiomas as indicators of tethered spinal cords. Pediatrics. 1989;83:977–80.
35. Frieden IJ, Reese V, Cohen D. PHACE syndrome. The association of posterior fossa brain malformations, hemangiomas, arterial anomalies, coarctation of the aorta and cardiac defects, and eye abnormalities. Arch Dermatol. 1996;132:307–11.
36. Metry D, Heyer G, Hess C, et al. Consensus Statement on Diagnostic Criteria for PHACE syndrome. Pediatrics. 2009;124:1447–56. Epub 2009 Oct 26.
37. Paltiel HJ, Burrows PE, Kozakewich HP, et al. Soft-tissue vascular anomalies: utility of US for diagnosis. Radiology. 2000;214:747–54.
38. Meyer JS, Hoffer FA, Barnes PD, et al. Biological classification of soft-tissue vascular anomalies: MR correlation. AJR Am J Roentgenol. 1991;157:559–64.
39. Burrows PE, Laor T, Paltiel H, et al. Diagnostic imaging in the evaluation of vascular birthmarks. Dermatol Clin. 1998;16:455–88.
40. Greene AK, Rogers GF, Mulliken JB. Management of parotid hemangioma in 100 children. Plast Reconstr Surg. 2004;113:53–60.
41. Margileth AM, Museles M. Cutaneous hemangiomas in children. Diagnosis and conservative management Jama. 1965;194:523–6.
42. Hermans DJ, Boezeman JB, Van de Kerkhof PC, et al. Differences between ulcerated and non-ulcerated hemangiomas, a retrospective study of 465 cases. Eur J Dermatol. 2009;19:152–156. Epub 2008 Dec 23.
43. Waner M, Suen JY. The natural history of hemangiomas. New York, NY: Wiley-Liss; 1999.
44. Leaute-Labreze C. Dumas de la Roque E, Hubiche T, et al: propranolol for severe hemangiomas of infancy. N Engl J Med. 2008;358:2649–51.
45. Leaute-Labreze C, Taieb A. [Efficacy of beta-blockers in infantile capillary haemangiomas: the physiopathological significance and therapeutic consequences]. Ann Dermatol Venereol. 2008;135:860–862. Epub 2008 Nov 20.

46. Buckmiller LM, Munson PD, Dyamenahalli U, et al. Propranolol for infantile hemangiomas: early experience at a tertiary vascular anomalies center. Laryngoscope. 2010;120:676–81.
47. Bagazgoitia L, Torrelo A, Gutierrez JC, et al. Propranolol for infantile hemangiomas. Pediatr Dermatol. 2011;28:108–114. doi: 1https://doi.org/10.1111/j.1525-1470.2011.01345.x. Epub 2011 Mar 8.
48. Storch CH, Hoeger PH. Propranolol for infantile haemangiomas: insights into the molecular mechanisms of action. Br J Dermatol. 2010;163:269–274. Epub 2010 May 8.
49. Sommers Smith SK, Smith DM. Beta blockade induces apoptosis in cultured capillary endothelial cells. In Vitro Cell Dev Biol Anim. 2002;38: 298–304.
50. Zhang D, Ma Q, Shen S, et al. Inhibition of pancreatic cancer cell proliferation by propranolol occurs through apoptosis induction: the study of beta-adrenoceptor antagonist's anticancer effect in pancreatic cancer cell. Pancreas. 2009;38:94–100.
51. Cushing SL, Boucek RJ, Manning SC, et al. Initial experience with a multidisciplinary strategy for initiation of propranolol therapy for infantile hemangiomas. Otolaryngol Head Neck Surg. 2011;144:78–84.
52. Maisel AS, Motulsky HJ, Insel PA. Propranolol treatment externalizes beta-adrenergic receptors in guinea pig myocardium and prevents further externalization by ischemia. Circ Res. 1987;60:108–12.
53. Harrison DC, Meffin PJ, Winkle RA. Clinical pharmacokinetics of antiarrhythmic drugs. Prog Cardiovasc Dis. 1977;20:217–42.
54. Holland KE, Frieden IJ, Frommelt PC, et al. Hypoglycemia in children taking propranolol for the treatment of infantile hemangioma. Arch Dermatol. 2010;146:775–8.
55. Pope E, Chakkittakandiyil A. Topical timolol gel for infantile hemangiomas: a pilot study. Arch Dermatol. 2010;146:564–5.
56. George ME, Sharma V, Jacobson J, et al. Adverse effects of systemic glucocorticosteroid therapy in infants with hemangiomas. Arch Dermatol. 2004;140:963–9.
57. Boon LM, MacDonald DM, Mulliken JB. Complications of systemic corticosteroid therapy for problematic hemangioma. Plast Reconstr Surg. 1999;104:1616–23.
58. Blei F, Chianese J. Corticosteroid toxicity in infants treated for endangering hemangiomas: experience and guidelines for monitoring. Int Pediatr. 1999;14:146–53.
59. Barlow CF, Priebe CJ, Mulliken JB, et al. Spastic diplegia as a complication of interferon Alfa-2a treatment of hemangiomas of infancy. J Pediatr. 1998;132:527–30.
60. Greenberger S, Boscolo E, Adini I, et al. Corticosteroid suppression of VEGF-A in infantile hemangioma-derived stem cells. N Engl J Med. 2010;362:1005–13.
61. Marler JJ, Mulliken JB. Plastic surgery. Philadelphia: Elsevier; 2009.
62. Dubois J, Garel L. Imaging and therapeutic approach of hemangiomas and vascular malformations in the pediatric age group. Pediatr Radiol. 1999;29:879–93.
63. Haisley-Royster C, Enjolras O, Frieden IJ, et al. Kasabach-Merritt phenomenon: a retrospective study of treatment with vincristine. J Pediatr Hematol Oncol. 2002;24:459–62.
64. Perez J, Pardo J, Gomez C. Vincristine—an effective treatment of corticoid-resistant life-threatening infantile hemangiomas. Acta Oncol. 2002;41: 197–9.
65. Sie KC, McGill T, Healy GB. Subglottic hemangioma: ten years' experience with the carbon dioxide laser. Ann Otol Rhinol Laryngol. 1994;103:167–72.
66. Fishman SJ, Burrows PE, Leichtner AM, et al. Gastrointestinal manifestations of vascular anomalies in childhood: varied etiologies require multiple therapeutic modalities. J Pediatr Surg. 1998;33:1163–7.
67. Fishman SJ, Fox VL. Visceral vascular anomalies. Gastrointest Endosc Clin N Am. 2001;11:813–834, viii.
68. Mulliken JB, Rogers GF, Marler JJ. Circular excision of hemangioma and purse-string closure: the smallest possible scar. Plast Reconstr Surg. 2002;109:1544–1554; discussion 1555.
69. Boon LM, Enjolras O, Mulliken JB. Congenital hemangioma: evidence of accelerated involution. J Pediatr. 1996;128:329–35.
70. Marler JJ, Fishman SJ, Upton J, et al. Prenatal diagnosis of vascular anomalies. J Pediatr Surg. 2002;37:318–26.
71. Elia D, Garel C, Enjolras O, et al. Prenatal imaging findings in rapidly involuting congenital hemangioma of the skull. Ultrasound Obstet Gynecol. 2008;31:572–5.
72. Berenguer B, Mulliken JB, Enjolras O, et al. Rapidly involuting congenital hemangioma: clinical and histopathologic features. Pediatr Dev Pathol. 2003;6:495–510.
73. Enjolras O, Mulliken JB, Boon LM, et al. Noninvoluting congenital hemangioma: a rare cutaneous vascular anomaly. Plast Reconstr Surg. 2001;107:1647–54.
74. Boon LM, Fishman SJ, Lund DP, et al. Congenital fibrosarcoma masquerading as congenital hemangioma: report of two cases. J Pediatr Surg. 1995;30:1378–81.
75. Christison-Lagay ER, Burrows PE, Alomari A, et al. Hepatic hemangiomas: subtype classification and development of a clinical practice algorithm and registry. J Pediatr Surg. 2007;42:62–67; discussion 67–68.
76. Morris J, Abbott J, Burrows P, et al. Antenatal diagnosis of fetal hepatic hemangioma treated with maternal corticosteroids. Obstet Gynecol. 1999;94:813–5.

77. Marsciani A, Pericoli R, Alaggio R, et al. Massive response of severe infantile hepatic hemangioma to propanolol. Pediatr Blood Cancer. 2010;54:176.
78. Kassarjian A, Zurakowski D, Dubois J, et al. Infantile hepatic hemangiomas: clinical and imaging findings and their correlation with therapy. AJR Am J Roentgenol. 2004;182:785–95.
79. Patrice SJ, Wiss K, Mulliken JB. Pyogenic granuloma (lobular capillary hemangioma): a clinicopathologic study of 178 cases. Pediatr Dermatol. 1991;8:267–76.
80. Browning JC, Eldin KW, Kozakewich HP, et al. Congenital disseminated pyogenic granuloma. Pediatr Dermatol. 2009;26:323–7.
81. Kirschner RE, Low DW. Treatment of pyogenic granuloma by shave excision and laser photocoagulation. Plast Reconstr Surg. 1999;104:1346–9.
82. Kasabach H, Merritt K. Capillary hemangioma with extensive purpura: report of a case. Am J Dis Child. 1940;59:1063–70.
83. Enjolras O, Gelbert F. Superficial hemangiomas: associations and management. Pediatr Dermatol. 1997;14:173–9.
84. Sarkar M, Mulliken JB, Kozakewich HP, et al. Thrombocytopenic coagulopathy (Kasabach-Merritt phenomenon) is associated with Kaposiform hemangioendothelioma and not with common infantile hemangioma. Plast Reconstr Surg. 1997;100:1377–86.
85. Jones EW, Orkin M. Tufted angioma (angioblastoma). A benign progressive angioma, not to be confused with Kaposi's sarcoma or low-grade angiosarcoma. J Am Acad Dermatol. 1989;20:214–25.
86. Martinez-Perez D, Fein NA, Boon LM, et al. Not all hemangiomas look like strawberries: uncommon presentations of the most common tumor of infancy. Pediatr Dermatol. 1995;12:1–6.
87. Hall GW. Kasabach-Merritt syndrome: pathogenesis and management. Br J Haematol. 2001;112:851–62.
88. Rodriguez V, Lee A, Witman PM, et al. Kasabach-Merritt phenomenon: case series and retrospective review of the mayo clinic experience. J Pediatr Hematol Oncol. 2009;31:522–6.
89. Seo SK, Suh JC, Na GY, et al. Kasabach-Merritt syndrome: identification of platelet trapping in a tufted angioma by immunohistochemistry technique using monoclonal antibody to CD61. Pediatr Dermatol. 1999;16:392–4.
90. Gruman A, Liang MG, Mulliken JB, et al. Kaposiform hemangioendothelioma without Kasabach-Merritt phenomenon. J Am Acad Dermatol. 2005;52:616–22.
91. Fahrtash F, McCahon E, Arbuckle S. Successful treatment of kaposiform hemangioendothelioma and tufted angioma with vincristine. J Pediatr Hematol Oncol. 2010;32:506–10.
92. Gidding CE, Kellie SJ, Kamps WA, et al. Vincristine revisited. Crit Rev Oncol Hematol. 1999;29:267–87.
93. Chang E, Boyd A, Nelson CC, et al. Successful treatment of infantile hemangiomas with interferon-alpha-2b. J Pediatr Hematol Oncol. 1997;19:237–44.
94. Harper L, Michel JL, Enjolras O, et al. Successful management of a retroperitoneal kaposiform hemangioendothelioma with Kasabach-Merritt phenomenon using alpha-interferon. Eur J Pediatr Surg. 2006;16:369–72.
95. Hammill AM, Wentzel M, Gupta A, et al. Sirolimus for the treatment of complicated vascular anomalies in children. Pediatr Blood Cancer. 2011;28:23124.
96. Blatt J, Stavas J, Moats-Staats B, et al. Treatment of childhood kaposiform hemangioendothelioma with sirolimus. Pediatr Blood Cancer. 2010;55:1396–8.
97. Enjolras O, Mulliken JB, Wassef M, et al. Residual lesions after Kasabach-Merritt phenomenon in 41 patients. J Am Acad Dermatol. 2000;42:225–35.
98. Christison-Lagay ER, Fishman SJ. Vascular anomalies. Surg Clin North Am 86:393–425, x;2006.
99. Brouillard P, Vikkula M. Genetic causes of vascular malformations. Hum Mol Genet. 2007;16:R140–149. Epub 2007 Jul 31.
100. Limaye N, Boon LM, Vikkula M. From germline towards somatic mutations in the pathophysiology of vascular anomalies. Hum Mol Genet. 2009;18:R65–74.
101. Sadler TW. Langman's medical embryology. Philadelphia: Lippincott Williams & Wilkins; 2004.
102. Folkman J, D'Amore PA. Blood vessel formation: what is its molecular basis? Cell. 1996;87:1153–5.
103. Wang HU, Chen ZF, Anderson DJ. Molecular distinction and angiogenic interaction between embryonic arteries and veins revealed by ephrin-B2 and its receptor Eph-B4. Cell. 1998;93:741–53.
104. Ramsauer M, D'Amore PA. Getting Tie(2)d up in angiogenesis. J Clin Invest. 2002;110:1615–7.
105. Karpanen T, Alitalo K. Molecular biology and pathology of lymphangiogenesis. Annu Rev Pathol. 2008;3:367–97.
106. Rodriguez-Niedenfuhr M, Papoutsi M, Christ B, et al. Prox1 is a marker of ectodermal placodes, endodermal compartments, lymphatic endothelium and lymphangioblasts. Anat Embryol (Berl). 2001;204:399–406.
107. Oliver G, Srinivasan RS. Lymphatic vasculature development: current concepts. Ann N Y Acad Sci. 2008;1131:75–81.
108. Banerji S, Ni J, Wang SX, et al. LYVE-1, a new homologue of the CD44 glycoprotein, is a lymph-specific receptor for hyaluronan. J Cell Biol. 1999;144:789–801.
109. Hong YK, Harvey N, Noh YH, et al. Prox1 is a master control gene in the program specifying lymphatic endothelial cell fate. Dev Dyn. 2002;225:351–7.
110. Karkkainen MJ, Haiko P, Sainio K, et al. Vascular endothelial growth factor C is required for sprouting of the first lymphatic vessels from embryonic veins. Nat Immunol. 2004;5:74–80. Epub 2003 Nov 23.

111. Jacobs AH, Walton RG. The incidence of birthmarks in the neonate. Pediatrics. 1976;58:218–22.
112. Smoller BR, Rosen S. Port-wine stains. A disease of altered neural modulation of blood vessels? Arch Dermatol. 1986;122:177–9.
113. Breugem CC, Alders M, Salieb-Beugelaar GB, et al. A locus for hereditary capillary malformations mapped on chromosome 5q. Hum Genet. 2002;110:343–347. Epub 2002 Mar 2.
114. Eerola I, Boon LM, Mulliken JB, et al. Capillary malformation-arteriovenous malformation, a new clinical and genetic disorder caused by RASA1 mutations. Am J Hum Genet. 2003;73:1240–1249. Epub 2003 Nov 24.
115. Tan OT, Sherwood K, Gilchrest BA. Treatment of children with port-wine stains using the flashlamp-pulsed tunable dye laser. N Engl J Med. 1989;320:416–21.
116. van der Horst CM, Koster PH, de Borgie CA, et al. Effect of the timing of treatment of port-wine stains with the flash-lamp-pumped pulsed-dye laser. N Engl J Med. 1998;338:1028–33.
117. Chapas AM, Eickhorst K, Geronemus RG. Efficacy of early treatment of facial port wine stains in newborns: a review of 49 cases. Lasers Surg Med. 2007;39:563–8.
118. Amitai DB, Fichman S, Merlob P, et al. Cutis marmorata telangiectatica congenita: clinical findings in 85 patients. Pediatr Dermatol. 2000;17: 100–4.
119. Kienast AK, Hoeger PH. Cutis marmorata telangiectatica congenita: a prospective study of 27 cases and review of the literature with proposal of diagnostic criteria. Clin Exp Dermatol. 2009;34:319–323. Epub 2009 Jan 12.
120. Fujita M, Darmstadt GL, Dinulos JG. Cutis marmorata telangiectatica congenita with hemangiomatous histopathologic features. J Am Acad Dermatol. 2003;48:950–4.
121. Vogel AM, Paltiel HJ, Kozakewich HP, et al. Iliac artery stenosis in a child with cutis marmorata telangiectatica congenita. J Pediatr Surg. 2005;40: e9–12.
122. McDonald J, Damjanovich K, Millson A, et al. Molecular diagnosis in hereditary hemorrhagic telangiectasia: findings in a series tested simultaneously by sequencing and deletion/duplication analysis. Clin Genet. 2011;79:335–344. doi: 10.1111/j.1399--0004.2010.01596.x. Epub 2010 Dec 16.
123. McAllister KA, Grogg KM, Johnson DW, et al. Endoglin, a TGF-beta binding protein of endothelial cells, is the gene for hereditary haemorrhagic telangiectasia type 1. Nat Genet. 1994;8: 345–51.
124. Johnson DW, Berg JN, Baldwin MA, et al. Mutations in the activin receptor-like kinase 1 gene in hereditary haemorrhagic telangiectasia type 2. Nat Genet. 1996;13:189–95.
125. Shovlin CL. Hereditary haemorrhagic telangiectasia: pathophysiology, diagnosis and treatment. Blood Rev. 2010;24:203–219. Epub 2010 Sep 25.
126. Govani FS, Shovlin CL. Hereditary haemorrhagic telangiectasia: a clinical and scientific review. Eur J Hum Genet 2009;17:860–871. Epub 2009 Apr 1.
127. Lee JH, Paull TT. ATM activation by DNA double-strand breaks through the Mre11-Rad50-Nbs1 complex. Science. 2005;308:551–554. Epub 2005 Mar 24.
128. de la Torre L, Carrasco D, Mora MA, et al. Vascular malformations of the colon in children. J Pediatr Surg. 2002;37:1754–7.
129. Baskerville PA, Ackroyd JS, Lea Thomas M, et al. The Klippel-Trenaunay syndrome: clinical, radiological and haemodynamic features and management. Br J Surg. 1985;72:232–6.
130. Kulungowski AM, Fox VL, Burrows PE, et al. Portomesenteric venous thrombosis associated with rectal venous malformations. J Pediatr Surg. 2010;45: 1221–7.
131. Limaye N, Wouters V, Uebelhoer M, et al. Somatic mutations in angiopoietin receptor gene TEK cause solitary and multiple sporadic venous malformations. Nat Genet. 2009;41:118–24. Epub 2008 Dec 14.
132. Jones N, Iljin K, Dumont DJ, et al. Tie receptors: new modulators of angiogenic and lymphangiogenic responses. Nat Rev Mol Cell Biol. 2001;2: 257–67.
133. Maisonpierre PC, Suri C, Jones PF, et al. Angiopoietin-2, a natural antagonist for Tie2 that disrupts in vivo angiogenesis. Science. 1997;277: 55–60.
134. Suri C, Jones PF, Patan S, et al. Requisite role of angiopoietin-1, a ligand for the TIE2 receptor, during embryonic angiogenesis. Cell. 1996;87: 1171–80.
135. Vikkula M, Boon LM, Carraway KL 3rd, et al. Vascular dysmorphogenesis caused by an activating mutation in the receptor tyrosine kinase TIE2. Cell. 1996;87:1181–90.
136. Calvert JT, Riney TJ, Kontos CD, et al. Allelic and locus heterogeneity in inherited venous malformations. Hum Mol Genet. 1999;8:1279–89.
137. Boon LM, Mulliken JB, Enjolras O, et al. Glomuvenous malformation (glomangioma) and venous malformation: distinct clinicopathologic and genetic entities. Arch Dermatol. 2004;140:971–6.
138. Barnes CM, Huang S, Kaipainen A, et al. Evidence by molecular profiling for a placental origin of infantile hemangioma. Proc Natl Acad Sci U S A. 2005;102:19097–102. Epub 2005 Dec 19.
139. Brouillard P, Boon LM, Mulliken JB, et al. Mutations in a novel factor, glomulin, are responsible for glomuvenous malformations ("glomangiomas"). Am J Hum Genet. 2002;70(4):866-74. Epub 2002 Feb 13.

140. Oranje AP. Blue rubber bleb nevus syndrome. Pediatr Dermatol. 1986;3:304–10.
141. Barlas A, Avsar E, Bozbas A, et al. Role of capsule endoscopy in blue rubber bleb nevus syndrome. Can J Surg. 2008;51:E119–20.
142. Puig S, Casati B, Staudenherz A, et al. Vascular low-flow malformations in children: current concepts for classification, diagnosis and therapy. Eur J Radiol. 2005;53:35–45.
143. Smithers CJ, Vogel AM, Kozakewich HP, et al. An injectable tissue-engineered embolus prevents luminal recanalization after vascular sclerotherapy. J Pediatr Surg. 2005;40:920–5.
144. Berenguer B, Burrows PE, Zurakowski D, et al. Sclerotherapy of craniofacial venous malformations: complications and results. Plast Reconstr Surg. 1999;104:1–11; discussion 12–5.
145. Fishman SJ, Smithers CJ, Folkman J, et al. Blue rubber bleb nevus syndrome: surgical eradication of gastrointestinal bleeding. Ann Surg. 2005;241:523–8.
146. Fishman SJ, Shamberger RC, Fox VL, et al. Endorectal pull-through abates gastrointestinal hemorrhage from colorectal venous malformations. J Pediatr Surg. 2000;35:982–4.
147. Liu AS, Mulliken JB, Zurakowski D, et al. Extracranial arteriovenous malformations: natural progression and recurrence after treatment. Plast Reconstr Surg. 2010;125:1185–94.
148. Revencu N, Boon LM, Mulliken JB, et al. Parkes Weber syndrome, vein of Galen aneurysmal malformation, and other fast-flow vascular anomalies are caused by RASA1 mutations. Hum Mutat. 2008;29:959–65.
149. Burrows PE, Mulliken JB, Fishman SJ, et al. Pharmacological treatment of a diffuse arteriovenous malformation of the upper extremity in a child. J Craniofac Surg. 2009;20:597–602.
150. Jacob AG, Driscoll DJ, Shaughnessy WJ, et al. Klippel-Trenaunay syndrome: spectrum and management. Mayo Clin Proc. 1998;73:28–36.
151. Smithers CJ, Fishman SJ. Vascular anomalies. Philadelphia: Elsevier Saunders; 2004.
152. Alomari AI. Characterization of a distinct syndrome that associates complex truncal overgrowth, vascular, and acral anomalies: a descriptive study of 18 cases of CLOVES syndrome. Clin Dysmorphol. 2008;18:1–7.
153. Sapp JC, Turner JT, van de Kamp JM, et al. Newly delineated syndrome of congenital lipomatous overgrowth, vascular malformations, and epidermal nevi (CLOVE syndrome) in seven patients. Am J Med Genet A. 2007;143A:2944–58.
154. Tan WH, Baris HN, Burrows PE, et al. The spectrum of vascular anomalies in patients with PTEN mutations: implications for diagnosis and management. J Med Genet. 2007;44:594–602. Epub 2007 May 25.
155. Hobert JA, Eng C. PTEN hamartoma tumor syndrome: an overview. Genet Med. 2009;11:687–94.

54 Tumors of the Head and Neck

Tomoaki Taguchi, Toshiharu Matsuura, and Yoshiaki Kinoshita

Abstract

Tumors of the head and neck in neonate, which pediatric surgeons encounter, are limited. They can be divided into three categories based on clinical manifestations; (1) Frontonasal mass, (2) Tumor in the oral cavity, and (3) cervical mass.

Keywords

Head and neck tumours • Newborn surgery • Classification • Management

Tumors of the head and neck in neonate, which pediatric surgeons encounter, are limited. They can be divided into three categories based on clinical manifestations; (1) Frontonasal mass, (2) Tumor in the oral cavity, and (3) cervical mass.

A frontonasal mass in a newborn (congenital midline nasal mass) is rare anomaly, with an incidence of 1 in 20,000–40,000 live births [1]. The common forms are dermoid cysts, encephalocoeles, nasal gliomas, and congenital hemangioma [2]. The newborn who presents with a midline frontonasal mass often poses a diagnostic challenge to the clinician. The development of the frontonasal region or anterior neuropore is complex. Understanding the developmental anatomy of the anterior neuropore and postnatal maturation will serve the pediatric surgeon well when it comes to imaging frontonasal masses [3]. The most pressing issue is whether the mass extends intracranially. There can be also many differential diagnoses. An accurate diagnosis permits proper management and prevents potentially life-threatening intracranial complications. Other frontonasal masses in the newborn include hemangiomas, myofibromatosis, hairy or teratoid polyp, fibroma, lipoma, lipoblastoma, and rarely malignancies such as fibrosarcoma, rhabdomyosarcoma, primitive neuroectodermal tumor (PNET), and hematopoietic tumors such as granulocytic sarcoma [3].

Oral tumor of newborn is represented by congenital epuris [4]. It is important to stress that clinicians should know differential diagnoses of growths in the oral cavities of newborns, including hemangioma, lymphangioma, fibroma, granuloma, rhabdomyosarcoma, osteogenic and chondrogenic sarcomas, fore-

T. Taguchi, MD, PhD (✉) • T. Matsuura, MD, PhD
Y. Kinoshita, MD, PhD
Department of Pediatric Surgery, Graduate School of Medical Sciences, Kyushu University, 3–1–1 Maidashi, Higashi-ku, Fukuoka 812–8582, Japan
e-mail: taguchi@pedsurg.med.kyushu-u.ac.jp

P.D. Losty et al. (eds.), *Rickham's Neonatal Surgery*, https://doi.org/10.1007/978-1-4471-4721-3_54

gut duplication cyst [5] as treatment modalities will be different for each case. The clinical presentation of congenital oral tumors can be impressive due to their size and aggressive appearance. Although in the case described the lesion was small, a considerable anxiety and apprehension by the parents could be observed. Therefore, if no spontaneous regression is observed, surgical intervention should be performed as soon as possible to benefit both infant and family well-being. Periodic review of oral soft-tissue pathology can help pediatric dentists to promptly identify common and rare abnormalities affecting infants and to plan the best recommended intervention.

A cervical mass in the newborn includes teratoma, neuroblastoma (primary or metastatic), rhabdomyosarcoma, fibromatosis colli, hemangioma, foregut duplication cyst, branchiogenic cyst, and vascular and lymphatic malformation [6]. In some cases, presenting symptoms are airway obstruction and feeding difficulty. In some cases antenatally diagnosed, the ex utero intrapartum treatment (EXIT) and the operation on placental support (OOPS) are indicated for airway management at birth [7].

54.1 Nasal Glioma (Figs. 54.1, 54.2)

54.1.1 Historical Notes and Incidence

Schmidt was the first scientist to describe the comprehensive nature of the nasal glioma in 1900 [8]. However, the term he used is a misnomer [9]. Nasal gliomas are not true neoplasms; they originate from ectopic glial tissue left extracranially following abnormal closure of the nasal and frontal bone during embryonic development [3]. Therefore, some authors recommend using the term 'glial heterotopia' instead [9]. They have a 3:1 male predominance, with no familial or hereditary predisposition and no malignant potential [10]. The tumor growth rate is consistent with the patient's body growth [10].

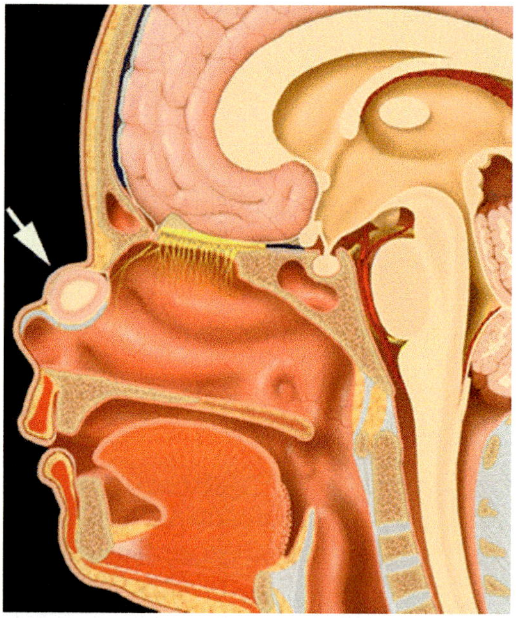

Fig. 54.1 Nasal glioma. Sagittal color plate demonstrates a nasal glioma presenting as a frontonasal mass (*arrow*). Approximately 60% of nasal gliomas are extranasal and 30% intranasal [3]

54.1.2 Pathology and Embryology

Nasal gliomas generally present at birth, rarely in adults, as a mass without associated nasal symptoms. About 60% of gliomas are extranasal, 30% are intranasal, and 10% are mixed lesions [11]. Extranasal gliomas are firm, incompressible masses that often occur along the nasomaxillary suture or near the glabella. The overlying skin may have telangiectasia, and they may easily be confused with haemangiomas. Histologically, nasal gliomas are composed of astrocytes and neuroglial cells, embedded in fibrous and vascular connective tissue [11]. They have no true capsule and mitosis is rarely noted. Multinucleated or gemistocytic astrocytes may be present but it is rare to find neurons. A fibrous stalk representing a relic of the intracranial connection can be found in 15% of cases [12]. Pathologically, these tumefactions are composed of dysplastic, neuroglial tissue and fibrovascular tissue.

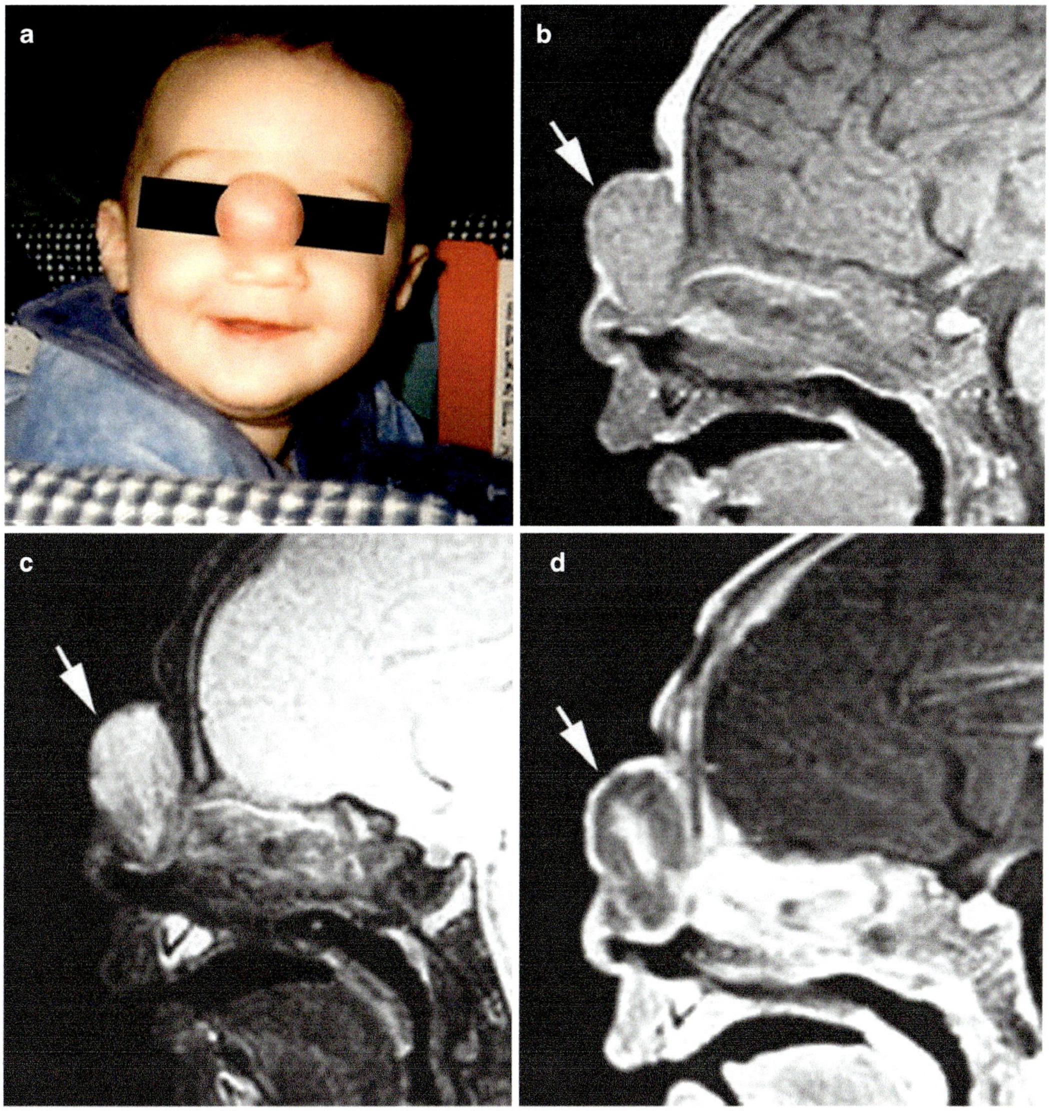

Fig. 54.2 (**a**) Extranasal glioma in a infant boy with a bulbous frontonasal mass. a Clinical photo shows a reddish frontonasal mass that enlarged with crying [3]. MRI imaging of Extranasal glioma in a infant boy with a bulbous frontonasal mass. (**b**) Sagittal T1-W image demonstrates a large frontonasal mass that is slightly hyperintense to brain (*arrow*). (**c**) Sagittal T2-W image shows hyperintensity within the extranasal glioma (*arrow*). (**d**) Sagittal T1-W image following MR contrast medium administration shows central enhancement of the nasal glioma (*arrow*) [3]

54.1.3 Clinical Picture

Nasal gliomas are one form of the congenital midline nasal masses that usually present at birth as a firm subcutaneous lump with red or bluish discoloration, lying on one side of the nasal bridge [13]. The nasal bridge may be broadened and the space between the eyes may be widened. Intranasal gliomas usually present as a pale mass with septal deviation or nasal obstruction. They often arise from the lateral nasal wall or, less often, from the nasal septum.

In all gliomas, pulsation or expansion of the lesions is absent during crying, coughing, straining or even compressing the jugular vein (Furstenberg's test). These tumors are well circumscribed, often bluish or reddish in color and often described as having a telangiectatic surface. Therefore, they are often misdiagnosed initially as capillary hemangiomas [14]. By virtue of their nasal location, they typically present with nasal airway obstruction [3].

MRI is the preferred method of evaluating all masses of the nasal dorsum, medial canthal region, and nasal cavity [3]. As mentioned, the initial clinical assessment of nasal glioma might be that of a probable hemangioma. MRI can typically distinguish these two masses.

54.1.4 Treatment

Surgical excision is the mainstay of treatment and is required for a definitive histopathological diagnosis [13]. A thorough preoperative imaging study must be performed prior to any attempt at removal of the glioma. The extent of the surgery is dictated by the exact size, location, and contents of the lesion. For pure extranasal gliomas, an external incision using either a vertical elliptical midline incision or a horizontal incision over the dorsum of the nose can yield equally good cosmetic results [11]. Some authors recommend a conservative and cosmetic incision using an external rhinoplasty approach, because nasal gliomas are benign and rarely recurrent [9]. For pure intranasal gliomas, a transnasal endoscopic approach is recommended for complete removal of the intranasal mass with no postoperative facial deformity [9]. Around 15–20% of nasal gliomas have a fibrous stalk connecting to the subarachnoid space of the brain [12]. Severe complications such as meningitis or a brain abscess can be avoided if the lesions are removed at an early stage. A neurosurgeon should be consulted whenever the tumor communicates with the brain, as a craniotomy may be necessary.

54.2 Nasal Dermal Sinus (Epidermoid or Dermoid Cyst) (Figs. 54.3, 54.4)

54.2.1 Pathology and Embryology

During fetal development of the anterior neuropore (the midline dural diverticulation that extends through the foramen cecum and protrudes through the prenasal space, terminating at the osteocartilaginous junction of the nasal bridge) typically undergoes complete regression, leaving behind the small blind foramen known as the foramen cecum. Incomplete separation of the dura (neuroectoderm) from the skin can lead to a pulling in dermal elements into the regressing dural tract. Dermal sinus and congenital inclusion cysts (epidermoid and dermoid) are possible outcomes [3].

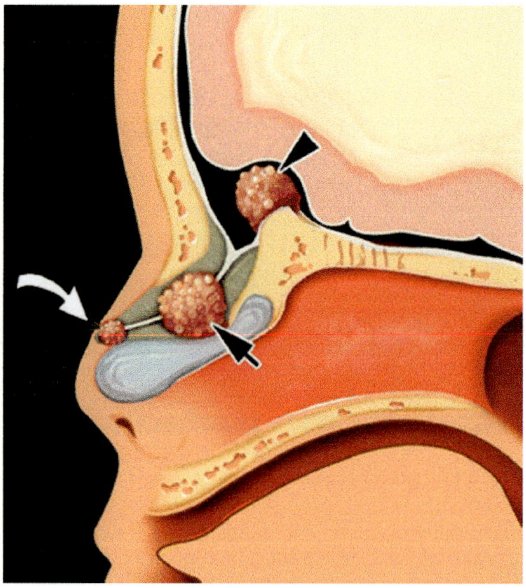

Fig. 54.3 Nasal dermal sinus. Sagittal color graphic depicts the possible spectrum of congenital cysts (epidermoid and dermoid) in a patient with nasal dermal sinus. The patient might present with a nasal dorsum pit, and underlying this might be a sinus. Epidermoid or dermoid cysts can be found anywhere from the subcutaneous nasal root region (*curved arrow*), to the deep sinus tract (*arrow*), to intracranially (*arrowhead*). The intracranial component might occur at the foramen cecum, adjacent to the crista galli, interhemispherically, or adjacent to the anterior third ventricle (courtesy AMIRSYS) [3]

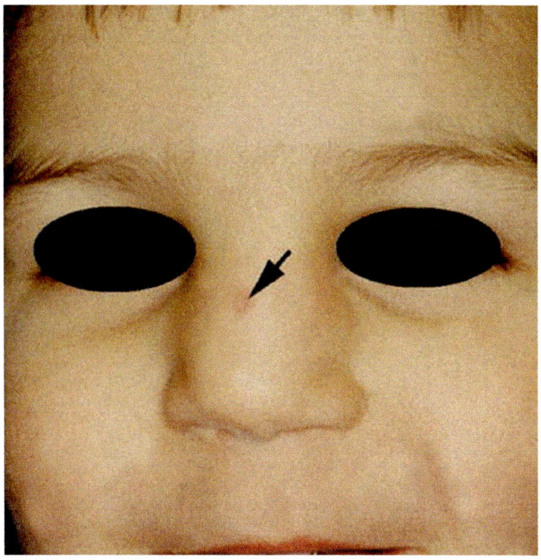

Fig. 54.4 Nasal dermal sinus and epidermoid. This infant boy presented with a draining mid-nasal pit (*arrow*). Note the broad, full nasal bridge and mild hypertelorism [3]

The epidermoid cyst represents a collection of desquamated epithelium (skin) lacking deeper dermal appendages. The dermoid cyst is composed of keratin debris and skin appendages such as sweat glands. Dermoid cysts in the frontonasal region comprise approximately 8% of all head and neck dermoids. These frontonasal inclusion cysts can occur anywhere along the course of the regressing embryologic dural tract. This includes the subcutaneous region of the nasal bridge from the glabella superiorly to the tip of the nose inferiorly, the nasal septum, and the prenasal space. Additionally, epidermoid and dermoid cysts might be found intracranially at the level of the foramen cecum and adjacent to the crista galli. There are also reports of intracranial epidermoid and dermoid cysts occurring adjacent to the anterior margin of the third ventricle.

54.2.2 Clinical Picture and Treatment

Half of the children have a dimple or pit over the nasal bridge [3]. This is usually found at the osteocartilaginous junction but can occur anywhere from the glabella to the tip of the nose. Hairs occasionally emanate from the pit, as may sebaceous discharge. A subcutaneous mass can be palpated over the nasal bridge in 30% of the patients. Approximately 50% have a broad nasal bridge and hypertelorism. The health history might be positive for meningitis caused by skin-colonizing organisms. This is strong evidence of an intracranial connection. In 80% of patients with nasal dermal sinus, the tract and associated epidermoid and/or dermoid cysts are extracranial. Craniofacial malformations have also been reported in patients with nasal dermal sinus [15]. As with any anomaly of the anterior neuropore, the most pressing clinical question is the possible connection between the clinically evident frontonasal abnormality and the intracranial compartment. In most practices, MRI has supplanted CT as the first choice and typically the only preoperative imaging study necessary in the evaluation of newborns and infants with congenital frontonasal masses and in the assessment of clinical findings suspicious for anterior neuropore anomalies without a mass. Surgical treatment is considered to be performed by pediatric neurosurgeons.

54.3 Congenital Anterior Cephaloceles (Frontonasal and Frontoethmoidal)

(Figs. 54.5, 54.6)

54.3.1 Pathology and Embryology

The pathogenesis of anterior cephaloceles is primarily based on a disturbance in the separation of neural and surface ectoderm at the site of final closure of the rostral neuropore during the final phase of neurulation in the fourth week of gestation [3]. An insufficient occurrence of apoptosis might cause this disturbance of separation [16]. Cephalocele denotes a defect in the skull and dura with an extension of intracranial contents. Categories of cephaloceles include: the herniation of meninges (meningocele); CSF,

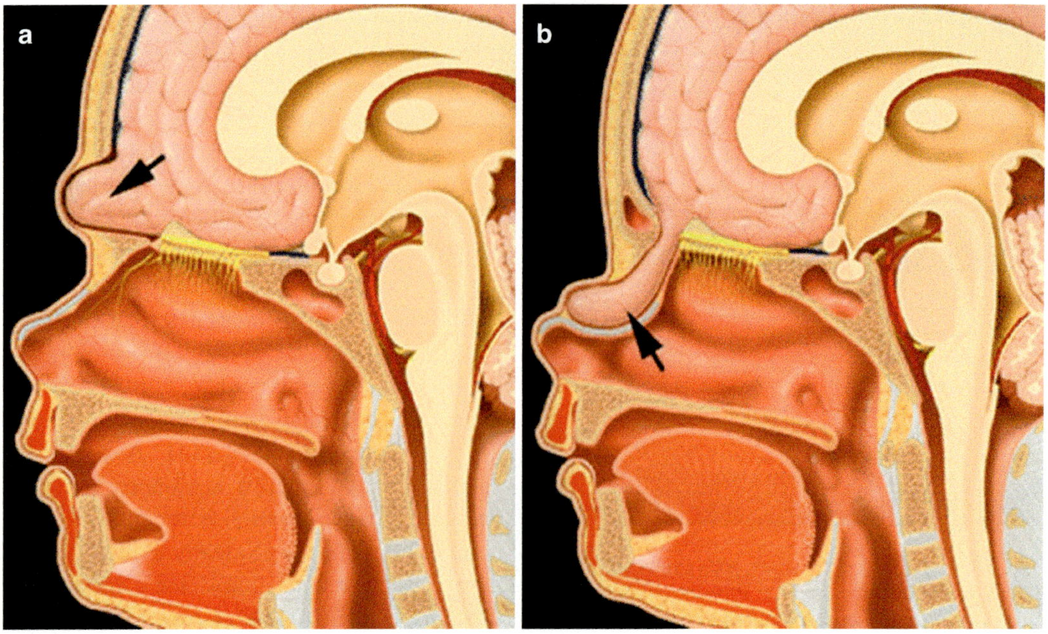

Fig. 54.5 Anterior cephaloceles, frontonasal cephalocele. (**a**) Sagittal color plate shows protrusion of meninges and brain through a frontal defect corresponding to the embryologic fonticulus frontalis (*arrow*). Frontoethmoidal cephalocele. (**b**) Sagittal color plate demonstrates protrusion of brain tissue through the foramen cecum, expanding the prenasal space and extending to the nasal bridge (*arrow*) (courtesy AMIRSYS) [3]

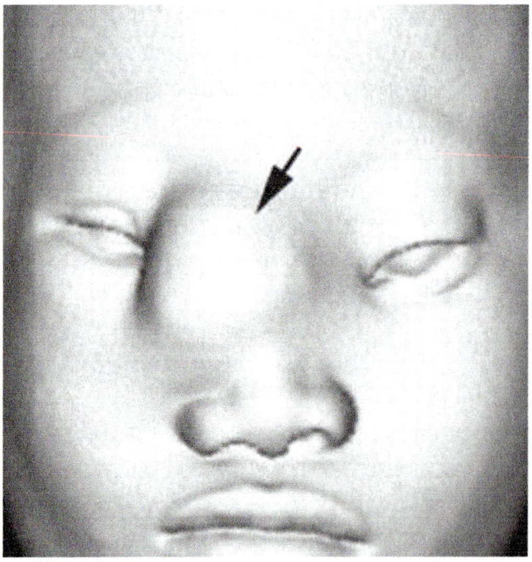

Fig. 54.6 Frontoethmoidal cephalocele in a infant boy presenting with a frontonasal mass that enlarges with crying. Surface-rendered 3-D CT demonstrates a large frontonasal mass (*arrow*). Note the associated hypertelorism [3]

meninges and brain (meningoencephalocele); atretic cephalocele, most common in the parietal-occipital area representing a form fruste of cephalocele consisting of dura, fibrous tissue, and dysplastic neural tissue; and glioceles, which consist of glial-lined cysts containing CSF [16].

54.3.2 Clinical Picture and Treatment

The frontonasal cephalocele projects through the fonticulus frontalis, and the frontoethmoidal cephalocele projects through the foramen cecum into the prenasal space. The sincipital cephalocele is usually suspected in the newborn or infant with an externally visible frontonasal mass. Frontonasal cephaloceles present with a mass at the glabella. Frontoethmoidal cephaloceles typically present with a mass at the nasal root or intranasally. Broadening of the nasal bridge and hypertelorism is often seen with anterior cephaloceles. The cephalocele commonly enlarges with crying and with jugular compression (positive Furstenberg sign). MR is the tool of choice when assessing a suspected anterior cephalocele. Frontonasal cephaloceles demonstrate a sub-skin mass in the region of the glabella at the location of the embryonic fonticulus frontalis. The mass will show continuity with the intracranial brain. Continuity of herniated tissue and/or fluid with the brain is crucial to the diagnosis. Surgical treatment is considered to be performed by pediatric neurosurgeons.

54.4 Hemangioma (Fig. 54.7)

54.4.1 Incidence and Pathology

Infantile hemangiomas are benign tumors of vascular endothelial cells and are the most common benign tumor of infancy. They occur in up to 10%

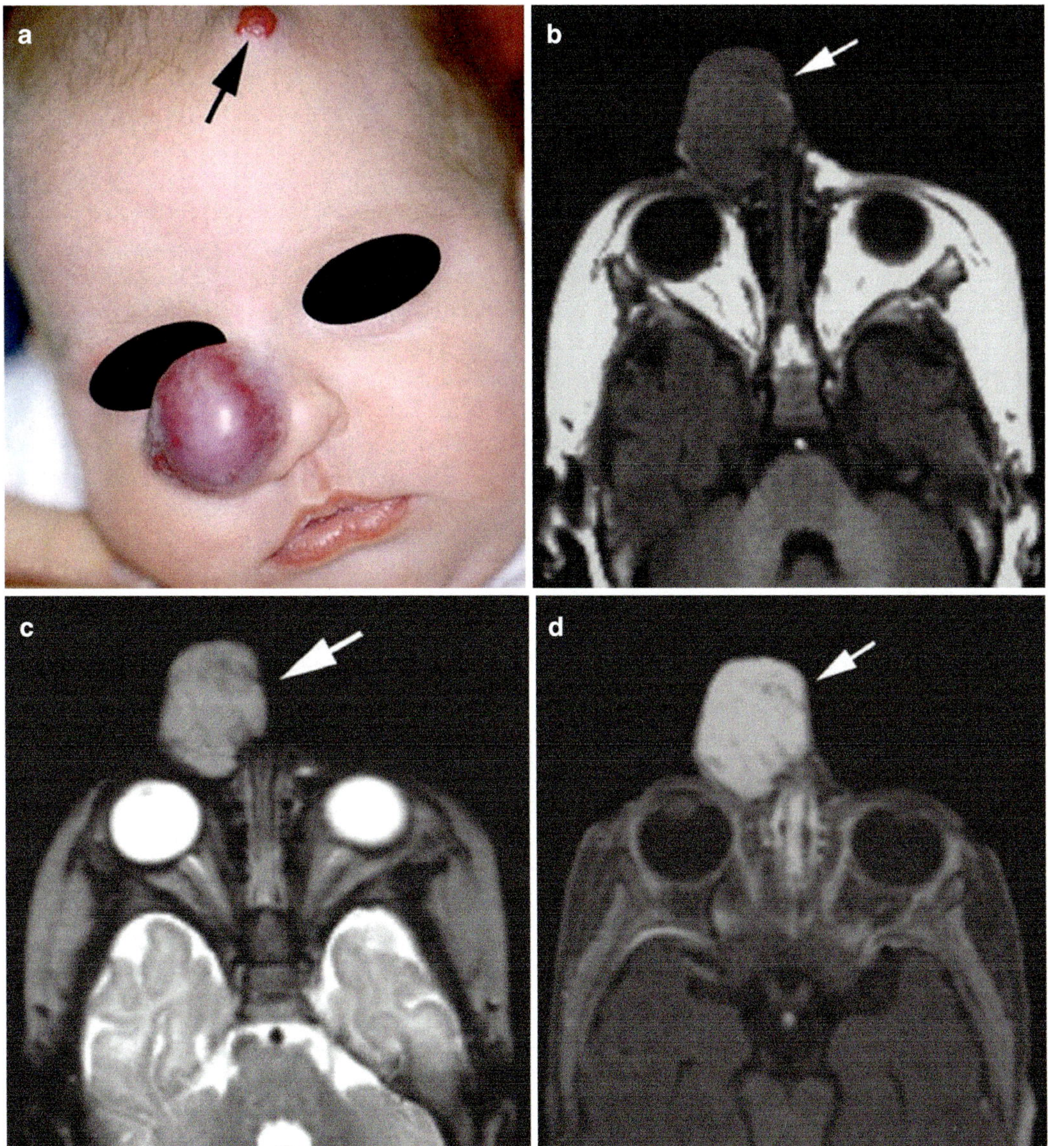

Fig. 54.7 Infantile hemangioma in a infant boy with a protuberant frontonasal mass. (**a**) Clinical photo demonstrates a large reddish-purple frontonasal mass. Note the scalp line hemangioma (*arrow*). (**b**) Axial T1-W image shows a lobulated frontonasal mass with slight T1 hyperintensity (*arrow*). (**c**) Axial T2-W image demonstrates a well-marginated hyperintense mass (*arrow*). (**d**) Axial T1-W image following MRI contrast medium administration shows robust enhancement of the hemangioma (*arrow*) [3]

of liveborn white infants with a low incidence in children of Asia and Africa descent [17, 18]. There is a 3:1 higher incidence in female infants and increased occurrence (23%) in premature, low-birth weight babies and in those whose gestation is complicated by placental abdominalities. Most hemangiomas are sporadic, solitary, and localized cutaneous lesions. However, there are reports of rare familial cases with a pattern of transmission that suggests autosomal dominant inheritance. These familial cases are often associated with other vascular anomalies. In addition, approximately 20% of the cases consist of multiple lesions. Pathologically, these unencapsulated proliferative vascular neoplasms are composed of thin-walled capillary-size vascular spaces with thin fibrous septa. These tumors have a distinct proliferative growth phase (during the first year) and an involutional phase (after the first year) [19]. Large facial hemangiomas (greater than 4 cm) can have associated central nervous system malformations.

54.4.2 Clinical Picture

Hemangiomas may differ in type, presenting as plaque-like segmental lesions or tumor-like focal lesions and deep or superficial lesions. About 80% of hemangiomas are located in the head and neck regions. Facial hemangiomas tend to occur at or close to boundaries of discrete developmental units of the face, suggesting that they may occur as a result of early craniofacial developmental events. Depending on the depth of these lesions, the overlying skin will have either a crimson, scarlet, or bluish hue. There is a clinical overlap between frontonasal capillary hemangioma and the nasal glioma. Both might present with a bluish or reddish mass.

MRI is the modality best suited to differentiate from other abnormalities.

Most hemangiomas are relatively small and pose only minor clinical problems, but approximately 20% do become clinically significant and require treatment. This may be a result of their aggressive growth and/or their location close to vital structures that they can invade, impairing function, and thus threatening the child's life. Complications include ulceration and hemorrhage, infection, and high output cardiac failure. Hemangiomas are often disfiguring and can have significant psychological/emotional impact on the affected child. This causes many parents to seek treatment rather than wait for the natural evolution to occur.

54.4.3 Treatment

Apart from the two extremes of clinical management (i.e., waiting for involution or surgical resection), complications or parental concerns may indicate treatment. Current treatment aims at inducting or accelerating the natural involution process. The most widely used option, oral/systemic or local corticosteroid treatment, has a reasonable success rate, although the reason for its efficacy is not well understood. In addition, benefits are only significant if treatment is administered in the proliferative phase. Therefore, it must be initiated early and at appropriate doses to avoid significant adverse effects. Life-threatening cases may be treated with intravenous vincristine and cyclophosphamide. Recombinant interferon alfa has also been used but is not always effective and should be avoided because of neurologic toxicity. There are reports of success in treating hemangiomas locally/intralesionally with the immune response modifier imiquimod, with becaplermin (recombinant platelet-derived growth factor) and with bleomycin. Most recently, Leaute-Labreze et al. report the treatment of severe hemangiomas associated with cardiac complications with the non-selective B-blocker propranolol [20]. A subsequent trial in children without such complications was also successful, resulting in stabilization and later regression of the lesions. Propranolol may work via vasoconstruction, decreased expression of proangiogenic factors, or by triggering apoptosis of endothelial cells. Some hemangiomas may require a combination of treatments.

In the last several years, much has been learned about molecular features of hemangioma and hemangioma-derived endothelial cells cultured in vitro, and many pathogenetic mechanisms have been proposed. The recent findings that antibodies against VEDF prevent the activation of VEGFR2 signaling in hemangioma endothelial cells, suggest that anti-VEGF reagents may be effective in hemangioma treatment [21]. Recently, Bender et al. conducted a phase I pediatric clinical trial using the VEGF neutralizing antibody bevacizumab (BV) in children with various solid tumors to determine toxicity [22]. As a result, BV could easily be further titrated for use in children of up to 3 years of age for the treatment of aggressively growing hemangiomas.

54.5 Rhabdomyosarcoma (Fig. 54.8)

Congenital presentation of rhabdomyosarcoma is very uncommon. Out of a total of 3217 patients enrolled in the Intergroup Rhabdomyosarcoma Study (IRS) only 14 patients (0.4%) were less than 1 month old at the time of diagnosis [23]. The head, neck and trunk are the predominant sites in neonatal rhabdomyosarcoma [24]. The diagnosis of congenital rhabdomyosarcoma suggests the possible intrauterine development of this tumor. In infants aged less than 1 year, Lobe et al. noted a higher frequency of embryonal/botryoid and poorly differentiated histological types [23]. There is no direct correlation between age at diagnosis and survival. Although, age is not a prognostic indicator in disease progression, neonates with rhabdomyosarcoma have a guarded prognosis due to direct or secondary complications of chemotherapy, radiotherapy and surgery on their underdeveloped organ systems. Treatment should be risk directed and based primarily on extent of disease. Multi-drug, multicycle, dose intensive chemotherapy combined with radiotherapy and wide surgical resection when feasible has shown to improve survival of children with head and neck rhabdomyosarcoma [25]. Initial surgical resection can be considered in patients with low risk localized embryonal non-orbital non-parameningial head and neck rhabdomyosarcoma. Clinical stage of the disease is the best indicator of survival. Surgeryshould be done as the first treatment, if it causes no functional or esthetic harm, followed by systemic chemotherapy. Rdiotherapy is indaicated for the alveolar subtype of rhanbomyosarcomas or for patients with residual tumors following the first treatment.

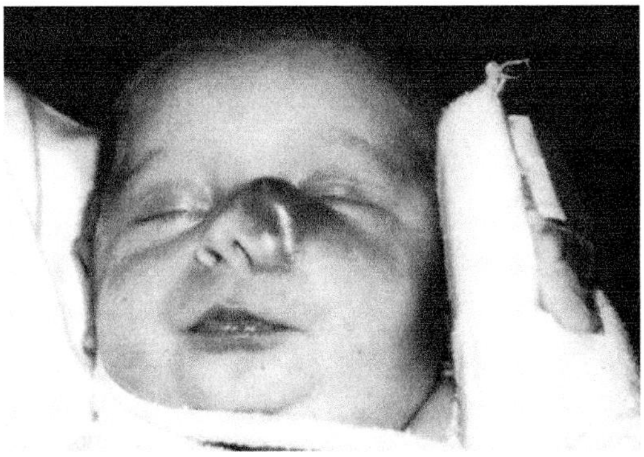

Fig. 54.8 Eighteen-day-girl infant with left paranasal rhabdomyosarcoma [25]

54.6 Myofibromatosis (Fig. 54.9)

54.6.1 Historical Notes and Incidence

Infantile myofibromatosis of the head and neck is reported as rare, but as pathologists become more familiar with histological features, this disorder may be increasingly seen by clinicians. Myofibromatosis was first described in 1954 by Stout as "congenital generalized fibromatosis", a term he chose to designate a disseminated disease of multiple nodular lesions in newborns [26]. Stout is also credited with recognizing that fibromatoses, although locally invasive, multicentric, and often aggressive, could be distinguished from fibrosarcoma, a malignant neoplasm with metastatic potential. For many years, the standard treatment of all types was aggressive, wide local resection, based on a review by Conley et al. of 40 cases of fibromatosis, including ten children younger than 15 years [27]. Subsequently, Chung and Enzinger argued for the classification of infantile myofibromatosis as a distinct lesion, based on its unique clinical and staining characteristics consistent with myofibroblastic origin [28].

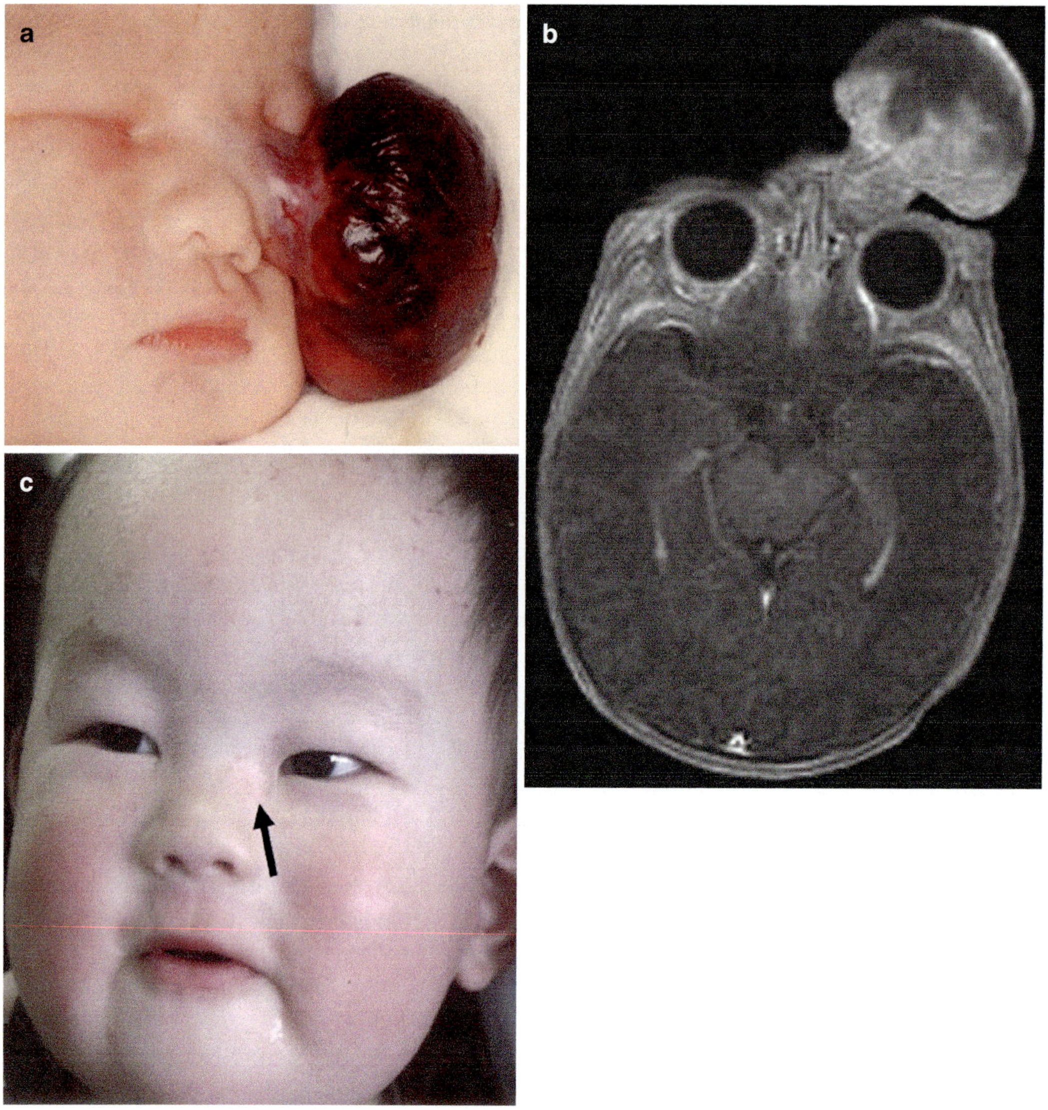

Fig. 54.9 Infantile myofibromatosis, solitary (**a**) 0-day, boy, A dark red-colored mass (5 x 4.5 x 4 cm in size) protrudes from the left alar nasal sulcus (**b**) MRI shows no invasion to the orbita. (**c**) After 1 year, cosmetic performance is satisfactory (An *arrow* shows very small scar) [29]

54.6.2 Pathology

Most nodules appeared grossly as distinct, circumscribed nodules with staining characteristics between fibroblasts and smooth muscle. Immunohistochemical stainings show the characteristic immunoprofile of myofibroma, consisting of positive immunoreactivity for vimentin and actin and negative immunoreactivity for desmin or S-100 protein. The specimens demonstrated characteristic spindle-shaped cells arranged in bundles or fascicles. There is great variability from low to high cellutarity within each specimen. A few specimens demonstrated central areas of massive cell death and necrosis, consistent with regression.

Some authors report that these lesions tend to be locally aggressive, with infiltrative growth and a strong tendency to recur after excision, whereas other reports suggest a benign character with spontaneous regression. The overall prognosis is excellent, with the exception of generalized forms involving the viscera. The generalized form is most often seen in neonates and may be fatal due to the involvement of vital structures. Both multicentric and solitary lesions may be inherited as an autosomal recessive or autosomal dominant disorder.

54.6.3 Clinical Picture

Nearly half of patients presented with a single dermal or subcutaneous nodule. The remaining patients exhibited a mass in the aerodigestive tract, including the oral cavity, oropharynx, or nasopharynx. In general, examination revealed a nontender, well-circumscribed mass. The presence of the other symptoms correlated with the size and location of the mass. The morbidity of myofibromatosis depends chiefly on the site of the lesion. Lesions in certain locations may never be diagnosed if they regress without causing symptoms.

Myofibroma is usually a solitary lesion with relatively benign features that occasionally can become aggressive.

54.6.4 Treatment

Conservative surgical excision is recommended as primary management for tumors that affect vital functions or cause growth anomalies. Cosmetic deformities sometimes become indications for resection. Watchful waiting may be appropriate if the lesion does not affect the function or growth of neighboring vital structures. In several case reports, tumors were described that underwent complete spontaneous regression. Fukazawa et al. provided evidence for greatly increased cell apoptosis in two patients with myofibroma and proposed that spontaneous regression may be mediated by massive cell death [29]. However, factors triggering apoptosis and tumor regression are unknown.

54.7 Lipoblastoma

These are rare benign mesenchymal tumors of embryonal fat that occur in newborns, infants and children. In the review of 32 patients with head and neck lipoblastoma of children, only one case was newborn [30]. Typically, lipoblastomas present before 3 years of age [31]. Male to female ratio is 2.1:1 [30]. The most common presenting symptoms are painless enlarging neck mass and respiratory distress. MRI is the imaging modality most capable of diagnosing. CT scan was often used, but due to the similarity of lipoblastoma to lymphangioma on these images, this madality rarely leads to the correct diagnosis. Conservative complete excision with preservation of vital structures is recommended.

54.8 Foregut Duplication Cysts

54.8.1 Incidence

The estimated incidence of alimentary tract duplications is 1:4500, approximately one-thirds of which are foregut duplication cysts. Foregut duplication cysts most commonly occur in the chest and abdomen. While foregut duplication cysts may occur anywhere from the mouth to the anus, occurrence in the head and neck is uncommon, with approximately 65 reported cases by 1997. The oral cavity is the most common location in the head and neck [32].

54.8.2 Pathology and Embryology

Foregut duplication cysts are benign developmental anomalies that contain foregut derivatives. Traditionally, there are three criteria that must be met to make a diagnosis of foregut duplication cysts: they must (1) be covered by a smooth muscle layer, (2) contain epithelium derived from the foregut, and (3) be attached to a portion of the foregut. Duplication cysts are lined by one or more types of epithelium: gastric mucosa, ciliated respiratory-type epithelium, stratified squamous epithelium, and simple cuboidal epithelium. All types of cysts may show squamous metaplasia, mucosal ulceration, inflammation, and necrosis, making distinction between the cysts sometimes impossible. Based on their epithelial type and other features, foregut duplication cysts may appear to closely resemble airway, esophagus, or small intestine. Therefore, the term foregut duplication cyst includes bronchogenic cyst, esophageal duplication cyst, and enteric duplication cyst.

54.8.3 Clinical Picture

The neonatal patients present with respiratory distress due to airway obstruction from the mass or feeding problems [32]. Foregut duplication cysts of the head and neck, although uncommon, should be included in the differential diagnosis of cystic head and neck lesions. Preoperative imaging is recommended to differentiate these lesions from other congenital cystic head and neck mass, namely, ranula, mucocele, piriform cyst, thyroglossal duct cyst, dermoid cyst, epidermal cyst, lymphangioma, cystic teratoma,

54.8.4 Treatment

Surgical intervention in the form of simple excision at least with complete removal of the mucosal lining is both diagnostic and therapeutic. If the cyst is left untreated, there is the potential for complications to develop. Malignant transformation has been reported to occur in long-standing foregut duplication cysts of the head and neck [33].

54.9 Congenital Epuris (Fig. 54.10)

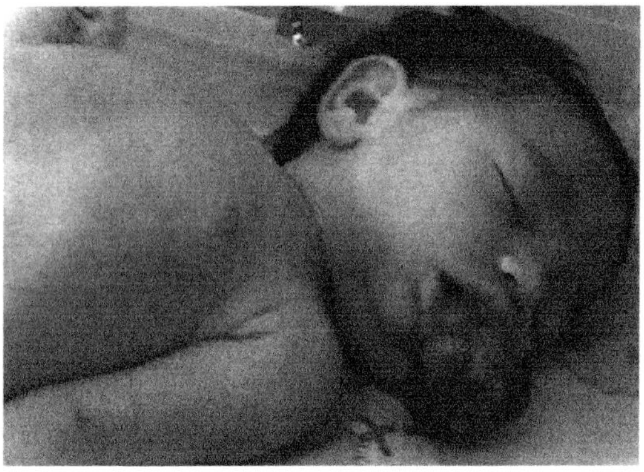

Fig. 54.10 Congenital epuris. Protruded pedunculated, pinkish red tumors in the mouse of new born [4]

54.9.1 Historical Notes and Incidence

Congenital epulis of the newborn is a rare tumour which is usually benign. The first description of a case is attributed to Neumann in 1871, hence it is also known as Neumann tumor [34]. Epulis is also known as a congenital gingival granular cell tumor because of its histological features. Since 1871, 216 cases have been reported. Epulis has a female predilection with 8:1 ratio with a Caucasian predisposition. Epulis is usually benign tumor and arises from the mucosa of the gingival and most frequently located on the anterior maxillary alveolar ridge and usually occurs as a single mass although 10% cases occur as multiple [4].

54.9.2 Pathology and Embryology

Microscopic examination shows a central mass of granular cells. This mass is surrounded by a stratified squamous mucosa. The histogenesis of the tumor is unknown. The exact histiogenesis is still uncertain; it is now thought to originate from primitive mesenchymal cells of neural crest origin. Histologically, congenital epuris shows highly vascularized fibrous tissue with nests of polygonal cells with large clear and granular cytoplasm and a small nucleus, with a normal overlying epithelium. Congenital epuris shows positive staining for vimentin either either in the intercellular spaces or in the cytoplasm of granular cells, which can be explained by the abundance of collagen and its precursors. Positive reaction for desmin, a 53kd fibrillar protein, is a specific marker of muscle cells [35].

54.9.3 Clinical Picture

Epulis clinically appears as a pedunculated protuberant pink tumor with smooth or lobulated surface, sometimes protruding from the mouse. The basis of the tumor is the alveolar mucosa. The size varies from a few millimetres to 9 cm in diameter. A larger lesion may interfere with respiration or feeding. In cases with large lesions mechanical oral and nasal obstruction can impair fetal deglutition and neonatal respiratory efforts resulting in polyhydramnios prenatally or respiratory impairment postnatally. After birth, the tumor normally does not increase in size. Malignant transformation has not been reported [4].

54.9.4 Treatment

Spontaneous regression has been reported in a few cases. However, surgical excision is generally indicated due to interference with feeding or respiration. Recurrence of the tumor after surgery has not been reported yet. The recommended treatment is prompt surgical resection. A "watchful waiting" procedure can be followed because small lesion spontaneous involution can occur, although this is rare. Of the more than 200 cases of CE of the newborn reported in the English literature, there have been eight case reports that have documented spontaneous regression. It may be concluded that if a CE lesion is less than 2 cm in its largest dimensions and the lesion does not interfere with respiration or feeding, non-surgical management of the lesions ought to be considered. The advantage of conservative management of such cases is to avoid exposure of general anesthesia in a neonate for a lesion which is known to be benign and will not recur [36].

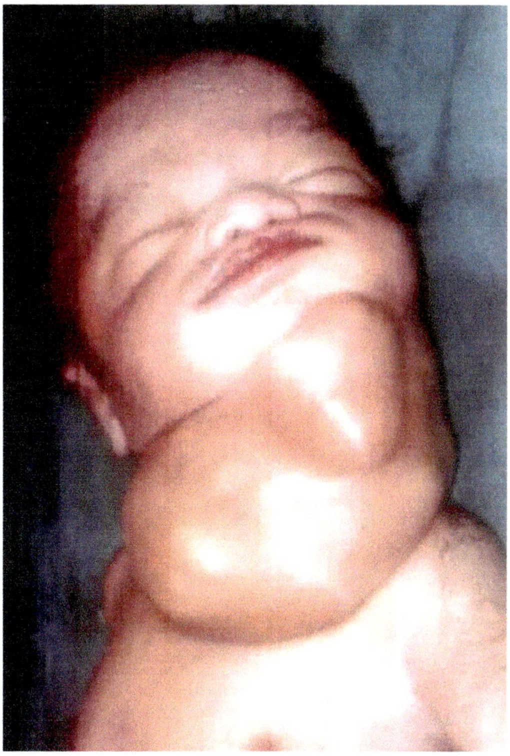

Fig. 54.11 Giant dervical teratoma in 0 day male newborn [40]

Table 54.1 Anatomical location of fetal and neonatal teratomas [37]

Anatomical location	No.	%
Sacrococcygeal teratoma	214	40
Intracranial teratoma	71	13.3
Cervical teratoma	70	13.1
Oropharygeal and nasopharyngeal teratoma	41	8
Cardiac teratoma	40	7.5
Gastric teratoma	14	2.6
Orbital teratoma	13	2.4
Mediastinal teratoma	13	2.4
Facial teratoma	8	1.5
Miscellaneous	17	3

54.10 Germ Cell Tumors (Fig. 54.11)

Germ cell tumors are relatively common in the fetus and neonate and are the leading neoplasms in some perinatal reviews. Germ cell tumors are a varied group of benign and malignant neoplasms occurring in the perinatal period. They are found in various sites, both gonadal and extragonadal, the latter in midline locations such as the sacrococcygeal area, retroperitoneum, mediastinum, neck, and intracranial region (Table 54.1) [37]. Most germ cell tumors of the fetus and neonate are histologically benign and are classified as either mature or immature teratomas [38]. *Yolk sac tumor* (endodermal sinus tumor) is the leading malignant germ cell tumor of the perinatal period and throughout childhood [38].

54.11 Cervical Teratoma

54.11.1 Incidence and Pathology

Cervical teratomas account for approximately 13% of neonatal teratomas [37]. The histologic appearance of these masses is varied because all three germinal layers are represented. Often immature neural elements are identified, especially in the solid portion of the tumor, suggesting neuroectodermal origin [39].

54.11.2 Clinical Picture

Airway compromise is the most serious postnatal complication of giant cervical teratoma [39], and prenatal diagnosis is crucial, allowing for early recognition of neck masses that obstruct the airway. A prenatal ultrasound can identify the characteristic appearance of multiloculated cystic mass originating most commonly from the anterolateral aspect of the fetal neck. Polyhydroamnios and rarely nonimmune hydrops are associated with this condition. The other conditions that need to be considered for a mass at this site include cystic hygroma (lymphangioma), cervical goiter, cervical sarcomas and neuroblastoma.

54.11.3 Treatment and Prognosis

Polyhydramnios and prematurity were associated with a poor outcome. Fetal death in utero was attributed to an effect of the tumor. The chances of survival in live born neonates is related to pulmonary hypoplasia as the result of in utero airway obstruction, the extent of neonatal airway obstruction, and the degree of pulmonary immaturity [37]. Survival with *cervical teratoma* depends on the size of the tumor and extent of the involved tissues, with respiratory compromise being the main cause of subsequent morbidity and mortality. EXIT and OOPS are indicated for airway management at birth [7]. After delivery and stabilization, early resection is the recommended treatment of *cervical teratomas* because affected neonates may have acute airway obstruction or lose a previously secure orotracheal airway within hours or days after delivery [40]. Moreover, resection is the most effective method of achieving total control of the airway. Immediate surgical intervention has reduced the significant mortality rates in newborns with cervical teratoma from more than 80% in nonoperative cases to less than 10% in operative cases. [40]. Neonates with cervical teratomas generally have a good outcome provided that the tumor is resectable. Although yolk sac tumor components were present in only 1 of 70 (1.4%) of cervical teratomas, it also removes the risk of malignant change, which occurs at much higher rates in patients with cervical teratomas not diagnosed or treated until later childhood or beyond, a situation perhaps analogous to sacrococcygeal teratomas [40].

Currently, there are no definite chemotherapy guidelines for neonates with cervical teratomas. Azizkhan et al. [40] recommend that chemotherapy should be given only in infants with disseminated metastases (that have not differentiated) and those who have invasive tumors and residual tumor after resection. Long-term follow-up with imaging and α-fetoprotein determinations are additional recommendations.

54.12 Epignathi and Nasopharingeal Teratoma

Some *epignathi* and *nasopharngeal* teratomas are so large and extensive that they are incompatible with life and therefore inoperable, which explains the high mortality rate [38]. The most common presenting findings here were a mass, respiratory distress, polyhydramnios, and dysphagia. Surgical resection of pharyngeal teratomas results in cure but is not without serious and sometimes fatal complications [41]. Radical disfiguring surgery, which could result in impairment of speech and swallowing or massive fatal hemorrhage, is contraindicated in the neonate [41]. Larger tumors may require multiple-operative procedures to obtain an optimal result. Before proceeding to surgical excision, it is imperative to rule out the existence of intracranial extension. The demonstration of hydrocephalus or an intracranial mass in fetuses and neonates with epignathi should facilitate counselling and prevent inappropriate intervention in cases in which the prognosis is very poor [42]. The neonates who were operated on did much better than fetuses who had no resections.

54.13 Facial Teratoma

Some *facial teratomas* are located superficially within the soft tissues of the face and head, whereas others are more extensive involving the underlying maxilla, orbit, or the intracranial cavity [43]. Large tumors may cause polyhydramnios and dystocia requiring cesarian section for delivery. Superficially (extracranial) located teratomas are associated with a good outcome. In the review by Isaacs, all eight of the facial teratomas, including the one fetus, were cured after surgical resection [37].

References

1. Grzegorczyk V, Brasseur-Daudruy M, Labadie G, Cellier C, Verspyck E. Prenatal diagnosis of a nasal glioma. Pediatr Radiol. 2010;40:1706–9.
2. Gatillo M. Congenital abnormalities of the nose: CT and MR findings. AJR Am J Roentgenol. 1994;162:1211–7.
3. Hedlund G. Congenital frontonasal masses: developmental anatomy, malformations, and MR imaging. Pediatr Radiol. 2006;36:647–62.
4. Eghbalian F, Monsef A. Congenital epuris in the newborn, review of the literature and a case report. J Pediatr Hematol Oncol. 2009;31:198–9.
5. Kanotra S, Kanotra SP, Paul J. Congenital epuris, review of literature. J Laryngol Otol. 2006;120:148–50.
6. Tantiwongkosi B, Goske MJ, Steele M. Congenital solid neck mass: a unique presentation of Langerhans cell histiocytosis. Pediatr Radiol. 2008;38:575–8.
7. Neidich MJ, Prager JD, Clark SL, Elluru RG. Comprehensive airway management of neonatal head and neck teratomas. Otolaryngol Head Neck Surg. 2011;144:257–61.
8. Schmidt MB. Ueber seltene Spaltbildungen im Bereich des mittleren Stirnfortsatzes. Arch Pathol Anat Physiol Klin Med. 1900;162:340–70.
9. Rahbar R, Resto VA, Robson CD, Perez-Atayde AR, Goumnerova LC, McGill TJ, Healy GB. Nasal glioma and encephalocele: diagnosis and management. Laryngoscope. 2003;113:2069–77.
10. Puppala B, Mangurten HH, McFadden J, Lygizos N, Taxy J, Pellettiere E. Nasal glioma presenting as neonatal respiratory distress. Definition of the tumor mass by MRI. Clin Pediatr (Phila). 2009;29:49–52.
11. Uzunlar AK, Osma U, Yilmaz F, Topeu I. Nasal glioma: report of two cases. Turk J Med Sci. 2001;31:| 87–90.
12. Barkovich AJ, Vandermarck P, Edwrds MS, Cogen PH. Congenital nasal mass: CT and MR imaging features in 16 cases. AJNR Am J Neuroradiol. 1991;12:105–16.
13. Ma K, Cheung KL. Nasal glioma. Hong Kong Med J. 2006;12:477–9.
14. Hoeger PH, Schaefer H, Ussmueller J, Helmke K. Nasal glioma presenting as capillary haemangioma. Eur J Pediatr. 2001;160:84–7.
15. McQuown SA, Smith JD, Gallo AE Jr. Intracranial extension of nasal dermoids. Neurosurgery. 1983;12:531–5.
16. Hoving EW, Vermeij-Keers C. Frontoethomoidal encephaloceles, a study of their pathogenesis. Pediatr Neurosurg. 1997;27:246–56.
17. Mulliken JB, Glowacki J. Hemangiomas and vascular malformations in infants and children: a classification based on endothelial characteristics. Plast Reconstr Surg. 1982;69:412–22.
18. Hideno A, Nakajima S. Earliest features of the strawberry mark in the newborn. Br J Dermatol. 1972;87:138–44.
19. Boye E, Jinnin M, Olsen BR. Infantile hemangioma: challenges, new insights and therapeutic promise. J Craniofac Surg. 2009;20:678–84.
20. Léauté-Labrèze C, Dumas de la Roque E, Hubiche T, Boralevi F, Thambo JB, Taïeb A. Propranolol for severe hemangiomas of infancy. N Engl J Med. 2008;358:2649–51.
21. Jinnin M, Medici D, Park L, Limaye N, Liu Y, Boscolo E, Bischoff J, Vikkula M, Boye E, Olsen BR. Suppressed NFAT-dependent VEGFR1 expression and constitutive VEGFR2 signaling in infantile hemangioma. Nat Med. 2008;14:1236–46.
22. Glade Bender JL, Adamson PC, Reid JM, Xu L, Baruchel S, Shaked Y, Kerbel RS, Cooney-Qualter EM, Stempak D, Chen HX, Nelson MD, Krailo MD, Ingle AM, Blaney SM, Kandel JJ, Yamashiro DJ; Children's Oncology Group Study. Phase I trial and pharmacokinetic study of bevacizumab in pediatric patients with refractory solid tumors: a Children's Oncology Group Study. J Clin Oncol. 2008;26:399–405.
23. Lobe TE, Wiener ES, Hays DM, Lawrence WH, Andrassy RJ, Johnston J, Wharam M, Webber B, Ragab A. Neonatal rhabdomyosarcoma: the IRS experience. J Pediatr Surg. 1994;29:1167–70.

24. Dillon PW, Whalen TV, Azizkhan RG, Haase GM, Coran AG, King DR, Smith M. Neonatal soft tissue sarcoma: the influence of pathology on treatment and survival. The Children Cancer Group Surgical Committee. J Pediatr Surg. 1995;30:1038–41.
25. Chigurupati R, Alfatooni A, Myall RMT, Hawkins D, Oda D. Orofacial rhabdomyosarcoma in neonates and young children: a review of literature and management of four cases. Oral Oncol. 2002;38:508–15.
26. Stout AP. Juvenile fibromatosis. Cancer. 1954;7:953–78.
27. Conley J, Healey WV, Stout AP. Fibromatosis of the head and neck. Am J Surg. 1966;112:609–14.
28. Chung EB, Enzinger FM. Infantile myofibromatosis. Cancer. 1981;48:1807–18.
29. Fukasawa Y, Ishikura H, Takada A, Yokoyama S, Imamura M, Yoshiki T, Sato H. Massive apoptosis in infantile myofibromatosis: a putative mechanism of tumor regression. Am J Pathol. 1994;144:480–5.
30. Pham NS, Poirier B, Fuller SC, Dublin AB, Tollefson TT. Pediatric lipoblastoma in the head and neck: A systematic review of 48 reported cases. Int J Pediatr Otorhinolaryngol. 2010;74:723–8.
31. Dogan R, Kara M, Firat P, Gedikoglu G. An usual tumor of the neck and mediastinum: lipoblastomatosis resulting in paraparesis. Eur J Cardiothorac Surg. 2007;31:325–7.
32. Kieran SM, Robson CD, Nose V, Rahbar R. Foregut duplication cysts in the head and neck. Presentation, diagnosis, and management. Arch Otolaryngol Head Neck Surg. 2010;136:778–82.
33. Volchok J, Jaffer A, Cooper T, Al-Sabbagh A, Cavalli G. Adenocarcinoma arising in a lingual foregut duplication cyst. Arch Otolaryngol Head Neck Surg. 2007;133:717–9.
34. Neumann E. Congenital epuris. Arch Heilk. 1871;12:189–90.
35. Leocata P, Bifaretti G, Saltarelli S, Corbacelli A, Ventura L. Congenital (granular cell) epuris of the newborn: a case report with immunohistochemical study on the histogenesis. Ann Saudi Med. 1999;19:527–9.
36. Ritwik P, Brannon RB, Musselman RJ. Spontaneous regression of congenital epuris: a case report and review of the literature. J Med Case Reports. 2010;4:331–4.
37. Isaacs H Jr. Perinatal (fetal and neonatal) germ cell tumors. J Pediatr Surg. 2004;39:1003–13.
38. Isaacs H Jr. Tumors. In: Gilbert-Barness E, editor. Potter's pathology of the fetus and infant, vol. 2. St Louis: Mosby; 1997. p. 1242–339.
39. Batra P, Saha A. Images in clinical practice. Congenital cervical teratoma. Indian Pediatr. 2006;43:549.
40. Azizkhan RG, Haase GM, Applebaum H, Dillon PW, Coran AG, King PA, King DR, Hodge DS. Diagnosis, management, and outcome of cervicofacial teratomas in neonates: A Childrens Cancer Group Study. J Pediatr Surg. 1995;30:312–6.
41. Valente A, Grant C, Orr JD, et al. Neonatal tonsillar teratoma. J Pediatr Surg. 1988;23:364–6.
42. Smith NM, Chambers SE, Billson VR, Laing I, West CP, Bell JE. Oral teratoma (epignathus) with intracranial extension. A report of two cases. Perinat Diagn. 1993;13:945–52.
43. Wilson JW, Gehweiler JA. Teratoma of the face associated with a patent canal extending into the cranial cavity (Rathke's pouch) in a three-week-old child. J Pediatr Surg. 1970;5:349–59.

55 Cystic Hygroma and Lymphatic Malformations

Shigeru Ono

Abstract

Lymphatic malformations (LMs) are uncommon congenital low-flow vascular anomalies previously referred to as lymphangiomas or cystic hygromas. The terminology of vascular and lymphatic lesions needs to be standardized. Vascular and lymphatic lesions, in general, have been notoriously difficult for pathologists to diagnose and classify because of the large number of entities and their variants, and their frequently overlapping clinical and histopathologic features. This problem has been compounded by imprecise terminology with various names referring to the same lesion or, conversely, a particular term denoting different entities. Recently, the International Society for the Study of Vascular Anomalies (ISSVA), an organization comprised of specialists in various disciplines interested in vascular anomalies, approved a novel classification of vascular lesions that distinguishes malformations from tumors and provides an easily understood and concise nomenclature.

Keywords

Cystic hygroma • Lymphatic malformations • Management • Sclerotherapy Outcome

Lymphatic malformations (LMs) are uncommon congenital low-flow vascular anomalies previously referred to as lymphangiomas or cystic hygromas. The terminology of vascular and lymphatic lesions needs to be standardized. Vascular and lymphatic lesions, in general, have been notoriously difficult for pathologists to diagnose and classify because of the large number of entities and their variants, and their frequently overlapping clinical and histopathologic features. This problem has been compounded by imprecise terminology with various names referring to the same lesion or, conversely, a particular term denoting different entities. Recently, the International Society for the Study of Vascular Anomalies (ISSVA), an organization comprised of specialists in various disciplines interested in vascular anomalies, approved a novel classification

S. Ono, MD, PhD
Pediatric Surgery, Jichi Medical University, Tochigi, Japan
e-mail: o-shige@jichi.ac.jp

P.D. Losty et al. (eds.), *Rickham's Neonatal Surgery*, https://doi.org/10.1007/978-1-4471-4721-3_55

Table 55.1 The International Society of the Study of Vascular Anomalies classification of lymphatic malformations

Lymphatic malformations (LMs)
Common (cystic) LMs
Macrocystic LMs
Microcystic LMs
Mixed cystic LMs
Generalized lymphatic anomaly (GLA)
LM in Gorham-Stout disease
Channel-type LM
Primary lymphedema
Others

of vascular lesions that distinguishes malformations from tumors and provides an easily understood and concise nomenclature [1]. The ISSVA Classification of Vascular Anomalies was recently updated in 2014, in which LMs has been classified into Simple Vascular Malformations, and further classified as shown in Table 55.1 [2]. According to some reports, the terms such as hemangioma or lymphangioma should be abandoned. The suffix -oma implies a tumor, including neoplasm. Indeed, LMs is a malformative lesion, sometimes with a tumor-like shape, but not a real tumor pathologically. For this reason, the classification accepted by ISSVA eliminates the term lymphangioma, and recommends instead the use of the term lymphatic malformation.

55.1 Classification of LMS

Many different classifications for LMs have been proposed in the literature, and these are sometimes confused because of overlapping clinical or histological features. Historically, lymphangioma has been classified into three groups: (1) lymphangioma simplex, composed of capillary-sized, thin-walled lymphatic channels; (2) cavernous lymphangioma; and (3) cystic lymphangioma (hygroma), composed of cysts from a few millimeters to several centimeters in diameter [3]. Although some previous investigators divided LMs into cystic, cavernous, and mixed types, the differences between these types in the literature are obscure. The most common LM classification scheme is based on the mean size of the cystic lesions. Lesions with a diameter greater than 1 cm are considered macrocystic (previously referred to as cystic lymphangioma or cystic hygroma), while lesions with a diameter less than 1 cm are considered microcystic (previously referred to as cavernous lymphangioma). Lesions containing both macroscopic and microscopic components can be referred to as mixed type [4–7]. As described above, the updated ISSVA classification of LMs has been acceptable (Table 55.1). When the size of the cervical macrocystic LMs is large, the term "cystic hygromas" is often used even now. LMs sizes are determined mainly by ultrasonography or magnetic resonance imaging (MRI). The classification of LMs is important clinically from the point of view of response to therapy (see below) [8, 9].

55.2 Embryology

LMs result from abnormal connections between the lymphatic and venous systems or from the abnormal development of lymphatic vessels [10]. The lymphatic system develops at the end of the fifth week as individual endothelial outgrowths from the venous system. Most recent reports regard lymphangioma as a lymphatic malformation that arises from sequestrations of lymphatic tissue that fail to communicate normally with the lymphatic system between 6 and 9 weeks gestation [10, 11]. Failure of the jugular lymphatic sacs to connect to and drain into the jugular veins leads to lymphatic fluid stasis and the development of single or numerous fluid-filled lesions in various locations of the neck. These abnormal remnants of anomalies may have a cavity in which to proliferate, and may accumulate vast amounts of fluid, which accounts for their cystic appearance. This hypothesis is most reasonable mechanism thus proposed for the formation of LMs, especially cervical cystic hygroma [11]. However, this theory fails to explain the often invasive character of the lesions.

55.3 Clinical Features

The approximate incidence of LMs is between 1 and 6000–16,000 live births [12]. No sexual or racial predictions have been demonstrated [4]. About 50% of LMs often manifest at birth and over 90% are diagnosed by at least the end of the second year of life. With modern advances in prenatal ultrasonography, the number of cases of prenatally diagnosed of LMs has increased [13–15]. LMs have recently been one of the most common prenatally diagnosed anomalies of the neck. It is relatively easy to detect large masses composed of macrocystic or microcystic LMs using ultrasonography or MRI. With ultrasonography single or multiple sonolucent cysts with or without several septa can typically be found. In our experience, 10 of 124 children (8%) with LMs could be diagnosed prenatally with ultrasonography or MRI. Especially in severe complicated cases with respiratory or circulatory morbidity, there would be some usefulness in perinatal management, including intubation or tracheostomy. Moreover, prenatal diagnosis of LMs could enable elective delivery and appropriate postnatal management, leading to improved prognosis of the condition [15]. Prenatal diagnosis of LMs would be also important for complicated cases with cardiac anomalies and/or chromosomal abnormalities when counseling parents.

Any part of the body served by the lymphatic system may be affected. Most of macrocystic LMs appear in the neck or axillary regions, whereas microcystic types show a predilection for the face, tongue, trunk, extremities, or retroperitoneal regions. In our experience, over 70% of macrocystic LMs were located in the neck and axillary region, and 70% of LMs in the neck and axillary region were of the macrocystic type. In contrast, microcystic LMs were more common than macrocystic LMs in the other sites, especially the face, tongue, and extremities. These correlations between site and type of LMs affect the treatment strategy for LMs.

LM masses are clinically poorly defined, and are usually soft and compressible with almost normal skin color (Fig. 55.1). LMs have the potential for rapid enlargement as a result of trauma, hemorrhage, or infection. The incidence of spontaneous infection has been reported ranged from 7 to 30% with bacteria [16]. LMs are histologically benign regardless of their type or location; however, they often expand into surrounding tissues, such as the trachea, major vessels and nerves, and can become life-threatening in some cases [17]. As mentioned above, MRI is particularly useful for the evaluation of the type and extension of LMs involving the neck, axillary, thorax, retroperitoneum, and extremities. MRI is also valuable for evaluating the involvement of surrounding tissues and the complex vascular lesions of LMs [18].

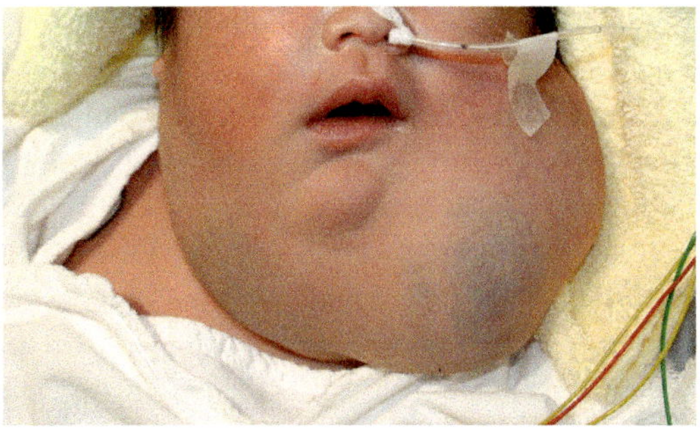

Fig. 55.1 Huge cervical microcystic lymphatic malformations (Cystic hygroma) in neonate

55.4 Treatment Strategies for LMS

All treatment strategies are based on a thorough initial assessment to detect the degree of functional impairment and/or disfigurement. Treatment options for LMs include observation, aspiration, sclerotherapy, and surgical excision. A wait-and-see strategy is recommended at least for 2 or 3 months after birth in asymptomatic patients, because there is a possibility of spontaneous regression of the lesion, reported in 12.5% of patients regardless of size and location [19].

Traditionally, surgical resection was the first-choice treatment strategy for LMs. However, complete resection of LMs is often impossible because it is technically difficult or unfeasible to remove all involved lesions and preserve the important surrounding structures. Surgical resection of LMs can be also associated with various complications and some morbidity [20, 21]. Incomplete resection may be followed by refractory lymphorrhea, wound infection, and high incidence of lesion recurrence. With regard to lymphorrhea, a recently developed instrument incorporating a vessel sealing system may be useful to reduce or prevent the leakage of lymphatic fluid. In some cases, with LMs of the tongue or extremities, partial surgical resection of the lesion to reduce its volume may be effective and useful for improvement of quality of life as will be described in further detail below.

Sclerotherapy is a widely accepted nonsurgical treatment strategy, and with recent advances is able to shrink the size of LMs, especially those of the macrocystic type [22, 23]. Various agents have been used in sclerotherapy of LMs, such as OK-432 [24], bleomycin [25, 26], doxycycline [6], fibrin sealant [27], Ethibloc [28], alcohol [29], Pingyangmycin [30], and hypertonic saline [31].

For macrocystic LMs, sclerotherapy with the use of OK-432 seems to be a widely accepted first-line treatment because of its safety profile and dramatic efficacy in shrinking the size of LMs [4, 7, 32]. However, there are few reports that have fully clarified the sclerosing mechanism of these agents [33]. In patients with macrocystic LMs, OK-432 injection therapy resulted in statistically significant complete or marked shrinkage of the lesion in over 80% of patients without any side effects. In contrast, OK-432 therapy was not so effective in patients with microcystic LMs, with complete or marked shrinkage in only 34% of patients (Table 55.2). It is interesting to note that the average number of OK-432 injections for microcystic LMs was higher than that for the macrocystic type. This suggests that some cases of microcystic LMs required repeat injections of OK-432 to achieve a clinical response. Since microcystic LMs are composed of multiple small cysts, diffusion of injected OK-432 and the evoked chemical reactions would be limited locally. Therefore, we advocate that OK-432 injection should be performed at least several times and at several sites for patients with microcystic LMs even if a clinical response is not obtained after the initial injection.

Table 55.2 Results of OK-432 therapy for lymphatic malformations in 124 children

Types of LMs	No. of patients	Complete or marked shrinkage	Slight shrinkage or no response
Macrocystic	42	34 (81%)[a]	8 (19%)[a]
Microcystic	82	28 (34%)[a]	54 (66%)[a]

LMs lymphatic malformations
[a]$p < 0.005$

Some reports have demonstrated over 80% efficacy of sclerotherapy with bleomycin for macrocystic LMs [25, 26]. Bleomycin was initially developed as an anti-tumor agent by Umezawa in 1966 [34]. Bleomycin has antineoplastic activity in a variety of malignant tumors. In addition, bleomycin incites a mild inflammatory effect on the endothelial cells composing the LM cyst walls. Although minor transient side effects such as fever, local cellulitis or induration, and skin discoloration have been reported, the major concern with bleomycin administration is the potential risk of interstitial pneumonia and pulmonary fibrosis [25, 35].

Other sclerosants for LMs have also yielded relatively good results in the treatment for macrocystic LMs, although in small series. However, sclerosing therapies could hardly be expected to achieve a dramatic effect in most cases of diffuse microcystic LMs. The results of OK-432 injection therapy for microcystic LMs are also not satisfactory, with an efficacy rate of 34% in our experience. Nonetheless, the efficacy of the other aforementioned sclerosing agents is not as pronounced as that of OK-432 in the treatment of microcystic LMs [29]. Most studies have confirmed that results with microcystic LMs are inferior to those with macrocystic LMs [22]. Therefore, the optimal treatment strategy for LMs in children is still controversial, especially for microcystic LMs; however, these sclerotherapy with certain agents should be considered when thinking about a long-term strategy for large microcystic LMs.

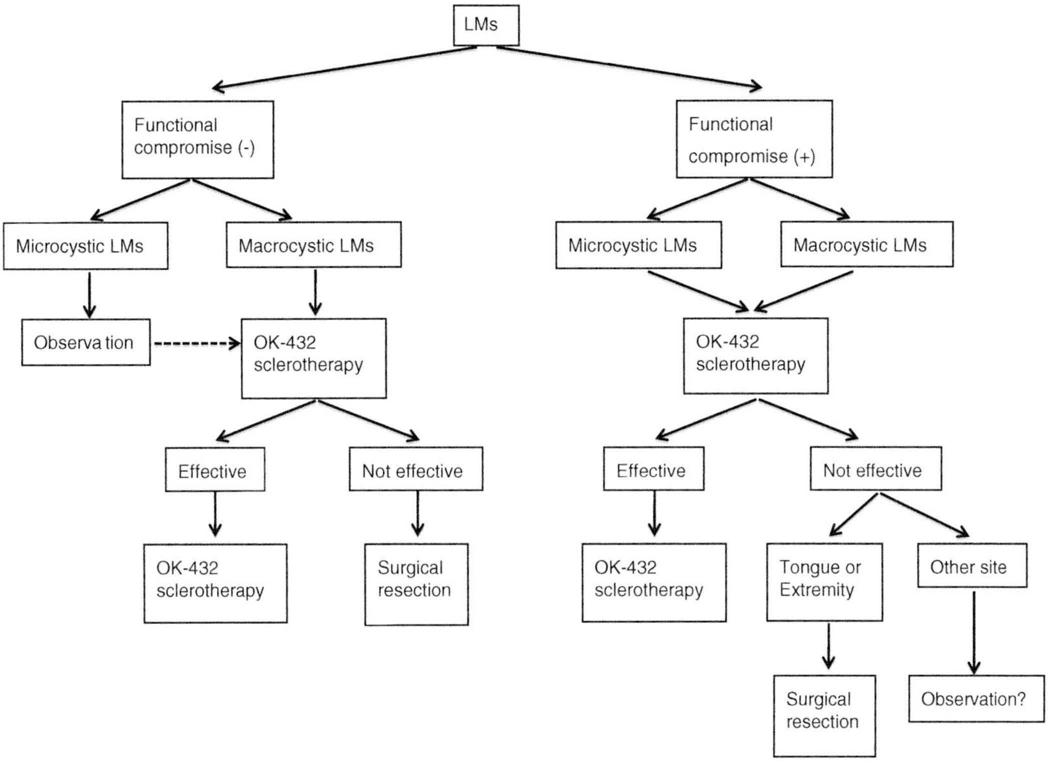

Fig. 55.2 The treatment algorithm for lymphatic malformations

Even if a wait-and-see strategy can be recommended in many cases of uneventful LMs in neonates and infants, the proliferative growth of such lesions requires an adequate treatment indication. LMs that persist lifelong require treatment in the majority of cases, especially when clinical symptoms occur. Based on individual parameters such as the diameter, location, or growth behavior, different therapeutic options as sclerotherapy and/or surgical intervention can be performed. None of those treatment concepts, however, represents the only treatment method of choice. The treatment algorithm for LMs is proposed and illustrated in Fig. 55.2.

55.5 OK-432 Injection Therapy

OK-432, an inactivated preparation of a low-virulence strain of group A *Streptococcus pyogenes* of human origin pretreated with benzylpenicillin G and heat preparation, is an effective sclerosing agent [36] (Picibanil, Chugai Pharmaceutical Co., Tokyo, Japan). With regard to the mechanism of the sclerosing action of OK-432, we speculate that OK-432 induces an inflammatory response at the site of injection that leads to sclerosis and occlusion of the sites of lymphatic leakage from LMs. Alternatively, OK-432-induced inflammation could also lead to increased resorption and/or drainage of excessive lymphatic fluid from LMs by opening new channels [37]. These two mechanisms may be mutually causing the shrinkage of LMs. Therefore, it is important that local inflammation with fever occurs after OK-432 injection to achieve clinical improvement in terms of LM size reduction. We have adopted OK-432 injection therapy for both macrocystic and microcystic LMs as an initial treatment since 1987 [24].

OK-432 injection therapy is routinely performed as the first-line treatment for all cases of macrocystic and microcystic LMs. If there is a clinical response of inflammation, repeat injections are performed every 6–8 weeks for several months. Even if there is no evidence of clinical improvement after the initial injection, OK-432 is injected at least two times or more. The degree of response to OK-432 therapy is divided into the following four categories according to the size of the LM after treatment: complete shrinkage (almost disappeared), marked shrinkage (50% or greater shrinkage), slight shrinkage (less than 50%) and no response [38].

If there is slight or no shrinkage in response to OK-432 injection therapy, surgical resection is attempted later, especially for cases involving the tongue or extremities.

55.6 Protocol of OK-432 Therapy for LMS

OK-432 is usually injected under general anesthesia in neonates and infants and in cases where the LM is located on the tongue or face. In patients aged more than 10 years, OK-432 is injected under local anesthesia. OK-432 is prepared by diluting 0.1 mg of OK-432 stock solution in 10 mL of normal saline with contrast medium. The cystic fluid is aspirated, and should be examined to confirm the diagnosis of LM. The fluid should be thin and tan in color. An equal volume of diluted OK-432 is then injected through the same lesion. The maximum volume of OK-432 solution injected at one time is 20 mL (0.2 mg), regardless of the volume of fluid aspirated from the lesion. For patients in which aspiration of intralesional fluid is difficult, e.g. those with microcystic LMs, the OK-432 solution is injected into the lesion at several sites. Extension of OK-432 within the lesion and microscopic communication between the components of multicystic LMs are confirmed under X-ray fluoroscope. Repeat injections of OK-432 are performed every 6–8 weeks for several cycles when there is evidence of clinical improvement. Even with no clinical response, it is recommended that OK-432 be injected at least two or three times in each patient [39].

55.7 Outcomes of Nonsurgical Treatment (OK-432 Sclerotherapy)

It has been demonstrated that OK-432 sclerotherapy would be safe and effective as the choice of treatment of LMs with significance in macrocystic type [4, 5, 7, 8, 32, 39–42]. In the literature, the number of OK-432 injections per patient ranged from 1 to 18, with an average of 2.0–4.3 [8, 41, 42]. The average number of OK-432 injections was 1.8 for macrocystic LMs and 6.2 for microcystic LMs [7]. This suggests that some cases of microcystic LMs required repeated injections of OK-432 to achieve a clinical response. Since microcystic LMs are composed of multiple small cysts, diffusion of injected OK-432 and chemical reactions evoked would be limited locally. Therefore, for patients with microcystic LMs, OK-432 injection should be performed at least several times and at several sites even if a clinical response is not obtained after the initial injection. The overall outcomes of OK-432 therapy are shown in Table 55.2. Complete or marked shrinkage of the lesions was found in 81% (34/42) of patients with macrocystic LMs. In contrast, only 34% (28/82) of patients with microcystic LMs showed complete or marked shrinkage following OK-432 injection therapy. OK-432 injection therapy was significantly more effective for macrocystic LMs than microcystic LMs ($p < 0.001$).

The relationship between LM locations, types and resection after OK-432 injection is shown in Table 55.3. Surgical resection of LMs following OK-432 injection therapy, including either complete or partial resection but not incisional biopsies, was performed in 22% (27/124) of patients. Lesions requiring surgical resection were most commonly located in the extremities (43%, 6/14) or the tongue (38%, 6/16). Surgical resection following OK-432 therapy was required least frequently for LMs in the neck and axillary region (2%, 1/41) and the retroperitoneum (0%, 0/6). Moreover, most of the patients (89%, 24/27) who underwent surgical LM resection had microcystic LMs. Microcystic LMs were significantly

Table 55.3 Relationship between location and type of lymphatic malformations and resection after OK-432 injection in 124 children

Locations of LMs	No. of patients	No. of cases with resection after OK-432 injection (%)	Types of LMs	
			Macrocystic	Microcystic
Face	26	7 (27)	1	6
Tongue	16	6 (38)	0	6
Neck & Axilla	41	1 (2)	0	1
Trunk	21	7 (33)	1	6
Retroperitoneum	6	0 (0)	0	0
Extremities	14	6 (43)	1	5
Total	124	27 (22)	3[a]	24[a]

It means that Microcystic LMs were significantly more likely to require surgical resection after OK-432 therapy when compared to macrocystic LMs (Macrocystic were 3/42 and Microcystic were 24/82, respectively)($p < 0.005$)
LMs lymphatic malformations
[a]$p < 0.005$

more likely to require surgical resection after OK-432 therapy when compared to macrocystic LMs ($p < 0.005$).

55.8 Surgical Treatment

Surgical treatment, including complete resection of LMs, may still be one of the treatments of choice for macrocystic LMs. The incidence of postoperative complications, including seromas, hematomas, wound infection or abscess, and nerve damage, is over 30% [20, 43]. Since advancement in sclerotherapy with OK-432 or bleomycin in macroscopic LMs has demonstrated significant efficacy, the role of surgical resection is more limited. However, if a poor response to OK-432 injection is recognized, surgical excision might be considered next. Based on the size, site, and type of LM, surgical excision should be considered following sclerotherapy for patients with LMs. In particular, when the LM occurs in the extremities, tongue, or trunk, we have tended to resect following an unsuccessful trial of OK-432 injection therapy [39].

Total surgical resection may be incomplete in most cases of microcystic LMs because they commonly extend into the surrounding tissues. Some severe complications, such as refractory lymphatic leakage, lymphatic fluid retention, and infection, may occur after partial resection of LMs. Moreover, incomplete excision is frequently associated with recurrence or further growth of LMs. Therefore, it is necessary and important to consider the indications for surgical excision of LMs, based on the site and type of LM as well as the clinical response to OK-432 injection. Some studies have reported that surgical excision of microcystic LMs following OK-432 therapy achieved satisfactory volume reduction with minimal complications [9, 40]. Recently, new technological hemostatic device, the Vessel Sealing System (VSS), is used widely in general and head and neck surgery. It is an electrothermal bipolar device that can provide excellent hemostasis by denaturing the collagen and elastin in vessel walls and lymphatic lumens and reforming them into a hemostatic seal [44]. VSS is also used to perform partial resection of refractory microcystic LMs, making it easy to maneuver intraoperatively and achieve excellent postoperative results without lymphatic leakage or fluid collection [45]. Surgical treatment strategies should be based on clinical responses of initial sclerotherapy and individualized according to site and type of LMs.

Management of LMs involving the tongue is also controversial and challenging. There is no consensus regarding treatment of LM-induced macroglossia, and children with this condition may have functional issues with speech difficulties, dysphagia, and dental problems (Fig. 55.3). Airway obstruction and obstructive

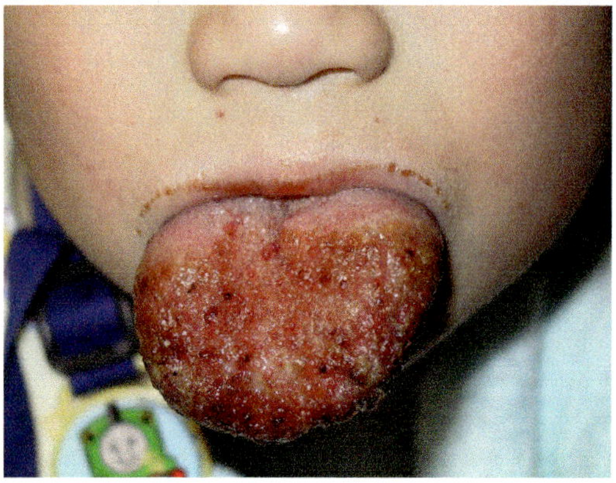

Fig. 55.3 Macroglossia induced lymphatic malformations with difficulty of mouth closure

sleep apnea followed by recurrent tongue trauma with bleeding pain or mucosal changes are the most common indications for treatment of LMs involving the tongue. Acutely enlarging LMs with tongue involvement are treated with steroids and antibiotics, and refractory bleeding from mucosal blebs would be managed with cautery, ablation, or laser therapy [46–48]. Reduction surgery for LM-induced macroglossia is used to reduce dental trauma to the tongue with associated refractory bleeding [49]. The preferred methods of tongue reduction are superficial laser ablation and surgical excision. The most commonly used procedures for surgical tongue reduction are anterior wedge and midline keyhole reduction [50].

55.9 Choice of New Therapies

New therapies as non-surgical treatment for LMs, especially diffuse microcystic or recurrent LMs, are come across occasionally in some case reports. Oral administration of sildenafil, propranolol, and sirolimus has been reported to be effective for LMs [51–53]. Sildenafil is phosphodiesterase inhibitors that have recently emerged as a potential treatment modality for lymphatic malformations [51, 54]. Although propranolol is known to have efficacy in the treatment for infantile hemangioma, recent studies have reported having a potential of treatment efficacy for some cases with LMs, especially including mixed vascular component [52]. Sirolimus is an mTOR inhibitor that reported having the efficacy in the treatment of refractory LMs. In a newborn with LMs of the neck with significant respiratory involvement and diffuse lymphangiomatosis, the treatment with sirolimus was found to be very effective, with complete resolution of the disease, good tolerability with no adverse events [53, 55]. These therapies should be estimated with prospective and randomized studies in the near future.

55.10 Massive Pleural Effusion and Ascites

The most prevalent clinical manifestation of LMs is the exertion of a mass effect on surrounding tissue, but in some cases the accumulation of large amounts of lymphatic fluid in the pleural or abdominal cavities may lead to respiratory distress. Diffuse microcystic LMs, in particular, can result in large chylous pleural effusions or chylous ascites that are often refractory to treatment. Chylous fluid collections develop when the lymphatic system becomes obstructed or disrupted, and can arise in a variety of clinical conditions, including malignancy, blunt trauma, liver cirrhosis, or surgical intervention in adults, and trauma, obstruction, or lymphatic abnormalities in children [56]. Lymphatic abnormalities in children include mainly LMs, which can give rise to physiologically compromising pleural effusions and ascites leading to respiratory distress (Figure 55.4).

Conventional conservative management of patients with LM-induced chylous pleural effusions or chylous ascites involves observation and feeding with medium-chain triglyceride-supplemented milk (MCT milk) [57]. However, MCT milk has only a minimal effect on pleural effusions or ascites associated with LMs. The thoracoscope- or laparoscope-guided direct injection of OK-432 is one of the optional treatment procedures for controlling chylous pleural effusion and chylous ascites associated with diffuse microcystic LMs. Although the role of OK-432 in the treat-

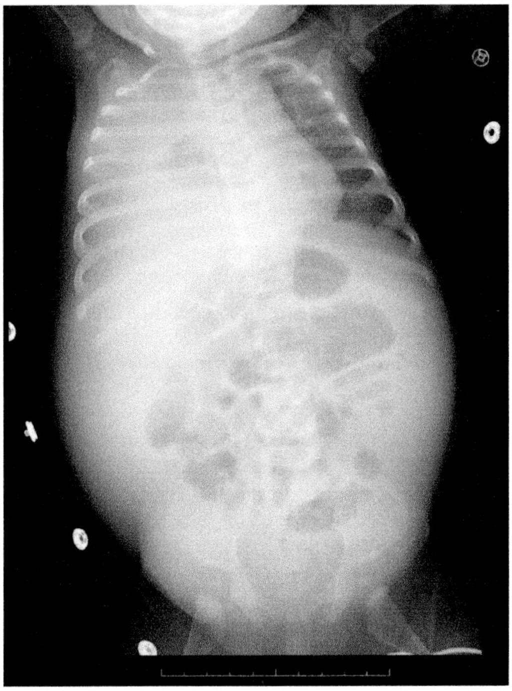

Fig. 55.4 Thoracoabdominal X-ray showing right pleural effusion and massive ascites associated with diffuse microcystic lymphatic malformations

ment of LM-induced pleural effusion or chylous ascites is unclear, the successful treatment of patients with microcystic LMs and pleural effusion or ascites using OK-432 injection therapy has been reported [58]. It is speculated that OK-432 induces an inflammatory response at the site of injection that leads to sclerosis and occlusion of the sites of lymphatic leakage. Alternatively, OK-432-induced inflammation could lead to increased resorption or drainage of lymph fluid. These two mechanisms are not mutually exclusive.

Conservative management strategies, such as dietary control, MCT milk, somatostatin, and diuretics, should be tried unless complications resulting from the fluid collections are life threatening [57, 59–62]. If these methods fail, surgical interventions such as therapeutic paracentesis and drainage should be considered. If these surgical approaches are also ineffective, the direct injection of OK-432 into the LMs under thoracoscope or laparoscope guidance is recommended. This technique should be considered for patients with refractory lymphatic fluid collections in the pleural or abdominal cavities caused by diffuse microcystic LMs.

References

1. Enjolras O, Mulliken JB. Vascular tumors and vascular malformations (new issues). Adv Dermatol. 1997;13:375–423.
2. Wassef M, Blei F, Adams D, et al. Vascular anomalies classification: recommendations from the international society for the study of vascular anomalies. Pediatrics. 2015;136:e203–14.
3. Landing BH, Farber S. Tumors of the cardiovascular system, Sec 3. Atlas of tumor pathology, vol 7. Washington, DC: United States Armed Forces Institute of Pathology, 1956. p. 124–35.
4. Poldervaart MT, Breugem CC, Speleman L, Pasmans S. Treatment of lymphatic malformations with OK-432 (Picibanil): Review of the literature. J Craniofac Surg. 2009;20:1159–62.
5. Sichel JY, Udassin R, Gozal D, et al. OK-432 therapy for cervical lymphangioma. Laryngoscope. 2004;114:1805–9.
6. Shiels WE II, Kenney BD, Caniano DA, Besner GE. Definitive percutaneous treatment of lymphatic malformations of the trunk and extremities. J Pediatr Surg. 2008;43:136–40.
7. Giguère CM, Bauman NM, Sato Y, Burke DK, Greinwald JH, Pransky S, et al. Treatment of lymphangiomas with OK-432 (Picibanil) sclerotherapy: a prospective multi-institutional trial. Arch Otolaryngol Head Neck Surg. 2002;128:1137–44.
8. Ogita S, Tsuto T, Nakamura K, Degichi E, Iwai N. OK-432 therapy in 64 patients with lymphangioma. J Pediatr Surg. 1994;29:784–5.
9. Okazaki T, Iwatani S, Yanai T, Kobayashi H, Kato Y, Marusasa T, Lane GJ, Yamataka A. Treatment of lymphangioma in children: our experience of 128 cases. J Pediatr Surg. 2007;42:386–9.
10. Gallagher PG, Mahoney MJ, Gosche JR. Cystic hygroma in the fetus and newborn. Semin Perinatol. 1999;23:341–56.
11. Chervenak FA, Isaacson G, Blakemore KJ, Breg WR, Hobbins JC, Berkowitz RL, Tortora M, Mayden K, Mahoney MJ. Fetal cystic hygroma. Cause and natural history. N Engl J Med. 1983;309:822–5.
12. McGill TJ, Mulliken JB. Vascular anomalies of the head and neck. In: Cummings CW, Friedrickson JM, Harker LA, et al., editors. Otolaryngology–head and neck surgery, vol 1. 2nd ed. St. Louis: Mosby; 1993. p. 333–46.
13. Zanotti SD, LaRusso S, Coulson C. Prenatal sonographic diagnosis of axillary cystic lymphangiomas. J Clin Ultrasound. 2001;29:112–5.
14. Goldstein I, Leibovitz Z, Noi-Nizri M. Prenatal diagnosis of fetal chest lymphangioma. J Ultrasound Med. 2006;25:1437–40.

15. Suzuki N, Tsuchida Y, Takahashi A, Kuroiwa M, Ikeda H, Mohara J, et al. Prenatally diagnosed cystic lymphangioma in infants. J Pediatr Surg. 1998;33:1599–604.
16. Wiswell TE, Miller JA. Infections of congenital cervical neck masses associated with bacteremia. J Pediatr Surg. 1986;21:173–4.
17. Feins NR. Lymphatic disorders. In: O'Neill Jr JA, et al., editors. Pediatric surgery. 5th ed. St Louis: Mosby; 1998. p. 1973–81.
18. Legiehn GM, Heran MK. Classification, diagnosis, and interventional radiologic management of vascular malformations. Orthop Clin North Am 2006; 37:435,74, vii–viii.
19. Perkins JA, Maniglia C, Magit A, Sidhu M, Manning SC, Chen EY. Clinical radiographic findings in children with spontaneous lymphatic malformation regression. Otolaryngol Head Neck Surg. 2008;128:772–7.
20. Smith RJH. Lymphatic malformations. Lymphat Res Biol. 2004;2:25–31.
21. Hancock BJ, St-Vil D, Luks FI, et al. Complications of lymphangiomas in children. J Pediatr Surg. 1992;27:220–6.
22. Lee BB, Kim YM, Seo JM, Hwang JH, et al. Current concepts in lymphatic malformation. Vasc Endovascular Surg. 2005;39:67–81.
23. Perkins JA, Mannin SC, Tempero RM, Cunningham MJ, Edmonds JL, Hoffer FA, Egbert MA. Lymphatic malformations: review of current treatment. Otolaryngol Head Neck Surg. 2010;142:795–803.
24. Ogita S, Tsuto T, Tokiwa K, Takahashi T. Intracystic injection of OK-432: a new sclerosing therapy for cystic hygroma in children. Br J Surg. 1987;74:690–1.
25. Orford J, Barker A, Thonell S, King P, Murphy J. Bleomycin therapy for cystic hygroma. J Pediatr Surg. 1995;30:1282–7.
26. Okada A, Kubota A, Fukazawa M, Imura K, Kamata S. Injection of bleomycin as a primary therapy of cystic lymphangioma. J Pediatr Surg. 1992;27:440–3.
27. Castañón M, Margarit J, Carrasco R, Vancells M, Albert A, Morales L. Long-term follow-up of nineteen cystic lymphangiomas treated with fibrin sealant. J Pediatr Surg. 1999;34:1276–9.
28. Riche MC. Traitement ono chirurgical des lymphangiomas kystiques. Ann Otolaryngol. 1986;103:67–70.
29. Alomari AI, Karian VE, Lord DJ, Padua HM, Burrows PE. Percutaneous sclerotherapy for lymphatic malformations: A retrospective analysis of patient-evaluated improvement. J Vasc Interv Radiol. 2006;17:1639–48.
30. Luo QF, Gan YH. Pingyangmycin with triamcinolone acetonide effective for treatment of lymphatic malformations in the oral and maxillofacial region. J Craniomaxillofac Surg. 2013;41:345–9.
31. Dubois J, Garel L, Abela A, Laberge L, Yazbeck S. Lymphangiomas in children: percutaneous sclerotherapy with an alcoholic solution of zein. Radiology. 1997;204:651–4.
32. Laranne J, Keski-Nisula L, Rautio R, Rautiainen M, Airaksinen M. OK-432 (Picibanil) therapy for lymphangioma in children. Eur Arch Otorhinolaryngol. 2002;259:274–8.
33. Ogita S, Tsuto T, Nakamura K, Deguchi E, Tokiwa K, Iwai N. OK-432 therapy for lymphangioma in children: Why and how does it work? J Pediatr Surg. 1996;31:477–80.
34. Umezawa H. Recent studies on biochemistry and action of bleomycin. In: Carter SK, Crooke ST, Umezawa H. editors. Bleomycin. current status and new developments. New York: Academic; 1978. p. 15–20.
35. Muir T, Kirsten M, Fourie P, et al. Intralesional bleomycin injection (IBI) treatment for haemangioma and congenital vascular malformations. Pediatr Surg Int. 2004;19:766–73.
36. Ishida N, Hoshino T. A Streptcoccal preparation as a potent biological response modifier OK-432. 2nd ed. Amsterdam: Excerpta Medica; 1985. p. 1–5.
37. Tuchihashi Y, Ogita S. Histopathological study of the effect of OK-432 on lymphangioma of an infant. J Kyoto Pref Univ Med. 1993;102:1055–60.
38. Tanigawa N, Shimomatsuya T, Takahashi K, Inomata Y, Tanaka K, Satomura K, et al. Treatment of cystic hygroma and lymphangioma with the use of bleomycin fat emulsion. Cancer. 1987;60:741–9.
39. Ogita S, Tsuto T, Deguchi E, Tokiwa K, Nagashima M, Iwai N. OK-432 therapy for unresectable lymphangiomas in children. J Pediatr Surg. 1991;26:263–70.
40. Boardman SJ, Cochrane LA, Roebuck D, Elliott MJ, Hartley BEJ. Multimodality treatment of pediatric lymphatic malformations of the head and neck using surgery and sclerotherapy. Arch Otolaryngol Head Neck Surg. 2010;136:270:276.
41. Smith RJH, Bruke DK, Sato Y, Poust RI, Kimura K, Bauman NM. OK-432 therapy for lymphangiomas. Arch Otolaryngol Head Neck Surg. 1996;122:1195–9.
42. Rautio R, Keski-Nisula L, Laranne J, Laasonen E. Treatment of lymphangiomas with OK-432 (Picibanil). Cardiovasc Intervent Radiol. 2003;26:31–6.
43. Ninh TN, Tx N. Cystic hygroma in children: a report of 126 cases. J Pediatr Surg. 1974;9:191–5.
44. Heniford BT, Matthews BD, Sing RF, Backus C, Pratt B, Greene FL. Initial results with an electrothermal bipolar vessel sealer. Surg Endosc. 2001;15:799–801.
45. Ono S, Tsuji Y, Baba K, Usui Y, Yanagisawa S, Maeda K. A New strategy for the treatment of refractory microcystic lymphangioma. Surg Today. 2014;44:1184–7.
46. Roy S, Reyes S, Smith LP. Bipolar radiofrequency plasma ablation (Coblation) of lymphatic malformations of the tongue. Int J Pediatr Otorhinolaryngol. 2009;73:289–93.
47. Ryu NG, Park SK, Jeong HS. Low power radiofrequency ablation for symptomatic microcystic lymphatic malformation of the tongue. Int J Pediatr Otorhinolaryngol. 2008;72:1731–4.
48. Leboulanger N, Roger G, Caze A, Enjolras O, Denoyelle F, Garabedian EN. Utility of radiofre-

quency ablation for hemorrhagic lingual lymphangioma. Int J Pediatr Otorhinolaryngol. 2008;72:953–8.
49. Jian XC. Surgical management of lymphangiomatous or lymphangiohemangiomatous macroglossia. J Oral Maxillofac Surg. 2005;63:15–9.
50. Bloom DC, Perkins JA, Manning SC. Management of lymphatic malformations and macroglossia: results of a national treatment survey. Int J Pediatr Otorhinolaryngol. 2009;73:1114–8.
51. Swetman GL, Berk DR, Vasanawala SS, et al. Sildenafil for severe lymphatic malformations. N Engl J Med. 2012;366:384–6.
52. Ozeki M, Kanda K, Kawamoto N, et al. Propranolol as an alternative treatment option for pediatric lymphatic malformation. Tohoku J Exp Med. 2013;229:61–6.
53. Akyuz C, Atas E, Varan A. Treatment of a tongue lymphangioma with sirolimus after failure of surgical resection and propranolol. Pediatr Blood Cancer. 2014;61:931–2.
54. Singh P, Mundy D. Giant neonatal thoraco-abdominal lymphatic malformations treated with sildenafil: A case report and review of the literature. J Neonatal Perinatal Med. 2013;6:89–92.
55. Laforgia N, Schettini F, De Mattia D, et al. Lymphatic malformation in newborns as the first sign of diffuse lymphangiomatosis: successful treatment with sirolimus. Neonatology. 2016;109:52–5.
56. Aalami OO, Allen DB, Organ CH Jr. Chylous ascites: a collective review. Surgery. 2000;128:761–78.
57. Weinstein LD, Scanlon GT, Hersh T. Chylous ascites. Management with medium-chain triglycerides and exacerbation by lymphangiography. Am J Dig Dis. 1969;14:500–9.
58. Ono S, Iwai N, Chiba F, Furukawa T, Fumino S. OK-432 therapy for chylous pleural effusion or ascites associated with lymphatic malformations. J Pediatr Surg. 2010;45:e7–10.
59. Huang Q, Jiang ZW, Jiang J, et al. Chylous ascites: treated with total parenteral nutrition and somatostatin. World J Gastroenterol. 2004;10:2588–91.
60. Collard JM, Laterre PF, Boemer F, et al. Conservative treatment of postsurgical lymphatic leaks with somatostatin-14. Chest. 2000;117:902–5.
61. Cochran WJ, Klish WJ, Brown MR, et al. Chylous ascites in infants and children: A case report and literature review. J Pediatr Gastroenterol Nutr. 1985;4:668–73.
62. Cardenas A, Chopra S. Chylous ascites. Am J Gastroenterol. 2002;97:1896–900.

Liver Tumors

56

Jörg Fuchs and Steven W. Warmann

Abstract

Primary malignant liver tumours are rare and account for 1–2% of all solid tumours in childhood.

Hepatoblastoma (HB) is a rare solid tumor in infancy and toddlers that accounts for approximately 55% of all malignant liver tumours. The incidence is approximately 1 case per 1,000,000 children. The description of morphological and histological differences between HB and hepatocellular carcinoma (HCC) was a major discovery under the aspects of treatment efficiency and outcome for the children. The observation of an increased HB incidence in children born before 28 weeks gestation (birth weight below 1500 g) compared to children born at term is difficult to explain. The exposure of endogenous metabolites, hormones, as well as exogenous toxic substances e.g. drugs could influence the tumour development of dividing hepatoblasts.

Keywords

Liver tumors • Newborns • Classification • Staging • Surgery • Outcomes.

56.1 Malignant Liver Tumours

56.1.1 Malignant Epithelial Tumors: Hepatoblastoma and Hepatocellular Carcinoma

56.1.1.1 Pathology

Primary malignant liver tumours are rare and account for 1–2% of all solid tumours in childhood [1].

Hepatoblastoma (HB) is a rare solid tumor in infancy and toddlers that accounts for approximately 55% of all malignant liver tumours. The

J. Fuchs, MD (✉) • S.W. Warmann, MD
Department of Pediatric Surgery and Pediatric Urology, University Children's Hospital, University of Tuebingen, TuebingenHoppe-Seyler-Str. 03, Tuebingen 72076, Germany
e-mail: joerg.fuchs@med.uni-tuebingen.de

P.D. Losty et al. (eds.), *Rickham's Neonatal Surgery*, https://doi.org/10.1007/978-1-4471-4721-3_56

incidence is approximately 1 case per 1,000,000 children. The description of morphological and histological differences between HB and hepatocellular carcinoma (HCC) was a major discovery under the aspects of treatment efficiency and outcome for the children. The observation of an increased HB incidence in children born before 28 weeks gestation (birth weight below 1500 g) compared to children born at term is difficult to explain. The exposure of endogenous metabolites, hormones, as well as exogenous toxic substances e.g. drugs could influence the tumour development of dividing hepatoblasts [2–4].

Different histological classifications have been proposed over the last decades. Currently HB are commonly subdivided into three subgroups according to the SIOPEL Liver Tumor Study Group classification (Table 56.1) [5].

The growth pattern of HB is unifocal in 85%; 15% of all tumors show a multifocal growth pattern. Characteristics of the epithelial tumor compounds range from anaplastic to embryonal and further on to well differentiated fetal cells. Therefore, the group of epithelial HB comprises purely fetal, embryonal, mixed embryonal/fetal, macrotrabecular, and small cell undifferentiated (SCUD) subtypes. The macrotrabecular subtype is a transition form to HCC and is commonly found in older children.

The subgroup of mixed epithelial/mesenchymal HB can be further subdivided into tumors with or without teratoid features. Mixed HB may contain osteoid, fully developed bones, muscle cells, and other tissues. In teratoid HB structures resembling germ cell tumours have been observed.

In contrast to fetal and embryonal HB exist so called highly malignant transitional liver cell tumours (TLCT). Most of these tumors are very aggressive and occur in older children or young adolescents. In the literature this entity is discussed controversly. These tumors are considered as being compositions of immature blastemal cells in combination with the classical features of all other liver tumors cells. Additionally, other new tumor entities of the liver such as desmoplastic nested spindle cell tumours have been described in few case reports [6].

Table 56.1 Classification of HB according to the SIOPEL Study Group

Wholly epithelial type
Fetal/pure fetal subtype
Embryonal/mixed fetal and embryonal subtype
Macrotrabecular subtype
Small cell undifferentiated subtype
Mixed epithelial and mesenchymal type
Without teratoid features
With teratoid features
HB, not otherwise specified

Hepatocellullar carcinomas (HCC) show a slightly decreased incidence over the last 20 years. The incidence is approximately 0.5 per 1,000,000 children above the age of 10 years, with a somewhat higher occurrence in the Asian population. One reason might be the immunization of infants against perinatal transmission of hepatitis B virus infection. From the epidemiological point of view we can distinguish between two groups of HCC: those developing in the context of advanced chronic liver diseases (α[alpha]-1-antitrypsin deficiency, hereditary tyrosinemia, chronic cholestatic disease and long term use of TPN) and children who develop sporadic tumors. The histological features of HCC are similar in children and adults. HCC cells are larger and more polymorphic than HB cells and include bile pigment as typical pattern. The most common genetic alteration is mutation of p53. Nearly 25% of all pediatric HCC belong to the fibrolamellar subtype (polygonal cells nested in a dense fibrous stoma). Pediatric HCC are characterized by low levels of cyclin D1 and a higher frequency of LOH 13q [7].

56.1.1.2 Clinical Presentation

Liver tumours in children most commonly present with a right upper quadrant mass as leading symptom. Unfortunately, by the time of detection, most of these lesions have grown to an enormous size. Approximately 20% of the children with HB and up to 40% with HCC have lung metastases at diagnosis. Further typical clinical signs of malignant epithelial liver tumors in children are abdominal distension, sometimes abdominal pain including vomiting or nausea, and loss of body weight. Anaemia is often present. Sometimes the patients present with paraneoplastic symptoms such as pubertas precox [8]. HB is the most common tumor in the age group below 5 years with an incidence peak between 2 and 3 years.

In contrast, HCC occur in patients between 5 and 20 years of age. HB is regularly found in association with several syndromes including Wiedemann-Beckwith, hemihypertrophia, or familiar adenomatous polyposis (FAP) [9].

Both tumor entities show an elevated serum α[alpha]-fetoprotein level in more than 85%. HB with an initial α[alpha]-fetoprotein level below 100 μg/L have a poor prognosis [10]. Other laboratory parameters are often normal. Especially serum bilirubin levels are physiologic, transaminases may be slightly elevated. In HB the thrombocyte count can be increased to over $500 \times 10^9/l$ [11].

56.1.1.3 Diagnostics

Availability and repeatability are the reason for the wide use of ultrasound scan. This investigation allows the description of tumour extension and also judgement of tumor response during chemotherapy. Sometimes HB are difficult to distinguish from the regular liver parenchyma because of the almost equal echogenicity [12]. The advantage of Doppler studies lies in the excellent assessability of borders between tumour and vessels under the aspect of moveable planes and tumor involvement (e.g. portal vein or hepatic vein). This applies in particular to the visualization of flow irregularities as well as small and localized portal or cava vein thrombi. Results from this investigation are especially helpful for the surgeon to estimate the type of liver resection [8].

Multislice CT scan and/or MRI are gold standard of the diagnostic in HB and HCC. These investigations are a roadmap for staging with a special focus on the PRETEXT- system (Fig. 56.1) and also an essential part for risk

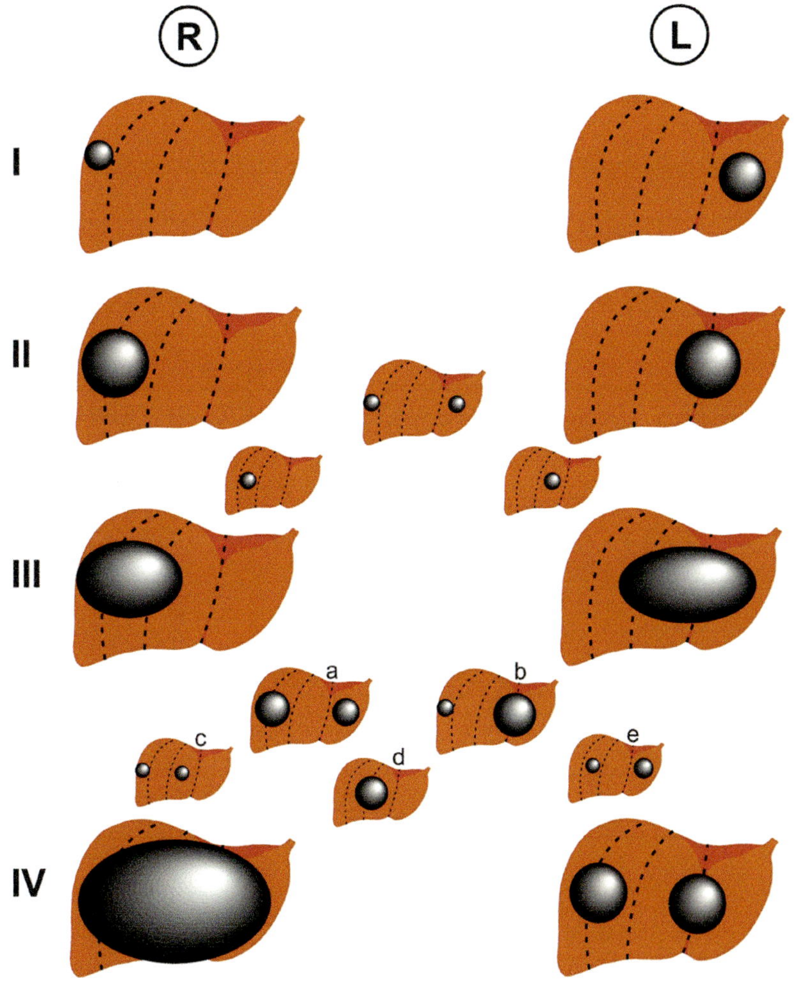

Fig. 56.1 PRETEXT staging system according to the SIOPEL Liver Study Group

stratification. The advantage of MRI is the absence of ionizing radiation. Furthermore, Angio-MRI is an excellent tool for reconstruction of the venous and arterial anatomy.

However, there exists also the possibility of computer-aided evaluation of imaging data using software assistants (for example MeVis LiverAnalyzer and MeVis Liver Explorer). These tools allow three-dimensional visualisation of liver tumors including all liver segments together with virtual simulation of liver resections. Further advantages of this system are establishment of detailed virtual risk analyses according to the liver segments, vessels, and biliary structures together with assessment of functional aspects based on the volume estimation of the liver remnant (Fig. 56.2) [13].

Thoracic CT scan is indicated in every pediatric epithelial malignant liver tumor in order to exclude lung metastases and as part of correct staging.

Conventional angiography is usually not necessary and plays a role only for interventional treatment options such as chemo-embolisation or intra-arterial application of chemotherapy in selected unresectable cases after chemotherapy.

The possible role of PET-CT or PET-MRI scan in the primary diagnostic workup of liver tumors or in the diagnostic of metastases or relapses has not yet been clarified. These modern tools should be analyzed in further studies [14].

56.1.1.4 Staging and Risk Stratification

Currently there exist three different staging systems for liver tumors in childhood. The well-known TNM classification system plays a historical role and is used in several national and international trials for HCC [15]. Meanwhile, we distinguish between the pre-operative

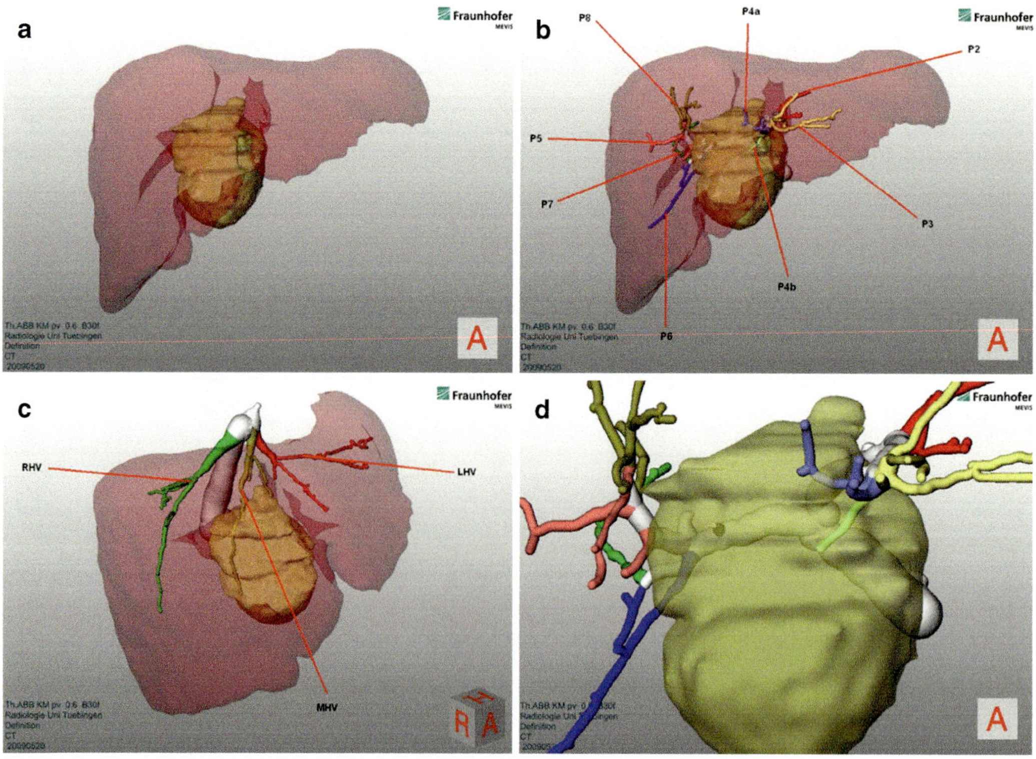

Fig. 56.2 3D reconstruction of a central liver tumor in a 4 year-old boy with central HB before mesohepatectomy. (**a**) Liver and tumor. (**b**) Anatomy of portal venous branches. (**c**) Hepatic veins. (**d**) Detailed view on tumor and portal veins

PRETEXT-system introduced by the SIOPEL group and the postoperative staging system according the Children's Cancer Study Group:

Stage I: Completely resected tumor
Stage II: Microscopic residual tumor
Stage III: Macroscopic residual tumor
Stage IV: Distant metastases

The main advantage of the PRETEXT (Pre Treatment Extent of Disease)-system is the standardized preoperative judgement of the tumor extension including risk stratification with a prognostic impact. The PRETEXT staging is based on Couinaud's system of liver segments which are grouped into four sections. In the original system, the caudate lobe or segment one was ignored. Additionally, the PRETEXT system describes the extension of disease beyond the liver, defining status v as affection of the inferior cava vein or hepatic veins, p as portal vein involvement, e as extrahepatic disease, and m as presence of metastases [16]. In 2007 Roebuck et al. added new relevant factors for risk stratification to the PRETEXT-system [17]. New parameters are caudate lobe involvement (C), tumor focality (F), and tumor rupture with different subdivisions [17]. The disadvantage of this system is the possibility of over-staging the liver tumor, probably as a result of the difficulty to distinguish between displacement and infiltration of liver parenchyma by the tumour. Another relevant issue is the weakness of standardisation of the radiological technique. This is relevant for unilocular tumors staged as PRETEXT III and IV with regard to the subsequent decision between tumor resection and liver transplantation [18].

In contrast, the postoperative staging system is exact and based on histological examination of the completeness of the liver tumor resection. Meanwhile both systems are used in different international trials under the aspects of evidence based comparison of treatment results.

Until recently, HB have been divided into two risk groups: the low (standard) risk group and the high risk group. The differences of characterisation of the risk groups within the treatment protocols are marginal. There is an agreement that high risk HB fulfil one or more of the following criteria:

- Mutifocality of the tumor
- Invasion of large vessels
- Distant metastases
- Lymph node involvement or extrahepatic disease
- Serum α[alpha]-fetoprotein level below 100 μg/1

All other tumors have been regarded as low or standard risk HB [19, 20]. This system has also been used for HCC in children. Based on the risk stratification children with liver tumors receive different regimens of chemotherapy. All children with high risk liver tumors receive delayed surgery after primary chemotherapy.

Until now, the prognostic significance of molecular findings, histology, or logarithmic α[alpha]-fetoprotein decline is still controversial. Neither the age of the children, sex and histological subtype, nor molecular genetic parameters such as LOH 11p15, DNA ploidy, and β[beta]-catein expression are significant prognostic factors for survival [21–24].

As a novel initiative the CHIC (Childhood Hepatic malignancies International Collaboration) Group has recently created a global approach to risk stratification in children with HB based on a data acquisition and interpretation combining the experiences with over 1600 patients from several international multicentre trials. Based on their analyses the authors proposed four risk groups: very low, low, intermediate, and high. This new stratification will be used as basis for adapted treatment protocols as well as for the prospective international cooperative study "Pediatric Hepatic International Tumor Trial (PHITT)". [25, 26].

56.1.1.5 Treatment

Chemotherapy. 40–60% of all liver tumors are unresectable at the time point of diagnosis and 10–20% of the children present with primary lung

Table 56.2 Relevance of preoperative chemotherapy for the resectability of liver tumors [31, 35, 86]

Entity	Response (%)	Resectabilitiy
Low risk HB	90	>90
High risk HB	74–84	64–70
HCC	46–49	36–47

metastases. The efficiency of chemotherapy in HB and HCC is proven and plays a key role for a successful treatment (Table 56.2) [27–29]. Different chemoherapy regimens are applied in HB depending on the respective stratification. Various cytotoxic drugs are used within the different international trials including cisplatin, doxorubicin, vincristin, 5-fluorouracil, irinotecan, cyclophosphamid, and carboplatin. In a randomized study the SIOPEL group could demonstrate that cisplatin monotherapy achieves similar results (complete resection rates and survival) in children with standard risk HB compared to those receiving combined doxorubicin/cisplatin treatment. This important analysis is an example for the success of reducing toxicity in standard tumors and thus preventing late effects (secondary malignancies, cardiomyopathy) [28, 30–32].

The treatment of high risk HB and relapsed HB is a challenge and requires an international collaboration in order to realize statistically relevant analyzes. High dose chemotherapy with stem cell rescue could not improve resection rates or treatment results.

The efficiency of chemotherapy in HCC is not yet clear. Several studies could show that these tumors respond to cisplatin and doxorubicin (PLADO) or cisplatin, 5-fluorouracil, and vincristin regimens. The response rate is approximately 50% in pediatric HCC treated with chemotherapy. In contrast, the response rate observed in adults is 0–33% [33]. Currently, an international study analyses the efficiency of cisplatin and doxorubicin together with the multikinase inhibitor sorafenib on HCC based on observations in adults. First results show a better response rate in comparison to conventional chemotherapy resulting in a higher rate of complete tumor resection. However, for the final judgment of response and survival rates the data are preliminary.

Surgery. Surgical procedures in pediatric liver tumors range from biopsy to extended liver resection and liver transplantation.

In the SIOPEL protocols ***tumor biopsy*** is recommended for risk stratification and biological reasons [34]. According to the German Liver Tumor Study Protocol tumor biopsy is not necessary in the age group between 6 months and 3 years as well as in cases presenting with the combination of typical radiological findings and elevated α[alpha]-fetoprotein level. In the CCSG-group primary surgery of low risk liver tumors is allowed [34–36].

Complete ***tumor resection*** is the main prognostic factor for survival in pediatric malignant liver tumors. The anatomical liver resection should be realized whenever possible because of a lower local recurrence rate [37, 38]. There exist different types of anatomical and non- anatomi-

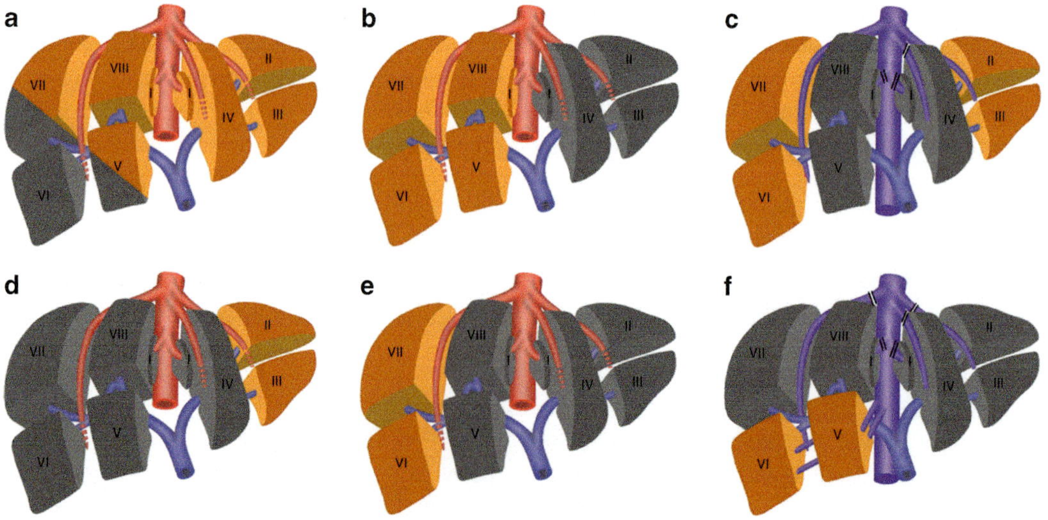

Fig. 56.3 Types of liver resections (resected portion in grey). (**a**) "Wedge resection". (**b**) Left hemihepatectomy. (**c**) Central hepatectomy ("mesohepatectomy"). (**d**) Right trisectionectomy. (**e**) Left trisectionectomy. (**f**) Atypical extended hepatectomy

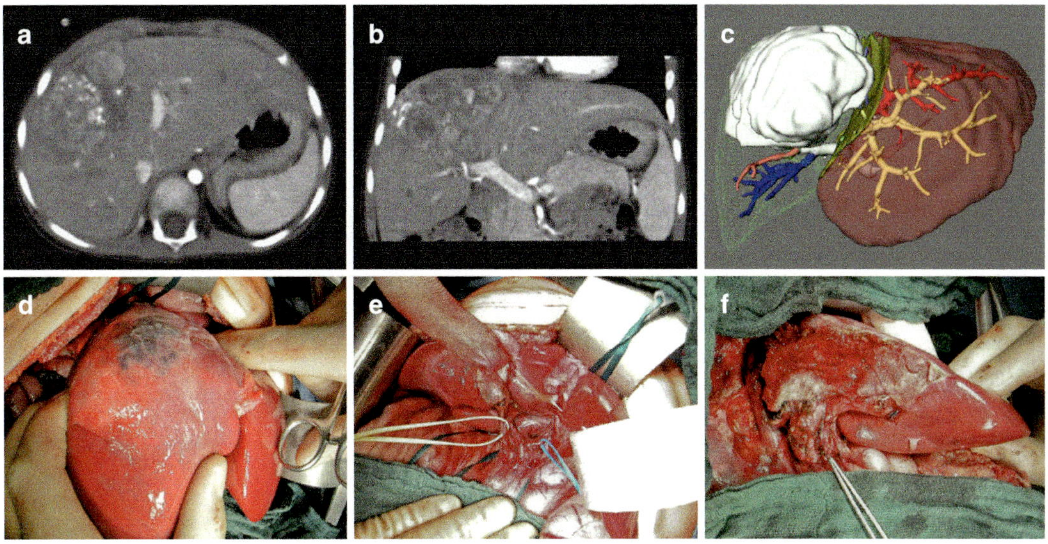

Fig. 56.4 Right TSE in a 2 year-old boy with stage I HB, NED after 6 years. (**a, b**) Tumor after chemotherapy (CT scan). (**c**) 3D reconstruction with simulation of virtual resection. (**d**) Intraoperative situs. (**e**) Dissection of porta hepatis. (**f**) Status after right TSE

cal liver resections (Fig. 56.3). In contrast to the adult population liver cirrhosis is an uncommon coexisting disease in children, also in those with HCC. Therefore, it is possible to remove up to over 80% (extended liver resection or trisegmentectomy) of the liver parenchyma without relevant liver dysfunction (Fig. 56.4) [39].

The standard approach for liver resection is the transverse laparotomy or a three-cornered, star-shaped incision when wider access is needed. The first step is the complete mobilisation of the liver. This is a precondition for achieving a free operative field and for the control of possible bleeding complications. Some surgeons prefer the preparation of vascular exclusion using loops or clamps in order to reduce the blood loss during the parenchymal phase of liver resection. Total vascular isolation is realized using the Pringle Manoeuvre; clamping of the supra- and intrahepatic cava vein is necessary in selected cases such as tumor involvement of the cava vein or hepatic veins, or in extended liver resections [40].

Usually, the Pringle manoeuvre is sufficient for reducing the blood loss during liver surgery by temporarily clamping the vascular structures within the hepatoduodenal ligament. Clamping is well tolerated for 30 min without postoperative liver dysfunctions. Vascular exclusion is possible for up to 60 min in selected cases; however, most surgeons recommend an "intermittent" form of Pringle's manoeuvre with short phases of reperfusion [41].

There exist several tools for the transsection or division of the liver parenchyma such as CUSA, harmonic knife, water-Jet, Laser devices or the conventional finger fracture technique. However, a precise knowledge of liver anatomy and tumor conditions rather is most important for the management of liver parenchyma and complete tumor resection.

Hemihepatectomies are indicated in children with PRETEXT I and II tumors. In unilocular tumors staged as PRETEXT III and IV, there is a controversial discussion between extended tumor resection versus ***liver transplantations***. Several authors could show, that children with such constellations have a good outcome (5 year overall survival above 80%) after extended right or left hepatectomies, mesohepatectomies, and extended atypical left hepatectomies [42, 43]. Otherwise, the results of primary liver transplantation are remarkable in unifocal and multifocal PRETEXT III and IV tumors (5 year overall survival above 75%) (Fig. 56.5) [42–44].

Further challenges in the surgical treatment of liver tumors are vascular involvement of hepatic,

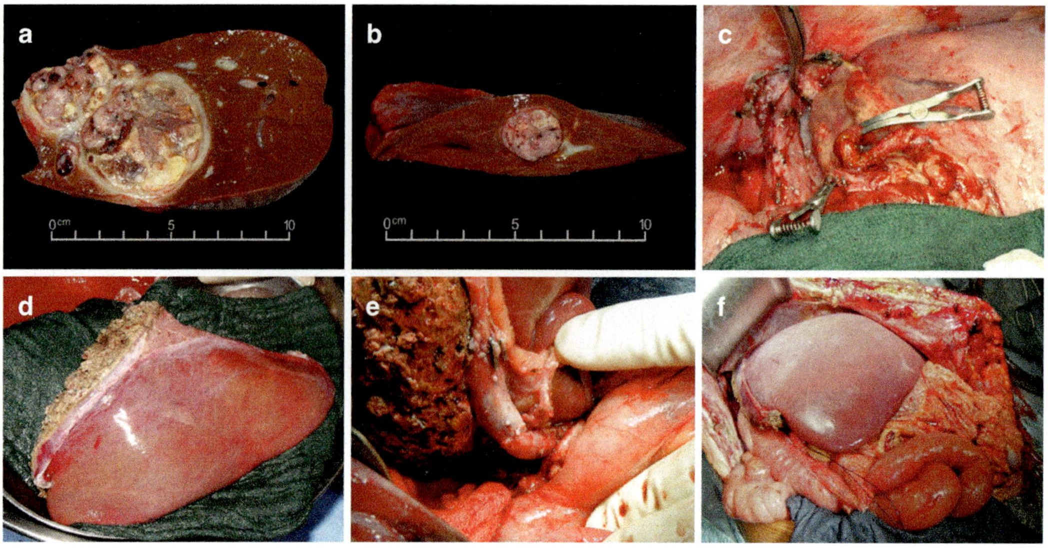

Fig. 56.5 Liver transplantation in a 6 year-old boy with multifocal Transsitional Cell Tumor, stage IV. (**a**, **b**) Macroscopic view of multiple tumor lesions within resected specimen. (**c**) Status after hepatectomy. (**d**) Donor liver (segments II/III). (**e**) Portal vein anastomosis during liver transplantation. (**f**) Status after transplantation showing a well perfused organ

cava, or portal vein and pre-existing extrahepatic disease. In these cases radical surgical procedures are indicated and include liver resection under cardiopulmonary bypass in selected cases. The number of cases is very limited and a clear treatment recommendation is difficult [45]. The German Liver Tumor Study Group HB99 analyzed the data of high risk HB with and without involvement of major hepatic vessels. On one hand there was a difference in overall and event free 3-year survival in both groups, on the other hand the data showed that radical surgery with reconstruction of large vessels can lead to an improved survival in selected cases.

The SIOPEL III study demonstrated the positive impact of liver transplantation in children with multifocal HB. Although there is a controversial discussion about the detailed indication of liver transplantation in HB and HCC, this procedure is recommended in all multifocal liver tumors without extrahepatic disease [46]. Pre-existing lung metastases are not a contraindication for liver transplantation in HB; however, they should be cleared after chemotherapy or be surgically removed prior to transplantation. The results of primary liver transplantations are significantly better than results of rescue transplantations [44, 47]. However, all relevant data in this field are based on retrospective analyses. Meanwhile a world wide database for these highly complex tumors has been established for prospectively judging the long term outcome (PLUTO—Pediatric Liver Unresectable Tumor Observatory) [48].

The Milan criteria (single tumor below 5 cm in diameter; or less than three lesions below 3 cm in diameter, absence of macrovascular invasion and extrahepatic disease) were developed for adult HCC. These criteria have been expanded to come closer to the "up-to-seven" recommendation, where the summary of the largest tumor size and the numbers of tumor nodules should not exceed seven. Nevertheless, the relevance of these criteria has not yet been clarified for children. Some authors report on survival of children with more than three nodules and larger tumors after liver transplantation. Accordingly, some oncologists recommend liver transplantation in children showing response to neoadjuvant chemotherapy regardless of macrovascular invasion and extrahepatic disease. In the end, these constellations are often controversially discussed without clear concept.

56.1.1.6 Treatment of Lung Metastases

Primary lung metastases occur in almost 20% of children with ***hepatoblastoma***. These children are regarded as high risk patients and are usually treated with an intensified chemotherapy regimen [49]. Primary hepatoblastoma lung metastases generally respond sufficiently to chemotherapy and often disappear completely. All relevant international trails recommend surgical treatment of lung metastases persisting after initial chemotherapy as well as an aggressive surgical management of lung relapses. In some situations, patients benefit from a simultaneous resection of lung metastases together with the hepatic resection of the liver tumor in a single stage approach [50]. Because of the possible need for a liver transplantation [51, 52], metastasectomy should especially be performed in cases of PRETEXT III tumors with involvement of hepatic/portal vein or in children with PRETEXT IV tumors and persistent nodules after several cycles of chemotherapy. However, the number of respective patients is low and in contrast to other embryonal tumors the determination of independent prognostic factors with statistical power is difficult in this subgroup. Otherwise serum α[alpha]-fetoprotein level is an available tumor marker in hepatoblastoma patients for the judgment of follow up and detection of relapses. This also applies in lung metastases. Serum α[alpha]-fetoprotein levels can be used for distinguishing between benign and malignant lesions. Metastatic disease in hepatoblastoma is combined with a poorer outcome. Most reports on the relevance of lung metastases surgery in hepatoblastoma have an anecdotal character. The SIOPEL Study group could significantly improve their treatment results over three study periods. In the SIOPEL-3 HR study the 3 year event free survival was 56% and the overall survival was 62% (71 study patients with metastases) [32].The SIOPEL experiences underline the relevance of radical surgery in combination with intensified chemotherapy in cases of metastatic disease.

56.1.1.7 Chemoembolization, Radiofrequency Ablation, and Cryoablation

The experiences with hepatic artery chemoembolization (HACE) for children with liver tumors are limited. After a temporary occlusion of the tumor supplying artery, different cytotoxic drugs are applied (cisplatin, doxorubicin, mitomycin) every 2–4 weeks until tumor become surgically resectable. In approximately 30–40% of all cases the tumor resection was reported feasible. A tolerable toxicity has been described. However, this method is an experimental treatment option and only indicated in selected cases with an unresectable status after chemotherapy and when there is a contraindication for liver transplantation [53–55].

Radiofrequency ablation is used effectively in adults with recurrent HCC or other metastatic lesions in the liver below 3 cm in diameter. There exist no series in pediatric populations; this technique may be useful for ablation in cases of local recurrences. The technique can be used percutaneously, laparoscopically, or as open approach under ultrasound guidance. Another option is the cryoablation with liquid nitrogen or argon gas units (temperature below 160 °C). Both techniques are a reasonable alternative for selected patients [56].

56.1.1.8 Prognosis

The prognosis of children with HB has been significantly improved over last two decades due to a better risk stratification with selective treatment concepts. Meanwhile the 5 year overall survival of children with standard or low risk HB is nearly 90% in all international trials [57]. Microscopic tumor rests do not influence the prognosis significantly [30, 35, 58]. High risk tumors are a major challenge. The 5-year overall survival of patients with lung metastases is 65–70% and the event free survival is 55–63% including all treatment options such as liver transplantation and intensified chemotherapy. Only 33% of the children with an initial AFP below 100 μg/l survive after 3 years [32]. The introduction of liver transplantation improved the outcome of children with high risk tumors [59]. It is remarkable that the 5-year overall survival in children with primary liver transplantation is 85% whereas it is 40% in patients undergoing rescue liver transplantation for incomplete tumor resection or tumor recurrence [60].

Children with initially completely resectable HCC have a good prognosis and benefit from adjuvant chemotherapy. The 5-year overall survival ranges between 70 and 80%. In contrast, children with advanced HCC (stage III or/and PRETEXT III) have a poor outcome with a 5-year overall survival of 15–20% [33, 61]. There are almost no survivors in the group of children with stage IV HCC. For the last two subgroups new therapeutic strategies are needed. In contrast to earlier studies the fibrocellular variant does not seem to have a better prognosis than the other HCC [62]. Presence of lung metastases and macrovascular invasion are among the strongest predictors for tumor recurrence within the transplanted liver. Therefore, the indications for liver transplantation in children with HCC have to be analyzed in a world wide data bank such as PLUTO for better definition of indications for liver transplantation. Finally, due to the preliminary data the effect of sorafenib on the outcome of children with HCC cannot yet be definitely judged [63].

56.1.2 Liver Sarcoma

Undifferentiated embryonal sarcomas of the liver (UESL) account for 5–10% of malignant liver tumors in children. The histological appearance is mesenchymal but can at the same time be characterized by a morphological diversity. Tumor cells often are spindle-shaped with an ill-defined outline. By now there is no specific immunohistochemical expression marker [64, 65]. A link between this entity and mesenchymal hamartoma of the liver is currently being controversially discussed [66].

Clinical presentation combines abdominal pain and a mass of the upper right abdomen. Diagnostic workup regularly reveals a discrepancy of internal architecture between Ultrasound and CT scan [67].

Chemosensitivity has been observed in some tumors, but complete surgical resection represents the central prognostic factor of treatment for children with UESL. However, this might be difficult to accomplish in some cases because of complex tumor extension or possible vascular invasion.

Despite the introduction of multimodal treatment approaches the outcome of patients is still unfavorable. Overall survival rates (approximately 20% after 5 years) are impaired by the occurrence of local relapses or secondary distant metastases.

Angiosarcoma of the liver usually affects adults and is rarely seen in children. The rarity of this tumor in the pediatric population makes the diagnosis of angiosarcoma in patients younger than 21 years a difficult proposition. As part of the group of vascular hepatic tumors, this entity presents predominantly with an abdominal mass. However the whole spectrum of clinical appearances of hepatic vascular tumors might be observed including high-output cardiac failure and Kasabach-Merritt-Syndrome. Histologically, tumors display hyperchromatic epitheloid or spindle-shaped cells which contain mitotic activity. Cells are commonly positive for the endothelial marker CD31.

Distinguishing hepatic angiosarcoma from other hepatic vascular tumors might be difficult and requires open biopsy in cases of uncertainty. Because of the aggressive behavior, a radical surgical approach including liver transplantation is justified in this entity [68].

56.1.3 Malignant Rhabdoid Tumor of the Liver

Malignant rhabdoid tumors (MRT) of the liver are rare and associated with a poor prognosis. Histologically they show an epitheloid differentiation and express cytokeratin and vimentin. Recent reports suggest that germ line and acquired mutations of the INI1 gene are present in MRTs and this is associated with absence of immunostaining for INI1 in the tumor tissue. The prognosis of this tumor is poor, however, successful treatment results with combined chemotherapy (ICE and VDC) together with secondary complete resection have been reported [69].

56.1.4 Infantile Choriocarcinoma

This rare but highly aggressive malignancy arises from the trophoblastic cells of the placenta. It is regularly associated with anemia and hepatomegaly. Serum β[beta]-HCG levels are usually elevated and can be used for diagnostic workup as well as for follow up. Tumors are highly vascularized. Mortality is high because of a rapid tumor progression. Several cases of successful treatment approaches have been reported, usually combining multimodal neoadjuvant chemotherapy and secondary complete resection [70, 71].

56.2 Benign Liver Tumors

56.2.1 Hemangioma

Hemangioma is the most common benign liver tumor of infancy and childhood; in over 80% of cases the diagnosis is made within the first 6 months of live. It occurs slightly more often in girls than in boys [72]. The exact incidence of liver hemangioma is difficult to judge since many tumors don't cause symptoms and are therefore not diagnosed. Also, many lesions do not require surgery or non-surgical treatment.

56.2.1.1 Pathology

Hemangioma may occur unifocally or multifocally within the liver. In accordance with the current classification of pediatric vascular tumors, liver hemangioma are sub-divided into lesions with or without spontaneous regression. The expression of Glucose Transporter Protein 1 (GLUT-1) allows differentiating between the two subgroups. The term "hemangioendothelioma of the liver" should not be longer used.

56.2.1.2 Clinical Presentation and Diagnostic Workup

In some cases the diagnosis is established prenatally. It is sometimes associated with a fetal hydrops. Liver hemangiomas are possibly associated with cutaneous hemangiomas. The leading post-natal symptom is a distended abdomen. A possibly life-threatening high output cardiac failure is present in up to 15% of cases. Without treatment this can lead to death in approximately 80% of cases. In 15–60% of cases hemangioma are detectable on other parts of the body, namely skin, pancreas, bones, and others (Fig. 56.6). Children are at risk of developing critical clinical conditions such as Kasabach-Merritt-Syndrome.

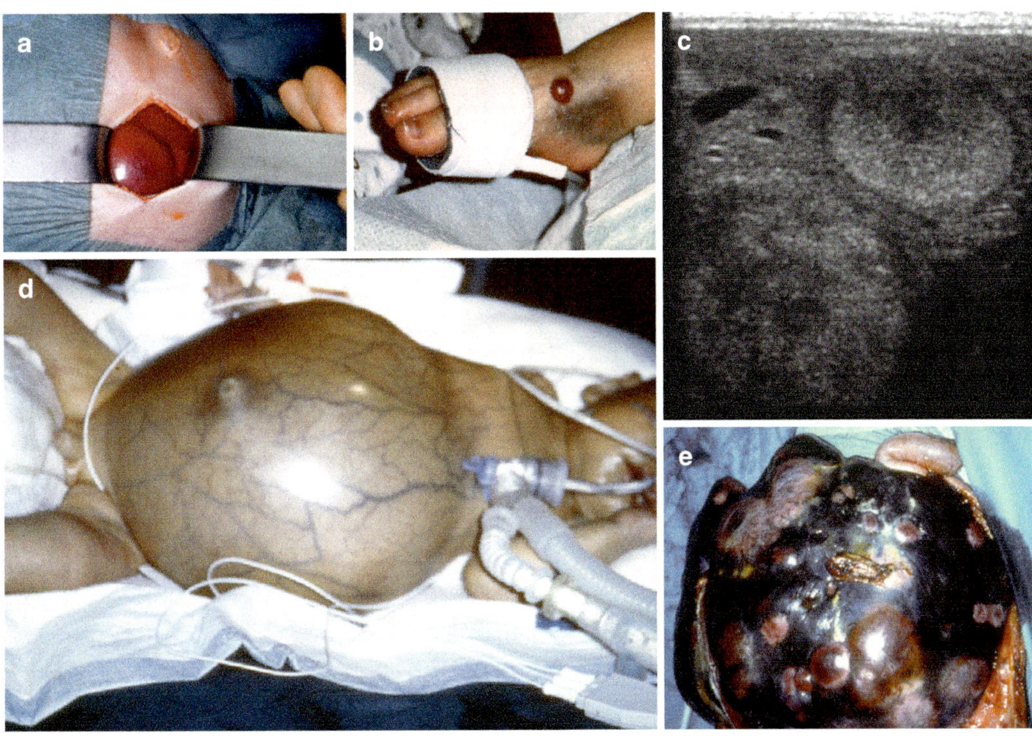

Fig. 56.6 Hemangiomatosis in a 6 month-old boy with multifocal involvement of liver segments. (**a**) Primary biopsy of a solid area. (**b**–**d**) Subsequent rapid tumor progress despite conservative treatment. (**e**) Intraoperative aspect during hepatectomy and liver transplantation (The child survived without evidence of disease)

Anaemia is present in over 50% of patients, approximately 20% develop hyperbilirubinaemia; elevation of serum transaminases can also occur. Furthermore, serum α[alpha]-fetoprotein can be increased making delineation of malignant epithelial liver tumors difficult.

Doppler sonography is the determining diagnostic tool regularly displaying hyperechogenic and increasingly perfused areas, an increased velocity within the hepatic artery (up to 100–200 cm/s), and a calibre change of the abdominal aorta at the celiac trunk-level [73]. Occasionally, the appearance might resemble solid nodules which should be clarified histologically. Regression is a regularly observed development in liver hemangioma. Indicators are size reduction, reduction of perfusion parameters, or calcification.

Computed tomography (CT) scan or Angio-Magnet Resonance Imaging (MRI) are important additional tools which have their relevance in the context of differential diagnoses. Angiography is mainly reserved for interventional treatment approaches.

56.2.1.3 Therapy

Depending on the clinical presentation, therapeutic options display a wide variation ranging from simple observation to liver transplantation.

Typical small asymptomatic nodules within the parenchyma can be observed since they are associated with a high probability for spontaneous regression. In contrast, symptomatic children require prompt treatment which often includes intensive care measures. Management of cardiac failure is hereby the initial therapeutic aim.

Medical treatment approaches for hepatic hemangioma include administration of high dose steroids (for example Prednisolon 2–5 mg/kg/day for 4 weeks), α[alpha]-interferon (1–33 mU/m^2/day), or β[beta]-blocker [74]. However, experiences concerning treatment of liver hemangioma in children using the latter are thus far limited. Success rates of steroids have been reported as being up to 25%; interferon therapy seems more successful (success rates 50–80%) [75].

Supra-selective embolization of liver hemangioma represents an alternative to surgery which can successfully be applied in bilobar processes as well. It has already been used in newborns or infants; experienced specialists use the approach via femoral vein, oval foramen, and descending aorta to the hepatic artery [76].

Surgery is indicated in unilobar lesions and preferably consists of anatomical resection. Ligation of the right or left hepatic artery represents an alternative to interventional approaches although there is no supra-selectivity and a higher risk for liver necrosis. Liver transplantation serves as ultima ratio in cases of multifocal hamangiomas with critical and/or progressive clinical course.

Today, a staged approach is commonly used as basis for the treatment of hepatic hemangioma; Fig. 56.7 displays a proposed system. The relevance of chemotherapy as well as irradiation is currently regarded as low since there are several other treatment options.

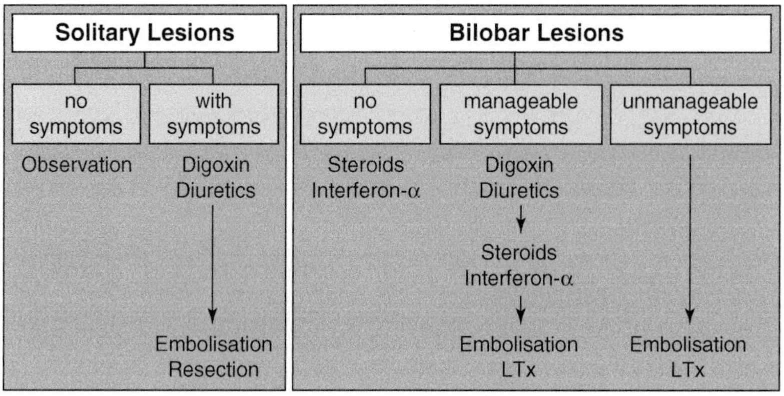

Fig. 56.7 Management of liver hemangioma

56.2.2 Hamartoma

Mesenchymal Hamartomas of the liver are the second most common benign liver tumor. In 85% of cases they are diagnosed in children below of 2 years of age; boys are more often affected than girls [77].

56.2.2.1 Pathology

The lesions are mostly cystic, might however also appear peduncular within the parenchyma. The cysts are lined with epithelium as well as endothelium. Whether they represent real tumors or rather hamartuous malformations is a still ongoing debate.

56.2.2.2 Clinical Presentation and Diagnostic

Leading symptom is a distended abdomen with a palpable mass in projection of the liver. Classical unspecific symptoms include vomiting, anaemia, or loss of appetite. If affected, newborns are often in critical clinical conditions displaying respiratory distress syndrome. In some cases when hydrops is present, the diagnosis of liver hamartoma can be established antenatally.

There are no typical tumor markers or other specific serum parameters. Differentiation of hamartoma from hemangioma or malignant epithelial tumors is possible using imaging analyses (Ultrasound, CT scan, MRI). Echogenic nodules and multicystic fluid-filled septated lesions are typical radiological findings in hepatic hamartoma [78].

56.2.2.3 Therapy

Surgical resection is the treatment of choice in hepatic hamartoma. Liver transplantation has to be considered in cases of bilobar affection because marsupilation and debulking are both associated with high rates of tumor recurrence.

Furthermore, there is a relevant risk of malignant transformation into undifferentiated embryonal sarcoma. In rare cases spontaneous regression has been observed following biopsy of the lesions [79].

56.2.2.4 Prognosis

Prognosis of hepatic hamartoma is excellent after complete resection. However, relevant intra- and postoperative complications have been described which must not be neglected [78].

56.2.3 Adenoma

Hepatic adenomas in children are rare. Associations with maternal intake of contraceptives or corticoids, but also with diabetes mellitus and disorders of glycogen metabolism have been observed. Cytologically, adenomas are hardly distinguishable from normal hepatocytes. The microscopic lobular architecture is lacking in adenomas.

These tumors sometimes cause upper abdominal pain and subsequent diagnostic workup reveals the mass within the liver. At ultrasound, adenomas are commonly isodens with sporadic inhomogeneous areas caused by haemorrhage. Definite diagnostic workup should be performed using CT scan and/or MRI. In some cases differentiation from focal nodular hyperplasia or highly differentiated hepatocellular carcinoma (HCC) is impossible and biopsy becomes necessary in order to achieve a definite diagnosis [80]. Because of relevant associated risks (intratumoral or intraabdominal haemorrhage, malignant transformation) complete resection of the tumor is recommended.

56.2.4 Focal Nodular Hyperplasia (FNH)

This tumor occurs in up to 3% of the adult population which makes it a quite common liver lesion. Only a small number of cases have been reported in children. The age maximum lies between 7 and 14 years. A correlation with intake of contraceptives has been discussed. However, the exact aetiology of these tumors is still unclear. FNH occur increasingly as secondary tumor after various malignant diseases [81, 82]. Diagnosis is often made by chance in the workup of other

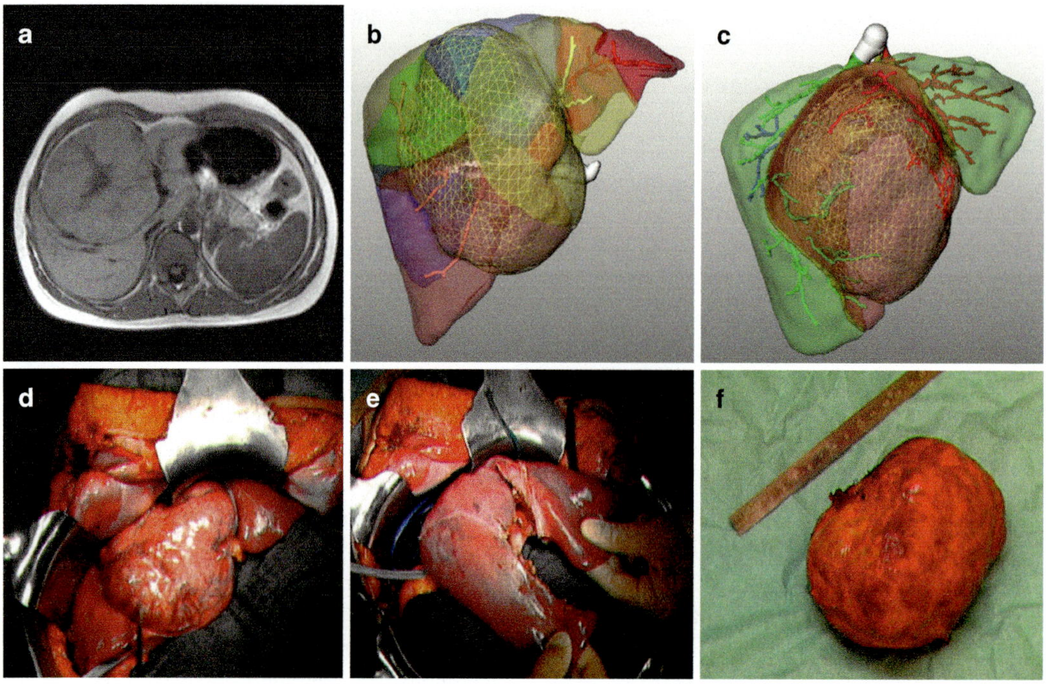

Fig. 56.8 Focal nodular hyperplasia (FNH) in a 12 year-old girl. (**a**) MRI scan showing the centrally located tumor. (**b**) 3D reconstruction of liver with portal venous segmentation and tumor. (**c**) Virtual simulation of central hepatectomy. (**d**) Intraoperative situs. (**e**) Intraoperative view after mesohepatectomy. (**f**) Resected specimen

pathologies. Morphologically, there is a central region of fibrosis, usually with vessels of increased diameter. Hepatocytes are cytologically unsuspicious; however, they don't display the typical lobular architecture of the liver.

Ultrasound plays a prominent role within the diagnostic workup. Hepatic scintigraphy (HIDA-scan) and MRI are important especially for excluding differential diagnoses. Most authors suggest the surgical resection of the lesions since simultaneous existence of HB/HCC has been described [83, 84] (Fig. 56.8). However, a wait-and-see-strategy has also been described [85].

References

1. Perilongo G, Shafford EA. Liver tumours. Eur J Cancer. 1999;35(6):953–8.
2. Jaing TH, Hung IJ, Lin JN, Lien RI, Hsueh C, Lu CS. Hepatoblastoma in a child of extremely low birth weight. Am J Perinatol. 2002;19(3):149–53.
3. Hadzic N, Finegold MJ. Liver neoplasia in children. Clin Liver Dis. 2011;15(2):443–62.
4. Spector LG, Ji H, Ross JEA. Hepatoblastoma incidence and very low birth weight in the US, 1981–1999. Am J Epidemiol. 2003;157(11):S15.
5. Zimmermann A. Pediatric liver tumors and hepatic ontogenesis: Common and distinctive pathways. Med Pediatr Oncol. 2002;39(5):492–503.
6. Hill DA, Swanson PE, Anderson K, et al. Desmoplastic nested spindle cell tumor of liver: report of four cases of a proposed new entity. Am J Surg Pathol. 2005;29(1):1–9.
7. Gupta AA, Gerstle JT, Ng V, et al. Critical review of controversial issues in the management of advanced pediatric liver tumors. Pediatr Blood Cancer. 2011;56(7):1013–8.
8. Wang JD, Chang TK, Chen HC, et al. Pediatric liver tumors: initial presentation, image finding and outcome. Pediatr Int. 2007;49(4):491–6.
9. Thomas D, Pritchard J, Davidson R, McKiernan P, Grundy RG, de Goyet JD. Familial hepatoblastoma and APC gene mutations: renewed call for molecular research. Eur J Cancer. 2003;39(15):2200–4.
10. Murray MJ, Nicholson JC. Alpha-fetoprotein. Arch Dis Child Educ Pract Ed. 2011;96(4):141–7.
11. von Schweinitz D. Management of liver tumors in childhood. Semin Pediatr Surg. 2006;15(1):17–24.
12. Al-Hussein HA, Graham EM, Tekes A, Huisman TA. Pre- and postnatal imaging of a congenital hepatoblastoma. Fetal Diagn Ther. 2011;30(2):157–9.

13. Warmann SW, Schenk A, Schaefer JF et al. Computer-assisted surgery planning in children with complex liver tumors identifies variability of the classical Couinaud classification. J Pediatr Surg. 2016;51(11):1801–6. doi: 10.1016/j.jpedsurg.2016.05.018.
14. Sironi S, Messa C, Cistaro A, et al. Recurrent hepatoblastoma in orthotopic transplanted liver: detection with FDG positron emission tomography. AJR Am J Roentgenol. 2004;182(5):1214–6.
15. Meyers RL, Katzenstein HM, Malogolowkin MH. Predictive value of staging systems in hepatoblastoma. J Clin Oncol. 2007;25(6):737–8.
16. Aronson DC, Schnater JM, Staalman CR, et al. Predictive value of the pretreatment extent of disease system in hepatoblastoma: results from the International Society of Pediatric Oncology Liver Tumor Study Group SIOPEL-1 study. J Clin Oncol. 2005;23(6):1245–52.
17. Roebuck DJ, Olsen O, Pariente D. Radiological staging in children with hepatoblastoma. Pediatr Radiol. 2006;36(3):176–82.
18. Meyers RL, Rowland JR, Krailo M, Chen Z, Katzenstein HM, Malogolowkin MH. Predictive power of pretreatment prognostic factors in children with hepatoblastoma: a report from the Children's Oncology Group. Pediatr Blood Cancer. 2009;53(6):1016–22.
19. von Schweinitz D. Identification of risk groups in hepatoblastoma—another step in optimising therapy. Eur J Cancer. 2000;36(11):1343–6.
20. Brown J, Perilongo G, Shafford E, et al. Pretreatment prognostic factors for children with hepatoblastoma results from the International Society of Paediatric Oncology (SIOP) Study SIOPEL 1. Eur J Cancer. 2000;36(11):1418–25.
21. von Schweinitz D, Kraus JA, Albrecht S, Koch A, Fuchs J, Pietsch T. Prognostic impact of molecular genetic alterations in hepatoblastoma. Med Pediatr Oncol. 2002;38(2):104–8.
22. Yeh YA, Rao PH, Cigna CT, Middlesworth W, Lefkowitch JH, Murty VVVS. Trisomy 1q, 2, and 20 in a case of hepatoblastoma: Possible significance of 2q35-q37 and 1q12-q21 rearrangements. Cancer Genet Cytogenet. 2000;123(2):140–3.
23. Taniguchi K, Roberts LR, Aderca IN, et al. Mutational spectrum of beta-catenin, AXIN1, and AXIN2 in hepatocellular carcinomas and hepatoblastomas. Oncogene. 2002;21(31):4863–71.
24. Zerbini MCN, Sredni ST, Grier H, et al. Primary malignant epithelial tumors of the liver in children: A study of DNA content and oncogene expression. Pediatr Dev Pathol. 1998;1(4):270–80.
25. Czauderna P, Haeberle B, Hiyama E, et al. The Children's Hepatic tumors International Collaboration (CHIC): Novel global rare tumor database yields new prognostic factors in hepatoblastoma and becomes a research model. Eur J Cancer. 2016;52:92–101.
26. Meyers RL, Maibach R, Hiyama E, Häberle B, Krailo M, Rangaswami A, Aronson DC, Malogolowkin MH, Perilongo G, von Schweinitz D, Ansari M, Lopez-Terrada D, Tanaka Y, Alaggio R, Leuschner I, Hishiki T, Schmid I, Watanabe K, Yoshimura K, Feng Y, Rinaldi E, Saraceno D, Derosa M, Czauderna P. Risk-stratified staging in paediatric hepatoblastoma: a unified analysis from the Children's Hepatic tumors International Collaboration. Lancet Oncol. 2017;18(1):122–131.
27. Katzenstein HM, Rigsby C, Shaw PH, Mitchell TL, Haut PR, Kletzel M. Novel therapeutic approaches in the treatment of children with hepatoblastoma. J Pediatr Hematol Oncol. 2002;24(9):751–5.
28. Perilongo G, Shafford E, Maibach R, et al. Risk-adapted treatment for childhood hepatoblastoma. final report of the second study of the International Society of Paediatric Oncology—SIOPEL 2. Eur J Cancer. 2004;40(3):411–21.
29. Haberle B, Bode U, von Schweinitz D. Differentiated treatment protocols for high- and standard-risk hepatoblastoma—An interim report of the German liver tumor study HB 99. Klin Padiatr. 2003;215(3):159–65.
30. Malogolowkin MH, Katzenstein H, Krailo MD, et al. Intensified platinum therapy is an ineffective strategy for improving outcome in pediatric patients with advanced hepatoblastoma. J Clin Oncol. 2006;24(18):2879–84.
31. Perilongo G, Maibach R, Shafford E, et al. Cisplatin versus cisplatin plus doxorubicin for standard-risk hepatoblastoma. N Engl J Med. 2009;361(17):1662–70.
32. Zsiros J, Maibach R, Shafford E, et al. Successful treatment of childhood high-risk hepatoblastoma with dose-intensive multiagent chemotherapy and surgery: final results of the SIOPEL-3HR study. J Clin Oncol. 2010;28(15):2584–90.
33. Katzenstein HM, Krailo MD, Malogolowkin MH, et al. Fibrolamellar hepatocellular carcinoma in children and adolescents. Cancer. 2003;97(8):2006–12.
34. Schnater JM, Kuijper CF, Zsiros J, Heij HA, Aronson DC. Pre-operative diagnostic biopsy and surgery in paediatric liver tumours—the Amsterdam experience. Eur J Surg Oncol. 2005;31(10):1160–5.
35. Fuchs J, Rydzynski J, von Schweinitz D, et al. Pretreatment prognostic factors and treatment results in children with hepatoblastoma—A report from the German Cooperative Pediatric Liver Tumor Study HB 94. Cancer. 2002;95(1):172–82.
36. Parikh B, Jojo A, Shah B, Bansal R, Trivedi P, Shah MJ. Fine needle aspiration cytology of hepatoblastoma: a study of 20 cases. Indian J Pathol Microbiol. 2005;48(3):331–6.
37. Czauderna P, Otte JB, Aronson DC, et al. Guidelines for surgical treatment of hepatoblastoma in the modern era—recommendations from the Childhood Liver Tumour Strategy Group of the International Society of Paediatric Oncology (SIOPEL). Eur J Cancer. 2005;41(7):1031–6.
38. Fuchs J, Rydzynski J, Hecker H, et al. The influence of preoperative chemotherapy and surgical technique in the treatment of hepatoblastoma—A report from the German Cooperative Liver Tumour Studies HB 89 and HB 94. Eur J Pediatr Surg. 2002;12(4):255–61.

39. Schnater JM, Aronson DC, Plaschkes J, et al. Surgical view of the treatment of patients with hepatoblastoma—Results from the first prospective trial of the International Society of Pediatric Oncology Liver Tumor Study Group (SIOPEL-1). Cancer. 2002;94(4):1111–20.
40. Pritchard J, Stringer M. Outcome and complications after resection of hepatoblastoma. J Pediatr Surg. 2004;39(11):1744–5.
41. Szavay PO, Luithle T, Warmann SW, Geerlings H, Ure BM, Fuchs J. Impact of pedicle clamping in pediatric liver resection. Surg Oncol. 2008;17(1):17–22.
42. Guerin F, Gauthier F, Martelli H, et al. Outcome of central hepatectomy for hepatoblastomas. J Pediatr Surg. 2010;45(3):555–63.
43. Superina RA, Bambini D, Filler RM, Almond PS, Geissler G. A new technique for resecting 'unresectable' liver tumors. J Pediatr Surg. 2000; 35(9):1294–9.
44. Fuchs J, Cavdar S, Blumenstock G et al. POST-TEXT III and IV Hepatoblastoma: Extended hepatic resection avoids liver transplantation in selected cases. Ann Surg. 2017;266(2):318–23.
45. Oldhafer KJ, Fuchs J, Steinhoff G, Mildenberger H. Extended liver resection in children under circulatory arrest and "low flow" cardiopulmonary bypass. Chirurg. 2000;71(6):692–5.
46. Barrena S, Hernandez F, Miguel M, et al. High-risk hepatoblastoma: results in a pediatric liver transplantation center. Eur J Pediatr Surg. 2011;21(1):18–20.
47. Stringer M, Pimpalwar A, Tovar J, Iyer Y, Tam P. Strategy for Hepatoblastoma management: Transplant versus nontransplant surgery—Discussion. J Pediatr Surg. 2002;37(2):245.
48. Otte JB, Meyers R. PLUTO first report. Pediatr Transplant. 2010;14(7):830–5.
49. Perilongo G, Brown J, Shafford E, et al. Hepatoblastoma presenting with lung metastases—Treatment results of the first cooperative, prospective study of the International Society of Paediatric Oncology on Childhood Liver Tumors. Cancer. 2000;89(8):1845–53.
50. Urla C, Seitz G, Tsiflikas I, et al. Simultaneous Resection of High-risk Liver Tumors and Pulmonary Metastases in Children. Ann Surg. 2015;262(1):e1–3.
51. Otte JB, de Ville DG, Reding R. Liver transplantation for hepatoblastoma: indications and contraindications in the modern era. Pediatr Transplant. 2005;9(5):557–65.
52. Otte JB. de Ville dG. The contribution of transplantation to the treatment of liver tumors in children. Semin Pediatr Surg. 2005;14(4):233–8.
53. Czauderna P, Zbrzezniak G, Narozanski W, Korzon M, Wyszomirska M, Stoba C. Preliminary experience with arterial chemoembolization for hepatoblastoma and hepatocellular carcinoma in children. Pediatr Blood Cancer. 2006;46(7):825–8.
54. Malogolowkin MH, Stanley P, Steele DA, Ortega JA. Feasibility and toxicity of chemoembolization for children with liver tumors. J Clin Oncol. 2000;18(6):1279–84.
55. Tashjian DB, Moriarty KP, Courtney RA, Bean MS, Steele DA. Preoperative chemoembolization for unresectable hepatoblastoma. Pediatr Surg Int. 2002;18(2–3):187–9.
56. Goering JD, Mahvi DM, Niederhuber JE, Chicks D, Rikkers LF. Cryoablation and liver resection for noncolorectal liver metastases. Am J Surg. 2002;183(4):384–9.
57. Schnater JM, Kohler SE, Lamers WH, von Schweinitz D, Aronson DC. Where do we stand with hepatoblastoma? Cancer. 2003;98(4):668–78.
58. Sasaki F, Matsunaga T, Iwafuchi M, et al. Outcome of hepatoblastoma treated with the JPLT-1 (Japanese Study Group for Pediatric Liver Tumor) protocol-1: A report from the Japanese Study Group for Pediatric Liver Tumor. J Pediatr Surg. 2002;37(6):851–6.
59. Stringer MD. The role of liver transplantation in the management of paediatric liver tumours. Ann R Coll Surg Engl. 2007;89(1):12–21.
60. Otte JB, Pritchard J, Aronson DC, et al. Liver transplantation for hepatoblastoma: results from the International Society of Pediatric Oncology (SIOP) study SIOPEL-1 and review of the world experience. Pediatr Blood Cancer. 2004;42(1):74–83.
61. Katzenstein HM, Krailo MD, Malogolowkin MH, et al. Hepatocellular carcinoma in children and adolescents: Results from the Pediatric Oncology Group and the Children's Cancer Group intergroup study. J Clin Oncol. 2002;20(12):2789–97.
62. Czauderna P. Adult type vs. childhood hepatocellular carcinoma—Are they the same or different lesions? Biology, natural history, prognosis, and treatment. Med Pediatr Oncol. 2002;39(5):519–23.
63. Hutten M, Lassay L, Sachs B, et al. Successful topical treatment of sorafenib-induced hand-foot skin reaction in a child with hepatocellular carcinoma. Pediatr Dermatol. 2009;26(3):349–50.
64. Leuschner I, Schmidt D, Harms D. Undifferentiated sarcoma of the liver in childhood: morphology, flow cytometry, and literature review. Hum Pathol. 1990;21(1):68–76.
65. Lack EE, Schloo BL, Azumi N, Travis WD, Grier HE, Kozakewich HP. Undifferentiated (embryonal) sarcoma of the liver. Clinical and pathologic study of 16 cases with emphasis on immunohistochemical features. Am J Surg Pathol. 1991;15(1):1–16.
66. Shehata BM, Gupta NA, Katzenstein HM, et al. Undifferentiated embryonal sarcoma of the liver is associated with mesenchymal hamartoma and multiple chromosomal abnormalities: a review of eleven cases. Pediatr Dev Pathol. 2011;14(2):111–6.
67. Moon WK, Kim WS, Kim IO, et al. Undifferentiated embryonal sarcoma of the liver: US and CT findings. Pediatr Radiol. 1994;24(7):500–3.
68. Geramizadeh B, Safari A, Bahador A, et al. Hepatic angiosarcoma of childhood: a case report and review of literature. J Pediatr Surg. 2011;46(1):e9–11.
69. Jayaram A, Finegold MJ, Parham DM, Jasty R. Successful management of rhabdoid tumor of the liver. J Pediatr Hematol Oncol. 2007;29(6):406–8.

70. Szavay PO, Wermes C, Fuchs J, Schrappe M, Flemming P, Von SD. Effective treatment of infantile choriocarcinoma in the liver with chemotherapy and surgical resection: a case report. J Pediatr Surg. 2000;35(7):1134–5.
71. Hanson D, Walter AW, Dunn S, Rittenhouse DW, Griffin G. Infantile choriocarcinoma in a neonate with massive liver involvement cured with chemotherapy and liver transplant. J Pediatr Hematol Oncol. 2011;33(6):e258–60.
72. Weinberg AG, Finegold MJ. Primary hepatic tumors of childhood. Hum Pathol. 1983;14(6):512–37.
73. Sato M, Ishida H, Konno K, et al. Liver tumors in children and young patients: sonographic and color Doppler findings. Abdom Imaging. 2000;25(6):596–601.
74. Horii KA, Drolet BA, Frieden IJ, et al. Prospective study of the frequency of hepatic hemangiomas in infants with multiple cutaneous infantile hemangiomas. Pediatr Dermatol. 2011;28(3):245–53.
75. Szymik-Kantorowicz S, Kobylarz K, Krysta M, et al. Interferon-alpha in the treatment of high-risk haemangiomas in infants. Eur J Pediatr Surg. 2005;15(1):11–6.
76. Warmann S, Bertram H, Kardorff R, Sasse M, Hausdorf G, Fuchs J. Interventional treatment of infantile hepatic hemangioendothelioma. J Pediatr Surg. 2003;38(8):1177–81.
77. von Schweinitz D. Neonatal liver tumours. Semin Neonatol. 2003;8(5):403–10.
78. Stringer MD, Alizai NK. Mesenchymal hamartoma of the liver: a systematic review. J Pediatr Surg. 2005;40(11):1681–90.
79. Fuchs J, Schweinitz DV, Feickert HJ. Acute respiratory distress syndrome following resection of a mesenchymal hamartoma of the liver. Med Pediatr Oncol. 1999;32(2):151–3.
80. Takayasu H, Motoi T, Kanamori Y, et al. Two case reports of childhood liver cell adenomas harboring beta-catenin abnormalities. Hum Pathol. 2002;33(8):852–5.
81. Bouyn CI, Leclere J, Raimondo G, et al. Hepatic focal nodular hyperplasia in children previously treated for a solid tumor. Incidence, risk factors, and outcome. Cancer. 2003;97(12):3107–13.
82. Towbin AJ, Luo GG, Yin H, Mo JQ. Focal nodular hyperplasia in children, adolescents, and young adults. Pediatr Radiol. 2011;41(3):341–9.
83. Gutweiler JR, Yu DC, Kim HB, et al. Hepatoblastoma presenting with focal nodular hyperplasia after treatment of neuroblastoma. J Pediatr Surg. 2008;43(12):2297–300.
84. Lautz T, Tantemsapya N, Dzakovic A, Superina R. Focal nodular hyperplasia in children: clinical features and current management practice. J Pediatr Surg. 2010;45(9):1797–803.
85. Reymond D, Plaschkes J, Luthy AR, Leibundgut K, Hirt A, Wagner HP. Focal nodular hyperplasia of the liver in children: review of follow-up and outcome. J Pediatr Surg. 1995;30(11):1590–3.
86. Czauderna P, Mackinley G, Perilongo G, et al. Hepatocellular carcinoma in children: results of the first prospective study of the Internantional Society of Pediatric Oncology group. J Clin Oncol. 2002;20(12):2798–804.

Neuroblastoma

57

Joshua N. Honeyman and Michael P. La Quaglia

Abstract

Neuroblastoma is a common solid tumor of infancy and childhood. It is uniquely characterized by a distinct natural history and prognosis in infants compared with older children. Whereas older children often experience rapidly progressive disease with a poor prognosis, many infants have indolent tumors that may exhibit only minimal progression over time or may even regress entirely. While the prognosis for infants with neuroblastoma is typically optimistic, patients still require multimodal therapy, ideally provided by institutions with expertise in the treatment of pediatric cancers.

Keywords

Neuroblastoma • Newborn • Staging • Surgical management • Outcomes

57.1 Introduction

Neuroblastoma is a common solid tumor of infancy and childhood. It is uniquely characterized by a distinct natural history and prognosis in infants compared with older children. Whereas older children often experience rapidly progressive disease with a poor prognosis, many infants have indolent tumors that may exhibit only minimal progression over time or may even regress entirely. While the prognosis for infants with neuroblastoma is typically optimistic, patients still require multimodal therapy, ideally provided by institutions with expertise in the treatment of pediatric cancers.

57.2 History

In 1864, Rudolf Virchow published a description of a patient with an abdominal glioma, providing the first account of what would eventually be known as neuroblastoma [1]. It was not until 1901, when William Pepper described a series of infants with large abdominal tumors that spread to the liver but spared bone [2], that the infantile phenotype of neuroblastoma was first identified; years later, these same patients would be defined as having stage 4S disease [3]. In 1907, Sir Robert

J.N. Honeyman, MD • M.P. La Quaglia, MD (✉)
Department of Surgery, Memorial Sloan Kettering Cancer Center, 1275 York Avenue, New York, NY 10065, USA
e-mail: laquaglm@mskcc.org

P.D. Losty et al. (eds.), *Rickham's Neonatal Surgery*, https://doi.org/10.1007/978-1-4471-4721-3_57

Hutchinson described a very different metastatic pattern for the same primary tumor—specifically, to the skull and orbits [4]. Three years later, James Homer Wright was the first to recognize the tumor as being of primitive neural cell origin, to describe the classic bone marrow involvement, and to use the term "neuroblastoma" [5]. The phenomenon of tumor maturation and differentiation, another significant component of the infantile presentation of neuroblastoma, was reported by Cushing and Wolbach in 1927 [6].

More recently, molecular aspects of neuroblastoma have been elucidated and correlated with clinical risk stratification of patients. In the 1950s, catecholamine metabolites were first identified as potential tumor markers [7]. Starting in the 1970s [8], a series of papers described the genetic and genomic aspects of neuroblastoma. In 1983, the N-*myc* oncogene was implicated in the pathogenesis of neuroblastoma [9], and since then, the amplification of N-*myc* has been found to be of significant prognostic importance. Therapeutically, the treatment of patients with neuroblastoma has been enhanced by molecular targeted treatments [10] and immunotherapy [11], which have been developed based on a greater understanding of the biochemical characteristics of neuroblastoma.

57.3 Epidemiology

Neuroblastoma is the most common pediatric extracranial solid tumor, accounting for 5% of all childhood cancers [12, 13]. While the median age at diagnosis is 2 years, 40% of cases occur in infants (age <12 months). In this age group, it is the single most common tumor overall, representing 25% of all cancers diagnosed in the first year of life [13, 14].

In the United States, the age-adjusted incidence of neuroblastoma in infants is 54.1 per million, compared with 7.3 cases per million children under age 20 [13]. During the period from 1974 to 1991, infants experienced a 3.1% average annual increase in incidence. The increase was higher in boys (4.1%) than in girls (2%).

The incidence of neuroblastoma in Europe is comparable, where 52.6 cases occur per million infants [15]. In addition, the incidence of neuroblastoma in infants increased from 35.4 cases per million in 1978 to 57.8 cases per million in 1997. The European data also demonstrate a slightly higher incidence in male infants than in female infants (54.6 vs. 50.5 cases per million).

A review of international registries suggests that the overall incidence of neuroblastoma is highest in affluent regions with predominantly white Caucasian populations, including the United States, Canada, Europe, Israel, Australia, and New Zealand. In the first year of life, the incidence ranges from 25 to 50 cases per million, representing 30% of all cases of neuroblastoma [16, 17]. A Japanese review of neuroblastoma occurring within the first month of life found an average incidence of 1 case per 210,000 live births [18].

Multiple studies have been undertaken to identify population risk factors for development of neuroblastoma, but there have been no clear causative or correlative factors identified. Areas of particular interest have included parental exposure to occupational and environmental toxins [19–24], but to date, no definitive associations have been determined. Patterns of community infections have also not correlated with neuroblastoma incidence [25].

In infants, several maternal factors have been identified that are associated with neuroblastoma in infancy, including intrapartum maternal anemia, neonatal respiratory distress, and 1-min Apgar score less than 7 [26]. Another review of birth records and cancer registries identified maternal hypertension and an age younger than 20 years to be associated with infant neuroblastoma [27]. In infants 6 months of age and younger, neuroblastoma was correlated with high birth weight, heavier maternal gestational weight gain, maternal hypertension, advanced maternal age, ultrasound, and respiratory distress. In contrast, risk of neuroblastoma in older infants correlated with low birth weight, but heavier maternal gestational weight was protective [28].

57.4 Molecular and Genetic Pathogenesis

The elucidation of genetic factors associated with neuroblastoma began with the identification of neuroblastoma pedigrees and the validation of inherited patterns of disease. A family history of the disease is present in about 1–2% of new cases [29–31], and siblings of index cases have a standardized incidence ratio of 9.7 [32]. While few pedigrees have been reported in the literature, the identification of these patient clusters first implicated a potentially heritable genetic component to the pathogenesis of neuroblastoma [29].

Additional observational data that demonstrate a genetic component of neuroblastoma include its occasional association with other congenital anomalies, both inherited and sporadic. A predisposition to neuroblastoma has been found with disorders of neural crest development, including congenital central hypoventilation syndrome [33], Hirschsprung disease [34, 35], and neurofibromatosis type 1 [36], as well as overgrowth syndromes such as Beckwith-Wiedemann [37]. Other associations have been described, including tuberous sclerosis, Friedrich ataxia, dermatomyositis, Soto syndrome, and cystic fibrosis.

In the 1970s, observations of genetic susceptibility led Knudson and Strong to propose a mutational model for neuroblastoma [31, 38] that expanded upon their previous work developing a two-hit model of tumorigenesis in retinoblastoma [39].

The molecular biology of neuroblastoma has been explored from many perspectives, from cytogenetics to genomics, genetics, and proteomics. Cytogenetic studies in particular have provided an early window into the underlying abnormalities in the function and organization of the neuroblastoma cell. DNA ploidy status of neuroblastic tumors is a significant predictor of outcome [40], particularly in infants [41]. Most aggressive, unfavorable tumors, as well as most neuroblastoma cell lines, are near-diploid or tetraploid, with genetic alterations in the form of amplifications, deletions, and translocations. In contrast, favorable tumors are typically hyperdiploid or tetraploid, with chromosomal duplications.

The most common genetic abnormality in primary neuroblastoma is a gain of genetic material from chromosome 17q [42–44], occurring in over half of tumors. This can occur via unbalanced 1;17 translocations, translocations involving other chromosomes, or the gain of a whole chromosome. While the gain of chromosome 17q in hyperdiploid tumors is associated with better overall prognosis, 17q gain has been associated with worse outcome [45, 46].

Another frequent genetic abnormality in neuroblastoma is deletion in chromosome 1p [8, 47]. Loss of heterozygosity (LOH) at 1p has been seen in over 25% of tumors, and the consistently deleted portion maps to 1p36.2–36.3 [48–50]. Although LOH at 1p has been found to correlate with features of high-risk disease [48, 51, 52], its independent prognostic utility is more relevant to event-free survival than to mortality.

Chromosomal abnormalities at 11q and 14q also occur in neuroblastoma. LOH at chromosome 11q is frequent, occurring in 30% of primary tumors [53, 54]. This chromosomal abnormality is associated with lower rates of N-*myc* amplification and may correlate with worse outcome in patients with non-N-*myc*–amplified tumors. Alterations of chromosome 14q are less common, occurring in approximately 25% of primary tumors [55]. Deletions in 14q have been correlated with LOH at 11q. LOH at 11q and 1p are independently associated with worse outcome [56], as are single-nucleotide polymorphisms at chromosome band 6p22 [57].

Neuroblastoma is closely associated with the amplification of the N-*myc* oncogene, which is normally expressed in the developing nervous system and other tissues. It encodes a nuclear phosphoprotein that acts as a transcriptional regulator. N-*myc*, which is located on the short arm of chromosome 2 (2p24.1), was first cloned in 1983 from a neuroblastoma cell line [9]. Amplification can reach levels of 50–400 copies [58], and involves a region of approximately 130 kilobases [59].

The consequences of N-*myc* amplification have been demonstrated in both cell lines [60, 61] and animal models [62], where the overexpression of *myc* is sufficient for malignant transformation. However, in tumors without N-*myc* amplification, the role of this oncogene has not been fully characterized.

The clinical significance of N-*myc* amplification in neuroblastoma has been clarified over the past three decades. First associated with advanced stage in untreated primary tumors [63], N-*myc* amplification was subsequently associated with rapid disease progression and worse overall prognosis [64]. As a result of its prognostic significance, N-*myc* amplification is included in all risk stratification schemes for neuroblastoma patients.

Neurotrophin signaling pathways, which play a role in the neuronal development, have also been implicated in the pathogenesis of neuroblastoma. The *TRK* gene family encodes receptors for neurotrophin, or nerve growth factor. Three specific high-affinity neurotrophin receptor genes have been identified (*TRKA*, *TRKB*, and *TRKC*), each with its own pattern of association. TrkA is the high-affinity receptor for nerve growth factor, which drives the differentiation of neural cells. *TRKA* expression is inversely related to disease stage and N-*myc* amplification status. Thus, high *TRKA* expression is associated with favorable neuroblastomas [65, 66]. TrkB binds brain-derived neurotrophic factor and neurotrophin-4, promoting cell growth and survival. In contrast to *TRKA*, *TRKB* expression is correlated with advanced disease stage and N-*myc* amplification status [67]. TrkC binds neurotrophin-3. *TRKC* expression is strongly correlated with *TRKA* expression [68] and, thus, is also associated with a favorable prognosis [69, 70].

57.5 Histopathology

Neuroblastic tumors originate from the neural crest–derived sympathetic nervous system and adrenal gland. Anatomically, they can arise anywhere along the sympathetic ganglia or in the adrenal medulla. The two predominant cell types identified in neuroblastic tumors are neuroblasts, which are primitive neural cells that are typically precursors to neurons and glia, and Schwann cells, which form the neuronal stroma. In the characteristic "rosette" structure, clearly visible tumor nuclei surround the fibrillary cytoplasm. (Fig. 57.1) The relative distribution of these cells within a single tumor is of significant prognostic importance and is a component of the classification systems described below.

Neuroblastoma is one of a spectrum of peripheral neuroblastic tumors that also includes ganglioneuroma and ganglioneuroblastoma, and multiple histopathologic classification schemes have been developed to differentiate these tumors. In 1984, Shimada and colleagues proposed an age-based tumor classification system for neuroblastoma [71]. The five features evaluated in the Shimada classification system were the degree of

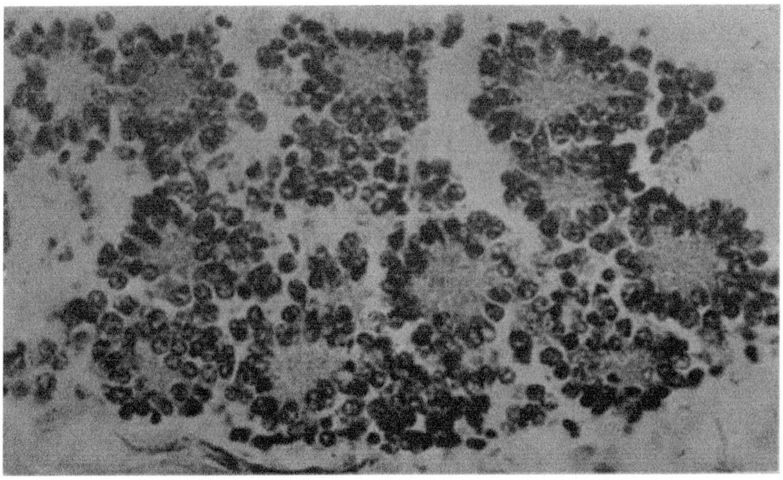

Fig. 57.1 Neuroblastoma histology featuring classic 'rosettes' from James Homer Wright's 1910 review [5]. Image ©1910 Rockefeller University Press. Originally published in J Exp Med. 12:556–561. Used with permission

neuroblast differentiation, the extent of Schwannian stromal development, the mitosis-karyorrhexis index (MKI), the presence or absence of a nodular pattern, and the patient's age at diagnosis. The MKI is determined by counting the number of cells in mitosis and in karyorrhexis. The latter cells demonstrate condensed and fragmented nuclear material with condensed and eosinophilic cytoplasm.

Since 1994, the International Neuroblastoma Pathology Committee (INPC) has standardized the terminology and diagnostic criteria for peripheral neuroblastic tumors, adopting a modified Shimada classification system [72, 73]. The INPC system for neuroblastic tumors includes four pathologic categories: neuroblastoma; ganglioneuroblastoma, intermixed; ganglioneuroma; and ganglioneuroblastoma, nodular. Tumors are then subclassified as either favorable or unfavorable.

Neuroblastoma is defined as Schwannian stroma-poor and is categorized under three specific subtypes: differentiating, poorly differentiated, and undifferentiated. Differentiating neuroblastoma contains neuroblasts with abundant neutrophil and 5% or more of the cells exhibiting differentiation. Poorly differentiated neuroblastoma contains neuroblastic cells with a background of neutrophils. Undifferentiated neuroblastoma is a rare subtype containing undifferentiated neuroblastic cells; these tumors often require additional testing beyond histopathologic analysis to confirm the diagnosis.

Ganglioneuroblastoma is classified as intermixed or nodular. The intermixed tumors are Schwannian stroma-rich and feature incomplete neuronal maturation with foci of neuroblastic cells in varying degrees of differentiation. Nodular tumors contain macroscopic, hemorrhagic neuroblastomatous nodules that coincide with a background of ganglioneuroma or ganglioneuroblastoma, intermixed.

Ganglioneuroma is a Schwannian stroma-dominant tumor with two subtypes: maturing and mature. These subtypes are distinguished based on the degree of differentiation of the ganglion cells present within the tumor.

Beyond defining clinically significant pathologic groupings, the purpose of the INPC system is to determine prognostically meaningful groups. Table 57.1 shows the favorable and unfavorable prognostic groups for neuroblastoma, as described by both the original Shimada system and the INPC classification. Ganglioneuroblastoma, intermixed, as well as ganglioneuroma are considered favorable histologies, regardless of the patient's age. Ganglioneuroblastoma, nodular, is stratified based on the classification of the tumor's nodular component.

The significance of age group in both the original Shimada classification and the INPC system underscores the fundamentally different biology observed in infants with neuroblastoma compared with older children.

Table 57.1 Prognosis based on histopathologic grouping [72]

Prognostic group	Age group (years)	INPC	Shimada (original)
Favorable	<1.5	Poorly differentiated or differentiating and low or intermediate MKI tumor	Stroma-poor; favorable
	1.5–5	Differentiating and low MKI tumor	Stroma-poor; favorable
Unfavorable	<1.5	Undifferentiated tumor	Unfavorable
		High MKI tumor	Unfavorable
	1.5–5	Undifferentiated or poorly differentiated tumor	Unfavorable
		Intermediate or high MKI tumor	Unfavorable
	≥5	All tumors	Unfavorable

From Shimada H, Ambros IM, Dehner LP, et al. The International Neuroblastoma Pathology Classification (the Shimada system). *Cancer* 1999; 86(3):364–372. Used with permission

MKI mitosis-karyorrhexis index

57.6 Staging and Risk Grouping

Since the mid-twentieth century, multiple staging systems have been developed to provide a means of clinically grouping and stratifying neuroblastoma patients based on their overall risk. These systems have been used to guide treatment and to monitor patients enrolled in clinical trials. The effort to consolidate the disparate staging systems into an internationally accepted prognostic staging system resulted in the development of the International Neuroblastoma Staging System (INSS) in 1988 [74].

The INSS was most recently revised in 1993. The major revisions included a redefinition of the midline (the vertebral column), a clarification of inclusion criteria for stage 4S disease (upper limit of 10% bone marrow involvement and age <1 year), and a general recommendation for the use of metaiodobenzylguanidine (MIBG) scintigraphy scanning to evaluate the extent of disease [75] (Table 57.2).

A commonly cited limitation of the INSS classification system is its reliance on intraoperative findings. During the initial evaluation of a patient, particularly in the setting of clinical trials, it became clear that a new staging system that relied on preoperative findings was needed. The International Neuroblastoma Risk Group (INRG) developed its own pretreatment risk classification system based on a series of image-defined risk factors [76] (Table 57.3).

Table 57.2 International Neuroblastoma Staging System [75]

Stage	Description
1	Localized tumor with complete gross excision, with or without microscopic residual disease; representative ipsilateral lymph nodes negative for tumor microscopically (nodes attached to and removed with the primary tumor may be positive)
2A	Localized tumor with incomplete gross excision; representative ipsilateral nonadherent lymph nodes negative for tumor microscopically
2B	Localized tumor with or without complete gross excision, with ipsilateral nonadherent lymph nodes positive for tumor. Enlarged contralateral lymph nodes must be negative microscopically
3	Unresectable unilateral tumor infiltrating across the midline,[b] with or without regional lymph node involvement; or localized unilateral tumor with contralateral regional lymph node involvement; or midline tumor with bilateral extension by infiltration (unresectable) or by lymph node involvement
4	Any primary tumor with dissemination to distant lymph nodes, bone, bone marrow, liver, skin, and/or other organs (except as defined for stage 4S)
4S	Localized primary tumor (as defined for stage 1, 2A, or 2B), with dissemination limited to skin, liver, and/or bone marrow[a] (limited to infants <1 year of age)

From Brodeur GM, Pritchard J, Berthold F, et al. Revisions of the International Criteria for Neuroblastoma Diagnosis, Staging, and Response to Treatment. J Clin Oncol. 1993; 11(8): 1466–1477. Used with permission

[a]Marrow involvement in stage 4S should be minimal, ie, <10% of total nucleated cells identified as malignant on bone marrow biopsy or on marrow aspirate. More extensive marrow involvement would be considered to be stage 4. The MIBG scan (if performed) should be negative in the marrow

[b]The midline is defined as the vertebral column. Tumors originating on one side and crossing the midline must infiltrate to or beyond the opposite side of the vertebral column

Table 57.3 International Neuroblastoma Risk Group Staging System [76]

Stage	Description
L1	Localized tumor not involving vital structures as defined by the list of image-defined risk factors and confined to one body compartment
L2	Locoregional tumor with presence of one or more image-defined risk factors
M	Distant metastatic disease (except stage MS)
MS	Metastatic disease in children younger than 18 months with metastases confined to skin, liver, and/or bone marrow

From Monclair T. Brodeur GM, Ambros PF, et al. The International Neuroblastoma Risk Group (INRG) Staging System: An INRG Task Force Report. J Clin Oncol. 2009; 27(2):298–303. Used with permission

As an adjunct to staging systems, risk groupings provide additional guidance for treatment planning. Different risk stratification systems take into account not only the INSS stage, but also the underlying biology and histopathologic characteristics of the tumor.

The Children's Oncology Group has established the most widely accepted risk groupings in North America. It stratifies patients into high-, intermediate-, and low-risk groups based on INSS stage, age, N-*myc* amplification status, INPC category, and DNA ploidy. This risk stratification system is used for Children's Oncology Group trials [77] (Table 57.4).

In 2009, the INRG also developed and published a risk stratification system based on their preoperative staging system [78] (Table 57.5).

Neuroblastoma in infants has two distinct personalities. The first, which is frequently associated with stages 3 and 4 and exhibits N-*myc* amplification, closely resembles the disease in older children and is characterized by aggressive growth and metastatic spread. The other, classified as stage 4S, has a more indolent biology and is characterized by spontaneous regression and optimistic prognosis with even minimal therapy [16]. Infants with disseminated disease who do not meet all the criteria for stage 4S disease are necessarily classified as having stage 4 disease.

The metastatic distribution for stage 4S disease includes the liver, bone marrow, skin, and lymph nodes. Aspirates of the bone marrow must have <10% malignant cells. The natural history of 4S disease includes complete maturation and regression, even in the setting of advanced disease [16, 79, 80]. Factors associated with spontaneous regression in stage 4S disease include triploidy, lack of N-*myc* amplification, and no LOH. Patients with N-*myc*–amplified tumors were found to have worse event-free survival than patients with non–N-*myc*-amplified tumors [81]. Moreover, patients with non–N-*myc*-amplified tumors have been shown to have a favorable prognosis, even in the setting of reduced systemic treatment [82, 83].

However, there is also a subgroup of patients with stage 4S disease who have rapidly progressive intra-abdominal disease. Such infants are at an increased risk of respiratory compromise and disseminated intravascular coagulation, so a more

Table 57.4 Children's Oncology Group Neuroblastoma Risk Grouping [77]

INSS stage	Age (years)	N-*myc* status	INPC category	DNA ploidy	Risk group
1	0–21	Any	Any	Any	Low
2a/b	<1 year	Any	Any	Any	Low
	1–21	Nonamplified	Any	—	Low
	1–21	Amplified	Favorable	—	Low
	1–21	Amplified	Unfavorable	—	Low
3	<1	Nonamplified	Any	Any	Intermediate
	<1	Amplified	Any	Any	High
	1–21	Nonamplified	Favorable	—	Intermediate
	1–21	Nonamplified	Unfavorable	—	High
	1–21	Amplified	Any	—	High
4	<1.5	Nonamplified	Any	Any	Intermediate
	<1	Amplified	Any	Any	High
	1.5–21	Any	Any	—	High
4S	<1	Nonamplified	Favorable	>1	Low
	<1	Nonamplified	Any	1	Intermediate
	<1	Nonamplified	Unfavorable	Any	Intermediate
	<1	Amplified	Any	Any	High

From *Neuroblastoma treatment (PDQ)*. Bethesda, MD: National Cancer Institute; National Institutes of Health. Available at: http://www.cancer.gov/cancertopics/pdq/treatment/neuroblastoma/HealthProfessional/Page3#Section_14. Accessed February 20, 2012

Table 57.5 International Neuroblastoma Risk Group (INRG) Consensus Pretreatment Classification Schema [78]

INRG stage	Age (months)	Histologic category	Grade of tumor differentiation	N-*myc* status	11q aberration	DNA ploidy	Pretreatment risk group
L1/L2		GN maturing; GNB intermixed					(A) Very low
L1		Any except above		NA			(B) Very low
				Amp			(K) High
L2	<18	Any except above		NA	No		(D) Low
					Yes		(G) Intermediate
	≥18	GNB nodular; neuroblastoma	Differentiating	NA	No		(E) Low
					Yes		(H) Intermediate
			Poorly differentiated or undifferentiated				
				Amp			(N) High
M	<18					Hyperdiploid	(F) Low
	<12					Diploid	(I) Intermediate
	12–18					Diploid	(J) Intermediate
	<18						(O) High
	≥18						(P) High
MS	<18			NA	No		(C) Very low
					Yes		(Q) High
				Amp			(R) High

From Cohn SL, Pearson ADJ, London WB, et al. The International Neuroblastoma Risk Group (INRG) Classification System: An INRG Task Force Report. J Clin Oncol. 2009;27(2):289–297

GN ganglioneuroma, *GNB* ganglioneuroblastoma, *Amp* amplified, *NA* not amplified aggressive chemotherapeutic treatment strategy may be necessary to ameliorate this risk [16].

Neonates diagnosed with neuroblastoma generally have the same favorable prognosis as older infants [79, 84]. However, there is some evidence that patients younger than 2 months may have a worse prognosis and that patients older than 6 months may require more aggressive therapy [85].

57.7 Fetal Neuroblastoma

Due to the increased use of prenatal ultrasound, more infants with neuroblastoma are receiving the diagnosis prenatally. In one series from the United Kingdom Children's Cancer Study Group, 15% of patients (5/33) were diagnosed based on prenatal ultrasound [79]. In a study of the Italian Neuroblastoma Registry, 20% of newborns (27/134) were diagnosed prenatally [84].

A multi-institutional series of fetal neuroblastoma suggested expectant management with serial ultrasounds for uncomplicated pregnancies [86]. These infants typically have a favorable prognosis based on early-stage and low-risk molecular classification [87]. Surgery is typically curative, although many investigators propose a trial of observation alone in carefully selected patients [87–89].

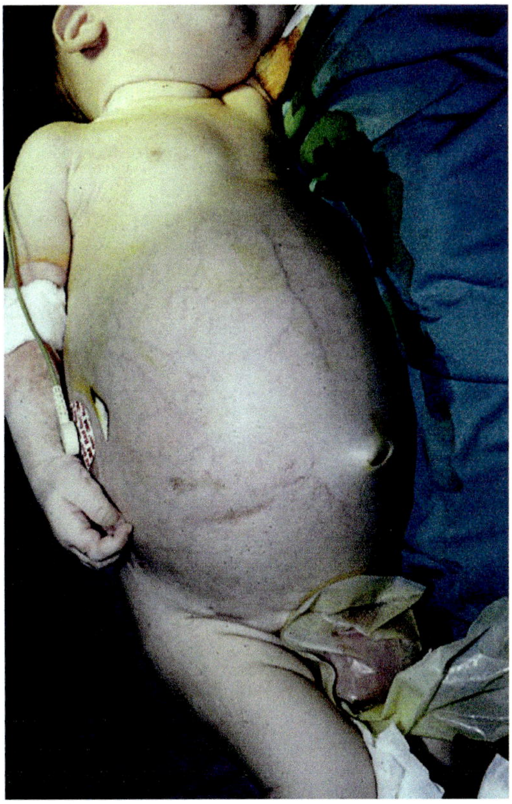

Fig. 57.2 Infant with massive liver involvement from stage 4S neuroblastoma [122]. Image courtesy of Brian H. Kushner, MD, Memorial Sloan-Kettering Cancer Center, New York, NY. ©2004 Society of Nuclear Medicine. Originally published in J Nucl Med. 2004 Jul;45(7):1172–88

57.8 Clinical Presentation

The clinical presentation of neuroblastoma is dictated by a series of factors, including the location of the primary tumor, the burden of metastatic disease, the age of the patient, and the metabolic activity of the tumor. A neuroblastic tumor can arise from anywhere within the sympathetic nervous system and the adrenal medulla. The specific location of the tumor may influence the timing of presentation and the local symptoms present at diagnosis. The metastatic burden, the age of the patient, and the metabolic activity of the tumor can also affect the clinical appearance.

The most common site for primary neuroblastoma is the abdomen. Three-quarters of neuroblastomas occur in the abdomen, the vast majority of which arise from within the adrenal gland. Of all tumors diagnosed within the first month of life, 90% are adrenal in origin [89]. Patients with these tumors can present with abdominal pain, abdominal distention, and bowel or urinary dysfunction. A large abdominal mass in infants more often represents extensive hepatic metastatic disease than a large primary tumor. These large masses can cause compressive symptoms, leading to respiratory distress and requiring emergency surgical resection. (Fig. 57.2).

After the abdomen, the posterior mediastinum is the second most common site of primary neuroblastoma. Infants with these tumors can be symptomatic at presentation, or in some infants, these tumors are found incidentally on chest radiographs

[90]. Upper mediastinal and cervical tumors can arise in patients with Horner's syndrome. Because of their low risk of metastasis, cervical tumors are associated with favorable prognosis [91]. However, given their location, complete surgical resection of locoregional disease may be difficult. Symptoms associated with these tumors may include Horner's syndrome.

Neuroblastoma can also arise in the pelvis, most commonly from the organ of Zuckerkandl. Infants with these tumors may present with a lower midline mass or a mass on rectal examination. Symptoms may include bowel or bladder dysfunction, pain, or weakness [92].

Metastatic tumors in infants are often found in the liver, bone, and subcutaneous tissue. Characteristically, subcutaneous metastases often have a blue color, leading to their description as "blueberry muffin" lesions. Bony orbital metastases can present with periorbital ecchymoses and proptosis. Bone marrow involvement can result in anemia. Because of the growth pattern of neuroblastic tumors along radicular nerves, tumors can invade the epidural space. Spinal disease may present with lower-extremity weakness and pain, as well as cord compression.

Infants may also present with paraneoplastic syndromes. Neuroblastomas often secrete catecholamines, but these are typically precursor molecules that are not adrenergically active. Catecholamine release can, however, cause hypertension and tachycardia. Neuroblastomas have also been reported to secrete vasoactive intestinal peptide, which can trigger chronic watery diarrhea.

Another paraneoplastic disorder associated with neuroblastoma is opsomyoclonus ("dancing eyes, dancing feet"). Symptoms of opsomyoclonus include truncal ataxia and rapid irregular eye movements.

57.9 Diagnosis and Initial Evaluation

A detailed history and physical examination are essential in the preliminary assessment of a patient with neuroblastoma. The history can provide information about the extent of disease, potential paraneoplastic disorders, and comorbid conditions. The physical examination should include a thorough assessment of the primary tumor site, whether abdominopelvic, mediastinal, or cervical. Evaluation of palpable lymph node basins, liver, orbits, and skull is essential when examining a patient who may have neuroblastoma. In addition, a complete neurologic examination should be performed to rule out any tumor involvement of the spine.

The initial evaluation of neuroblastoma should also include a complete laboratory and radiologic workup. The necessary studies will vary based on the individual patient, but certain studies are necessary for all patients to ensure proper clinical staging and risk stratification. Furthermore, since some patients will undergo aggressive chemotherapeutic and surgical interventions, it is important to obtain baseline metabolic data.

In addition to basic laboratory investigations, including complete blood count, metabolic panel, and coagulation studies, blood tests for lactate dehydrogenase, ferritin, neuron-specific enolase, and ganglioside GD2 should also be performed because of the potential prognostic significance of these serum markers.

Since most neuroblastomas maintain the necessary enzymes for catecholamine synthesis, metabolites of this pathway are excreted in the urine, and they can be readily detected. Urinary levels of homovanillic acid and vanillylmandelic acid are elevated in the majority of neuroblastoma cases. Thus, these levels can assist in the initial diagnosis of neuroblastic tumors, as well as provide information about the metabolic activity of the tumor. Urinary homovanillic acid and vanillylmandelic acid levels have also been correlated with the degree of tumor differentiation and may be used to assess treatment response and monitor patients for recurrence.

Radiologic assessment of neuroblastoma serves three purposes: confirmation of diagnosis, establishment of primary disease site, and evaluation of metastatic disease. Although the basic imaging evaluation typically includes obtaining plain radiographs of the chest and abdomen, cross-sectional imaging is the most important modality for surgical planning.

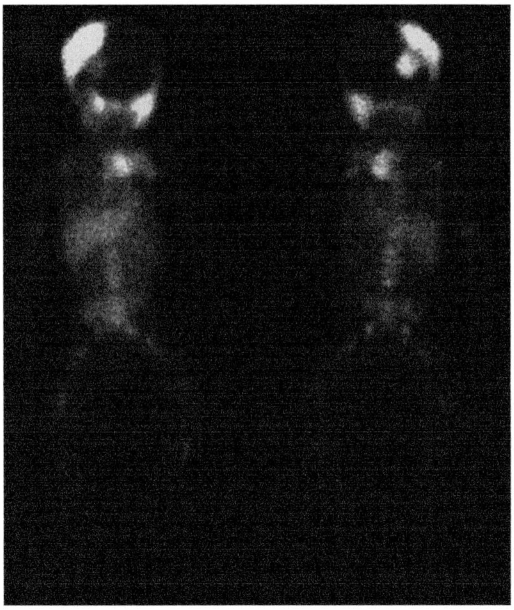

Fig. 57.3 MIBG scan of an infant with neuroblastoma involving the posterior mediastinum, bone marrow, right parietal skull, and left sphenoid [122]. Image courtesy of Brian H. Kushner, MD, Memorial Sloan-Kettering Cancer Center, New York, NY. ©2004 Society of Nuclear Medicine. Originally published in J Nucl Med. 2004 Jul;45(7):1172–88

Metaiodobenzylguanidine (MIBG) scintigraphy is an increasingly important component of the radiologic evaluation of neuroblastic tumors. MIBG is a radiolabeled structural homolog of noradrenaline that shows preferential uptake in adrenergic tumors such as neuroblastomas and pheochromocytomas. Iodine-123–labeled MIBG (^{123}I-MIBG) is currently the most sensitive and specific scintigraphic method for evaluating metastatic disease, so its routine use in the evaluation of new patients with neuroblastoma is recommended. In patients with MIBG-negative neuroblastic tumors, who represent approximately 10% of new patients, a bone scan using technetium-99m (^{99m}Tc)-diphosphonate can be used to evaluate for osteolytic lesions. (Fig. 57.3).

Bilateral bone marrow aspiration is another important component of the initial staging of neuroblastoma. While standard histologic assessment is essential, the addition of immunohistochemical and cytologic techniques provides greater sensitivity and can offer additional molecular insights that will aid in the initial evaluation of the patient. Histologic evaluation may reveal either classic rosettes, composed of clumps of tumor cells, or individual tumor cells.

Multiple immunohistochemical markers are useful in the diagnosis of neuroblastoma [73]. Markers that are typically positive in neuroblastoma include neuron-specific enolase, chromogranin A, synaptophysin, tyrosine hydroxylase, protein gene product 9.5, ganglioside GD2, and NB84. Markers that are typically negative in neuroblastoma include actin, desmin, low-molecular-weight cytokeratin, leukocyte common antigen, and vimentin.

57.10 Surgical Management

Surgery plays an essential role in the diagnosis, staging, and therapy of neuroblastoma. For patients with suspected neuroblastoma, initial tissue diagnosis is crucial for accurate tumor classification and molecular risk stratification. Except in those patients in whom the primary tumor is small and more easily resected, an incisional biopsy is usually the first step in the surgical management of neuroblastoma.

The primary goal of the initial biopsy is to obtain an adequate amount of high-quality tissue for histopathologic, molecular, and genetic analysis. Minimizing the invasiveness of this procedure is essential to shorten the time to chemotherapy initiation. To facilitate future surgery, the incision should be oriented along the planned incision for the definitive resection. Also, in anticipation of systemic therapy, vascular access for chemotherapy can be placed at the time of initial biopsy.

Subsequent surgical management of infants with neuroblastoma depends on clinical presentation. The most significant factor for achieving local tumor control is resection of the primary tumor along with removal of any involved regional lymph nodes. Patients with low-risk, localized neuroblastoma can be treated effectively with surgery alone [93], achieving survival rates as high as 94–98% [94, 95].

Although gross total resection has been correlated with outcome in neuroblastoma [96–98], prognosis is most dependent on the underlying biology of the tumor, not the extent of resection [99]. Resection of the primary tumor in patients with metastatic disease may improve outcome if the metastases can also be controlled [100], although, again, the underlying biology of the metastatic tumors is more important to overall survival than resection status [101]. In low risk infants, complete resection is not always necessary [102], and patients with stage 4S tumors may not require resection at all [103].

Patients with high risk neuroblastoma may benefit from neoadjuvant chemotherapy, since resection of the primary tumor prior to chemotherapy is associated with increased rates of treatment-related complications [104], and neoadjuvant chemotherapy increases resection rates for the primary tumor [105].

Indicators of resectability in abdominal disease include tumors that do not cross the midline and tumors that cross the midline without vessel encasement. Aggressive surgical intervention in patients without these indicators has not been shown to improve outcomes. These patients warrant adjuvant therapies prior to resection, which may allow for downstaging of the primary tumor.

As mentioned above, the INRG staging system uses image-defined surgical risk factors to classify patients [76]. While vessel encasement is commonly encountered during attempted resection, and the INRG considers vessel encasement to be a risk factor for worse outcome, some series have demonstrated that visceral vessel encasement does not preclude gross total resection [106].

57.11 Chemotherapy

Chemotherapy plays a significant role in the management of disseminated neuroblastoma, as well as of high- and intermediate-risk disease. Multiagent therapy is the mainstay of treatment. In the neoadjuvant setting, chemotherapy is particularly useful to decrease the total tumor burden. For patients with disease that is initially deemed unresectable, preoperative chemotherapy can increase the possibility of gross total resection.

In patients with high-risk neuroblastoma, systemic treatment has trended toward the use of higher dose intensities. In these patients, myeloablative chemotherapy has been shown to improve outcomes [107, 108]. However, even in these patients, efforts have been made to reduce the total exposure to chemotherapy [109]. Infants with advanced-stage disease have also been found to benefit from a reduction or elimination of chemotherapy [110].

In patients with intermediate- and low-risk neuroblastoma, efforts have been made to reduce total exposure to chemotherapy, because these patients generally have good overall survival and because of the increased awareness of the long-term toxicities of chemotherapy. Many of these patients can be cured with surgery alone. Reduced doses and duration of chemotherapy did not have a detrimental effect in patients with intermediate-risk neuroblastoma without N-*myc* amplification [111].

The most common chemotherapeutic regimen for patients with intermediate-risk disease is a combination of cisplatin, cyclophosphamide, doxorubicin, and etoposide. In patients with high-risk disease, systemic treatment usually requires a different set of chemotherapeutic agents, including cyclophosphamide, ifosfamide, cisplatin, vincristine, doxorubicin, melphalan, etoposide, teniposide, and topotecan.

57.12 Radiation Therapy

Neuroblastoma is a radiosensitive tumor, and while external-beam radiation therapy is not curative, it can help control local disease. In patients with high-risk neuroblastoma, radiation therapy has been shown to reduce the risk of local relapse with doses ranging from 15 to 30 Gy, delivered in 1.5- to 3.0-Gy fractions, depending on tumor size, patient age, and tumor location.

Radiation therapy also has applications in the acute setting, such as in infants with massive hepatic disease. While usually not indicated in stage 4S neuroblastoma, radiation therapy may be used on an emergency basis for patients suffering respiratory distress from large hepatic metastases who did not respond to initial chemotherapy. In the emergency setting, radiation therapy may also play a role in controlling tumors that extend into the spinal canal. While it may provide rapid control of expanding tumors when combined with laminectomy, radiation therapy also increases the risk of vertebral damage and growth arrest.

In appropriately equipped centers, intraoperative radiation therapy is an important treatment option in patients with high-risk, locally recurrent, or persistent neuroblastoma [112–114]. This technique allows for the delivery of higher doses of radiation to the tumor bed while sparing the surrounding normal tissues.

External-beam radiation therapy is also a powerful tool in the palliation of end-stage disease, particularly in providing relief from painful bone metastases.

57.13 Other Therapies

Immunomodulatory agents and immunotherapeutics have promising roles in the future of neuroblastoma therapy. The tumor-associated disialoganglioside GD2 is found on the surface of most neuroblastoma cells, and monoclonal antibodies against GD2 have shown promise in the treatment of neuroblastoma. Targeted monoclonal antibody therapies can exploit the intrinsic pathways of antibody-dependent cellular cytotoxicity, or they can be conjugated to toxins or to diagnostic markers, such as radionuclides (e.g., ^{131}I). Treatment of high-risk neuroblastoma with a combination of granulocyte macrophage–colony stimulating factor, interleukin-2, and an anti-GD2 antibody has been shown to be effective in early clinical trials [115].

MIBG provides another means for the targeted delivery of beta-emitting radionuclides to neuroblastoma cells. The tissue specificity of MIBG increases tumor exposure while reducing overall systemic toxicity. ^{131}I-MIBG has been used as an adjuvant treatment in combination with chemotherapy and bone marrow transplantation for high-risk neuroblastoma.

Retinoic acid derivatives, specifically 13-*cis*-retinoic acid, have been shown to slow the growth of high-risk neuroblastoma, induce differentiation, and improve survival when used in combination with myeloablative chemotherapy and radiation [107, 108].

57.14 Screening

The observation that mortality varies inversely with patient age, combined with the diagnostic utility and noninvasive nature of urine metanephrine testing, prompted the introduction of population-wide infant screening protocols for neuroblastoma. However, population screening for neuroblastoma in infants remains a controversial issue.

In Japan, a nationwide screening protocol for neuroblastoma was introduced in 1984, which required the testing of urinary vanillylmandelic acid levels in all 5-month-old infants. While screening did have a marginally positive effect on survival, there was a concomitant increase in the overall incidence of neuroblastoma [116]. The additional cases that were detected included a number of low-grade tumors that would not otherwise have become clinically apparent. Consequently, the inclusion of these additional low-grade tumors improved the calculated survival rates. The Japanese screening program was halted in 2003 pending further review of the data.

An aggressive screening protocol in Quebec, Canada, in which all children born during a 5-year period were offered screening for urine metanephrines at 3 weeks and 6 months of age, did not result in a reduction of mortality due to neuroblastoma [117]. A similar screening protocol in Germany offered urine screening to children at 1 year of age. Again, there was no demonstrable mortality benefit [118].

Currently, there are no widely accepted methods of population-based screening of infants for neuroblastoma. For such a screening protocol to be successful, it must yield increases in overall survival while avoiding the overdiagnosis of tumors that are not clinically significant. Advances in our understanding of the molecular biology of neuroblastoma may provide insights that lead to better screening methods.

57.15 Survival and Late Effects

Survival trends in infant populations with neuroblastoma are typically positive. In Europe, 5-year overall survival increased from 37% between 1978 and 1982 to 66% for the period between 1993 to 1997 [15]. This far outpaced the rates of survival in older children, who experienced an increase from 21 to 45% during the same period.

In results published by the Childhood Cancer Survivor Study [119], the cumulative incidence of chronic health conditions in survivors of neuroblastoma was 41.4% at 20-year follow-up. Neurologic symptoms were most common and included weakness, sensory deficits, and pain. In the same study population, the cumulative incidence of secondary malignancies was 7% at 30 years after the original neuroblastoma diagnosis [119].

While patients with stage 4S disease typically have good oncologic outcomes, they remain at an increased risk of long-term sequelae. In a single-center study, 20% of patients had long-term disease- or treatment-related effects [120].

In patients with advanced-stage neuroblastoma (stages 3 and 4), late complications have been found in up to 95% of childhood survivors [121]. Complications ranged from hearing loss, primary hypothyroidism, ovarian failure, musculoskeletal abnormalities, and pulmonary abnormalities.

Because of these health-related late complications of neuroblastoma and its treatment, survivors may also be at risk for social and economic sequelae. Long-term follow-up of patients with neuroblastoma is essential to ensure good oncologic outcomes, as well as to address any long-term complications.

References

1. Virchow RLK. Die krankhaften Geschwulste; dreissig Vorlesungen, gehalten wahrend des Wintersemesters 1862–1863 an der Universitat zu Berlin. Berlin: Hirschwald; 1863.
2. Pepper W. A study of congenital sarcoma of the liver and suprarenal. Am J Med Sci. 1901;121:287–99.
3. D'Angio GJ, Evans AE, Koop CE. Special pattern of widespread neuroblastoma with a favourable prognosis. Lancet. 1971;1:1046–9.
4. Hutchison R. On suprarenal sarcoma in children with metastasis in the skull. Quart J Med. 1907;1:33–41.
5. Wright JH. Neurocytoma or neuroblastoma, a kind of tumor not generally recognized. J Exp Med. 1910;12:556–61.
6. Cushing H, Wolbach SB. The transformation of a malignant paravertebral sympathicoblastoma into a benign ganglioneuroma. Am J Pathol. 1927;3:203–216.7.
7. Mason GA, Hart-Mercer J, Millar EJ, Strang LB, Wynne NA. Adrenaline-secreting neuroblastoma in an infant. Lancet. 1957;273:322–5.
8. Brodeur GM, Sekhon G, Goldstein MN. Chromosomal aberrations in human neuroblastomas. Cancer. 1977;40:2256–63.
9. Schwab M, Alitalo K, Klempnauer KH, Varmus HE, Bishop JM, Gilbert F, Brodeur G, Goldstein M, Trent J. Amplified DNA with limited homology to myc cellular oncogene is shared by human neuroblastoma cell lines and a neuroblastoma tumour. Nature. 1983;305:245–8.
10. Matthay KK, DeSantes K, Hasegawa B, Huberty J, Hattner RS, Ablin A, Reynolds CP, Seeger RC, Weinberg VK, Price D. Phase I dose escalation of 131I-metaiodobenzylguanidine with autologous bone marrow support in refractory neuroblastoma. J Clin Oncol. 1998;16:229–36.
11. Kushner BH, Kramer K, Cheung NK. Phase II trial of the anti-G(D2) monoclonal antibody 3F8 and granulocyte-macrophage colony-stimulating factor for neuroblastoma. J Clin Oncol. 2001;19:4189–94.
12. Li J, Thompson TD, Miller JW, Pollack LA, Stewart SL. Cancer incidence among children and adolescents in the United States, 2001–2003. Pediatrics. 2008;121:e1470–7.
13. Linabery AM, Ross JA. Trends in childhood cancer incidence in the U.S. (1992–2004). Cancer. 2008;112:416–32.
14. Kenney LB, Miller BA, Ries LA, Nicholson HS, Byrne J, Reaman GH. Increased incidence of cancer in infants in the U.S.: 1980–1990. Cancer. 1998;82:1396–400.
15. Spix C, Pastore G, Sankila R, Stiller CA, Steliarova-Foucher E. Neuroblastoma incidence and survival in European children (1978–1997): report from the Automated Childhood Cancer Information System project. Eur J Cancer. 2006;42:2081–91.
16. Nickerson HJ, Matthay KK, Seeger RC, Brodeur GM, Shimada H, Perez C, Atkinson JB, Selch M, Gerbing RB, Stram DO, Lukens J. Favorable biology and outcome of stage IV-S neuroblastoma with supportive care or minimal therapy: a Children's Cancer Group study. J Clin Oncol. 2000;18:477–86.
17. Stiller CA, Parkin DM. International variations in the incidence of neuroblastoma. Int J Cancer. 1992;52:538–43.

18. Tsuchida Y, Ikeda H, Iehara T, Toyoda Y, Kawa K, Fukuzawa M. Neonatal neuroblastoma: incidence and clinical outcome. Med Pediatr Oncol. 2003;40:391–3.
19. MacCarthy A, Bunch KJ, Fear NT, King JC, Vincent TJ, Murphy MFG. Paternal occupation and neuroblastoma: a case-control study based on cancer registry data for Great Britain 1962–1999. Br J Cancer. 2010;102:615–9.
20. Moore A, Enquobahrie DA. Paternal occupational exposure to pesticides and risk of neuroblastoma among children: a meta-analysis. Cancer Causes Control. 2011;22:1529–36.
21. Olshan AF, De Roos AJ, Teschke K, Neglia JP, Stram DO, Pollock BH, Castleberry RP. Neuroblastoma and parental occupation. Cancer Causes Control. 1999;10:539–49.
22. Michalek AM, Buck GM, Nasca PC, Freedman AN, Baptiste MS, Mahoney MC. Gravid health status, medication use, and risk of neuroblastoma. Am J Epidemiol. 1996;143:996–1001.
23. Kerr MA, Nasca PC, Mundt KA, Michalek AM, Baptiste MS, Mahoney MC. Parental occupational exposures and risk of neuroblastoma: a case-control study (United States). Cancer Causes Control. 2000;11:635–43.
24. Bunin GR, Ward E, Kramer S, Rhee CA, Meadows AT. Neuroblastoma and parental occupation. Am J Epidemiol. 1990;131:776–80.
25. Nyari TA, Dickinson HO, Parker L. Childhood cancer in relation to infections in the community during pregnancy and around the time of birth. Int J Cancer. 2003;104:772–7.
26. Bluhm E, McNeil DE, Cnattingius S, Gridley G, Ghormli El L, Fraumeni JF. Prenatal and perinatal risk factors for neuroblastoma. Int J Cancer. 2008;123:2885–90.
27. Johnson KJ, Puumala SE, Soler JT, Spector LG. Perinatal characteristics and risk of neuroblastoma. Int J Cancer. 2008;123:1166–72.
28. McLaughlin CC, Baptiste MS, Schymura MJ, Zdeb MS, Nasca PC. Perinatal risk factors for neuroblastoma. Cancer Causes Control. 2009;20: 289–301.
29. Kushner BH, Gilbert F, Helson L. Familial neuroblastoma. Case reports, literature review, and etiologic considerations. Cancer. 1986;57:1887–93.
30. Maris JM, Kyemba SM, Rebbeck TR, White PS, Sulman EP, Jensen SJ, Allen C, Biegel JA, Brodeur GM. Molecular genetic analysis of familial neuroblastoma. Eur J Cancer. 1997;33:1923–8.
31. Knudson AG, Strong LC. Mutation and cancer: neuroblastoma and pheochromocytoma. Am J Hum Genet. 1972;24:514–32.
32. Friedman DL, Kadan-Lottick NS, Whitton J, Mertens AC, Yasui Y, Liu Y, Meadows AT, Robison LL, Strong LC. Increased risk of cancer among siblings of long-term childhood cancer survivors: a report from the childhood cancer survivor study. Cancer Epidemiol Biomarkers Prev. 2005;14:1922–7.
33. Amiel J, Laudier B, Attié-Bitach T, Trang H, de Pontual L, Gener B, Trochet D, Etchevers H, Ray P, Simonneau M, Vekemans M, Munnich A, Gaultier C, Lyonnet S. Polyalanine expansion and frameshift mutations of the paired-like homeobox gene PHOX2B in congenital central hypoventilation syndrome. Nat Genet. 2003;33:459–61.
34. Moore SW. The contribution of associated congenital anomalies in understanding Hirschsprung's disease. Pediatr Surg Int. 2006;22:305–15.
35. Maris JM, Chatten J, Meadows AT, Biegel JA, Brodeur GM. Familial neuroblastoma: a three-generation pedigree and a further association with Hirschsprung disease. Med Pediatr Oncol. 1997;28:1–5.
36. Kushner BH, Hajdu SI, Helson L. Synchronous neuroblastoma and von Recklinghausen's disease: a review of the literature. J Clin Oncol. 1985;3:117–20.
37. DeBaun MR, Tucker MA. Risk of cancer during the first four years of life in children from The Beckwith-Wiedemann Syndrome Registry. J Pediatr. 1998;132:398–400.
38. Knudson AG, Meadows AT. Developmental genetics of neuroblastoma. J Natl Cancer Inst. 1976;57:675–82.
39. Knudson AG. Mutation and cancer: statistical study of retinoblastoma. Proc Natl Acad Sci U S A. 1971;68:820–3.
40. Brodeur GM, Maris JM, Yamashiro DJ, Hogarty MD, White PS. Biology and genetics of human neuroblastomas. J Pediatr Hematol Oncol. 1997;19:93–101.
41. Look AT, Hayes FA, Nitschke R, McWilliams NB, Green AA. Cellular DNA content as a predictor of response to chemotherapy in infants with unresectable neuroblastoma. N Engl J Med. 1984;311:231–5.
42. Gilbert F, Feder M, Balaban G, Brangman D, Lurie DK, Podolsky R, Rinaldt V, Vinikoor N, Weisband J. Human neuroblastomas and abnormalities of chromosomes 1 and 17. Cancer Res. 1984;44:5444–9.
43. Savelyeva L, Corvi R, Schwab M. Translocation involving 1p and 17q is a recurrent genetic alteration of human neuroblastoma cells. Am J Hum Genet. 1994;55:334–40.
44. Van Roy N, Laureys G, Cheng NC, Willem P, Opdenakker G, Versteeg R, Speleman F. 1;17 translocations and other chromosome 17 rearrangements in human primary neuroblastoma tumors and cell lines. Genes Chromosomes Cancer. 1994;10:103–14.
45. Bown N, Cotterill S, Lastowska M, O'Neill S, Pearson AD, Plantaz D, Meddeb M, Danglot G, Brinkschmidt C, Christiansen H, Laureys G, Speleman F, Nicholson J, Bernheim A, Betts DR, Vandesompele J, Van Roy N. Gain of chromosome arm 17q and adverse outcome in patients with neuroblastoma. N Engl J Med. 1999;340:1954–61.
46. Bown N, Lastowska M, Cotterill S, O'Neill S, Ellershaw C, Roberts P, Lewis I, Pearson AD. U.K. Cancer Cytogenetics Group and the U.K. Children's Cancer Study Group 17q gain in neuroblastoma predicts adverse clinical outcome. U.K. Cancer Cytogenetics Group and the U.K. Children's Cancer Study Group. Med Pediatr Oncol. 2001;36:14–9.

47. Brodeur GM, Green AA, Hayes FA, Williams KJ, Williams DL, Tsiatis AA. Cytogenetic features of human neuroblastomas and cell lines. Cancer Res. 1981;41:4678–86.
48. Maris JM, White PS, Beltinger CP, Sulman EP, Castleberry RP, Shuster JJ, Look AT, Brodeur GM. Significance of chromosome 1p loss of heterozygosity in neuroblastoma. Cancer Res. 1995;55:4664–9.
49. White PS, Maris JM, Beltinger C, Sulman E, Marshall HN, Fujimori M, Kaufman BA, Biegel JA, Allen C, Hilliard C. A region of consistent deletion in neuroblastoma maps within human chromosome 1p36.2–36.3. Proc Natl Acad Sci U S A. 1995;92:5520–4.
50. White PS, Maris JM, Sulman EP, Jensen SJ, Kyemba SM, Beltinger CP, Allen C, Kramer DL, Biegel JA, Brodeur GM. Molecular analysis of the region of distal 1p commonly deleted in neuroblastoma. Eur J Cancer. 1997;33:1957–61.
51. Maris JM, Guo C, Blake D, White PS, Hogarty MD, Thompson PM, Rajalingam V, Gerbing R, Stram DO, Matthay KK, Seeger RC, Brodeur GM. Comprehensive analysis of chromosome 1p deletions in neuroblastoma. Med Pediatr Oncol. 2001;36:32–6.
52. Caron H, van Sluis P, de Kraker J, Bökkerink J, Egeler M, Laureys G, Slater R, Westerveld A, Voûte PA, Versteeg R. Allelic loss of chromosome 1p as a predictor of unfavorable outcome in patients with neuroblastoma. N Engl J Med. 1996;334:225–30.
53. Brinkschmidt C, Poremba C, Christiansen H, Simon R, Schäfer KL, Terpe HJ, Lampert F, Boecker W, Dockhorn-Dworniczak B. Comparative genomic hybridization and telomerase activity analysis identify two biologically different groups of 4s neuroblastomas. Br J Cancer. 1998;77:2223–9.
54. Lastowska M, Nacheva E, McGuckin A, Curtis A, Grace C, Pearson A, Bown N. Comparative genomic hybridization study of primary neuroblastoma tumors. United Kingdom Children's Cancer Study Group. Genes Chromosomes Cancer. 1997;18:162–9.
55. Thompson PM, Seifried BA, Kyemba SK, Jensen SJ, Guo C, Maris JM, Brodeur GM, Stram DO, Seeger RC, Gerbing R, Matthay KK, Matise TC, White PS. Loss of heterozygosity for chromosome 14q in neuroblastoma. Med Pediatr Oncol. 2001;36:28–31.
56. Attiyeh EF, London WB, Mossé YP, Wang Q, Winter C, Khazi D, McGrady PW, Seeger RC, Look AT, Shimada H, Brodeur GM, Cohn SL, Matthay KK, Maris JM. Children's Oncology Group Chromosome 1p and 11q deletions and outcome in neuroblastoma. N Engl J Med. 2005;353:2243–53.
57. Maris JM, Mossé YP, Bradfield JP, Hou C, Monni S, Scott RH, Asgharzadeh S, Attiyeh EF, Diskin SJ, Laudenslager M, Winter C, Cole KA, Glessner JT, Kim C, Frackelton EC, Casalunovo T, Eckert AW, Capasso M, Rappaport EF, McConville C, London WB, Seeger RC, Rahman N, Devoto M, Grant SFA, Li H, Hakonarson H. Chromosome 6p22 locus associated with clinically aggressive neuroblastoma. N Engl J Med. 2008;358:2585–93.
58. Seeger RC, Wada R, Brodeur GM, Moss TJ, Bjork RL, Sousa L, Slamon DJ. Expression of N-myc by neuroblastomas with one or multiple copies of the oncogene. Prog Clin Biol Res. 1988;271:41–9.
59. Reiter JL, Brodeur GM. MYCN is the only highly expressed gene from the core amplified domain in human neuroblastomas. Genes Chromosomes Cancer. 1998;23:134–40.
60. Schwab M, Varmus HE, Bishop JM. Human N-myc gene contributes to neoplastic transformation of mammalian cells in culture. Nature. 1985;316:160–2.
61. Small MB, Hay N, Schwab M, Bishop JM. Neoplastic transformation by the human gene N-myc. Mol Cell Biol. 1987;7:1638–45.
62. Weiss WA, Aldape K, Mohapatra G, Feuerstein BG, Bishop JM. Targeted expression of MYCN causes neuroblastoma in transgenic mice. EMBO J. 1997;16:2985–95.
63. Brodeur GM, Seeger RC, Schwab M, Varmus HE, Bishop JM. Amplification of N-myc in untreated human neuroblastomas correlates with advanced disease stage. Science. 1984;224:1121–4.
64. Seeger RC, Brodeur GM, Sather H, Dalton A, Siegel SE, Wong KY, Hammond D. Association of multiple copies of the N-myc oncogene with rapid progression of neuroblastomas. N Engl J Med. 1985;313:1111–6.
65. Nakagawara A, Arima M, Azar CG, Scavarda NJ, Brodeur GM. Inverse relationship between trk expression and N-myc amplification in human neuroblastomas. Cancer Res. 1992;52:1364–8.
66. Nakagawara A, Arima-Nakagawara M, Scavarda NJ, Azar CG, Cantor AB, Brodeur GM. Association between high levels of expression of the TRK gene and favorable outcome in human neuroblastoma. N Engl J Med. 1993;328:847–54.
67. Nakagawara A, Azar CG, Scavarda NJ, Brodeur GM. Expression and function of TRK-B and BDNF in human neuroblastomas. Mol Cell Biol. 1994;14:759–67.
68. Svensson T, Rydén M, Schilling FH, Dominici C, Sehgal R, Ibáñez CF, Kogner P. Coexpression of mRNA for the full-length neurotrophin receptor trk-C and trk-A in favourable neuroblastoma. Eur J Cancer. 1997;33:2058–63.
69. Rydén M, Sehgal R, Dominici C, Schilling FH, Ibáñez CF, Kogner P. Expression of mRNA for the neurotrophin receptor trkC in neuroblastomas with favourable tumour stage and good prognosis. Br J Cancer. 1996;74:773–9.
70. Yamashiro DJ, Liu XG, Lee CP, Nakagawara A, Ikegaki N, McGregor LM, Baylin SB, Brodeur GM. Expression and function of Trk-C in favourable human neuroblastomas. Eur J Cancer. 1997;33:2054–7.
71. Shimada H, Chatten J, Newton WA, Sachs N, Hamoudi AB, Chiba T, Marsden HB, Misugi K. Histopathologic prognostic factors in neuroblastic

tumors: definition of subtypes of ganglioneuroblastoma and an age-linked classification of neuroblastomas. J Natl Cancer Inst. 1984;73:405–16.
72. Shimada H, Ambros IM, Dehner LP, Hata J, Joshi VV, Roald B, Stram DO, Gerbing RB, Lukens JN, Matthay KK, Castleberry RP. The International Neuroblastoma Pathology Classification (the Shimada system). Cancer. 1999;86:364–72.
73. Shimada H, Ambros IM, Dehner LP, Hata J, Joshi VV, Roald B. Terminology and morphologic criteria of neuroblastic tumors: recommendations by the International Neuroblastoma Pathology Committee. Cancer. 1999;86:349–63.
74. Brodeur GM, Seeger RC, Barrett A, Berthold F, Castleberry RP, D'Angio G, De Bernardi B, Evans AE, Favrot M, Freeman AI. International criteria for diagnosis, staging, and response to treatment in patients with neuroblastoma. J Clin Oncol. 1988;6:1874–81.
75. Brodeur GM, Pritchard J, Berthold F, Carlsen NL, Castel V, Castelberry RP, De Bernardi B, Evans AE, Favrot M, Hedborg F. Revisions of the international criteria for neuroblastoma diagnosis, staging, and response to treatment. J Clin Oncol. 1993;11:1466–77.
76. Monclair T, Brodeur GM, Ambros PF, Brisse HJ, Cecchetto G, Holmes K, Kaneko M, London WB, Matthay KK, Nuchtern JG, von Schweinitz D, Simon T, Cohn SL, Pearson ADJ, Task Force INRG. The International Neuroblastoma Risk Group (INRG) staging system: an INRG Task Force report. J Clin Oncol. 2009;27:298–303.
77. Neuroblastoma treatment (PDQ). Bethesda: National Cancer Institute; National Institutes of Health. http://www.cancer.gov/cancertopics/pdq/treatment/neuroblastoma/HealthProfessional/Page3#Section_14. Accessed Feb. 20, 2012.
78. Cohn SL, Pearson ADJ, London WB, Monclair T, Ambros PF, Brodeur GM, Faldum A, Hero B, Iehara T, Machin D, Mosseri V, Simon T, Garaventa A, Castel V, Matthay KK, Task Force INRG. The International Neuroblastoma Risk Group (INRG) classification system: an INRG Task Force report. J Clin Oncol. 2009;27:289–97.
79. Moppett J, Haddadin I, Foot AB. Neonatal neuroblastoma. Arch Dis Child Fetal Neonatal Ed. 1999;81:F134–7.
80. Haas D, Ablin AR, Miller C, Zoger S, Matthay KK. Complete pathologic maturation and regression of stage IVS neuroblastoma without treatment. Cancer. 1988;62:818–25.
81. Schmidt ML, Lukens JN, Seeger RC, Brodeur GM, Shimada H, Gerbing RB, Stram DO, Perez C, Haase GM, Matthay KK. Biologic factors determine prognosis in infants with stage IV neuroblastoma: A prospective Children's Cancer Group study. J Clin Oncol. 2000;18:1260–8.
82. De Bernardi B, Gerrard M, Boni L, Rubie H, Cañete A, Di Cataldo A, Castel V, Forjaz de Lacerda A, Ladenstein R, Ruud E, Brichard B, Couturier J, Ellershaw C, Munzer C, Bruzzi P, Michon J, Pearson ADJ. Excellent outcome with reduced treatment for infants with disseminated neuroblastoma without MYCN gene amplification. J Clin Oncol. 2009;27:1034–40.
83. Rubie H, De Bernardi B, Gerrard M, Cañete A, Ladenstein R, Couturier J, Ambros P, Munzer C, Pearson ADJ, Garaventa A, Brock P, Castel V, Valteau-Couanet D, Holmes K, Di Cataldo A, Brichard B, Mosseri V, Marquez C, Plantaz D, Boni L, Michon J. Excellent outcome with reduced treatment in infants with nonmetastatic and unresectable neuroblastoma without MYCN amplification: results of the prospective INES 99.1. J Clin Oncol. 2011;29:449–55.
84. Gigliotti AR, Di Cataldo A, Sorrentino S, Parodi S, Rizzo A, Buffa P, Granata C, Sementa AR, Fagnani AM, Provenzi M, Prete A, D'Ippolito C, Clerico A, Castellano A, Tonini GP, Conte M, Garaventa A, De Bernardi B. Neuroblastoma in the newborn. A study of the Italian Neuroblastoma Registry. Eur J Cancer. 2009;45:3220–7.
85. De Bernardi B, Pianca C, Boni L, Brisigotti M, Carli M, Bagnulo S, Corciulo P, Mancini A, De Laurentis C, Di Tullio MT. Disseminated neuroblastoma (stage IV and IV-S) in the first year of life. Outcome related to age and stage. Italian Cooperative Group on Neuroblastoma. Cancer. 1992;70:625–33.
86. Jennings RW, LaQuaglia MP, Leong K, Hendren WH, Adzick NS. Fetal neuroblastoma: prenatal diagnosis and natural history. J Pediatr Surg. 1993;28:1168–74.
87. Acharya S, Jayabose S, Kogan SJ, Tugal O, Beneck D, Leslie D, Slim M. Prenatally diagnosed neuroblastoma. Cancer. 1997;80:304–10.
88. Granata C, Fagnani AM, Gambini C, Boglino C, Bagnulo S, Cecchetto G, Federici S, Inserra A, Michelazzi A, Riccipetitoni G, Rizzo A, Tamaro P, Jasonni V, De Bernardi B. Features and outcome of neuroblastoma detected before birth. J Pediatr Surg. 2000;35:88–91.
89. Nuchtern JG. Perinatal neuroblastoma. Semin Pediatr Surg. 2006;15:10–6.
90. Adams GA, Shochat SJ, Smith EI, Shuster JJ, Joshi VV, Altshuler G, Hayes FA, Nitschke R, McWilliams N, Castleberry RP. Thoracic neuroblastoma: a Pediatric Oncology Group study. J Pediatr Surg. 1993;28:372–7. discussion 377–8
91. Abramson SJ, Berdon WE, Ruzal-Shapiro C, Stolar C, Garvin J. Cervical neuroblastoma in eleven infants—a tumor with favorable prognosis. Clinical and radiologic (US, CT, MRI) findings. Pediatr Radiol. 1993;23:253–7.
92. Haase GM, O'Leary MC, Stram DO, Lukens JN, Seeger RC, Shimada H, Matthay KK. Pelvic neuroblastoma—implications for a new favorable subgroup: a Children's Cancer Group experience. Ann Surg Oncol. 1995;2:516–23.
93. Nitschke R, Smith EI, Shochat S, Altshuler G, Travers H, Shuster JJ, Hayes FA, Patterson R,

McWilliams N. Localized neuroblastoma treated by surgery: a Pediatric Oncology Group Study. J Clin Oncol. 1988;6:1271–9.
94. Perez CA, Matthay KK, Atkinson JB, Seeger RC, Shimada H, Haase GM, Stram DO, Gerbing RB, Lukens JN. Biologic variables in the outcome of stages I and II neuroblastoma treated with surgery as primary therapy: a Children's Cancer Group study. J Clin Oncol. 2000;18:18–26.
95. De Bernardi B, Conte M, Mancini A, Donfrancesco A, Alvisi P, Tomà P, Casale F, Cordero di Montezemolo L, Cornelli PE, Carli M. Localized resectable neuroblastoma: results of the second study of the Italian Cooperative Group for Neuroblastoma. J Clin Oncol. 1995;13:884–93.
96. La Quaglia MP, Kushner BH, Su W, Heller G, Kramer K, Abramson S, Rosen N, Wolden S, Cheung NKV. The impact of gross total resection on local control and survival in high-risk neuroblastoma. J Pediatr Surg. 2004;39:412–7.
97. O'Neill JA, Littman P, Blitzer P, Soper K, Chatten J, Shimada H. The role of surgery in localized neuroblastoma. J Pediatr Surg. 1985;20:708–12.
98. Haase GM, Wong KY, deLorimier AA, Sather HN, Hammond GD. Improvement in survival after excision of primary tumor in stage III neuroblastoma. J Pediatr Surg. 1989;24:194–200.
99. Shorter NA, Davidoff AM, Evans AE, Ross AJ, Zeigler MM, O'Neill JA. The role of surgery in the management of stage IV neuroblastoma: a single institution study. Med Pediatr Oncol. 1995;24:287–91.
100. Le Tourneau JN, Bernard JL, Hendren WH, Carcassonne M. Evaluation of the role of surgery in 130 patients with neuroblastoma. J Pediatr Surg. 1985;20:244–9.
101. Castel V, Tovar JA, Costa E, Cuadros J, Ruiz A, Rollan V, Ruiz-Jimenez JI, Perez-Hernández R, Cañete A. The role of surgery in stage IV neuroblastoma. J Pediatr Surg. 2002;37:1574–8.
102. Kaneko M, Iwakawa M, Ikebukuro K, Ohkawa H. Complete resection is not required in patients with neuroblastoma under 1 year of age. J Pediatr Surg. 1998;33:1690–4.
103. Guglielmi M, De Bernardi B, Rizzo A, Federici S, Boglino C, Siracusa F, Leggio A, Cozzi F, Cecchetto G, Musi L, Bardini T, Fagnani AM, Bartoli GC, Pampaloni A, Rogers D, Conte M, Milanaccio C, Bruzzi P. Resection of primary tumor at diagnosis in stage IV-S neuroblastoma: does it affect the clinical course? J Clin Oncol. 1996;14:1537–44.
104. Shamberger RC, Smith EI, Joshi VV, Rao PV, Hayes FA, Bowman LC, Castleberry RP. The risk of nephrectomy during local control in abdominal neuroblastoma. J Pediatr Surg. 1998;33:161–4.
105. Adkins ES, Sawin R, Gerbing RB, London WB, Matthay KK, Haase GM. Efficacy of complete resection for high-risk neuroblastoma: a Children's Cancer Group study. J Pediatr Surg. 2004;39(6):931.
106. Rich BS, McEvoy MP, Kelly NE, Oh E, Abramson SJ, Price AP, Cheung NKV, La Quaglia MP. Resectability and operative morbidity after chemotherapy in neuroblastoma patients with encasement of major visceral arteries. J Pediatr Surg. 2011;46:103–7.
107. Matthay KK, Villablanca JG, Seeger RC, Stram DO, Harris RE, Ramsay NK, Swift P, Shimada H, Black CT, Brodeur GM, Gerbing RB, Reynolds CP. Treatment of high-risk neuroblastoma with intensive chemotherapy, radiotherapy, autologous bone marrow transplantation, and 13-cis-retinoic acid. Children's Cancer Group. N Engl J Med. 1999;341:1165–73.
108. Matthay KK, Reynolds CP, Seeger RC, Shimada H, Adkins ES, Haas-Kogan D, Gerbing RB, London WB, Villablanca JG. Long-term results for children with high-risk neuroblastoma treated on a randomized trial of myeloablative therapy followed by 13-cis-retinoic acid: a Children's Oncology Group study. J Clin Oncol. 2009;27:1007–13.
109. Kushner BH, Kramer K, LaQuaglia MP, Modak S, Yataghene K, Cheung NKV. Reduction from seven to five cycles of intensive induction chemotherapy in children with high-risk neuroblastoma. J Clin Oncol. 2004;22:4888–92.
110. Kushner BH, Kramer K, LaQuaglia MP, Modak S, Cheung NKV. Liver involvement in neuroblastoma: the Memorial Sloan-Kettering Experience supports treatment reduction in young patients. Pediatr Blood Cancer. 2006;46:278–84.
111. Baker DL, Schmidt ML, Cohn SL, Maris JM, London WB, Buxton A, Stram D, Castleberry RP, Shimada H, Sandler A, Shamberger RC, Look AT, Reynolds CP, Seeger RC, Matthay KK. Children's Oncology Group Outcome after reduced chemotherapy for intermediate-risk neuroblastoma. N Engl J Med. 2010;363:1313–23.
112. Rich BS, McEvoy MP, LaQuaglia MP, Wolden SL. Local control, survival, and operative morbidity and mortality after re-resection, and intraoperative radiation therapy for recurrent or persistent primary high-risk neuroblastoma. J Pediatr Surg. 2011;46:97–102.
113. Gillis AM, Sutton E, Dewitt KD, Matthay KK, Weinberg V, Fisch BM, Chan A, Gooding C, Daldrup-Link H, Wara WM, Farmer DL, Harrison MR, Haas-Kogan D. Long-term outcome and toxicities of intraoperative radiotherapy for high-risk neuroblastoma. Int J Radiat Oncol Biol Phys. 2007;69:858–64.
114. Kunieda E, Hirobe S, Kaneko T, Nagaoka T, Kamagata S, Nishimura G. Patterns of local recurrence after intraoperative radiotherapy for advanced neuroblastoma. Jpn J Clin Oncol. 2008;38:562–6.
115. Yu AL, Gilman AL, Ozkaynak MF, London WB, Kreissman SG, Chen HX, Smith M, Anderson B, Villablanca JG, Matthay KK, Shimada H, Grupp SA, Seeger R, Reynolds CP, Buxton A, Reisfeld RA, Gillies SD, Cohn SL, Maris JM, Sondel PM. Children's Oncology Group Anti-GD2 antibody

with GM-CSF, interleukin-2, and isotretinoin for neuroblastoma. N Engl J Med. 2010;363:1324–34.
116. Yamamoto K, Ohta S, Ito E, Hayashi Y, Asami T, Mabuchi O, Higashigawa M, Tanimura M. Marginal decrease in mortality and marked increase in incidence as a result of neuroblastoma screening at 6 months of age: cohort study in seven prefectures in Japan. J Clin Oncol. 2002;20:1209–14.
117. Woods WG, Gao RN, Shuster JJ, Robison LL, Bernstein M, Weitzman S, Bunin G, Levy I, Brossard J, Dougherty G, Tuchman M, Lemieux B. Screening of infants and mortality due to neuroblastoma. N Engl J Med. 2002;346:1041–6.
118. Schilling FH, Spix C, Berthold F, Erttmann R, Fehse N, Hero B, Klein G, Sander J, Schwarz K, Treuner J, Zorn U, Michaelis J. Neuroblastoma screening at one year of age. N Engl J Med. 2002;346:1047–53.
119. Laverdière C, Liu Q, Yasui Y, Nathan PC, Gurney JG, Stovall M, Diller LR, Cheung NK, Wolden S, Robison LL, Sklar CA. Long-term outcomes in survivors of neuroblastoma: a report from the Childhood Cancer Survivor Study. J Natl Cancer Inst. 2009;101:1131–40.
120. Levitt GA, Platt KA, De Byrne R, Sebire N, Owens CM. 4S neuroblastoma: the long-term outcome. Pediatr Blood Cancer. 2004;43:120–5.
121. Laverdière C, Cheung NKV, Kushner BH, Kramer K, Modak S, LaQuaglia MP, Wolden S, Ness KK, Gurney JG, Sklar CA. Long-term complications in survivors of advanced stage neuroblastoma. Pediatr Blood Cancer. 2005;45:324–32.
122. Kushner BH. Neuroblastoma: a disease requiring a multitude of imaging studies. J Nucl Med. 2004;45:1172–88.

Neonatal Soft Tissue Sarcomas

58

Timothy N. Rogers and Helen L. Rees

Abstract

Soft tissue lesions in neonates are relatively common. They cause concern for parents and can also present diagnostic difficulties for health professionals. Fortunately most are benign and usually vascular or developmental in origin. However, a small number of these lesions are found to be malignant and can present significant challenges in terms of management and may carry a poor prognosis. Therefore it is important to develop an approach to the diagnosis and management of all soft tissue lesions that will allow such tumours to be distinguished from the more common benign lesions.

Keywords

Neonatal soft tissue sarcoma • Classification • Surgical management • Outcomes

58.1 Introduction

Soft tissue lesions in neonates are relatively common. They cause concern for parents and can also present diagnostic difficulties for health professionals. Fortunately most are benign and usually vascular or developmental in origin [1]. However, a small number of these lesions are found to be malignant and can present significant challenges in terms of management and may carry a poor prognosis. Therefore it is important to develop an approach to the diagnosis and management of all soft tissue lesions that will allow such tumours to be distinguished from the more common benign lesions.

Soft tissue sarcomas are a heterogeneous group of tumours showing different pathways of differentiation depending on the putative cell of origin. They mainly derive from muscle, connective and supportive tissues, vascular and adipose tissues and can therefore arise at almost any anatomical site including superficial and deep soft tissues and within internal organs

T.N. Rogers, MBBCh, FCS(SA), FRCS(Paed) (✉)
Bristol Royal Hospital for Children, Upper Maudlin Street, Bristol BS2 8BJ, UK
e-mail: Timothy.Rogers@UHBristol.nhs.uk

H.L. Rees, FRCPCH
Medical Oncology,
Bristol Royal Hospital for Children, Bristol, UK

P.D. Losty et al. (eds.), *Rickham's Neonatal Surgery*, https://doi.org/10.1007/978-1-4471-4721-3_58

such as kidney and liver. By far the commonest subtype in children is rhabdomyosarcoma (RMS) with the remaining subtypes being grouped together as "non-rhabdomyosarcoma" (non-RMS) tumours, more commonly presenting in the adult population. RMS are generally categorised according to prognosis and site whilst the non-RMS tumours are classified by tissue of origin.

There are a number of issues which must be considered when a diagnosis of soft tissue sarcoma is made in a neonate. Firstly some malignant soft tissue tumours will behave differently in the neonate compared with their natural history in older children or adults, despite being histologically identical. In addition, delivery of multimodality therapies to neonates offers unique challenges and therefore it is important to consider the management of these tumours in the context of the age of the patient rather than just the histological diagnosis.

In this chapter we will include discussion around the epidemiology, histopathology, biology and clinical aspects of neonatal soft tissue sarcomas as well as appropriate management of this rare group of tumours. As well as those tumours historically described within the soft tissue sarcoma family we will also discuss malignant peripheral nerve sheath tumours, malignant rhabdoid tumours and the locally aggressive group of myofibroblastic lesions derived from mesenchymal tissue [2, 3].

58.2 Epidemiology

The incidence of malignancy occurring during the neonatal period (first 28 days of extra-uterine life) is over three times that of other paediatric age groups [4]. However, neonatal malignancy remains rare. In the United States, 130 neonates/year or 36.5 per 1 million live births over the neonatal period are diagnosed with cancer [5, 6]. It is worth noting that the definition of a congenital neoplasm is not consistent. Some describe neoplasms diagnosed up to 3 months after birth as being congenital. These congenital neoplasms account for 0.5–2% of all childhood neoplasms with a prevalence of 1.7–13.5 per 100,000 live births [7]. Others define congenital tumours as those recorded at birth or observed during the first week of life [8].

The commonest malignancy to present in the neonatal period is neuroblastoma. Other tumours presenting during this period include germ cell tumours, renal tumours, intracranial tumours, hepatic tumours and soft tissue sarcomas. Soft tissue sarcomas make-up 11% of malignancies diagnosed in the neonatal period [9]. Fifty percent of neonatal soft tissue sarcomas are diagnosed at birth with the remainder presenting during the first 4 weeks of life [9]. Rarely these tumours are identified on antenatal ultrasound.

Over the past 40 years, collaborative groups have studied some of these rare paediatric malignancies in the context of clinical trials where continued improved outcomes have been achieved. The Intergroup Rhabdomyosarcoma Study Group (IRSG) studies 1–4 showed that out of 3217 paediatric RMS treated in these trials only 14 (0.4%) were diagnosed in the neonatal period [10]. Overall soft tissue sarcomas represent about 8% of all childhood malignancies and by far the commonest histological subtype across all age ranges is rhabdomyosarcoma. However, only 2% of soft tissue sarcomas present in the neonatal period.

Neonatal soft tissue sarcomas can be broadly divided into three histologically distinct subgroups; rhabdomyosarcoma represents over a third of patients with the heterogeneous group of "other" non-rhabdomyosarcoma soft tissue sarcomas and congenital infantile fibrosarcoma making up the rest [9]. The United Kingdom National Registry of Childhood Tumours for infants born 1988–2007 and diagnosed in the first 4 weeks of life reflects this distribution (Table 58.1, see Table 52.1 in Chap. 52). In this National Registry the incidence of neonatal sarcoma was 2.6 per million live births.

Table 58.1 Epidemiology of neonatal tumours (see Table 52.1 in Chap. 52)

	Male	Female	Total
Rhabdomyosarcoma	9	4	13
Fibrosarcoma	3	7	10
Malignant haemangiopericytoma	1	0	1
Mesenchymal chondrosarcoma	1	0	1
Extrarenal rhabdoid	0	5	5
Peripheral PNET	2	0	2
Malignant haemangioendothelioma	1	0	1
Epithelioid sarcoma	1	0	1
Soft tissue sarcoma NOS (not otherwise specified)	1	2	3
Total sarcomas	19	18	37
Total cancers	183	211	394

Data from National Registry of Childhood Tumours for infants born 1988–2007 and diagnosed in the first 4 weeks of life

Table 58.2 Histological subtypes of soft tissue sarcomas described in the neonatal period

Frequency	Histological subtype
Most commonly occurring	Rhabdomyosarcoma Infantile fibrosarcoma
Others	Malignant peripheral nerve sheath tumour (2) Alveolar soft part sarcoma Malignant rhabdoid tumour of soft tissues Malignant ectomesenchymoma (13) Epithelioid hemangioendothelioma Malignant haemangioendothelioma Leiomyosarcoma (2) Epithelioid sarcoma Clear cell sarcoma of soft tissue (2) Malignant mesenchymal sarcoma (9) Angiosarcoma (9) Chondrosarcoma (9) Primitive sarcoma (9) Peripheral neuroectodermal tumour Malignant haemangiopericytoma

Sarcomas accounted for 9.4% of all cancers in neonates.

58.3 Histopathology

Soft tissue sarcomas constitute a heterogeneous group of tumours with over 70 histological sub types of sarcoma recognised. It is very important to make an accurate histological diagnosis as the management and outcomes vary considerably between subtypes. Table 58.2 shows a list of soft tissue sarcomas documented in the literature as arising in the neonatal period [3, 11, 12]. RMS, the most common sarcoma seen in childhood, is further subdivided into a number of histological subtypes based on prognosis. The more common subtypes include embryonal rhabdomyosarcoma (ERMS) and alveolar rhabdomyosarcoma (ARMS). RMS will be discussed in more detail later. There are a few sarcomas where there are no documented cases arising in neonates to be found following a thorough review of the literature. These subtypes include synovial sarcoma, desmoplastic small round cell tumour, undifferentiated sarcoma of the liver and low-grade fibromyxoid sarcoma.

58.4 Genetics and Biology

Advancing knowledge and understanding about the biological features of tumours has allowed us to begin to characterise the behaviour of soft tissue sarcomas as well as many other types of tumours. Increasingly this knowledge is contributing not only to making the diagnosis but also towards planning the treatment of that patient. Recent molecular studies have provided us with a battery of cytogenetic abnormalities that can be detected almost routinely when a tumour is investigated by the pathologist. In many tumours there are a variety of abnormalities including chromosomal translocations, inversions, gene amplification and gene rearrangements. Several childhood sarcomas bear reciprocal chromosomal translocations which correlate with specific tumour

Table 58.3 Common cytogenetic abnormalities found in soft tissue sarcomas

Histology	Translocation/cytogenetic abnormalities	Fusion Gene
Alveolar rhabdomyosarcoma (ARMS)	t(2;12)(q35;q14) t(1;12)(q36;q14)	PAX3/FOXO1A PAX7/FOXO1A
Embryonal rhabdomyosarcoma (ERMS)	Gain of chromosomes: 2,8,11,12,13, 20 LOH at 11p25	
Congenital infantile fibrosarcoma (CIF)	t(12;15)(q13;q25) Trisomy: 8,11,17 and 20	NTRK3/ETVG (TEL)
Ewings/PNET	t(11;22)(q24;q12) t(11;22)(q22;q12) t(17;22)(q12;q12) t(7;22)(p22;q12)	EWS/FLI1 EWS/ERG EWS/E1AF EWS/ETV1
Desmoplastic small round cell tumours (DSRCT)	t(11;22)(q13;q12)	EWS/WT1
Clear cell sarcoma (CCS)	t(12;22)(q13;q12)	EWS/ATS1
Inflammatory myofibroblastic tumours	t(1;2)(q25;p23) t(2;19)(p23;q23)	TPM3/ALK TPM4/ALK
Alveolar soft part sarcoma	t(X;17)(p11;q25)	TEL/ASPL
Synovial sarcoma (SS)	t(X;18)(p11;q11)	SYT/SSX1 SYT/SSX2 SYT/SSX4
Malignant rhabdoid tumours (MRT)	Loss of INI1 on q22	

types. Table 58.3 shows some of the more common cytogenetic abnormalities which can be identified in a variety of soft tissue sarcomas. This list includes some tumours which have not been reported in the neonatal age group. In order to continue our pursuit of knowledge around the biological behaviour of all solid tumours, it is essential that we continue to collect fresh tissue at biopsy or resection for cytogenetic analysis which can be performed using both FISH (fluorescent in situ hybridisation) and RT-PCR (reverse transcription polymerase chain reaction). In many cases, the significance of the genetic abnormality is not clear. However, in other instances, such as for ARMS bearing the fusion gene PAX3-FOX01A, we have known for a number of years that these tumours carry a worse prognosis [13].

58.5 Specific Tumour Types

58.5.1 Rhabdomyosarcoma

ERMS does not have structural chromosomal rearrangements but rather has frequent chromosome gains. The most notable gains in ERMS are to chromosomes 2, 8, 11, 12, 13, and 20 [14–16]. Loss of heterozygosity (LOH) at 11p15 (the Beckwith—Wiedemann region) is a frequent abnormality in ERMS [17]. This is also the location for the IGF-2 gene. LOH leads to an overexpression of the IGF-2 gene and this event is proposed to play a part in the pathogenesis of ERMS [18]. Approximately 85% of ARMS carry the characteristic reciprocal translocation t(2;13)(q35;q14) resulting in the formation of *PAX3-FOX01A which codes for a chimeric transcription factor. A variant translocation* t(1;13)(p36;q14) which occurs in approximately 10% of ARMS, gives rise to *PAX7-FOX01A fusion protein and is thought to carry a better prognosis* [13]. The molecular disruptions caused by these translocations are well characterised and involve three developmentally important transcription factors, PAX3, PAX7 and FOX01A (formerly FKHR). These translocations rearrange the transcription factors PAX3 and PAX7, and juxtapose these genes with FOX01A (formerly FKHR), a member of the fork head transcription factor family. The juxtaposition of

PAX3/7 and FOX01A causes transcriptional upregulation.

Recently there has been some interesting work investigating the difference between fusion positive and fusion negative ARMS. Williamson et al. performed gene expression analysis on over 200 histologically verified RMS. The tumours were divided into ERMS, fusion positive ARMS and fusion negative ARMS. They were able to show convincingly that ERMS and ARMS fusion-negative are one and the same; that is, they arise in the same locations and have a comparable frequency of metastases—distinct from ARMS fusion-positive. Most importantly, they have indistinguishable outcomes with therapies that were not stratified for histological subtype. This piece of work may allow us already to consider how we stratify treatment based on molecular investigations [19].

58.5.2 Infantile Fibrosarcoma

The majority of congenital infantile fibrosarcomas (CIF) carry the characteristic t(12;15)(p13;q26) translocation which gives rise to an ETV6-NTRK3 fusion gene [20]. The t(12;15)(p13;q25) fuses the *ETV6 (TEL)* gene from chromosome 12q13 with the 15q25 neurotrophin-3 receptor gene, *NTRK3 (TRKC)*. Fusion transcripts are expressed in tumour cells and encode for the ETV6-NTRK3 fusion protein. This protein has a role in activation of the P13-Akt pathway which is involved in cell survival. This translocation is identical to that seen in cellular mesoblastic nephroma, with a similar histology [21]. This fusion has not been described in adult fibrosarcoma. In addition, trisomies of chromosomes 8, 11, 17 and 20 are consistently found in infantile fibrosarcomas, and again are also described in the cellular form of CMN [21].

58.5.3 Malignant Rhabdoid Tumour

In malignant rhabdoid tumours the INI1 (SMARCB1) gene on chromosome 22q functions as a classic tumour suppressor gene. SMARCB1 acts as an epigenetic tumour suppressor which functions as a "gatekeeper" within the cell cycle. The presence of germline mutations (in up to 30% of patients) are correlated with manifestations at a very early age, synchronous and metachronous tumours at different locations, and poor prognosis [22].

58.5.4 Ewing's Sarcoma Family of Tumours

Ewing's sarcoma/soft tissue Primitive Neuro-Ectodermal Tumours (PNET) are characterised by translocations involving the EWS gene on chromosome 22. Amongst paediatric sarcomas, Ewing's sarcoma appears to have the greatest variety of fusion partners, resulting in considerable complexity in analysis and interpretation. T(11;22) involving the EWS gene on chromosome 22 and the FLI1 gene on chromosome is the most common translocation, present in 85–90% of Ewing's tumours. Approximately 5–10% of Ewing's sarcomas carry an alternate translocation (see Table 58.3) [21].

58.5.5 Desmoplastic Small Round Cell Tumour (DSRCT)

The molecular hallmark of DSCRT is a unique chromosomal translocation (t11;22)(p13:q12) resulting in a transcript EWS-WT1, which is diagnostic of this tumour. EWS is located on chromosome 22 at 22q12 whilst the Wilms tumour suppressor gene (WT1) is located on chromosome 11, at 11p13. This transcript encodes for a protein which acts as a transcriptional activator that fails to suppress tumour growth. Variant forms resulting from alternative splices are recognised and are more common in tumours arising in unusual sites [21].

58.5.6 Clear Cell Sarcoma of Soft Tissue

Clear cell sarcoma (CCS) of soft tissue is another example of a tumour bearing a translocation involving the EWS gene [21]. The t(12;22)(q13;q12) fuses EWS with the ATF1 gene on chromosome 12. However fusions associated with CCS are not specific and have also been associated with angiomatoid fibrous histiocytoma, which has a much more favourable prognosis [21].

58.5.7 Synovial Sarcoma

Synovial sarcomas (SS) are characterised as a group by the presence of a specific translocation t(X;18)(p11.2;q11.2). This translocation is considered the "gold standard" for the diagnosis of synovial sarcoma and is present in >95% of cases. The t(X;18)(p11.2;q11.2) translocation fuses the SSXT(SYT) gene from chromosome 18 with SSX1 (about 2/3 of cases), SSX2 (about 1/3 of cases) or SSX4 (rare cases) genes from the X chromosome. Cases with both SYT/SSX1 and SYT/SSX2 fusion transcripts have been described and the SYT/SSX1 transcript is reported to be significantly associated with biphasic Synovial sarcoma.

58.6 Genetic Predisposition Syndromes

A number of recognised genetic predisposition syndromes are associated with the development of soft tissue sarcomas. These include Beckwith-Weidemann syndrome, Li Fraumeni syndrome, retinoblastoma, neurofibromatosis type 1, Costello syndrome, Rubinstein-Taybi syndrome and Gorlin basal cell naevus syndrome. However, sarcomas developing in these clinical situations seldom present in the perinatal period. Nevertheless, it is important to recognise any potential genetic predisposition to cancer so that genetic counselling, screening, surveillance and timely treatment can be offered [23].

58.7 Clinical Presentation and Differential Diagnosis

Initial signs and symptoms depend on the site of the tumour, extension into surrounding tissue and the presence or not of metastases. Identification of neonatal soft tissue tumours may be made in the foetal period [24–27], at birth or within the first month of life. Routine antenatal ultrasound may identify a mass. Polyhydramnios, hydrops foetalis, obstructive uropathy or growth restriction can be associated with intra-uterine tumours [22, 23, 28]. Pre-natal MRI with planned post-natal MRI is the radiological investigation of choice to further characterise these tumours and inform decisions about obstetric and post-natal care [27]. If a mass is small at the time of routine obstetric ultra-

Table 58.4 Commonest presenting signs and symptoms by primary site

Primary site	Symptoms and signs
Skin and subcutaneous tissue	Asymptomatic mass Discoloured subcutaneous nodule Solid or semicystic swelling
Head and neck (including orbital, paranasal, nasopharyngeal and sinuses)	Painless or painful swelling Proptosis Ptosis Ophthalmoplegia Facial nerve palsy Other cranial nerve palsies Nasal discharge Trismus
Limbs	Painless swelling
CNS	Irritability Seizures Hydrocephalus
Abdomen/genito-urinary tract	Painless scrotal lesions Haematuria Vulval nodule Polypoid vaginal lesions Antenatal diagnosis of abdominal mass Postnatal diagnosis of abdominal mass Intestinal obstruction
Metastatic disease	Otherwise unexplained: Poor feeding Seizures Pain Irritability Pancytopenia

sound scanning or develops later in gestation, it may remain undetected until presenting as dystocia during natural delivery [27]. Presentation at delivery with obstructed labour has been described in congenital infantile fibrosarcoma [29].

Soft tissue sarcomas may be clinically and ultrasonographically mistaken for haemangiomas or vascular malformations which are the commonest soft tissue tumours diagnosed in early life [8, 30–32]. There are a few reports of angiosarcomas presenting in pre-existing complex vascular malformations [33]. It is important to recognise this possibility if a pre-existing lesion changes characteristics. (Table 58.4).

Cutaneous and subcutaneous sarcomas of the neonate can present as asymptomatic masses. They may be solid to semicystic, solitary or multiple, skin coloured or erythematous, blue or yellow, fungating or ulcerating.

Intra-Abdominal masses or retroperitoneal masses may be identified on antenatal scanning or on post-natal examination. Haemoperitoneum from an extensive intra-abdominal rhabdoid tumour has presented in an ex-premature corrected to term neonate with sudden abdominal distention, fall in haematocrit and irritability [22].

Neonatal surgeons need to be aware of the possibility that intestinal obstruction can in rare instances, be caused by intestinal tumours as this in turn may require a different surgical approach [34, 35]. When faced with this intra-operative finding, the surgeon should try to achieve a complete resection.

Non-neoplastic conditions of the scrotum are usually diagnosed clinically. However if a tumour is suspected then appropriate investigations must be undertaken as the correct oncological approach differs from the approach to commoner benign pathologies. If a tumour is not suspected and a direct scrotal approach made, then the risk will be that of contaminating the surgical field with tumour cells resulting in the need for re-resection.

Table 58.5 Differential diagnosis of lesions by primary site

Site	Benign	Malignant
Head and neck	Branchial cyst/ remnant	Teratoma
	Thyroglossal cyst	Neuroblastoma
	Lymphangioma	Leukaemia
	Haemangioma	Retinoblastoma
	Abscess	
	Dermoid cyst	
	Encephalocoele	
	Epulis	
	Congenital goitre	
	Sternomastoid tumour	
	Ectopic thyroid	
	Thymic cyst	
Skin and subcutaneous lesions	Haemangioma	Neuroblastoma
	Xanthoma	Leukaemia
	Other vascular anomaly	
Abdominal/ pelvic masses	Hydronephrosis	Neuroblastoma
	Ovarian cyst	Mesoblastic nephroma
	Vitello-intestinal remnant	Teratoma
	Urachal remnant	Nephroblastoma
	Lymphangioma	Hepatoblastoma
	Hepatic vascular	
	Renal cystic disease	
Scrotal masses	Hydrocoele	Germ cell tumour
	Hernia	Sarcoma
	Testicular torsion	
Vaginal/vulval lesions	Prolapsing ureterocoele	Sarcoma
	Condylomata	

58.8 Making the Diagnosis

58.8.1 Principles

When there is suspicion that a neonatal soft tissue lesion may be malignant then tissue diagnosis is essential. In this situation, consultation with a wider experienced team may be helpful. An experienced paediatric dermatologist can help to distinguish the commoner benign lesions from the rare atypical malignant ones and your local paediatric oncologists may be helpful to plan appropriate investigations such as imaging and tumour markers ahead of a biopsy. (Table 58.5).

58.8.2 Tumour Markers

Whilst there are no tumour markers specific for soft tissue sarcoma, exclusion of other tumours is always helpful. Therefore a single timepoint collection of urine for catecholamines will exclude neuroblastoma in the majority of cases and a normal AFP/BHCG (corrected for the age of the infant), will exclude germ cell tumours.

58.8.3 Imaging

Ultrasound of a suspicious lesion should be the first radiological investigation. Sonography can delineate whether a palpable abnormality is a mass, whether the mass is solid or cystic, and vascular characteristics of the lesion. For extensive or deep lesions, cross-sectional imaging is preferred and MRI has replaced CT in most cases. MRI will delineate the extent of the lesion, define local involvement of surrounding structures and demonstrate characteristics of the lesion. Malignant tumours often show an infiltrative growth pattern shown by encasement of neurovascular bundles and growth into surrounding structures such as joints and bone and these features can usually be identified and clearly documented on MRI. It is often appropriate to perform an MRI before biopsy so post-surgical changes do not distort the radiological appearance.

In addition to its diagnostic value, MRI is used to monitor post-operative complications as well as to evaluate response to therapy. Limitations of MRI include the inability to differentiate residual or recurrent disease from post-operative oedema, inflammation and haemorrhage. CT is superior to MRI in the evaluation of bone involvement; therefore, CT should be performed when osseous invasion is suspected. As part of a staging process once histopatholgical diagnosis is confirmed, a Technecium 99 m scan may be required to exclude bony metastases.

Distinction between different tumour subtypes is not always possible because they often have similar appearances, however there are sometimes features demonstrated on an MRI which point to a particular subtype of sarcoma. For example, rhabdomyosarcomas are usually isointense to muscle on T1-W, intermediate to high intensity on T2-W, and may have signal voids due to vessels having high flow velocity. Infantile Fibrosarcomas are similar to rhabdomyosarcomas on T1-W and T2-W imaging but their margins are usually poorly defined. Synovial sarcomas are usually also isointense on T1-W and hyperintense on T2-W imaging. Evidence of intra-tumoural haemorrhage may be present, and fluid-filled levels are seen in 20% of scans. These tumours can be predominantly cystic and therefore can be mistaken for a Baker's cyst, or a haematoma. Their appearance can also be similar to a ganglion [27, 36].

58.8.4 Biopsy

The history, examination and radiological evaluation of a soft tissue mass should provide sufficient clinical information for a differential diagnosis to be made ahead of a biopsy of the lesion. This is essential to ensure that the biopsy is taken and transported in the correct manner to the laboratory to allow the pathologist to make the diagnosis.

Incision biopsy is usually the appropriate initial surgical procedure. Excision biopsy should only be undertaken if a microscopically clear resection can be achieved without danger or mutilation. In an excisional biopsy, margins and specimen should be carefully marked to allow re-resection should the biopsy reveal a positive margin on histological assessment. Incision biopsy is also indicated if the regional lymph nodes are positive or there is metastatic disease.

In accessible sites open incisional biopsy is indicated. Longitudinal incisions are frequently better than horizontal incisions on areas such as an extremity. A biopsy to confirm malignancy requires that the biopsy tract be excised at the time of reoperation; if the biopsy site is inappropriately placed, a much larger subsequent excision would be required. In less accessible sites, multiple core-needle biopsies under ultrasound guidance may be appropriate. Endoscopic biopsies are appropriate for pelvic or paranasal tumours if technically feasible.

It is important to obtain sufficient tissue for histology, immunohistochemistry, cytogenetics, biological studies and for frozen storage/tissue banking. Prior discussion with the pathologist and pathology laboratory is essential so the specimen is processed correctly.

Biopsy of the regional lymph nodes is recommended where possible. Current trials have adopted a more aggressive approach to evaluating lymph nodes. Previously it was thought that lymph node involvement was rare. Of the patients whose lymph nodes were clinically negative but were biopsied anyway, 17% were found to have microscopic disease [37]. The utility of sentinel-lymph node mapping is being evaluated. For extremity tumours if sentinel lymph node mapping is not available, aggressive sampling is warranted.

58.9 Specific Tumour Types

58.9.1 Rhabdomyosarcoma

RMS is the commonest subtype of soft tissue sarcoma seen in the neonatal population. Rhabdomyosarcoma arises from embryonic mesenchymal cells that have the potential to differentiate into skeletal muscle. RMS and can be further divided into the following subgroups based on prognosis:

- Superior prognosis
  - Botryoid embryonal
  - Spindle
- Intermediate prognosis
  - Embryonal
- Poor prognosis
  - ARMS including
  - Solid variant
  - Undifferentiated

The subtypes most frequently found in neonates with rhabdomyosarcoma are embryonal, botryoid variant and undifferentiated rhabdomyosarcoma [10].

Rhabdomyosarcoma is one of the "small round blue-cell tumours" of childhood. Occasionally, these types of tumours can be difficult to differentiate. Rhabdomyosarcoma cells tend to have variable differentiation along the myogenesis pathway. The various rhabdomyosarcoma subtypes often have characteristic features that allow them to be distinguished histologically. For example, botryoid are classically described macroscopically as "grape-like" in appearance. Histopathologically, it is necessary to identify a cambium layer beneath an intact epithelium in at least one microscopic field to make this diagnosis. For the diagnosis of ARMS to be made, the characteristic "alveolar" pattern needs to be present even if just in a small focal area. However, in order to confirm the diagnosis of RMS immunohistochemistry must be performed as well as cytogenetic analysis to confirm the presence or not of chromosomal aberrations. The most sensitive and specific immunohistochemical test for RMS is for myogenin. Myogenin belongs to a group of myogenic regulatory proteins whose expression determines commitment and differentiation of primitive mesenchymal cells into skeletal muscle. The expression of myogenin has been demonstrated to be extremely specific for rhabdomyoblastic differentiation, which makes it a useful marker in the differential diagnosis of rhabdomyosarcomas from other malignant small round cell tumours of childhood. The percentage of cells expressing myogenin is significantly higher in alveolar than embryonal RMS [21]. As discussed previously (Genetics and Biology section) cytogenetic analysis using FISH and/or RTPCR should be routinely performed to look for evidence of translocation or chromosomal loss. This may further help to confirm a sub-classification of RMS which in turn will contribute to the decisions regarding treatment and prognosis.

RMS can arise anywhere in the body but the anatomical distribution does vary with patient age. The head, neck and trunk are the predominant sites in neonatal RMS [9]. In early childhood, head and neck and genito-urinary tumours predominate whereas in older children the proportion of extremity tumours with alveolar histology increases. Paratesticular RMS accounts for 12% of childhood scrotal tumours and usually presents between 4 and 5 years of age [38]. In childhood, paratesticular RMS accounts for 7% of RMS but only one paratesticular RMS has been described in the neonatal age group up to 2000.

Neonatal RMS carries a very poor prognosis unless it can be fully resected. The Children's Cancer Group reported on 11 neonates with RMS. Nine of these received chemotherapy to which they had a poor response and 2/11 were alive at the time of reporting, one with metastatic disease, and the other after total cystectomy. Two neonates received radiotherapy [39]. The results reported by the Intergroup Rhabdomyosarcoma Study Group were better with 6/14 patients surviving at 3 year follow-up. Seven died of disease and one died of chemotherapy-related toxicity [10].

Children below the age of 1 year have a poorer prognosis than older children. Whilst this may in part be due to biological factors, the difficulties in delivering multimodality treatment in this age group should not be underestimated.

58.9.2 Congenital Infantile Fibrosarcoma

Infantile fibrosarcoma is the most common soft tissue sarcoma diagnosed in infants under 1 year of age. Infantile fibrosarcomas make-up between 20 and 50% of malignant soft tissue tumours in neonates and infants. 30–50% are present at birth. Most report a male predominance. The predominant anatomic sites in neonates are the extremities (58%), trunk (25%), and head and neck (17%) [40]. They are subcutaneous lesions but can rarely occur in the mesentery, retroperitoneum or orbit [41]. Metastases are rare, occurring in less than 10% of cases with dissemination most commonly to the lungs.

Histologically these tumours are composed of spindle-cells arranged in bundles and fascicles, resulting in a characteristic "herring-bone" appearance. Unlike adult fibrosarcoma, infantile fibrosarcoma is often infiltrated by inflammatory cells, and tends to have less pleomorphism. Immunohistochemistry tends to be non-specific

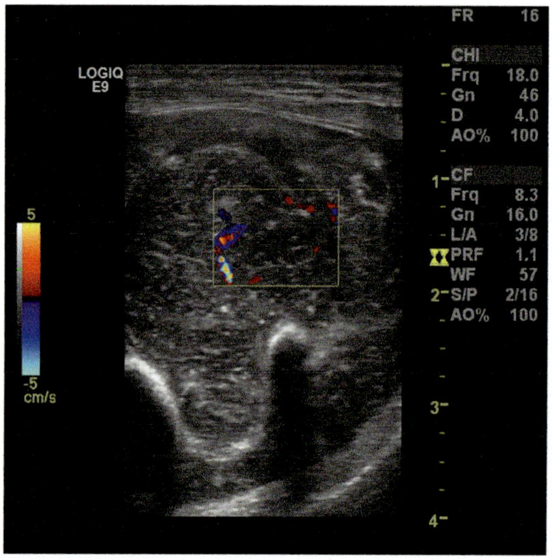

Fig. 58.1 Ultrasound at day 8 of life showing a large right calf mass

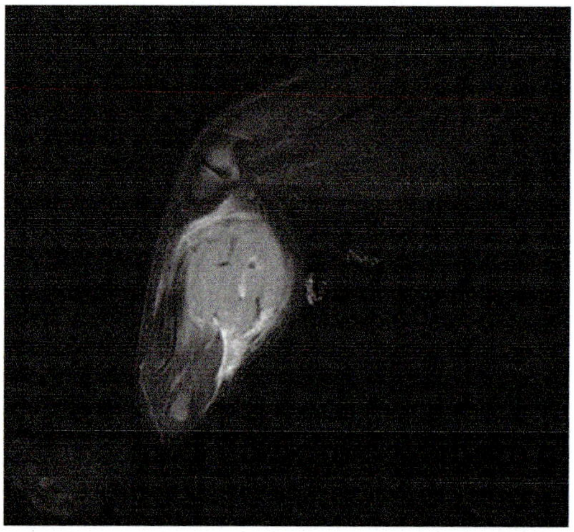

Fig. 58.2 MRI Sagittal STIR sequence at 15 days of life showing right calf mass involving neurovascular bundle and expanding between tibia and fibular bones

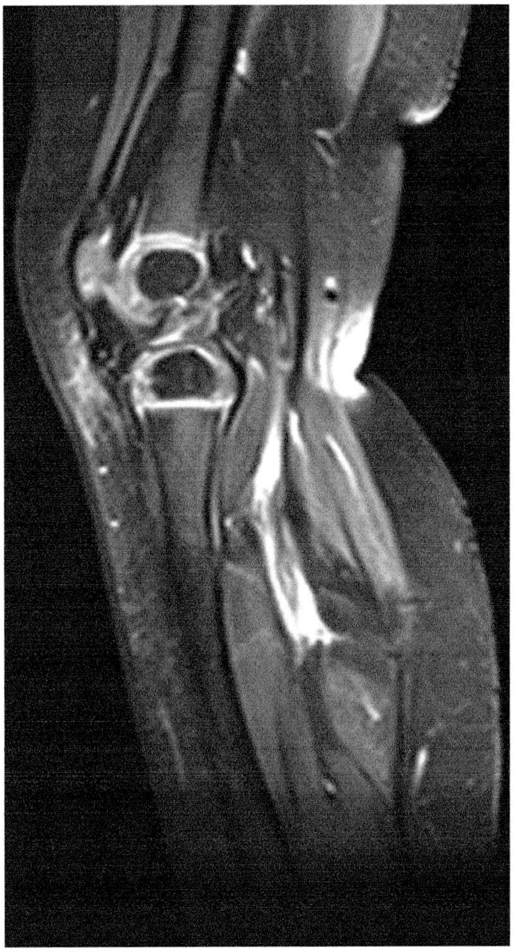

Fig. 58.3 MRI Sagittal STIR sequence 16 months after commencement of chemotherapy showing almost complete response to systemic therapy alone

[21]. The translocation t(12;15) and resulting fusion product are present in the infantile-type of fibrosarcoma but not in the adult-type.

Clinically they are violaceous firm tumours that enlarge rapidly, often within a few weeks or months. They can grow to become massive but conversely spontaneous regression has been reported.

Surgery is the mainstay of treatment if it can be achieved simply without mutilation. In those under 3 months of age a "wait and see" approach could be considered to allow for possible spontaneous regression. Infantile fibrosarcoma is chemosensitive and where a tumour is felt to be inoperable, chemotherapy can be tried to permit subsequent conservative surgery [11] (see Figs. 58.1, 58.2, and 58.3). Infantile fibrosarcoma has a much better prognosis than the adult form of fibrosarcoma with a 5 years survival estimated between 84 and 93%. The Children's Cancer Group reported that all 12 of their cases were disease free at a median follow-up of 6.6 years [9]. Local recurrence rates are high, ranging from 17 to 43% and often occur within the first few weeks after the initial excision. Even if local disease does recur, repeat surgical resection will result in cure in the majority of the cases. Therefore close follow-up is essential to allow earlier intervention in the event the disease returns locally [32].

58.9.3 Extracranial Malignant Rhabdoid Tumour (MRT)

Extracranial Rhabdoid tumours are highly aggressive malignant tumours of childhood. The tumour was given the name "rhabdoid" because microscopically it resembles a rhabdomyosarcoma although it does not show skeletal muscle markers by electron microscopy, immunoperoxidase, or cytogenetic studies. The most well-known extracranial site for rhabdoid tumours to occur is the kidney but tumours can be found elsewhere in soft tissues outside the CNS. Recently there has been recognition that rhabdoid tumours of the kidney and CNS are identical or closely related in terms of the characteristic genetic abnormalities [42]. It is less clear whether the non-renal extracranial rhabdoid tumours share the same histogenic origins as their renal and CNS counterparts. Therefore appropriate cytogenetic analysis on tumours with these histological features is essential.

Some cases of malignant rhabdoid tumours have been reported at birth and a few more in the first month of life [43]. In the perinatal period the extrarenal non-CNS site predominates. When the tumour occurs *in utero,* it is more likely to present at birth with multiple metastases and a rapidly progressive, downhill clinical course ending in early death. Rupture of the tumour *in utero* causing a severe foetal anaemia has been described. Rhabdoid tumour may present with subcutaneous nodules resembling the "blueberry muffin" lesion more commonly associated with neuroblastoma before discovery of the primary tumour. 75% of patients have metastases at diagnosis [22, 42]. The tumour metastasizes to multiple sites such as the skin, placenta, bones, lungs, lymph nodes, brain and liver.

The histological diagnosis of rhabdoid tumour is based on identifying the characteristic rhabdoid tumour cell and the presence of a deletion or mutation of the INI1 gene located on chromosome 22q11. The INI1 gene (SMARCB1) on chromosome 22q functions as a classic tumour suppressor gene. The observation that mice, which have only one functioning copy of the INI1 gene present, are predisposed to MRT supports this premise [44]. Germline mutations of INI1 have been documented in patients with more than one primary tumour within the CNS and kidney and therefore the presence of MRT in a neonate requires the additional consideration of genetic investigation and counselling for the family.

Treatment is multimodal with surgery, chemotherapy with or without radiotherapy. Cure generally is achieved only in cases of localised disease. Chemotherapy usually results in a partial but not durable response and is often administered to simplify the tumour resection or reduce the radiation field.

Regardless of location, all rhabdoid tumours are highly aggressive and have a universally poor prognosis.

58.9.4 Desmoplastic Small Round Cell Tumour

Desmoplastic small round cell tumour (DSRCT) is a highly aggressive tumour that mainly affects young adults, and has a strong male predilection. Occasionally the histological diagnosis may be challenging if the immunohistochemistry is inconclusive or the fibrous stroma is poorly represented in a small biopsy [21]. However, the translocation t(11;22)(p13;q12) which results in the chimeric fusion transcript EWS-WT1, characterises this tumour. Therefore, once again, appropriate cytogenetic analysis, should be requested where the clinical features might suggest this diagnosis.

58.9.5 Malignant Ectomesenchymoma

Malignant ectomesenchymomas are usually diagnosed in the first 3 years of life. Surgery is the mainstay of treatment and survival correlates with resectability. These tumours are treated in a similar way to high-risk rhabdomyosarcomas [45].

58.9.6 Ewing's Sarcoma Family of Tumours

Ewing's sarcoma or soft tissue PNETs are a group of tumours that arise from pluripotential neural crest cells. Histologically they have small round blue cells and characteristically Homer-Wright rosettes. PNETs have varying degrees of neuroectodermal differentiation [21]. PNETs are highly aggressive and have a high local recurrence rate. Common sites of metastasis are lung, bone, and liver. Wide excision is performed, but if this is not feasible then amputation should be considered. Chemotherapy usually precedes definitive surgery and adjuvant radiotherapy may be useful in the presence of microscopically positive surgical margins [8].

58.9.7 Synovial Sarcoma

Synovial sarcoma (SS) is the most common non-rhabdomyosarcoma soft tissue sarcoma (NRSTS) in childhood. Despite its name it does not arise from the synovium but from the soft tissue in close proximity to it. As discussed previously over 90% of SS carry the characteristic reciprocal t(x; 18)(p11.2;q11.2).SS typically presents as a painless mass located near a joint, but can present as acute arthritis or joint contracture. Synovial sarcomas have been reported in a wide variety of anatomical sites, including visceral organs and the head and neck. They may appear as purely cystic and are the most common malignant tumour to be mistaken for a benign lesion.

58.9.8 Epithelioid Sarcoma

Epithelioid sarcoma is a rare tumour that primarily affects adolescents and young adults but does occur in neonates [31]. It most commonly presents as a superficial lesion in the distal extremities, particularly the hands, and although typically indolent in behaviour, carries a high risk of recurrence and late metastasis. A "proximal" form of epithelioid sarcoma has been described, that has a propensity to occur in the perineum, pelvis and genitourinary tract. It is more aggressive than the classic form of epithelioid sarcoma. Cytogenetically, epithelioid sarcomas have shown non-specific chromosomal gains and deletions.

58.9.9 Malignant Peripheral Nerve Sheath Tumour (MPNST)

Malignant peripheral nerve sheath tumours arise from cells differentiating towards those of the peripheral nerve sheath. They occur rarely in the neonatal period but have been described causing neonatal intestinal obstruction [34]. Complete surgical resection offers the only chance for cure as these tumours are not usually chemosensitive. Overall MPNST carries a poor prognosis but there is a suggestion that survival for patients less than 1 year may be better than in older patients [46].

58.9.10 Clear Cell Sarcoma of Soft Tissue

Clear cell sarcoma of soft tissue (CCS) almost always arises in deep soft tissues, closely related to aponeuroses and tendons of the extremities. CCS is primarily a tumour of adolescents and young adults, and is unusual in children younger than 10. CCS is the most common malignancy of the ankle and foot in adolescents with up to 75% arising in the extremity. Early diagnosis with wide local excision offers the best chance of cure with a 5-year survival ranging from 47 to 63% [47].

58.9.11 Low-Grade Fibromyxoid Sarcoma

This neoplasm displays a deceptively bland microscopic appearance, and yet carries a significant risk of metastases, with a propensity for a long latent period before metastases develop. It occurs primarily in young adults, but 19% of cases are seen in children [21].

58.9.12 Hemangioendothelioma

Hemangioendotheliomas (HE) includes a variety of neoplasms of vascular origin. Malignant Hemangioendotheliomas are considered to be angiosarcomas. Kaposiform HE, spindle cell HE and retiform HE are low-grade tumours, and should be treated by surgery alone. Epithelioid Hemangioendotheliomas (EHE) include two distinct subtypes, epithelioid hemangioendothelioma of soft-parts, and epithelioid hemangioendothelioma of bone, lung and liver. Treatment of these lesions is unclear as they do not usually respond to chemotherapy. Alpha-interferon treatment has been advocated and may work by an anti-angiogenic mechanism [48].

58.9.13 Haemangiopericytoma

Haemangiopericytomas are composed of mesenchymal cells derived from pericytes that occur in blood vessels. Haemangiopericytomas constitute 3% of pediatric soft tissue sarcomas. One neonate in Great Britain was diagnosed in the 20 year period 1988–2007. When occurring in the first year of life their behaviour is more benign and sometimes demonstrates spontaneous regression or maturation into a haemangioma. Treatment is wide local excision with chemotherapy reserved for incomplete resection [49].

58.9.14 Mesenchymal Chondrosarcoma

Mesenchymal chrondrosarcomas are rare aggressive tumours arising from soft tissues in about a third of cases. They are thought to originate from chondroblasts that have failed to develop into mature chondrocytes and have the appearance of primitive connective tissue cells. One neonate in Great Britain was diagnosed in the 20 year period 1988–2007.

58.9.15 Myofibroblastic Lesions and Aggressive Fibromatosis/Desmoid

58.9.15.1 Myofibromatosis

These lesions are benign and are derived from contractile myoid cells around blood vessels [50]. These tumours can be divided into three different entities:

1. Infantile myofibroma (solitary)
2. Multicentric myofibromatosis and
3. Multicentric myofibromatosis with visceral involvement.

There are no specific cytogenetic changes identified in this group of tumour. Solitary or multicentric lesion are most commonly found within subcutaneous tissues of the head and neck although can also be found on the extremities. Visceral lesions can occur within any of the major organs such as liver and heart. These lesions can often grow rapidly to begin with but usually settle down and can regress spontaneously. Complete resection is curative but not always possible. Therefore when vital structures such as the heart, lungs, pleura, mesentery, liver and even the central nervous system are involved, surgical resection can be challenging if not impossible and this form of the disease carries a very poor prognosis [51–53].

58.9.15.2 Inflammatory Myofibroblastic Tumours

These tumours usually involve the abdomen or lungs and behave in a benign manner. However they can be locally invasive particularly in the abdomen and recur in about 25% of cases. Again they can be multifocal in origin and can prove fatal if they involve a large portion of the bowel mesentery. Resection with a clear histological margin is the treatment of choice. Chemotherapy, immunosuppressive therapy and radiotherapy are generally not effective.

58.9.15.3 Solitary Intestinal Fibromatosis

This is a rare cause of neonatal intestinal obstruction. This tumour is diagnosed at laparotomy and may appear as a circumferential firm white mass causing marked narrowing of the intestinal lumen. Solitary Intestinal Fibromatoses have been reported in both small and large bowel [54]. Spindle cell neoplasms originating from fibroblastic, myofibroblastic or smooth muscle cell origin have also been reported in the literature to cause intestinal obstruction in neonates [54]. These lesions are categorised as a variety of lesions including fibromatosis, fibrosarcoma, or leiomyosarcoma. Fibromatosis is a neoplastic proliferation of myofibroblasts and/or fibroblasts and therefore some of the reported cases of intestinal leiomyosarcoma may represent fibromatosis [54]. When fibromatosis is occurs as a solitary lesion the prognosis is excellent. In contrast, the generalised or multiple form of fibromatosis demonstrates a high rate of local recurrence and overall carries a worse prognosis [55].

58.9.15.4 Aggressive Fibromatosis or Desmoid Tumours

Aggressive fibromatosis (AF) are fibrous tissue proliferations that are locally aggressive, but do not metastasize. They tend to grow slowly and diffusely along fascial planes and lack a defined edge. Resection, although difficult, is the treatment of choice. When unresectable, there are a number of adjuvant therapies available to try. These range from non-cytotoxic agents such as anti-inflammatory agents/NSAIDs and Tamoxifen to chemotherapy agents such as doxorubicin or cyclophosphamide. These tumours grow slowly and therefore the treatment strategy involves prolonged exposure to therapy of between 12 and 18 months. For this reason methotrexate and vinblastine is a good low dose combination that is frequently adopted as it is effective and least toxic over time. There is a variable response to chemotherapy with approximately a 50% response rate. Local recurrence rate is reported to occur in between 25 and 75% of resected cases. Positive microscopic margins, large initial tumours and extremity/girdle tumours have the highest chance of recurrence [45].

58.9.16 Staging

Once a diagnosis of soft tissue sarcoma is made then the patient needs to be staged fully in order to assess the extent of disease and plan treatment. There are different staging classifications depending on whether the diagnosis is RMS or Non-RMS. In addition, the staging in the USA is slightly different to that used across Europe.

Non-Rhabdomyosarcoma soft tissue sarcomas are staged according to the TNM Classification. The staging process includes radiological assessment of the primary site, the drainage nodal basins, and distant sites looking for metastatic disease. Bone marrow aspirates and trephines identify the presence of metastatic disease in the marrow whilst patients with parameningeal primary tumours require a lumbar puncture to assess for presence of disease in the cerebrospinal fluid. (Table 58.6).

After surgical resection a post-surgical pTNM Classification uses the same variables with the designation complemented by histological findings. In the case of rhabdomyosarcomas, the stage designated at diagnosis as localised or metastatic and the treatment pathway is defined according to the risk stratification (see below). In addition there is an IRS grouping classification based on primary tumour status after surgical treatment or biopsy. (Table 58.7).

Table 58.6 TNM staging classification

T1	Tumour confined to tissue of origin
T2	Tumour extends beyond tissue of origin
a	≤5 cm in maximum diameter
b	>5 cm in maximum diameter
N0	No nodal involvement
N1	Nodal involvement
M0	No distant metastases
M1	Distant metastases

Table 58.7 IRS staging classification

IRS 1	Primary tumour macroscopically and microscopically completely removed
IRS 2	Primary tumour macroscopically removed but with proven or suspected microscopic residual disease
IRS 3	Macroscopic primary residual disease
IRS 4	Metastases or malignant non-regional nodes

58.10 Risk Stratification

Patients are stratified according to a number of variables that have been shown to predict the likelihood of recurrence. These variables include:

1. Primary tumour site,
2. tumour size,
3. age at diagnosis,

Table 58.8 Risk stratification for treatment of non-metastatic Rhabdomyosarcoma in Europe

Risk Group	Subgroups	Pathology	IRS Group	Site	Nodal stage	Size and age
Low	A	Favourable	1	Any	N0	Favourable
Standard	B	Favourable	1	Any	N0	Unfavourable
	C	Favourable	2, 3	Favourable	N0	Any
	D	Favourable	2, 3	Unfavourable	N0	Favourable
High	E	Favourable	2, 3	Unfavourable	N0	Unfavourable
	F	Favourable	2, 3	Any	N1	Any
	G	Unfavourable	1, 2, 3	Any	N0	Any
Very high	H	Unfavourable	1, 2, 3	Any	N1	Any

4. IRS grouping,
5. pathology,
6. nodal involvement
7. Presence of metastases.

The European paediatric soft tissue sarcoma group (EpSSG) risk stratification designates patients according to whether they are Low risk, Standard risk, High risk, Very high risk based on the variables listed above. For example favourable pathology would include all embryonal, botryoid and spindle cell RMS whilst alveolar subtype falls into unfavourable category (see Table 58.8). The patients are then stratified into a subgroup (A–H) and a treatment strategy is decided. The Intergroup Rhabdomyosarcoma study group (IRS) uses slightly different risk stratification with subgroups separated into low, intermediate and high risk.

58.11 Multimodality Therapy

General considerations in the delivery of chemotherapy to neonates with cancer include their body composition, body water, body surface area, and body weight. Physiological differences in renal and liver function, P450 enzyme activity, and nutritional requirements need to be taken into account in order to treat neonates effectively whilst minimizing treatment related toxicity [17]. Treatment should aim to limit any compromise to normal growth and development of the neonate. Extravasation injuries can be devastating therefore chemotherapy needs to be delivered into a central vein via reliable central venous access.

58.12 Primary Site Management

58.12.1 Surgical Management

The general principles of surgical management include complete wide excision of the primary tumour and surrounding uninvolved margins while preserving function. However, the surgical strategy needs to be informed by the histological diagnosis as some tumour types can afford a more conservative surgical approach or may require upfront chemotherapy before any definitive surgical procedure [56]. There are virtually no circumstances where it would be appropriate to embark on a "debulking" procedure. The quality of resection is often crucial to local control and is graded:

- R0—microscopically clear margin,
- R1—macroscopic resection with positive microscopic margins,
- R2—macroscopic tumour left at resection margin

Primary resection should only be undertaken if an R0 resection can be achieved without danger or mutilation. Generally an incision biopsy is appropriate if the regional nodes are involved and/or there are distant metastases.

Primary Re-Excision (PRE) is performed to achieve microscopic clearance in patients with residual tumour (certain or doubtful) after primary operation, before other therapies, if this can be done without danger or mutilation. PRE should be considered, even if the margins are apparently normal, if the initial resection was not a "cancer" operation (i.e. malignancy was not suspected at initial excision).

Secondary Operation. The aim is to achieve an R0 resection of residual tumour after neoadjuvant chemotherapy. Marginal resection R1 may be acceptable depending on the histological type of soft tissue tumour, particularly infantile fibrosarcoma. If neoadjuvant chemotherapy (or chemotherapy and radiotherapy) have been unsuccessful then mutilating surgery may be indicated.

Reconstructive surgical options need to be considered before the primary tumour is treated. This is done in conjunction with a reconstructive plastic, orthopaedic or urologic surgeon as the case dictates.

58.12.2 Radiotherapy

Radiotherapy delivered to neonates carries a very high morbidity and is generally avoided if at all possible. It is destructive to normal tissues within the radiotherapy field and interferes significantly with normal growth. In addition having radiotherapy poses a significant risk for development of second malignancies in later life. In order to limit the morbidity, brachytherapy at certain sites using intracavitary or interstitial implants is being used in older children in the management of bladder/prostate and head and neck soft tissue sarcomas [57, 58].

58.12.3 Site-Specific Surgical Treatment

The surgical treatment of soft tissue sarcomas is site-specific, and will be discussed by individual site.

58.12.3.1 Head and Neck

Complete surgical resection is difficult but may be appropriate after neoadjuvant chemotherapy. Histological diagnosis will influence the need for a radical local therapy approach. For example, infantile fibrosarcoma may respond to chemotherapy alone and not require complete resection. Conversely, treatment of rhabdomyosarcoma requires complete resection to offer the best chance of cure. Parameningeal sites pose the greatest difficulty. Radiotherapy is initially withheld in neonates because of the high associated morbidity. The planning of reconstructive surgery needs to be done ahead of resection.

58.12.3.2 Orbital Rhabdomyosarcoma

Biopsy is usually the only local therapy required although occasionally enucleation or exenteration may be needed.

58.12.3.3 Vagina

Chemotherapy alone may be sufficient treatment. Conservative local resection may be feasible to resect the tumour. In older girls, intra-cavitory brachytherapy after ovarian transposition is often preferable.

58.12.3.4 Bladder/Prostate

Cystoscopy and biopsy should be the initial procedure. Primary resection is seldom indicated and only for small tumours in the fundus of the bladder. Neoadjuvant chemotherapy followed by conservative surgery and radiotherapy (external beam or brachytherapy) may be appropriate. If this is not feasible then exenterative surgery should be considered.

58.12.3.5 Paratesticular Rhabdomyosarcoma

Orchidectomy should be through an inguinal incision with ligation of the cord at internal ring. With very large tumours a scrotal approach may be appropriate keeping the tunica vaginalis intact.

58.12.3.6 Extremities

Wide local excision is usually indicated. Again, histological diagnosis will influence the need for a radical local therapy approach. Frozen sections of resection margins can inform intra-operative surgical decisions. Amputation may need consideration because the radiotherapy effects on growth and function may deliver a poorer result than amputation.

Conclusion

Neonatal soft tissue sarcomas are a rare heterogeneous group of tumours. A growing understanding of their differing biological characteristics in the context of multinational cooperative studies will continue to improve the treatment strategies offered. The aim to improve survival outcomes in poor prognosis tumours and minimise treatment morbidity in those with favourable tumours will continue. Early involvement of a multidisciplinary team is key to appropriate management.

References

1. Minard-Colin V, Orbach D, Martelli H, Bodemer C, Oberlin O. [Soft tissue tumors in neonates]. Arch Pediatr 2009;16(7):1039–48.
2. Spicer RD. Neonatal sarcoma. Early Hum Dev. 2010;86(10):633–6.
3. Sultan I, Casanova M, Al-Jumaily U, Meazza C, Rodriguez-Galindo C, Ferrari A. Soft tissue sarcomas in the first year of life. Eur J Cancer. 46(13):2449–56.
4. Reis LA, Hankey BF, Miller BA, et al. Cancer statistics review 1973–1988. Bethesda: NIH Publication; 1991.
5. Reaman G. Special considerations for the infant with cancer. In: Rizzo PA, Poplack DG, editors. Principles and practice of pediatric oncology. Philadelphia: Lippincott; 1989. p. 263–74.
6. Bader JL, Miller RW. US cancer incidence and mortality in the first year of life. Am J Dis Child. 1979;133(2):157–9.
7. Kazan-Tannus JF, Levine D. Imaging of fetal tumors. Ultrasound Clin. 2007;2(2):245–63.
8. Daw JL, Wiedrich TA, Bauer BS. Congenital primitive neuroectodermal tumor of the hand: a case report. J Hand Surg [Am]. 1997;22(4):743–6.
9. Dillon PW, Whalen TV, Azizkhan RG, Haase GM, Coran AG, King DR, et al. Neonatal soft tissue sarcomas: the influence of pathology on treatment and survival. Children's Cancer Group Surgical Committee. J Pediatr Surg. 1995;30(7):1038–41.
10. Lobe TE, Wiener ES, Hays DM, Lawrence WH, Andrassy RJ, Johnston J, et al. Neonatal rhabdomyosarcoma: the IRS experience. J Pediatr Surg. 1994;29(8):1167–70.
11. Braun P, Fernandezmontes J, Calatayud A. Congenital infantile fibrosarcoma: Report of four cases and review of the literature. Eur J Radiol Extra. 2007;61(1):33–9.
12. Ferrari A, Miceli R, Meazza C, Zaffignani E, Gronchi A, Piva L, et al. Soft tissue sarcomas of childhood and adolescence: the prognostic role of tumor size in relation to patient body size. J Clin Oncol Off J Am Soc Clin Oncol. 2009;27(3):371–6.
13. Sorensen PH, Lynch JC, Qualman SJ, Tirabosco R, Lim JF, Maurer HM, et al. PAX3-FKHR and PAX7-FKHR gene fusions are prognostic indicators in alveolar rhabdomyosarcoma: a report from the Children's Oncology Group. J Clin Oncol. 2002;20(11):2672–9.
14. Wang-Wuu S, Soukup S, Ballard E, Gotwals B, Lampkin B. Chromosomal analysis of sixteen human rhabdomyosarcomas. Cancer Res. 1988;48(4):983–7.
15. Dietrich CU, Jacobsen BB, Starklint H, Heim S. Clonal karyotypic evolution in an embryonal rhabdomyosarcoma with trisomy 8 as the primary chromosomal abnormality. Genes Chromosomes Cancer. 1993;7(4):240–4.
16. Bridge JA, Liu J, Weibolt V, Baker KS, Perry D, Kruger R, et al. Novel genomic imbalances in embryonal rhabdomyosarcoma revealed by comparative genomic hybridization and fluorescence in situ hybridization: an intergroup rhabdomyosarcoma study. Genes Chromosomes Cancer. 2000;27(4):337–44.
17. Loh WE Jr, Scrable HJ, Livanos E, Arboleda MJ, Cavenee WK, Oshimura M, et al. Human chromosome 11 contains two different growth suppressor genes for embryonal rhabdomyosarcoma. Proc Natl Acad Sci U S A. 1992;89(5):1755–9.
18. Zhan S, Shapiro DN, Helman LJ. Activation of an imprinted allele of the insulin-like growth factor II gene implicated in rhabdomyosarcoma. J Clin Invest. 1994;94(1):445–8.
19. Williamson D, Missiaglia E, de Reynies A, Pierron G, Thuille B, Palenzuela G, et al. Fusion gene-negative alveolar rhabdomyosarcoma is clinically and molecularly indistinguishable from embryonal rhabdomyosarcoma. J Clin Oncol. 2010;28(13):2151–8.
20. Knezevich SR, McFadden DE, Tao W, Lim JF, Sorensen PH. A novel ETV6-NTRK3 gene fusion in congenital fibrosarcoma. Nat Genet. 1998;18(2):184–7.
21. Pawel BR. Recent advances in the molecular diagnosis of paediatric soft tissue sarcomas. Diagn Histopathol. 2011;17(1):25–35.
22. Malhotra Y, Fitzgerald TN, Jubinsky PT, Harper H, Silva CT, Zambrano E, et al. A unique case of rhabdoid tumor presenting as hemoperitoneum in an infant. J Pediatr Surg. 2011;46(1):247–51.
23. Loh ML. In: Taeusch HW, Ballard RA, Gleason CA, eds. Avery's diseases of the newborn: Neoplasia. 8th ed. Philadelphia: Elsevier Saunders; 2004. 1664 p.
24. Dolkart LA, Reimers FT, Kuonen CA. Intrathoracic congenital fibrosarcoma. A case report. J Reprod Med. 1995;40(5):391–3.
25. Michigami T, Yamato H, Mushiake S, Nakayama M, Yoneda A, Satomura K, et al. Hypercalcemia associated with infantile fibrosarcoma producing parathyroid hormone-related protein. J Clin Endocrinol Metab. 1996;81(3):1090–5.
26. Tadmor OP, Ariel I, Rabinowitz R, Ne'eman Z, Stark M, Newman M, et al. Prenatal sonographic appearance of congenital fibrosarcoma. J Clin Ultrasound. 1998;26(5):276–9.
27. Ozcan Umit Aksoy KE, Atilla D, Canan E. Diagnosis of congenital fibrosarcoma facilitated by pre- and postnatal MRI. J Radiol Extra. 2010;74(3):e65–8.
28. Scheier M, Ramoni A, Alge A, Brezinka C, Reiter G, Sergi C, et al. Congenital fibrosarcoma as cause for fetal anemia: prenatal diagnosis and in utero treatment. Fetal Diagn Ther. 2008;24(4):434–6.
29. Nonaka D, Sun CC. Congenital fibrosarcoma with metastasis in a fetus. Pediatr Dev Pathol. 2004;7(2):187–91.
30. Chigurupati R, Alfatooni A, Myall RW, Hawkins D, Oda D. Orofacial rhabdomyosarcoma in neonates and young children: a review of literature and management of four cases. Oral Oncol. 2002;38(5):508–15.
31. Gupta H, Davidoff AM, Rao BN, Jenkins JJ, Spunt SL. Neonatal epithelioid sarcoma: a distinct clinical entity? J Pediatr Surg. 2006;41(7):e9–e11.
32. Asgari M, Rubin BP, Hornung RL. Neonate with a fibrosarcoma and consumptive coagulopathy. J Am Acad Dermatol. 2004;50(2 Suppl):S23–5.
33. Al Dhaybi R, Agoumi M, Powell J, Dubois J, Kokta V. Lymphangiosarcoma complicating extensive con-

genital mixed vascular malformations. Lymphat Res Biol. 2010;8(3):175–9.
34. Lee YJ, Moon H, Park ST, Ha WS, Choi SG, Hong SC, et al. Malignant peripheral nerve sheath tumor arising from the colon in a newborn: report of a case and review of the literatures. J Pediatr Surg. 2006;41(2):e19–22.
35. Ein SH, Beck AR, Allen JE. Colon sarcoma in the newborn. J Pediatr Surg. 1979;14(4):455–7.
36. Stein-Wexler R. MR imaging of soft tissue masses in children. Radiol Clin North Am. 2009;47(6):977–95.
37. Neville HL, Andrassy RJ, Lobe TE, Bagwell CE, Anderson JR, Womer RB, et al. Preoperative staging, prognostic factors, and outcome for extremity rhabdomyosarcoma: a preliminary report from the Intergroup Rhabdomyosarcoma Study IV (1991-1997). J Pediatr Surg. 2000;35(2):317–21.
38. Cakmak O, Karaman A, Cavusoglu YH, Oksal A. Paratesticular rhabdomyosarcoma in a neonate. J Pediatr Surg. 2000;35(4):605–6.
39. Reaman GH. Special considerations for the infant with cancer. In: Rizzo PA, Poplack DG, editors. Principles and practice of pediatric oncology. Philadelphia: Lippincott; 1989. p. 263–74.
40. Blocker S, Koenig J, Ternberg J. Congenital fibrosarcoma. J Pediatr Surg. 1987;22(7):665–70.
41. Petra Braun JGF-M, Calatayud AV. Congenital infantile fibrosarcoma: Report of four cases and review of the literature. Eur J Radiol Extra. 2007;61(1):33–9.
42. Isaacs H Jr. Fetal and neonatal rhabdoid tumor. J Pediatr Surg. 2010;45(3):619–26.
43. Dominey A, Paller AS, Gonzalez-Crussi F. Congenital rhabdoid sarcoma with cutaneous metastases. J Am Acad Dermatol. 1990;22(5 Pt 2):969–74.
44. Roberts CW, Galusha SA, McMenamin ME, Fletcher CD, Orkin SH. Haploinsufficiency of Snf5 (integrase interactor 1) predisposes to malignant rhabdoid tumors in mice. Proc Natl Acad Sci U S A. 2000;97(25):13796–800.
45. EPSSG. A protocol for localized non-rhabdomyosarcoma soft tissue sarcomas. Phase 3 clinical trial STS 2006.03. 2005.
46. Hayes-Jordan AA, Spunt SL, Poquette CA, Cain AM, Rao BN, Pappo AS, et al. Nonrhabdomyosarcoma soft tissue sarcomas in children: is age at diagnosis an important variable? J Pediatr Surg. 2000;35(6):948–53; discussion 53–4
47. Malchau SS, Hayden J, Hornicek F, Mankin HJ. Clear cell sarcoma of soft tissues. J Surg Oncol. 2007;95(6):519–22.
48. Ferrari A, Miceli R, Meazza C, Zaffignani E, Gronchi A, Piva L, et al. Soft tissue sarcomas of childhood and adolescence: the prognostic role of tumor size in relation to patient body size. J Clin Oncol. 2009;27(3):371–6.
49. Ping-Yi Hsu W-MH, Huang H-Y, Chen C-Y, Chou H-C, Tsao P-N, Hsieh W-S. Congenital hemangiopericytoma in a neonate. J Formos Med Assoc. 2006;105(3):247–51.
50. LeBoit PE, Burg G, Weedon D, Sarasain A. (Eds.): World Health Organization Classification of Tumours. Pathology and Genetics of Skin Tumours. IARC Press: Lyon 2006
51. Ang P, Tay YK, Walford NQ. Infantile myofibromatosis: a case report and review of the literature. Cutis. 2004;73(4):229–31.
52. Wiswell TE, Davis J, Cunningham BE, Solenberger R, Thomas PJ. Infantile myofibromatosis: the most common fibrous tumor of infancy. J Pediatr Surg. 1988;23(4):315–8.
53. Roggli VL, Kim HS, Hawkins E. Congenital generalized fibromatosis with visceral involvement. A case report. Cancer. 1980;45(5):954–60.
54. Chang WW, Griffith KM. Solitary intestinal fibromatosis: a rare cause of intestinal obstruction in neonate and infant. J Pediatr Surg. 1991;26(12):1406–8.
55. Arets HG, Blanco C, Thunnissen FB, Heineman E. Solitary intestinal fibromatosis as a cause of bile vomiting in a neonate. J Pediatr Surg. 2000;35(4):643–5.
56. Orbach D, Rey A, Cecchetto G, Oberlin O, Casanova M, Thebaud E, et al. Infantile fibrosarcoma: management based on the European experience. J Clin Oncol. 2010;28(2):318–23.
57. Blank LE, Koedooder K, Pieters BR, van der Grient HN, van de Kar M, Buwalda J, et al. The AMORE protocol for advanced-stage and recurrent nonorbital rhabdomyosarcoma in the head-and-neck region of children: a radiation oncology view. Int J Radiat Oncol Biol Phys. 2009;74(5):1555–62.
58. Martelli H, Haie-Meder C, Branchereau S, Franchi-Abella S, Ghigna MR, Dumas I, et al. Conservative surgery plus brachytherapy treatment for boys with prostate and/or bladder neck rhabdomyosarcoma: a single team experience. J Pediatr Surg. 2009;44(1):190–6.

Renal Tumours

59

Robert Carachi

Abstract

Renal neoplasms are rare in the newborn and account for only 8% of neonatal tumours. Congenital mesoblastic nephroma (CMN), first described by Kastner in 1921, is the most common renal tumour in the neonate. It is also known as a fetal renal hamartoma, mesenchymal hamartoma of infancy, or lipomyomatous hamartoma.

Keywords

Newborn renal tumors • Congenital mesoblastic nephroma

59.1 History

Renal neoplasms are rare in the newborn and account for only 8% of neonatal tumours. Congenital mesoblastic nephroma (CMN) first described by Kastner in 1921 [1], is the most common renal tumour in the neonate. It is also known as a fetal renal hamartoma, mesenchymal hamartoma of infancy, or lipomyomatous hamartoma.

59.2 Incidence and Epidemiology

It has an incidence of 2.8% of all renal tumours of childhood, with a mean age of presentation of 3.4 months in contrast to an average age of 3 years in Wilms' tumours [2]. Its frequency is 22.8% of all primary tumours in children 1 year old or less [3]. The majority of renal neoplasms originating in the fetus and found during the first weeks of life, differ in structure and in biological behaviour from a nephroblastoma. In the CCG Neonatal Study there were 25 neonatal renal neoplasms of which 17 were CMN and the rest were Wilms' tumours [4]. A review of neonatal Wilms' tumours in the national Wilms' tumour register identified 15 cases out of 6832 patients with an incidence of 0.16% demonstrating how rare malignant renal neoplasms are in neonates.

59.3 Pathology

Bolande and associates, in 1967, recognised CMN as a unique lesion that could be distinguished

R. Carachi, MBE, MD, PhD, FRCS(Gla)
University of Glasgow, Glasgow, Scotland
e-mail: robert.carachi@glasgow.ac.uk

P.D. Losty et al. (eds.), *Rickham's Neonatal Surgery*, https://doi.org/10.1007/978-1-4471-4721-3_59

clinically and pathologically from true congenital Wilms' tumour by its benign clinical behaviour, a preponderance of mesenchymal derivatives and lack of the malignant epithelial components typical of Wilms' tumour [5]. A definite infiltrative tendency distinguishes CMN from hamartomas with more limited growth potential. CMN is usually solid, unilateral and can attain a very large size like a uterine fibroid.

Histological differentiation is that of a spindle cell neoplasm with interlacing bundles of fibroblasts and myofibroblasts. Tumour types have irregular interdigitating margins in the perirenal fat and wide margins of excision are desirable for complete removal. Incomplete removal results in tumour recurrence which happens within a year of resection in most instances [6].

Atypical and more aggressive mesoblastic nephromas tend to be soft, fleshy tumours with areas of gross haemorrhage and necrosis and are more cellular without recognisable normal glomeruli or tubules.

Another variant is a congenital cystic mesoblastic nephroma (cellular variant) which can present as a unilocular haemorrhagic cyst. This can be detected antenatally and mis-diagnosed as a haematoma in the kidney. The lining of the wall of this cyst shows a typical cellular rim comprising of mitotically active small round and spindle-shaped cells giving the diagnosis of CMN [7].

Gaillard and colleagues recently reported pathological and molecular characteristics of CMN in 35 cases [8]. Based on cellular criteria, 14 were classified as classical, 4 as partly cellular and 17 as cellular CMN. The mean ages were 24, 11 and 70 days, respectively. There were 13 intrarenal tumours (stage I), but 9 classical, 3 partly cellular and 5 cellular CMNs extended to the perirenal fat (stage II) and 5 cellular tumours ruptured (stage III). In order to assess cellular proliferative activity, silver staining of nucleolar organiser region (Ag-NOR) proteins was performed on 19 CMNs. The number of Ag-NOR dots per cell was significantly lower in classical and partly cellular CMN than in cellular CMN, whatever the stage.

Within the cellular CMNs, the mean number of Ag-NOR dots was statistically higher in the single case that recurred with fatal outcome. The number of Ag-NOR dots, DNA content measurements, the histological subclassification, and the presence or absence of tumour at the surgical margins, may be useful features in selecting those patients who will benefit from further treatment after nephrectomy.

59.4 Cytogenetics

A characteristic chromosomal translocation, t(12;15)(p13;q25) has been described which results in fusion of the ETV6 (TEL) gene from 12p13 with the NRTK3 neurtrophin-3 receptor gene (TRKC) from 15q25. This results in a chimeric RNA which is characteristic of both infantile fibrosarcoma and the cellular variant of congenital mesobhlastic nephroma. This suggests a close relation between these two conditions [9].

Human epidermal growth factor receptors (HER) play a critical role in the branching morphogenesis of renal tubules. In addition HER2 expression in Wilms' tumour had been assessed and its role in tumorgenesis has been established. Amplification and over expression increases the metastatic potential of a tumour and promotes chemoresistance [10].

59.5 Tumour Markers

It has been reported that abnormal renin production and hypertension are common features of CMN. Several investigators have reported distinctive patterns of immunoreactive renin staining, suggesting that mesoblastic nephromas are a source of increased renin production producing hypertension [11, 12].

The most intense staining for renin was observed within areas of recognisable cortex trapped within the tumour. Renin was localised in cells in the walls of vessels running up to the glomeruli.

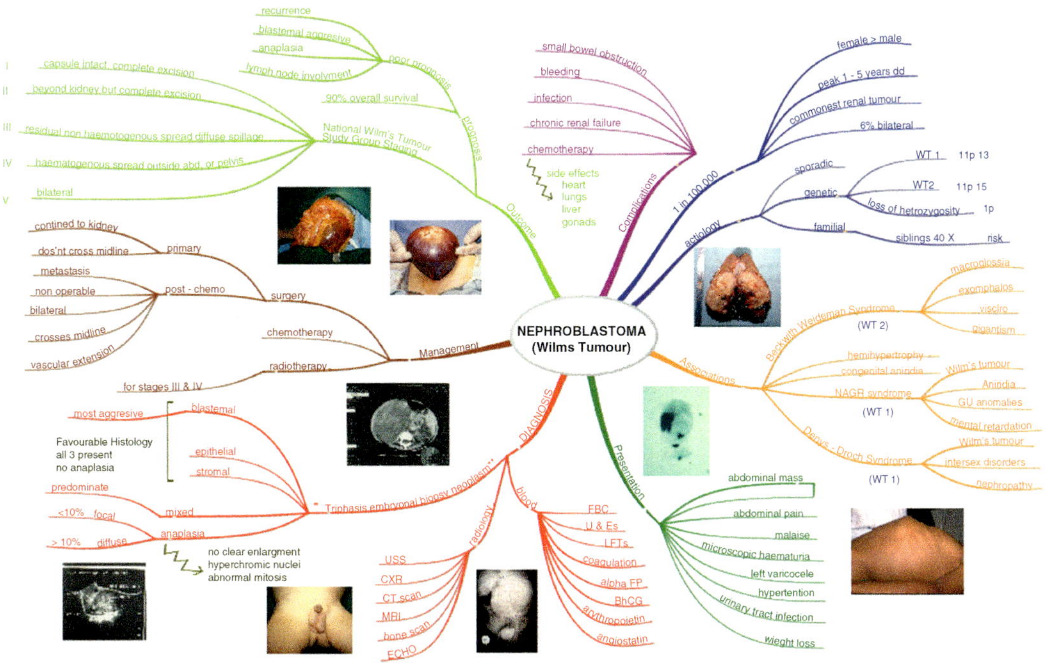

Fig. 59.1 Mind map. Practical Problems in Pediatric Surgery—An Atlas and Mind Maps. Eds. R. Keilani, R. Carachi, D. Gupta, E. Broadis, S. Sharma. Jaypee Brothers, ISBN 978 81 8448 723 7

59.6 Clinical Features

Although prenatal ultrasound is capable of detecting renal neoplasms in utero, there is no specific sonographic characteristics that can differentiate a CMN from a Wilms' tumour. Both tumours present as a palpable abdominal mass in the neonate. Males outnumber females by 2 to 1 with CMN and both sexes are equally affected by Wilms' tumours.

The newborn usually presents with a large, non-tender abdominal mass. Maternal polyhydramnios and prematurity are frequently seen although the reason for this is unclear. Male to female ratio ranges from 1.8:1 to 3:1 [6, 12] Hypertension has been recognised as a presenting feature, and there is an association between preoperative hypertension and cardiac arrest during surgery [6]. Some patients present with haematuria. In the congenital cystic mesoblastic nephroma variant the patient may present with a haemorrhagic problem. Recently mind maps have been introduced to explain in a didactic fashion the clinical features, investigations, differential diagnosis and management of CMN and Wilms' tumour (Fig. 59.1).

Detailed antenatal ultrasound scans may pick up a solid tumour of the kidney. Plain films of the abdomen show a large, soft-tissue abdominal mass that is rarely calcified. Sonography demonstrates the solid nature and renal origin of the mass and most commonly shows a mixed echogenic intrarenal mass.

CMN should easily be distinguished from more common renal masses in the newborn [13]—hydronephrosis or multicystic kidney—which are sonolucent. MRI scans give detailed imaging of the renal tumour and its surrounding structures.

59.7 Treatment

Nephrectomy of this benign tumour is curative without the need for supplementary radiation or adjuvant chemotherapy. Even when there has been intraoperative rupture, excisional surgery is curative, and local recurrence is rare. Distant metastasis has been reported but is extremely uncommon [14]. In a review of 38 patients with the cellular variant of mesoblastic nephroma showed that seven children had recurrence and three died. Pathologically positive surgical margins were the only statistically significant predictor of recurrent disease. Frozen section may help in obtaining tumour-free margins during surgery. Recent studies on molecular biology may shed further light on tumour behaviour and add criteria for further therapy after surgery.

59.7.1 Preoperative Preparation

Blood samples are obtained for a full blood count, group and crossmatch. Tumour markers renin, active renin, and inactive renin should also be assayed because these tumours have been documented as producing high levels of these hormones [12]. Erythropoietin levels should also be assayed. Careful monitoring and control of blood pressure is required to prevent dangerous perioperative fluctuations. A central venous cannula for intravenous infusion is inserted into the neck vein or subclavian vein as well as an arterial cannula to monitor blood pressure.

59.7.2 Operative Technique

59.7.2.1 Position

The patient is placed supine with a roll under the lumbar spine to create a lordosis.

59.7.2.2 Incision

An upper transverse muscle-cutting incision from the flank across the midline provides adequate exposure. *Laparotomy and exposure of the renal pedicle.*

The abdomen is entered, taking care not to cut into the tumour while incising the abdominal wall muscles. The small intestine is displaced towards the opposite side and covered with moist packs. The liver and the opposite kidney are inspected for the presence of any other disease. This is very rare in this condition. Free fluid is sampled and sent for cytology.

The colon overlying the tumour is retracted medially and the posterior peritoneum lateral to the colon is incised and reflected forward to the midline. Tumour handling should be minimised in hypertensive patients to prevent excessive release of renin. The inferior vena cava and renal veins are both palpated for the presence of tumour. The ureter is identified and a tape is passed around it. It is traced as far down as possible into the pelvis, ligated with 3–0 chromic catgut and divided. Next the gonadal vessels are ligated and divided. Before mobilisation of the tumour, abdominal packs are used to isolate the operative site from the rest of the abdominal cavity. This is to prevent any dissemination of tumour if there is spillage during the time of surgery. The renal vein is doubly ligated and divided. The renal artery is exposed and transfixed with non absorbable sutures.

The para-aortic lymph glands, together with surrounding tissue, are dissected off the aorta and inferior vena cava and labelled carefully. The tumour is removed from the posterior abdominal wall using finger dissection. The excised specimen should contain kidney, Gerota's fascia, fat from the lumbar fossa and para-aortic lymph glands.

After removal of the tumour, haemostasis is obtained with diathermy coagulation or suture ligatures. No drain is required.

59.7.2.3 Postoperative Care

Postoperative recovery following resection of mesoblastic nephroma is rapid. Nephrectomy of this benign tumour is curative. If on histology the tumour is found to be Wilms', it should be treated in accordance with the degree of involvement as outlined in the National Wilms' Tumour Study Programs.

59.7.2.4 Complications

The main complication of CMN is rupture of the tumour during surgery. Howell and colleagues reported intra-operative rupture in 20% of their cases [6]. In practice this is extremely rare despite intra-operative rupture, excellent subsequent relapse-free survival has been reported within tumour.

References

1. Kastner K. Nierensarckon ber einem siebenmonatlichen. Fotus Ztschn Path. 1921;25:1.
2. Crom DB, Wilimas HA, Green AA, et al. Malignancy in the neonate. Med Pediatr Oncol. 1989;17:101–4.
3. Campbell AN, Chan HSL, O'Brien A, et al. Malignant tumours in the neonate. Arch Dis Childh. 1987;62:19–23.
4. Ritchey ML, Azizkhan RG, Beckwith JB, et al. Neonatal Wilms' tumour. J Pediatr Surg. 1995;30:| 856–9.
5. Bolande RP, Brough AJ, Izant RJ. Congenital mesoblastic nephroma of infancy. A report of 8 cases and the relationship to Wilms' tumour. Pediatrics. 1967;40:272–8.
6. Howell CG, Otherson HB, Kiviat NE, et al. Therapy and outcome in 51 children with mesoblastic nephroma. A report of the National Wilms' Tumour Study J Pediatr Surg. 1982;17:826–31.
7. Murthi S, Carachi R, Howatson A. Congenital cystic mesoblastic nephroma (cellular variant), (Unilocular, haemorrhagic). Personal Communication.
8. Gaillard D, Bouvier R, Sonsino E, et al. Nucleolar organizer regions in congenital mesoblastic nephroma. Pediatr Pathol. 1992;12:811–21.
9. Shamberger RC. Renal tumors. In: Carachi R, Grosfeld JL, Azmy AF, editors. The surgery of childhood tumors, 2nd edn. Berlin: Springer; 2008.
10. Salem M, Kinoshita Y, Tajiri T, et al. Association between the HER2 expression and histological differentiation in Wilms tumor. Pediatr Surg Int. 2006;22:891–6.
11. Yokomori K, Hori T, Takemura T, et al. Demonstration of both primary and secondary reninism in renal tumours in children. J Pediatr Surg. 1988;23: 403–9.
12. Malone PS, Duffy PG, Ransley PG, et al. Congenital mesoblastic nephroma, renin production and hypertension. J Pediatr Surg. 1989;24:599–600.
13. Kirks DR, Kaufman RA. Function with mesoblastic nephroma: imaging—pathologic correlation. Pediatr Radiol. 1989;19:136–9.
14. Heidelberger KP, Ritchy ML, Dauser RC, et al. Congenital mesoblastic nephroma metastatic to brain. Cancer. 1993;72:2499–505.

Ovarian and Genital Tract Neoplasms

60

Carmen Capito, Daniel Orbach,
and Sabine Sarnacki

Abstract

Neonatal tumors occur every 12,500–27,500 live births and ovarian and female genital tract tumors are reported as rare cases in the literature.

Ovarian tumor is an exceptional condition in neonates and, in contrast to older children, sex-cord-stromal tumors are the most frequently reported symptomatic neoplasms.

Considering gynecological neoplasms, a vaginal bleeding in a female neonate should always alert on the risk of vaginal malignant neoplasm with rhabdomyosarcoma and malignant germ cell tumors as the first tumoral types encountered.

Neonatal tumors occur every 12,500–27,500 live births and ovarian and female genital tract tumors are reported as rare cases in the literature.

Ovarian tumor is an exceptional condition in neonates and, in contrast to older children, sex-cord-stromal tumors are the most frequently reported symptomatic neoplasms.

Considering gynecological neoplasms, a vaginal bleeding in a female neonate should always alert on the risk of vaginal malignant neoplasm with rhabdomyosarcoma and malignant germ cell tumors as the first tumoral types encountered

Keywords

Neonatal ovarian tumors • Gynaecological tract neoplasms • Vaginal tumors • Surgical management • Outcomes

C. Capito, MD • S. Sarnacki, MD, PhD (✉)
Department of Pediatric Surgery, AP-HP, Hôpital Necker Enfants-Malades, Université Paris Descartes, 149 Rue de Sèvres, 75015 Paris, France
e-mail: sabine.sarnacki@aphp.fr

D. Orbach, MD
Department of Pediatric, Adolescent, Young Adult, Institut Curie, Paris, France

60.1 Neonatal Ovarian Tumors

60.1.1 Introduction

Ovarian lesions encountered in prenatal and early postnatal period are predominantly benign and mainly represented by functional ovarian cysts

P.D. Losty et al. (eds.), *Rickham's Neonatal Surgery*, https://doi.org/10.1007/978-1-4471-4721-3_60

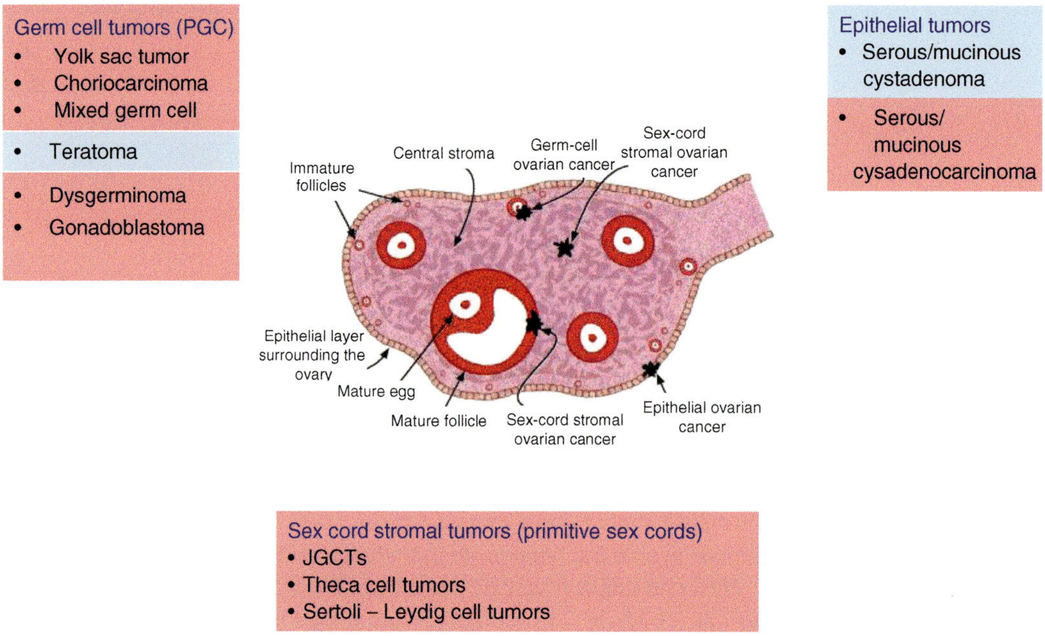

Fig. 60.1 Classification of ovarian tumors

(Fig. 60.1). Considering the entire pediatric age group, ovarian tumors represent nearly 50% of all ovarian masses [1]. Among them, 90% are benign [2]. Three major histopathological groups are recognized [3]. The most frequent is represented by germ cell tumors (60–70%) with teratoma as the major entity and a median age of occurrence of 9 years [4]. This type can be seen in neonates and particularly in its cystic form. A second group is composed by epithelial cell tumors (10–20%) such as cystadenoma and cystadenocarcinoma. These tumors have never been reported in neonates and are mostly seen in adolescence and adulthood. The last group is sex-cord-stromal tumors (10%), very heterogeneous and includes fibro-thecoma, juvenile granulosa cell tumors (JGCT), Sertoli and/or Leydig cell tumors (SLCT) and unclassified sex-cord-stromal tumors [5, 6]. Whereas SLCT and thecomas predominate during adolescence, JGCT predominantly develop during infancy and childhood at a median age of 7 years [7].

Neonatal presentations of ovarian neoplasms have been rarely reported and as in older children, germ cells tumors are expected to be the most frequent type encountered. But these neoplasms and specifically teratomas will rarely be symptomatic in the neonatal period because of their small size explaining why sex-cord-stromal tumors are the symptomatic type the most frequently reported [8–11].

60.1.2 Pathological Entities Encountered in Neonates

Sex-cord-stromal ovarian tumors (SCST) are developed from the peri-ovocytic follicular and stromal cells [1, 5, 12, 13]. Three major histological entities are classically described. Granulosa cell tumor is the most frequent subtype in this group and originates from the granulosa cells of the ovarian follicle. In this subtype, the main steroid secretion is estradiol [7, 14–17] which induces isosexual precocious puberty in girls. In the literature, up to 70% of juvenile granulosa cell tumor of prepubertal occurrence display an estradiol secretion leading to precocious puberty [16–18]. Fibro-thecoma originates from the stromal cells of the ovary that will give rise to the future theca. This type, very rare in the pediatric age group, rarely displays hormonal secretion with almost exclusively androgen secretion and rarely estrogen secretion, as it derivates from stromal cells. The last subtype is Sertoli-Leydig cell tumor (SLCT). One third of these SLCT induce virilization, but more than 50% have no endocrine manifestations [19]. In case of pure Sertoli tumor, isosexual precocious puberty is a frequent condition [20]. Considering the similarities between Leydig and theca cells in one hand and Sertoli and granulosa cells in the other hand, it is hypothesized that SLCT originate from an ovarian-testicular "trans-differentiation" of unknown mechanism [13]. The physiopathology of those three subtypes is not clear [5, 13, 17, 19, 20] but this illustrates well the peculiar framework of neonatal ovarian tumors and the tight relations between development anomalies and tumorigenesis [21]. Recently, SCST and particularly SLCT were reported to be associated to germline-inactivating DICER1 mutations (mapped to chromosome 14q) as a part of the tumor spectrum of the DICER1 pleuropulmonary blastoma familial tumor predisposition syndrome. This implies that constitutional genetic screening for DICER1 mutations is now mandatory when an ovarian neoplasm is found to be a SLCT as it could be the initial clinical presentation of DICER1 mutations within a family [22].

Germ cell tumors (GCT) comprise highly malignant GCT (yolk sac tumors, choriocarcinoma, embryonal carcinoma, mixed GCT and dysgerminoma), moderately malignant lesions (immature teratoma) and benign lesions (gonadoblastoma and mature teratoma). Their aetiology is unknown and the cell of origin is believed to be the totipotent germ cells [23, 24] These cells develop among the endodermal cells of the yolk sac near the origin of the allantois and migrate to the gonadal ridges during the first month of development. It is thus hypothesized that GCT are developmental tumors arising from a pathological undifferentiated cell that remains within the gonad since the end of ovarian embryogenesis and proliferate slowly, until tumoral lesion becomes evident for diagnosis. The same hypothesis is done for extragonadic locations of GCTs. Curiously the incidence of the different histological subtypes varies according to the anatomical initial location and also the age at diagnosis. In the neonatal period, mature teratoma is mostly encountered in the sacrococcygeal sites (which concern mostly female) [23, 24]. Malignant subtypes and particularly yolk sac tumors are generally encountered in older children after 1 year of age, except for the genital tract location.

60.1.3 Presentation and Differential Diagnosis

Three major modes of revelation can be seen:

- Clinical signs of abnormal hormonal secretion
- Radiological lesions diagnosed fortuitously or during follow up of prenatal pelvic cystic lesion
- Palpable abdominal mass or other rare situations

60.1.3.1 Clinical Signs of Atypical Hormonal Secretion

In case of sex cord stromal tumors, almost 70% produce steroids. Specific signs of abnormal hormonal impregnation at this age can thus reveal them: premature pubarche (Fig. 60.2), breast enlargement, vaginal bleeding or virilization at birth. Prenatal presentation of this type of tumor has been rarely reported [8, 9] and virilized genitalia at birth was reported in one case [9].

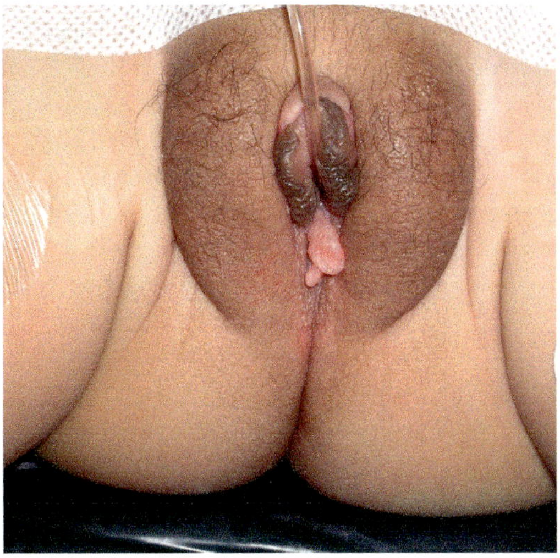

Fig. 60.2 Premature pubarche at birth associated with a prenatal ovarian sex cord stromal tumor

Differential diagnosis of isosexual precocious puberty in neonates is the so called "mini-puberty" occurring during the first 3–4 months of the child development. This mini-puberty state is generally associated with mild signs of hormonal impregnation such as small breast enlargement, acne eruption and possible vaginal bleeding. A pelvic ultrasound evaluation will easily allow this differential diagnosis.

60.1.3.2 Radiological Lesions Diagnosed Fortuitously or During Follow Up of Prenatal Pelvic Cystic Lesion

All these tumors can present as abdominal solid and/or cystic masses. If solid or mixed solid cystic masses are easily attributed to organic lesions needing surgical management, difficulties are essentially encountered with exclusive cystic lesions during neonatal period. Indeed, ovarian cyst is a frequent situation encountered during prenatal diagnosis. Functional cysts are due to foetal impregnation by maternal steroid secretion. These cysts are mainly simple but maybe sometimes complicated (associated ovarian torsion, haemorrhage). Nevertheless, they require precise postnatal follow up until normalization of ovarian images is achieved. This is supported by few series of prenatal ovarian cysts where cases of mature teratomas [25, 26] were identified after surgical removal of a persisting prenatal cyst. This suggests that an ovarian cyst diagnosed prenatally and persisting after breastfeeding weaning or more generally after 6 months should be considered as a potential ovarian tumor [27].

60.1.3.3 Palpable Abdominal Mass or Other Rare Presentations

Diagnosis of an ovarian tumor in the neonatal period as an abdominal mass is exceptional. One case of neonatal Meig's syndrome has been reported associated with a mature teratoma [11].

60.1.4 Management and Prognosis

60.1.4.1 Preoperative Management

The major issue challenging the surgeon is to be able to perform conservative surgery for benign lesions but also to strictly follow the rules of carcinologic surgery for malignant lesions. The intrinsic contradiction between both approaches underlines the need for a diagnosis of the malignant or benign nature of the lesion before surgery. Because of the problem of potential peritoneal spreading of malignant cells, percutaneous cytopunction or fine needle biopsy is not recommended. Diagnosis relies on two main features at this age: imaging and biological markers evolution (AFP, HCG). Interpretation of normal values of AFP in neonatal period is sometimes difficult due to physiological high levels until the age of 1 year. Absence of spontaneous decrease during follow-up must be a sign of alert.

60.1.4.2 Radiological Features

Whereas ultrasound exam is the best way to detect the lesion, pelvic CT or ideally MRI allows a reliable location of the lesion in the gonad (Fig. 60.3). It also permits an accurate description of the components of the lesion orienting on the histological subtype. Indeed, MRI disclosing heterogeneous tumors with different tissue component such as adipose tissue or calcifications will be very specific of germ cell tumors and particularly mature teratoma. Regarding the most frequent malignant lesion encountered in the neonatal period, i.e. SCST, it is usually a solid or mixed lesion but pure cystic lesions have been described in oldest girls [28].

Metastatic spreading is rare in the pediatric age group and has never been reported in neonates. Nevertheless, pretherapeutic work up should include

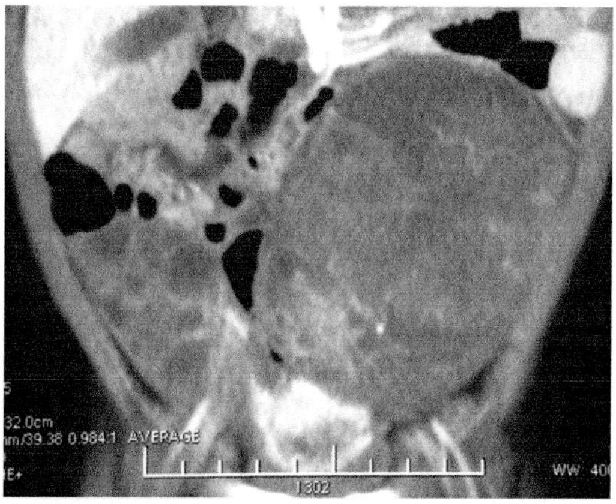

Fig. 60.3 CT image of a bilateral ovarian sex cord stromal tumor in a neonate

thoraco-abdominal CT if a malignant histology is suspected looking for retroperitoneal lymph nodes enlargement and lung or liver metastasis.

60.1.4.3 Biological Markers

The biological markers according to the histological subtype are listed below.

- Sex cord stromal tumors
- Juvenile granulosa cell tumors: antimullerian hormone (AMH), inhibin B, estradiol (70%), rarely testosterone
- Sertoli Leydig tumors: testosterone, estrogen and in some cases a moderate production of AFP is possible [6, 29]
- Germ cell tumors
- Yolk sac or endodermal sinus tumor: alphafoetoprotein (AFP). The interpretation of this marker is difficult in the neonatal period regarding the elevated level of this marker at birth, with a slow decrease during the first year of life. Interpretation relies thus on kinetic more than absolute level (normal level < 10 ng/mL after 1 year of life) (Table 60.1).
- Choriocarcinoma or GCT with a choriocarcinoma component: β-HCG, total HCG
- Embryonal carcinoma: non secreting tumors even if in some cases AFP may be slowly elevated especially in case of mixed tumour,
- Dysgerminoma: non secreting even if low level of β(beta) HCG may be observed
- Mature and immature teratoma: markers are by definition normal

Table 60.1 AFP level until normalization

	AFP level (ng/mL)	Standard deviation
Premature	134,734	41,444
Newborn	48,406	34,718
2 weeks	33,113	32,503
1 month	9452	12,610
2 months	323	278
3 months	88	87
4 months	74	56
5 months	46,5	19
6 months	12,5	9,8
7 months	9,7	7,1
8 months	8,5	5,5

60.1.4.4 Surgical Procedure

In case of SCST or suspected malignant GCT, total ovariectomy is recommended with adnexectomy if the fallopian tube is involved. Considering mature teratoma, the estimated risk of metachronous contralateral teratoma is around 10%. Thus partial surgery, when possible, is recommended if this subtype is radiologically suspected. If post operative pathological analysis reveals a part of malignant contingent, a second procedure will be performed in order to complete the ovariectomy. A strict follow-up is recommended to detect early metachronous lesion. In all cases, the rule is to avoid any tumor effraction during surgery because the sanction will be adjuvant chemotherapy with high risks for these young patients. Thus, it is mandatory to avoid a laparoscopic approach to remove the lesion in these paediatric ovarian tumors since even apparent mature teratoma can have a small content of malignant subtypes with undetectable levels of biological markers. The surgical treatment of ovarian lesions in girls is performed by a supra-pubic approach, which allows the exteriorization and treatment of the lesion. Before this step, a laparoscopic exploration is mandatory in order to perform the staging of the tumor including: obtain a sample of ascitis or peritoneal washing (in the absence of ascitis) for cytology and inspect the peritoneal surfaces (including diaphragmatic domes), the abdominal organs, with special attention to the contralateral ovary, pelvic and retroperitoneal lymph node and liver. Biopsy of any suspicious areas should be performed and omentectomy if the omentum (or parts of it) is abnormal. Adjuvant chemotherapy is exceptionally necessary in this age group as complete surgical resection is generally obtained.

60.1.4.5 Prognosis

Prognosis in this specific age group is unknown as the onset of malignant tumor of the ovary in the neonatal period is an exceptional condition. However, providing a non metastatic disease at diagnosis and a complete resection of the lesion without tumor effraction, long term prognosis should be as good as their older counterpart, meaning around 88% and more than 90% long term survival rates for respectively sex cord stromal tumors [7, 13] and malignant germ cell tumors [30].

60.2 Neonatal Genital Tract Tumors

60.2.1 Introduction

Tumors of the genital tract are very rare but classically diagnosed in infants. Different entities are encountered with by frequency: rhabdomyosarcoma, malignant germ cell tumors and other rare entities such as clear cell adenocarcinoma; this last subtype being diagnosed later in life [31]. Their primitive location can be the vulva, the vagina or the uterus cervix. Prognosis of these tumors relies on the local tumor control obtained nowadays with less radical surgical management than in past decades [32, 33]. Recent therapeutic regimens combine chemotherapy, conservative surgery and in some cases local radiation therapy (essentially brachytherapy).

60.2.2 Pathological Entities Encountered in Neonates and Their Molecular Characteristics

Rhabdomyosarcoma (RMS) is the most common soft tissue sarcoma in childhood and also the most frequent tumor of the paediatric female genital tract [31–35]. The tumor arises from mesenchymal derivated cells and histologically resembles normal fetal muscle. Vagina is the most frequent localization encountered in the neonatal period. RMS are classified in two main subtypes in the pediatric population: embryonal and alveolar. The recent improvement in cytogenetic characterization of these two subtypes has improved the differential diagnosis [36] which is of great importance as alveolar RMS is associated with a more aggressive disease pattern and a higher mortality.

Embryonal RMS neoplasms are typically comprised of spindle shaped cells, with a stromal rich appearance [36]. Botryoid tumors, which are a particular form of embryonal RMS with a grape-like aspect, occur almost exclusively in the bladder or vagina of infants and young children. These embryonal RMS are characterized by a loss of maternal imprinting (loss of heterozygosity) at the 11p15 locus, a region harbouring the insulin-like growth factor 2 (IGF2) gene, H19 and P57, the latter being two tumor suppressor genes [36]. These tumor types tend to occur in the younger age group and account for almost two third of all RMS. Recent analysis have found a new recurrent VGLL2-related fusion transcript in "infantile RMS" that encourage to search all rare transcripts in addition to classical ones at this age to help diagnosis [37].

Alveolar RMS is typically comprised of small round densely packed cells, arranged around spaces resembling pulmonary alveoli. These subtypes of RMS tumors harbour distinguishing chromosomal translocation marker, with typically t(2;13)(q35;q14, 36). This translocation creates a fusion protein (PAX3-FOX01) that is thought to be responsible at least in part for its malignant phenotype [38, 39]. A variant translocation t(1;13) leading to the fusion protein PAX7-FOX01, can also be seen with a slightly better prognosis [36]. Alveolar RMS is more frequently diagnosed in older children considering the urogenital tract.

Although mostly sporadic, some syndromes can predispose to development of RMS in childhood such as Neurofibromatosis type 1, Li-Fraumeni, Costello and Beckwith-Wiedemann syndromes.

Malignant germ cell tumor (GCT). Vagina remains a rare primary location of GCT (3–8% of all GCT) and in contrast to the ovary, germ cells tumors encountered in genital tract location are mainly malignant ones, with yolk sac tumors accounting for almost all the cases [31, 36, 40, 41]. They are supposed to derive from an aberrant migration of totipotent germ cells, like other extra gonadal germ cells tumors. Most of these tumors will be secreting ones (AFP).

Clear cell carcinoma of the vagina was related to prenatal exposure to diethylstilboestrol during the first trimester of pregnancy. Since this treatment is no longer used, this tumor type has disappeared in the diagnosis algorithm of young girls vaginal tumors. Anyway, some recent studies seem to advocate a transgenerational effect of this treatment via epigenetic transmission [42]. This should then be kept in mind even extremely rare.

60.2.3 Presentation and Differential Diagnosis

60.2.3.1 Presentation

Recent large review by Fernandez Pineda et al. [31] has highlighted the frequency of the symptoms in vaginal tumors as follow:

- Bleeding or blood tinged discharge from the vagina (61%)
- Protruding mass (39%) (Fig. 60.4)

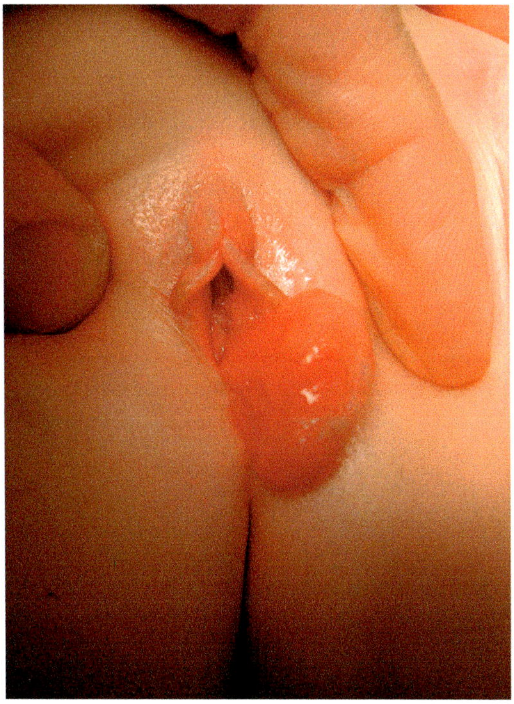

Fig. 60.4 Embryonal bifocal tumor (vaginal and bladder) revealed by a protruding mass in a 5 months old baby

Considering vulvar tumor, the diagnosis is suspected by local examination with the discovery of a mass bulging in the perineum.

Uterus tumors are generally diagnosed in older children because of delayed symptoms before diagnosis. This may partially explain their worst prognosis. In a large series by Martelli et al. [32], median age at diagnosis for vulvovaginal rhabdomyosarcoma was 21 months (range, 9 months to 15.6 years) whereas for uterus RMS, it was 15 years (range, 10 months to 16.6 years). Bleeding remains the most reliable sign in this location.

Neonatal rhabdomyosarcomas have generally aggressive biologic behaviour as 50% of the patients reported in some large series [43, 44] had widespread disease at the time of diagnosis. Metastatic disease can appear in the lungs, lymph nodes, liver, bone marrow, bone, and brain. However this seems not to be the case in the specific urogenital tract location [32, 35].

60.2.3.2 Differential Diagnosis

Differential diagnosis of vaginal blood discharge in neonatal period remains hormonally induced genital bleeding that can occur during the so called "mini-puberty" of the first 3–4 months of the child development or in case of secreting sex cord stromal tumors. The absence of associated signs of hormonal impregnation will point on genital tract neoplasm and ultrasound, pelvic MRI and/or vaginoscopy will confirm the diagnosis.

60.2.4 Management and Prognosis

60.2.4.1 Imaging and Histological Studies

As most of vaginal GCT are secreting Yolk Sac tumors (YST), the first exam must be blood analysis of biological markers (AFP, β-HCG, total HCG). Normal physiological level in the neonatal period of these markers should also be taken into account. Initial management of these tumors should then include histological diagnosis and evaluation of the disease extension. Surgical biopsies remain the gold standard in order to obtain enough materials for immunohistochemical and molecular biology studies especially if blood markers are negative. This will be performed under general anaesthesia and the procedure will include a vaginoscopy and a cystoscopy. Both explorations are mandatory as extension to the adjacent tract can occur and rare cases of true double locations have been observed (personal observation). As one part of the tissue harvested must be rapidly frozen for molecular studies it is important to carefully prepare this surgical procedure. If a complete resection can be achieved without large mutilation, this should be attempted. Otherwise a central catheter should be placed at the end of the procedure in order to rapidly start chemotherapy treatment.

Complementary investigations include abdominal ultrasound, thoraco-abdominal CT or MRI (Figs. 60.5 and 60.6), bone scintigraphy and bone marrow aspirate if bone metastases are suspected.

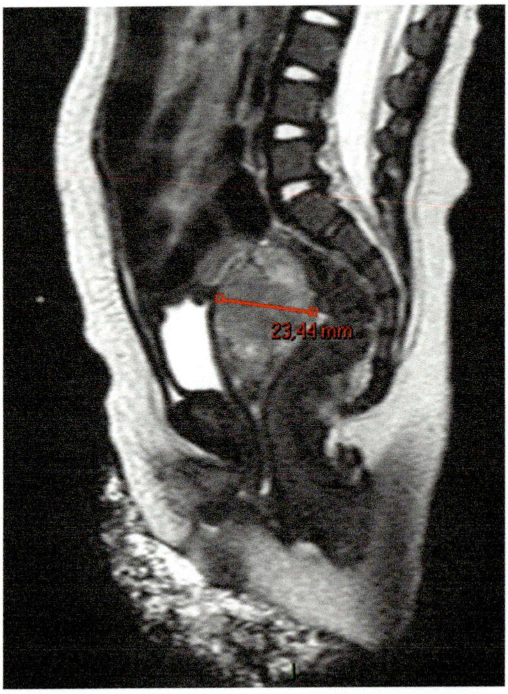

Fig. 60.5 Secreting vaginal yolk sac tumor in a 8 months girl, AFP 3268 UI/mL – Pelvic MRI, T2 weighted sequence

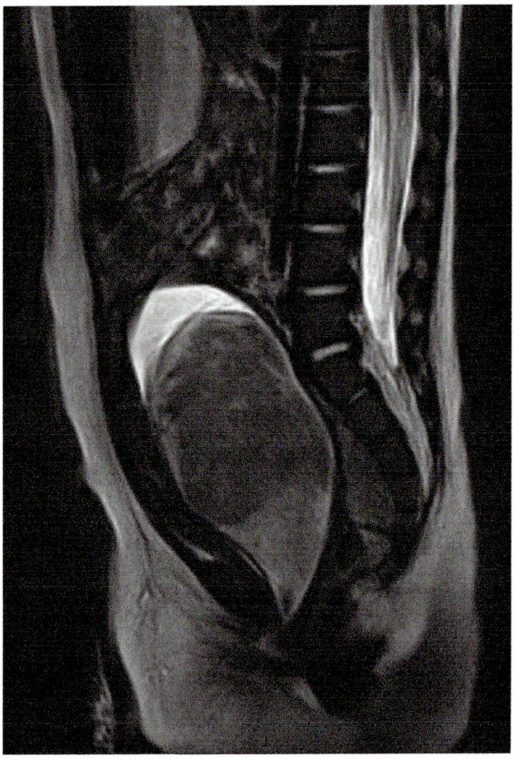

Fig. 60.6 Pelvic MRI of a vaginal rhabdomyosarcoma—T2 weighted sequence

60.2.4.2 Therapeutic Strategies

The treatment regimen proposed should take into account the particularities of the young age of the patient. Indeed, immaturity of enzymatic processes for drug metabolism, and risks of unacceptable long-term morbidity should always be kept in mind. Thus, in contrast to older children, external radiation therapy will never be proposed in neonates. A local radiation therapy (brachytherapy) will be reserved to infants with residual disease or after relapse.

First line treatment combines chemotherapy and surgery and their chronology will be dictate by the stage at presentation, the location of the primary tumor, the resectability at each step of treatment, the expected morbidity of the operative procedure and the histological characteristics of the lesion. The most effective and less deleterious chemotherapy regimen in neonatal rhabdomyosarcoma associates vincristine and actinomycin D. Cyclophophamide is reserved to advanced disease [32, 35, 45, 46]. For neonatal malignant germ cell tumors, the regimen associates carboplatine and etoposide.

Regarding the surgical treatment, the strategy is different between vaginal GCT and urogenital RMS. In both cases, iterative urogenital endoscopies are performed along the treatment protocol to better plan the modalities of the surgical resection. It is important to explore both the urinary and genital tract to appreciate the extension of the disease but also because potential double location (vagina and bladder) of RMS is possible (personal observation). Whereas treatment could be achieved without surgery in urogenital RMS when complete imaging defined remission is obtained after chemotherapy, surgical resection of the primary location is always mandatory in vaginal GCT. In this latter case, efficiency of neoadjuvant chemotherapy usually allows to avoid mutilating surgery and to propose partial colpectomy. For urogenital RMS, surgical local treatment could be completed by local brachytherapy and thus mutilating surgery is exceptional. Ovarian transposition should then be considered if brachytherapy is decided [35].

Follow up consists of periodical endoscopies under general anaesthesia and repeated MRI (every 3 months during the first 2 years of follow up and twice a year after). Relapse, if occurring, is essentially local and will benefit of extensive surgery whatever importance of mutilation rather than external radiation therapy which exposed to higher morbidity in this age group [35]. Whereas the options for reconstructive surgery (vaginoplasty, bladder reconstruction) will be exposed to parents before mutilating surgical treatment, this will be proposed after complete oncological remission.

60.2.4.3 Prognosis

Genital tract locations are known to be of better prognosis regarding the overall prognosis of rhabdomyosarcoma. This prognosis seems more or less identical to older children with a long term survival rate of 70% [32, 35]. More accurately, infants with embryonal histology and complete surgical resection have a cure rates higher than 90% [45] and those with metastatic disease at diagnosis a long-term survival rates under 25% [44, 45]. At this opposite, vaginal malignant germ cell tumors in these locations have an overall good prognosis provided that early diagnosis is made and multidisciplinary care is provided [40, 47, 48].

References

1. Cass DL, Hawkins E, Brandt ML, Chintagumpala M, Bloss RS, Milewicz AL, et al. Surgery for ovarian masses in infants, children, and adolescents: 102 consecutive patients treated in a 15-year period. J Pediatr Surg. 2001;36(5):693–9.
2. von Allmen D. Malignant lesions of the ovary in childhood. Semin Pediatr Surg. 2005;14(2):100–5.
3. Schultz KA, Sencer SF, Messinger Y, Neglia JP, Steiner ME. Pediatric ovarian tumors: a review of 67 cases. Pediatr Blood Cancer. 2005;44(2):167–73.
4. De Backer A, Madern GC, Oosterhuis JW, Hakvoort-Cammel FG, Hazebroek FW. Ovarian germ cell tumors in children: a clinical study of 66 patients. Pediatr Blood Cancer. 2006;46(4):459–64.
5. Young RH. Sex cord-stromal tumors of the ovary and testis: their similarities and differences with consideration of selected problems. Mod Pathol. 2005;18(Suppl 2):S81–98.
6. Schneider D, Orbach D, Cecchetto G, Stachowicz-Stencel T, Brummel B, Brecht I, et al. Ovarian sertoli Leydig cell tumours in children and adolescents: an analysis of the European Cooperative Study Group on Pediatric Rare Tumors (EXPeRT). Eur J Cancer. 2015;51(4):543–50.
7. Schneider DT, Calaminus G, Harms D, Gobel U. Ovarian sex cord-stromal tumors in children and adolescents. J Reprod Med. 2005;50(6):439–46.
8. Capito C, Flechtner I, Thibaud E, Emond S, Kalfa N, Jaubert F, et al. Neonatal bilateral ovarian sex cord stromal tumors. Pediatr Blood Cancer. 2009;52(3):401–3.
9. Nitzsche K, Kamin G, Dittert DD, Bier A, Distler W. [Fetal juvenile granulosa cell tumor with hermaphroditism verus—prenatal diagnosis, management and outcome]. Ultraschall Med. 2009;30(4):404–7.
10. Rauber G, Duprez A, Bardaji O. [Ruptured neonatal ovarian cyst with theca cells]. Arch Anat Pathol (Paris). 1964;12:221–4.
11. Tsakiri SP, Turk CA, Lally KP, Garg K, Morris B. Atypical Meigs' syndrome in a neonate with ovarian torsion associated with an ovarian dermoid cyst. Pediatr Surg Int. 2005;21(5):407–9.
12. Meizner I, Levy A, Katz M, Maresh AJ, Glezerman M. Fetal ovarian cysts: prenatal ultrasonographic detection and postnatal evaluation and treatment. Am J Obstet Gynecol. 1991;164(3):874–8.
13. Schneider DT, Janig U, Calaminus G, Gobel U, Harms D. Ovarian sex cord-stromal tumors—

a clinicopathological study of 72 cases from the Kiel Pediatric Tumor Registry. Virchows Arch. 2003;443(4):549–60.
14. Bonnevalle M, Mazingue F, Nelken B, Vaast P, Lecomte-Houcke M, Debeugny P. [Precocious pseudo-puberty in granulosa cell tumor in children less than 1 year old. 2 cases]. Chir Pediatr. 1990;31(1):32–4.
15. Cronje HS, Niemand I, Bam RH, Woodruff JD. Granulosa and theca cell tumors in children: a report of 17 cases and literature review. Obstet Gynecol Surv. 1998;53(4):240–7.
16. Merras-Salmio L, Vettenranta K, Mottonen M, Heikinheimo M. Ovarian granulosa cell tumors in childhood. Pediatr Hematol Oncol. 2002;19(3):145–56.
17. Zaloudek C, Norris HJ. Granulosa tumors of the ovary in children: a clinical and pathologic study of 32 cases. Am J Surg Pathol. 1982;6(6):503–12.
18. Plantaz D, Flamant F, Vassal G, Chappuis JP, Baranzelli MC, Bouffet E et al. [Granulosa cell tumors of the ovary in children and adolescents. Multicenter retrospective study in 40 patients aged 7 months to 22 years]. Arch Fr Pediatr. 1992;49(9):793–8.
19. Truss L, Dobin SM, Rao A, Donner LR. Overexpression of the BCL2 gene in a Sertoli-Leydig cell tumor of the ovary: a pathologic and cytogenetic study. Cancer Genet Cytogenet. 2004;148(2):118–22.
20. Oliva E, Alvarez T, Young RH. Sertoli cell tumors of the ovary: a clinicopathologic and immunohistochemical study of 54 cases. Am J Surg Pathol. 2005;29(2):143–56.
21. Virgone C, Cecchetto G, Ferrari A, Bisogno G, Donofrio V, Boldrini R, et al. GATA-4 and FOG-2 expression in pediatric ovarian sex cord-stromal tumors replicates embryonal gonadal phenotype: results from the TREP project. PLoS One. 2012;7(9):e45914. https://doi.org/10.1371/journal.pone.0045914. Epub 2012 Sep 24
22. Faure A, Atkinson J, Bouty A, O'Brien M, Levard G, Hutson J, et al. DICER1 pleuropulmonary blastoma familial tumour predisposition syndrome: what the paediatric urologist needs to know. J Pediatr Urol. 2016;12(1):5–10.
23. Isaacs H Jr. Perinatal (fetal and neonatal) germ cell tumors. J Pediatr Surg. 2004;39(7):1003–13.
24. Lakhoo K. Neonatal teratomas. Early Hum Dev. 2010;86(10):643–47.
25. Heling KS, Chaoui R, Kirchmair F, Stadie S, Bollmann R. Fetal ovarian cysts: prenatal diagnosis, management and postnatal outcome. Ultrasound Obstet Gynecol. 2002;20(1):47–50.
26. Mittermayer C, Blaicher W, Grassauer D, Horcher E, Deutinger J, Bernaschek G, et al. Fetal ovarian cysts: development and neonatal outcome. Ultraschall Med. 2003;24(1):21–6.
27. Dolgin SE. Ovarian masses in the newborn. Semin Pediatr Surg. 2000;9(3):121–7.
28. Gittleman AM, Price AP, Coren C, Akhtar M, Donovan V, Katz DS. Juvenile granulosa cell tumor. Clin Imaging. 2003;27(4):221–4.
29. Gui T, Cao D, Shen K, Yang J, Zhang Y, Yu Q, et al. A clinicopathological analysis of 40 cases of ovarian Sertoli-Leydig cell tumors. Gynecol Oncol. 2012;127(2):384–9.
30. Billmire D, Vinocur C, Rescorla F, Cushing B, London W, Schlatter M, et al. Outcome and staging evaluation in malignant germ cell tumors of the ovary in children and adolescents: an intergroup study. J Pediatr Surg. 2004;39(3):424–9.
31. Fernandez-Pineda I, Spunt SL, Parida L, Krasin MJ, Davidoff AM, Rao BN. Vaginal tumors in childhood: the experience of St. Jude Children's Research Hospital. J Pediatr Surg. 2011;46(11):2071–5.
32. Martelli H, Oberlin O, Rey A, Godzinski J, Spicer RD, Bouvet N, et al. Conservative treatment for girls with nonmetastatic rhabdomyosarcoma of the genital tract: a report from the Study Committee of the International Society of Pediatric Oncology. J Clin Oncol. 1999;17(7):2117–22.
33. Spicer RD. Neonatal sarcoma. Early Hum Dev. 2010;86(10):633–6.
34. Groff DB. Pelvic neoplasms in children. J Surg Oncol. 2001;77(1):65–71.
35. Magne N, Oberlin O, Martelli H, Gerbaulet A, Chassagne D, Haie-Meder C. Vulval and vaginal rhabdomyosarcoma in children: update and reappraisal of Institut Gustave Roussy brachytherapy experience. Int J Radiat Oncol Biol Phys. 2008;72(3):878–83.
36. Merlino G, Helman LJ. Rhabdomyosarcoma—working out the pathways. Oncogene. 1999;18(38):5340–8.
37. Alaggio R, Zhang L, Sung Y, Huang S, Chen C, Bisogno G, et al. A molecular study of Pediatric spindle and sclerosing Rhabdomyosarcoma: identification of novel and recurrent VGLL2-related fusions in infantile cases. Am J Surg Pathol. 2016;40(2):224–35.
38. Linardic CM. PAX3-FOX01 fusion gene in rhabdomyosarcoma. Cancer Lett. 2008;270(1):10–8.
39. Naini S, Etheridge KT, Adam SJ, Qualman SJ, Bentley RC, Counter CM, et al. Defining the cooperative genetic changes that temporally drive alveolar rhabdomyosarcoma. Cancer Res. 2008;68(23):9583–8.
40. Arafah M, Zaidi SN. A case of yolk sac tumor of the vagina in an infant. Arch Gynecol Obstet. 2012;285(5):1403–5.
41. Watanabe N, Okita H, Matsuoka K, Kiyotani C, Fujii E, Kumagai M, et al. Vaginal yolk sac (endodermal sinus) tumors in infancy presenting persistent vaginal bleeding. J Obstet Gynaecol Res. 2010;36(1):213–6.
42. Kalfa N, Paris F, Soyer-Gobillard M, Daures J, Sultan C. Prevalence of hypospadias in grandsons of women exposed to diethylstilbestrol during pregnancy: a multigenerational national cohort study. Fertil Steril. 2011;95(8):2574–7.
43. Dillon PW, Whalen TV, Azizkhan RG, Haase GM, Coran AG, King DR, et al. Neonatal soft tissue sarcomas: the influence of pathology on treatment and survival. Children's Cancer Group Surgical Committee. J Pediatr Surg. 1995;30(7):1038–41.

44. Grosfeld JL, Weber TR, Weetman RM, Baehner RL. Rhabdomyosarcoma in childhood: analysis of survival in 98 cases. J Pediatr Surg. 1983;18(2):141–6.
45. Crist WM, Anderson JR, Meza JL, Fryer C, Raney RB, Ruymann FB, et al. Intergroup rhabdomyosarcoma study-IV: results for patients with nonmetastatic disease. J Clin Oncol. 2001;19(12):3091–102.
46. Minard-Colin V, Orbach D, Martelli H, Bodemer C, Oberlin O. [Soft tissue tumors in neonates]. Arch Pediatr. 2009;16(7):1039–48.
47. Lacy J, Capra M, Allen L. Endodermal sinus tumor of the infant vagina treated exclusively with chemotherapy. J Pediatr Hematol Oncol. 2006;28(11):768–71.
48. Mauz-Korholz C, Harms D, Calaminus G, Gobel U. Primary chemotherapy and conservative surgery for vaginal yolk-sac tumour. Maligne Keimzelltumoren Study Group. Lancet. 2000;355(9204):625.

Sacrococcygeal Teratoma

61

Dhanya Mullassery and Paul D. Losty

Abstract

Sacrococcygeal tumour (SCT) is the commonest neoplasm seen in the newborn. A 'teratoma' (derived from the Greek language meaning "Monster")—is best defined as a neoplasm arising from primitive tissues which originated from all three embryonic germ cell layers—endoderm. Mesoderm and ectoderm. SCT occurs in 1:30,000–40,000 births according to recent publications emerging from the UK and Europe (Ayed et al. Prenat Diagn. 35: 1037–47, 2015; Pauniaho et al. Acta Paediatr. 102:e251–6, 2013). There is often a female preponderence (3:1) except in familial cases of SCT which may have an equal gender distribution (M:F = 1).

Keywords

Sacrococcygeal teratoma • Prenatal diagnosis staging • Surgery • Outcomes

61.1 Introduction

Sacrococcygeal tumour (SCT) is the commonest neoplasm seen in the newborn. A 'teratoma' (derived from the Greek language meaning "Monster")—is best defined as a neoplasm arising from primitive tissues which originated from all three embryonic germ cell layers—endoderm. Mesoderm and ectoderm. SCT occurs in 1:30,000–40,000 births according to recent publications emerging from the UK and Europe [1, 2]. There is often a female preponderence (3:1) except in familial cases of SCT which may have an equal gender distribution (M:F = 1).

D. Mullassery PhD, FRCS(Paed)
P.D. Losty, MD, FRCS(Paed), FEBPS (✉)
Institute of Translational Medicine, Alder Hey Children's Hospital NHS Foundation Trust, University of Liverpool, Liverpool, UK
e-mail: paul.losty@liverpool.ac.uk

61.2 Pathology

Primordial germ cells originating in the region of the yolk sac of the developing human migrate to the genital ridge on the posterior abdominal wall at 4–5 weeks gestation [3]. Arrested or aberrant cell migration is thought to result in the development of totipotent germ cell tumours often at midline anatomical sites. Tumours may therefore contain hair, teeth, neural and gastrointestinal

P.D. Losty et al. (eds.), *Rickham's Neonatal Surgery*, https://doi.org/10.1007/978-1-4471-4721-3_61

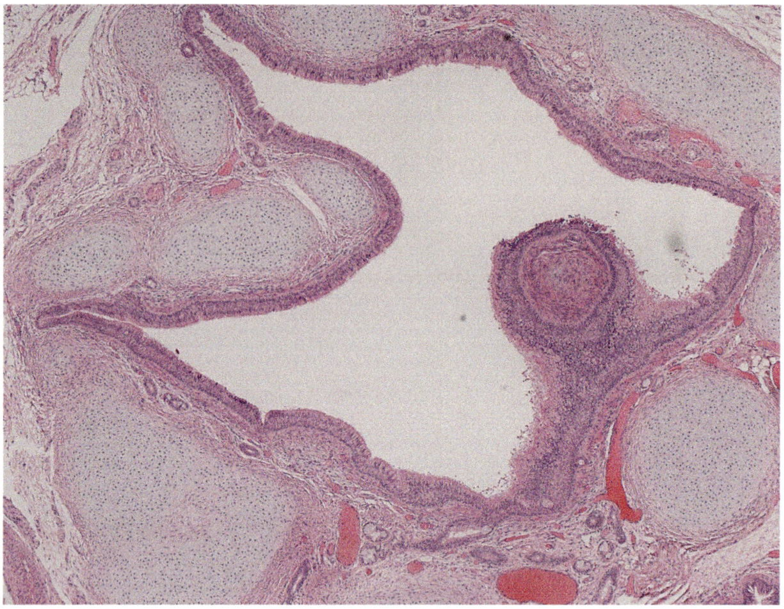

Fig. 61.1 Histology sacrococcygeal tumour specimen. Pathology shows SCT tumour with central cystic areas surrounded by respiratory type epithelium with lobules of cartilage, connective tissue including blood vessels and adipose tissue

like tissues (Fig. 61.1). Most sacrococcygeal lesions (95%) are mature 'benign' or 'immature' teratomas with 5% belonging to the malignant spectrum of endodermal sinus tumours (EST)]. A small number of patients (5%) may harbour metastastic disease at primary presentation. Risks of malignancy are reported to be significantly greater in SCT tumours which are often less apparent externally and those also encountered in older patients that may present beyond the typical neonatal period. Altman proposed that the higher malignancy rate(s) encountered in older infants is likely a reflection of delayed diagnosis with consequent histological transformation of occult lesions.

61.3 Fetus with SCT

The diagnosis of SCT is most often made in the fetal period with the routine use of obstetrical screening ultrasound [4]. Some 70–80% of SCTs are now detected by prenatal sonography. Real time ultrasound is useful in monitoring growth characteristics of SCT tumours which may have haemodynamic consequences for fetal well being. Rapidly growing lesions may contribute to a 'vascular steal' phenomenon arising in the fetus with risks of 'in utero' death from hydrops and 'maternal mirror' syndrome—a pre-eclamptic associated illness developing in mothers with severe hypertension and proteinuria. Prenatal SCT detection should always prompt a careful search for other anomalies present in up to 15–30% cases. These may include haemangioma(s), chromosomal disorders, anorectal, urologic, spinal meningocoele, orthopaedic and cardiac pathologies. Mothers should be offered amniocentesis to exclude these chromosomal disorders such as trisomy(s) 13, 18, and 21. Fetal MRI can be deployed in selected cases to view definition of anatomy with tumour extension into the pelvis or abdominal cavity(s) readily seen on magnetic resonance imaging. These fetal medicine studies may influence the site and mode of planned delivery [4, 5].

A recent publication from Finland reported a high mortality (33%) for antenatally detected SCT after excluding termination of pregnancies [2]. This emphasises the crucial need for prenatal counselling by an expert team [4]. The strongest predictors for fetal death are placentomegaly with hydrops a marker of cardiac failure in the fetus. This is related to anaemia occurring in the fetus resultant from haemorrhage into tumour. Maternal polyhydramnios contributes to early rupture of membranes and premature birth. The histological identification of anterior pituitary gland like tissues in pathology sections of SCT lends speculation to the role of vasoactive substances released by the tumour contributing to fluid retention in the fetus and hydrops.

Although several fetal intervention procedures have been advocated for SCT ranging from simple amnioreduction to fetal tumour resection clinical experience is strictly limited to only a few centres worldwide and is associated with procedure related morbidity with risk of preterm labour [4]. Minimally invasive techniques that have been promoted include laser, radiofrequency ablation, thermocoagulation and tumour embolisation using coils or alcohol [6]. Recent work has suggested improved outcomes for 'vascular' ablation (objective here to target the tumour's feeding vessels) compared to 'interstitial' ablation (goal to directly ablate the tumour itself) in these high risk groups [6, 7].

Elective delivery with C-section hysterotomy near term (>37 weeks) is best advocated for neoplasms >5 cm in size to avoid obstructed vaginal labour with its risks of tumour rupture and fetal death. In those fetuses with impending hydrops, early C-section is advisable as soon as fetal lung maturity is established i.e. >30 weeks gestation [4, 8]. This may also be achievable in premature 'high risk' cases by maternal antenatal corticosteroid administration a practice we have occasionally employed in Liverpool with some success.

61.4 Newborn Presentation

In the newborn a "monstrous" like neoplasm is readily observed at the base of the spine within the buttock region that frequently displaces the normal external anatomy of the anal orifice (Figs. 61.2 and 61.3). Large tumours can have pelvic or abdominal cavity extension that may obstruct the urinary tract resulting in hydronephrosis. Likewise large tumours may interfere with bladder and bowel emptying from birth by compression of vital anatomy.

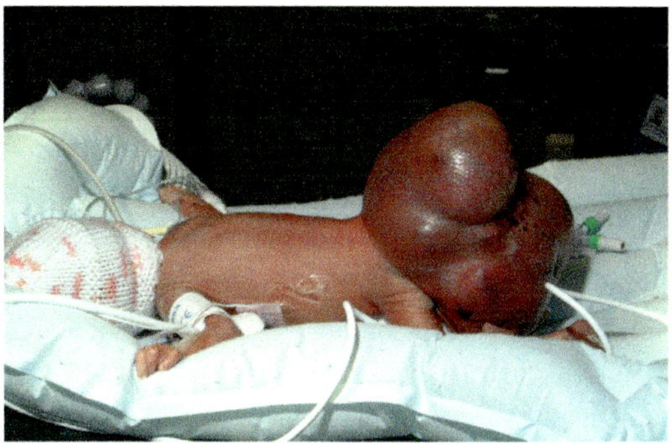

Fig. 61.2 Premature female infant with large sacrococcygeal teratoma

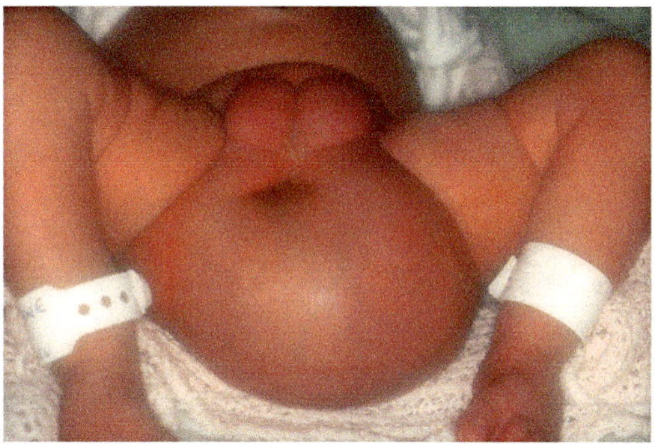

Fig. 61.3 Term newborn with large tumour displacing the normal anatomical site of the anal orifice

61.5 Associated Conditions

Associated conditions are reported in up to one third of patients most commonly involving the urogenital system including hydronephrosis and vesicoureteric reflux [9, 10]. Others mentioned earlier include anorectal malformations, myelomeningocele, hip dysplasia and sometimes lung hypoplasia. The most common and well known syndrome linked with SCT is the Currarino triad [11]. Trisomy(s)—13, 18, and 21 are excluded by offering prenatal screening. Currarino syndrome defines the co-existence of a presacral mass lesion, sacral bony defect and anal stenosis [11]. The condition is transmitted in an autosomal dominant pattern with identifiable mutations in the homeobox family of genes—MNX1 formerly HLXB9 [11, 12].

61.6 Investigations after Birth

An abdominopelvic ultrasound is the first recommended screening investigation ordered. Magnetic resonance imaging can provide very clear definition of Altman stage to plan operative strategy [13]. Serum tumour markers—alpha fetoprotein (AFP) and beta human chorionic gonadtropin (B-HCG) levels are routinely obtained and measured. AFP is greatly elevated in fetal life (100, 000 IU or higher). AFP half -life varies considerably in early postnatal life with levels reaching normal values by 12 months of age. AFP and HCG should be routinely assayed in follow up visits post resection to monitor and detect tumour recurrence.

61.7 Staging

Altman (1973) surveyed members of the Surgical Section of The American Academy of Pediatric Surgical and proposed the following staging classification (Fig. 61.4) [13].

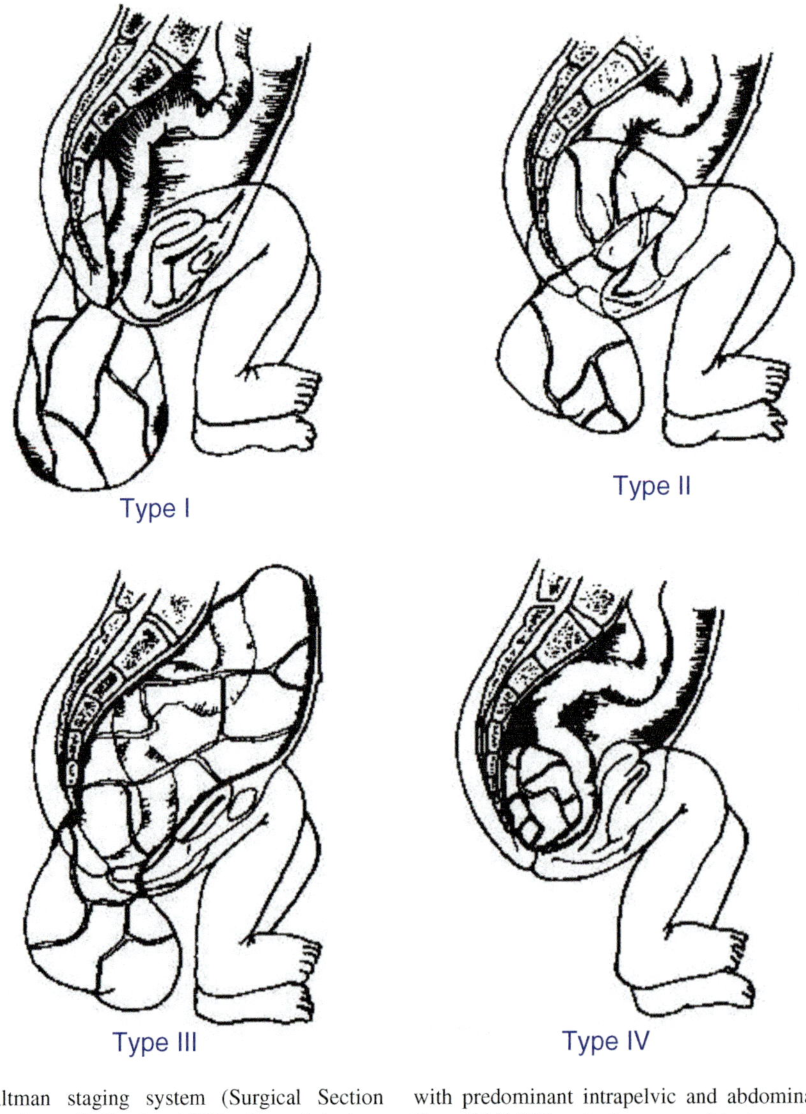

Fig. 61.4 Altman staging system (Surgical Section American Academy Pediatrics 1973). Type I lesions (46.7% of reported cases) predominantly external tumours, Type II (34.7%) external tumours with intrapelvic extension, Type III (8.8%) tumours visible externally with predominant intrapelvic and abdominal extension, Type IV (9.8%) entirely presacral lesions. Adapted from Altman RP, Randolph JG, Lilly JR. Sacrococcygeal teratoma; American Academy of Pediatric Surgery Survey 1973. J Pediatr Surg. 1974; 9: 389–398

Table 61.1 CCG/POG staging system for malignant extra gonadal germ cell tumours

Stage	Description
I	Complete resection at any site, coccygectomy for SCT, negative tumour margins, tumour markers negative or positive
II	Microscopic residual, lymph nodes negative, tumour markers negative or positive
III	Gross residual or biopsy only, retroperitoneal nodes negative or positive, tumour markers negative or positive
IV	Distant metastases including liver

Type 1: predominantly external with minimal presacral component
Type 2: presenting externally with significant intrapelvic extension
Type 3: apparent externally but predominant mass pelvic extending into abdomen
Type 4: presacral with no external presentation

The CCG/POG staging system for malignant extra gonadal germ cell tumours is shown in Table 61.1.

61.8 Postnatal Management

Following patient work up early elective resection of SCT is planned (in the absence of metastatic disease)—where complete resection is judged feasible from imaging studies. Neoadjuvant chemotherapy is administered in cases of malignancy where metastatic disease is evident or the primary tumour is deemed initially unresectable. Modern chemotherapy regimes for malignant extra gonadal germ cell tumours include platinum based therapy (carboplatin or cisplatin), etoposide and bleomycin (PEB or JEB) in association with vinblastin and ifosfamide for high risk tumours.

Operation for SCT entails gross tumour resection with coccygectomy [14, 15]. The surgeon must also pay particular attention to meticulous reconstruction of the pelvic floor to ensure preservation of bladder and bowel function along with aesthetic buttock wound closure. Blood should be cross matched, coagulation profile(s) checked, arterial line monitoring secured and a urinary catheter inserted to monitor renal function. The author routinely inserts an internal jugular central venous catheter (Broviac) before commencing tumour resection to ensure the anaesthetist has adequate circulatory access for blood, platelet products or pharmacologic agents (e.g. inotropes) if necessary. Broad spectrum antibiotics should be routinely administered. The patient is placed in a prone 'sky-diver' position with the shoulders and pelvis supported with the aid of rolls. A Chevron incision (or modified Chevron/midline PSARP in small lesions) is commenced after outlining the operative field with a skin marking pen (Fig. 61.5). Care should be taken to preserve as much skin as possible at the commencement of the operation. Excess or redundant skin can be trimmed after tumour resection. Resection aided by bipolar diathermy proceeds with great attention to avoid tumour spill or rupture with efforts to secure and ligate the middle sacral vessels and resection of the coccyx. As the resection proceeds a suitably sized Hegar dilator positioned in the rectum aids its ready identification. The tumour is then carefully freed from its lateral and inferior attachments avoiding injury to the internal and external anal sphincter complex. Reconstruction of the pelvic floor is aided with use of a muscle nerve stimulator. The thinned out levator ani are sutured to the perichondrium of the anterior surface of the sacrum which brings the displaced anus into a more normal anatomical position. The gluteal muscles are reconstructed in the midline and the overlying skin defect closed with fine interrupted absorbable sutures (Fig. 61.6). Large lesions (Altman I and II) extending into the pelvis may be adequately resected with a Chevron perineal approach. Abdominal tumour extension (Altman III) if desired may be first approached through an infraumbilical incision to isolate and secure feeding vessels. The patient may then be turned with temporary abdominal wound closure achieved with an adhesive steridrape. The Chevron perineal stage of the operation is continued with tumour resection and coccygectomy. Recent reports emphasise the importance of surgical aesthetics with avoidance of unsightly scars as many SCT patients are female. Modified elliptical posterior sagittal incisions which can then be closed in the midline can provide cosmetically superior results [10]. Principles of surgical oncology should be strictly adhered to and it must be remembered that the coccyx should always be

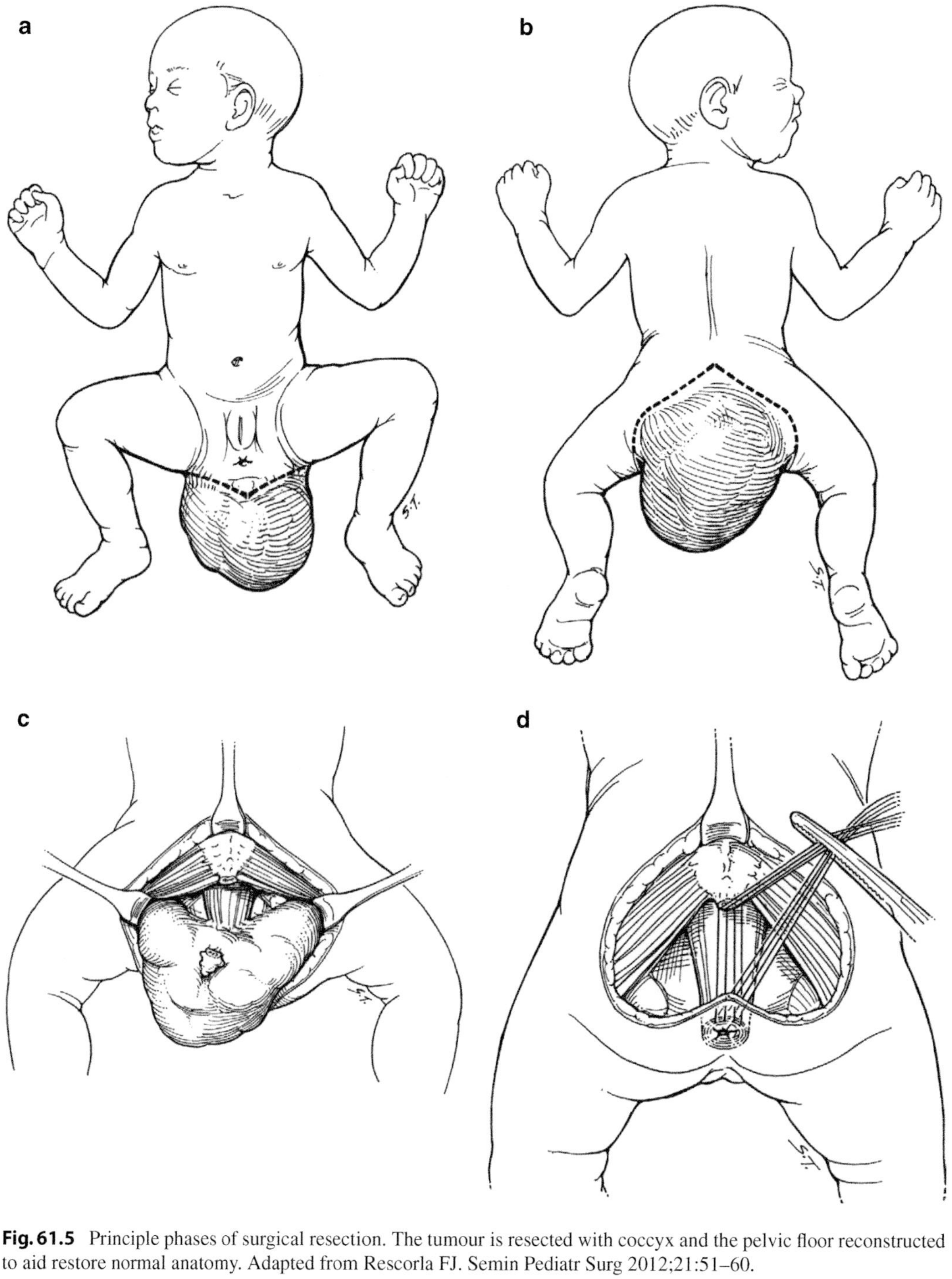

Fig. 61.5 Principle phases of surgical resection. The tumour is resected with coccyx and the pelvic floor reconstructed to aid restore normal anatomy. Adapted from Rescorla FJ. Semin Pediatr Surg 2012;21:51–60.

excised with the tumour mass to reduce risks of recurrence [10].

The major intraoperative risks for the patient and attending surgeon is exsanguinating haemorrhage usually from sacral vessels feeding the tumour. Several methods have been suggested to control or ligate the median sacral artery before mobilising the tumour. Bentley first reported ligation of the median sacral artery before attempting to resect SCT tumours [15]. Lindahl

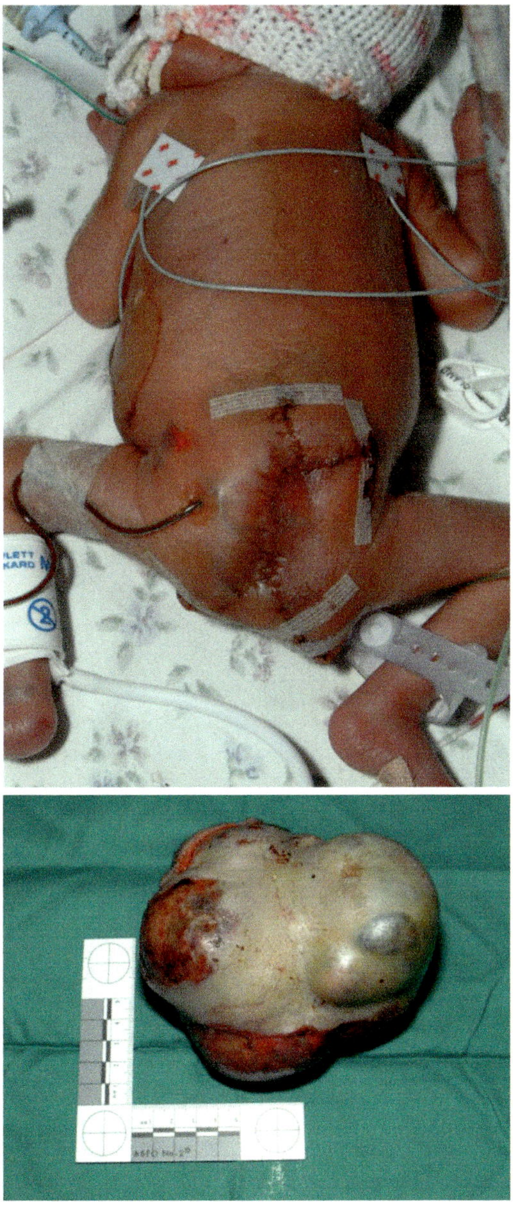

Fig. 61.6 Infant (Fig. 61.2 photo) immediately after surgery with resected tumour

also advocated use of an aortic snare to minimise risk of haemorrhage during resection of a giant lesion in a newborn [16]. Minimally invasive surgery has been deployed in a similar fashion to obtain vascular control of large Altman stage tumours. Interventional radiology with angiography and embolization has likewise been successfully utilised to occlude feeding vessels prior to resection of a large SCT [17]. Altman IV lesions (not often seen in newborns) are resected using a posterior saggital approach.

61.9 Prognosis and Outcomes

Poor prognosis for those detected antenatally will include in utero deaths, need for fetal intervention and early perinatal fatalities [4, 18]. Tumour volume to fetal weight ratio (TFR >0.12) and solid tumour volume to estimated fetal weight index (STVI >0.16) have recently been proposed as prognostic indicators for impending fetal cardiac failure, hydrops and mortality of the fetus before 32 weeks gestation [19, 20]. Benachi et al. suggested a prognostic staging classification based on SCT tumour diameter (>10 cm) with the presence of pronounced vascularity, cardiac failure and rapid growth resulting in 58% mortality in a "high risk" group [21].

The primary cause(s) for postnatal deaths in SCT patients are exsanguinating haemorrhage and malignant disease. Thirty day postoperative mortality rate(s) for SCTs are estimated at 5–6%, mainly from haemorrhage, coagulopathy and prematurity. Further scrutiny of SCT mortality figure(s)–(up to 15% in some published studies)—also shows primary tumour malignancy or disease recurrence(s) as risk factors [20–25].

An overall survival rate of 95% should be achieved for most benign lesions in the newborn period managed in experienced surgical centres [25]. In patients harbouring malignant tumours 87% survival is attainable with the new platinum based chemotherapy regimens [23, 24]. Distant metastases to multiple organ sites is a strong prognostic factor for poor survival especially so in those few infants who do not benefit from neo-adjuvant chemotherapy [23, 24].

Incomplete resection of tumour is a well documented risk factor for local recurrence [24]. Recurrences in up to 11% of cases after SCT operations are detailed. Recurrent lesions may be mature or immature teratomas or endodermal sinus tumours. Malignant recurrences have been observed even after previous resection of benign tumours. These are thought to result from very small foci of malignant cells residing in a

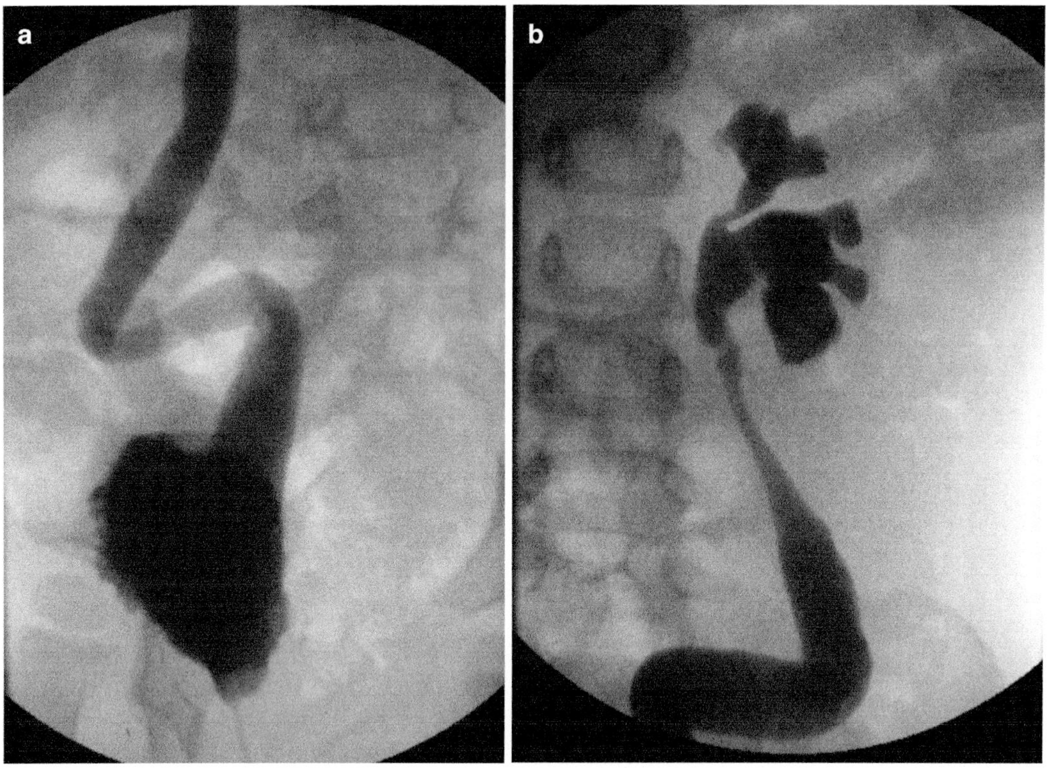

Fig. 61.7 Voiding cystogram showing neuropathic bladder with vesicoureteric reflux in a female patient some months after surgical resection of an Altman Stage III sacrococcygeal tumour

predominantly benign looking lesion. Recurrences can occur weeks, months or many years after primary resection which emphasises the need for vigilant long term follow up with monitoring tumour markers aided by surveillance ultrasound imaging [25]. Treatment for a benign recurrence is 'red-do' surgical resection. Malignant recurrences need a combination of treatment modalities—chemotherapy and 're-do' resection. Survival metrics for an SCT recurrence are of the order of 86% [24].

Data reporting functional outcome(s) after operation for SCT have become increasingly important. Bladder and bowel continence problems have been recorded in up to 30–40% of survivors [25–28]. It is not clear whether this is primarily linked to the tumour itself compressing/stretching pelvic organs and vital nerves or secondary/iatrogenic to acquired pelvic dysautonomia after surgical operation. Some published reports cite a higher prevalence of functional deficits in patients who have had large Altman type II and III tumours. Bowel and bladder disturbance require an individualized co-ordinated patient care plan. Investigations should include US imaging (pre and post micturition urine volume), urodynamics, voiding cystography (Fig. 61.7) and anorectal manometry where feasible. Clean intermittent catheterisation, rectal enemas/suppositories and in older patients (>5 years) the ACE procedure (appendicostomy stoma) may be required. Studies now also note a significant proportion of adult survivors with impaired sexual function and quality of life issues [27]. These findings serve to highlight the need for comprehensive long term follow up clinics to measure the success of selected management programmes. Publications also report a high incidence (10–40%) of cosmetically unacceptable scars of particular concern in young girls and boys with obvious psychological impact on self esteem and body image. Finally with many paediatric surgical centres in the UK, Europe and elsewhere perhaps treating no more than one or two new cases per year a debate could be made for centralising care to improve patient outcomes [25].

References

1. Ayed A, Tonks A, Lander A, Kilby M. A review of pregnancies complicated by congenital sacrococcygeal teratoma in the West Midlands region over an 18-year period: population-based, cohort study. Prenat Diagn. 2015;35:1037–47.
2. Pauniaho SL, Heikinheimo O, Vettenranta K, et al. High prevalence of sacrococcygeal teratoma in Finland—a nationwide population-based study. Acta Paediatr. 2013;102:e251–6.
3. Gray SW, Skandalakis JE. Embryology for surgeons. Philadelphia: Saunders; 1972.
4. Hedrick HL, Flake AW, Crombleholme TM, et al. Sacrococcygeal teratoma: prenatal assessment, fetal intervention and outcome. J Pediatr Surg. 2004;39:430–8.
5. Danzer E, Hubbard AM, Hedrick HL, et al. Diagnosis and characterization of fetal sacrococcygeal teratoma with prenatal MRI. AJR Am J Roentgenol. 2006;187:W350–W356.6.
6. Van Mieghem T, Al-Ibrahim A, Deprest J, et al. Minimally invasive therapy for fetal sacrococcygeal teratoma: case series and systematic review of the literature. Ultrasound Obstet Gynecol. 2014;43:611–9.
7. Sananes N, Javadian P, Britto IS, et al. Technical aspects and effectiveness of percutaneous fetal therapies for large sacrococcygeal teratomas—a cohort study and a literature review. Ultrasound Obstet Gynecol. 2015;47:712–9.
8. Roybal JL, Moldenhauer JS, Khalek N, et al. Early delivery as an alternative management strategy for selected high-risk fetal sacrococcygeal teratomas. J Pediatr Surg. 2011;46:1325–32.
9. Cost NG, Geller JI, Le LD, et al. Urologic comorbidities associated with sacrococcygeal teratoma and a rational plan for urologic surveillance. Pediatr Blood Cancer. 2013;60:1626–9.
10. Le LD, Alam S, Lim FY, Keswani SG, Crombleholme TM. Prenatal and postnatal urologic complications of sacrococcygeal teratomas. J Pediatr Surg. 2011;46:1186–90.
11. Currarino GCD, Votteler T. Triad of anorectal, sacral and presacral anomalies. AJR Am J Roentgenol. 1981;137:395.
12. Dirix M, van Becelaere T, Berkenbosch L, et al. Malignant transformation in sacrococcygeal teratoma and in presacral teratoma associated with Currarino syndrome: a comparative study. J Pediatr Surg. 2015;50:462–4.
13. Altman RP, Randolph JG, Lilly JR. Sacrococcygeal teratoma: American Academy of Pediatrics Surgical Section Survey—1973. J Pediatr Surg. 1974;9:389–98.
14. Jan IA, Khan EA, Yasmeen N, Orakzai H, Saeed J. Posterior sagittal approach for resection of sacrococcygeal teratomas. Pediatr Surg Int. 2011;27:545–8.
15. Bentley J. Coccygeal teratoma. Operative Surg. 1968;V:824–9.
16. Lindahl H. Giant sacrococcygeal teratoma: a method of simple intraoperative control of hemorrhage. J Pediatr Surg. 1988;23:1068–9.
17. Cowles RA, Stolar CJ, Kandel JJ, Weintraub JL, Susman J, Spigland NA. Preoperative angiography with embolization and radiofrequency ablation as novel adjuncts to safe surgical resection of a large, vascular sacrococcygeal teratoma. Pediatr Surg Int. 2006;22:554–6.
18. Akinkuotu AC, Coleman A, Shue E, et al. Predictors of poor prognosis in prenatally diagnosed sacrococcygeal teratoma: a multiinstitutional review. J Pediatr Surg. 2015;50:771–4.
19. Rodriguez MA, Cass DL, Lazar DA, et al. Tumor volume to fetal weight ratio as an early prognostic classification for fetal sacrococcygeal teratoma. J Pediatr Surg. 2011;46:1182–5.
20. Shue E, Bolouri M, Jelin EB, et al. Tumor metrics and morphology predict poor prognosis in prenatally diagnosed sacrococcygeal teratoma: a 25-year experience at a single institution. J Pediatr Surg. 2013;48:1225–31.
21. Benachi A, Durin L, Vasseur Maurer S, et al. Prenatally diagnosed sacrococcygeal teratoma: a prognostic classification. J Pediatr Surg. 2006;41:1517–21.
22. Huddart SN, Mann JR, Robinson K, et al. Sacrococcygeal teratomas: the UK Children's Cancer Study Group's experience. I Neonatal Pediatr Surg Int. 2003;19:47–51.
23. Gobel U, Schneider DT, Calaminus G, et al. Multimodal treatment of malignant sacrococcygeal germ cell tumors: a prospective analysis of 66 patients of the German cooperative protocols MAKEI 83/86 and 89. J Clin Oncol. 2001;19:1943–50.
24. Derikx JP, De Backer A, van de Schoot L, et al. Factors associated with recurrence and metastasis in sacrococcygeal teratoma. Br J Surg. 2006;93:1543–8.
25. Gabra HO, Jesudason EC, McDowell HP, Pizer BL, Losty PD. Sacrococcygeal teratoma—a 25-year experience in a UK regional center. J Pediatr Surg. 2006;41:1513–6.
26. Malone PS, Spitz L, Kiely EM, et al. The functional sequelae of sacrococcygeal teratoma. J Pediatr Surg. 1990;25:679–80.
27. Rintala R, Lahdenne P, Lindahl H, et al. Anorectal function in adults operated for a benign sacrococcygeal teratoma. J Pediatr Surg. 1993;28:1165–7.
28. Partridge EA, Canning D, Long C, et al. Urologic and anorectal complications of sacrococcygeal teratomas: prenatal and postnatal predictors. J Pediatr Surg. 2014;49:139–42.

Part IX

Urology

62 Management of Impaired Renal Function in the Newborn

Henry Morgan and Caroline Ann Jones

Abstract

The neonatal kidney can adapt to the usual physiological processes occurring after birth and allow homeostatic regulation to transfer from the placenta to the kidney. However during this period of transition the neonatal kidney is vulnerable. It is less able to withstand stress such as hypotension, hypoxia or hypovolaemia which will result in a decrease in kidney function. It is therefore not unexpected that the incidence of acute renal failure in children is highest in the neonatal period, with an incidence similar to adult patients. This is more pronounced in the more immature infants. Improvements in perinatal and neonatal medicine have increased the survival chances of critically ill neonates. However mortality and morbidity rates remain significant for those newborns who have suffered from a kidney injury with a reported incidence of death in 25–50%.

Keywords

Renal function • Newborn renal physiology • Renal failure • Peritoneal dialysis • Outcomes

62.1 Introduction

The neonatal kidney can adapt to the usual physiological processes occurring after birth and allow homeostatic regulation to transfer from the placenta to the kidney. However during this period of transition the neonatal kidney is vulnerable. It is less able to withstand stress such as hypotension, hypoxia or hypovolaemia which will result in a decrease in kidney function. It is therefore not unexpected that the incidence of acute renal failure in children is highest in the neonatal period, with an incidence similar to adult patients [1]. This is more pronounced in the more immature infants. Improvements in perinatal and neonatal medicine have increased the survival chances of critically ill neonates. However mortality and morbidity rates remain significant for those newborns who have suffered from a kidney injury with a reported incidence of death in 25–50% [2, 3].

H. Morgan, MB, ChB, MRCPCH (✉)
C.A. Jones, MBChB, FRCPCH, MD
Department of Paediatric Nephrology, Alder Hey Children's NHS Foundation Trust, Liverpool, UK
e-mail: henry.morgan@alderhey.nhs.uk

P.D. Losty et al. (eds.), *Rickham's Neonatal Surgery*, https://doi.org/10.1007/978-1-4471-4721-3_62

For practical purposes the term 'renal impairment' is used to describe any reduction in kidney function. This chapter will primarily address changes in the glomerular filtration rate (GFR), which occurs as a consequence of kidney injury in the neonatal surgical unit. A reduction in GFR results in acidosis, hyperkalaemia and an accumulation of waste products. These metabolic changes have an adverse effect on cellular function and post-operative recovery. Specific, isolated, disorders of neonatal renal tubular function such as Bartter's Syndrome and Neonatal Oxalosis are beyond the scope of this chapter.

Malformations of the kidneys and renal tract are the most commonly detected antenatal anomaly. These kidneys are more vulnerable to the various nephrotoxic injuries associated with surgical treatment. An understanding of neonatal renal function will aid the clinician in the appropriate management of fluid, electrolyte, nutritional and acid-base disturbances in the neonate with surgical problems. This chapter will help the clinician to identify those patients with renal impairment, which can be a particular challenge in the neonate. There is a high incidence of non-oliguric renal failure [2] which may be manifest only by a creatinine increase within the normal range for an older child. Guidance will be given on appropriate nutritional, fluid and electrolyte management, avoidance of potential complications from nephrotoxic medication in order to optimise surgical recovery. The indication for renal replacement therapy and practical consideration regarding dialysis in newborn children will be considered.

62.2 Normal Renal Function in the Newborn

Nephrogenesis starts at gestational age week five and nephrons are functional at week eight. From approximately 10 weeks gestation the foetus produces increased amounts of urine, which is the main constituent of amniotic fluid. By 36 weeks gestation nephrogenesis is complete and each kidney has approximately 1,000,000 functional nephrons [4]. No new nephrons are able to form after this period and kidney growth is a result of an increase in length and cell number of existing nephrons. In utero the kidneys do not contribute to foetal homeostasis which is performed by foetal-maternal exchange across the placenta.

62.2.1 Glomerular Filtration Rate

Glomerular filtration rate is low after birth and is closely correlated to gestational age. It is approximately 5 mL/min/1.73 m^2 in neonates of 28 weeks gestation and 10–20 mL/min/1.73 m^2 in term infants. Post natally there is a rapid increase in GFR with a two fold increase occurring in the first 2 weeks of life. The increase in GFR is a result of haemodynamic factors and renal maturation. Following birth haemodynamic factors, including an increase in cardiac output, fall in renal vascular resistance and increase in mean arterial blood pressure, lead to an increase in renal blood flow. GFR will thus increase in absolute terms, even if the proportion of renal blood flow that is filtered remains unchanged. The proportion of renal blood flow that is filtered also increases. Structural changes in the glomerular capillary bed increase the basement membrane surface area available for filtration and GFR rises. Adult values of GFR, 80–120 mL/min/1.73m^2 (a 5–10-fold increase compared newborns) are usually reached by 1–2 years [5].

Nephrogenesis is directly proportional to gestational age which may explain the lower GFR seen in the more premature infants. Plasma creatinine is usually higher in the more premature infants and does not fall steadily from birth, but rises in the first few days of life, reaching a peak and then falling to an equilibrium. This effect is more pronounced with increasing prematurity [6]. This is most likely to be due to tubular 'back leak' of creatinine across the immature tubules and may not represent true renal impairment [7].

Formal measurement of GFR, using a fully filtered, non-secreted, tracer, such as Cr^{51} EDTA, is invasive and expensive. Creatinine is usually used as a measure of GFR, but may not be accurate in the neonate. Creatinine may be falsely elevated if the patient has a high bilirubin and the biochemical analyser does not correct for non-creatinine chromogens, including medication. The Schwartz formula can be used to estimate GFR once the plasma creatinine has stabilised [8]. Estimated GFR = body length (cm) × K/creatinine (μmol/l) The constant K is 33 for term infants and 24 for low birth weight infants [9]. Reference ranges for normal creatinine may vary between different laboratories, depending on the analyser, but are between 30 and 58 μmol/l in infants age 0–2 weeks and 20–48 μmol/l in infants age 2–26 weeks. As already indicated foetal kidneys do not contribute to the excretion, thus the neonate's creatinine at birth reflects maternal plasma creatinine values and is not a measure of neonatal renal function.

62.2.2 Water Homeostasis

In early postnatal life there is a reduction in total body water, extracellular water and extracellular sodium and chloride. This loss of extracellular volume is readily apparent as the postnatal weight loss, which is greater in the more immature infants where a weight loss of up to 10% can occur. This is caused by the inability of the neonatal kidney to generate concentrated urine. Maximal urine concentration in the first week of life is about 700 mosmol/kg compared with 1000–1200 mosmol/kg in an adult. The metabolic demand for urine concentrating ability is high. In utero this burden is carried out by the placenta. It takes time for postnatal adaptations to occur. Neonates consume large volumes of dilute fluid, in the form of breast milk, relative to the body size. (Breast milk contains ~10 mmol/L sodium.) This high free water intake reduces the need for a significant urine concentrating capacity. The main clinical consequence of a low urine concentrating capacity is the risk of water depletion and hypernatraemia if insufficient fluids are provided.

Conversely the ability to excrete excess water following the administration of hypotonic fluid is limited by the low neonatal glomerular filtration rate. Thus increasing the likelihood of fluid overload and hyponatraemia in these circumstances.

Insensible water loss is also greater in the neonate as a result of increased trans-epidermal water loss. Trans-epidermal water loss is inversely correlated with gestational age as a result of a large ratio of surface area to weight and is also affected by environmental factors including temperature, relative humidity and air circulation. Fluid prescriptions need to be adjusted for increased insensible water losses particularly in the premature infant exposed to phototherapy and overhead heaters. Although the range of fluid intake that can be tolerated is wide, the limits can be reached when renal function is impaired.

62.2.3 Sodium Homeostasis

At birth there is a limited capacity to excrete a sodium load or conserve sodium if there is a sodium restriction. In the first week of life fractional sodium excretion is high and this is greater in the more immature infants. This results in a fall in the plasma sodium and chloride and relatively high urinary sodium to plasma sodium. Again this may be explained by the high metabolic requirement for this active process and resulting limited sodium and chloride reabsorption in the neonatal kidney. Intravenous fluids should ensure the correct sodium content to avoid plasma sodium falling. Conversely foetal sodium excretion is usually less than 10% of the intake in premature infants. Colonic sodium reabsorption decreases with increasing gestational and postnatal age and may help to counterbalance urinary sodium loss.

Causes of hyponatraemia occurring shortly after birth include excessive hypotonic fluid given to the mother and inadequate sodium content of neonatal feed or intravenous fluid. Antidiuretic hormone is also released in response to neonatal pathology, including asphyxia, which results in excessive water reabsorption. Causes of hyponatraemia occurring later include inadequate sodium content of the neonatal feed or intravenous fluid with the more immature infant being less able to adapt. Excessive sodium losses from the gastrointestinal tract including patients with short bowel syndrome and an ileostomy or patients with upper gastrointestinal losses are also at an increased risk of developing hyponatraemia. Excess renal tubular sodium losses may occur in patients with intrinsic renal pathology, including dysplasia but in the neonatal surgical unit may be more common in the recovery phase of acute renal failure or following the diuretic phase after treatment for an obstructive uropathy such as posterior urethral valves.

62.2.4 Potassium Homeostasis

The rate of potassium excretion in the neonate is low and the tubules are less able to respond to a potassium load than an older child. Plasma potassium in the more immature infants is greater than in term infants and is also increased by hypoxia, metabolic acidosis, catabolic state, potassium administration, oliguric renal failure and reduced potassium secretion by the immature distal nephron.

62.2.5 Tubular Function

Tubular function matures later than glomerular function and reaches maturity by 1 year of age. The increase in tubular glucose reabsorption in infancy and childhood parallels the increase in GFR. Glycosuria is commoner in neonates and is higher in the more immature infants. Likewise aminoaciduria is more common in the neonate. The degree of aminoaciduria is variable between different amino acids. These factors need to be considered when interpreting amino acid profiles for metabolic conditions [10]. Phosphate reabsorption is greater in the neonate than in older infants and children. This is to achieve a positive phosphate balance for bone accretion.

62.3 Impaired Renal Function in the Newborn

The low GFR of the neonatal kidney helps to explain why it is vulnerable to periods of stress resulting in renal impairment. It limits the newborns ability to adapt to haemodynamic changes, such as hypotension, hypovolaemia and vasoactive drugs, and more readily accumulates non-excreted waste products (elevated creatinine) and the other associated features of renal impairment. It is also less able to adapt to injury from hypoxia or nephrotoxic drugs. The neonate with an acute surgical condition is likely to be exposed to more than one of these factors and is consequently at risk of renal impairment. Table 62.1 lists some causes of renal impairment according to the timing of the renal injury. Causes may also divided into pre-renal, intrinsic-renal and post-renal (obstruction to urine flow). This aides management strategies.

Table 62.1 Causes of neonatal renal impairment

Antenatal vascular injury
• Maternal medication—ACE inhibitors, NSAIDs
• Twin-twin transfusion
• Co-twin death
Renal tract congenital abnormalities
• Obstructive uropathy—Posterior urethral valves
• Polycystic kidney disease—Autosomal recessive
• Renal hypo—Dysplasia
• Renal agenesis
• Renal tubular dysgenesis
• Diffuse mesangial sclerosis
• Congenital nephrotic syndrome (Finnish type)
Acquired postnatal renal injury
• Shock
• Dehydration
• NEC with third space losses
• Cardiac failure
• Cardiopulmonary bypass, ECMO
• DIC
• Vascular thrombosis—Umbilical artery and venous cannulation
• Perinatal asphyxia
• Infection—Pyelonephritis, congenital infections, fungal UTI +/− obstruction
• Closure of abdominal wall defects
• Nephrotoxic medication—Indomethacin (PDA), ACEi (cardiac failure), aminoglycosides, vancomycin, amphotericin

62.3.1 Pre-renal

Preterm neonates with reduced renal perfusion, from a reduced circulating volume, account for approximately one third of cases of impaired renal function [11] A true circulation volume contraction or a decrease in the effective circulating volume may be present. Renal hypoperfusion reduces GFR, which is manifested by an increase in plasma creatinine, as there is less blood available to be filtered at the glomerulus. Adaptive mechanisms include the Renin, Angiotensin, Aldosterone system, which increases renal vascular resistance to support blood pressure and perfusion to other vital organs. GFR is maintained by alteration in glomerular afferent and efferent arteriolar tone, increasing glomerular hydrostatic pressure. In this way total renal blood flow is reduced but the proportion filtered is increased thus maintaining GFR. Urea is disproportionally reabsorbed and then recirculated in order to improve urine concentrating ability. This reduces urine output, helping to maintain circulating volume. The kidney avidly retains sodium, the main cation of the extracellular fluid, which helps to maintain ECF volume and circulating volume. These two features lead to the characteristic pattern of a low urine sodium concentration (<10 mmol/l) and concentrated urine (>plasma osmolality) observed in pre renal impairment. As a temporary measure GFR can be reduced in order to protect vital organs against the low circulating volume. Correcting the underlying disturbance in circulating volume will return renal function to normal.

62.3.2 Intrinsic-Renal

If renal hypoperfusion persists renal tubular cells suffer from a hypoxic/ischaemic injury leading to Acute Tubular Necrosis (ATN). In this setting GFR is further reduced by sloughing of tubular epithelial cells forming casts in the tubular lumen and obstructing urine flow. Local reduction of 'single nephron GFR' is activated by the macular densa registering a high solute flow in the distal nephron. This reduction prevents excessive solute loss but if widespread will reduce overall GFR. Creatinine may filter back across the damaged tubule. Inappropriately high urine sodium levels, in the presence of low circulating volume are seen as sodium can no longer be avidly reabsorbed by the injured tubular epithelial cells. Clinically ATN may be identified by a persistent elevation of creatinine despite improvement of circulating volume.

Restoration of renal perfusion will enable tubular cells to recover. The length of time before recovery is variable. Patients may require dialysis for several weeks and still eventually recover complete renal function. Acute cortical necrosis occurs following more prolonged or severe ischemia and results in long term renal impairment.

In the neonatal surgical unit necrotising enterocolitis increases the relative risk of renal impairment and is associated with more severe renal impairment [12]. Nephrotoxic injury from medication is a significant cause of intrinsic renal impairment. Other causes of intrinsic renal disease resulting in neonatal renal impairment include Renal Dysplasia, Hypoplasia and Autosomal Recessive Polycystic Kidney Disease. Neonates who do not have renal tract anomalies but do have other major anatomical or genetic abnormality have a higher incidence of renal impairment [12]. Neonates who have undergone cardiac surgery or with severe birth asphyxia are at particular risk [13].

62.3.3 Post-renal

The commonest cause of obstructive renal disease in the neonate is secondary to posterior urethral valves. Other causes include sacrcoccygeal teratoma, urethral atresia and a neuropathic bladder. Spina bifida is a well recognised cause of neuropathic bladder which may present difficulties in the neonatal period. The majority of VACTERL patients (92%) have bladder involvement that requires urological intervention [14]. Mild renal pelvis dilatation may indicate obstructive renal pathology in a patient with oliguric renal impairment because the kidney cannot 'generate' sufficient urine flow to lead to significant hydronephrosis. This situation needs careful consideration and may result in intervention such as nephrostomy.

62.4 Evaluation of the Newborn with Renal Impairment

The term renal impairment is a term used to describe any reduction in glomerular or tubular function. There has been an increased effort to standardise the definitions for renal impairment, to improve the ability to compare studies, predict clinical course and improve outcome. Long term renal impairment is described as Chronic Kidney Disease (CKD). This has little significance in the neonatal surgical unit but does have some relevance when considering the long term outcome of the children. Acute changes in GFR, whether baseline levels are normal or not, are classified as Acute Kidney Injury (AKI), synonymous with the previous term 'acute renal failure'. The pRIFLE classification was proposed in 2007 to classify acute kidney injury in children [15]. This stratified patients according to those at **R**isk, **I**njury, **F**ailure, **L**oss & **E**nd stage renal disease. This followed the RIFLE classification initially introduced for the recognition of AKI in adults in 2004 [16]. These scoring systems use two clinical parameters to stratify patients in severity of their kidney injury. Firstly the change in serum creatinine, both absolute and relative changes, and secondly urine output. Table 62.2 shows an abbreviated comparison between these systems indicating the scale of changes. The value of these systems is significant, They have shown that AKI has a negative impact upon survival. It is pertinent to note that patients not only die from AKI but suffer from functional changes in other organs as a consequence of reduced renal function.

Unfortunately this classification has not been validated in the neonates. Currently the diagnosis of acute kidney injury is dependent on a change in serum creatinine as a marker of GFR and the presence of oliguria. A change in serum creatinine may not occur until 25–50% of the kidney function is lost and may overestimate renal function at a lower GFR because of the tubular secretion of creatinine. Conversely serum creatinine will underestimate GFR if the analyser does not correct for non-creatinine chromogens, including bilirubin. This is particularly relevant for neonates who are jaundiced. There is a wide distribution of normal serum creatinine in the neonate, which as previously discussed is dependent on prematurity and age. The presence of oliguria will not identify those infants with polyuric renal failure. In neonates, there is up to a 40% incidence of non-oliguric renal impairment. Oliguric renal failure is associated with a higher mortality rate than non-oliguric renal failure [2]. Despite these difficulties the underlying principles remain valid for newborn children, and can be used to identify patients at risk of, or who have developed, renal impairment.

Urinary biomarkers of AKI, including neutrophil gelatinase-associated lipocalin (NGAL) kidney injury molecule (KIM-1) and urinary interleukin-18 are currently being explored for their ability to diagnose AKI early in the disease process [17]. These biomarkers are currently being validated as a useful clinical tool in neonates, who are at risk of AKI from cardiopulmonary bypass surgery [13]. Genetic risk factors for renal impairment from various nephrotoxic insults have been investigated [18, 19]. but these are not yet clinically useful.

Antenatal sonography may detect structural renal tract abnormalities and raise the concern that the child will be born with a degree of renal impairment. At present there is no readily available way to estimate renal function prior to birth. The classic example of this is the baby with oligohydramnios and abnormal kidneys (e.g. Autosomal Recessive Polycystic Kidney Disease). They may not have sufficient urine output and amniotic fluid for adequate lung development but still have a urine output adequate to avoid renal replacement therapy for a considerable period [20].

62.5 Management

Following the diagnosis of renal impairment, understanding the pathogenesis will enable the infant to receive the appropriate treatment. A careful physical examination should be undertaken with close attention to hydration status and circulating volume. An accurate weight is the best guide to changes in overall hydration status. The urine should be collected and analysed for urinalysis, microscopy and microbial culture and electrolytes. Urinary electrolyte concentrations can be used to help differentiate pre-renal and intrinsic-renal impairment. Meaningful interpretation can be made on random, spot urine specimens. A low

Table 62.2 Classification of Acute Kidney Injury (AKI) in children in comparison to adult.

	Adult				Children		
AKIN staging		AKIN/RIFLE	RIFLE		pRIFLE		
Stage	Serum creatinine	Urine output (common to both)	Class	SCR or GFR	Class	eGFR	Urine output
I	↑SCr by >0.3 mg/dL or ↑SCr by >150–200%	<0.5 mL/kg/l/h x > 6 h	Risk	↑SCr by 150% or ↓GFR by 25%	Risk	↓eGFR by 25%	<0.5 mL/kg/h × 8 h
II	↑SCr by >200–300%	<0.5 mL/kg/L/h x > 12	Injury	↑SCr by 200% or ↓GFR by 50%	Injury	↓eGFR by 50%	<0.5 mi/kg/h × 16 h
III	↑SCr by >300% or SCr > 4.0 mg/dL with acute rise of at least 0.5 mg/dL	<0.3 mL/kg/L/h >24 or anuria × 12 h	Failure	↑SCr by 300% or SCr > 4.0 mg/dL with acute rise of 0.5 mg/dL or↓GFR by 75%	Failure	↓eGFR by 75% or <35 mL/min per 1.73 m^2	<0.3 mL/kg/h × 24 h or anuric × 12 h
			Loss	Failure × > weeks 4	Loss	Failure × > 4 weeks	
			ESRD	Failure × > 3 months	ESRD	Failure × > 3 months	

AKIN, Acute Kidney Injury Network, For AKIN classification: an acute (within 48 h) reduction in kidney function is required.
(p)RIFLE (pediatric) risk injury failure loss ESRD, *ESRD* end-stage renal disease, *SCr* serum creatinine, *GFR* glomerular filtration rate, *eGFR* estimated glomerular filtration rate

urinary sodium concentration (<10 mmol/1) and low fractional excretion of sodium ((Urine sodium × serum creatinine)/(serum sodium × urine creatinine) <1%) suggests pre-renal impairment. Blood should be sent for sodium, potassium, chloride, bicarbonate, urea, creatinine, calcium, phosphate, magnesium, albumin and total protein. A renal ultrasound scan should always be performed.

The management of renal impairment requires attention to, fluid balance and electrolyte homeostasis. Low urine output renal impairment is not frequently present in neonates, which greatly facilitates conservative treatment. Conversely if urine output is restricted there is a very significant challenge, particularly to provide sufficient calories for growth.

62.5.1 Fluid Management

Standard neonatal fluid guidelines (for infants with normal renal function) provide an acceptable starting point from which to modify according to clinical circumstance [11, 21]. In the presence of renal impairment the guiding principle is that intake and output must be balanced. Each fluid prescription must be individualised. Fluid administration must be directed by fluid losses including insensible water losses (evaporative) of 30 mL/kg/day (or 20 mL/kg/day if ventilated) [22] Urine output, gastrointestinal losses and surgical drain losses should be replaced with equal volumes. Strict recording of fluid balance and daily weighing is required.

If pre-renal impairment is suspected a fluid challenge of 10–20 mL/kg over 1–2 h of isotonic saline solution should be given. Another fluid challenge can be given followed by furosemide 1–2 mg/kg. This should result in an improvement in urine output if the diagnosis of pre-renal failure is correct. If there is no improvement following two fluid boluses and the infant is no longer considered to be hypovolaemic further fluid volumes must be carefully considered to avoid fluid overload, cardiac failure and pulmonary oedema.

Management is greatly facilitated if urine output is maintained. It is reasonable to try and promote this with the cautious use of diuretics. Their toxicity must be balanced against the low chance of benefit. Diuretics are beneficial in controlling oedema associated with mild renal impairment (Table 62.2. 'Risk' & 'Injury' classification.) but rarely improves the volume of urine passed in significant renal impairment (Table 62.2. 'Failure', 'Loss' or 'ESRD' classification).

62.5.2 Nutrition and Growth

In general infants with renal impairment should be feed to the same recommended nutrient intake as for healthy infants. Calorie intake targets are 120–150 kcal/kg/day to avoid the infant becoming catabolic which may result in an increase in urea and acidosis. Dietary protein restriction in not recommended and should be the same recommended intake as for healthy infants to allow growth. Energy intake is difficult to achieve in the oliguric neonate who is dependent on milk or parenteral nutrition. In significant renal impairment daily weight loss of 0.2–1% of body weight may be expected beyond the first week [22]. If sufficient calories cannot be achieved, within an acceptable timescale, because of oliguria then dialysis should be considered to allow a greater volume of feed to be administered. An accurate fluid balance will help differentiate an increase in weight secondary to fluid retention, in the oliguric infant, from nutritional growth.

Poor weight gain may be secondary to sodium wasting which is common in infants with renal hypodysplasia and following treatment of obstructive uropathy. Breast milk and normal infant formula contain approximately 7–10 mmol/l of sodium. In renal impairment although the volume of fluid intake may be matched, by urine output & insensible losses, the kidneys may not be able to reduce urinary sodium to a correspondingly low concentration and a negative sodium balance will result. Sodium chloride supplements, starting at 1 mmol/kg/day in divided doses, should be given and may improve growth.

62.5.3 Electrolytes

Significant alterations in serum sodium concentrations may occur without neurological compromise in newborn infants. Hyponatraemia is frequently seen in fluid overloaded infants. The treatment here is fluid (water) restriction. Again, it is not possible to be precise about the volume of 'fluid restriction'. The principle is to achieve a negative water balance, thus output must be greater than input. Careful recording of fluid balance (e.g. weighing nappies), daily (or twice daily weight), clinical examination and frequent measurement of electrolytes will indicate whether the therapeutic goal is being achieved. Rarely the emergency treatment of symptomatic hyponatraemia will require the infusion of hypertonic saline to more quickly increase plasma osmolality, restore intracellular volume and reduce cerebral swelling.

Neonates are remarkably resistant to the effect of hyperkalaemia. Preterm infants may tolerate a serum potassium concentration up the 7 mmol/l without cardiac symptoms [23]. In this paper only 25% of patients with a serum potassium above 8 mmol/l had a cardiac arrhythmia. A frequent problem is artefactual hyperkalaemia from mechanical haemolysis during capillary blood sampling. Care must be taken to avoid being falsely reassured when haemolysis is reported and the potassium is elevated. A rise in creatinine, fall in plasma bicarbonate or calcium suggest true hyperkalaemia.

Hyperkalaemia can lead to cardiac rhythm disturbance because of its depolarising effect on the cells of the cardiac conducting pathway. The potassium level at which this occurs is dependent upon acid base variables and other electrolytes, notably calcium. Significant ECG changes are often a late development (Long PR, increased QRS duration) and require prompt treatment [24]. Intravenous calcium gluconate has an immediate stabilising effect on the myocardium. Sodium bicarbonate, to reduce acidosis, can be quickly and easily administered. Nebulised and intravenous salbutamol have appreciable effect upon reducing plasma potassium levels. Insulin and dextrose is useful for life threatening hyperkalaemia but may result in significant hypoglycaemia in newborn infants.

All these measures have only a temporary effect on blood potassium levels, by shifting potassium into cells. Reducing potassium intake is essential. Breast milk and normal infant formula can be exchanged for a low potassium infant milk such as Renastart. Ion exchange resins (Kayexalte and Calicium Resonium) have limited use in the emergency setting and are not without complications, particularly in post operative patients [25]. If the source of potassium cannot quickly be rectified hyperkalaemia associated with renal impairment frequently requires the initiation of dialysis.

Renal tubular unresponsiveness to aldosterone results in hyperkalaemia, hyponatraemia, dehydration and metabolic acidosis. This 'transient psuedohypoaldosteronism' is seen in patients with abnormal renal tracts, such as posterior urethral valves or vesicoureteric reflux, and urinary tract infection [26]. The biochemical features of this condition are indistinguishable from salt wasting congenital adrenal hyperplasia. Aggressive fluid resuscitation with 0.9% sodium chloride and correction of acidosis with sodium bicarbonate will correct hyperkalaemia. The reduced renal tubular response to aldosterone may persist for a long period after surgical correction [27]. Weight gain and electrolytes should be monitored for at least a year [28].

Acidosis due to renal impairment can be buffered by sodium bicarbonate supplements at a dose of 1 mmol/kg/day. Hypocalcaemia must be corrected when treating acidosis to avoid a fall in ionised calcium and tetany or seizures.

Electrolyte abnormalities may be associated with medication [29]. Particular attention should be paid to phosphate, used for the treatment of osteopenia of prematurity or as an enema for constipation. Phosphate containing medication should be avoided when the GFR is below 60 mL/min/1.73 m^2 [30]. to avoid hyperphosphatemia and hypocalcaemia.

The return of normal renal function may be associated with a diuretic phase. This period of excessive urine output requires close attention to fluid and electrolyte balance. It is useful to consider that normal breast milk and infant formula contains about 7–10 mmol/l of sodium. In neutral water balance, a daily intake of 150 mL/kg/day will be associated with ~30 mL/kg/day transepidermal loss (almost entirely free water) and 120 mL/kg/day urine. This urine will contain ~12 mmol/l to stay in neutral sodium balance.

Persistently higher urine sodium levels, in the setting of recovering renal function, suggest salt wasting and may need supplementation.

62.5.4 Drug Handling

The dynamic processes of growth, development and renal maturation that occur in the neonate influence the dosing regimens of drugs during early life and childhood. Kidney size, as a percentage of body weight, rises to a maximum at 5 years and then falls steadily until adulthood [11]. This may be one explanation as to why children are usually administered a higher dose of a renal excreted drug, when corrected for size, than adults to achieve targeted therapeutic concentrations.

Knowledge of specific transporters involved in renal drug clearance will enable adjustment of therapeutic doses that avoid toxicity. Several drug are excreted via the same renal pathway as organic acids. The secretion of organic acids is low during the neonatal period and increases over the first few years of life as a result of increasing GFR, increased number of transporter sites and increased metabolic capacity. Organic acid secretion reaches its maximum in the first few weeks of life and then falls to adult levels [31]. Immaturity of the organic anion transport system is more pronounced in the preterm infant. Organic anions frequently administered to the neonate include benzyl penicillin, folic acid, phenobarbitone, ACE inhibitors, antiviral drugs and non-steroidal anti-inflammatory drugs [32]. The neonatal kidney has a greater ability to secrete organic cations than organic anions. Organic cations that may be administered to the neonate include amiloride, morphine and noradrenaline [32].

The weight of the liver relative to the body size is also greater in the infant and younger child than adult. Developmental changes in drug handling are also dependent on the maturation of other hepatic functions such as cytochrome P450 enzymes. Drug toxicity may occur if the P450 enzyme activates the parent drug into its reactive metabolite at a faster rate than the renal excretion pathway. Toxicity may be decreased if renal clearance that removes the active metabolite matures earlier than the P450 enzyme that inactivates the parent drug. To determine optimal therapeutic doses and avoid potential drug interactions the handling of drugs by the developing kidney and liver need to be understood.

Thus particular care should be taken with the dosing of all medication in the presence of known, or suspected renal impairment. Aminoglycosides are frequently administered to neonates with suspected or proven sepsis. A Cochrane review supports the once daily dosing schedule of gentamicin for the beneficial effect on microbial killing without an increase in nephrotoxicity compared to the traditional multiple dose schedule [30, 33]. However, this dosing schedule has not been proven to be safe in the neonate with renal impairment. We recommend a single standard dose (2.5 mg/kg) with close monitoring of therapeutic levels to ensure a trough level below 2 mg/L is reached before a further dose is administered.

Evidence of severe and irreversible renal insufficiency after prenatal exposure to NSAID's has resulted in these drugs being avoided during pregnancy [34]. NSAID's reduce renal perfusion by inhibiting prostaglandins that are vasodilatory. NSAID's, such as Indomethacin, are used for the treatment of patent ductus areteriosus. Other nephrotoxic medication that is frequently encountered in the neonatal surgical unit are Angiotensin Converting Enzyme inhibitors (Captopril, Lisinopril) used for the treatment of congenital heart disease and cardiac failure.

There is no specific medical therapy to improve renal function. The use of low dose dopamine for the prevention or treatment of renal failure in neonates remains controversial [11, 22]. There is little evidence to strongly support its use in the absence of low blood pressure requiring inotropic support. There is some emerging evidence to suggest a benefit from theophylline to prevent AKI following birth asphyxia [35–37]. Treatment appears to reduce frequency of significantly elevated creatinine levels and markers of renal dysfunction. Long term effects were not reported.

62.5.5 Hypertension

Blood pressure in neonates increases with gestational age, post-conceptual age and birth weight [38]. The centile charts produced from this study can be used to define if an infants blood pressure is above the 95th percentile and considered to be hypertensive. These centile charts produce data for infants aged 24–42 weeks gestation. For older infants and children the percentile charts generated from the second Task Force are the most useful [39].

The commonest causes of hypertension in the neonate are renovascular and renal parenchymal disease. Umbilical artery catheter-associated thromboembolism should be considered as a cause of 'renovascular' hypertension in the neonatal ICU [40]. It is therefore important to assess the blood pressure in neonates with nephro-urological conditions **and** also in neonates with abdominal masses or hydronephrosis causing compression of the renal arteries.

Measurement of blood pressure in the NICU is usually performed by an indwelling arterial line. If automated oscillometric devices are used it is important to select the correct cuff size and use the upper limb as normative data is generally obtained from measurements in the right upper arm. An alternative method, which we prefer, is the Doppler technique by skilled nursing staff.

Hypertension in the surgical neonate is usually detected by routine monitoring of vital signs. Classical symptoms and signs include unexplained tachyapnea, irritability, lethargy, failure to thrive and in the more severe case congestive heart failure.

Hypertension in the surgical neonate may require the use of intravenous agents, which have a short half life, and allow the drug to be titrated against the blood pressure to avoid too rapid a reduction in blood pressure leading to cerebral ischaemia and haemorrhage. Intermittently administered intravenous agents, such as hydralazine, may be of use in the neonate with moderate hypertension, who are unable to tolerate oral medication.

Oral antihypertensives are often considered for infants with mild hypertension. An ACE inhibitor should not be used if there is any concern that the neonate has renovascular disease and with caution if the neonate has deranged renal function. The calcium channel blocker Amlodipine is a vasodilator that is available in a suspension and is usually well tolerated in the neonate. It is important that the neonate is not volume depleted before administering a vasodilator as this can result in an unexpected fall in blood pressure. Surgical intervention may be required for patients with an obstructive uropathy or abdominal mass.

62.5.6 Renal Replacement Therapy

62.5.6.1 Peritoneal Dialysis

Renal replacement therapy is indicated when conservative therapy fails to control complications of renal impairment, such as electrolyte and acid-base abnormalities but more commonly progressive fluid overload. Peritoneal dialysis (PD) remains the renal replacement modality of choice. PD provides fluid and solute removal, dependent upon the volume, osmolality and dwell time of the dialysis fluid in the peritoneal space. The major limitation for peritoneal dialysis is related to abdominal pathology. Peritoneal dialysis is unlikely to succeed in a patient with bowel perforation, for example as a consequence of necrotising enterocolitis., Success in this situation is rare with reported attempts representing 'last ditch' attempts in extreme situations [41]. PD can be successfully performed after abdominal surgery and the creation of enterostomies. [Personal Observations] Extra-renal anomalies can significantly complicate the renal course. Patients with VACTERL anomalies are less likely to have peritoneal dialysis because of abdominal surgery [14].

Access to the peritoneal cavity is usually through a Tenckhoff catheter. There are a range of catheters available with different configurations, such as straight, coiled or swan-necked. They may have 1 or 2 'cuffs' for securing to the subcutaneous tissues. None have proven benefits for providing acute, short term dialysis [42]. Insertion technique is important to reduce catheter related malfunction. In neonates the thin abdominal wall increases the likelihood of leaking dialysis fluid around the catheter. Catheters can be successfully placed using a percutaneous seldinger technique. In our institution short term PD catheters are placed percutaneously. Long term catheters are placed surgically with a subcutaneous tunnel. Peritoneal dialysis catheters with two cuffs requiring a subcutaneous tunnel are recommended for those infants who may need long-term dialysis. This reduces the risk of recurrent peritonitis. These catheters are best placed by an experienced surgeon dedicated to their long term management. The cardiothoracic surgeon place catheters via a trans-diaphragmatic route, at the time of cardiac surgery in patients who are considered at risk for AKI.

There are no accurate automated devices for delivering PD to small children because of the low dialysate volumes required. Manual 'exchanges' of dialysis fluid can be easily managed in the intensive care environment. Standard practice is to start with an initial volume of 10 mL/kg exchanged every hour. This can be progressively increased up to 40 mL/kg. Higher volumes may compromise respiratory function, by splinting the diaphragm. Cardiac function may be compromised, in critically unwell infants, by a reduction in cardiac return through compression to the vena cave. Pericatheter leakage of dialysis fluids is also more likely with larger volumes particularly in the infant with little subcutaneous or oedematous tissues. Small infants, of almost any weight, can be successfully managed, achieving adequate fluid removal, with low volumes (10 mL/kg) PD. [43]

Standard, commercially prepared dialysis fluid is suitable for the majority of patients. Some infants with liver impairment may not metabolise the lactate in these solutions to bicarbonate and failure to control acidosis. Commercial solutions are available with both lactate and bicarbonate buffers. 'Home made' preparations of dialysis fluid using entirely bicarbonate may be required if acid-base homeostasis cannot be maintained.

The most significant challenge remains the 'mechanical' problem of obstruction to fluid flow either during filling or commonly during drainage of dialysate. Small infants can rapidly accumulate significant fluid volumes if several cycles do not drain adequately.. Various PD techniques have been reported to improve PD drainage and include change in the infant's position [44, 45].

62.5.6.2 Blood Based Dialysis

There are several forms of extracorporeal renal replacement therapy. Each has subtle advantages they may be appropriate depending on the clinical situation. Conventional haemodialysis, in which waste product and fluid removal usually occursover a 3–4 h session corrects metabolic abnormalities quickly. This is useful for the treatment on hyperammonemia from urea cycle disorders. Infants are usually unable to tolerate haemodialysis because of the relatively large extracorporeal circuit and the physiological stress associated with fluid removal of a short time. Extracorporeal circuit volumes of more than 10–15% of patient's body weight should be primed with blood.

Continuous therapies, with waste product and fluid removal taking place over a 24 h period, provide more stability. Haemofiltration, dialysis or a combination of both can be employed. Blood is usually taken and returned via a large gauge venous catheter in one of the major vessels. Thus providing the acronym CVVHF (continuous veno-veno haemofiltration). The significant technical challenge with these techniques is vascular access. Even very small infants can be managed provided vascular access can be achieved; At least 6 French catheter is usually required [46]. There are machines that can deliver blood based renal replacement therapy to very small infants, but they are not yet widespread [47]. Using conventional machines the rate of technical complications is low [48]. Although there is a trend towards lower survival rates in infants less than 3 kg [48]. Maintaining vascular access and loss of central veins is a limiting factor for the long term use of blood based dialysis therapies in neonates.

62.6 Long Term Outcome

Neonates who have had an episode renal impairment require follow up. There is limited data on the long term risk of neonatal renal failure [49]. However an underlying principle of the kidney's response to injury supports the need to monitor children. When the number of nephrons is reduced the remaining nephrons increase their GFR in order to compensate. However the compensatory mechanisms within the glomeruli damages the glomerular capillary walls and leads to progressive glomerulosclerosis, proteinuria, hypertension and chronic kidney disease [50]. This phenomena has been demonstrated paediatric patients. Neonates with congenital abnormalities, such as the VACTERAL anomaly, have a greater risk that the renal impairment will continue beyond the neonatal period [14, 51]. Patients who have an elevated creatinine for more than 3 months are classified as having Chronic Kidney Disease. Babies who require long term dialysis are a particular challenge. Although 12% may recover native renal function 25–50% may die before the age of 5 years [52, 53] The presence of oliguria is associated with lower patient survival.

Conclusion

Renal impairment is common in the neonatal period. Frequently the cause is multifactorial with a 'pre-renal' component. Infants may have underlying renal tract abnormalities. For the majority of patients treatment is conservative. Attention to electrolyte abnormalities can maximise the opportunities to achieve adequate nutrition. This will have a beneficial effect on post operative recovery. Active conservative management might avoid the need for dialysis. Renal replacement therapy, primarily peritoneal dialysis is possible and can provide the necessary bridge to renal transplantation in those infants with end stage renal failure. Hard end points regarding renal outcome are lacking but the majority of newborns are likely to have good levels of renal function.

References

1. Moghal NE, Brocklebamk JT, Meadow SR. A review of acute renal failure in children: incidence, etiology and outcome. Clin Nephrol. 1998;49(2):91–5.
2. Agras PI, Tarcan A, Baskin E, Cengiz N, Gurakan B, Saatci U. Acute renal failure in the neonatal period. Ren Fail. 2004;26(3):305–9.
3. Korallkar R, Ambalavanan N, Levitan EB, McGwin G, Goldstein S, Askenaz D. Acute kidney injury reduces survival in very low birth weight infants. Pediatr Res. 2011;69(4):354–8.
4. Solhaug MJ, Bolger PM, Jose P. The developing kidney and environmental toxins. Pediatrics. 2004;113:1084–91.
5. Aperia A, Broberger O, Thodenius K, Zetterström R. Development of renal control of salt and fluid homeostasis during the first year of life. Acta Pediatr Scand. 1975;64:393–8.
6. Cuzzolin L, Fanos V, Pinna B, di Mrzio M, Perin M, Tramontozzi P, Tonetto P, Cataldi L. Postnatal renal function in preterm newborns: a role of diseases, drugs and therapeutic interventions. Pediatr Nephrol. 2006;21:931–8.
7. Matos P, Duarte-Silva M, Drukker A, Guignard JP. Creatinine reabsorption by the newborn rabbit kidney. Pediatr Res. 1998;44:639–41.
8. Schwartz GJ, Feld LG, Langdorf DJ. A simple estimate of glomerular filtration rate in full-term infants during the first year of life. J Pediatr. 1984;104:849–54.
9. Brion LP, Fleishchman AR, McCarron C, Schwarz GJ. A simple estimate of glomerular filtration rate in low birth weight infants during the first year of life: non-invasive assessments of body composition and growth. J Pediatr. 1986;109:698–707.
10. Zelikovic I, Chesney RW. Development of renal amino-acid transport systems. Semin Nephrol. 1989;9:49–55.
11. Yaffe SI, Aranda JV, Kauffman RE, editors. Neonatal and pediatric pharmacology: therapeutic principles in practice (Chapter 3). 3rd ed. Philadelphia: Lippincott Williams and Wilkins; 2005. p. 20–31.
12. Sweet DH, Bush KT, Nigam SK. The organic anion transporter family: from physiology to ontogeny and the clinic. Am J Physiol. 2001;281:F197–205.
13. Chen N, Aleska K, Woodland C, Rieder M, Koren G. Ontogeny of drug elimination by the human kidney. Pediatr Nephrol. 2006;21:160–8.
14. Peruzza L, Gianoglio B, Porcellini MG, Coppo R. Neonatal end stage renal failure associated with maternal ingestion of cyclo-oxygenase-type-1 selective inhibitor nimesulphide as tocolytic. Lancet. 1999;354:1615.
15. Andreoli SP. Acute renal failure in the newborn. Semin Perinatol. 2004;28(2):112–23.
16. Walker MW, Clark RH, Spitzer AR. Elevation in plasma creatinine and renal failure in premature neonates without major anomalies: terminology, occurrence and factors associated with increased risk. J Perinatol. 2011;31(3):199–205.

17. Parikh CR, Devarajan P, Zappitelli M, Sint K, Thiessen-Philbrook H, Li S, Kim RW, Koyner JL, Coca SG, Edelstein CL, Shlipak MG, Garg AX, Krawczeski CD, TRIBE-AKI Consortium. Postoperative biomarkers predict acute kidney injury and poor outcomes after pediatric cardiac surgery. J Am Soc Nephrol. 2011;22(9):1737–47.
18. Moghal NE, Embleton ND. Management of acute renal failure in the newborn. Semin Fetal Neonatal Med. 2006;11(3):207–13.
19. Ahn SY, Mendoza S, Kaplan G, Reznik V. Chronic kidney disease in the VACTERL Association: clinical course and outcome. Pediatr Nephrol. 2009;24(5):1047–53.
20. Akcan-Arikan A, Zappitelli M, Loftis LL, Washburn KK, Jefferson LS, Goldstein SL. Modified rIFLE criteria in critically ill children with acute kidney injury. Kidney Int. 2007;71:1028–35.
21. Bellorno R, Ronco C, Kellum JA, Mehta RL, Palevsky P. Acute renal failure-definition, outcome measures, animal models, fluid therapy and information technology needs: the Second International Consensus Conference of the Acute Dialysis Quality Initiative (ADQI) group. Crit Care. 2004;8:R204–12.
22. Ashkenazi DJ, Ambalavanan N, Goldstein SL. Acute kidney injury in critically ill newborns: what do we know? What do we need to learn? Pediatr Nephrol. 2009;24:265–74.
23. Nobilis A, Kocsis I, Tóth-Heyn P, Treszl A, Schuler A, Tulassay T, Vásárhelyi B. Variance of ACE and AT1 receptor gene does not influence the risk of neonatal acute renal failure. Pediatr Nephrol. 2001;16(12):1063–6.
24. Treszl A, Tóth-Heyn P, Kocsis I, Nobilis A, Schuler A, Tulassay T, Vásárhelyi B. Interleukin genetic variants and the risk of renal failure in infants with infection. Pediatr Nephrol. 2002;17(9):713–7.
25. Guay-Woodford LM, Desmond RA. Autosomal recessive polycystic kidney disease: the clinical experience in North America. Pediatrics. 2003;111:1072–80.
26. Gouyon JB, Guignard JP. Management of acute renal failure in newborns. Pediatr Nephrol. 2000;14(10–11):1037–44.
27. Fukuda Y, Kojima T, Ono A, Matsuzaki S, Iwase S, Kobayashi Y. Factors causing hyperkalemia in premature infants. Am J Perinatol. 1989;6(1):76–9.
28. Masilamani K, van der Voort J. The management of acute hyperkalaemia in neonates and children. Arch Dis Child. 2012;97:376–80.
29. Gerstman BB, Kirkman R, Platt R. Intestinal necrosis associated with postoperative orally administered sodium polystyrene sulfonate in sorbitol. Am J Kidney Dis. 1992;20:159–61.
30. Fujinaga S, Ohtomo Y, Someya T, Shimizu T, Yamashiro Y. Transient pseudohypoaldosteronism complicating acute renal failure in an infant with vesico-ureteral reflux and pyelonephritis. Pediatr Int. 2009;51(5):744–6.
31. Bülchmann G, Schuster T, Heger A, Kuhnle U, Joppich I, Schmidt H. Transient pseudohypoaldosteronism secondary to posterior urethral valves—a case report and review of the literature. Eur J Pediatr Surg. 2001;11(4):277–9.
32. Marra G, Goj V, Appiani AC, Dell Agnola CA, Tirelli SA, Tadini B, Nicolini U, Cavanna G, Assael BM. Persistent tubular resistance to aldosterone in infants with congenital hydronephrosis corrected neonatally. J Pediatr. 1987;110(6):868–72.
33. Dissaneewate S, Vachvanichsanong P. Severe hyperphosphatemia in a newborn with renal insufficiency because of an erroneous medical prescription. J Ren Nutr. 2009;19(6):500–2.
34. British National Formulary for Children. www.bnfc.org.uk.
35. Rao SC, Srinivasjois R, Hagan R, Ahmed M. One dose per day compared to multiple doses per day of gentamicin for treatment of suspected or proven sepsis in neonates. Cochrane Database Syst Rev. 2011;(11):CD005091.
36. Jenik AG, Ceriani Cernadas JM, Gorenstein A, Ramirez JA, Vain N, Armadans M, Ferraris JR. A randomized, double-blind, placebo-controlled trial of the effects of prophylactic theophylline on renal function in term neonates with perinatal asphyxia. Pediatrics. 2000;105(4):E45.
37. Bakr AF. Prophylactic theophylline to prevent renal dysfunction in newborns exposed to perinatal asphyxia—a study in a developing country. Pediatr Nephrol. 2005;20(9):1249–52.
38. Bhat MA, Shah ZA, Makhdoomi MS, Mufti MH. Theophylline for renal function in term neonates with perinatal asphyxia: a randomized, placebo-controlled trial. J Pediatr. 2006;149(2):180–4.
39. Zubrow AB, Hulman S, Kushner H, Falkner B. Determinants of blood pressure in infants admitted to neonatal intensive care units: a prospective multicentre study. J Perinatal. 1995;15:470–9.
40. National High Blood Pressure Education Program Working Group on High Blood Pressure in Children and Adolescents. The fourth report on the diagnosis, evaluation, and treatment of high blood pressure in children and adolescents. Pediatrics. 2004;114(2 Suppl 4th Report):555–76.
41. Neal WA, Reynolds JW, Jrvis CW, Williams HJ. Umbilical artery catheterisation: demonstration of arterial thrombosis by aortography. Pediatrics. 1972;50:506–13.
42. Canpolat FE, Vurdakok M, Vigit S, Tekinalp G. Can peritoneal dialysis be used in preterm infants with gastrointestinal perforation? Pediatr Int. 2010;52(5):834–5.
43. Cribbs RK, Greenbaum LA, Heiss KF. Risk factors for early peritoneal dialysis catheter failure in children. J Pediatr Surg. 2010;45(3):585–9.
44. Golej J, Kitzmueller E, Hermon M, Boigner H, Burda G, Trittenwein G. Low-volume peritoneal dialysis in

116 neonatal and paediatric critical care patients. Eur J Pediatr. 2002;161(7):385–9.
45. Yu JE, Park MS, Pai KS. Acute peritoneal dialysis in very low birth weight neonates using a vascular catheter. Pediatr Nephrol. 2010;25(2):367–71.
46. Kostic D, Rodrigues AB, Leal A, Metran C, Nagaiassu M, Watanabe A, Ceccon ME, Tannuri U, Koch VH. Flow-through peritoneal dialysis in neonatal enema-induced hyperphosphatemia. Pediatr Nephrol. 2010;25(10):2183–6.
47. Goldstein SL. Overview of pediatric renal replacement therapy in acute kidney injury. Semin Dial. 2009;22(2):180–4.
48. Everdell NL, Coulthard MG, Crosier J, Keir MJ. A machine for haemodialysing very small infants. Pediatr Nephrol. 2005;20(5):636–43.
49. Symons JM, Brophy PD, Gregory MJ, McAfee N, Somers MJ, Bunchman TE, Goldstein SL. Continuous renal replacement therapy in children up to 10 kg. Am J Kidney Dis. 2003;41(5):984–9.
50. Hsu CW, Symons JM. Acute kidney injury: can we improve prognosis? Pediatr Nephrol. 2010;25(12):2401–12.
51. Brenner BM, Lawler EV, Mackenzie HS. The hyperfiltration theory: a paradigm shift in nephrology. Kidney Int. 1996;49(6):1774–7.
52. Carey WA, Talley LI, Sehring SA, Jaskula JM, Mathias RS. Outcomes of dialysis initiated during the neonatal period for treatment of end-stage renal disease: a north American Pediatric renal trials and collaborative studies special analysis. Pediatrics. 2007;119(2):e468–73.
53. Rheault MN, Rajpal J, Chavers B, Nevins TE. Outcomes of infants <28 days old treated with peritoneal dialysis for end-stage renal disease. Pediatr Nephrol. 2009;24(10):2035–9.

Newborn Urinary Tract Infections 63

Colin Jones and Joshua Kausman

Abstract

Urinary tract infection (UTI) is among the most common bacterial infections affecting newborns. Urinary tract infection can cause septicaemia or chronic ill health with failure to thrive and is often an indication of an underlying urinary tract malformation.

Keywords

Urinary tract infection • Newborns • Management • Outcomes

63.1 Introduction

Urinary tract infection (UTI) is among the most common bacterial infections affecting newborns. Urinary tract infection can cause septicaemia or chronic ill health with failure to thrive and is often an indication of an underlying urinary tract malformation.

C. Jones, MBBS, FRACP, PhD
Department of Nephrology, Royal Children's Hospital, Melbourne, VIC, Australia

J. Kausman, MBBS, FRACP, PhD (✉)
Department of Nephrology, Royal Children's Hospital, Melbourne, VIC, Australia

University of Melbourne, Parkville, VIC 3010, Australia

Department of Nephrology, Murdoch Childrens Research Institute, Parkville, VIC 3010, Australia
e-mail: joshua.kausman@rch.org.au

63.2 Epidemiology and Risk Factors

Neonatal epidemiologic studies have shown that the prevalence of UTI in term infants varies between 0.1 and 1% with a male to female ratio of between 2 and 6 to 1 [1]. Premature infants have a prevalence of 4–25%. The prevalence of UTI in febrile infants under the age of 3 months presenting to emergency departments is up to 20–30% and boys outnumber girls [2–5]. After the age of 3 months the prevalence of UTI in febrile children falls to around 8% in females and 2% in male children [2]. UTI are uncommon in the first 72 h of life [5].

Certain risk factors affect the prevalence of neonatal UTI. Breast feeding has a protective role in this group [4]. Hospital-acquired urinary infections are more common in infants having other infectious diseases (meningitis, omphalitis, pneumonia and generalised sepsis), treatment with broad spectrum antibiotics, mechanical ventilation, parenteral nutrition and those treated using intravascular and

P.D. Losty et al. (eds.), *Rickham's Neonatal Surgery*, https://doi.org/10.1007/978-1-4471-4721-3_63

urinary catheters [1, 4, 5]. The occurrence of more than one of these risk factors increased the risk of UTI 11 times [5]. One study found maternal bacteriuria at the time of vaginal delivery resulted in colonization of the foreskin and female perineum in neonates and 24% developed bacteriuria with clinical pyelonephritis in 3% [6].

The presence of underlying urinary tract malformations is more common in neonates with urinary infection and more so in nosocomial acquired infection than in community-acquired urinary infection with vesico-ureteric reflux being found in almost 50% of the former and 25% of the latter [1].

63.2.1 Antenatal Abnormalities

The advent of almost routine antenatal scanning at 18 weeks' gestation has led to the detection of approximately 1 in 200 infants having an increased anterior-posterior renal pelvis diameter (APD, >5 mm at any gestation). Postnatal follow-up studies have not shown an increased frequency of UTI in infants with mild to moderate degrees of APD (up to 15 mm) where the hydronephrosis was isolated (i.e. no ureteric, renal cortical or bladder abnormality) even where the infants were not treated with antibiotics [7]. In more severe cases antibiotics have usually been given in a prophylactic manner and UTI have mainly been detected outside the early infancy period [8, 9].

63.2.2 Circumcision

Wiswell et al. [10] found the incidence of UTI in circumcised male infants was 0.11% compared to 1.12% in uncircumcised infants, but the protective effect seems to fall off after infancy. The risk of circumcision is haemorrhage, injury to the glans penis and local infection. The complication rate can be as high as 4% although complications are less common in experienced hands (0.2%) [11]. Thus, 1000 circumcisions may prevent 91 UTI but be associated with 2–40 complications.

The effect of circumcision is presumably related to decreasing the density of bacterial growth and faecal contamination of the urethral meatus. The reduction in UTI with circumcision is one of the stronger pieces of evidence for an ascending route of infection, rather than haematogenous spread, although the latter is said to be more common in the neonatal period than at older ages.

63.3 Diagnosis

63.3.1 Clinical

Non-specific symptoms are the rule in the presentation of a neonate with urinary infection. While fever, vomiting and failure to thrive cover the symptoms the majority of neonates have no specific diagnostic symptoms and irritability, temperature instability, respiratory distress with apnoea or failure to clear secretions are commonly found. While the blood pressure is usually normal, hypotension with tachycardia is common. The newborn may be jaundiced or there may have been an increase in the serum bilirubin, and the hyperbilirubinaemia may be conjugated, unconjugated or mixed. Hepatosplenomegaly may be found. Infection may be asymptomatic. The frequency of symptoms of urinary tract infection in a series of 301 neonates is listed in Table 63.1 [1]. The presentation varies so much because the developmental status of the neonate does not allow specific localizing features that are present at later ages and reflects the systemic response to infection at this age. This results in the majority of urine infections being diagnosed on the basis of a "septic work-up" rather than specifically targeting urine infection as the cause of the neonate's symptoms.

Table 63.1 Frequency of symptoms (%) in neonates with urinary tract infections [1]

Symptom	Community acquired	Nosocomial
Fever	67.6	39.2
Poor feeding	27	13.7
Vomiting	22.4	21.5
Failure to thrive	15.6	11.7
Jaundice	13.7	13.7
Diarrhoea	2	0

The occurrence of meningitis with urinary tract infection is common and examination and culture of the CSF should be made before starting treatment for UTI in this age group. Similarly, a blood culture should be performed. Leucocytosis on blood film examination and a raised CRP are usually found, but the absence of these abnormalities does not disprove the diagnosis.

63.3.2 Rapid Diagnostic Techniques

Microscopy for bacteria with Gram stain has the highest accuracy for rapid detection of urinary tract infection (sensitivity 91% and specificity 96%) but requires laboratory facilities. Phase contrast microscopy is simple and more reliable than standard microscopy [12]. It is a useful adjunct to urine culture and can help discriminate false positive cultures from clean catch urines. The finding of epithelial squamous cells indicates a poorly collected sample and the absence of leukocyturia in a sample with mixed growth or low colony count on culture may indicate a contaminated sample.

Urinalysis for leukocyte esterase is positive in 19–90% of neonates with urine infection, and urinary nitrite, while more specific for urine infection is only present in 10–60% of urine infections [13]. Thus, even achieving the highest success rates for rapid diagnosis and taking the prevalence rates for urine infection into account, a positive test for both nitrites and leukocyte esterase in a child under 3 months of age predicts 90% of urine infections. This is not good enough for clinical purposes as the diagnosis of urine infection would be missed in a significant number of ill infants.

63.3.3 Urine Culture

The diagnosis is dependent upon urinary culture. The two methods for urine culture that are reliable and accurate are catheter sampling and suprapubic aspiration (see Table 63.2) [14–16].

Table 63.2 Comparison of methods of urine collection

Urine collection method	Advantages	Disadvantages
Paediatric bag	Widespread use in primary care paediatrics because considered convenient Collection of urine from infant or toddler at low risk for UTI (not febrile and no known urological abnormality) Only results of <10^8 cfu/L[a] are useful in excluding UTI	Contamination with skin flora common Should not be used where immediate antibiotic treatment is required
Clean catch	Non-invasive Method of choice in infants and toddlers where risk of UTI thought to be low Good correlation with SPA/MSU/CSU (can be collected within 1 h) A result of >10^8 cfu/L[a] indicates infection Squamous epithelial cells indicate contamination	Perceived to be difficult to collect (majority of samples collected in 40 min)
Catheter sample	Usually results in collection of sample of urine Invasive—poor acceptance by parents and second choice to SPA in infants and toddlers Reasonable for diagnosis especially if 1st drops of urine are discarded Difficult with phimosis >10^3 cfu/L taken to indicate infection	Difficult in neonates with some anatomical abnormalities (e.g. posterior urethral valve)
Suprapubic aspirate	Gold standard as avoids contamination Less invasive than CSU Method of choice in neonates with high risk of UTI Any growth significant	'Dry tap' relatively common (confirmation of a full bladder on ultrasound can reduce this)

[a]Quantitative analysis of urine was introduced by Kass [14] recognizing that most UTI's had colony counts 100–1000 times 10^8/1. Significant numbers of asymptomatic premature and term neonates and infants have counts greater than this number in bag or clean catch samples (proven by negative SPA cultures [15, 16]). Conversely there is a time in the development of UTI when the count will be lower

63.3.4 Microbiology

The aetiological agent varies markedly between community- and hospital-acquired infection [1, 15, 17]. In neonates presenting with community-acquired UTI Escherichia coli accounts for 75–90% of pathogens isolated. Klebsiella is frequent (4–15%), and Enterococci and all gram negative enteric bacteria are represented. Infrequent causes are gram positives other than the enterococcus and Candida. Causes of nosocomial UTI comprise a lesser percentage of E. coli, and a greater percentage of Klebsiella, Enterobacter, Enterococci and Candida. Pseudomonas and Proteus species are more frequently isolated in infants with complicated anatomical malformations and in those neonates who have had surgical procedures, especially where foreign materials (e.g. urinary stents) have been left *in situ*. Approximately 5% of children have two organisms isolated. Viral causes of infection have been thought to be rare in neonates who are not immunosuppressed.

Some factors make E. coli that cause UTI more virulent. Certain polysaccharide antigens (K1, K2, K12 and K13) are found more often in neonates with upper tract infection and fimbriated E. coli that attach to glycolipids of the P blood group are more common causes of pyelonephritis in neonates who do not have vesicoureteric reflux. These restricted serotypes adhere to the urothelium avidly, resist serum bactericidal activity and cause increased inflammatory activity (for instance, increased CRP) [18, 19].

63.4 Treatment

63.4.1 Initial Treatment

The newborn with urinary infection will often present as a septic infant with signs such as hypotension, tachycardia and decreased conscious state, and there is frequently vomiting. These neonates may require resuscitation with IV boluses of normal saline and the use of ionotropic agents and intensive care monitoring may be necessary. Even in the well neonate intravenous therapy is always advised to ensure effective absorption of antibiotic.

The electrolytes and creatinine are usually normal. A common finding where obstruction of the urinary tract is an issue, and sometimes without findings of obstruction, is hyponatraemia, hyperkalaemia and normal anion gap metabolic acidosis. This finding can be attributed to failure of collecting duct function with salt wasting and non-responsiveness to aldosterone—a form of hyperkalaemic Type 4 renal tubular acidosis. It usually responds to rehydration and antibiotic treatment rapidly. Where severe hyponatraemia (serum sodium less than 120 mmol/L) is found with a long history (over a week) of symptoms care must be taken to raise the serum sodium slowly (less than 0.5 mmol/L/h) to avoid neurological injury such as central pontine myelinolysis and demyelination of the extrapontine myelin-bearing neurons [7].

Once the urine, blood and CSF cultures and have been obtained a decision on acute antibiotic treatment must be made. The intravenous antibiotics used acutely are listed in Table 63.3. The usual choice is a penicillin (to cover the enterococcus) and an aminoglycoside. The aminoglycoside should be given slowly, over an hour, and blood levels and creatinine monitored. If there is renal impairment cefotaxime may be substituted for the aminoglycoside. Institutional sensitivities of organisms isolated may differ and the regime may need to be modified. The urine culture should be sterile after 48 h treatment. Non response to treatment should lead to reculture of the urine and renal ultrasonography searching for infection with obstruction of urinary drainage or abscess formation, both of which may require surgical drainage and prolonged antibiotic use. Intravenous antibiotics are used for 7–10 days in the usual instance.

63.4.2 Prophylactic Antibiotics

After acute treatment the infant may be placed on prophylactic antibiotics given once each night.

Table 63.3 Antibiotic treatment of urinary tract infection

Acute treatment			
Intravenous benzylpenicillin	30–50 mg/kg/12 h in 1st week of life; 6 hourly after 1st week of life		
And			
Intravenous gentamicin	Wt <1200 g 5 mg/kg given 48 hourly 0–7 days, then 36 hourly 8–30 days, then 24 hourly >30 days of age Wt 1200–2500 g 5 mg/kg 36 hourly 0–7 days, then 24 hourly >7 days Term neonate after 1st week of life: 8 mg/kg day 1, 6 mg/kg day 2 and after Give IV over 1 h Monitoring: trough level <1 mg/1 taken on 3rd day and serum creatinine 3rd day Renal impairment: same dose but redose when trough level <1 ng/mL		
Prophylactic treatment			
1st month of life	Trimethoprim	3 mg/kg/day	
>1 month of age	Co-trimoxazole	0.25 mL/kg/night	40/200 mg/5 mL
	Nitrofurantoin	1–2 mg/kg/night	
	Cephalexin	5 mg/kg/night	

The antibiotics usually used for prophylaxis are listed in Table 63.3. These antibiotics are excreted in the urine, achieve high urinary concentrations and are well tolerated over long periods of time without inducing excessive microbiological changes in the gut (leading to the emergence of resistant organisms or candidiasis). They are usually given until the results of imaging tests are available, and may be used for prolonged periods with the aim of reducing the risk of further UTI. This has been an area of medical controversy but systematic review of higher quality studies has shown a significant reduction in the risk of repeat urine cultures by 50%.

63.5 Investigations

Investigations are aimed at excluding obstructive urinary tract lesions, determining whether there are significant underlying urinary tract malformations and assessing renal injury. The extent of investigation necessary after a first neonatal urinary tract infection has become an area of medical controversy, centred on the role of the cystourethrogram.

All centres perform a renal ultrasound. Most importantly the possibility of obstruction is detected. Secondly, the presence, site, size and shape of the kidneys can be determined. However small lesions can be missed: in the age group under 5 years, only 15% of abnormalities found on DMSA scan ('scars/dysplasia') will be seen on ultrasound examination. The ureters are not visualized unless enlarged. The finding of hydronephrosis or hydroureter leads to further nuclear medical imaging (discussed below) to diagnose obstructive lesions of the urinary tract.

A spinal ultrasound is useful in the first weeks of life for examination of the spinal cord and should be done with bladder abnormalities or if there is abnormality of the spine such as a deep sacral pit.

A spinal radiograph should be done if the sacrum cannot be palpated.

The radiological examination of the urethra and bladder, using a cystourethrogram, was performed in most centres as a routine on neonates until the last decade. However, this investigation is performed less frequently than in the past because the demonstration of vesicoureteric reflux (VUR) does not alter management at many centres. Thus, in the absence of abnormalities of the kidneys, ureters or bladder on ultrasound examination it is often not performed as a routine. This is discussed further below.

Nuclear medicine investigations with technetium-99 m-labelled radioisotopes are useful for a number of purposes.

The *DTPA* radionuclide is injected intravenously, is filtered by the glomerulus and then is neither secreted nor absorbed by the tubule of the kidney. Like creatinine or inulin, it can be used to obtain an accurate measure of the glomerular filtration rate.

The *Mag 3* scan has largely replaced the DTPA scan because, in addition to some glomerular filtration, the isotope is mainly secreted by the proximal tubular cells into the urine so that the signal to background ratio is higher than in the DTPA scan. This is particularly useful in infants in the first 3 months of life when the glomerular filtration rate is low. Both of these investigations are useful for diagnosing the presence of obstruction to urinary flow from the kidneys to the bladder, for determining the 'split' of kidney function (between the right and left kidneys), and for estimating overall renal function.

The *DMSA* radionuclide is filtered by the glomerulus and taken up by the proximal tubular cells. Scanning takes place when it has been taken up by these cells, which are in the renal cortex. Lack of uptake gives a defect on the scan and this can be due to either transient impairment of the tubular cell function (e.g. following acute inflammation with pyelonephritis for a period of up to 3–4 months) or absence of kidney tissue (renal 'scarring/dysplasia').

Delayed uptake of any of these three radionuclides may occur in conditions where perfusion to the kidney is abnormal (e.g. renal artery stenosis in a unilateral case or dehydration in a bilateral case).

The ongoing management depends on the results of investigations. A flow diagram of possibilities is shown in Fig. 63.1.

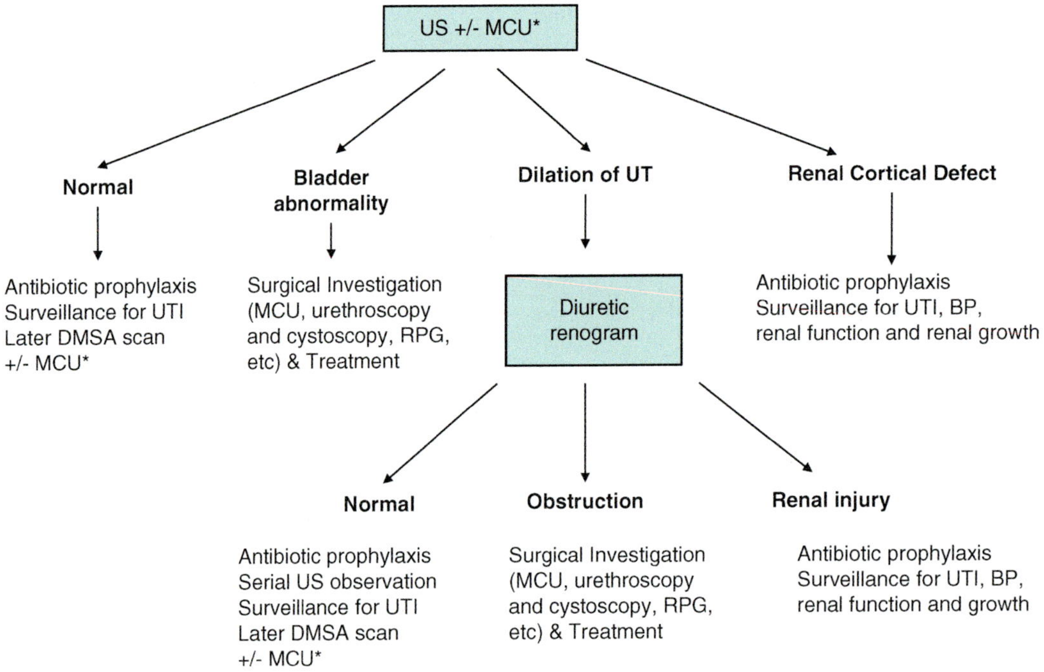

Fig. 63.1 A flow diagram of ongoing management following a proven urinary tract infection. A normal ultrasound does not exclude scarring. This age is chosen for convenience. Boys uncommonly get recurrent infections after 1 year; girls commonly have recurrent infection until about 3 years. Follow-up includes a yearly blood pressure check. The finding of a normal DMSA scan normalizes the risk of developing hypertension. *MCU* micturating cystourethrogram, *US* ultrasound, *VUR* vesicoureteric reflux, *BP* blood pressure, *RPG* retrograde pyelogram. Where indicated by asterisk (*) the results of the MCU do not influence the authors' treatment or investigation of UTI

63.6 Urinary Tract Infection and Normal Renal Ultrasound

If the neonate responds to antibiotics there is no need to perform another urine culture at the end of treatment. Prophylactic antibiotics may be continued for 6–12 months. Long-term follow-up is essential unless DMSA scan is normal. The authors' preferred practice is to follow the infant through childhood clinically and to do a DMSA scan around the age of 5 years. If the scan is normal the child is discharged, and if abnormal the child continues with follow-up for detection of hypertension or development of proteinuria.

63.7 The Diagnosis of Vesicoureteric Reflux

Vesicoureteric reflux (VUR) is a common disorder, affecting 40% of children under 1 year of age who are investigated for a first urinary tract infection. The diagnosis is made by cystourethrogram in neonates.

Vesicoureteric reflux is often a familial trait affecting up to between 30 and 50% of first-degree relatives of index cases. In some cases, it is associated with renal abnormality (variously referred to as renal scarring, dysplasia, reflux-associated nephropathy), excessive dilatation and tortuosity of the ureter, occurrence on the contralateral side and abnormalities of bladder function including premature detrusor contractions (causing urgency symptoms and wetting at older ages) and poor bladder emptying. Higher grades of VUR are associated with higher recurrence rates of UTI.

The treatment of VUR has been controversial. Controlled trials have shown no advantage of either anti-reflux surgery or antibiotic prophylaxis in preventing urinary infections, hypertension, renal injury or renal failure [20–23]. In fact, it is not clear whether these treatments, in turn, are better than episodic treatment of urine infection alone. Much of the renal injury leading to renal failure in a small number of patients with VUR is congenital and the significance of acquired injury is debated [24]. An increasing amount of embryological and genetic data have accumulated that relate congenital abnormalities of the kidney and urinary tract (CAKUT) to vesicoureteric reflux and renal dysplasia and conditions that resemble scarring on radiological or nuclear imaging [25]. Thus, the aim of treatment of VUR is as much or more about prevention of symptomatic UTI, as prevention of renal injury. Attention to reducing and treating precipitating factors for UTI, the use of antibiotic treatment in a prophylactic or episodic manner and the selective use of antireflux surgery for patients with intractable symptoms form the basis of treatment [26–28]. The authors' practice is to continue prophylactic antibiotic until the age of 6–12 months and then to reinstitute them if infections ensue on stopping the antibiotic. For troublesome cases in male infants circumcision can be useful as discussed earlier.

References

1. Sastre JB, Aparicio AR, Cotallo GD, Colomer BF, Hernandez MC. Grupo de Hospitales Castrillo 2007 Urinary tract infection in the newborn: clinical and radio imaging studies. Pediatr Nephrol. 22; 1735–41.
2. Craig JC, Irwig LM, Knight JF, Sureshkumar P, Roy P. Symptomatic urinary tract infections in preschool Australian children. J Paediatr Child Health. 1998;34:154–9.
3. Hanson S, Jodal U. Urinary tract infection. In: Barratt TM, Avner ED, Marmon WE, editors. Paediatric nephrology. Baltimore: Lippincott Williams & Wilkins; 1999. p. 835–50.
4. Levy I, Comarsca J, Davidovits M, et al. Urinary tract infection in preterm infants: the protective role of breast feeding. Pediatr Nephrol. 2009;24:527–31.
5. Falcao MC, Leone CR, D'Andrea RAP, Berardi R, Ono NA, Vaz FAC. Urinary tract infections in full-term newborn infants: risk factor analysis. Rev Hosp Clin Fac Med S Paulo. 2000;55:9–16.
6. Patrick MJ. Influence of maternal renal infection on the fetus and infant. Arch Dis Child. 1967;42:208–11.
7. Manz F, Kalhoff H, Remar T. Renal acid excretion in early infancy. Pediatr Nephrol. 1997;11:231–43.
8. Becker AM. Postnatal evaluation of infants with an abnormal antenatal renal sonogram. Curr Opin Pediatr. 2009;21:207–13.
9. Mallik M, Watson AR. Antenatally detected urinary tract abnormalities: more detection but less action. Pediatr Nephrol. 2008;23:897–900.
10. Wiswell TE, Smith FR, Bass JW. Decreased incidence of urinary tract infections in circumcised male infants. Pediatrics. 1985;75:901–3.

11. Craig J. Urinary tract infection. In: Isaacs D, Moxon ER, editors. A practical approach to pediatric infections. London: Churchill Livingstone; 1996. p. 235–7.
12. Vickers D, Ahmed T, Coulthard MG. Diagnosis of urinary tract infection in children: fresh urine microscopy or culture? Lancet. 1991;338:767–70.
13. Williams GJ, Macaskill P, Chan SF, Turner RM, Hodson E, Graig J. Absolute and relative accuracy of rapid urine tests for urinary tract infection in children: a meta-analysis. Lancet Infect Dis. 2010;10:240–50.
14. Kass EH. Asymptomatic infections of the urinary tract. Transactions of the Association of American Physicians. 1956;69:56–64.
15. Nelson JD, Peters PC. Suprapubic aspiration of urine in premature and term infants. Pediatrics. 1965;36:132–4.
16. Newman CG, O'Neill P, Parker A. Pyuria in infancy, and the role of suprapubic aspiration of urine in diagnosis of infection of urinary tract. Br Med J. 1967;2:277–9.
17. Klein JO, Long SS. Bacterial infections of the urinary tract. In: Remington JS, Klein JO, editors. Infections of the fetus and newborn infant. 3rd ed. Philidelphia: WB Saunders; 1995. p. 925–34.
18. de Man P. Bacterial attachment, inflammation and renal scarring in urinary tract infection. Weiner Medizinische Wochenschrift. 1991;141:537–40.
19. Connell I, Agace W, Klemm P, Schembri M, Marild S, Svanborg C. Type 1 fimbrial expression enhances Escherichia coli virulence for the urinaruy tract. Proc Nat Acad Sciences USA. 1996;93:9827–32.
20. Birmingham Reflux Study Group. Prospective trial of operative versus non-operative treatment of severe vesicoureteric reflux in children: five years observation. BMJ. 1987;295:237–41.
21. Olbing H, Caesson H, Ebel K, Seppanen U, Smellie J, Tamminem-Mobius T, Wikstad I. Renal scars and parenchymal thinning in children with vesico ureteral reflux: a 5-year report of the International Reflux Study in Children (European Branch). J Urol. 1992;148:1653–6.
22. Weiss R, Duckett J, Spitzer A. Results of a randomized clinical trial of medical versus surgical management of infants and children with grade III and IV primary vesicoureteral reflux (United States). J Urol. 1992;148:1667–73.
23. International Reflux Study Committee. Medical versus surgical treatment of primary vesico-uretereral reflux. Pediatrics. 1981;67:392–400.
24. Risdon RA, Yeung CK, Ransley P. reflux nephropathy in children submitted to unilateral nephrectomy: a clinicopathological study. Clin Nephrol. 1993;40:308–14.
25. Song R, Yosypiv IV. Genetics of congenital anomalies of the kidney and urinary tract. Pediatr Nephrol. 2011;26:353–64.
26. Mei C, Jia J, Lui Y, Dai B. Long term antibiotics for the prevention of recurrent urinary tract infection in children: a systematic review and meta-analysis. Arch Dis Child. 2010;95:499–508.
27. NICE. Urinary tract infection: diagnosis, treatment and long term management of urinary tract infection in children. London: National Institute for Health and Clinical Excellence; 2007. http://guidance.nice.org.uk/CG054
28. Wheeler D, Vimalochandra D, Hodson EM, Roy LP, Smith G, Craig JC. Antibiotics and surgery for vesicoureteric reflux: A meta-analysis of randomized controlled trials. Arch Dis Child. 2003;88:688–94.

Indications for Investigation of the Urinary Tract in the Newborn

64

Harriet J. Corbett and Helen Fiona McAndrew

Abstract

The urinary tract in the newborn may require investigation for a number of reasons. The urinary tract is the commonest system in which abnormalities are detected during antenatal ultrasonography (USS). The majority will have isolated hydronephrosis, with mild dilatation detected in as many as 1:100 pregnancies. Others will have more significant urological abnormalities thus investigation of the urinary tract is indicated to interpret the antenatal USS findings. Investigation is also indicated for those neonates presenting with urinary tract related symptoms. Equally, in neonates presenting with non-specific symptoms such as failure to thrive, poor feeding or prolonged jaundice, urinary tract pathology should be considered. Finally, there are neonates with congenital anomalies or syndromes with known associated uropathies who require further investigation. The range of such conditions or syndromes in which the urinary tract may be involved is extensive.

Keywords

Antenatal diagnosis • Urinary tract anomalies • Imaging • Management Outcomes

64.1 Introduction

The urinary tract in the newborn may require investigation for a number of reasons. The urinary tract is the commonest system in which abnormalities are detected during antenatal ultrasonography (USS). The majority will have isolated hydronephrosis, with mild dilatation detected in as many as 1:100 pregnancies [1, 2]. Others will have more significant urological abnormalities thus investigation of the urinary

H.J. Corbett, MD, FRCS(Paed) (✉)
H.F. McAndrew, MD, FRCS(Paed)
Regional Department of Paediatric Urology, Alder Hey Children's Hospital NHS Foundation Trust, Liverpool, UK
e-mail: harriet.corbett@alderhey.nhs.uk

P.D. Losty et al. (eds.), *Rickham's Neonatal Surgery*, https://doi.org/10.1007/978-1-4471-4721-3_64

tract is indicated to interpret the antenatal USS findings. Investigation is also indicated for those neonates presenting with urinary tract related symptoms. Equally, in neonates presenting with non-specific symptoms such as failure to thrive, poor feeding or prolonged jaundice, urinary tract pathology should be considered. Finally, there are neonates with congenital anomalies or syndromes with known associated uropathies who require further investigation. The range of such conditions or syndromes in which the urinary tract may be involved is extensive.

64.2 Antenatal Diagnosis

In most healthcare systems, modern day antenatal care includes a routine ultrasound scan (USS) seeking structural anomalies between 18 and 20 weeks of gestation [3]. The fetus is examined according to a routine protocol that includes measurement of the amniotic fluid volume. The renal tract examination should document the number and location of the kidneys and the presence and appearance of the bladder. The ureters would not normally be seen so visualisation of either ureter is notable. Other abnormal findings may include dilatation of the renal pelvis, caliectasis, absent or ectopic renal tissue, duplication anomalies, cysts, bladder abnormalities and oligohydramnios. Anomalies in other systems that may be of relevance to the urinary tract include spinal fusion defects such as myelomeningocele, or suspicion of the VACTERL complex.

The most frequently detected urological abnormality on antenatal USS is dilatation of the renal pelvis, which is also known as pelviectasis or hydronephrosis (antenatal hydronephrosis, ANH) [1, 2]. In many this finding will be transitory, but in the others ANH will be a marker of pathology in the urinary tract [1]. Not surprisingly, those with minor degrees of ANH will typically resolve whilst more severe ANH, especially when associated with calyceal dilatation, is more likely to persist postnatally [2]. Table 64.1, adapted from the recent Consensus Statement on the evaluation and management of antenatal hydronephrosis by the Society for Fetal Urology, outlines the aetiology of ANH and the most common causes [4]. Others diagnoses, such as prune belly syndrome, cystic kidney disease, congenital ureteric strictures and megalourethra are uncommon causes of ANH. The presence of abnormalities of renal echogenicity, cortico-medullary differentiation and parenchymal thickness should be noted since these make significant pathology more likely, as does the presence of oligohydramnios, chromosomal defects or multiple anomalies within other organ systems [4]. Overall, fetuses with an abnormality detected in the urinary tract on antenatal USS are predominantly male (male:female ratio of 2:1), particularly in fetuses subsequently found to have obstructive lesions [1].

Table 64.1 The aetiology of ANH

Aetiology	Incidence (%)
Transient hydronephrosis	41–88
Pelviureteric junction obstruction	10–30
Vesicoureteric reflux	10–20
Vesicoureteric junction obstruction/ megaureters	5–10
Ureterocele/ectopic ureter/duplex system	5–7
Multicystic dysplastic kidney	4–6
Posterior urethral valves/urethral atresia	1–2

Adapted from Nguyen HT, Herndon CD, Cooper C, Gatti J, Kirsch A, Kokorowski P, Lee R, Perez-Brayfield M, Metcalfe P, Yerkes E, Cendron M, Campbell JB. The Society for Fetal Urology consensus statement on the evaluation and management of antenatal hydronephrosis. J Pediatr Urol 2010:6:212–31; used with permission

The degree of dilatation of the renal pelvis may be assessed in a number of ways. The simplest grading system of mild, moderate or severe is quite subjective. The Society for Fetal Urology published a system based on *postnatal* appearance in 1993, for which reproducibility is only modest [5, 6]. A more objective, and frequently reported, technique records the transverse antero-posterior diameter (APD) of the renal pelvis at the level of the renal hilum (see Fig. 64.1) [7]. A number of factors influence the degree of ANH, including maternal hydration, the degree of fetal bladder distension and the gestational age at which the dilatation is detected [4]. An increasing degree of dilatation increases the significance, particularly at earlier gestation [7]. However, no single measurement separates normal from abnormal APD measurements. The consensus statement from the Society for Fetal Urology uses a simple grading of

ANH according to the APD and gives recommendations for subsequent prenatal evaluation (see Table 64.2) [4]. In more complex cases, such as those with unclear anatomy, antenatal Magnetic Resonance Imaging (MRI) may be considered (see Fig. 64.2). Severe cases should be discussed on a case-by-case basis, preferably within a multidisciplinary team. Fetal intervention, early delivery or even termination may be considered.

The antenatal scan findings guide the timing and degree of postnatal investigations, bearing in mind that in 30–50% hydronephrosis will persist postnatally and around 30% will be associated with a significant abnormality, particularly in those with more marked ANH [1, 4, 7]. The challenge is to determine which newborns have obstructing lesions and which have simple physiological dilatation. Postnatal USS undertaken at less than 24 h of age have a false negative rate, and this is thought to be due to neonatal dehydration [8]. Significant pathology may be missed in the first few days of life and, hence, very early ultrasound scans are not usually recommended for the majority of infants [8–10]. However, in newborns with bilateral dilation, unilateral dilatation in the presence of bladder abnormality or any uropathy associated with oligohydramnios or lung abnormality, the postnatal ultrasound should be done at 24–72 h of age. If the scan is normal it should be repeated after 3–7 days, and if the scan is still normal, a repeat scan at 4–6 weeks is recommended. In male infants, posterior urethral valves must be considered. A micturating cystourethrogram is usually required in such neonates, after a period of bladder decompression and once the renal function has stabilised.

For all other newborns, the initial postnatal USS should be done at 3–14 days. Again, if this scan is normal it should be repeated at 4–6 weeks of age. In those with an abnormal postnatal USS, further imaging will be indicated according to the antenatal and postnatal findings. The schedule

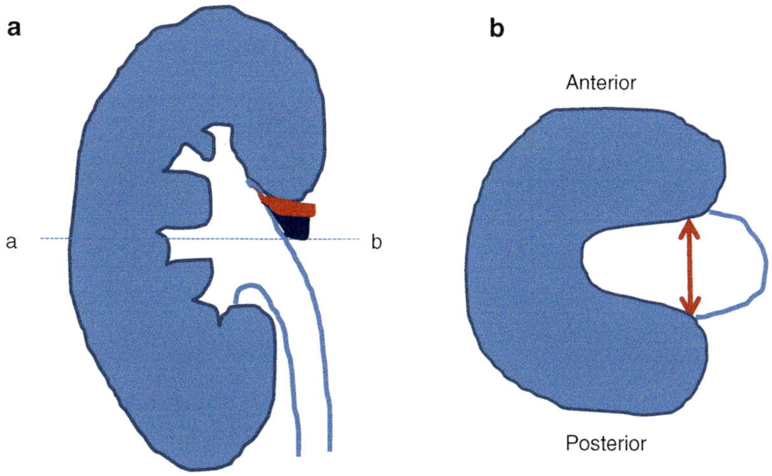

Fig. 64.1 (**a**) Longitudinal view of the kidney. The transverse measurement of the pelvis should be taken at the level of the renal hilum (a, b). (**b**) Transverse antero-posterior view of the kidney and pelvis showing where the APD should be measured (*arrow*)

Table 64.2 Recommendations for the ongoing prenatal evaluation of ANH

Time of detection of ANH	Severity of ANH	APD (mm)	Recommendations
2nd Trimester	Mild	<7	Consider 3rd trimester US
	Moderate	7–10	3rd Trimester US
	Severe	>10	Repeat US in 3–4 weeks
3rd Trimester	Mild	<9	Postnatal evaluation
	Moderate	9–15	Postnatal evaluation
	Severe	>15	Repeat US in 2–3 weeks

From Nguyen HT, Herndon CD, Cooper C, Gatti J, Kirsch A, Kokorowski P, Lee R, Perez-Brayfield M, Metcalfe P, Yerkes E, Cendron M, Campbell JB. The Society for Fetal Urology consensus statement on the evaluation and management of antenatal hydronephrosis. J Pediatr Urol 2010:6:212–31; used with permission

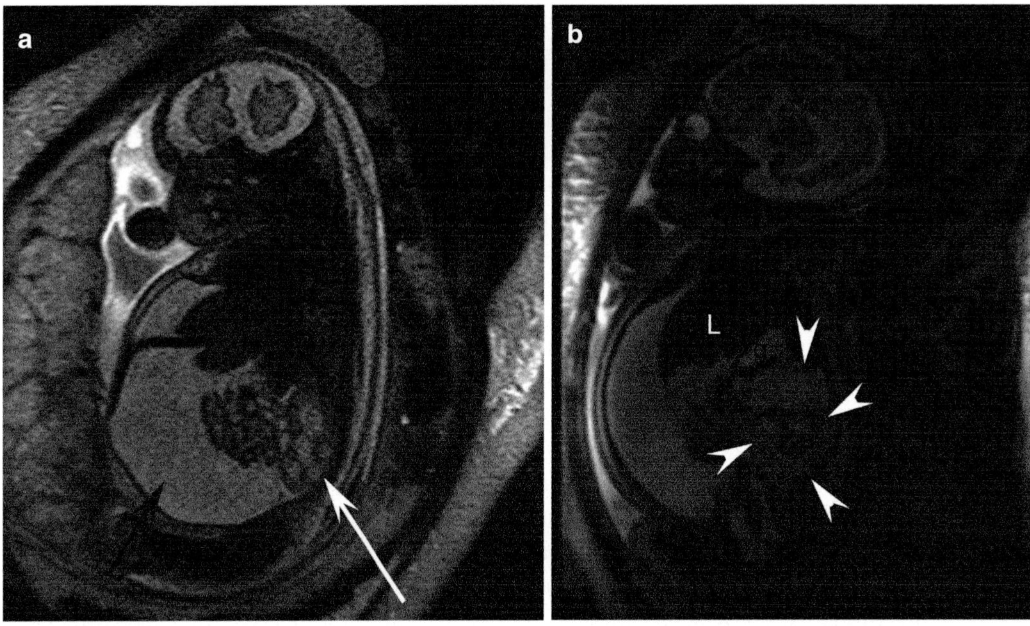

Fig. 64.2 Antenatal uropathy: (**a**, **b**) Sagittal heavily T2-weighted imaging of the fetal abdomen of a hydropic fetus showing a ascites (*black arrow*) and a hydronephrotic kidney (*white arrow*) with b contralateral multicystic dysplastic kidney (*arrowheads*), a loculated urinoma could give rise to similar appearances. Liver (*L*), gallbladder (*g*). Images courtesy of Dr. Gurdeep S. Mann, MRCP FRCR, Alder Hey Children's Hospital, Liverpool.

adopted by the Departments of Urology and Radiology at Alder Hey and the Fetal Medicine Unit and Department of Neonatolgy at Liverpool Women's Hospital is outlined in Fig. 64.3 (adapted from HK Dhillon [11, 12]).

Antibiotic prophylaxis should be given to infants considered to be at increased risk of urinary tract infection due to urinary stasis or vesicoureteric reflux. However, whilst a number of studies have documented the increased risk of UTI in neonates with ANH [13–15], no randomised controlled trials have proven the efficacy of antibiotic prophylaxis [4]; further, UTI are known to occur even with antibiotic prophylaxis. Despite this, most clinicians still deem it appropriate to give prophylactic antibiotics [4, 13–15].

64.3 Postnatal Presentation

Neonates may present with symptoms and/or signs indicative of urinary tract pathology, including an abdominal mass or distension, poor urinary stream, oliguria, or an abnormal appearance of the genitalia, perineum, umbilical cord or abdominal wall. Others will present with non-specific symptoms such as vomiting or sepsis due to urinary tract infection, and some will present with abnormal renal function (see Table 64.3 and Fig. 64.4) [16–19]. In addition, urinary tract pathology should be considered in neonates with failure to thrive, poor feeding or prolonged jaundice, as well as in those newborns presenting with respiratory compromise caused by pulmonary hypoplasia secondary to oligohydramnios [19].

Suspected urinary tract infection in neonates warrants prompt urine microscopy and culture; diagnosis should not be based on dipstick testing in this age group [16, 19]. A standard urine specimen is a 'clean catch' voided sample but this can be difficult to obtain, particularly in girls. Urine collection bags are commonly used but often yield indeterminate culture results so if a clean catch sample is unobtainable, urine should be sampled directly from the bladder by catheter or suprapubic aspiration [19, 20]. Pyuria of more than 5 white blood cells per high-power field or the presence of bacteria on microscopy is highly

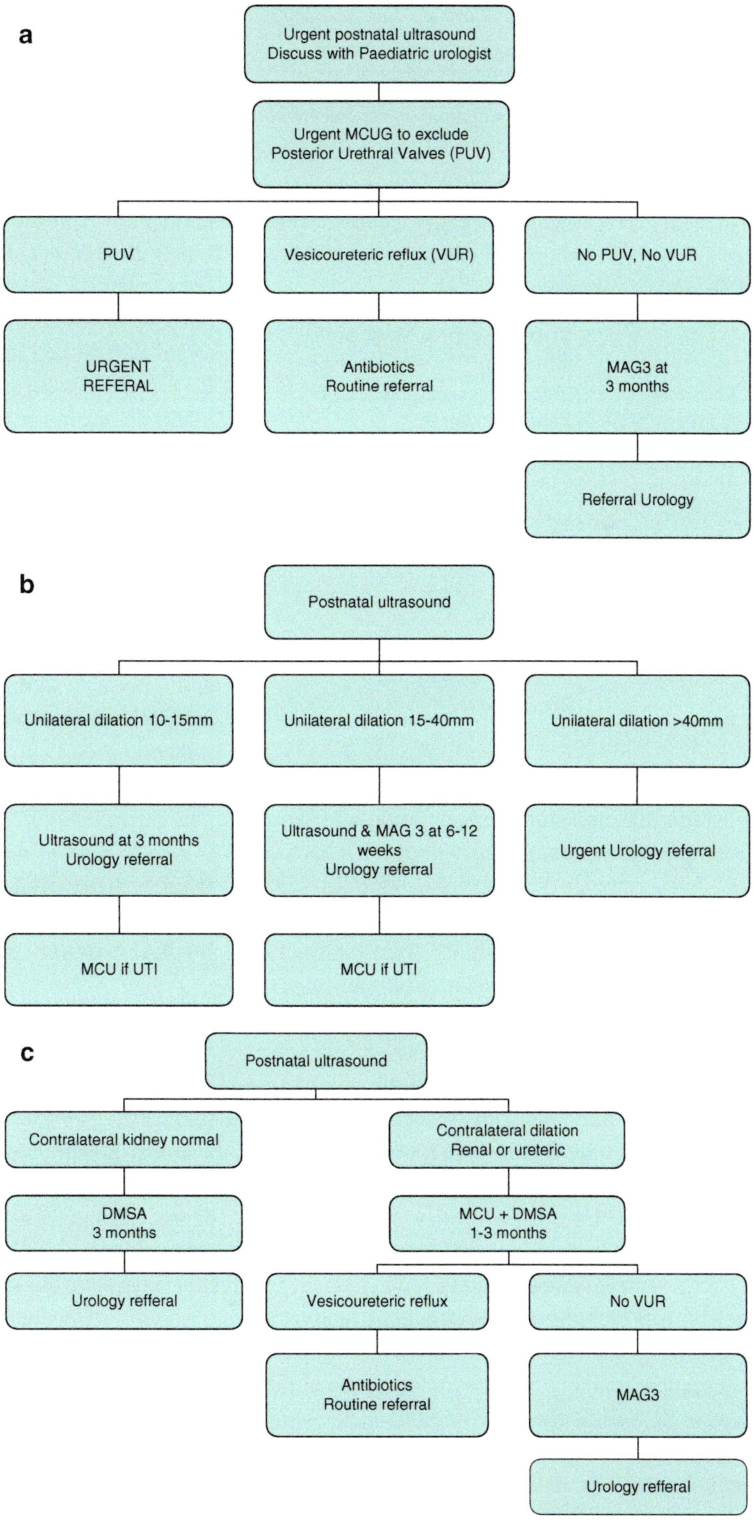

Fig. 64.3 *Protocol 1* (**a**): For (1) neonates with renal dilation with oligohydramnios or lung abnormality, (2) bilateral renal dilation or (3) unilateral renal dilation with ureteric dilation or bladder abnormality or abnormal contralateral kidney. *Protocol 2* (**b**): Isolated Unilateral renal dilation confirmed postnatally (if only has one kidney or bladder or ureteric abnormality, pre or postnatally see protocol 1). *Protocol 3* (**c**). Unilateral cystic kidney confirmed postnatally

Table 64.3 Postnatal signs of urinary tract pathology

Presenting feature	Diagnosis
Poor urinary stream	Bladder outlet obstruction e.g. posterior urethral valves, urethral abnormalities
Abdominal mass or distension	Hydronephrosis Enlarged bladder Vagina (hydrocolpos) e.g. urogenital sinus, persistent cloaca Neuroblastoma Urinary ascites Renal tumour e.g.Mesoblastic nephroma
Abnormal abdominal wall	Prune belly syndrome / eagle-Barrett syndrome Bladder or cloacal exstrophy
Abnormal umbilical cord	Urachal or allantoic anomalies
Abnormal perineum	Disorders of sexual development Urogenital sinus Persistent cloaca Ureterocele Spinal dysraphism
Haematuria	Urinary tract infection Renal vein thrombosis

suggestive of a UTI [20]. A pure growth of >10^5 bacteria/mL on culture in association with pyuria is diagnostic although a growth of >10^4 bacteria/mL from catheter or suprapubic samples is also highly suggestive of UTI. It is worth mentioning that in neonates with urinary tract obstruction above the bladder, the urine from the may be clean if the infection is contained within the obstructed part of the system. As such, a specimen may only be obtained when the obstruction is relieved. A high index of suspicion is therefore required and urgent USS is recommended.

Around 14% of infants with a urinary tract infection will have a previously undetected urinary tract anomaly, hence all such infants should undergo timely investigations [18]. Indeed, any newborn presenting with suspected urinary tract pathology must have an USS in the first instance; subsequent imaging will be guided by the clinical course as well as the USS findings [19]. A thorough history and examination is also mandatory, seeking clues to underlying pathology such as a poor urine stream, a family history of vesicoureteric reflux (VUR) or renal disease, constipation, an abdominal mass, poor growth, high blood pressure or an abnormal spine (see Table 64.3) [19].

Newborns with spinal dysraphism or congenital anomalies including anorectal malformations and the VACTERL association all require urinary tract screening with USS in the newborn period as associated anomalies are common [20–23]. Spinal dysraphism encompasses a wide spectrum of anomalies from the clinically obvious myelomeningocele through sacral agenesis to occult spinal cord tethering or syringomyelia. Cutaneous stigmata of spinal dysraphism include a hairy patch, sacral lipoma and an abnormal gluteal cleft [21]. USS can be used as a screening tool for abnormalites of the lower spinal cord in neonates but any abnormality suggestive of dysraphism warrants Mangetic Resonance Imaging (MRI) of the spine to delineate the anatomy in detail [24]. Such babies may have a neuropathic bladder so bladder emptying should be assessed in the newborn period. This is readily achieved by placing an alarmed pad in the nappy; the alarm is triggered when the baby voids and a portable ultrasound is used to ascertain the bladder's residual volume. Alternatively an intermittent catheter may be passed, any residual urine drained and the volume measured.

64.4 Imaging Modalities

64.4.1 Ultrasound Scan

Ultrasonography is the first choice of investigation as the scans are relatively easy to perform and involve no radiation, and as such can be repeated frequently (see Fig. 64.5) [4]. USS can show the anatomy in detail, although the scan findings will be dependent upon the degree of hydration, the degree of bladder filling and the experience of the sonographer. Doppler studies will give information regarding blood flow, particularly important in infants suspected to have pyelonephritis or at risk of renal vein thrombosis. And whilst USS are typically static scans, dynamic information can be captured if, for example, reflux is seen to occur during the Doppler scan. Portable scan machines can be taken to the cot or bed-side which is particularly useful in very sick infants or children. USS is operator dependant and therefore should be repeated whenever there is diagnostic doubt or unexpected clinical course.

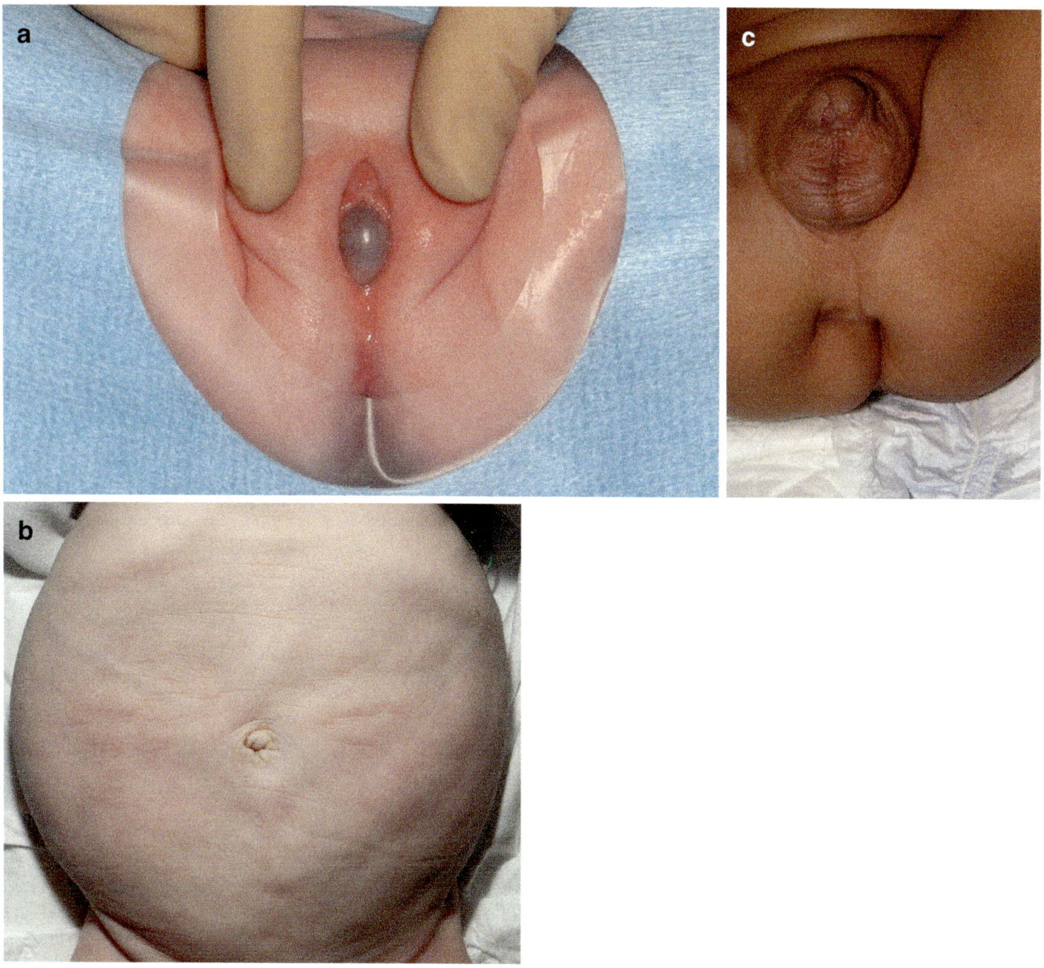

Fig. 64.4 Clinical examination findings that should prompt investigation of the urinary tract: (**a**) Caeco-ureterocele protruding through the urethra. (**b**) Prune belly syndrome. (**c**) Asymmetrical perineum in spinal dysraphism

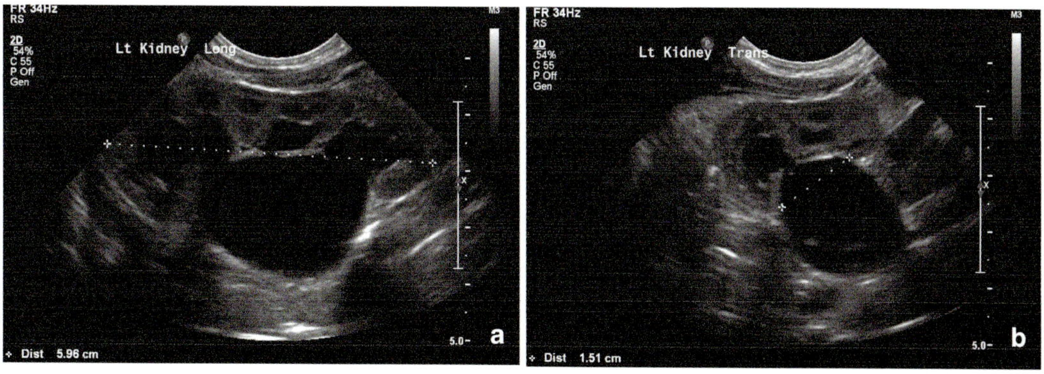

Fig. 64.5 Ultrasound scan in a neonate with significant hydronephrosis (**a**) longitudinal view (**b**) transverse view—the APD is 15 mm

64.4.2 Micturating or Voiding Cystourethrogram

The micturating (or voiding) cystourethrogram (MCUG or VCUG) is uncommonly required in the neonatal period. There is a risk of introducing infection during the study, so antibiotic cover should be considered particularly in neonates in whom intravenous administration is recommended. A MCUG is indicated for delineation of the anatomy of the lower urinary tract and diagnosis of bladder outflow obstruction and vesicoureteric reflux (VUR) (see Fig. 64.6). The study involves catheterisation, which will usually be per urethra but the study may be performed via a suprapubic catheter if clinical circumstances have required one. Water soluble contrast is slowly instilled via the catheter, with intermittent fluoroscopic screening to guide the dynamics of the study. The study should capture both filling and voiding phases; complete views of the male urethra are essential to look for posterior urethral valves.

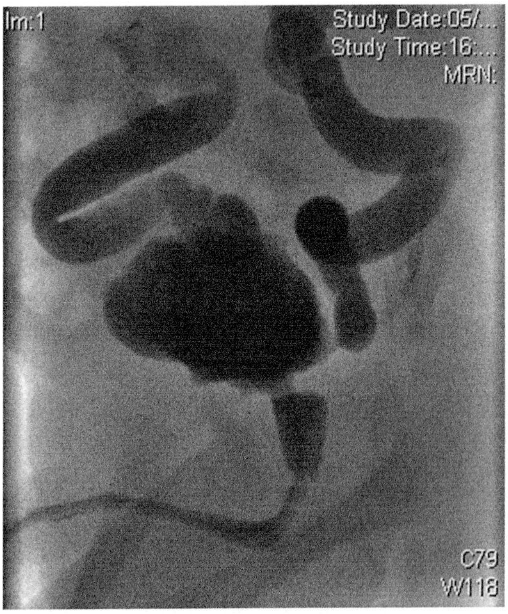

Fig. 64.6 Micturating cystourethrogram showing unilateral vesico-ureteric reflux and an enlarged posterior urethra secondary to Posterior Urethral Valves

64.4.3 Nuclear Medicine Imaging/ Isotope Scans

Renal isotope scans may be dynamic or static studies, using technetium-99 (Tc-99) bound to mercapto acetyl tri-glycerine (MAG3), dimercaptosuccinic acid (DMSA) or diethylenetriamine pentaacetic acid (DTPA). These studies are rarely utilised in the newborn period as the neonatal kidney is relatively immature. The European Society for Paediatric radiology recommends monitoring of the renal tract in the newborn with USS over 3 months prior to performing a renal isotope scan whilst in the USA, scans are rarely performed prior to 6 weeks of age [4]. Ideally all such scans should be performed in a standardised manner but many units will still use local protocols.

64.4.4 DMSA (Dimercaptosuccinic Acid) Scan

Dimercaptosuccinic acid binds to the cells of the proximal tubule, giving a static image of the renal parenchyma. In older children the scans are used primarily to identify focal defects or scars within the kidneys. In neonates DMSA scans have a high background count and there is a high degree of urinary excretion. DMSA scans may occasionally be required to confirm function where ultrasound raises the question of a need for neonatal intervention or when it is necessary to confirm or exclude acute pyelonephritis (see Fig. 64.7) [19].

64.4.5 MAG3 (Mercapto Acetyl Tri-Glycerine) Scan

Tri-mercaptoglycerine is chiefly bound to plasma proteins and is subject to tubular secretion. The scan provides dynamic information relating to the collecting system and drainage of the kidney. The parenchyma is also outlined reasonably well in the early stage of the scan and so the MAG3 serves to give an estimate of split function. The dose of radiation is low and for this reason a MAG3 scan may be used in the occasional newborn in whom information is required about drainage of the kidneys.

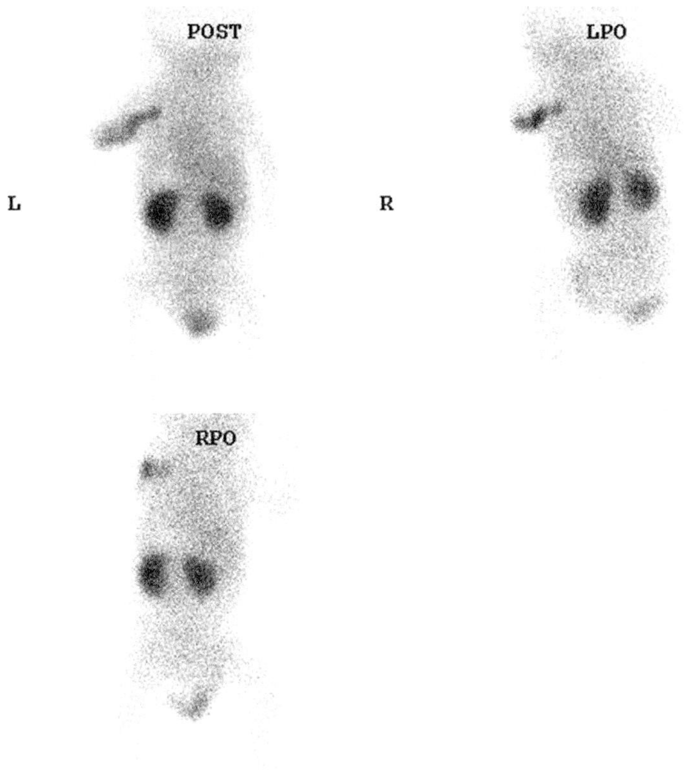

Fig. 64.7 Preterm infant with right nephrostomy in situ: DMSA showed a split function of Right 45%, Left 55%. (*POST* posterior, *LPO* left posterior oblique, *RPO* right posterior oblique)

64.4.6 DTPA (Diethylenetriamine Pentaacetic Acid)

DTPA is cleared by filtration, and in the immature neonatal kidney visualisation of the renal parenchyma is poor. It is of very limited use in infants and has largely been replaced by DMSA.

64.4.7 Magnetic Resonance Imaging (MRI)

MRI can give excellent anatomical information, and can be specifically targeted at the urinary tract through the MR urogram (MRU). The scans take a long time to acquire and for older children this will often require general anaesthesia. In infants however, scans may be acquired in 'natural' sleep, after a feed. As there is no radiation involved, MRU is becoming the investigation of choice if cross sectional imaging is required. However, MRU is rarely indicated in neonates due the quality of USS which, when combined with MCUG and nuclear medicine usually gives sufficient information.

64.4.8 Computed Tomography (CT)

CT scans provide useful cross-sectional information but at the expense of very high doses of radiation so are utilised infrequently in the newborn. Tumours are a rare indication.

64.5 Summary

Antenatally detected urinary tract anomalies are the commonest indication for urological investigations in the newborn. Ultrasound confirmation of the abnormality is followed by further investigations as indicated. Paediatric Urologists play a central role in this group as it is important not to over-investigate these newborns yet critical not to miss those with significant pathology. Neonates will all present postnatally with a wide range of symptoms and signs; once again the Paediatric Urologist must tailor the investigations accordingly.

References

1. Scott JE, Renwick M. Urological anomalies in the Northern Region Fetal Abnormality Survey. Arch Dis Child. 1993:68:22–6.
2. Sairam S, Al-Habib A, Sasson S, Thilaganathan B. Natural history of fetal hydronephrosis diagnosed on mid-trimester ultrasound. Ultrasound Obstet Gynecol. 2001;17:191–6.
3. NICE. Antenatal care: routine care for the healthy pregnant woman. National Institute for Clinical Excellence (NICE) Clinical guidelines. CG62: 2008. London: National Collaborating Centre for Women's and Children's Health.
4. Nguyen HT, Herndon CD, Cooper C, Gatti J, Kirsch A, Kokorowski P, Lee R, Perez-Brayfield M, Metcalfe P, Yerkes E, Cendron M, Campbell JB. The Society for Fetal Urology consensus statement on the evaluation and management of antenatal hydronephrosis. J Pediatr Urol. 2010;6:212–31.
5. Fernbach SK, Maizels M, Conway JJ. Ultrasound grading of hydronephrosis: introduction to the system used by the Society for Fetal Urology. Pediatr Radiol. 1993;23:478–80.
6. Keays MA, Guerra LA, Mihill J, Raju G, Al-Asheeri N, Geier P, Gaboury I, Matzinger M, Pike J, Leonard MP. Reliability assessment of Society for Fetal Urology ultrasound grading system for hydronephrosis. J Urol. 2008;180:1680–2.
7. Lee RS, Cendron M, Kinnamon DD, Nguyen HT. Antenatal hydronephrosis as a predictor of postnatal outcome: a meta-analysis. Pediatrics. 2006;118:586–93.
8. Laing FC, Burke VD, Wing VW, Jeffrey RB Jr, Hashimoto B. Postpartum evaluation of fetal hydronephrosis: optimal timing for follow-up sonography. Radiology. 1984;152:423–4.
9. Dejter SW Jr, Gibbons MD. The fate of infant kidneys with fetal hydronephrosis but initially normal postnatal sonography. J Urol. 1989;142:661–2.
10. Wiener JS, O'Hara SM. Optimal timing of initial postnatal ultrasonography in newborns with prenatal hydronephrosis. J Urol. 2002;168:1826–9.
11. Dhillon HK. Prenatally diagnosed hydronephrosis: the Great Ormond Street experience. Br J Urol. 1998;81(Suppl 2):39–44.
12. : Dhillon HK. Prenatal diagnosis (Chap. 10). In: Thomas DFM, Duffy PG, Rickwood AMK, editors. Essentials of paediatric urology, 2nd edn. London: Informa; 2008. p. 133–42.
13. Walsh TJ, Hsieh S, Grady R, Mueller BA. Antenatal hydronephrosis and the risk of pyelonephritis hospitalization during the first year of life. Urology. 2007;69:970–4.
14. Coelho GM, Bouzada MC, Lemos GS, Pereira AK, Lima BP, Oliveira EA. Risk factors for urinary tract infection in children with prenatal renal pelvic dilatation. J Urol. 2008;179:284–9.
15. Estrada CR, Peters CA, Retik AB, Nguyen HT. Vesicoureteral reflux and urinary tract infection in children with a history of prenatal hydronephrosis—should voiding cystourethrography be performed in cases of postnatally persistent grade II hydronephrosis? J Urol. 2009;181:801–6.
16. American Academy of Pediatrics Committee on Quality Improvement. Subcommittee on Urinary Tract Infection. Practice parameter: the diagnosis, treatment, and evaluation of the initial urinary tract infection in febrile infants and young children. Pediatrics. 1999;103:843–52.
17. Rudinsky SL, Carstairs KL, Reardon JM, Simon LV, Riffenburgh RH, Tanen DA. Serious bacterial infections in febrile infants in the post-pneumococcal conjugate vaccine era. Acad Emerg Med. 2009;16:585–90.
18. Hsieh MH, Madden-Fuentes RJ, Roth DR. Urologic diagnoses among infants hospitalized for urinary tract infection. Urology. 2009;74:100–3.
19. NICE. Urinary tract infection in children: Diagnosis, treatment and long-term management. National Institute for Clinical Excellence (NICE) Clinical guidelines. CG54:2007. London: National Collaborating Centre for Women's and Children's Health.
20. Crain EF, Gershel JC. Urinary tract infections in febrile infants younger than 8 weeks of age. Pediatrics. 1990;86:363–7.
21. Netto JM, Bastos AN, Figueiredo AA, Pérez LM. Spinal dysraphism: a neurosurgical review for the urologist. Rev Urol. 2009;11:71–81.
22. Kolon TF, Gray CL, Sutherland RW, Roth DR, Gonzales ET Jr. Upper urinary tract manifestations of the VACTERL Association. J Urol. 2000;163:1949–51.
23. Goossens WJ, de Blaauw I, Wijnen MH, de Gier RP, Kortmann B, Feitz WF. Urological anomalies in anorectal malformations in The Netherlands: effects of screening all patients on long-term outcome. Pediatr Surg Int. 2011;27:1091–7.
24. Azzoni R, Gerevini S, Cabitza P. Spinal cord sonography in newborns: anatomy and diseases. J Pediatr Orthop B. 2005;14:185–8.

Urinary Tract Obstruction and Dilatation

65

Anju Goyal

Abstract

Congenital anomalies of the kidney and urinary tract (CAKUT) has an incidence of 3–6 per 1000 birth and is a common cause of chronic kidney disease in children. While most CAKUT are believed to be sporadic, recent studies have suggested a high incidence (upto 50%) of CAKUT in families of index cases of urinary tract anomaly (Renkema et al. Nephrol Dial Transplant. 26:3843–51, 2011; Bulum et al. Pediatr Nephrol. 28:2143–7, 2013). This suggest a genetic basis and various genes such as HNF1 β[beta], PAX2, RET and ROBO2 have been implicated. Commonly CAKUT result in dilatation and/or obstruction of the urinary tract anywhere from the kidney down to the bladder and urethra. There can be isolated dilatation of the pelvicalyceal system (hydronephrosis [HDN]) or associated ureteric dilatation (hydroureteronephrosis [HDUN]) with or without bladder abnormality. HDN/HDUN can be secondary to obstructive or non-obstructive pathology. Obstruction is defined as 'some impedence to the flow of urine, which causes gradual and progressive damage to the kidney' (Dhillon. Essentials of paediatric urology. Informa Healthcare, p. 133–42, 2008). The non-obstructive dilatation can be due to vesico-ureteric reflux (VUR) or it can be non-obstructive, non-refluxing dilatation. Non-obstructive non-refluxing pathology, which is usually due to inherent dysplasia of the developing urinary tract, is more difficult to define and to differentiate from obstruction. Occasionally obstruction and reflux can coexist.

Keywords

Urinary tract anomaly • Prenatal diagnosis • Investigations • Surgical management • Outcomes

A. Goyal, MCh, FRCS(Paed)
Royal Manchester Children's Hospital,
Manchester, UK
e-mail: anju.goyal@cmft.nhs.uk

P.D. Losty et al. (eds.), *Rickham's Neonatal Surgery*, https://doi.org/10.1007/978-1-4471-4721-3_65

65.1 Introduction

Congenital anomalies of the kidney and urinary tract (CAKUT) has an incidence of 3–6 per 1000 birth and is a common cause of chronic kidney disease in children. While most CAKUT are believed to be sporadic, recent studies have suggested a high incidence (upto 50%) of CAKUT in families of index cases of urinary tract anomaly [1, 2]. This suggest a genetic basis and various genes such as HNF1 β[beta], PAX2, RET and ROBO2 have been implicated. Commonly CAKUT result in dilatation and/or obstruction of the urinary tract anywhere from the kidney down to the bladder and urethra. There can be isolated dilatation of the pelvicalyceal system (hydronephrosis [HDN]) or associated ureteric dilatation (hydroureteronephrosis [HDUN]) with or without bladder abnormality. HDN/HDUN can be secondary to obstructive or non-obstructive pathology. Obstruction is defined as 'some impedence to the flow of urine, which causes gradual and progressive damage to the kidney [3]. The non-obstructive dilatation can be due to vesico-ureteric reflux (VUR) or it can be non-obstructive, non-refluxing dilatation. Non-obstructive non-refluxing pathology, which is usually due to inherent dysplasia of the developing urinary tract, is more difficult to define and to differentiate from obstruction. Occasionally obstruction and reflux can coexist.

The landscape of neonatal urinary tract dilatation and obstruction anomalies has been transformed by the introduction of routine antenatal ultrasound (US) screening. A mid-trimester ultrasound scan to detect fetal structural anomalies has been undertaken in the UK since the 1980s. A fetal anomaly screening scan is offered to all pregnant women from 18 to 20(+6) weeks. High-resolution 2D ultrasound scan provides detailed assessment of urinary tract from early 2nd trimester onwards. It can detect renal pelvic (Fig. 65.1) and/or ureteric dilatation/anomaly and/or bladder distention (Fig. 65.2) along with other associated non urinary tract abnormalities. Many of the detected anomalies might never have come to attention clinically in childhood but often generates disproportionate parental anxiety during the pregnancy [4].

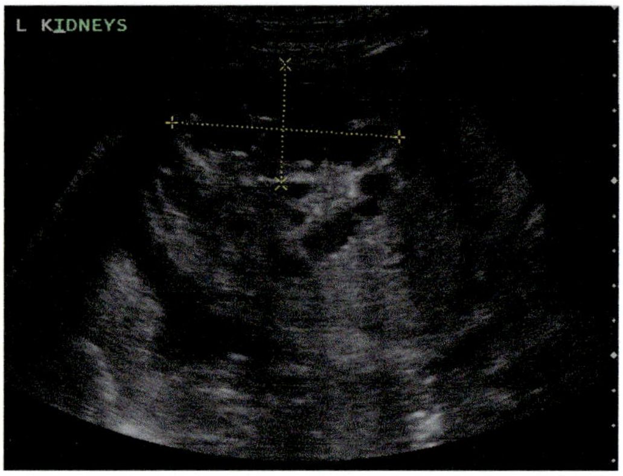

Fig. 65.1 Antenatal scan demonstrating left hydronephrosis

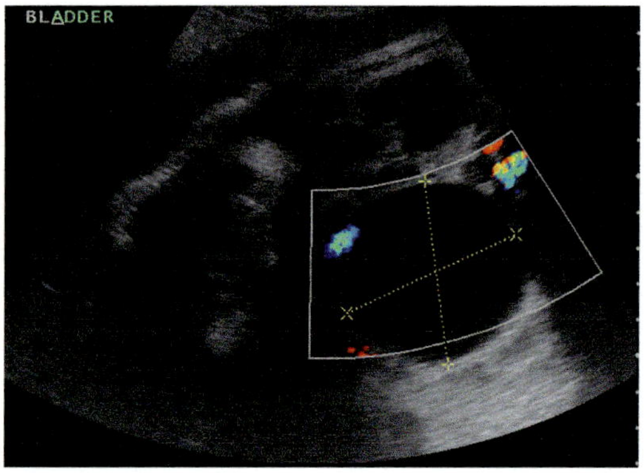

Fig. 65.2 Distended bladder on antenatal scan

Antenatal detection has created a whole new field in the practice of paediatric urology. It deals predominantly with healthy children with no obvious clinical problem who have a potential for morbidity in the form of urinary tract infection (UTI) and renal functional deterioration. There are management dilemmas as to how far to investigate in an apparently healthy child, especially where natural history of the abnormality is not clear and management may not yield satisfactory outcomes. This is especially brought to focus when managing cases with megaureter and non-specific renal pelvic dilatation. Natural history studies are limited. Some anomalies such as antenatal HDN and megaureter are better studied than others and this has led to majority of these being managed conservatively with careful monitoring [5].

Most neonates are asymptomatic at birth and have a benign pathology, which needs antibiotic prophylaxis, careful and optimally timed investigations and monitoring. In the medium term, only 7% of these antenatally detected anomalies require surgery [5]. A recent long-term outcome study demonstrated that one third each showed normalization, need of surgery or persistence of anomalies without need of surgery [6]. And further few of these such as those with posterior urethral valves (PUV), severe pelvi-ureteric junction (PUJ) obstruction and obstructing duplex ureterocoele, will require intervention in the neonatal period.

The challenge for the medical community is to differentiate those, which need treatment to prevent renal deterioration from those that are unlikely to have any consequences. In order to make this differentiation, the optimum level of investigations that a child should be subjected to, continue to be refined. As demonstrated by trends in management of HDN, the pendulum has swung from aggressive surgical correction to non-interventional observation for majority [5, 7].

65.2 Antibiotic Prophylaxis

Urinary tract dilatation and obstruction, on account of stasis of urine predisposes the child to urinary tract infection. In some pathology, prophylaxis has been proven to be helpful where as in others, the benefit is debatable. Antibiotic prophylaxis reduces the risk of UTI and prevents renal scarring in selected cases [8, 9]. Regardless of the need for intervention, antibiotic prophylaxis is started in most neonates with suspected urological anomaly while awaiting investigations and it remains the mainstay of urological management in a significant number of refluxing, obstructive and non-refluxing, non-obstructive pathologies. In our practice, trimethoprim at 2 mg/kg is the most commonly used antibiotic, followed by cefalexin.

65.3 Prenatally Detected Urinary Tract Anomalies and Their Antenatal Management

65.4 Incidence

A significant proportion of congenital urinary tract anomalies are diagnosed antenatally on detailed fetal anomaly scan done at 20 weeks gestation. About 20% of the anomalies are detected at a later gestation scan despite an apparently normal 20 weeks scan [5]. A small proportion escapes antenatal detection and may present in early infancy with symptoms of abdominal mass or UTI.

The reported incidence of antenatal urological anomalies is increasing due to improved detection. A variable incidence has been reported depending upon the threshold for diagnosing pelvicalyceal dilatation with most citing incidence of 1 in 100 or higher [4, 5, 10, 11]. A consensus statement by the Society for Fetal Urology (SFU) suggests that up to 5% of fetuses might be affected by HDN [12]. Most of these are mild dilatation and incidence of significant uropathy is around 1 in 500 [4].

The most commonly detected anomalies are—non-specific dilatation (NSD) of pelvicalyceal system (48.6%), VUR (12%), PUJ obstruction (10.6%), multicystic dysplastic kidney (MCDK) (6%) [5]. Apart from urinary tract dilatation, antenatal screening may detect—absence of kidney, absence of bladder, renal dysplasia, amniotic fluid volume increase or decrease, associated other system anomalies such as haematocolpos, etc. (Table 65.1). Though antenatal findings suggest the possible diagnosis, it is not always accurate and hence prognostic predictions are fraught with pitfalls. Any advice about antenatal intervention or progression or otherwise of pregnancy has to be very cautious with recognition of limitations of imaging techniques [13].

Table 65.1 Features and possible aetiology of antenatally detected urinary tract dilatation/pathology

Pathology	Features on antenatal scans	Aetiology
Upper urinary tract pathology	Renal pelvic dilatation	Non specific dilatation, PUJ obstruction, duplex kidney
	Ureteric dilatation ± Renal pelvic dilatation	Megaureter (obstructed or non-obstructed), Vesico-ureteric reflux, duplex kidney
	Other renal pathologies	Renal aplasia, dysplasia, MCDK, duplex
Lower urinary tract pathology	Bladder distention ± renal pelvic and ureteric dilatation	PUV, Isolated Megacystis, Neuropathic bladder (unusual), urethral atresia
	Bladder not seen	Bladder exstrophy / Cloacal exstrophy
Entire urinary tract malformation	Renal pelvic and ureteric dilatation along with bladder distention	PUV, Prune belly syndrome, Megacystis megaureter syndrome, MMIHS
Associated with complex urogenital tract malformations	Usually renal pelvic and ureteric dilatation ± bladder distention	Cloacal anomaly, Vaginal atresia, Urogenital sinus, Imperforate anus

65.5 Antenatal Investigations

Most antenatally detected anomalies require monitoring during pregnancy with ultrasound scan. The frequency of monitoring depends upon the severity of pathology. In unilateral renal dilatation follow up scan at 30–32 weeks gestation would suffice but in bilateral PCS dilatation or solitary kidney, serial scans at 4 weekly intervals are required (see Fig. 65.3a). In case of associated oligohydramnios, referral to specialist fetal therapy unit must be made. In selected cases such as when kidneys are not seen clearly due to maternal habitus or low liquor volume, magnetic resonance (MR) scan of fetus may be helpful to assess anatomy. In some instances, when pathology detected might warrant consideration of termination, MR may be done to be absolutely sure of the pathology—such as in cloacal exstrophy [13]. Depending upon the findings of antenatal scan, other investigations such a karyotyping, amniotic fluid analysis might be required. There is up to 22% reported incidence of chromosomal abnormalities in antenatal lower urinary tract obstruction (LUTO) [14–17].

65.6 Antenatal Intervention

Intervention can be diagnostic or therapeutic. Alternatively it may be termination of pregnancy (TOP). TOP is recommended only if bilateral severe renal dysplasia/solitary dysplastic kidney with or without oligohydramnios or in very severe anomalies with poor quality of life such as cloacal exstrophy.

Antenatal intervention is most commonly considered in cases of LUTO because if untreated, it carries a mortality of up to 45% mainly due to the severe oligohydramnios and resulting pulmonary hypoplasia [18]. One third of survivors may develop end-stage chronic renal impairment [19]. Because of this prognosis, there is a termination rate of up to 50% in severe LUTO [20, 21]. LUTO is amenable to therapeutic fetal intervention and it is considered if there is predicted poor prognosis with some anticipated salvage consequent to intervention. The aim of therapeutic antenatal intervention is prevention of renal failure and pulmonary hypoplasia. The prognostic criteria for case selection for intervention include echogenicity of kidneys and liquor volume. Biochemistry of fetal urine gives information about the prognosis but a systematic review [22] demonstrated that none of the analytes of fetal urine yielded clinically significant accuracy to predict poor postnatal renal function. Also fetal urine for analysis is obtained by vesicocentesis, which carries its own risk; hence it is not routinely performed. As a preparation for therapeutic intervention, it is mandatory to perform a detailed anomaly scan, determine fetal sex and offer fetal karyotyping.

There are different modalities of therapeutic intervention. Though fetal cystoscopy, open shunt insertion and repeated vesicocentesis have been utilised [23, 24], percutaneous vesico-amniotic shunt (VAS) placement is the most commonly used modality. VAS involves the placement of a double pig-tailed catheter under ultrasound guidance and local anaesthesia, with the distal end in the fetal bladder and the proximal end in the amniotic cavity to allow drainage of fetal urine. Since the first report of VAS in human fetuses in 1982 [25], many case series have suggested that

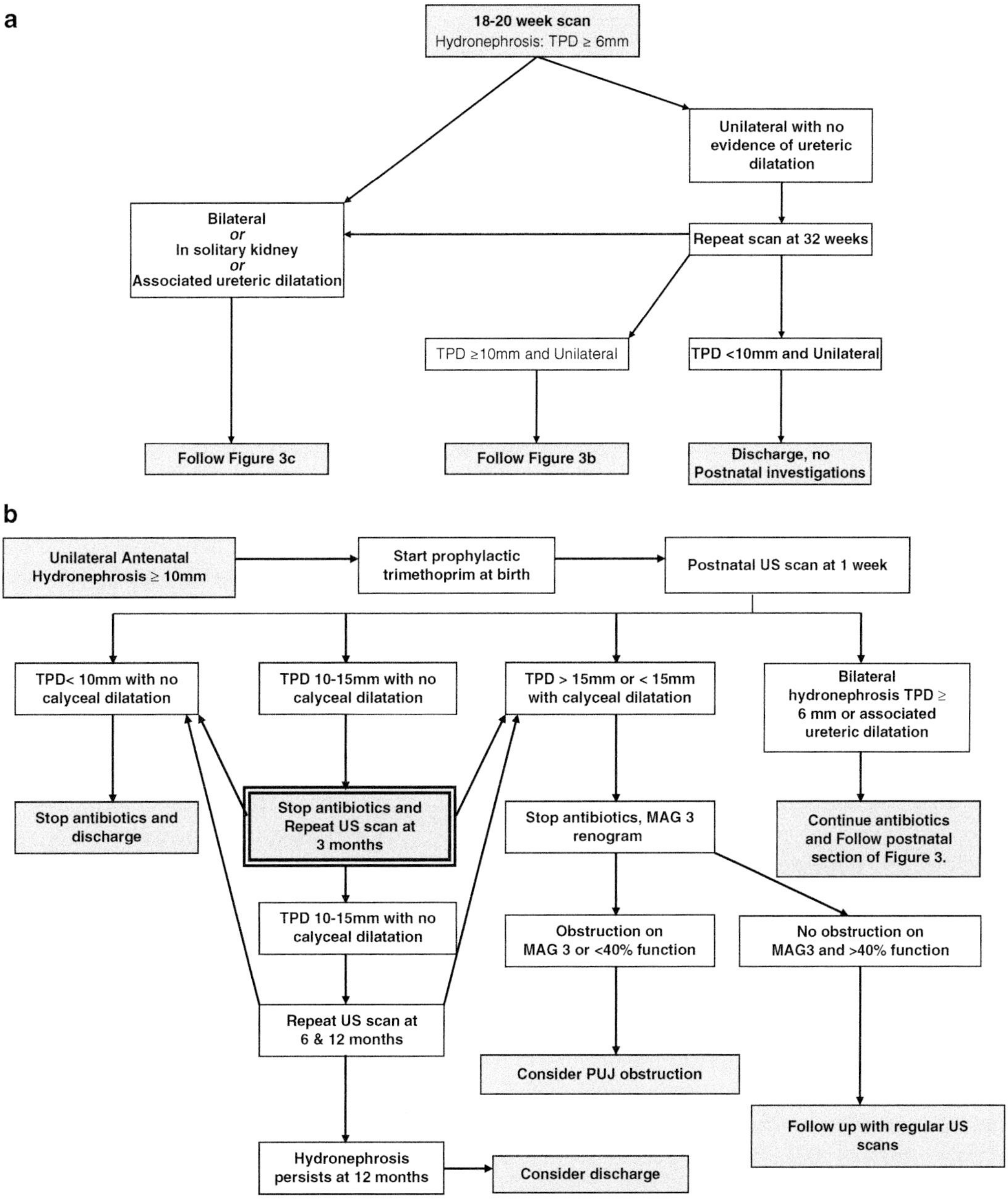

Fig. 65.3 Institutional management protocol for antenatal hydronephrosis. (**a**) Antenatal scan findings and pathway for management, (**b**) Postnatal management for unilateral hydronephrosis, (**c**) Pathway for bilateral hydronephrosis, hydronephrosis in a solitary kidney or associated ureteric dilatation

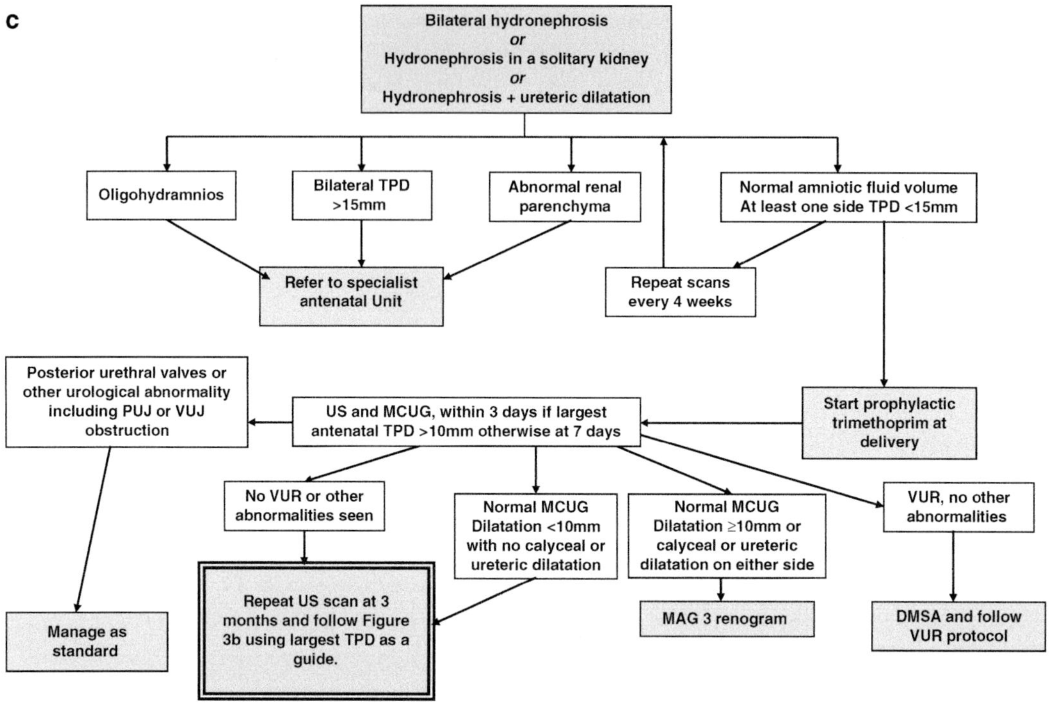

Fig. 65.3 (continued)

survival could be improved with this [26]. VAS has a significant incidence of complications: shunt displacement/occlusion (upto 34%), preterm labour, chorioamnionitis, traumatic injury and fetal/neonatal death [27]. Despite initial promise of good results, outcomes have not been very positive and VAS is not in vogue any more. Systematic review of observational studies showed a role for VAS in reduction of perinatal mortality but long-term mortality and morbidity remains high. It suggests that amelioration of oligohydramnios by shunting reduces mortality due to pulmonary hypoplasia, but the renal damage is not reversible [27]. A multi centre randomised controlled trial (PLUTO—The Percutaneous shunting in Lower Urinary Tract Obstruction) conducted by The University of Birmingham, UK compared in-utero VAS with conservative management [28]. The as-treated analysis of 31 pregnancies showed that fetuses that underwent bladder shunting had a three-time higher chance of postnatal survival than non-shunted fetuses, though very few survived with normal renal function. These findings are in line with results from studies in animals, which have shown that renal damage occurs rapidly after the onset of obstruction and might be only partly reversible [29]. The dysplastic changes seen in fetal kidneys are probably a different pathological process, rather than just a consequence of obstruction [30].

65.7 General Principles of Postnatal Management

A thorough clinical examination of the newborn remains very relevant. The necessity of investigations is clear when a neonate presents with symptoms of UTI or mass or urinary stream problems. However formulating a rational investigation protocol for antenatally detected anomalies that is appropriate and is tailored to the urgency of concerned pathology is more difficult. The aim is to investigate urgently those, which are likely to result in infection or nephron damage if left untreated. Others can be investigated at a pace that is suitable for the child, family and is likely to give best information. Fig. 65.3a–c shows the pro-

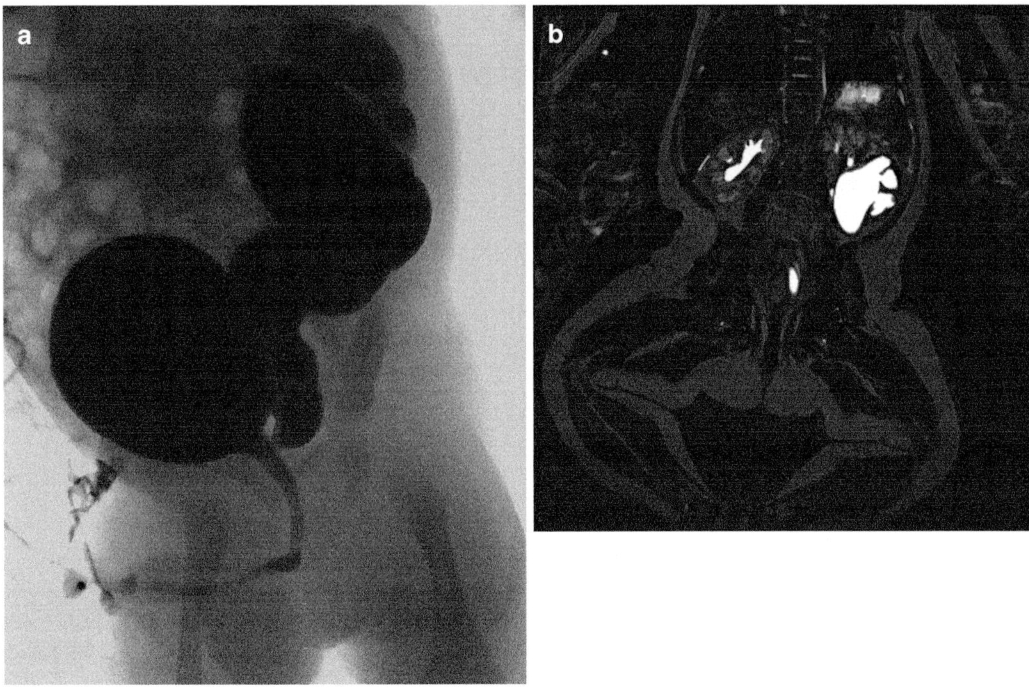

Fig. 65.4 (**a**) MCUG showing left VUR in an apparently simplex system but is actually lower pole reflux in duplex kidney, (**b**) MR scan showing left duplex in the same patient

tocol for investigation and management of antenatally detected hydronephrosis at our institute.

Due to renal immaturity, a nuclear medicine scan in first 2 months might not give accurate information about renal function and drainage. Similarly an ultrasound scan done in first 48 hours may miss important pathology as diuresis is not established as yet. Hence in most cases ultrasound should be delayed till at least 1 week of age. The indication for earlier ultrasound in first 2–3 days would be palpable mass, bilateral HDN or HDN in a solitary kidney or suspected LUTO. Micturating cystourethrogram (MCUG) is being used more selectively now whereas earlier it was performed in most cases with HDN and MCDK. MCUG is warranted in cases of suspected LUTO or if there is any ureteric dilatation. Bilateral HDN in boys even in the absence of ureteric dilatation could be due to LUTO and should be investigated with MCUG. An MR scan may be helpful to delineate anatomy in selected cases such as in duplex kidneys (Fig. 65.4a, b), horseshoe kidney, etc.

65.8 Multicystic Dysplastic Kidney

MCDK constitutes 6% of the antenatally detected anomalies. Overall Incidence has been estimated at 1 in 2400. Previously most common presentation was postnatally with abdominal mass but now most are detected antenatally.

MCDK develops due to failure of induction of metanephric blastema by the ureteric bud leading to replacement of whole kidney with multiple non-communicating cysts with no discernible parenchyma. There may be associated ureteric atresia, dilatation of ureter or ureterocoele. Confirmation is done with a postnatal ultrasound (Fig. 65.5a). If there are multiple cysts with big central cyst then a PUJ obstruction with huge pelvicalyceal dilatation (Fig. 65.5b) must be considered in differential diagnosis. Differentiation can be made with a DMSA scan which shows no function in a MCDK.

Natural history of MCDK is well documented [31]. Based on the natural history stud-

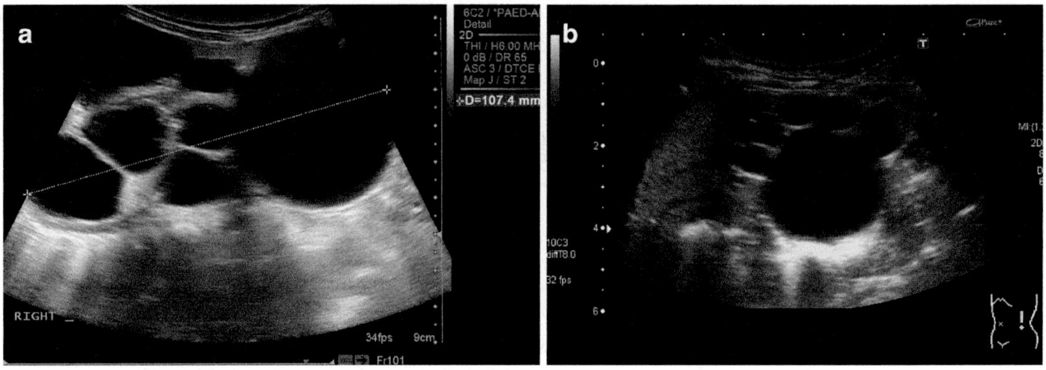

Fig. 65.5 (**a**) MCDK with multiple non-communicating cysts on US, (**b**) MCDK with dominant medial cyst mimicking severe PUJ obstruction

ies, significant changes in investigations and management have happened in last 2 decades. In MCDK there is associated VUR with reported incidence of contralateral reflux being 4.5–20% and ipsilateral reflux is present in 3–16%. It was a standard practice to do a MCUG to assess for reflux. However, it is an invasive investigation involving radiation and risk of UTI. Reflux is however low grade and mostly clinically inconsequential. Hence MCUG is no longer routinely recommended [31–34]. It may be considered in selected cases when there is contralateral kidney pathology or ureteric dilatation or family history of VUR or if there is UTI in infancy.

MCDK are managed conservatively with monitoring of blood pressure, urinalysis for protein, Glomerular Filteration Rate (GFR) estimation and follow up US to check for MCDK involution and contralateral kidney growth. Spontaneous complete involution rate is 60% at 10 years [31]. Nephrectomy is no longer recommended. Hitherto, one of the rationales for nephrectomy was to prevent risk of hypertension, malignancy and the argument that removing MCDK allowed child to be discharged from follow up. However large long-term studies have identified small but important risk of contralateral pathology (PUJ obstruction, Vesico-Ureteric Junction (VUJ) obstruction, VUR, abnormal echogenicity with low GFR) mandating follow up in early childhood regardless [29].

65.9 Isolated Pelvicalyceal Dilatation

Hydronephrosis in newborn does not equate with obstruction. Pelvicalyceal system (PCS) dilatation can be due to non-specific dilatation (NSD) or PUJ obstruction [5]. In NSD there is no hold up on MAG3 scan. While some NSD are result of fetal polyuria and resolve with time, others are consequent to kinks, folds and narrowings at PUJ, which straighten/settle over time. About 50% of antenatal PCS dilatation is transient and post natal ultrasound scan is normal. In PUJ obstruction there is delayed drainage on MAG3 scan. These are more difficult to manage, as they are a different entity to PUJ obstruction presenting later in childhood with symptoms. The standard investigations for diagnosing obstruction such as MAG3 scan and severity of dilatation on ultrasound are not applicable to this group [35, 36]. Evidence of obstructive injury to kidney in the form of decrease in function of >10% and increasing hydronephrosis, is currently the accepted way of differentiating between those needing surgery and those who can be managed conservatively. Only 22–30% of PUJ obstructions require surgical intervention [5, 35] and intervention is rarely required in neonatal period. Most neonates can be investigated as per the protocol shown (Fig. 65.3 b). Only indication for urgent investigations would be in cases of severe dilatation bilaterally or in a solitary kidney (Fig. 65.3c). Even severe unilateral hydronephrosis can be observed safely non-operatively with regular imaging (Fig. 65.6a, b)

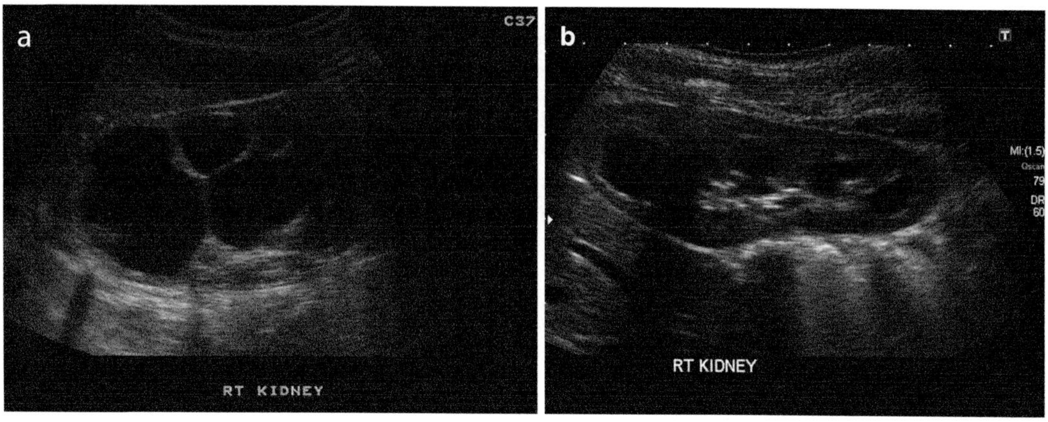

Fig. 65.6 (**a**) Severe PCS dilatation SFU grade 4, (**b**) Same patient, PCS dilatation now improved on conservative management

Table 65.2. SFU grading of Hydronephrosis

Grade	Characteristics of central renal echo complex
0	Closely apposed
1	Slight separation
2	Further separation; one or few calyces may be visualized
3	Pelviectasis and fluid filled calyces seen throughout kidney
4	Grade 3 with parenchyma over calyces thinned

and need for intervention seems to be independent of initial severity of HDN, degree of renal function and renogram pattern [35].

Thirty years after commencement of antenatal detection and management, we are still debating the indications and timing of surgical intervention. Protocols and guidelines in various centres are derived from natural history studies, which had arbitrary cut-off points for surgical interventions; hence many current indications continue to be arbitrary.

Hydronephrosis can be graded on the basis of pelvic dilatation assessed as transverse anteroposterior diameter (TAPD) with separate specific reference to calyceal dilatation and cortical thinning. Society for Fetal Urology (SFU) recommends grading on the basis of dilatation and renal cortex thickness [37] (Table 65.2). Only grades 3 and 4 are felt to be clinically significant with respect to obstruction. In our centre and in most UK centres, radiologists prefer to assess hydronephrosis with TAPD. A new classification system—Urinary Tract Dilation (UTD) Classification System has been proposed which can be applied both prenatally and postnatally [38].

Two most debated aspects of antenatal HDN are initial assessment protocol of antenatal HDN and indication for intervention in PUJ obstruction.

65.10 Assessment of Antenatal HDN

Different parameters have been proposed. The maximum antero-posterior diameter at the hilum in the transverse plane (TAPD) is the crucial measurement. After detection of isolated HDN on 20 weeks scan, it is recommended that repeat scan should be done around 30 weeks gestation. TAPD at this scan correlates closely with the need for surgery [39] and hence is the basis of postnatal management. Some including our institution protocol (Fig. 65.3a–c) recommend no postnatal scanning for those who have TAPD of less than 10 mm on >30 week scan. But with this cut-off parameter, a small proportion of urologically significant anomalies (mostly non-dilating reflux but some PUJ obstruction) may be missed. Hence some recommend at least one postnatal scan for those with TAPD more than or equal to 7 mm [5].

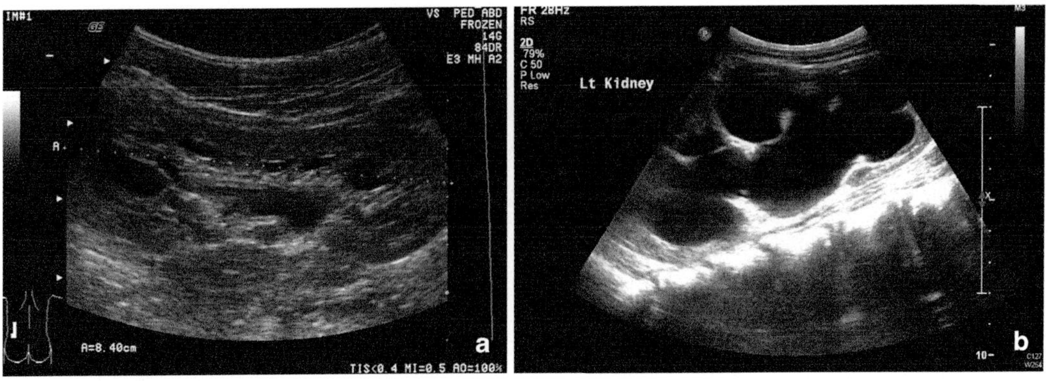

Fig. 65.7 (**a**) Ultrasound scan showing PCS dilatation which settled on conservative management and thus discharged, (**b**) Same patient presented 3 days later with acute obstruction and pain

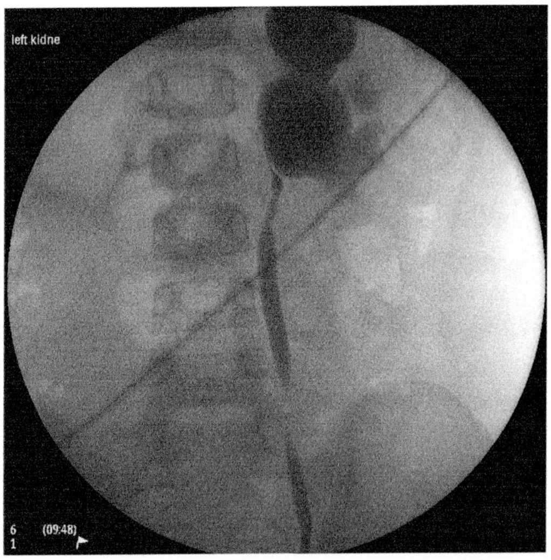

Fig. 65.8 Retrograde pyelogram demonstrating narrowing at the PUJ

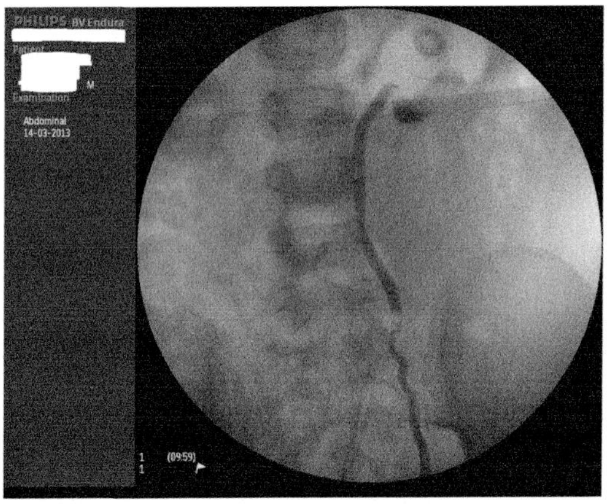

Fig. 65.9 Retrograde pyelogram showing a kink at the PUJ due to aberrant lower pole vessel

It is important that postnatal ultrasound should be viewed in light of antenatal scans. If antenatal scans showed huge dilatation but postnatal scans do not, they should be viewed with suspicion and a further ultrasound scan should definitely be performed. MCUG is usually indicated if there is any ureteric or bladder dilatation and is usually done few weeks after birth. An urgent MCUG should be considered in first week of life, in cases of bilateral dilatation or dilatation in a solitary kidney and should be adequately covered with antibiotics. When indicated, MAG 3 scan should be performed at 2–3 months of age. Again it may be indicated earlier in bilateral/solitary kidney cases.

Early natural history studies of PCS dilatation [35, 40–42] demonstrated that majority of these can be managed conservatively. A very small proportion of antenatal HDN that has resolved fully or partially may develop obstruction at a later date (Fig. 65.7a, b) and families should be counselled about it at the time of discharge from follow up.

65.11 Pelvi-Ureteric Junction Obstruction

PUJ obstruction is the most commonly detected anomaly on antenatal scans after NSD. It is defined as PCS dilatation with impaired drainage on MAG3 scans. It can be unilateral or bilateral. It is more common in males and left side is more common. About 10% may be bilateral [5]. Occasionally there may be a familial predisposition with cases found in different generations and in siblings.

Usually there is an intrinsic PUJ narrowing of variable length (Fig. 65.8), rarely it may be due to aberrant lower pole vessel (Fig. 65.9). In intrinsic PUJ, the proximal ureter is bound to the lower renal pelvis by flimsy adhesions. Once the ureter is dissected free, it is usual to find a narrow segment, 2–10 mm in length immediately below the pelvi-ureteric junction and that urine does not escape from the renal pelvis until an incision is carried proximally above the narrow segment [43]. PUJ usually shows histological features of narrowing with decreased smooth muscle and increased collagen and elastin.

PUJ obstruction usually remains asymptomatic despite increasing dilatation. Very rarely it may present in infancy with mass, UTI, sepsis, hypertension or haematuria.

65.12 Diagnosis and Indication for Intervention in PUJ Obstruction

Initial assessment is with an US and MAG3. Delayed drainage pattern or a non-draining curve should not be taken as a mark of obstruction [36]. Peters [44] has defined obstruction as "a condition of impaired urinary drainage which, if uncorrected, will limit the ultimate functional potential of a developing kidney." The dilemma facing urologists managing these patients is that are we loosing nephrons because we are waiting for too long [45] or are we intervening when we did not need to. Certainly the trend over the years is more towards conservative management following results from natural history studies. Dynamic functional MR is being investigated for its utility to provide more accurate assessment of obstruction [46].

65.12.1 Management

The most commonly accepted indications for intervention are: serial ultrasound scans showing increasing PCS dilatation, MAG3 scan showing deterioration in kidney function by >10% and symptoms of UTI/haematuria or echogenic fluid in pelvis on US (Fig. 65.10). Intervention if the differential renal function on first assessment is below 40% is debatable [35].

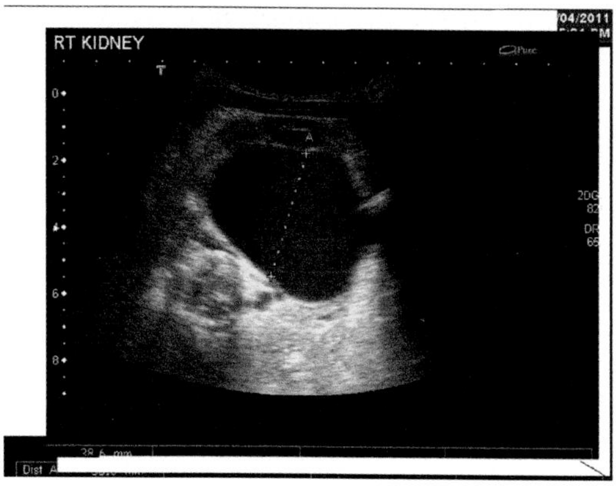

Fig. 65.10 Echogenic debris on US in a child with PUJ obstruction

Anderson Hynes pyeloplasty is the standard procedure performed. Occasionally if there is some uncertainty about the level of obstruction, a retrograde pyelogram can be done on the table to delineate anatomy better before proceeding to pyeloplasty (Fig. 65.11a, b). Though laparoscopic/robotic pyeloplasty is gaining acceptance and becoming more common in older children, open surgery is still the procedure of choice in infants. If there is massive pelvic dilatation, a reduction of pelvis is important to prevent kinking at the PUJ. In our practice, a transanastomotic stent is kept and patient is usually discharged the next day of the operation. Stent is removed approximately 6 weeks later.

A percuatenous nephrostomy may occasionally be done before pyeloplasty when there is poor function or if there is presentation with pyonephrosis. Post-nephrostomy nuclear medicine scan will provide better assessment of function to guide towards nephrectomy or pyeloplasty. If there is an acute presentation with pain which does not settle, emergency stent insertion might be considered but proceeding straight to emergency pyeloplasty is another option.

Post operative scans if done early often show preoperative level of PCS dilatation causing

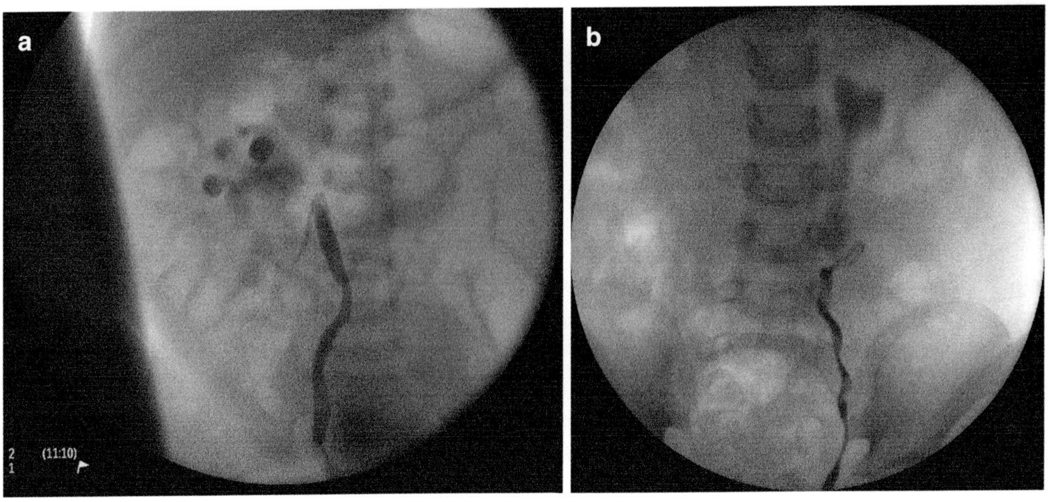

Fig. 65.11 Retrograde pyelogram. (**a**) narrowing at the PUJ, (**b**) mid-ureteric stricture

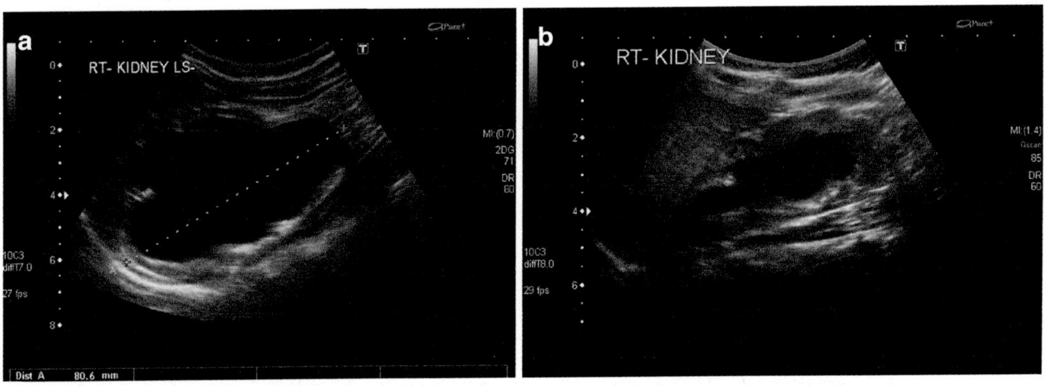

Fig. 65.12 Post pyeloplasty imaging. (**a**) US scan 4 weeks following stent removal demonstrating severe PCS dilatation, (**b**) repeat scan after 10 weeks showing that dilatation has settled without any intervention

unnecessary anxiety. It takes some time for dilatation to settle down. For this reason we defer follow up scan till about 3 months following removal of stent (Fig. 65.12a, b).

65.12.2 Vesico-Ureteric Reflux

Vesico-ureteric reflux is the retrograde flow of urine from the bladder up into the ureter and upper urinary tract. Postnatally VUR usually present as UTI. Prenatally diagnosed VUR refers to a diagnostic sequence in which the dilatation of the fetal urinary tract initiates postnatal investigations confirming VUR. An indicator of reflux on antenatal scan is ureteric dilatation. A significant proportion of infantile VUR escape antenatal detection and present with UTI [47]. Prenatal VUR constitutes 12–15% of all prenatal HDN and the protocol for investigation of antenatal HDN determines the proportion of VUR in any series. Prenatal VUR tends to be more in males and higher grade and bilateral and is known to follow a benign course [5, 48–51]. Approximately 80% is in males [51, 52]. Prenatal VUR is bilateral in 60–80% [47, 49, 51, 52]. Upto 50% VUR is grade IV and V [50, 52].

Bilateral high-grade reflux in boys is a distinct entity, which is known to have a high rate of spontaneous resolution. Up to 30% of grade 4 and 5 VUR resolve in first year of life. Transient functional urethral obstruction has been suggested as a cause for high grade VUR in males [53]. VUR can be primary due to an anatomical abnormality of the vesico-ureteric junction, which weakens the normal anti-reflux mechanism. Secondary VUR is associated with abnormal bladder such as the neuropathic bladder, posterior urethral valves or anatomical variants such as duplex kidneys.

65.12.3 Investigations

MCUG is the gold standard investigation for VUR and allows grading (Fig. 65.13). A DMSA scan informs about the kidney function and any scarring or global dysplasia. Global atrophy might be seen without any UTI and is usually associated with high-grade reflux and is reflective of intrinsic developmental anomaly of the renal units [48, 50]. UTI usually results in focal scarring [51]. Follow-up is usually with US and DMSA. In our unit we do not do a formal assessment of VUR resolution. If the child is infection free on antibiotic prophylaxis, a trial of discontinuation is given at attainment of potty training. A proportion of HDN due to low grade VUR picked up antenatally may never have presented postnatally [54]. There is a trend towards a more select approach to MCUG in antenatal HDN due to low yield in NSD without ureteric dilatation. Rather than exposing every child with HDN to the invasive procedure of MCUG, indications have been rationalised and we advocate it only in cases with dilated ureter or bilateral HDN (see Fig. 65.3c). This approach tends to detect high grades of VUR which are clinically relevant [5].

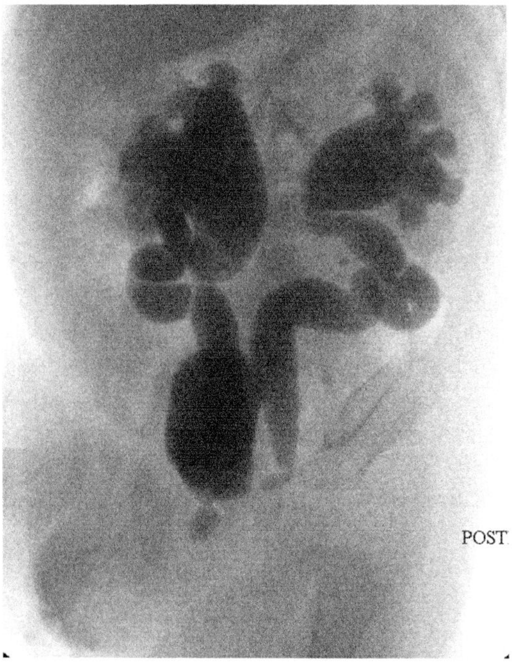

Fig. 65.13 MCUG demonstrating bilateral grade 5 VUR

65.12.4 Treatment

The goal of management of VUR is to prevent UTI. Antibiotic prophylaxis is the mainstay of VUR management for all grades. Evidence for this has been limited but some good observational, long term studies have provided insight into the best treatment options for VUR and provided evidence base for current management. In children with non-dilating reflux, antibiotic prophylaxis is an option but its efficacy is not established [55]. Recently Swedish reflux trial demonstrated that in dilating reflux, antibiotic prophylaxis result in a significant decrease in infection rate and scarring [8, 9].

All grades of VUR have a tendency for spontaneous resolution with up to 3/4th improving or resolving [47, 48, 50–52]. Recurrent UTI and bladder dysfunction predicts non-resolution [47, 48]. 16–52% breakthrough infection rate has been reported in prenatal VUR while on antibiotic prophylaxis [47, 48, 50, 51, 56]. Up to 20% have recurrent UTI.

A surgical intervention is rarely required in infancy. For recurrent UTI in boys, circumcision reduces the risk. An endoscopic correction of reflux may be done in cases of recurrent UTI. In high grade reflux—ureteric reimplantation can be done but is technically difficult in infants; ureterostomy or vesicostomy can be a temporary option [51].

65.12.5 Primary Non-refluxing Megaureter

Primary non-refluxing megaureter is mostly detected antenatally. It may be obstructed or non-obstructed and the distinction between them is very difficult. VUJ obstruction constitutes

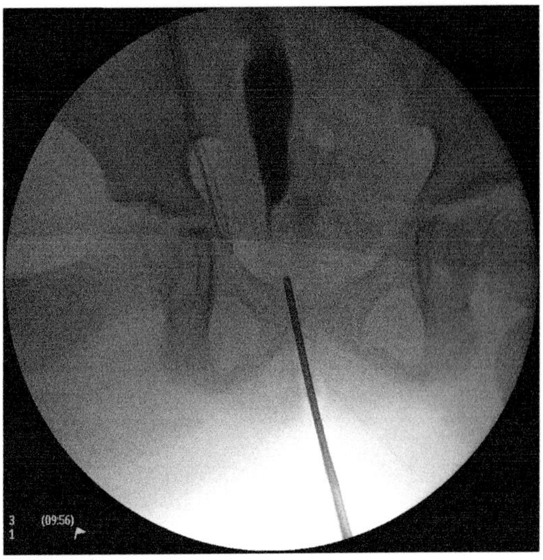

Fig. 65.14 Retrograde study showing an adynamic segment of the lower ureter in a megaureter

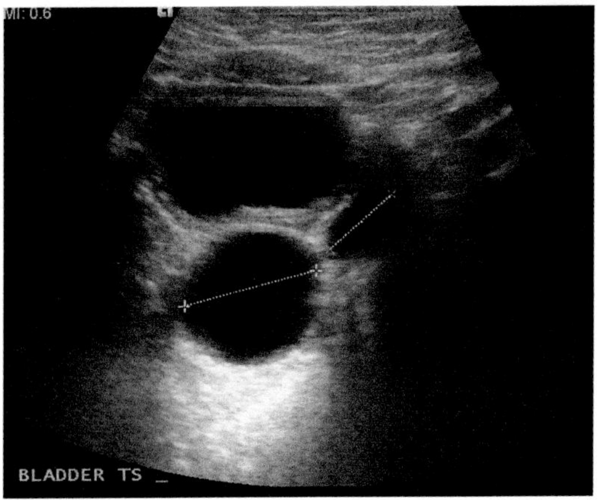

Fig. 65.15 Bilateral dilated ureters behind the bladder

2.3% of all antenatally detected urinary tract anomalies [5]. Most are asymptomatic but some may present with UTI. Non-refluxing megaureter has an incidence of about 1 in 1500 with a male preponderance and is more common on the left [57–59]. It can be bilateral in 13–42% of cases [58, 59].

The obstruction may be functional with an adynamic segment at the VUJ (Fig. 65.14) or may be due to narrow VUJ. Histological studies of the VUJ show increased collagen with reduction in muscle component [60]. The pathology is thought to result from congenital defective vascular development at the vesicoureteric junction [60]. Other mechanism might be dysplastic development of the entire ureter and PCS. Spontaneous resolution in majority supports a maturational causation [61, 62].

Ultrasound (Fig. 65.15) and MAG3 (Fig. 65.16) scans give anatomical and functional details. A MAG3 may show draining kidney in the presence of obstruction if area of interest in drawn over the kidney as the isotope is draining into the dilated ureter. A MCUG rules out VUR. An MR urogram might be done to evaluate further if needed. Similar to dilemmas in PCS dilatation management, the most important challenge is to define and identify obstruction in megaureter. Nevertheless, the relevant pathophysiology is stasis of urine. The walls of dilated ureter cannot coapt to generate effective peristalsis leading to stasis related complications such as infection and stone formation.

Antibiotic prophylaxis needs to be commenced at birth. The concept of management has changed from surgical intervention to close observation. Currently 70—90% can be managed conservatively [58, 63]. Conventional surgical option is ureteric reimplantation. However despite ureteric reimplant, the ureteric and PCS dilatation might not improve due to developmental dysplasia of the system. Minimally invasive procedures such as stent insertion, balloon dilatation and cutting balloon endoureterotomy of VUJ have been reported with variable success rates [64–69]. The rationale for stenting is that a period of drainage would allow the ureteric dilatation to come down to such an extent that following removal of the stent effective peristalsis would continue [58]. However, sometimes the narrow VUJ may not allow a guidewire insertion precluding endourological intervention. Occasionally an ureterostomy may be required if obstruction is leading to sepsis. A refluxing reimplantation is another option in infants [70]. There is a great debate on the best interventional modality.

Even more keenly debated is the indication for surgical intervention. Most commonly agreed indications include renal function deterioration on nuclear medicine scan and development of

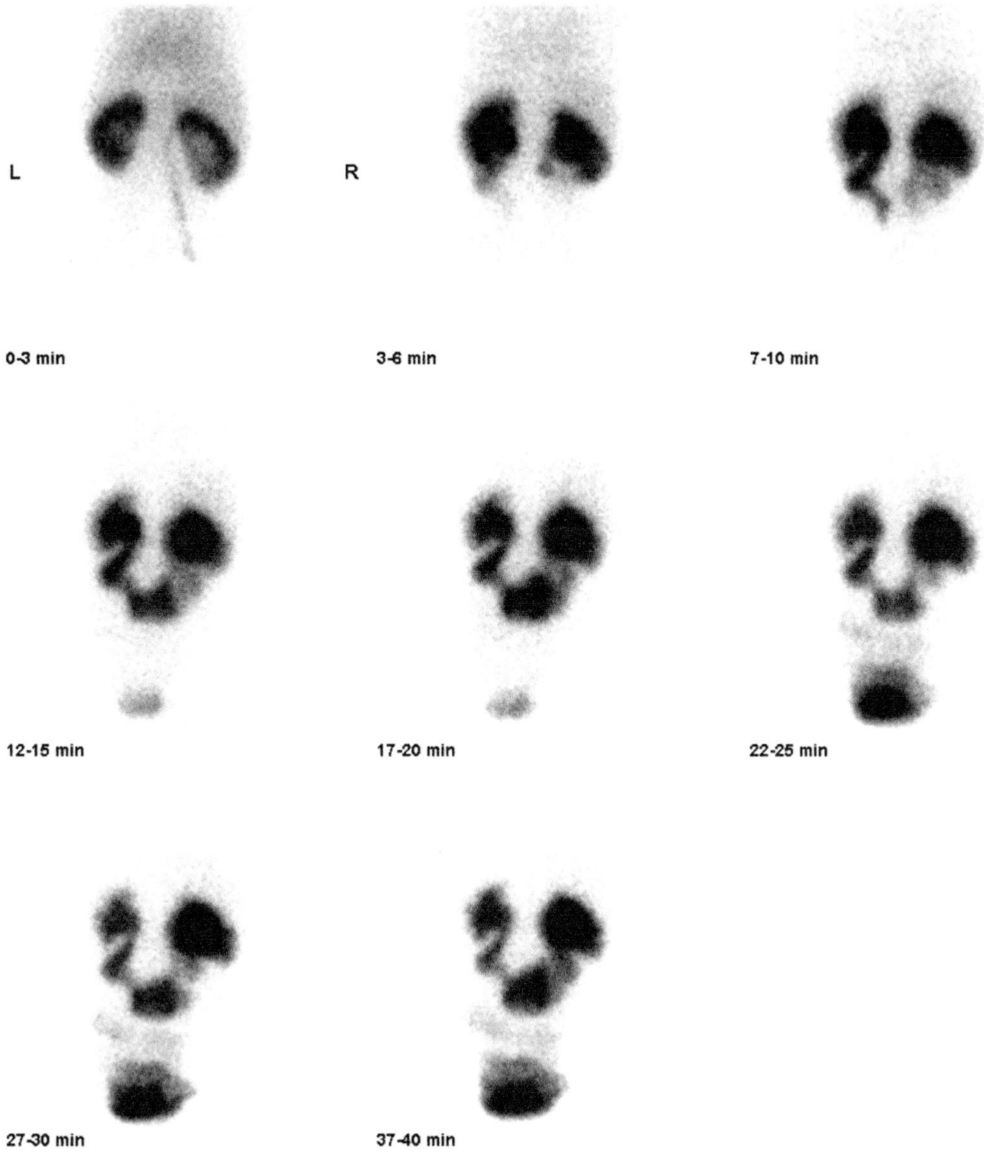

Fig. 65.16 MAG 3 scan showing bilateral megaureters

symptoms such as UTI or pain [57, 58, 63]. An increasing hydronephrosis or hydroureter can be monitored closely. A recent long term observational study from our institute [58] confirmed that conservative management is highly successful especially when the ureteric diameter was less than 10 mm with virtually all resolving completely. When ureter was more than 10 mm size, complete resolution is not common and 25% developed complications. Still the majority remains asymptomatic.

65.12.6 Duplication Anomalies

They constitute 2.6% of antenatally detected anomalies [5]. The commonly identified features are hydronephrosis, dilated ureter, duplex appearance and ureterocoele. But majority of duplication anomalies are uncomplicated where there is no associated dysplasia or dilatation and they remain undetected.

Those that are detected on antenatal scans or which present postnatally have either dysplastic/

dilated one moiety or both. Upper moiety is usually associated with obstruction due to ureterocoele or narrow VUJ. Upper moiety ureter may have an ectopic opening outside the bladder. Lower moiety is usually associated with VUR and rarely PUJ obstruction.

Duplication anomalies rarely cause symptoms in infancy. A large ureterocoele (Fig. 65.17) may give rise to obstructive bladder symptoms. Child may present with sepsis/pyonephrosis of the dilated obstructed upper pole or have UTI due to refluxing lower pole. Girls may present with wetting due to ectopic ureter opening in urethra, perineum or vagina but it is usually noted after potty training. Boys with ectopic ureter are never incontinent as opening is always above the sphincter but may present with UTI/epididymo-orchitis when ectopic ureter is opening into the vas/seminal vesicle.

Antibiotic prophylaxis is commenced at birth. Ultrasound delineates the anatomy. MCUG is done to assess for reflux. A MAG 3/DMSA scan should be done in 2–3 months time. In complex cases a MR scan may be done (Fig. 65.18).

Ureterocoele associated with a dilated upper pole may be non-obstructive and can be managed non-operatively [71]. Intervention is required early if the obstructed upper pole gets infected. An urgent endoscopic incision of ureterocoele relieves the obstruction [72–75]. Ureterocoele incision may prove to be the definitive management in 2/3rd of patients. In our series of 39 patients who had incision of ureterocoele, further surgery was necessary in only 13%. Incision may result in reflux into the upper pole. Heminephrectomy is the treatment of choice when the function of upper moiety is poor. If there is reasonable function then excision of ureterocoele with ureteric reimplantation is an option [75, 76]. If there is persistent obstruction/infection in infancy following incision of ureterocoele or if obstruction is due to narrow VUJ without associated ureterocoele, then an urgent ureterostomy may need to be done. Another option is to do uretero-ureterostomy but non-refluxing lower pole is the prerequisite [77].

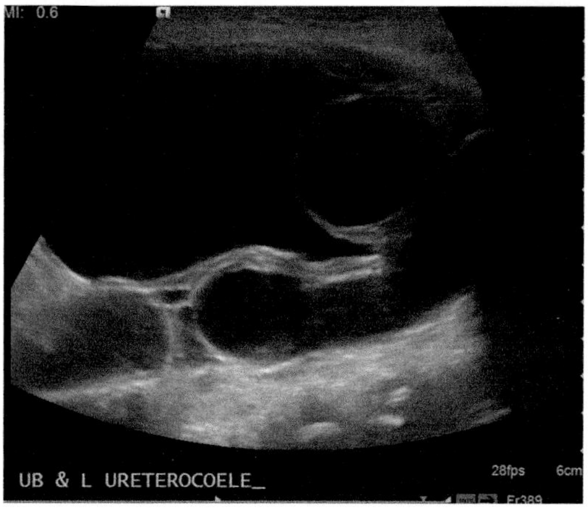

Fig. 65.17 A large ureterocoele obstructing the bladder neck on US

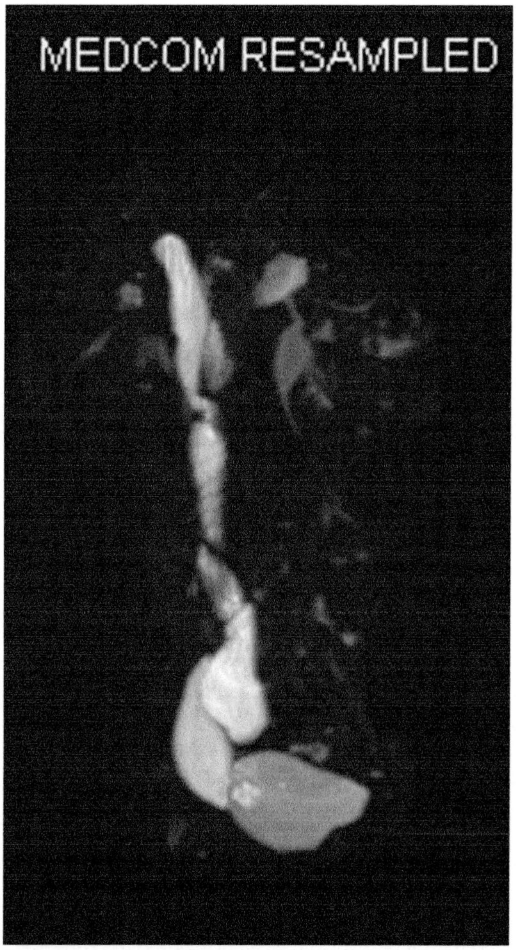

Fig. 65.18 MR urogram demonstrating an ectopic ureter associated with cryptic upper pole

VUR associated with lower pole is managed with antibiotic prophylaxis. It can be treated endoscopically or with ureteric reimplantation if there are recurrent UTI despite antibiotics. If lower pole is dysplastic with poor function then lower pole heminephrectomy can be carried out, preferably laparoscopically.

65.12.7 Megacystis

A large bladder may be detected on antenatal scans and its presence along with findings of HDN commonly suggest lower urinary tract obstruction, which is predominantly due to posterior urethral valves and urethral atresia. A small proportion is due to non-obstructive pathology such as isolated megacystis, megacystis associated with severe dilating VUR (also called Megacystis Megaureter Syndrome (MMS)) [74], Megacystis Microcolon Intestinal Hypoperistalsis Syndrome (MMIHS) and Prune Belly syndrome (PBS). Isolated megacystis is a distinct entity where a large bladder exists without VUR or any obstructive pathology (Fig. 65.19) and may be detected antenatally [78, 79].

The pathophysiology of megacystis in MMS is proposed to be consequent to the inability of the bladder to stay empty completely after voiding due to reflux into extremely voluminous ureters [78]. But existence of isolated megacystis without VUR and detection of large bladder in MMS as early as 15 weeks of gestation [80] contests this theory. An alternative hypothesis is that it is due to dysplasia of the developing urinary tract, which can range from involvement of the kidney (HDN), ureters (megaureter), bladder (isolated megacystis), whole urinary tract (MMS, PBS), to involving the gastrointestinal tract (MMIHS).

In megacystis, a MCUG to assess bladder volume and VUR is done (Fig. 65.20a, b). Urodynamic study gives information on bladder storage and emptying function. The bladder is usually large capacity, hypotonic and may have poor emptying (Fig. 65.21). DMSA scan informs about the degree of renal dysplasia.

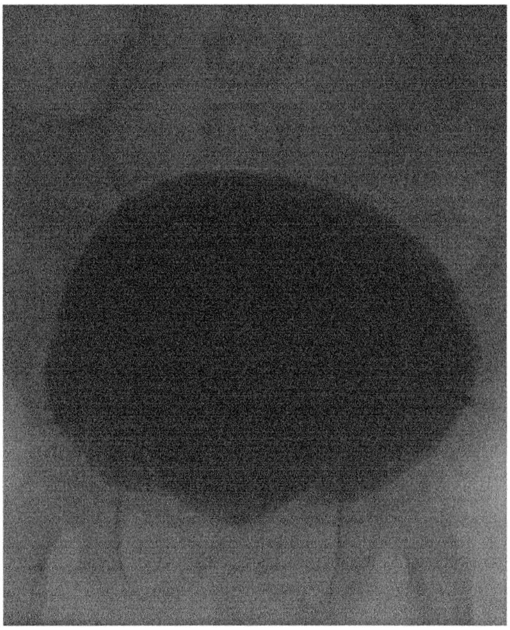

Fig. 65.19 Large bladder—isolated megacystis

65.12.8 Management

The concept of management has evolved from surgical reduction of bladder [81] to antireflux surgery [82] to conservative management. Long-term outcome series are lacking. The prognosis depends upon the extent of inherent dyplasia of the system including kidneys. Management goals are prevention of infection by ensuring complete bladder emptying. Surprisingly, a good proportion has good bladder emptying but a minority might require ISC. Our series [83] demonstrate that bladder dynamics tend to stabilise over time as long as UTI's can be prevented by antibiotic prophylaxis and complete bladder emptying. A few went on to develop deterioration of bladder dynamics and these had poor bladder emptying.

65.12.9 Posterior Urethral Valves

Posterior urethral valves are an important cause of antenatally detected and postnatally presenting lower urinary tract obstruction which carries a 50% fetal and neonatal mortality [18]. PUV is a congenital obstructive uropathy where there is

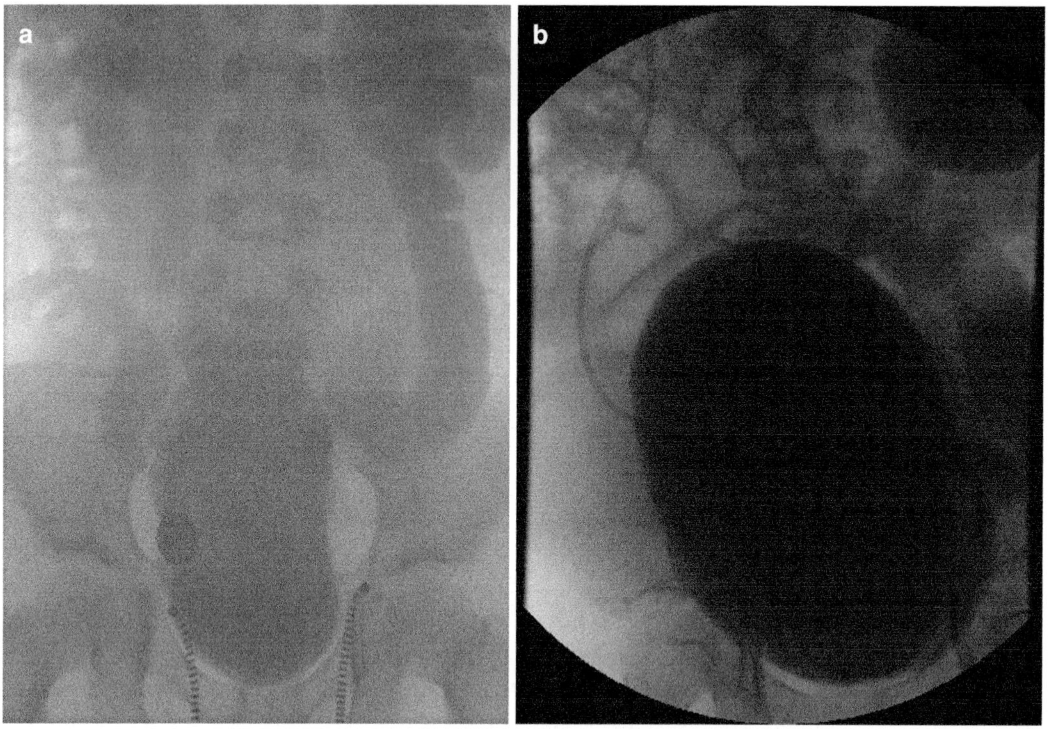

Fig. 65.20 Megacystis megaureter syndrome. (**a**) bilateral VUR, (**b**) unilateral VUR

obstruction in the posterior urethra and there is associated variable developmental dysplasia of the entire urinary tract. An incidence of 1 in 5000 live births has been reported. Anecdotally its incidence has been thought to be declining because of antenatal detection and subsequent terminations. But a recent study refutes this assumption [84]. It is an important cause of renal failure in paediatric population. UK Renal registry shows that obstructive uropathy accounts for 15% of end stage renal disease (ESRD) and that PUV is responsible for 25–30% of paediatric renal transplants [85]. There is a known association with Downs syndrome [86, 87]. A familial predisposition to PUV is rare but it may be associated with other CAKUT in family members [1, 2].

65.12.10 Pathology

Historically Young classified PUV into 3 types—Type 1, II and III [88]. But this classification is not accepted any more. Typical valves are mucosal folds, which arise from the lower end of verumontanum and go down to meet in midline anteriorly and cause obstruction to antegrade flow and correspond to type I valve. Rarely one may find a transverse membrane across the urethra immediately below the verumontanum with a centrally or eccentrically sited aperture (Type III). Type II valves are not recognized as a pathology. Dewan [89] postulated the concept of congenital obstructing posterior urethral membrane (COPUM) and proposed that typical configuration of valve results from rupture of this membrane by a catheter. But this configuration can be seen in uncatheterised urethra as well. Embryologically valves result from abnormal integration of wolffian ducts into the developing urethral wall. It is an early event and can be detected in early second trimester.

There may be minimal involvement of upper urinary tract or there may be associated disordered development of entire urinary tract resulting in dysplastic kidneys and ureters with thickened hypertrophied bladder. In some cases

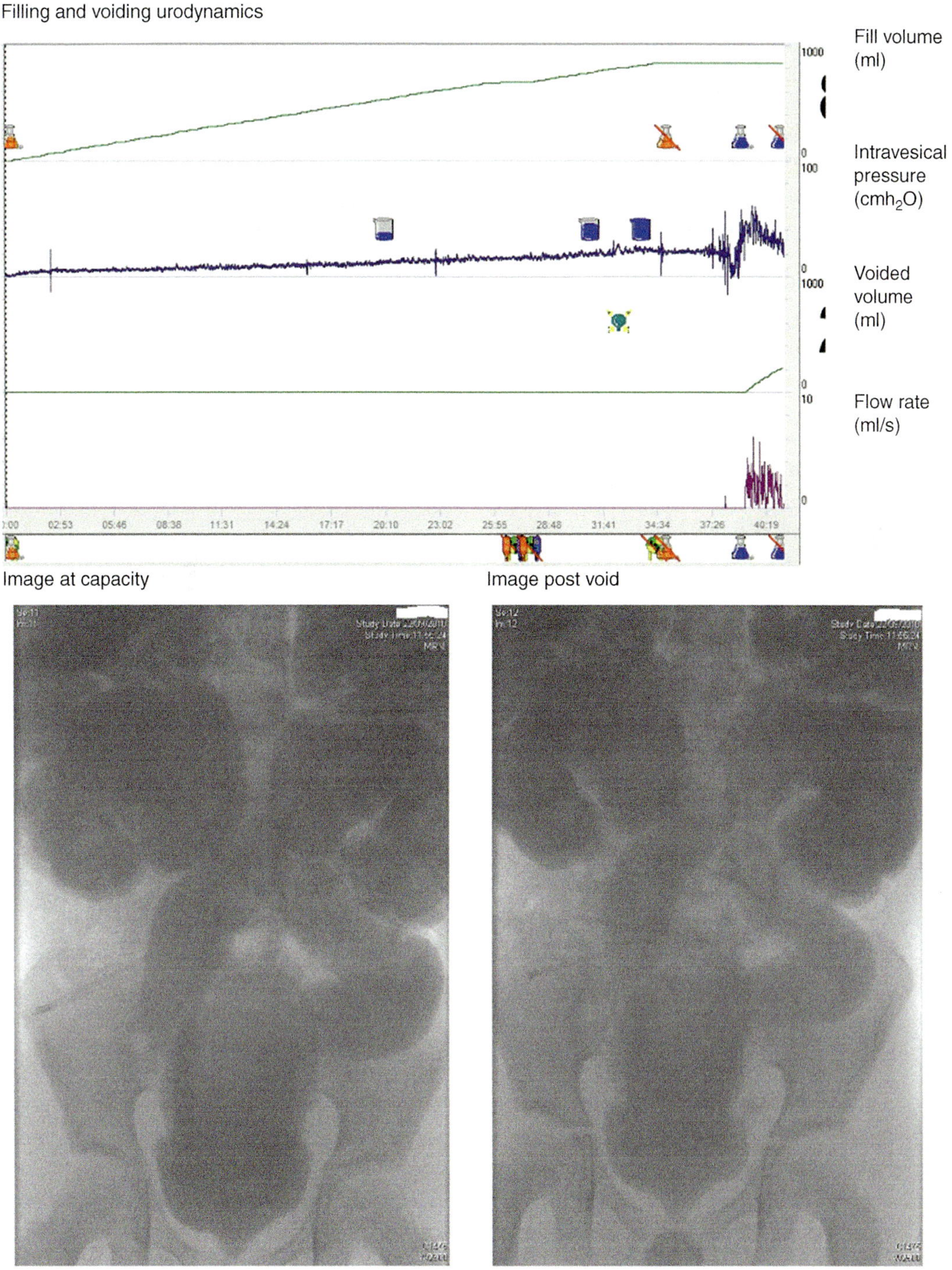

Fig. 65.21 Urodynamic study in a 7 year old boy with MMS showing 850 ml capacity with bilateral VUR, compliance of 55 mls/cm of H_2O and poor emptying

only one kidney might be dysplastic with very poor function and almost normal function on other side—termed Vesico-Ureteric Reflux and Dysplasia (VURD) syndrome. In mild variant of PUV, both kidneys might be well developed with only bladder distension. VUR is present in 40–60% cases and is bilateral in half of these.

65.12.11 Clinical Presentation

Antenatal detection is the most common presentation with two-third of PUV detected to have abnormal findings on prenatal scans though specific diagnosis of LUTO has been made in only 3/4th of these [90]. Rest present postnatally with poor urinary stream, large bladder, UTI's. A few still present with sepsis and renal failure. A good urinary stream does not exclude posterior urethral valves. Very occasionally child may present with urinary ascites either due to leak from bladder or more commonly from kidney and this is protective for renal development. Those who have had antenatal intervention may get ascites due to displacement of the bladder stent into peritoneal cavity.

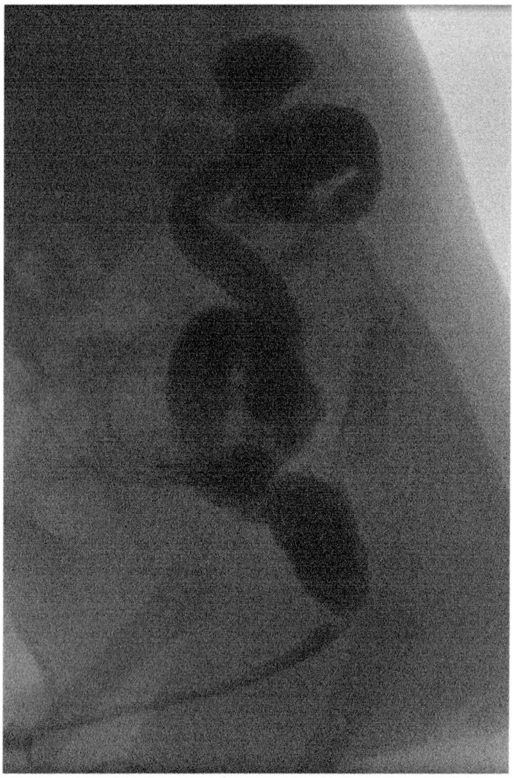

Fig. 65.22 Dilated and elongated posterior urethra along with VUR on MCUG in a neonate with posterior urethral valves

65.12.12 Diagnosis and Investigations

On antenatal scans, a keyhole sign is suggestive of PUV. Spectrum of findings may include bilateral HDUN, unilateral HDN, bilateral HDN with no ureteric dilatation or only bladder dilatation. Similar features on postnatal ultrasound supports diagnosis but definitive diagnosis is made on MCUG, which shows a dilated elongated posterior urethra with or without associated trabeculated bladder and VUR (Fig. 65.22). Bladder neck may be prominent leading to impression of constriction at the bladder neck.

Cystoscopy provides the final answer and the valves are best observed endoscopically with the tip of the cystoscope situated approximately 1 cm distal to the verumontanum. With antegrade flow through the proximal urethra obtained by opening the draining channel and stopping the flow of irrigation fluid, the valve margins can be seen to co-apt in the midline [43].

65.12.13 Management

Antibiotic prophylaxis is started after birth in antenatally detected or postnatally suspected cases. The urinary tract is obstructed from the first trimester of gestation and catheterisation can usually wait until transfer to a specialist paediatric surgical centre. Negotiation of catheter past the valves may be slightly awkward or more commonly it can curl in the dilated posterior urethra. It is not uncommon to damage the urethra when balloon is blown in the urethra by an inexperienced person. If it is imperative that child be urgently catheterised in the non-specialist unit to relieve obstruction, then a fine polythene catheter is safer than a balloon catheter.

These patients should be ideally be jointly managed along with a paediatric nephrologist as the neonate needs close monitoring of electrolytes, acid-base balance, fluid balance and renal function due to associated renal dysplasia and tubular dysfunction. Catheterisation results in post-obstructive diuresis and appropriate fluids should be supplemented, usually orally. A period of catheterisation stabilises the renal function. A MCUG under appropriate antibiotic cover should be done to confirm the valves and assess the bladder and VUR. If there is UTI or sepsis, appropriate antibiotic management should be instituted.

Once renal function is stabilised, resection can be attempted with a 9 Fr resectoscope and in older patients. 11/13 Fr resectoscope can be used. A diathermy hook or a cold knife may be used and valve may be ablated at 5 and 7 o'clock position or at 12 o'clock position. Nd YAG and Ho YAG [91, 92] laser have also been used for valve ablation with claims of lower risk of stricture. Where urethra does not accept a resectoscope or one is not available, a ureteric catheter or a cold knife can be utilised through a cystoscope to ablate the valves. Post-operative catheter drainage for a short duration may be employed if there is some trauma or oedema to urethra during the ablation but is not necessary. A post-operative MCUG or check cystoscopy to check completion of ablation is optional.

Further follow up is with regular monitoring of renal function, DMSA scan and US.

65.12.14 Bladder in PUV

Typically the bladder may be small capacity and poorly compliant with detrusor overactivity. Bladder dysfunction in PUV may progress from detrusor overactivity to normal function to low compliance and in later stages detrusor hypocontractility [93]. Short term anti-cholinergic therapy may be warranted in initial stages and usually results in improvement. Most bladders normalize with time. However some bladders go on to develop valve bladder syndrome. Valve bladder syndrome is characterized by persisting or progressive HDUN in the absence of obstruction [93–95]. This is attributed to constant bladder overdistention due to a combination of polyuria and incomplete emptying, bladder insensitivity and VUR. Polyuria due to renal dysplasia and consequent concentration defect is known to be present in 60% of PUV [96]. Resolution of valve bladder after renal transplant supports the role of polyuria in aetiopathogenesis of valve bladder. Where renal function dose not warrant transplant, ensuring effective bladder emptying by regular voiding, double voiding and overnight catheterisation has been reported to have good outcomes [94]. In severe cases, bladder augmentation or urinary diversion might be required.

65.12.15 Urinary Diversion

A short term urinary diversion may occasionally be required when a premature baby's urethra is unable to accept a resectoscope; a suprapubic catheter may be inserted or a temporary vesicostomy might be fashioned.

After valve ablation if there is recurring UTI and poor renal function and accurate assessment of obstruction at the VUJ is precluded by dysplastic dilated urinary tract, ureterostomy may provide relief. A low, loop ureterostomy can be done easily via a Pfannensteil incision and will allow some bladder cycling as well. It can be simply reversed. An end ureterostomy will warrant reimplantation at closure. A high ureterostomy may be preferred if very dilated tortuous ureters are causing stagnation of urine with recurrent UTI's, as it ensures the best unobstructed drainage of urine. Once done, ureterostomy is best left for at least 1 year or preferably 2 years to allow growth of kidney without any obstruction and UTI. There have been concerns about bladder dysfunction due to non-cycling of urine but in our experience bladder function quickly recovers after ureterostomies are closed. A vesicostomy has the advantage of bladder cycling and is preferable to ureterostomy under appropriate circumstances where obstruction at the VUJ is not an issue.

65.13 Long Term Outcomes

65.13.1 Renal Failure

Development of renal failure depends on the degree of urinary tract dysplasia at birth. If kidneys are dysplastic then they are more likely to develop ESRD. Further continuing damage may occur due to persistent obstruction, VUR, UTI or bladder dysfunction. Historically 1/3rd developed renal failure but better management has led to improved results with latest data suggesting that only 13% progress to ESRD [97, 98]. 31% of PUV have severe bladder dysfunction which can contribute to it [99].

65.13.2 Sexual Function and Fertility

Many factors in PUV can affect sexual function including renal failure, bladder neck procedure, abnormal reflux into ejaculatory system leading to epididymo-orchitis, and cryptorchidism. While concerns have been raised about fertility and sexual function, a recent long-term study of 67 adult PUV patients did not show any particular difference compared to normal controls regarding fertility, and erections [99, 100]. Again abnormal sperm parameters have been identified by few studies, but no significant semen abnormality has been identified and reported fertility is comparable to controls [101].

65.13.3 VUR

VUR tends to resolve after ablation of valve and is managed with antibiotic prophylaxis. Ureteric reimplantation is rarely required. Circumcision is protective against infection and should be considered as first line of management for recurrent UTI. But when VUR is associated with poorly functioning kidney as in VURD (Fig. 65.23a, b), it tends to persist causing recurrent UTI and requires nephrectomy.

65.13.4 Urinary Incontinence

Patients with posterior urethral valves achieve daytime and night-time urinary continence significantly later than their healthy peers [102]. Continued urinary incontinence might be a consequence of bladder dysfunction or rarely may be related to sphincter damage during valve ablation. Urethral stricture may also occur after valve resection.

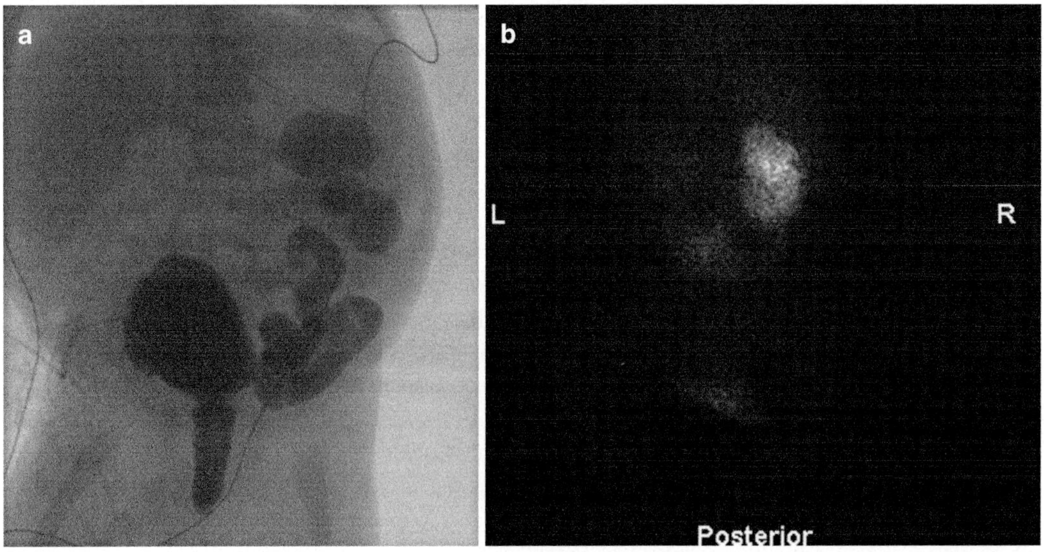

Fig. 65.23 VURD syndrome in PUV. (**a**) Left high grade reflux, (**b**) no function on the side of reflux on DMSA

References

1. Renkema KY, Winyard PJ, Skovorodkin IN, et al. Novel perspectives for investigating congenital anomalies of the kidney and urinary tract (CAKUT). Nephrol Dial Transplant. 2011;26:3843–51.
2. Bulum B, Ozçakar ZB, Ustüner E, et al. High frequency of kidney and urinary tract anomalies in asymptomatic first-degree relatives of patients with CAKUT. Pediatr Nephrol. 2013;28:2143–7.
3. DFM T. Upper tract obstruction (Chapter 6). In: DFM T, Duffy PG, AMK R, editors. Essentials of paediatric urology. 2nd ed. London: Informa Healthcare; 2008. p. 73–92.
4. Dhillon GK. Antenatal hydronephrosis (Chapter 10). In: DFM T, Duffy PG, AMK R, editors. Essentials of paediatric urology. 2nd ed. London: Informa Healthcare; 2008. p. 133–42.
5. Mallik M, Watson AR. Antenatally detected urinary tract abnormalities: more detection but less action. Pediatr Nephrol. 2008;23:897–904.
6. Nef S, Neuhaus TJ, Spartà G, et al. Outcome after prenatal diagnosis of congenital anomalies of the kidney and urinary tract. Eur J Pediatr. 2016;175:667–76.
7. James CA, Watson AR, Twining P, Rance CH. Antenatally detected urinary tract abnormalities: changing incidence and management. Eur J Pediatr. 1998;157:508–11.
8. Brandstrom P, Esbjorner E, Herthelius M, et al. The Swedish reflux trial in children: III. Urinary tract infection pattern. J Urol. 2010;184:286–91.
9. Brandstrom P, Neveus T, Sixt R, et al. The Swedish reflux trial in children: IV. Renal damage. J Urol. 2010;184:292–7.
10. Thomas DFM. Prenatal diagnosis. What do we know of long-term outcomes? J Pediatr Urol. 2010;6:204–11.
11. Hsieh MH, Lai J, Saigal CS. Urologic Diseases in America Project. Trends in prenatal sonography use and subsequent urologic diagnoses and abortions in the United States. J Pediatr Urol. 2009;5:490–4.
12. Nguyen HT, Herndon CD, Cooper C, et al. The Society for Fetal Urology consensus statement on the evaluation and management of antenatal hydronephrosis. J Pediatr Urol. 2010;6:212–31.
13. Goyal A, Fishwick J, Hurrell R, Cervellione RM, Dickson AP. Antenatal diagnosis of bladder/cloacal exstrophy: challenges and possible solutions. J Pediatr Urol. 2012;8:140–4.
14. Sebire NJ, Von Kaisenberg C, Rubio C, Snijders RJM, and Nicolaides KH. Foetal megacystis at 10-14 weeks of gestation. Ultrasound Obstet Gynaecol 1996: 8: 387–390
15. Favre R, Kohler M, Gasser B, Muller F, Nisand I. Early fetal megacystis between 11 and 15 weeks of gestation. Ultrasound Obstet Gynecol. 1999;14:402–6.
16. Liao AW, Sebire NJ, Geerts L, Cicero S, Nicolaides KH. Megacystis at 10-14 weeks of gestation: chromosomal defects and outcome according to bladder length. Ultrasound Obstet Gynecol. 2003;21:338–41.
17. Al-Hazmi H, Dreux S, Delezoide AL, et al. Outcome of prenatally detected bilateral higher urinary tract obstruction or megacystis: sex-related study on a series of 709 cases. Prenat Diagn. 2012;32:649–54.
18. Freedman AL, Johnson MP, Gonzalez R. Fetal therapy for obstructive uropathy: past, present, future? Pediatr Nephrol. 2000;14:167–76.
19. Parkhouse HF, Barratt TM, Dillon MJ, et al. Long term outcome of boys with posterior urethral valves. Br J Urol. 1988;62:59–62.
20. Cromie WJ, Lee K, Houde K, Holmes L. Implications of prenatal ultrasound screening in the incidence of major genitourinary malformations. J Urol. 2001;165:1677–80.
21. Lee J, Kimber C, Shekleton P, Cheng W. Prognostic factors of severe foetal megacystis. ANZ J Surg. 2010;81:552–5.
22. Morris RK, Quinlan-Jones E, Kilby MD, Khan KS. Systematic review of accuracy of fetal urine analysis to predict poor postnatal renal function in cases of congenital urinary tract obstruction. Prenat Diagn. 2007;27:900–11.
23. Ruano R. Fetal surgery for severe lower urinary tract obstruction. Prenat Diagn. 2011;31:667–74.
24. Morris RK, Malin GL, Khan KS, Kilby MD. Systematic review of the effectiveness of antenatal intervention for the treatment of congenital lower urinary tract obstruction. BJOG. 2010;117:382–90.
25. Robyr R, Benachi A, Daikha-Dahmane F, Martinovich J, Dumez Y, Ville Y. Correlation between ultrasound and anatomical findings in fetuses with lower urinary tract obstruction in the first half of pregnancy. Ultrasound Obstet Gynecol. 2005;25:478–82.
26. Harrison MR, Ross N, Noall R, de Lorimier AA. Correction of congenital hydronephrosis in utero. I. The model: fetal urethral obstruction produces hydronephrosis and pulmonary hypoplasia in fetal lambs. J Pediatr Surg. 1983;18:247–56.
27. Clark TJ, Martin WL, Divakaran TG, Whittle MJ, Kilby MD, Khan KS. Prenatal bladder drainage in the management of fetal lower urinary tract obstruction: a systematic review and meta-analysis. Obstet Gynecol. 2003;102:367–82.
28. Morris RK, Malin GL, Quinlan-Jones E, et al. Percutaneous vesicoamniotic shunting in Lower Urinary Tract Obstruction (PLUTO) Collaborative Group. Percutaneous vesicoamniotic shunting versus conservative management for fetal lower urinary tract obstruction (PLUTO): a randomised trial. Lancet. 2013;382:1496–506.
29. Kitagawa H, Pringle KC, Koike J, et al. Vesicoamniotic shunt for complete urinary tract obstruction is partially effective. J Pediatr Surg. 2006;41:394–402.

30. Berman DJ, Maizels M. The role of urinary obstruction in the genesis of renal dysplasia. A model in the chick embryo. J Urol. 1982;128:1091–6.
31. Aslam M. Watson AR; Trent & Anglia MCDK Study Group. Unilateral multicystic dysplastic kidney: long term outcomes. Arch Dis Child. 2006;91:820–3.
32. Ismaili K, Avni FE, Alexander M, Schulman C, Collier F, Hall M. Routine voiding cystourethrography is of no value in neonates with unilateral multicystic dysplastic kidney. J Pediatr. 2005;146:759–63.
33. Kuwertz-Broeking E, Brinkmann OA, Von Lengerke HJ, et al. Unilateral multicystic dysplastic kidney: experience in children. BJU Int. 2004;93:388–92.
34. Goyal A and Hennayake S. Routine voiding cystourethrogram in multicystic dysplastic kidney: Rationalising its use. Presented at British Association of Paediatric Surgeons, 54th Annual International Conference, Edinburgh, 2007.
35. Ulman I, Jayanthi VR, Koff SA. The long-term followup of newborns with severe unilateral hydronephrosis initially treated nonoperatively. J Urol. 2000;164:1101–5.
36. Gordon I, Dhillon HK, Gatanash H, Peters AM. Antenatal diagnosis of pelvic hydronephrosis: assessment of renal function and drainage as a guide to management. J Nucl Med. 1991;32:1649–54.
37. Fernbach SK, Maizels M, Conway JJ. Ultrasound grading of hydronephrosis: introduction to the system used by the Society of Fetal Urology. Pediatr Radiol. 1993;23:478–80.
38. Nguyen HT, Benson CB, Bromley B, et al. Multidisciplinary consensus on the classification of prenatal and postnatal urinary tract dilation (UTD classification system). J Pediatr Urol. 2014;10:982–98.
39. Policiano C, Djokovic D, Carvalho R, Monteiro C, Melo MA, Graça LM. Ultrasound antenatal detection of urinary tract anomalies in the last decade: outcome and prognosis. J Matern Fetal Neonatal Med. 2015;28:959–63.
40. Gordon I, Dhillon HK, Peters AM. Prenatally diagnosed hydronephrosis: the Great Ormond Street experience. Br J Urol. 1998;81(Suppl 2):39–44.
41. Dhillon HK. Antenatal diagnosis of renal pelvic dilatation--the natural history of conservative management. Pediatr Radiol. 1991;21:272–3.
42. Ransley PG, Dhillon HK, Gordon I, Duffy PG, Dillon MJ, Barratt TM. The postnatal management of hydronephrosis diagnosed by prenatal ultrasound. J Urol. 1990;144:584–7. discussion 593-4
43. AMK R. Urinary tract obstruction and dilatation in the newborn (Chapter 45). In: Rickham PP, Johnston JH, Lister J, Irvine IM, Irving IM, editors. Neonatal surgery. 3rd ed. Boston: Butterworth-Heinemann; 1990. p. 656–77.
44. Peters CA. Urinary tract obstruction in children. J Urol. 1995;154:1874–83.
45. Thornhill BA, Burt LA, Chen C, et al. Variable chronic partial ureteral obstruction in the neonatal rat: a new model of ureteropelvic junction obstruction. Kidney Int. 2005;67:42–52.
46. Grattan-Smith JD, Jones RA. MR urography: technique and results for the evaluation of urinary obstruction in the pediatric population. Magn Reson Imaging Clin N Am. 2008;16:643–60.
47. Sjöström S, Sillén U, Bachelard M, Hansson S, Stokland E. Spontaneous resolution of high grade infantile vesicoureteral reflux. J Urol. 2004;172:694–8. discussion 699
48. Upadhyay J, McLorie GA, Bolduc S, Bägli DJ, Khoury AE, Farhat W. Natural history of neonatal reflux associated with prenatal hydronephrosis: long-term results of a prospective study. J Urol. 2003;169:1837–41.
49. van Eerde AM, Meutgeert MH, de Jong TP, Giltay JC. Vesico-ureteral reflux in children with prenatally detected hydronephrosis: a systematic review. Ultrasound Obstet Gynecol. 2007;29:463–9.
50. Penido Silva JM, Oliveira EA, Diniz JS, Bouzada MC, Vergara RM, Souza BC. Clinical course of prenatally detected primary vesicoureteral reflux. Pediatr Nephrol. 2006;21:86–91.
51. Gordon AC, Thomas DFM, Arthur RJ, Irving HC, Smith SE. Prenatally Diagnosed Reflux: a follow–up study. Br J Urol. 1990;65:407–12.
52. Farhat W, McLorie G, Capolicchio G, et al. The natural history of neonatal vesicoureteral reflux associated with antenatal hydronephrosis. J Urol. 2000;164:1057–60.
53. Avni EF, Schulman CC. The origin of vesico-ureteric reflux in male newborns: further evidence in favour of a transient fetal urethral obstruction. Br J Urol. 1996;78:454–9.
54. Ismaili K, Avni FE, Hall M. Results of systematic voiding cystourethrography in infants with antenatally diagnosed renal pelvis dilation. J Pediatr. 2002;141:21–4.
55. Garin EH, Olavarria F, Garcia NV, et al. Clinical significance of primary vesicoureteral reflux and urinary antibiotic prophylaxis after acute pyelonephritis: a multicenter, randomized, controlled study. Pediatrics. 2006;117:626–32.
56. Evans K, Asimakadou M, Nwankwo O, et al. What is the risk of urinary tract infection in children with antenatally presenting dilating vesico-ureteric reflux? Pediatr Urol. 2015;11:93.e1–6.
57. Hodges SJ, Werle D, McLorie G, et al. Megaureter. ScientificWorldJournal. 2010;10:603–12.
58. Ranawaka R, Hennayake S. Resolution of primary non-refluxing megaureter: an observational study. J Pediatr Surg. 2013;48:380–3.
59. Shukla AR, Cooper J, Patel RP, et al. Prenatally detected primary megaureter: a role for extended followup. J Urol. 2005;173:1353–6.
60. Payabvash S, Kajbafzadeh AM, Tavangar SM, et al. Myocyte apoptosis in primary obstructive megaureters: the role of decreased vascular and neural supply. J Urol. 2007;178:259–64.

61. Shokeir AA, Nijman RJ. Primary megaureter: current trends in diagnosis and treatment. BJU Int. 2000;86:861–8.
62. Wilcox D, Mouriquand P. Management of megaureter in children. Eur Urol. 1998;34:73–8.
63. Chertin B, Pollack A, Koulikov D, et al. Long-term follow up of antenatally diagnosed megaureters. J Pediatr Urol. 2008;4:188–91.
64. Christman MS, Kasturi S, Lambert SM, et al. Endoscopic management and the role of double stenting for primary obstructive megaureters. J Urol. 2012;187:1018–22.
65. Farrugia MK, Steinbrecher HA, Malone PS. The utilization of stents in the management of primary obstructive megaureters requiring intervention before 1 year of age. J Pediatr Urol. 2011;7:198–202.
66. Carroll D, Chandran H, Joshi A, McCarthy LS, Parashar K. Endoscopic placement of double-J ureteric stents in children as a treatment for primary obstructive megaureter. Urol Ann. 2010;2:114–8.
67. Romero RM, Angulo JM, Parente A, Rivas S, Tardaguila AR. Primary obstructive megaureter: the role of high pressure balloon dilatation. J Endourol. 2014;28(5):517–23.
68. García-Aparicio L, Blázquez-Gómez E, Martin O, et al. Use of high-pressure balloon dilatation of the ureterovesical junction instead of ureteral reimplantation to treat primary obstructive megaureter: is it justified? J Pediatr Urol. 2013;9:1229–33.
69. Smeulders N, Yankovic F, Chippington S, Cherian A. Primary obstructive megaureter: cutting balloon endo-ureterotomy. J Pediatr Urol. 2013;9:692.e1–2
70. Lee SD, Akbal C, Kaefer M. Refluxing ureteral reimplant as temporary treatment of obstructive megaureter in neonate and infant. J Urol. 2005;173:1357–60.
71. Han MY, Gibbons MD, Belman AB, Pohl HG, Majd M, Rushton HG. Indications for nonoperative management of ureteroceles. J Urol. 2005;174:1652–5.
72. Jayanthi VR, Koff SA. Long-term outcome of transurethral puncture of ectopic ureteroceles: initial success and late problems. J Urol. 1999;162:1077–80.
73. Chertin B, Fridmans A, Hadas-Halpren I, Farkas A. Endoscopic puncture of ureterocele as a minimally invasive and effective long-term procedure in children. Eur Urol. 2001;39:332–6.
74. Smith C, Gosalbez R, Parrott TS, Woodard JR, Broecker B, Massad C. Transurethral puncture of ectopic ureteroceles in neonates and infants. J Urol. 1994;152:2110–2.
75. Castagnetti M, El-Ghoneimi A. Management of duplex system ureteroceles in neonates and infants. Nat Rev Urol. 2009;6:7–15.
76. de Jong TP, Dik P, Klijn AJ, Uiterwaal CS, van Gool JD. Ectopic ureterocele: results of open surgical therapy in 40 patients. J Urol. 2000;164:2040–3.
77. Prieto J, Ziada A, Baker L, Snodgrass W. Ureteroureterostomy via inguinal incision for ectopic ureters and ureteroceles without ipsilateral lower pole reflux. J Urol. 2009;181:1844–8.
78. Williams DI. Megacystis and Megaureter in children. Bull N Y Acad Med. 1959;35:317–27.
79. Paquin AJ Jr, Marshall VF, McGovern JH. The megacystis syndrome. J Urol. 1960;83:634–46.
80. Mandell J, Lebowitz RL, Peters CA, Estroff JA, Retik AB, Benacerraf BR. Prenatal diagnosis of megacystis-megaureter association. J Urol. 1992;148:1487–9.
81. Welch KJ, Steward W, Leibowitz RL. Non obstructive megacystis and refluxing megaureter in preteen enuretic boys with minimal symptoms. J Urol. 1975;114:449–54.
82. Willi UV, Lebowitz RL. The so-called megaureter-megacystis syndrome. AJR Am J Roentgenol. 1979;133:409–16.
83. Angotti R, Lewis MA, Goyal A. Megacystis megaureter syndrome: 20 years experience. Presented at annual meeting of the European Society for Pediatric Urology 2014.
84. Lloyd JC, Wiener JS, Gargollo PC, Inman BA, Ross SS, Routh JC. Contemporary epidemiological trends in complex congenital genitourinary anomalies. J Urol. 2013;190:1590–5.
85. Lewis MA, Shaw J, Sinha MD, et al. UK Renal Registry 12th Annual Report (December 2009): Chapter 14: demography of the UK paediatric renal replacement therapy population in 2008. Nephron Clin Pract. 2010(115):c279–88.
86. Kupferman JC, Stewart CL, Kaskel FJ, Fine RN. Posterior urethral valves in patients with Down syndrome. Pediatr Nephrol. 1996;10:143–6.
87. Kupferman JC, Druschel CM, Kupchik GS. Increased prevalence of renal and urinary tract anomalies in children with Down syndrome. Pediatrics. 2009;124:e615–21.
88. Young HH, Frontz WA, Baldwin JC. Congenital obstruction of the posterior urethra. J Urol. 1919;3:289.
89. Dewan PA, Keenan RJ, Morris LL, Le Quesne GW. Congenital urethral obstruction: Cobb's collar or prolapsed congenital obstructive posterior urethral membrane (COPUM). Br J Urol. 1994;73:91–5.
90. Malin G, Tonks AM, Morris RK, Gardosi J, Kilby MD. Congenital lower urinary tract obstruction: a population-based epidemiological study. BJOG. 2012;119:1455–64.
91. Mandal S, Goel A, Kumar M, et al. Use of holmium: YAG laser in posterior urethral valves: Another method of fulguration. J Pediatr Urol. 2013;9:1093–7.
92. Bhatnagar V, Agarwala S, Lal R, Mitra DK. Fulguration of posterior urethral valves using the Nd: YAG laser. Pediatr Surg Int. 2000;16:69–71.
93. Koff SA, Mutabagani KH, Jayanthi VR. The valve bladder syndrome: pathophysiology and treatment with nocturnal bladder emptying. J Urol. 2002;167:291–7.
94. Capitanucci ML, Marciano A, Zaccara A, La Sala E, Mosiello G, De Gennaro M. Long-term bladder function followup in boys with posterior urethral

valves: comparison of noninvasive vs invasive urodynamic studies. J Urol. 2012;188:953–7.
95. De Gennaro M, Capitanucci ML, Mosiello G, Caione P, Silveri M. The changing urodynamic pattern from infancy to adolescence in boys with posterior urethral valves. BJU Int. 2000;85:1104–8.
96. Dinneen MD, Duffy PG, Barratt TM, Ransley PG. Persistent polyuria after posterior urethral valves. Br J Urol. 1995;75:236–40.
97. Smith GH, Canning DA, Schulman SL, Snyder HM 3rd, Duckett JW. The long-term outcome of posterior urethral valves treated with primary valve ablation and observation. J Urol. 1996;155:1730–4.
98. DeFoor W, Clark C, Jackson E, Reddy P, Minevich E, Sheldon C. Risk factors for end stage renal disease in children with posterior urethral valves. J Urol. 2008;180:1705–8.
99. Woodhouse CR, Reilly JM, Bahadur G. Sexual function and fertility in patients treated for posterior urethral valves. J Urol. 1989;142:586–8.
100. Taskinen S, Heikkilä J, Santtila P, Rintala R. Posterior urethral valves and adult sexual function. BJU Int. 2012;110:E392–6.
101. Caione P, Nappo SG. Posterior urethral valves: long-term outcome. Pediatr Surg Int. 2011;27:1027–35.
102. Jalkanen J, Heikkilä J, Kyrklund K, Taskinen S. Controlled outcomes for achievement of urinary continence among boys treated for posterior urethral valves. J Urol. 2016;196:213–8.

Renal Cystic Disease and Vascular Lesions of the Adrenal and Kidney

66

Kelvin K.W. Liu and Michael W.Y. Leung

Abstract

Multicystic dysplastic kidney (MCDK) is the most common renal cystic disease in neonates. Autosomal recessive polycystic kidney disease (ARPKD) is an uncommon condition that can present in utero or early infantile period. Autosomal dominant polycystic kidney disease (ADPKD) and solitary renal cyst are rarely seen in newborns. Localized adrenal haemorrhage may occur in infants but massive haemorrhage is rare and is often confined to newborn. Renal vein thrombosis leading to haemorrhagic infarction has become much less common due to improved perinatal management. Renal artery thrombosis and stenosis are the main causes of renovascular hypertension in neonate

Keywords

Renal cystic disease • Adrenal lesions • Adrenal haemorrhage • Renal vein thrombosis • Renovascular hypertension • Management • Outcomes

66.1 Renal Cystic Disease

Multicystic dysplastic kidney (MCDK) is the most common renal cystic disease in neonates. Autosomal recessive polycystic kidney disease (ARPKD) is an uncommon condition that can present in utero or early infantile period. Autosomal dominant polycystic kidney disease (ADPKD) and solitary renal cyst are rarely seen in newborns.

66.1.1 Multicystic Dysplastic Kidney

Multicystic dysplastic kidney (MCDK) was first described by Schwarz in an infant with kidney replaced by a "bunch of grapes" [1] (Fig. 66.1). The incidence of MCDK is about 1 in 4000 live births with a male to female ratio of 3:2 [2, 3]. Left MCDK is slightly more common. Bilateral MCDK occurs in about 20% of cases leading to fetal loss, stillbirth

K.K.W. Liu, MBBCh, FRCS(Glas), FRACS, FRCS(Ed) (✉)
Division of Paediatric Surgery, Department of Surgery, United Christian Hospital, Hong Kong, China

M.W.Y. Leung, MBChB, FRCS(Ed, Paed), FCSHK
Division of Paediatric Surgery, Department of Surgery, Queen Elizabeth Hospital, Hong Kong, China
e-mail: liukwk@ha.org.hk

P.D. Losty et al. (eds.), *Rickham's Neonatal Surgery*, https://doi.org/10.1007/978-1-4471-4721-3_66

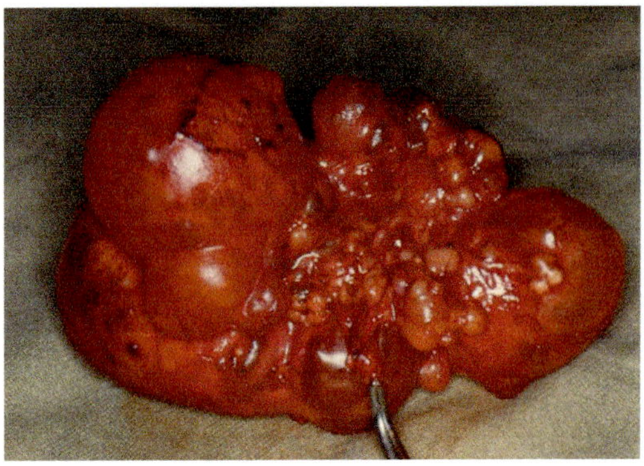

Fig. 66.1 Multicystic dysplastic kidney

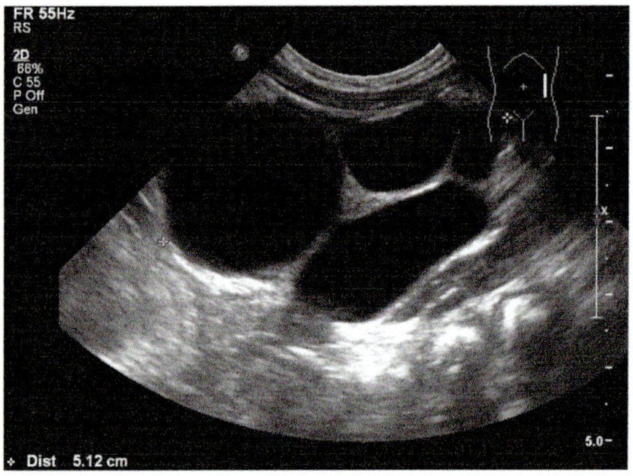

Fig. 66.2 Multicystic dysplastic kidney with almost complete replacement of renal parenchyma with cysts (Courtesy of Dr. Sunny Tse)

or early neonatal death as a result of oligohydramnios, pulmonary hypoplasia and renal failure [4].

66.1.1.1 Pathogenesis

MCDK is a variant of renal dysplasia. According to the ureteric bud theory of Mackie and Stephens, MCDK may be a consequence of abnormal induction of metanephric mesenchyme by the ureteric bud [5]. It is also hypothesized that MCDK can be caused by urinary tract obstruction during early gestational period [6].

Most MCDK occurs sporadically although familial occurrence has been reported. The *EYA1, SIX1 and PAX2* genes play important roles in ureteric bud development [7]. Mutations of these genes have been identified in Branchio-oto-renal syndrome and renal-coloboma syndrome associated with renal dysplasia [8–10]. In utero viral infections including cytomegalovirus may be associated with MCDK development [11].

66.1.1.2 Clinical Presentation and Diagnosis

Prenatal diagnosis by fetal ultrasound is the most common presentation of MCDK. Next to hydronephrosis, MCDK is the second most common aetiology of incidentally palpable abdominal mass in neonates. The two diagnoses can be differentiated by postnatal ultrasonography. The sonographic appearance of MCDK consists of haphazardly arranged multiple non-communicating cysts with variable size, separated by hyperechoic dysplastic stroma (Fig. 66.2). There is no pelvicaliceal structure. Atresia of the ureter can occur. When an isotope mercaptoacetyltriglycine (MAG3) dynamic diuresis renography or dimercaptosuccinic acid (DMSA) scintigraphy is performed, MCDK is non-functional and can be distinguished from other causes of hydronephrotic kidney (Fig. 66.3).

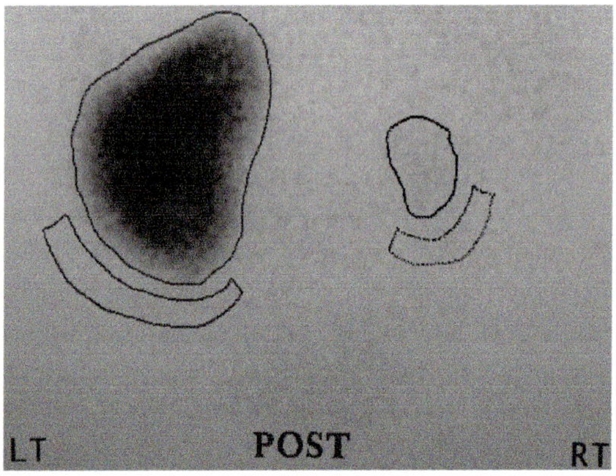

Fig. 66.3 Non functioning right kidney demonstrated on DMSA

The contralateral kidney can be abnormal. Vesicoureteric reflux (VUR) occurs in 4–43% of patients and pelviureteric junction (PUJ) obstruction can be found in up to 15% of cases [12–15]. As the contralateral kidney is the only functioning unit, its management is crucial. Micturition cystourethrography (MCUG) should be considered in MCDK patients [16]. Fortunately, majority of contralateral VUR is of low grade with tendency of spontaneous resolution [17].

66.1.1.3 Natural History

Less than 20% of prenatally diagnosed MCDK is clinically palpable [14]. Without antenatal detection, most patients with MCDK can be asymptomatic. Outcome of MCDK is variable. Spontaneous involution of MCDK can occur in up to 60% of patients, after a period of few months to 10 years [18, 19]. The involution velocity is higher in infancy period [20]. Small size of MCDK (<6 cm length) and presence of compensatory hypertrophy of contralateral kidney are positive predictors for complete involution [21, 22].

Urinary tract infection (UTI) is not common in MCDK as the associated ureteric atresia prevents ascending infection. The US National Multicystic Kidney Registry reported a UTI prevalence of 4.6% in 5 years follow-up [14].

The risk of developing hypertension is low in patients with MCDK. In a systemic review, Narchi reported six cases of hypertension developed in 1115 children [23]. Other series also suggested that the risk of hypertension development is lower than 3% on long term follow-up [14, 24]. Once hypertension has developed, conversion to normal blood pressure after nephrectomy can occur in only about one-third of cases [2, 25].

Concerning the risk of malignant change, there are case reports of Wilms tumour in patients with MCDK [26, 27]. The non-involuted intervening stroma of dysplastic kidney may be a focus for malignant degeneration. The higher prevalence of nodular renal blastema in these patients comparing with the general population may be related to the development of Wilms tumour [28]. However, in a systemic review of 26 studies for 1041 children with MCDK, none developed Wilms tumour [29]. Renal cell carcinoma and transitional cell carcinoma have been reported in adults with MCDK [30–32].

In conclusion, most children with unilateral MCDK do not have any long term consequences. However, the patients and parents should be informed of the implications of only one functioning kidney for lifetime.

66.1.1.4 Treatment

The role of nephrectomy in MCDK is controversial. In general, nephrectomy may need to be considered in cases of enlarged renal mass, persistent symptoms such as pain, development of complications including UTI or hypertension, suspicion of malignancy, concomitant surgery and poor compliance to long term follow-up. With recent advances in minimal invasive surgery, laparoscopic nephrectomy can be performed from either trans-peritoneal or retro-peritoneal route with evolution to single port operation [33, 34] (Fig. 66.4).

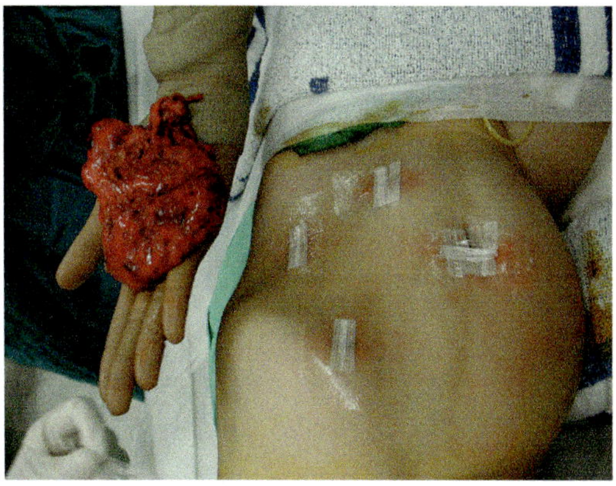

Fig. 66.4 Multicystic dysplastic kidney removed via trans-peritoneal laparoscopy

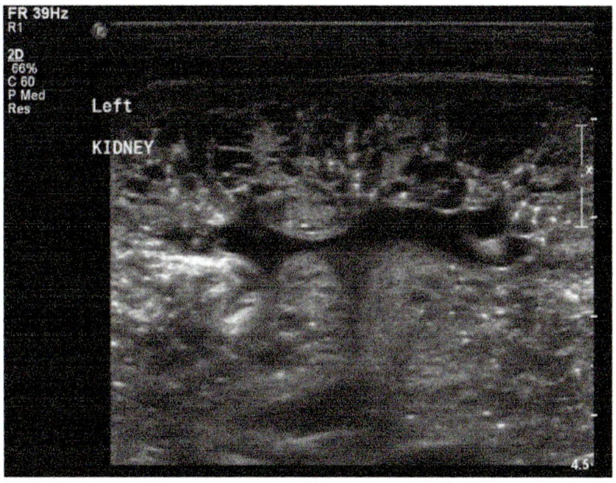

Fig. 66.5 Multiple cysts in autosomal recessive polycystic kidney (Courtesy of Dr. Sunny Tse)

66.1.2 Autosomal Recessive Polycystic Kidney Disease

Autosomal recessive polycystic kidney disease (ARPKD) occurs one in 10,000–40,000 live births [35]. It is previously also known as infantile polycystic kidney disease which is not an accurate terminology as some patients can present at late childhood [36]. A single gene, *Polycystic Kidney and Hepatic Disease 1 (PKHD1)*, mutation on chromosome 6p was identified to account for the disease [37]. The disease affects both kidneys and liver invariably, characterized by the cystic changes of renal collecting tubules and congenital hepatic fibrosis (CHF) [38] (Fig. 66.5). Age of presentation and severity of renal symptoms depend on the number of abnormally dilated collecting ducts involved [39]. Antenatal diagnosis of bilateral renal masses, oligohydramnios and Potter sequence is common [40]. In neonates, patients will present with bilateral flank masses, impaired renal function and respiratory insufficiency. Neonatal death is usually caused by pulmonary complications. More than 70% of patients can survive beyond neonatal period, with progression to end stage renal disease and hypertension. The renal collecting tubules are affected, resulting in polyuria and polydipsia [41]. For long term survivors, hepatic manifestation as a result of CHF by abnormal ductal plate development will cause symptoms of hepatosplenomegaly, cholangitis, portal hypertension and oesophageal variceal bleeding [39].

Postnatal USG should be performed in neonates suspicious of ARPKD. Bilateral homogenously enlarged kidneys are seen with hyperechogenicity and poor corticomedullary differentiation. Renal cysts are small in neonates, different from those in MCDK and autosomal dominant polycystic kidney disease (ADPKD) [42]. Macrocysts are more common in older patients [43]. Hepatic parenchymal hyperechoic texture, cyst formation and occasionally intrahepatic ductal dilatation resembling Caroli's disease are found. If portal hypertension develops in juvenile period, splenomegaly and reverse hepatic venous flow can be demonstrated. If USG findings are equivocal, more sensitive imaging studies including computed tomography (CT) and magnetic resonance imaging (MRI), should be considered [44].

Treatment of ARPKD is mainly supportive. Recent advances in neonatal intensive care especially ventilation support decrease neonatal mortality from pulmonary hypoplasia. Patients will require treatment for chronic renal failure and hypertension. As the patients grow older, treatment for hepatic complications such as portal hypertension are necessary.

66.1.3 Autosomal Dominant Polycystic Kidney Disease

Autosomal dominant polycystic kidney disease (ADPKD) is the most common inherited human renal disease affecting one in 400–1000 people [45]. The age of onset is usually in third to fifth decades. Neonatal and early infantile presentations can occur that are not clinically distinguishable from ARPKD [46].

In 85–90% of patients with ADPKD, mutation of *PKD1* gene on chromosome 16p occurs [45]. Mutation of *PKD2* gene on chromosome 4q is found in rest of cases [47].

Extra-renal cysts in liver and pancreas, cardiac and cerebral manifestations are rare in neonates. USG may show enlarged hyperechoic kidneys, presence of macrocysts and increased corticomedullary differentiation [48]. Similar to ARPKD, management of early onset ADPKD is mainly supportive.

66.1.4 Solitary Renal Cysts

Contrary to adult population, solitary renal cyst is uncommon in children and extremely rare in neonates. It can occur sporadically or exist in patients with urinary tract obstruction such as posterior urethral valve [49]. USG is useful to differentiate it from other neonatal renal cystic diseases and hydronephrosis. Treatment of isolated solitary renal cyst is usually conservative. Image guided percutaneous aspiration of cysts had been reported in symptomatic children with loin pain [50].

66.2 Vascular Lesions of the Adrenal and Kidney

66.2.1 Adrenal Haemorrhage

The adrenal gland is vulnerable to haemorrhage due to its large size and high vascularity [51, 52].

Localized adrenal haemorrhage may occur in infants and children under stress [53, 54]. This condition is more frequently seen in term infants delivered vaginally [51, 55–57]. Massive adrenal haemorrhage, however, is much rarer and is often confined to newborns [58].

66.2.1.1 Aetiology

Birth trauma, prolonged labor, intrauterine infection, perinatal asphyxia or hypoxia, large birth weight, septicaemia, haemorrhagic disorder and hypothrombinemia are the most common predisposing causes of adrenal haemorrhage [52, 53, 56, 59]. In term infants, it is often related to large size following a difficult and traumatic delivery whereas in premature infants, perinatal hypoxia is often the predisposing cause. However it can also occur spontaneously [59]. Prenatal occurrence has also been documented [60].

66.2.1.2 Clinical Features

Clinical features vary depending on the amount of blood lost. The most common clinical presentations are persistent jaundice and flank mass [51, 52, 56, 57, 61]. However, adrenal haemorrhage may also present with scrotal haematoma, anaemia, adrenal insufficiency, shock [51, 55, 56, 59, 62], and as an incidental finding [63]. Macroscopic haematuria can occur if there is associated vascular lesion affecting the kidney. Breakdown of the red blood cells in haematoma causes jaundice. Adrenal insufficiency due to adrenal haemorrhage is rare [51, 52, 56, 57, 63] and is usually seen in premature infants [64]. As the adrenal gland has a considerable regenerative capacity, most adrenal haemorrhage is not associated with significant adrenal insufficiency. When adrenal insufficiency occurs, prematurity and severe underlying diseases such as sepsis, disseminated intravascular coagulation, perinatal hypoxia and intraventricular haemorrhage are also potential causes. Cytokine-related suppression of adrenocorticotropic hormone or cortisol synthesis, inadequate perfusion of the adrenal gland, a limited adrenocortical reserve or immaturity of the hypothalamic-pituitaryadrenal axis may also contribute to the development of adrenal insufficiency [65].

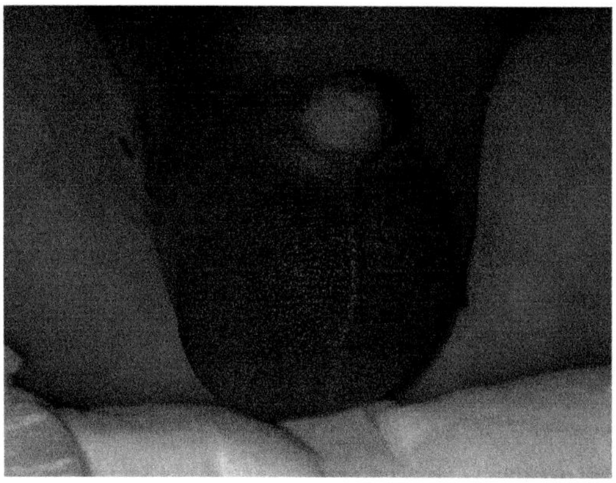

Fig. 66.6 Acute bluish discolouration and swelling of the right scrotum

Adrenal haemorrhage may present with swelling and bluish discoloration of the scrotum [51, 55, 56, 59, 62, 66] (Fig. 66.6). When adrenal haemorrhage occurs with rupture of the capsule, blood can easily reach the scrotum via the patent processus vaginalis or along the retroperitoneum [55, 62]. Swelling and discoloration of the scrotum in newborns may arise from other disorders, including torsion of the testis, epididymitis, scrotal or testicular edema, strangulated inguinal hernia and meconium peritonitis. Ultrasonography of the abdomen and scrotum should be performed in infants with scrotal swelling and ecchymosis to exclude adrenal haemorrhage [62]. If differential diagnosis between adrenal haemorrhage and torsion of the testis cannot be established, nuclear scanning or color Doppler analysis is required [62]. The right adrenal gland is the frequent (38–100%) site of adrenal haemorrhage [51–53, 55–57, 63]. This may be related to the direct drainage of the right adrenal vein into the inferior vena cava thus exposing the gland to the raised intravenous pressure that may occur during birth compression. Frequencies of 8–38% for bilateral adrenal haemorrhage have been reported [53, 56].

66.2.1.3 Diagnosis

Differential diagnosis of adrenal haemorrhage includes adrenal abscess, cystic neuroblastoma, cortical renal cyst, obstructed upper cortical renal cyst and an obstructed upper moiety of a duplicated kidney [67]. Measurement of urinary vanil-

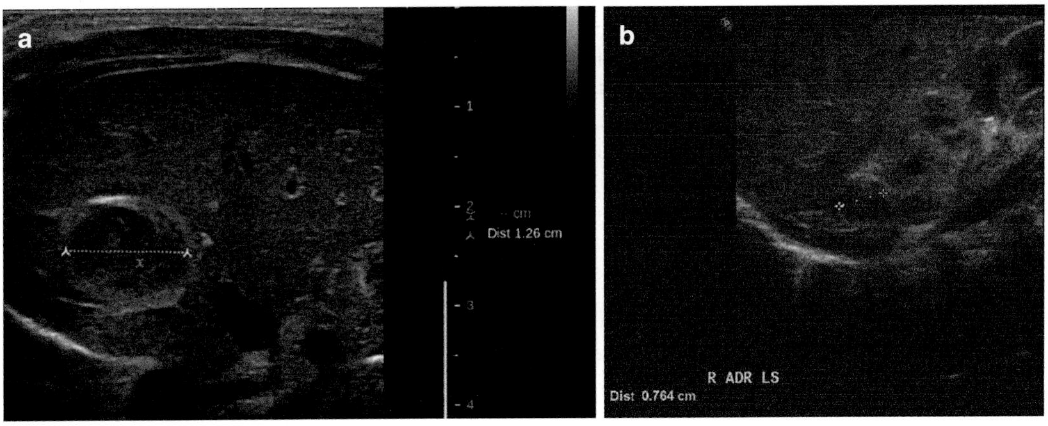

Fig. 66.7 Adrenal haemorrhage in a neonate (Courtesy of Professor Winnie Chu). Predominately cystic lesion with internal echoes over the right adrenal region. Interval reduction in size of the cystic lesion appearing more homogeneous and anechoic after 3 months

lylmandelic acid (VMA) levels assists in the differentiation of adrenal haemorrhage from neuroblastoma. The ultrasonographic appearance of adrenal haemorrhage depends on the age of haematoma, and this gradually resolves with time [61]. Diagnosis and follow-up of adrenal haemorrhage using ultrasonography is the most effective modality and avoids unnecessary laparotomy. Serial ultrasonography can demonstrate decrease in size and echogenity (Fig. 66.7), multiloculated cystic mass, calcifications and complete resolution of adrenal haemorrhage [55, 68]. Adrenal haemorrhage usually resolves between 3 weeks to 6 months [55–57, 59, 61]. For the case of neuroblastoma, the lesion remains solid in appearance and may enlarge over several weeks [51, 52]. In patients suggestive of adrenal insufficiency, cortisol and adrenocorticotropic hormone (ACTH) are measured and ACTH provocative test is performed. Rarely, adrenal haemorrhage may be associated with renal vein thrombosis. This may be due to the connection between the two venous systems or the same causative factor affecting both organs. It is therefore worthwhile to do imaging study to determine if the kidney has been affected by similar vascular lesion.

66.2.1.4 Treatment

Most cases of adrenal haemorrhage can be managed conservatively particularly in term infants. Occasionally blood transfusion for hypovolaemia, antibiotics for sepsis and hormonal treatment for bilateral involvement may be required. Most cases treated conservatively usually resolve with time. Occasionally the haematoma may calcify [69] and rarely becomes infected [70]. Surgery is seldom indicated except for dangerously high level of serum bilirubin or very extensive haemorrhage. Late sequelae of adrenal haemorrhage are uncommon.

66.2.2 Renal Vein Thrombosis

Renal vein thrombosis (RVT) leading to haemorrhagic infarction of the kidney was first described by Rayer [71] in 1837. It is predominantly a disease of the paediatric age group, primarily newborn infants [72, 73]. Between 60 and 75% of the cases are observed in the first month of life [72, 73] and about one third of all cases are diagnosed in the first week. Male infants are slightly more often affected than female. The number of surviving patients has increased, but at the same time, late complications are now being recognized with greater frequency [74–79].

66.2.2.1 Pathogenesis

It is now believed that the thrombus starts in an arcuate or interlobular vein, and it may spread in both directions to involve the renal cortex and to occlude the main renal vein [80]. The thrombus may extend into the vena cava. However, spread to involve the contralateral kidney is unusual. Bilateral renal involvements are usually caused by thrombi arising from each kidney. Microthrombi found in small caliber veins of other organs in young infants support a generalized disease.

66.2.2.2 Aetiology

RVT occasionally occurs in previously well babies but dehydration has been implicated most commonly [73, 81, 82]. Infants of diabetic mothers seem to be susceptible [83, 84], and it has been observed as a complication of congenital heart disease, nephrotic syndrome, acute blood loss, sepsis, shock, or asphyxia at birth [85]. These associated factors together with the sluggish perfusion in the neonatal kidney and the relative polycythaemia render the neonate susceptible to RVT [73, 82].

66.2.2.3 Clinical Manifestations

RVT has a wide range of clinical manifestations. The complex of flank mass, gross haematuria, and thrombocytopenia should always alert the possibility of RVT. Swelling and cyanosis of the legs are indicative of thrombus within the inferior vena cava. Bilateral loin swellings, severe oliguria, anuria and azotaemia suggest bilateral renal involvement. In the first month of life, haematuria has been reported in 64% of cases and in older children in 49% [73]. Vomiting, diarrhea, pallor, cyanosis or shock, and the clinical signs of metabolic acidosis, occur in some infants. Prenatal RVT is a less common entity and has been found incidentally on prenatal imaging [86, 87].

Although the biochemical findings can vary greatly, decreased renal function is usually indicated by an increase in serum creatinine and blood urea nitrogen concentrations. At the same time, the serum bicarbonate level is decreased. The level of plasma potassium is significantly increased in about one third of the patients. The serum sodium level is variable, ranging from normal to high or low concentrations.

Renal venous thrombosis can sometimes be confused with hydronephrosis or a tumour within the kidney or adjacent tissues. Although rare in infants, a mesoblastic nephroma or hamartoma is an important differential diagnostic consideration. Furthermore, neuroblastoma and cystic disease of the kidneys are also palpated as abdominal masses in the newborn period.

66.2.2.4 Diagnosis

The clinical diagnosis of RVT can be supported by ultrasonographic and radiologic examinations. The plain film of the abdomen may show enlarged renal outlines. Ultrasonography is the technique most commonly used in the evaluation of neonates with suspected RVT [88]. The ultrasound appearances depend on the stage at which the examination is performed and the extent of the thrombus. Initially the thrombi in the peripheral small renal veins appear as highly echogenic streaks which only persist for a few days. In the first week the affected kidney swells and becomes echogenic with prominent echopoor medullary pyramids. Later, the swelling increases and the kidney becomes heterogenous with loss of corticomedullary differentiation. Grey scale ultrasound readily demonstrates thrombus within the renal vein and inferior vena cava. Colour Doppler may demonstrate absent intrarenal and renal venous flow in the early stages of RVT. Computed tomography (CT) can demonstrate both renal anatomy and function and is of help in the evaluation of a thrombotic process within the kidney [89]. Renal scintigraphy that measures glomerular filtration rate and renal plasma flow have been used in newborn infants to diagnose RVT and to estimate the renal function in the initial assessment and in monitoring upon the return of function during therapy. Tc-99 m mercaptoacetyltriglycine (MAG3) renal scintigraphy provides superior images because of its greater extraction and faster clearance and this is especially helpful in the neonates who inherently have immature renal function [90]. Similarly, renal nuclear magnetic resonance may be useful in evaluating the kidney, and particularly RVT. This technique demonstrates the anatomy, as well as the function, of the kidney and also any disease in the retroperitoneum. The intravenous pyelogram (IVP) in many cases shows no or minimal function on one side while the other functions normally. Because of rather nonspecific and inconclusive findings, an IVP is of limited value in acute RVT. Renal angiography is an invasive study and is seldom required nowadays in the diagnosis of RVT.

66.2.2.5 Treatment

All children with RVT should be treated medically in the acute phase. Immediate treatment consists of correction of shock, metabolic acidosis, anaemia, sepsis, and cyanosis with or without hypoxia. Normal hydration must be achieved as soon as possible. If azotemia is present, fluid administration should be calculated to avoid overload. Anticoagulant therapy is still controversial [91, 92] Since extensive thrombosis is almost always present by the time of diagnosis, the usefulness of heparin is in doubt. Heparin probably should be used if RVT is diagnosed early [92] and in cases with evidence of intravascular coagulation or bilateral disease. If there is complete renal shutdown or the patient's condition deteriorates, early dialysis is beneficial. Haemodialysis is rarely used except in older patients with anuria. Surgery has only limited value in the treatment of RVT. Neither exploration of the kidney nor nephrectomy should be performed during the acute phase because the prognosis is generally favorable. Surgical intervention may be necessary in bilateral RVT, which usually also involves the inferior vena cava. Patients have recovered after thrombectomy [93], but even spontaneous recovery is known. Any other surgical procedure should be delayed for at least 4–6 months, when damage to the kidney can be defined more clearly after complete reevaluation and the appropriate procedure can be selected. Nephrectomy may be necessary for secondary complications such as hypertension, frequent infections of an atrophic kidney, or nephrotic syndrome.

66.2.2.6 Late Sequelae

Although the majority of neonates who receive supportive treatment can survive, structural or functional renal abnormalities are found in up to 90% of survivors [74–79]. Recanalization of occluded vessels or development of extensive collateral circulation may explain the functional recovery. There is a wide spectrum of complications including renal atrophy, renal tubular defects, growth retardation and hypertension. Hypertension seems to develop in only a few cases [74, 76]. It is usually accompanied by a high plasma renin level and is practically always relieved by nehrectomy. Recognition of these complications is important because early treatment can avoid many disturbing or debilitating diseases. The nephrotic syndrome has been diagnosed in older children with history of RVT. Present evidence favors the theory that the nephrotic syndrome is a precondition for the development of renal venous thrombosis rather than its late sequelae [94].

66.2.3 Renovascular Hypertension in Neonate

Hypertension in neonate may be seen in up to 2% of all infants cared for in neonatal intensive care unit [95]. It is increasingly recognized because of improved techniques of measurement and monitoring. Defining what is considered a normal blood pressure in newborn infants is a complex task. Studies in both term and preterm infants have demonstrated that blood pressure in neonates increases with both gestational and post-conceptual age, as well as with birth weight [95–97]. An infant's blood pressure is considered to be elevated if it falls above the upper limit of the 95% confidence interval for infants of similar gestational or post-conceptual age, size and gender.

The causes of hypertension in neonates are numerous, with the two largest categories being renovascular and other renal parenchymal diseases [98, 99]. Renal artery thrombosis accounts for 75% of cases of neonatal hypertension and renal artery stenosis for a further 18% [100]. Other renovascular problems may also lead to neonatal hypertension including renal vein thrombosis and diseases involving the renal artery either by direct involvement such as mid-aortic coarctation [101], idiopathic arterial calcification [102], congenital rubella infection [103], renal artery aneurysm [104], renal artery embolism [105], or by compression of the renal artery such as hydronephrotic kidneys and other abdominal masses.

Although apparently spontaneous renal artery thrombosis has been reported [106], majority of cases occur as a consequence of umbilical artery catheterization used in the management of critically ill infants. A clear association between use of umbilical arterial catheters and development of arterial thrombi was first reported by Neal et al. [107] The association between umbilical arterial catheter-associated thrombi and the development of neonatal hypertension was confirmed by others [108, 109] though the rate of thrombus formation has been much lower than that reported by Neal. Thus, it is possible that the cause of hypertension in such cases is related to thrombus formation at the time of line placement, probably related to disruption of the vascular endothelium of the umbilical artery. Such thrombi may then embolize to the kidneys, causing areas of infarction and increased renin release. Isolated renal arterial stenosis is mainly caused by fibromuscular dysplasia. Although the main renal artery may appear fairly normal on angiography but there may be significant branch vessel disease that can cause severe hypertension [110].

66.2.3.1 Clinical Presentation and Diagnostic Approach

In many infants, hypertension will be discovered on routine monitoring of vital signs. However, other classic presentations of neonatal hypertension have been described. Congestive heart failure and cardiogenic shock represent life-threatening consequences of hypertension [111]. In the less acutely ill infant, feeding difficulties, unexplained tachypnea, apnea, lethargy, irritability, or seizures may constitute symptoms of unsuspected hypertension. In older infants unexplained irritability or failure to thrive may be the only manifestations of hypertension. In case of renal artery thrombosis, haematuria, azotaemia and proteinuria are the cardinal features. It is important that blood pressure is being measured accurately so that hypertension will be correctly identified. In most acutely ill neonates, blood pressure is usually monitored directly via an indwelling arterial catheter either in the radial or umbilical artery. Automated, oscillometric devices are less invasive and the more common alternative method of blood pressure measurement in most NICUs.

The correct cause of neonatal hypertension is usually suggested by careful history and physical examination. Relevant laboratory tests and diagnostic studies are then performed to confirm/exclude other non-renovascular causes. Determination of plasma renin activity is frequently performed in the assessment of neonates with hypertension. Although renal arterial stenosis and thromboembolic phenomenon are typically considered high renin forms of hypertension, a peripheral renin level may not be elevated in some infants despite the presence of significant underlying pathology. Selective renin level may yield more accurate information. Ultrasound and Doppler sonography should be performed and may detect potential correctable causes of hypertension such as renal vein thrombosis, renal artery thrombosis and renal artery stenosis. Renal scintigraphy may demonstrate abnormalities of renal perfusion. For infants with extremely severe blood pressure elevation, angiography may be necessary. A formal angiogram offers the most accurate method of diagnosing renal arterial stenosis, particularly given the high incidence of intrarenal branch vessel disease in children with fibromuscular dysplasia [110]. In extremely small infants, it may be appropriate to defer angiography, managing the hypertension medically until the baby is large enough for an angiogram to be performed safely. Because of the invasiveness of conventional renal angiography, magnetic resonance angiography has been reported by some to be of use in evaluation of renovascular cause of neonatal hypertension [111, 112]. Similarly, computed tomography angiography has been reported to be of help in the diagnosis of renovascular hypertension [113, 114] (Fig. 66.8).

66.2.3.2 Treatment

Immediate and urgent treatment consists of correction of hypertension. An antihypertensive agent should be chosen that is most appropriate for the specific clinical situation. For the majority of acutely ill infants, particularly those with severe hypertension, continuous intravenous

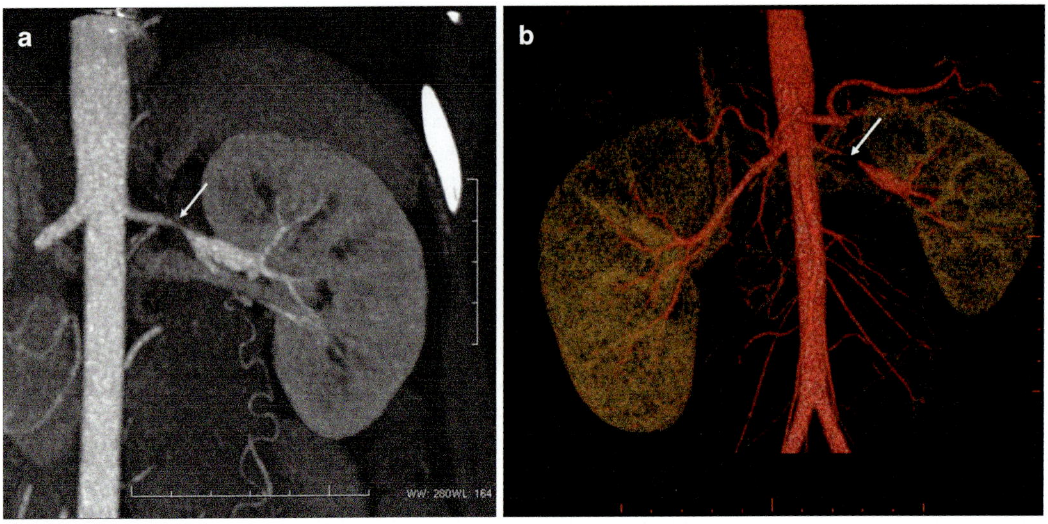

Fig. 66.8 Renovascular hypertension caused by renal artery stenosis (Courtesy of Professor Winnie Chu). (**a**) Coronal Reformat Contrast enhanced CT shows a focal stenosis (*arrow*) at the proximal left renal artery. (**b**) 3D volume rendering renal arteriogram shows again left renal artery stenosis (*arrow*) and relative smaller size of the left kidney when compared with the normal right side

infusion is the most appropriate approach. It is important to avoid too rapid a reduction in blood pressure [110] to avoid cerebral ischemia and hemorrhage, a problem that premature infants in particular are at increased risk. Surgery is indicated for treatment of neonatal hypertension due to renovascular cause in selected cases. For infants with renal arterial stenosis, it may be necessary to manage the infant medically until it has grown sufficiently to undergo definitive repair of the vascular abnormalities [115, 116]. Surgical reconstructive procedures include surgical dilatation, renal artery resection and reanastomosis, autologous or synthetic bypass grafts and autotransplantation. Good long term results have been reported but may sometimes result in primary or secondary nephrectomy [117, 118]. Percutaneous transluminal angioplasty for renal artery stenosis has been proven to be safe and effective in older children [119]. Generally good results outweigh the risks of recurrent stenosis and the rare but severe complications of dissection, rupture, bleeding, occlusion and aneurysm formation [119, 120]. Its successful use in neonate has also been reported [121]. For cases of severe hypertension with poor response to medical therapy, nephrectomy may have to be performed [122]. For cases of renal artery thrombosis that fail to respond to medical therapy, nephrectomy has to be performed as a lifesaving intervention [123, 124].

References

1. Schwartz J. An unusual unilateral multicystic kidney in an infant. J Urol. 1936;36:259.
2. Gordon AC, Thomas DFM, Arthur RJ, et al. Multicystic dysplastic kidney: is nephrectomy still appropriate? J Urol. 1988;140:1231–4.
3. Robson WL, Leung AK, Thomason MA. Multicystic dysplasia of the kidney. Clin Pediatr (Phila). 1995;34:32–40.
4. Al-Khaldi N, Watson AR, Zuccollo J, Twining P, Rose DH. Outcome of antenatally detected cystic dysplastic kidney disease. Arch Dis Child. 1994;70:520–2.
5. Mackie GG, Stephens FD. Duplex kidneys: a correlation of renal dysplasia with position of the ureteral orifice. J Urol. 1975;114:274–80.
6. Peters CA, Carr MC, Lais A, Retik AB, Mandell J. The response of the fetal kidney to obstruction. J Urol. 1992;148:503–9.
7. Murawski IJ, Gupta IR. Vesicoureteric reflux and renal malformations: a developmental problem. Clin Genet. 2006;69:105–17.
8. Buller C, Xu X, Marquis V, Schwanke R, Xu PX. Molecular effects of Eya1 domain mutations causing organ defects in BOR syndrome. Hum Mol Genet. 2001;10:2775–81.

9. Ruf RG, Xu PX, Silvius D, et al. SIX1 mutations cause branchio-oto-renal syndrome by disruption of EYA1-SIX1-DNA complexes. Proc Natl Acad Sci U S A. 2004;101:8090–5.
10. Amiel J, Audollent S, Joly D, et al. PAX2 mutations in renal-coloboma syndrome: mutational hotspot and germline mosaicism. Eur J Hum Genet. 2000;8:820–6.
11. Chan M, Hecht JL, Boyd T, Rosen S. Congenital cytomegalovirus infection: a cause of renal dysplasia? Pediatr Dev Pathol. 2007;10:300–4.
12. Aslam M, Watson AR. Unilateral multicystic dysplastic kidney: long term outcomes. Arch Dis Child. 2006;91:820–3.
13. Kuwertz-Broeking E, Brinkmann OA, Von Lengerke HJ, et al. Unilateral multicystic dysplastic kidney: experience in children. BJU Int. 2004;93:388–92.
14. Wacksman J, Phipps L. Report of the Multicystic Kidney Registry: preliminary findings. J Urol. 1993;150:1870–2.
15. John U, Rudnik-Schoneborn S, Zerres K, Misselwitz J. Kidney growth and renal function in unilateral multicystic dysplastic kidney disease. Pediatr Nephrol. 1998;12:567–71.
16. Flack CE, Bellinger MF. The multicystic dysplastic kidney and contralateral vesicoureteral reflux: protection of the solitary kidney. J Urol. 1993;150:1873–4.
17. Miller DC, Rumohr JA, Dunn RL, Bloom DA, Park JM. What is the fate of the refluxing contralateral kidney in children with multicystic dysplastic kidney? J Urol. 2006;172:1630–4.
18. Chiappinelli A, Savanelli A, Farina A, Settimi A. Multicystic dysplastic kidney, our experience in non-surgical management. Pediatr Surg Int. 2011;27:775–9.
19. Mansoor O, Chandar J, Rodriguez MM, et al. Long-term risk of chronic kidney disease in unilateral multicystic dysplastic kidney. Pediatr Nephrol. 2011;26:597–603.
20. Siqueira Rabelo EA, Oliveira EA, Silva JM, Oliveira DS, Colosimo EA. Ultrasound progression of prenatally detected multicystic dysplastic kidney. Urology. 2006;68:1098–102.
21. Rabelo EA, Oliveira EA, Silva GS, Pezzuti IL, Tatsuo ES. Predictive factors of ultrasonographic involution of prenatally detected multicystic dysplastic kidney. BJU Int. 2005;95:868–71.
22. Onal B, Kogan BA. Natural history of patients with multicystic dysplastic kidney-what followup is needed? J Urol. 2006;176:1607–11.
23. Narchi H. Risk of hypertension with multicystic kidney disease: a systematic review. Arch Dis Child. 2005;90:921–4.
24. Rudnik-Schoneborn S, John U, Deget F, Ehrich JH, Misselwitz J, Zerres K. Clinical features of unilateral multicystic renal dysplasia in children. Eur J Pediatr. 1998;157:666–72.
25. Husmann DA. Renal dysplasia: the risks and consequences of leaving dysplastic tissue in situ. Urology. 1998;52:533–6.
26. Oddone M, Marino C, Sergi C, et al. Wilms' tumor arising in a multicystic kidney. Pediatr Radiol. 1994;24:236.
27. Hosey YL, Anderson JH, Oudjhane K, Russo P. Wilms tumor and multicystic dysplastic kidney disease. J Urol. 1997;158:2256–60.
28. Beckwith JB. Should asymptomatic unilateral multicystic dysplastic kidneys be removed because of the future risk of neoplasia? Pediatr Nephrol. 1992;6:511.
29. Narchi H. Risk of Wilms' tumour with multicystic kidney disease: a systematic review. Arch Dis Child. 2005;90:147–9.
30. Rackley RR, Angermeier KW, Levin H, Pontes JE, Kay R. Renal cell carcinoma arising in a regressed multicystic dysplastic kidney. J Urol. 1994;152:1543–5.
31. Shirai M, Kitagawa T, Nakata H, Urano Y. Renal cell carcinoma originating from dysplastic kidney. Acta Path Jpn. 1986;36:1263.
32. Mingin GC, Gilhooly P, Sadeghi-Nejad H. Transitional cell carcinoma in a multicystic dysplastic kidney. J Urol. 2000;163:544.
33. Lima M, Ruggeri G, Molinaro F, Gargano T, Gregori G, Randi B. One-trocar-assisted nephrectomy (OTAN): initial experience and codification of a technique. Surg Endosc. 2011;26(4):1165–9. [Epub ahead of print]
34. Cabezalí Barbancho D, Gómez Fraile A, López Vázquez F, Aransay Bramtot A. Single-port nephrectomy in infants: Initial experience. J Pediatr Urol. 2011;7:396–8.
35. Shaikewitz ST, Chapman A. Autosomal recessive polycystic kidney disease: Issues regarding the variability of clinical presentation. J Am Soc Nephrol. 1993;3:1858–62.
36. Adeva M, El-Youssef M, Rossetti S, et al. Clinical and molecular characterization defines a broadened spectrum of autosomal recessive polycystic kidney disease (ARPKD). Medicine. 2006;85:1–21.
37. Guay-Woodford LM, Muecher G, Hopkins SD, et al. The severe perinatal form of autosomal recessive polycystic kidney disease maps to chromosome 6p21.1-p12: Implications for genetic counseling. Am J Hum Genet. 1995;56:1101–7.
38. Turkbey B, Ocak I, Daryanani K, et al. Autosomal recessive polycystic kidney disease and congenital hepatic fibrosis (ARPKD/CHF). Pediatr Radiol. 2009;39:100–11.
39. Blythe H, Ockenden B. Polycystic disease of the kidneys and liver presenting in childhood. J Med Genet. 1971;8:257–84.
40. Romero R, Cullen M, Jeanty P, et al. The diagnosis of congenital renal anomalies with ultrasound: II. Infantile polycystic kidney disease. Am J Obstet Gynecol. 1984;150:259–62.
41. Sweeney WE Jr, Avner ED. Diagnosis and management of childhood polycystic kidney disease. Pediatr Nephrol. 2011;26:675–92.
42. Avni FE, Guissard G, Hall M, et al. Hereditary polycystic kidney diseases in children: changing sonographic patterns through childhood. Pediatr Radiol. 2002;32:169–74.
43. Traubici J, Daneman A. High-resolution renal sonography in children with autosomal recessive

polycystic kidney disease. AJR Am J Roentgenol. 2005;184:1630–3.
44. Akhan O, Karaosmanoğlu AD, Ergen B. Imaging findings in congenital hepatic fibrosis. Eur J Radiol. 2007;61:18–24.
45. Gabow PA. Autosomal dominant polycystic kidney disease. N Engl J Med. 1993;329:332–42.
46. Fick GM, Johnson AM, Strain JD. Characteristics of very early onset autosomal dominant polycystic kidney disease. J Am Soc Nephrol. 1993;3:1863–70.
47. San Millán JL, Viribay M, Peral B, Martínez I, Weissenbach J, Moreno F. Refining the localization of the PKD2 locus on chromosome 4q by linkage analysis in Spanish families with autosomal dominant polycystic kidney disease type 2. Am J Hum Genet. 1995;56:248–53.
48. Brun M, Maugey-Laulom B, Eurin D, Didier F, Avni EF. Prenatal sonographic patterns in autosomal dominant polycystic kidney disease: a multicenter study. Ultrasound Obstet Gynecol. 2004;24:55–61.
49. Azmy AF, Ransley PG. Simple renal cysts in children. Ann R Coll Surg Engl. 1983;65:124–5.
50. Murthi GV, Azmy AF, Wilkinson AG. Management of simple renal cysts in children. J R Coll Surg Edinb. 2001;46:205–7.
51. Velaphi SC, Perlman JM. Neonatal adrenal hemorrhage: clinical and abdominal sonographic findings. Clin Pediatr (Phila). 2001;40:545–8.
52. Chang TA, Chen CH, Liao MF, Chen CH. Asymptomatic neonatal adrenal hemorrhage. Clin Neonatol. 1998;5:23–6.
53. Black J, Williams DI. Natural history of adrenal haemorrhage in the newborn. Arch Dis Child. 1973;48:183–90.
54. DeSa DJ, Nicholls S. Haemorrhagic necrosis of the adrenal gland in perinatal infants: a clinicopathological study. J Pathol. 1972;106:133–49.
55. Miele V, Galluzzo M, Patti G, Mazzoni G, Calisti A, Valenti M. Scrotal hematoma due to neonatal adrenal hemorrhage: the value of ultrasonography in avoiding unnecessary surgery. Pediatr Radiol. 1997;27:672–4.
56. Rumińska M, Welc-Dobies J, Lange M, Maciejewska J, Pyrzak B, Brzewski M. Adrenal hemorrhage in neonates: risk factors and diagnostic and clinical procedure. Med Wieku Rozwoj. 2008;12:457–62.
57. Chen CH, Chang TA. The value of ultrasound in the diagnosis and management of neonatal adrenal hemorrhage. Chin J Radiol. 1999;24:107–11.
58. Snelling CE, Erb IH. Haemorrhage and subsequent calcification of the adrenal. J Pediatr. 1935;6:22–41.
59. Duman N, Oren H, Gülcan H, Kumral A, Olguner M, Ozkan H. Scrotal hematoma due to neonatal adrenal hemorrhage. Pediatr Int. 2004;46:360–2.
60. Siegel BS, Shedd DP, Selzer R, Mark JBD. Adrenal haemorrhage in the newborn. JAMA. 1961;177:263–5.
61. Katar S, Oztürkmen-Akay H, Devecioğlu C, Taşkesen M. A rare cause of hyperbilirubinemia in a newborn: bilateral adrenal hematoma. Turk J Pediatr. 2008;50:485–7.
62. Huang CY, Lee YJ, Lee HC, Huang FY. Picture of the month. Neonatal adrenal hemorrhage. Arch Pediatr Adolesc Med. 2000;154:417–8.
63. Lee MC, Lin LH. Ultrasound screening of neonatal adrenal hemorrhage. Acta Paediatr Taiwan. 2000;41:327–30.
64. Mutlu M, Karagüzel G, Aslan Y, Cansu A, Ökten A. Adrenal hemorrhage in newborns: a retrospective study. World J Pediatr. 2011;7:355–7.
65. Watterberg KL. Adrenal insufficiency and cardiac dysfunction in the preterm infant. Pediatr Res. 2002;51:422–4.
66. Liu KW, Ku KW, Cheung KL, Chan YL. L. Chan. Acute scrotal swelling: a sign of neonatal adrenal haemorrhage. J Paediatr Child Health. 1994;30:368–9.
67. Bergami G, Malena S, Di Mario M, Fariello G. Echography in the follow-up of neonatal AH. The presentation of 14 cases. Radiol Med. 1990;79:474–8.
68. Wang CH, Chen SJ, Yang LY, Tang RB. Neonatal adrenal hemorrhage presenting as a multiloculated cystic mass. J Chin Med Assoc. 2008;71:481–4.
69. Perl S, Kotz L, Keil M, Patronas NJ, Stratakis CA. Image in Endocrinology: Calcified adrenals associated with perinatal adrenal hemorrhage and adrenal insufficiency. J Clin Endocrinol Metab. 2007;92(3):754.
70. Kutluk G, Cetinkaya F, Aytac DB, Caliskan CK. Bilateral adrenal abscesses as a complication of neonatal suprarenal hemorrhage. Pediatr Int. 2010;52(4):e207–8.
71. Rayer PFO. Traite des Maladies des Reins et des Alterations de Ia Secretion Urinaire. Paris, Bailliere, 1837; p. 591–9.
72. Belman AB. Renal vein thrombosis in infancy and childhood. Clin Pediatr. 1976;15:1033–44.
73. Arneil GC, MacDonald AM, Murphy AV, et al. Renal venous thrombosis. Clin Nephrol. 1973;1:119–31.
74. Smith JA Jr, Lee RE, Middleton RG. Hypertension in childhood from renal vein thrombosis. J Urol. 1979;122:389–90.
75. Rasoulpour M, McLean RH. Renal venous thrombosis in neonates. Am J Dis Child. 1980;134:276–9.
76. Evans DJ, Silverman M, Bowley NB. Congenital hypertension due to unilateral renal vein thrombosis. Arch Dis Child. 1981;56:306–8.
77. Mogan H, Beattie T, Murphy A. Renal venous thrombosis in infancy: long-term follow-up. Pediatr Nephrol. 1992;5:45–9.
78. Jobin J, O'Regan S, Kemay G, Mongeau J, Robitaille P. Neonatal renal vein thrombosis—long-term follow-up after conservative management. Clin Nephrol. 1982;17:36–40.
79. Keidan I, Lotan D, Gazit G, Boichis H, Reichman B, Linder N. Early neonatal renal vein thrombosis: long-term outcome. Acta Paediatr. 1994;83:1225–7.
80. Hepler AB. Thrombosis of the renal veins. J Urol. 1934;31:527–31.
81. Olson D. Renal vein thrombosis. Clinical pediatric nephrology. Lieberman E, editor. Philadelphia, JB Lippincott, 1st Ed, 1976, pp 372–380.

82. McFarland JB. Renal vein thrombosis in children. Q J Med. 1965;34:269–90.
83. Takeuchi A, Benirschke K. Renal vein thrombosis of the newborn and its relation to maternal diabetes. Biol Neonat. 1961;3:237–56.
84. Avery ME, Oppenheimer EH, Gordon HH. Renal vein thrombosis in newborn infants to diabetic mothers. N Engl J Med. 1957;256:1134–8.
85. Oliver WJ, Kelsch RC. Renal venous thrombosis in infancy. Pediatr Rev. 1982;4:61–6.
86. Fishman J, Joseph R. Renal vein thrombosis in utero: duplex sonography in diagnosis and follow-up. Pediatr Radiol. 1994;24:135–6.
87. Cozzolino DJ, Cendron M. Bilateral renal vein thrombosis in a newborn: a case of prenatal renal vein thrombosis. Urology. 1997;50(1):128–31.
88. Hibbert J, Howlett DC, Greenwood KL, Macdonald LM, Saunders AJS. The ultrasound appearances of neonatal renal vein thrombosis. Br J Radiol. 1997;70:1191–4.
89. Gatewood OMB. Renal vein thrombosis in patients with nephrotic syndrome: CT diagnosis. Radiology. 1986;159:117.
90. Sfakianakis GN, Vonorta K, Zilleruelo G, et al. Scintigraphy in acquired renal disorders. In: Freeman LM, editor. Nuclear medicine annual 1992. New York: Raven Press; 1992. p. 157–224.
91. Ross DL, Lubowitz H. Anticoagulation in renal vein thrombosis. Arch Intern Med. 1978;138:1349–51.
92. Nuss R, Hays T, Manco-Johnson M. Efficacy and safety of heparin anticoagulation for neonatal renal vein thrombosis. Am J Pediatr Hematol Oncol. 1994;16(2):127–31.
93. Thompson IM, Schneider R, Labadibi Z. Thrombectomy for neonatal renal vein thrombosis. J Urol. 1975;113:396–9.
94. Schrier RW, Gardenswartz MH. Renal vein thrombosis. Postgrad Med. 1980;67:83–93.
95. Flynn JT. Neonatal hypertension: diagnosis and management. Pediatr Nephrol. 2000;14:332–41.
96. Zubrow AB, Hulman S, Kushner H, Falkner B. Determinants of blood pressure in infants admitted to neonatal intensive care units: a prospective multicenter study. J Perinatol. 1995;15:470–9.
97. Georgieff MK, Mills MM, Gomez-Marin O, Sinaiko AR. Rate of change of blood pressure in premature and full term infants from birth to 4 months. Pediatr Nephrol. 1996;10:152–5.
98. Arar MY, Hogg RJ, Arant BS, Seikaly MG. Etiology of sustained hypertension in children in the southwestern United States. Pediatr Nephrol. 1994;8:186–9.
99. Singh HP, Hurley RM, Myers TF. Neonatal hypertension: incidence and risk factors. Am J Hypertens. 1992;5:51–5.
100. Adelman RD. Neonatal hypertension. Pediatr Clin North Am. 1978;25:99–110.
101. Sethna CB, Kaplan BS, Cahill AM, Velazquez OC, Meyers KEC. Idiopathic mid-aortic syndrome in children. Pediatr Nephrol. 2008;23:1135–42.
102. Milner LS, Heitner R, Thomson PD, Levin SE, Rothberg AD, Beale P, Ninin DT. Hypertension as the major problem of idiopathic arterial calcification of infancy. J Pediatr. 1984;105:934–8.
103. Dorman DC, Reye RDK, Reid RR. Renal-artery stenosis in the rubella syndrome. Lancet 1966;287(7441):790–792.
104. Rahill WJ, Molteni A, Hawking KM, Koo JH, Menon VA. Hypertension and narrowing of the renal arteries in infancy. J Pediatr. 1974;84:39–44.
105. Durante D, Jones D, Spitzer R. Neonatal arterial embolism syndrome. J Pediatr. 1976;89:978–81.
106. Woodard JR, Patterson JH, Brinsfield D. Renal artery thrombosis in newborn infants. Am J Dis Child. 1967;114:191–4.
107. Neal WA, Reynolds JW, Jarvis CW, Williams HJ. Umbilical artery catheterization: demonstration of arterial thrombosis by aortography. Pediatrics. 1972;50:6–13.
108. Merten DF, Vogel JM, Adelman RD, Goetzman BW, Bogren HG. Renovascular hypertension as a complication of umbilical arterial catheterization. Radiology. 1978;126:751–7.
109. Seibert JJ, Taylor BJ, Williamson SL, Williams BJ, Szabo JS, Corbitt SL. Sonographic detection of neonatal umbilical-artery thrombosis: clinical correlation. Am J Roentgenol. 1987;148:965–8.
110. Deal JE, Snell MF, Barratt TM, Dillon MJ. Renovascular disease in childhood. J Pediatr. 1992;121:378–84.
111. Mustafa AE, Bloom DA, Valentini RP, Mattoo TK, Imam AA. MR angiography in the evaluation of a renovascular cause of neonatal hypertension. Pediatr Radiol. 2006;36:158–61.
112. Cachat F, Bogaru A, Micheli JL, et al. Severe hypertension and massive proteinuria in a newborn with renal artery stenosis. Pediatr Nephrol. 2004;19:544–6.
113. Visrutaratna P, Srisuwan T, Sirivanichai C. Pediatric renovascular hypertension in Thailand: CT angiographic findings. Pediatr Radiol. 2009;39:1321–6.
114. Lam HS, Chu WCW, Lee CH, Wong W, Ng PC. Renal artery thrombosis and ischaemia presenting as severe neonatal hypertension. Arch Dis Child Fetal Neonatal Ed. 2007;92(4):F264.
115. Hendren WH, Kim SH, Herrin JT, Crawford JD. Surgically correctable hypertension of renal origin in childhood. Am J Surg. 1982;143:432–42.
116. Bendel-Stenzel M, Najarian JS, Sinaiko AR. Renal artery stenosis: long-term medical management before surgery. Pediatr Nephrol. 1995;10:147–51.
117. McTaggart SJ, Gulati S, Walker RG, Powell HR, Jones CL, Gelati S. Evaluation and long-term outcome of pediatric renovascular hypertension. Pediatr Nephrol. 2000;14:1022–9.
118. Stanley JC, Zelenock GB, Messina LM, Wakefield TW. Pediatric renovascular hypertension: a thirty-year experience if operative treatment. J Vasc Surg. 1995;21:212–26.

119. Tyagi S, Kaul UA, Satangi DK, Arora R. Percutaneous transluminal angioplasty for renovascular hypertension in children: initial and long term results. Pediatrics. 1997;99:44–9.
120. Courtel JV, Soto B, Niaudet P, Gagnadoux MF, Carteret M, Quignodon JF, et al. Percutaneous transluminal angioplasty of renal artery stenosis in children. Pediatr Radiol. 1998;28:59–63.
121. Daehnert I, Hennig B, Scheinert D. Percutaneous transluminal angioplasty for renovascular hypertension in a neonate. Acta Paediatr. 2005;94(8):1149–52.
122. Wilson DI, Appleton RE, Coulthard MG, Lee RE, Wren C, Bain HH. Fetal and infantile hypertension caused by unilateral renal artery disease. Arch Dis Child. 1990;65:881–4.
123. Kavaler E, Hensle TW. Renal artery thrombosis in the newborn infant. Urology. 1997;50(2):282–4.
124. Kiessling SG, Wadhwa N, Kriss VM, Iocono J, Desai NS. An unusual case of severe therapy-resistant hypertension in a newborn. Pediatrics. 2007;119(1):301–4.

Prune Belly Syndrome

67

John M. Hutson

Abstract
Prune Belly Syndrome (PBS) is a rare anomaly of the anterior abdominal wall, urinary tract and undescended testes. It is thought to be caused by transient obstruction of the urethra between 10 and 20 weeks of gestation, leading to massive dilatation of the bladder which resolves in the third trimester. The atrophic abdominal wall and cryptorchidism are secondary to the enlarged bladder. Management primarily requires treatment of the intraabdominal testes.

Keywords
Prune belly syndrome • Management • Outcomes

67.1 History

A case of congenital deficiency of the abdominal muscles, now known as prune belly syndrome, was recorded in the mid nineteenth century [1], but the first description of the association of the condition with urogenital tract anomalies was made by Parker in 1895 [2].

Prune belly syndrome (PBS) was previously called Eagle-Barrett or Triad syndrome, because it included the triad of congenital deficiency of the abdominal musculature, massive dilatation of the urinary tract and intra-abdominal undescended testes [3]. Stephens proposed that there was a defect in mesodermal development affecting the anterior abdominal wall, urinary tract and the genital tract of males [4, 5].

Development of antenatal ultrasonography has shown that the characteristic anomaly in midgestation is massive dilatation of the fetal bladder, which may be larger than the fetal head [6].

67.2 Epidemiology

This is a rare morphological anomaly in males, now easily identified on antenatal ultrasonography with an incidence of 1/25,000 [7]. In many centres, the number of live-born infants with PBS has decreased dramatically in recent years, because of selective termination of pregnancy. The anomaly is extremely rare in females, and is usually associated with massive dilatation of the

J.M. Hutson, BS, MD(Monash), MD, DSc(Melb)
University of Melbourne & Royal Children's Hospital, Parkville, VIC, Australia
e-mail: john.hutson@rch.org.au

P.D. Losty et al. (eds.), *Rickham's Neonatal Surgery*, https://doi.org/10.1007/978-1-4471-4721-3_67

urogenital tracts in a cloacal anomaly, or even more rarely, with massive abdominal distention associated with bowel obstruction such as meconium ileus caused by cystic fibrosis. In the latter case the other features are absent.

67.3 Pathogenesis

Opinions remain divided between a primary mesodermal disorder affecting the abdominal wall and pelvic organs on one hand and temporary obstruction of the male urinary tract in midgestation on the other [5, 8, 9].

Primary deficiency of mesodermal migration into the lower anterior abdominal wall has been proposed as the cause of bladder exstrophy and epispadias [10] and there is preliminary evidence that mutations in the P63 gene may be responsible [10]. However, this idea does not readily explain the massive dilatation of the bladder, which suggests distal obstruction (see below).

PBS has been reported as part of the Ectrodactyly-Ectodermal Dysplasia-Clefting Syndrome (EEC) where a mutation in the P63 gene (p R204W) has been identified [11]. Another gene associated with PBS is the hepatocyte nuclear factor-1β[beta] gene [12].

Megacystis-microcolon-intestinal hypoperistalsis syndrome (MMIHS) has an overlapping phenotype with PBS, and has been reported within the same family, consistent with a common genetic cause [13].

Most post-mortem studies of fetuses with PBS show some form of urethral obstruction, which may or may not have resolved by the time of examination [9]. A flap-like obstruction between the prostatic and penile urethra is a relatively common finding [14, 15], but severe phimosis has also been suggested as the cause [15]. Urethral atresia with complete obstruction at the level of the membraneous urethra is well-reported [16, 17].

In a detailed study of 21 PBS specimens and 23 specimens of posterior urethral valve (PUV) (Young types 1 and 3) there was an obvious difference in development of the seminal vesicles and ducts. In the PBS specimens the prostatic glands and seminal vesicles were atrophic, while in the PUV specimens the prostate and seminal vesicles were developed normally. These differences are consistent with a primary abnormality in the intermediate and lateral plate mesoderm in PBS, leading to Wolffian duct maldevelopment as well as defects in the abdominal wall musculature and urinary tract [18].

Deletion of the hepatocyte nuclear factor-1-β [beta] gene has been reported in association with PBS [19]. This is a transcription factor that is expressed in a number of tissues derived from the urogenital ridge including Wolffian duct, renal tubules and urethra, leading to the "renal cysts and diabetes" syndrome with mutations. Other reports of transient neonatal diabetes and PBS have been associated with DNA hypomethylation [20].

The massive enlargement of the fetal bladder in midgestation with resolution in the third trimester is characteristic of PBS, and is consistent with temporary bladder-outlet obstruction [21]. In a study of urethral diameters, as measured on micturating cystourethrograms, we were able to show that the anterior urethra was dilated in PBS, consistent with transient distal urethral obstruction [8, 9, 21] (Fig. 67.1).

67.4 Antenatal Presentation

Most babies with PBS are now diagnosed by antenatal ultrasonography because of the massive bladder enlargement at 15–20 weeks of gestation [17]. Because of the gross disturbance of the urinary tract and abdominal wall, as well as 25% have co-existing anomalies in the cardiovascular system, termination of pregnancy is a common outcome [7]. This trend has caused a significant drop in the number of live-born infants with PBS in many centres (Fig. 67.2).

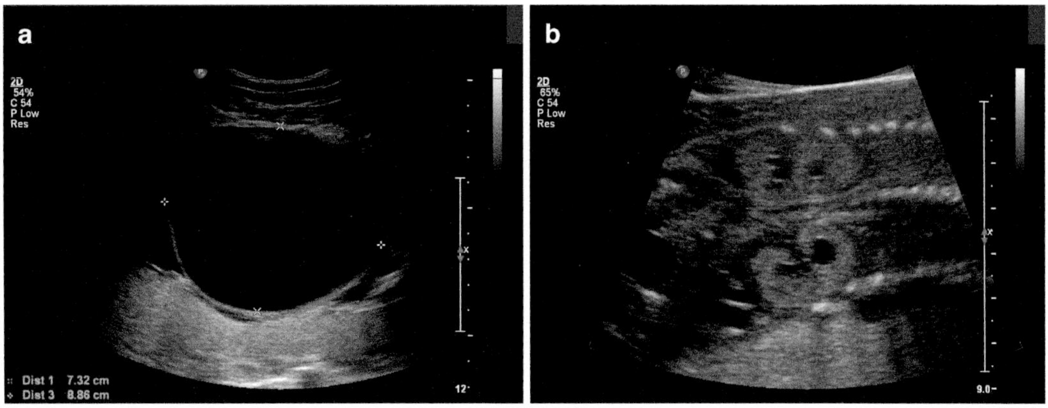

Fig. 67.1 (**a**) Antenatal ultrasound (20 + 4 weeks) showing massively dilated and tense bladder. (**b**) Echogenic kidneys with caliectasis

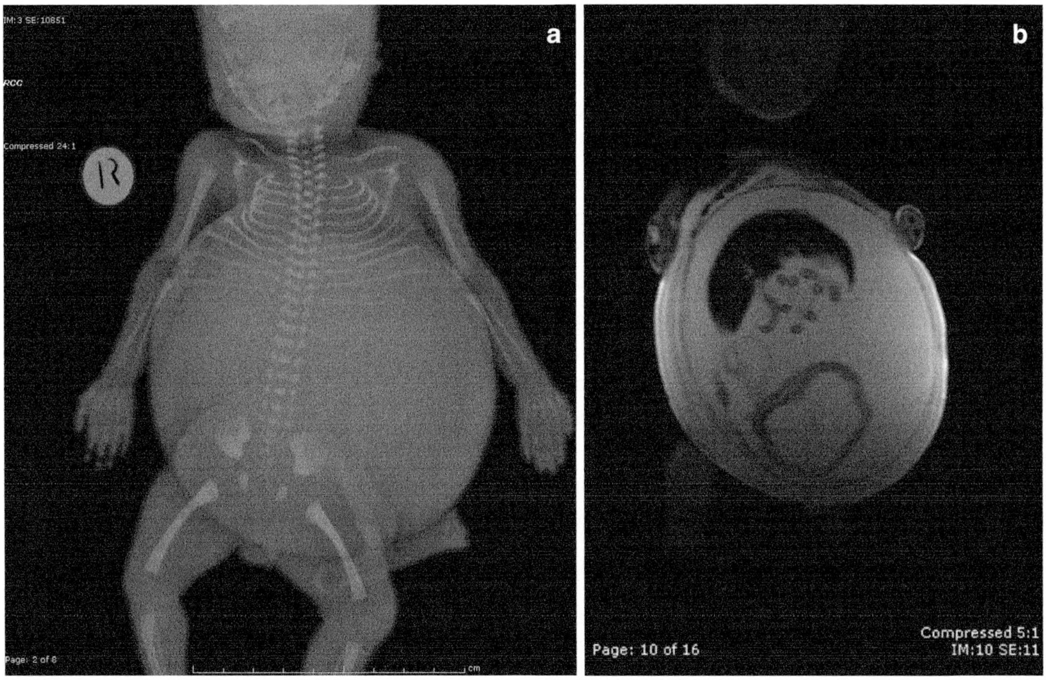

Fig. 67.2 (**a**) Postmortem X-ray of same foetus as shown in Fig. 67.1 after termination. The massively enlarged abdomen is obvious. (**b**) Postmortem MRI of same foetus showing thick-walled bladder, massive ascites and thin anterior abdominal wall

67.5 Clinical Presentation

67.5.1 Urinary Tract

The bladder is massively enlarged and there is often a urachal diverticulum extending to the umbilicus. The vesical muscle is hypertrophied but there is not usually any trabeculation. The urethra is dilated and there may be an associated enlargement of the utriculus. Megalourethra is relatively common.

The upper tracts show significant hydronephrosis and hydroureter, with high-grade vesicoureteric reflux being very common (Fig. 67.3).

Renal function is extremely variable, from normal at one extreme to renal failure at birth at the other. In the latter circumstance there may be oligohydramnios or anhydramnios and Potter facies.

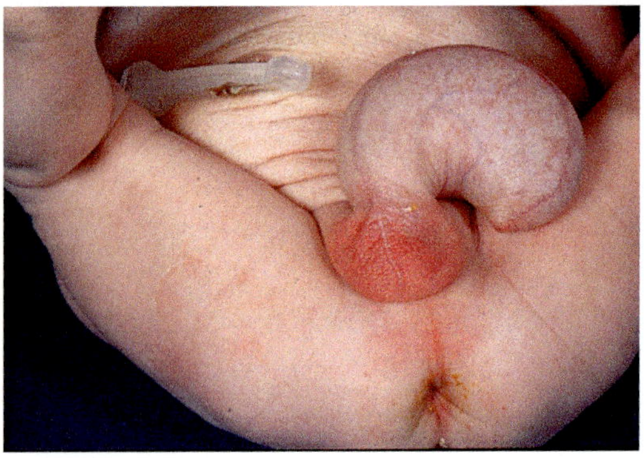

Fig. 67.3 Megalourethra in a newborn with prune belly syndrome, consistent with distal urethral obstruction in mid gestation. Note also the hypoplastic, empty scrotum

67.5.2 Genital Tract

The testes are impalpable, and are usually on the back of the bladder, which reached such a size in midgestation that the gubernaculum was (presumably) torn out of the inguinal abdominal wall. Hence the processus vaginalis is usually absent and there is no recognisable inguinal canal (Fig. 67.4) In other respects the testes are normal histologically and functionally, as the intra-abdominal cryptorchidism is caused by the enlarged bladder rather than a primary gonadal dysplasia. Postnatally, however, secondary degeneration of the testes will develop in the first year if orchidopexy is not carried out.

In the rare female neonate with PBS, there is usually a complex anorectal or cloacal anomaly leading to hydrometrocolpos and/or bladder outlet obstruction [22].

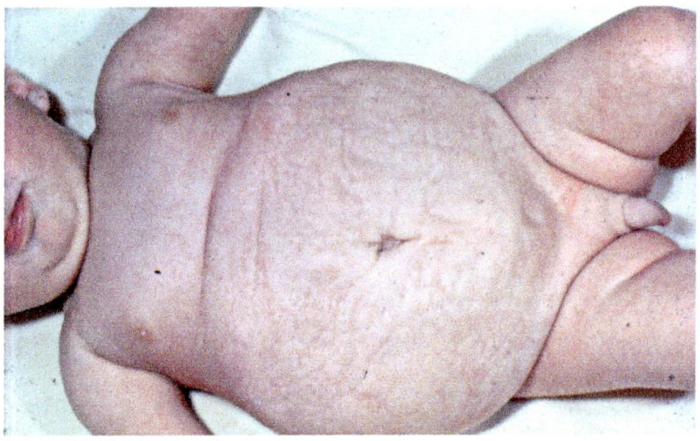

Fig. 67.4 The flabby, wrinkled anterior abdominal wall at birth that gives the condition its name, after decompression of the obstructed bladder in midgestation

67.5.3 Abdominal Wall

The thin and wrinkled anterior abdominal wall that is characteristic of PBS is quite variable depending on the maximum size of the bladder at 15–20 weeks of development (Fig. 67.1a). The area affected undergoes pressure atrophy so that the anterior muscles are replaced by a thin fibrous sheet. The most severely affected part is the central hypogastrium which is stretched most severely by the enlarged bladder. The epigastric component of the rectus abdominis and oblique muscles are relatively well preserved, as are the flanks. Secondary spinal deformity may accompany the wrinkled abdominal wall because the massive bladder enlargement may deform the fetal posture.

67.5.4 Orthopaedic Anomalies

Massive bladder enlargement in midgestation can be associated with congenital dysplasia and dislocation of the hips, as well as congenital amputation of the leg [23].

67.5.5 Cardiovascular Anomalies

Heart defects occur in about 25% of babies, although these are more likely caused by coincidental genetic anomaly rather than postural or pressure effects of the enlarged bladder [7].

67.6 Surgical Management

Most infants with PBS do not need surgical treatment of the dilated urinary tract, although the nephrologist may be involved to manage any renal insufficiency.

By contrast, the intra-abdominal testes need orchidopexy, which is usually carried out laparoscopically [24]. The timing of surgery should be the same as for other babies with impalpable testes: 6–12 months, on the premise that this has the best chance of preserving fertility [25].

Orchidopexy may be achieved by radical mobilisation of the testicular vessels laparoscopically, but a 2-stage Fowler-Stephens procedure may be required [26], with reasonable long-term results. The surgical details do not need to be described, as the procedures have been well documented elsewhere.

There is controversy about whether surgery is required for the abdominal wall. Many centres advocate total surgical reconstruction as initially championed in the 1970s [27, 28] and subsequently in recent decades [29, 30]. However, in some centres it has been found that minimal surgical intervention is required [31].

References

1. Frohlich F. Der Mangel der Muskeln, insbesondere der Seitenbauchmuskeln. Wurzburg: C.A. Zurn; 1839.
2. Parker RW. Absence of abdominal muscles in an infant. Lancet. 1895;1
3. Nunn IN, Stephens FD. The triad syndrome: a composite anomaly of the abdominal wall, urinary system and testes. J Urol. 1961;86:782–94.
4. Stephens F D. Morphology and embryogenesis of the triad. in: Congenital Malformations of the Urinary Tract. New York: Praeger; 1983. p. 497–8.
5. Wheatley JM, Stephens FD, et al. Prune-belly syndrome: ongoing controversies regarding pathogenesis and management. Semin Pediatr Surg. 1996;5(2):95–106.
6. Yiee J, Wilcox D. Abnormalities of the fetal bladder. Semin Fetal Neonatal Med. 2008;13(3):164–70.
7. Routh JC, Huang L, et al. Contemporary epidemiology and characterization of newborn males with prune belly syndrome. Urology. 2010;76(1):44–8.
8. Beasley SW, Bettenay F, et al. The anterior urethra provides clues to the aetiology of prune belly syndrome. Pediatr Surg Int. 1988;3:169–72.
9. Nijagal A, Sydorak RM, et al. Spontaneous resolution of prenatal megalourethra. J Pediatr Surg. 2004;39(9):1421–3.
10. Cheng W, Jacobs WB, et al. DeltaNp63 plays an anti-apoptotic role in ventral bladder development. Development. 2006;133(23):4783–92.
11. Janssens S, Defoort P, et al. Prune belly anomaly on prenatal ultrasound as a presenting feature of ectrodactyly-ectodermal dysplasia-clefting syndrome (EEC). Genet Couns. 2008;19(4):433–7.
12. Murray PJ, Thomas K, et al. Whole gene deletion of the hepatocyte nuclear factor-1beta gene in a patient with the prune-belly syndrome. Nephrol Dial Transplant. 2008;23(7):2412–5.
13. Levin TL, Soghier L, et al. Megacystis-microcolon-intestinal hypoperistalsis and prune belly: overlapping syndromes. Pediatr Radiol. 2004;34(12):995–8.
14. Volmar KE, Fritsch MK, et al. Patterns of congenital lower urinary tract obstructive uropathy: relation to abnormal prostate and bladder development and the prune belly syndrome. Pediatr Dev Pathol. 2001;4(5):467–72.
15. Volmar KE, Nguyen TC, et al. Phimosis as a cause of the prune belly syndrome: comparison to a more common pattern of proximal penile urethra obstruction. Virchows Arch. 2003;442(2):169–72.
16. van Velden DJ, de Jong G, et al. Fetal bilateral obstructive uropathy: a series of nine cases. Pediatr Pathol Lab Med. 1995;15(2):245–58.
17. Lopes H, Guedes L. Prune belly syndrome. Journal of Maternal-Fetal and Neonatal Medicine Conference. Spain: Granada; 2010.
18. Stephens FD, Gupta D. Pathogenesis of the prune belly syndrome. J Urol. 1994;152(6 Pt 2):2328–31.
19. Haeri S, Devers PL, et al. Deletion of hepatocyte nuclear factor-1-beta in an infant with prune belly syndrome. Am J Perinatol. 2010;27(7):559–63.
20. Laborie LB, Mackay DJ, et al. DNA hypomethylation, transient neonatal diabetes, and prune belly sequence in one of two identical twins. Eur J Pediatr. 2010;169(2):207–13.
21. Woods AG, Brandon DH. Prune belly syndrome. A focused physical assessment. Adv Neonatal Care. 2007;7(3):132–43. quiz 144–5
22. Giuliani S, Vendryes C, et al. Prune belly syndrome associated with cloacal anomaly, patent urachal remnant, and omphalocele in a female infant. J Pediatr Surg. 2010;45(11):e39–42.

23. Green NE, Lowery ER, et al. Orthopaedic aspects of prune belly syndrome. J Pediatr Orthop. 1993;13(4):496–501.
24. Saxena AK, Brinkmann OA. Unique features of prune belly syndrome in laparoscopic surgery. J Am Coll Surg. 2007;205(2):217–21.
25. Lambert SM, Caesar SR. Prune belly syndrome. 2009 American Urological Association (AUA) annual meeting Chicago. USA: Chicago; 2009.
26. Patil KK, Duffy PG, et al. Long-term outcome of Fowler-Stephens orchiopexy in boys with prune-belly syndrome. J Urol. 2004;171(4):1666–9.
27. Randolph JG. Total surgical reconstruction for patients with abdominal muscular deficiency ("prune-belly") syndrome. J Pediatr Surg. 1977;12(6):1033–43.
28. Woodard JR, Parrott TS. Reconstruction of the urinary tract in prune belly uropathy. J Urol. 1978;119(6):824–8.
29. Parrott TS, Woodard JR. The Monfort operation for abdominal wall reconstruction in the prune belly syndrome. J Urol. 1992;148(2 Pt 2):688–90.
30. McEvoy HC, Moss ALH. Prune belly syndrome and abdominal wall. Eur J Plast Surg. 2006;29(4):177–80.
31. McMullen ND, Hutson JM, et al. Minimal surgery in the prune belly syndrome. Pediatr Surg Int. 1988;3:51–4.

Disorders of Sex Development

68

John M. Hutson

Abstract

Disorders of sex development (DSD) are rare, complex anomalies of genital development that often present with an ambiguous genital appearance at birth. Rapid recognition and diagnosis are essential to prevent inappropriate gender assignment in the neonatal ward. After morphological and molecular assessment is complete a management plan is developed by a multidisciplinary team in the tertiary and/or quaternary referral centre.

Keywords

Intersex • Ambiguous genitalia • Disorders of sexual development • Surgical management, outcomes

68.1 Introduction

Disorders of sex development (DSD) are rare and complex anomalies affecting sexual differentiation, and cause significant stress for the new parents, as well as life-long issues for the patient. There have been rapid changes recently in the nomenclature and also in the approach to management, with the development of regional referral centres to permit multidisciplinary care at an appropriate level. Gender assignment and surgical intervention remain controversial, while legal issues now need to be considered in some societies. Meanwhile we have learnt more about the genes controlling normal sex development, and now understand the normal and abnormal embryology much better than previously.

68.2 History

Fascination with abnormalities of sexual differentiation is very ancient, as evident in the word "hermaphrodite" (from the Greek: hermaphroditos), used to describe the unfortunate individual with both male and female genital anatomy. Babies with ambiguous genitalia were thought to have "intersex", but there was little medical understanding of underlying disorders prior to the discovery of congenital adrenal hyperplasia (CAH) by Dr. Lawson Wilkins in Baltimore in 1953. There was an explosion of knowledge in the 1960s and 1970s, as surgical and medical ther-

J.M. Hutson, BS, MD(Monash), MD, DSc(Melb)
University of Melbourne and Royal Children's Hospital, Parkville, VIC, Australia
e-mail: john.hutson@rch.org.au

P.D. Losty et al. (eds.), *Rickham's Neonatal Surgery*, https://doi.org/10.1007/978-1-4471-4721-3_68

Table 68.1 Classification of DSD

Level of anomaly	XY	XX	Mixed chromosomes
Chromosome	46,XY DSD	46,XX DSD	Mixed chromosome DSD (aneuploidy) (Klinefelter/ Turner)
Gonad	MGD	Partial/complete	Partial/mixed
Development	Complete dysgenesis	Dysgenesis	Dysgenesis
Partial/complete/mixed	Partial dysgenesis Ovotesticular DSD Denys Drash syndrome Frasier WAGR	Ovotesticular DSD Denys Drash syndrome Frasier WAGR	Ovotesticular DSD
Abnormal Androgen action	Androgen biosynthesis defect Androgen insensitivity (receptor defect) (partial/complete)	Androgen excess (CAH)	
Syndromic and non-hormonal	Abdominal wall defect Anorectal/perineal anomalies Hypospadias	Abdominal wall defect Vaginal agenesis	

apies evolved. In the 1980s and 1990s the first cohort of adult patients with DSD began campaigning for better care, and patient-support groups appeared. Long-term follow-up studies began appearing in the last 10 years, and showed varied outcomes, from reasonable to poor, and this led to intense public scrutiny on the quality of care. There were calls for irreversible surgery to be delayed until children were old enough to make their own decisions. In some places all surgical intervention ceased. In 2004 a consensus meeting was held in Chicago to address some of the issues raised by the support groups, and this led to nomenclature change and articulation of a set of principles for management, which have been developed further since [1].

68.3 Classification

Following the 2004 consensus, a new classification was adopted, based on the underlying chromosomal status. The main groups are now called 46,XX DSD, 46,XY DSD, ovo-testicular DSD, mixed chromosomal DSD, 46, XY complete gonadal dysgenesis and 46, XX testicular DSD (Table 68.1).

68.4 Prognosis

Most forms of DSD cause abnormalities of sexual function and/or fertility, but are not fatal, except for congenital adrenal hyperplasia (CAH). In the latter case, a salt-losing adrenal crisis may occur in the second or third week of life, with the baby presenting with sudden vomiting and shock from lack of cortisol production by the adrenal glands. Glucocorticoid (and usually mineralocorticoid replacement therapy) is required for life, but overcomes this.

68.5 Epidemiology

Although uncomplicated hypospadias has an incidence of 1 in 100–200 live male births, more significant DSD occur rarely, at about 1 in 5000 live births. Most are recognised at or shortly after birth as having ambiguous genitalia, but some disorders do not present until after childhood, puberty or in adult life.

68.6 Genetics

The genetic regulation of sexual differentiation was unknown until the discovery of the sex-determining region on the Y-chromosome, now known as the SRY gene [2]. Recently it has been shown that SOX9 is one of the early downstream genes regulated by SRY, with SOX9 in turn stimulating FGF9 and down-regulating WNT4 and β-catenin to trigger development of a testis. In the absence of SRY, WNT4 activates β-catenin and blocks SOX9 and FGF9 to initiate ovarian development. Steroidogenic factor 1 (SF1) and Wilms tumour 1 (WT1) both have roles in early development of the ambisexual gonad.

Mutations in the gene DAX1 cause gonadal dysgenesis, although the mechanism is not yet determined, and no doubt many more genes will be found in future to have a role on testicular and ovarian differentiation.

Apart from the genes controlling gonadal development, mutations in the genes coding for steroid synthesis enzymes, particularly in the androgen pathway, are well known. These lead to 46,XY DSD with inadequate production of testosterone, with the common lesion being in 17β-hydroxysteroid dehydrogenase-3 (17β-HSD3), In this case the androgen levels may be too low to virilise prenatally, causing female external genitalia, so that the affected girl presents in early adolescence with primary amenorrhoea, virilisation, and palpable gonads in the inguinal region.

Anomalies in the androgen receptor gene interfere with androgen signalling and cause partial or complete androgen insensitivity syndrome. As the androgen receptor gene is on the X-chromosome, the inheritance is X-linked. In some families the mother is a heterozygote carrier, but spontaneous mutations are common. Another genetic anomaly in androgenic function is in the gene for 5α-reductase-2, the enzyme that converts testosterone to dihydrotestosterone (DHT) in peripheral tissues, especially the prostate and external genitalia. Infants with this anomaly are mostly found in societies with inbreeding, although subtle mutations may be more common than previously appreciated. Babies have ambiguous or feminine external anatomy, but increasing androgen production at puberty bypasses the need for conversion to DHT, leading to virilisation and, often, gender-change to male at puberty [3].

68.7 Embryology

The genital tract arises from the urogenital ridge that is formed from the intermediate mesoderm in the early embryo. Prior to the onset of sexual differentiation the mid section of the urogenital ridge contains the mesonephros (or "middle kidney", present from 4–8 weeks, the mesonephric (Wolffian) duct and the paramesonephric (Műllerian duct) and also the ambisexual gonad. The latter is colonised by germ cells migrating from the caudal stalk of the yolk sac between 3 and 5 weeks of development.

At 7–8 weeks, the SRY gene on the Y-chromosome activates a still mostly unknown chain of genetic signals to initiate development of a testis in a male embryo [2]. The testis begins making anti-Műllerian hormone (AMH; also called Műllerian inhibiting substance, MIS) from the Sertoli cells, and this is secreted down the mesonephric or Wolffian duct (which becomes the duct of the testis after the mesonephros regresses) to cause regression of the immediately adjacent ipsilateral Műllerian duct [4]. Testosterone is synthesised in the Leydig cells and secreted into the Wolffian duct to initiate its differentiation into epididymis, vas deferens and a distal bud that forms the seminal vesicle [5]. Testosterone is also secreted into the bloodstream

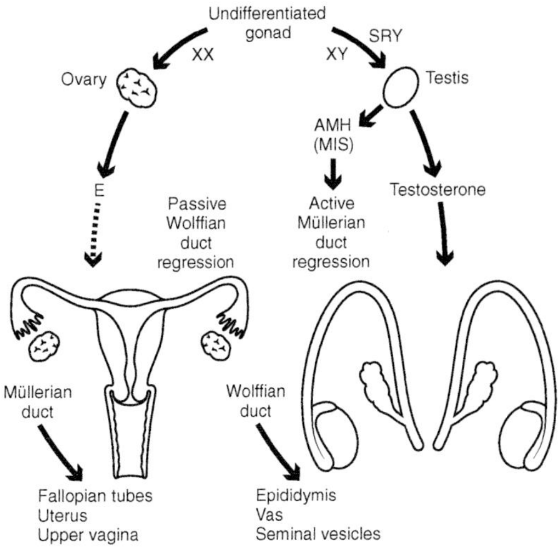

Fig. 68.1 Sexual differentiation of internal genitalia. At 7–8 weeks the undifferentiated gonad develops into an ovary or a testis. SRY gene on the Y-chromosome triggers testicular development. Testosterone (T) and anti-Műllerian hormone (AMH) produced by the testis are secreted down the mesonephric (Wolffian) duct to induce its preservation and development into epididymis, vas deferens and seminal vesicle (by T) and regression of the adjacent Műllerian duct (by AMH). In the female, ovaries develop that begin making oestrogen (E). As AMH is absent the Műllerian duct persists to form Fallopian tubes, uterus and upper vagina. In the absence of testosterone the Wolffian duct regresses and the lower vagina develops

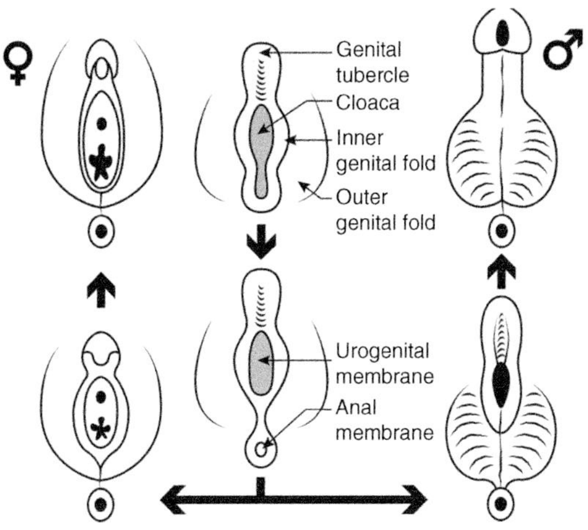

Fig. 68.2 External genital development requires testosterone to be converted to DHT, which triggers genital tubercle enlargement to form the penis, canalisation of the urethral plate to form the anterior urethra and fusion of the labial folds to make a scrotum. In the female, absence of DHT allows the lower vagina to develop, while there is apoptosis in the urethral plate to cause the natural bend in the clitoral shaft

to reach the future prostate and external genitalia. Between 8–12 weeks of gestation however, the serum levels are still low, so virilisation of the external genitalia at this time is mediated by conversion of testosterone itself. This local tissue conversion to DHT effectively increases the activity of testosterone 5–10-fold, enabling growth of the genital tubercle to form a penis, canalisation of the urethral plate to make the male anterior urethra, fusion of the outer genital folds to form the scrotum, and regression of the lower vaginal primordium which formed after the Műllerian ducts reached the cloaca. Coincidentally with lower vaginal involution, the DHT activates prostatic development (Fig. 68.1).

During this same period (8–12 weeks) the Leydig cells make another hormone, insulin-like hormone (Insl 3), which stimulates the genito-inguinal ligament (gubernaculum) to enlarge in males, thereby anchoring the developing testis to the future inguinal canal as the fetus enlarges [6, 7]. Later in development (25–35 weeks) testosterone controls the migration of the gubernaculum from the inguinal canal to the scrotum, enabling the testis to arrive in the scrotum shortly before birth (Fig. 68.2).

68.8 Associated Anomalies

Genital abnormalities caused by gonadal and hormonal defects form the primary group of DSD, but there are also a large group of abdominal wall and perineal anomalies that have associated deformities of the internal and external genitalia [8]. Defects in fusion of the Műllerian ducts are often accompanied by atresia, leading to the Rokitansky sequence, where there is atresia in one half of the unfused vagina and absence of the ipsilateral kidney.

Anorectal malformations may be associated with genital anomaly if the cutaneous fistula is in the vestibule or between the bifid scrotum [9]. Complete agenesis of the genital tubercle may also occur, leading to agenesis of the penis in boys, with the urethra opening into the anterior wall of the anal canal [10].

Abdominal wall defects affecting the pubic region lead to secondary genital anomaly when there is failure of fusion in the midline. These conditions include bladder exstrophy and epispadias, and the rare cloacal exstrophy, or OEIS association (omphalocele, exstrophy, imperforate anus and spinal anomaly).

One of the rarest anomalies of the genitalia is that associated with severe caudal regression, such as in sirenomelia, with hypoplastic fused lower limbs like a mermaid. Another extremely rare anomaly is partial duplication of the caudal embryo, where there may be duplication of the external genitalia.

Where the genital anomaly is caused by inappropriate hormone levels, there are a few recognisable multiple malformation syndromes. These include Smith-Lemli-Opitz syndrome with developmental delay and microphaly, hypotonia, fusion of the second and third toes with incomplete virilisation in boys [11]. Another syndrome is Denys-Drash syndrome, where the mutation has been found in the WT1 gene on chromosome 11. There are abnormalities in all the structures derived from the urogenital ridge, including the kidneys and the gonads. In 46,XY babies there is gonadal dysgenesis and the related ambiguous genitalia from incomplete virilisation, while the kidneys are predisposed to progressive glomerulosclerosis, causing renal failure in infancy. There is also a significant risk (75%) of developing Wilms tumour [12]. Different mutations in the WT1 gene can lead to Frasier syndrome, where the 46,XY fetus has complete or almost complete gonadal dysgenesis, leading to a female phenotype. The intra-abdominal streak gonads are at high risk of gonadoblastoma and there is also some focal glomerulosclerosis [13]. In yet another syndrome affecting the WT1 gene there is a major deletion of the chromosome 11p13, causing a cluster of anomalies called WAGR syndrome (Wilms tumour, aniridia, genitourinary anomalies, and retardation of development). The ocular anomaly is caused by the close relationship between WT1 and PAX6 on chromosome 11 [14].

ATRX syndrome is a disorder causing 46,XY DSD because a mutation in the gene for the chromatin-remodelling enzyme, helicase, which is on the X-chromosome. There is severe gonadal dysgenesis associated with developmental delay and thalassaemia, and a range of other defects.

Opitz syndrome is characterised by hypertelorism, hypospadias and a cleft between the larynx and trachea and the oesophagus, and occasionally oesophageal atresia [11].

The frequency of multiple malformation syndromes is high in babies with 46,XY DSD, and there is a significant risk of potentially fatal cardiac anomalies [15].

68.9 Antenatal Presentation

The increasing use of ultrasonography has led to predictions of gender of the fetus, based on the external anatomy. However, in DSD prenatal diagnosis is extremely uncommon except in those families with a previous infant with a DSD. In the most common of these circumstances, where there is a previous infant with CAH, the mother can be treated with dexamethasone to prevent virilisation in the fetus. When chorion villus biopsy at 10–12 weeks determines the gender, as well as whether or not the fetus is affected, the steroid treatment can be ceased in a male. Termination of pregnancy is possible in this circumstance but remains controversial.

68.10 Clinical Presentation

DSD present at birth in three broad categories: obviously ambiguous genitalia, a female phenotype with some clitoromegaly and an apparent male with hypospadias with or without undescended testes. The first situation is readily identified in the labour ward, and should trigger immediate referral to the DSD referral centre, while the latter two circumstances require significant skill and experience to determine the diagnosis (Fig. 68.3).

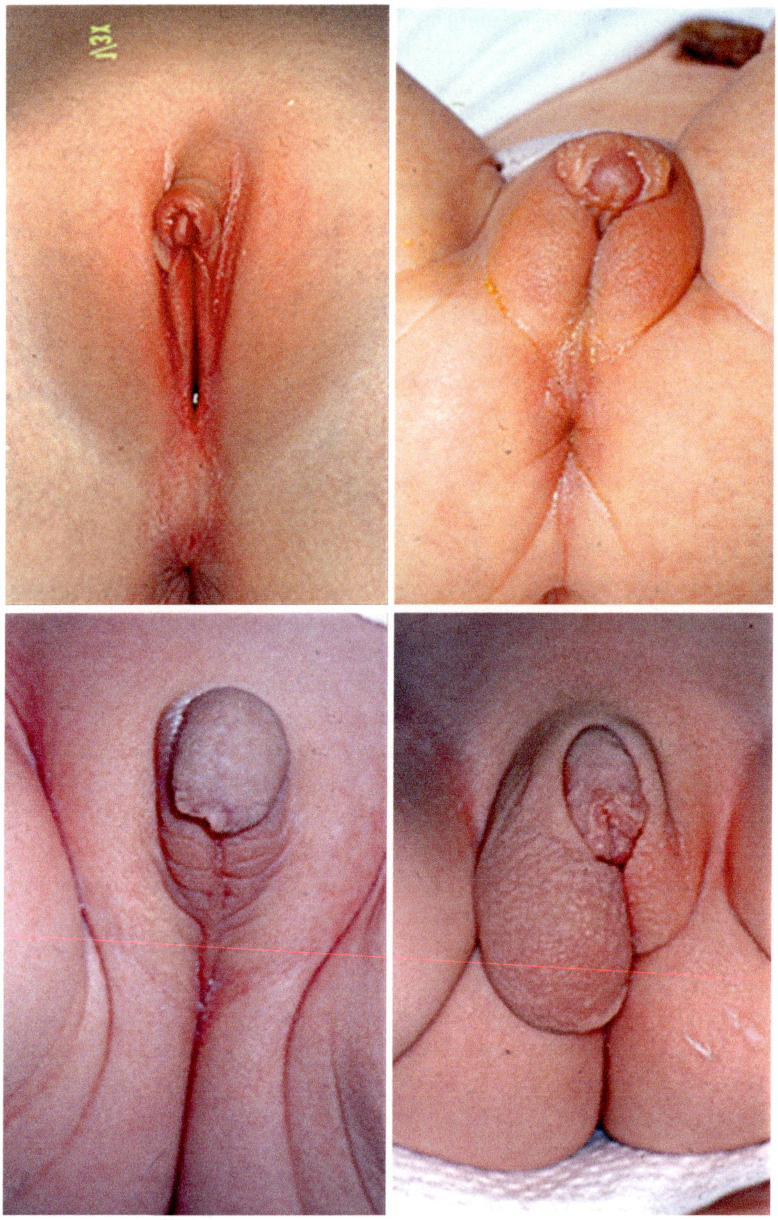

Fig. 68.3 The four broad categories of DSD: (1) apparent female phenotype with minor clitoral enlargement (CAH, Prader 1) (2) clearly ambiguous genitalia (CAH, Prader 2) (3) apparent male phenotype with "hypospadias", with absent testes (CAH, Prader 4) (4) apparent male phenotype with "hypospadias" with bifid scrotum and absent testis (45X, 46XY MGD)

The clinical examination includes a careful history of pregnancy and possible prenatal factors, as well as the family history. The physical examination is based on a deep understanding of the normal embryology, which allows a prediction of the underlying hormonal status from the anatomy. The first step is to establish the degree of masculinisation using the Prader scale (0—normal female to 5—normal male phenotype), which is an estimate of the amount of androgenic action (Fig. 68.4). The next step is to determine the status of the urogenital opening, which in ordinary hypospadias is smaller than the normal male urethral meatus, but in DSD is often a funnel-shaped opening. At the apex of the funnel the presence of bluish mucosal folds indicates the hymen, and hence the presence of the vagina where the genital and urinary tracts diverge. Then the presence and site of the gonads should be determined, which if palpable

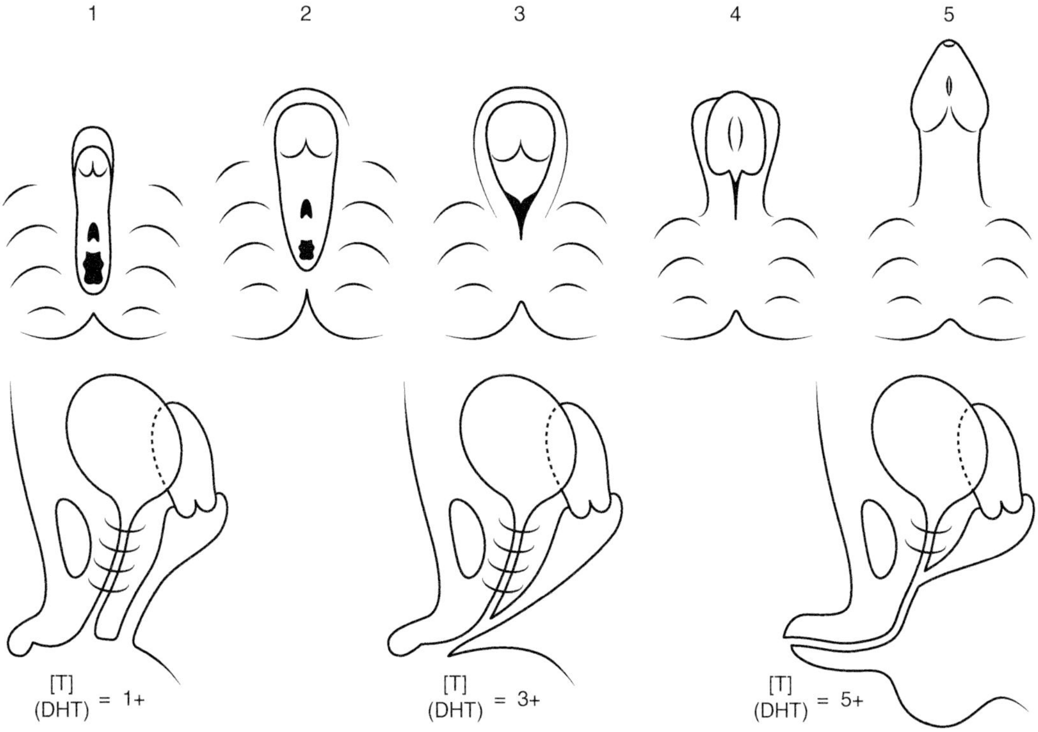

Fig. 68.4 (**a**) The Prader classification of the degree of virilisation of the external genitalia is from O (normal female) to 5 (normal male appearance). Prader 1 is clitoromegaly alone. Prader 2 is clitoromegaly and a funnel-shaped urogenital opening showing 2 orifices (urethra and vagina). Prader 3 is more virilised where only one opening is visible inside the urogenital opening. Prader 4 is more masculinised still, where the opening is on the proximal shaft of the enlarged phallus. The increasing virilisation from 1 to 5 is directly related to levels of androgens the fetus is exposed to, and also inversely related to the degree of regression of the developing lower vagina. (**b**) The regression of the lower part of the vagina is directly related to the amount of androgens present and the degree of external genital virilisation. From Hutson JM. The neonate with ambiguous genitalia. In Hutson JM, Warne GL, Grover SR (eds), Disorders of Sex Development. Springer-Verlag; Berlin, Heidelberg; 2012: 103–114; used with permission from Springer

are almost always testes. If the gonads are impalpable, the external inguinal ring should be felt to see if it is open, which may indicate the testes are within the inguinal canal. The final step in the clinical examination is to determine the status of the internal genital tract by rectal examination with the little finger. If a uterus is present, the cervix is palpable against the back of the pubic bone and feels like the eraser on the end of a pencil. Understanding how to interpret the clinical findings can be aided by using a set of rules based on the embryological processes (Table 68.2) [15].

Further investigations include pelvic ultrasonography to document the status of the internal genitalia. Then it is important to obtain a full karyotype, which might take several days, and an urgent fluorescent *in-situ* hydridisation (FISH) test to detect a Y-chromosome can be done within a few hours. Serum levels are obtained of the electrolytes (abnormal in CAH with hyponatraemia and hyperkalaemia), 17-hydroxyprogesterone, testosterone, FSH and LH. The serum level of AMH is also useful if available in the local laboratory. Second line tests include the hCG stimulation test to assess the androgenic synthesis pathway. An ACTH stimulation test can be useful to assess steroid hormone synthesis in both the adrenal gland and the testis. A 24-h urine collection enables the urinary steroid profile by gas chromatography and mass spectrometry, and will identify the

Table 68.2. Rules for diagnosis

Rule No.	Rule	Implication
1	Testes descend, ovaries don't	A palpable gonad is a testis
2	Testis descent + Mullerian ducts linked	A palpable gonad means Müllerian duct (on that side) is regressed
3	Uterus present = Sertoli cells poor/ absent (PR or ultrasound)	Persisting Müllerian ducts only occur in absent/dysgenetic testis (or rare PMDS)
4	Internal ducts mirror ipsilateral testis	MD/WD controlled by exocrine hormones from ipsilateral testis
5	Circulatory (adrenal) androgens cannot masculinise Wolffian duct	Endocrine levels too low and needs exocrine (high) levels
6	External genital development proportional to amount of effective androgens	Clitoral enlargement (erectile tissue) only caused by androgen exposure
7	External masculine development inversely proportional to lower vaginal regression	Vaginal remnant will be present in ambiguous genitalia
8	Masculinisation externally complete by 12 weeks but penis needs androgen up to 40 weeks	Absent androgens after this (in hypothalamic defects) cause micropenis
9	"hypospadias" assumes male gender Therefore only use if scrotum fused and testes descended	= Boy with normal hormone levels
10	Nonhormonal genital anomalies outside spectrum from male to female	Perineal anatomical anomalies include genitalia as well as other features

level of any enzyme defect in the steroid synthesis pathway.

A useful anatomical test to augment the pelvic ultrasonography is the urogenital sinugram, to outline the urogenital sinus and connection between urethra and vagina, and whether or not the cervix is present. The final test available in some referral centres, is molecular genetics to identify specific gene mutations.

68.11 Management

The medical and surgical approach to DSD first requires consideration of the degree of risk to the baby. Most importantly, there is a risk of death from adrenal failure in the second or third week of life if there is congenital adrenal hyperplasia (CAH) which is present in about half the affected babies. Where the baby has XY DSD, there is a risk of germ cell malignancy in the dysgenetic testis, as well as a significant risk of infertility and osteoporosis in adulthood from hormonal deficiency. In 46,XY DSD there is a risk of early onset renal failure or Wilms tumour if there is a WT1 mutation (Denys-Drash, Frasier, WAGR syndromes). In 46,XY DSD with incomplete virilisation the common urogenital sinus poses a risk of recurrent urosepsis if there is pooling of urine in the vaginal cavity. In all babies with a hormonal cause for DSD there is a risk of gender dysphoria in adolescence, as well as rejection by traumatised parents.

These potential risks have led to the development of a set of ethical principles on which to base the gender assignment and subsequent medical and surgical treatment plan for patients with DSD [16]. In the Royal Children's Hospital, Melbourne, these principles are now used by the ethics committee to oversee all decision-making for DSD patients, so that there is some external and transparent review of decisions that have lifelong consequences. The principles are: (1) Minimisation of physical harm to the child; (2) Minimisation of psycho-social harm to the child; (3) Maximising the potential for fertility; (4) Maximising opportunities for satisfying sexual relations, if required; (5) Keeping options open for the future; (6) Respecting the wishes and beliefs of the parents and (7) Considering the views of older children and adolescents where they are the patient.

Parents of babies with DSD suffer significant stress from the situation, and need not only definitive and frank information about the diagnosis, its implications and prognosis, but also counselling and support from a social worker and/or psychologist [17]. Another key requirement for reducing parental stress is a common message from all team members, so there is no confusion or contradictory views about the management plan.

The surgical treatment of DSD requires a high level of expertise because the operations are complex, and have life-long impact on the person if done poorly.

The surgical timing remains controversial, with proponents of early surgery in infancy (between 6/52 and 6/12) and those recommending delay until puberty, or at least until the patient is able to decide for themselves [18, 19]. In our own centre we still offer early surgery, as our long-term results support this approach [20–22].

Female genital reconstruction is the most controversial, because of a poor outcome for clitoral appearance and sensation, as well as persisting vaginal stenosis requiring revision in adolescence [18]. We have a 30-year history of performing the clitoroplasty with a specific technique that preserves neuronal and vascular supply to the glans clitoris by not dissecting the dorsal surface of the clitoris [23, 24]. This has given very reliable long-term results. For the vaginoplasty, we have found that more complex operations such as the Passerini procedure [25] or total urogenital mobilisation (TUM) [26] do not seem to be necessary as long as the posterior skin flap in a standard Y-V vaginoplasty is inserted high enough up the posterior vaginal wall, to overcome the congenital stenosis present in the lower third of the vagina secondary to the masculinisation.

Male genital reconstruction follows standard guidelines for hypospadias repair, although initial laparoscopy may be required to excise any streak gonad or ovotestis, as well as address the urogenital confluence. Most authors have advised excision of the redundant internal female genital tract in patients being raised as boys to prevent development of a urine-storing vagina after hypospadias repair. Recently, we have opted to merely disconnect the retained vagina from the urinary tract and leave it *in-situ*, based on the ethical principles described above, which recommend keeping options open for the future. There appears to be no measurable malignancy risk, but long-term follow-up will be essential to determine this.

68.12 Long-Term Follow-Up and Prognosis

Women with CAH have a reasonable prognosis for fertility, if the surgery allows normal sexual intercourse without significant discomfort. As hormone treatment of the adrenal defect improves the side-effects have decreased, with Cushing syndrome from excess steroid replacement now less common than previously. However, there remains a risk of polycystic ovaries as well as the residual anatomical or psychosocial issues.

In boys with 46,XY DSD fertility is lower, as poor androgenic function may prevent normal spermatogenesis, in addition to the anatomical defects where the vas deferens would normally enter the prostate to reach the posterior urethra. Sexual function, however, is still reasonable despite the small size of the penis, and the problem may be lessened with professional counselling. Fertility may be possible in some patients with the assistance of reproductive technology, if a viable sperm can be retrieved from the epididymis.

Gender dysphoria remains an issue for partial androgen insensitivity syndrome (PAIS), 5α-reductase-2 deficiency and 17β-hydroxysteroid dehydrogenase-3 deficiency. In patients with CAH who were commenced on steroid therapy at birth, gender dysphoria later in life is extremely rare and only occurs when the treatment is ceased, allowing physical (and mental) virilisation to recur.

Long-term outcomes from Royal Children's Hospital, Melbourne show a quality-of-life score in adulthood that is similar to patients with Hirschsprung disease or childhood-onset diabetes mellitus [21]. Outcome results from other centres show more varied results, perhaps reflecting a less cohesive and stable team that has been our strength for 3–4 decades [27].

The key requirement for optimal outcomes is a cohesive, multidisciplinary team in a quaternary referral centre, so that patients receive "best practice" treatment for their DSD. The appearance of Support Groups has enabled many issues to be addressed, as the groups perform an invaluable role for advocacy, distribution of information, lobbying and open communication with the medical team.

References

1. Hughes IA, Houk C, et al. Consensus statement on management of intersex disorders. Arch Dis Child. 2006;91(7):554–63.
2. Sinclair AH, et al. (1990) A gene from the human sex-determining region encodes a protein with homology to a conserved DNA-binding motif. Nature. 1990;346:(6281)240–4.
3. Imperato-McGinley J, Guerrero L, et al. Steroid 5alpha-reductase deficiency in man: an inherited form of male pseudohermaphroditism. Science. 1974;186(4170):1213–5.
4. Seifer DB, Maclaughlin DT. Mullerian inhibiting substance is an ovarian growth factor of emerging clinical significance. Fertil Steril. 2007;88(3):539–46.
5. Tong SY, Hutson JM, et al. Does testosterone diffuse down the wolffian duct during sexual differentiation? J Urol. 1996;155(6):2057–9.
6. Nef S, Parada LF. Cryptorchidism in mice mutant for Insl 3. Nat Genet. 1999;22(3):295–9.
7. Zimmerman S, Steding G, et al. Targeted disruption of the INSL3 gene causes bilateral cryprotchidism. Mol Endocrinol. 1999;13:681–91.
8. Stephens FD, Smith ED, Hutson JM. Congenital anomalies of the kidney, urinary and genital tracts. 2nd edn. Martin Dunitz, London. 2002.
9. Holschneider A, Hutson JM. Anorectal malformations in children. Berlin: Springer; 2006.
10. Srinivasan J, McDougall P, et al. When is 'intersex' not intersex? A case of penile agenesis demonstrates how to distinguish non-endocrine disorders in neonates with genital anomaly. J Paediatr Child Health. 2003;39(8):629–31.
11. Jones KL. Smith's recognizable patterns of human malformation. Philadelphia: W B Saunders; 1997.
12. Hutson JM, Werther G. Pseudohermaphroditism, glomerulopathy and Wilms' tumour (Drash syndrome): a case report. J Paediatr Child Health. 1990;26(4):227–9.
13. Hutson JM. The neonate with ambiguous genitalia. In: Hutson JM, Warne GL, Grover SR, editors. Disorders of sex development: an integrated approach to management. Springer-Verlag. Berlin: Heidelberg; 2012. p. 103–14.
14. Fischbach BV, Trout KL, et al. WAGR syndrome: a clinical review of 54 cases. Pediatrics. 2005;116(4):984–8.
15. Low Y, Deshpande AV, et al. Lethal comorbidity with genital anomaly in the infant. J Pediatr Urol. 2006;2(6):534–8.
16. Gillam, L. H., Hewitt, J.K. et al. Ethical principles an essential part of process in DSD care. Horm Res Paediatr. 2011;76(5):367–8.
17. Loughlin E. The family. In: Hutson JM, Warne GL, Grover SR, editors. Disorders of sex development: an integrated approach to management. Berlin: Springer; 2012.
18. Creighton SM, Minto CL, et al. Objective cosmetic and anatomical outcomes at adolescence of feminising surgery for ambiguous genitalia done in childhood. Lancet. 2001;358(9276):124–5.
19. Hrabovszky Z, Hutson JM. Surgical treatment of intersex abnormalities: a review. Surgery. 2002;131(1):92–104.
20. Lean WL, et al. Cosmetic and anatomic outcomes after feminizing surgery for ambiguous genitalia. J Pediatr Surg. 2005;40(12):1856–60.
21. Warne G, Grover S, et al. A long-term outcome study of intersex conditions. J Pediatr Endocrinol Metab. 2005;18(6):555–67.
22. Crawford JM, et al. Results from a pediatric surgical centre justify early intervention in disorders of sex development. Pediatr Surg Int. 2009;44(2):413–6.
23. Hutson J, Voigt R, et al. Girth-reduction clitoroplasty—a new technique: experience with 37 patients. Pediatr Surg Int. 1991;6:336–40.
24. Roberts JP, Hutson JM. Reduction of scrotalized skin improves the cosmetic appearance of feminising genitoplasty. Pediatr Surg Int. 1997;12(2–3):228–9.
25. Passerini-Glazel G. A new 1-stage procedure for clitorovaginoplasty in severely masculinized female pseudohermaphrodites. J Urol. 1989;142(2 Pt 2):565–8. discussion 572
26. Pena A. Total urogenital mobilization—an easier way to repair cloacas. J Pediatr Surg. 1997;32(2):263–8.
27. Warne GL. Long-term outcome of disorders of sex development. Sex Dev. 2008;2(4–5):268–77.

Male Genital Tract

69

Mike O'Brien

Abstract

Until the 12th week of gestation it is difficult to ascertain the sex of a human embryo based on the appearance of the external genitalia and yet the process is complete by 16–17 weeks. Our understanding of the complexity of the genetic and endocrinological interactions controlling this process continues to develop. There is emerging evidence that penile development has much in common with the development of limb buds. The developmental direction the indeterminate external genitalia take is driven by gonadal development which in turn is controlled by genetic sex determination. Though presented as sequential events, much of this happens in parallel. Between the 4th and 6th weeks the cloaca becomes divided into a posterior anorectal canal and an anterior urogenital sinus by the formation of the urorectal septum, the tip of which will eventually form the perineum. Simultaneously the mesoderm antero-lateral to the developing urogenital sinus expands to create the genital tubercle. When the cloacal membrane ruptures it exposes the floor of the urogenital sinus that will form the urethral plate. The mesoderm on either side of the urethral plate expands to form urogenital folds that extend into the genital tubercle. These are flanked by a pair of labioscrotal swellings. During the 6th week the urethral plate develops into a urethral groove which becomes the penile urethra as a result of fusion of the urogenital folds from proximal to distal, and is usually complete by 14 weeks. The formation of the glanular urethra is still under investigation and it is still unclear if it occurs by tubularization of the endoderm as in the penile urethra or through

M. O'Brien, PhD, FRCSI, FRCSI(Paed)
Department of Paediatric Urology,
Royal Children's Hospital,
Flemington Road, Melbourne, VIC 3052, Australia
e-mail: mike.obrien@rch.org.au

P.D. Losty et al. (eds.), *Rickham's Neonatal Surgery*, https://doi.org/10.1007/978-1-4471-4721-3_69

canalization of ectoderm distally. The prepuce itself develops as a result of ectodermal folding and cellular ingrowth resulting in the glans penis and inner prepuce sharing a common mucosal lining which gradually separates over years.

Keywords
Male genital tract • Newborns • Phimosis • Buried penis • Hypospadias Undescended testes • Varicocoele • Acute scrotum

69.1 Penis

69.1.1 Phimosis

Until the 12th week of gestation it is difficult to ascertain the sex of a human embryo based on the appearance of the external genitalia and yet the process is complete by 16–17 weeks. Our understanding of the complexity of the genetic and endocrinological interactions controlling this process continues to develop. There is emerging evidence that penile development has much in common with the development of limb buds [1]. The developmental direction the indeterminate external genitalia take is driven by gonadal development which in turn is controlled by genetic sex determination. Though presented as sequential events, much of this happens in parallel. Between the 4th and 6th weeks the cloaca becomes divided into a posterior anorectal canal and an anterior urogenital sinus by the formation of the urorectal septum, the tip of which will eventually form the perineum. Simultaneously the mesoderm anterolateral to the developing urogenital sinus expands to create the genital tubercle. When the cloacal membrane ruptures it exposes the floor of the urogenital sinus that will form the urethral plate. The mesoderm on either side of the urethral plate expands to form urogenital folds that extend into the genital tubercle. These are flanked by a pair of labioscrotal swellings. During the 6th week the urethral plate develops into a urethral groove which becomes the penile urethra as a result of fusion of the urogenital folds from proximal to distal, and is usually complete by 14 weeks. The formation of the glanular urethra is still under investigation and it is still unclear if it occurs by tubularization of the endoderm as in the penile urethra or through canalization of ectoderm distally [2]. The prepuce itself develops as a result of ectodermal folding and cellular ingrowth resulting in the glans penis and inner prepuce sharing a common mucosal lining which gradually separates over years.

The penile condition for which most medical opinion/intervention is sought is phimosis, which derives from the Greek phimoo (=muzzle) or phimos (=gag) and the suffix -osis (= process or state). Over the millenia since its original description by the Greeks it's meaning has been extended to include normal physiological states such as a non-retractile prepuce, residual glanulo-preputial adhesions and even 'excessive' or 'redundant' preputial length [3]. This unfortunate confounding with a genuine pathological process such as Balanitis Xerotica Obiterans has resulted in innumerable unnecessary circumcisions and even more unnecessary medical consultations. Rickwood's efforts to restrict the use of the term to BXO are doomed to fail and the more pragmatic approach is to adopt a classification into physiological or pathological phimosis.

Physiological phimosis describes normal anatomical findings that tend to disappear/resolve with growth. At birth a small minority of boys (4%) will have a foreskin that is fully retractable over the head of the penis, a further 54% will have a partially retractable foreskin but in the remaining 42% the glans is not at all visible [4]. The rate of separation of the glans and prepuce is exponential such that 20% of boys had a fully retractable foreskin by 6 months of age, 50% by 1 year, 80% by 2 years and 90% by 3 years. Oster took Gairdner's work and extended to older boys

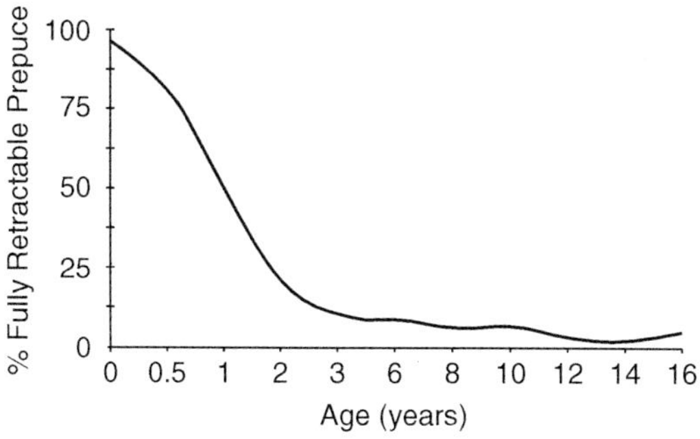

Fig. 69.1 Percentage of boys with a fully retractable foreskin [4, 5]

(see Fig. 69.1) and a significantly larger study population (>9500) of which a subset, 173 boys were reviewed annually for 7 years confirming that they had a similar trend to the graph for the overall population [5]. I would agree with Gairdner that the term 'preputial adhesions' is misleading as it implies that the glans and prepuce were previously separated and have adhered together. This misunderstanding perpetuates the false impression that forcible retraction of the prepuce from an early age is necessary for penile hygiene to clean a space that does not yet exist.

That said physiological phimosis is associated with some pathological and non-pathological processes. Smegma pearls are collections of shed epithelial cells, keratin and natural oils that accumulate in the developing space between the glans and prepuce and present as a mobile, non-tender, non-fluctuant swelling on the penis. Their formation contributes to the natural separation of the prepuce occasionally presenting as a non-offensive 'discharge'. Ballooning on micturition, especially if fusiform along the shaft of the penis, rather than spherical at the base as discussed below, is often a presenting complaint. Hutton and Babu found no evidence of obstructed urine flow when comparing uroflowmetry of uncircumcised boys when comparing those with and without ballooning [6]. After non-retractability the most common reason for referral for circumcision is recurring balanitis often misdiagnosed as recurrent UTIs when in fact it is posthitis! Posthitis is an inflammation of the prepuce, balanitis inflammation of the glans and balanoposthitis inflammation of both. The 'redundancy' of the foreskin encourages retention of urine subpreputially which then develops an ammoniacal dermatitis or inflammation which if left untreated may develop a secondary cellulitis. The initial posthitis, because of its association with dysuria is often diagnosed as a UTI, is best treated with topical barrier agents, simple hygiene advice and patient, parent and GP education.

Paraphimosis is an acquired condition thought to result from failure to reduce a tight foreskin that has been withdrawn over the glans and causes glanular oedema secondary to constriction which then makes spontaneous reduction unlikely. It tends to occur at the extremes of life in children whose foreskin has been retracted 'to clean', post sexual intercourse and in the elderly post urethral catheterization. It is a surgical emergency as failure to reduce has been associated with necrosis, gangrene and necrotising fasciitis. There are a number of treatment options including manual reduction with or without the aid of an ice glove, multiple needle punctures (The Dundee technique) to facilitate evacuation of oedema [7], injection of hyaluronidase or the topical application of granulated sugar [8]. All methods have been shown to work with no comparative studies to demonstrate superior efficacy of any individual technique [9]. That said topical osmotic agents (sugar etc.) take a long time to work and are probably best used where there is a delay in manual reduction [10]. Occasionally surgical intervention in the form of a dorsal slit is required especially where there is a delay in seeking medical attention. Once reduced there are mixed opinions on the merits or necessity of circumcision as recurrence of paraphimosis is notably uncommon.

The majority of cases of pathological phimosis can be attributed to Balanitis Xerotica Obliterans or BXO. More correctly known as penile lichen sclerosis it is a progressive sclerosing condition that affects the prepuce, glans and if left untreated, the urethra. It has a reported incidence of 0.07% [11]. Clinically it is distinguishable from physiological phimosis by virtue of the indurated pallor of the prepuce that prevents retraction of the foreskin in patients presenting in acute urinary retention or with a penile discharge.

However it is rare for referring doctors to make the diagnosis [12]. Its exact aetiology is unknown but it largely occurs in uncircumcised males thought possibly to be due to chronic irritation/inflammation from sub-preputial epithelial debris or an as yet unidentified infectious agent. In the paediatric population at least circumcision is curative in half [12] but may need supplementation with topical steroids especially if the glans/meatus is affected. Glanular lesions usually disappear within 6 months in >99% of patients [13]. Treatment with topical or intra-lesional steroid therapy may be sufficient in milder cases [14]. Topical steroid therapy alone was associated with resolution of symptoms and signs in 17% of boys with mild BXO after 3 months of therapy and this increased to 30% after 17 months [15].

The topical application of steroid ointment to treat both physiological and pathological phimosis has its origins here in Melbourne when proposed by Kikiros, Beasley and Woodward. Since that time there have been multiple publications of control trials of topical steroid versus placebo demonstrating statistically greater efficacy [16–18]. Despite this the optimal steroid treatment regimen has not been determined. Twice daily application appears to be as effective as three-times (without the need for application during the school day) with success rates approaching 85% [19]. Success is enhanced when application is coupled with routine preputial retraction. Topical steroid ointment has been shown to significantly more cost-effective than circumcision with potential annual savings in France in 2001 of 150 million Francs. One of the problems with topical steroid therapy is accurate dose application/administration sometimes resulting in non-compliance from steroid phobia, as has been demonstrated in up to a third of patients [20]. Of greater concern to physicians is over administration resulting in exogenous Cushing's syndrome or suppression of the hypothalamic-pituitary-adrenal axis. This has been demonstrated in infants treated with potent steroids for nappy rash i.e. a large area. Similarly absorption of preputially administered oestrogen cream has been shown to have systemic effects in a boy with phimosis [21]. However no evidence of H-P-A axis suppression was found in a study of topical Clobetasol [22]. Clobetasol proprionate is a Class I super potent topical steroid so the more commonly used Betamethasone valerate, a Class II or potent agent, should have even fewer side effects provided administered correctly.

69.1.2 Circumcision

For an operation to remove a few cm [2] of skin, practised for over 5000 years and carried out on over 1/3rd of the world's male population, circumcision still manages to generate a great deal of debate and controversy. No one knows exactly when circumcision was first practised. Sir Grafton Elliot Smith a British Egyptologist suggests it started over 15,000 years ago. Egyptian mummies as far back as 2300 BC were found to have been circumcised [23]. It has been demonstrated on 6000-year-old reliefs on the wall of the tomb of Ankh-Mahor at Saqqara near Cairo, Egypt [24]. There are many theories as to the origins of circumcision from a necessity in arid/desert regions to address the accumulation of sand under the prepuce through a humiliating 'branding' of slaves in ancient Egypt to a 'rite of passage' into adulthood [23]. Whatever the origins or indications circumcision continues to be performed amongst Jewish and Muslim cultures for religious reasons and for cultural reasons amongst some western societies.

In Judaism circumcision (*Brit Milah*) is a commandment (a *mitzvah*) from God representing a covenant between God and Abraham and all of Abraham's descendants—Genesis 17:10–14:

> 10. This is my covenant, which ye shall keep, between me and you and thy seed after thee; Every man child among you shall be circumcised.
>
> 11. And ye shall circumcise the flesh of your foreskin; and it shall be a token of the covenant betwixt me and you.
>
> 12. And he that is eight days old shall be circumcised among you, every man child in your generations, he that is born in the house, or bought with money of any stranger, which is not of thy seed.

> 13. He that is born in thy house, and he that is bought with thy money, must needs be circumcised: and my covenant shall be in your flesh for an everlasting covenant.
>
> 14. And the uncircumcised man child whose flesh of his foreskin is not circumcised, that soul shall be cut off from his people; he hath broken my covenant.

It is the father's obligation to perform the circumcision himself or as is more usual to appoint a *mohel* to carry it out. The rules and requirements are set out in the *Talmud* including the requirement that the entire glans be uncovered when the penis is flaccid [25]. In the UK *mohelim* are trained and regulated by the Initiation Society, under the guidance of the Chief Rabbi of Great Britain. Training takes 6 months, they have to see 40–50 before being permitted to perform one and have to pass a two-part practical and theoretical exam before being licensed. As has happened in those cultures that practice social circumcision there are people in the Jewish community who question its validity and relevance in modern society [26].

Among the six schools of Islam only one, the Shafiite school considers circumcision obligatory (*wajib*). The remaining five consider it to be recommended as a tradition (*Sunnah*) attributed to the Prophet Abraham [27]. Unlike Judaism a specific age, technique or person is not designated. This in part explains why, with the exception of bleeding, more complications are seen in circumcisions performed on Muslim boys than in Jewish boys.

It was in the nineteenth century that circumcision as a 'treatment' for widespread ills became increasingly common. Circumcision was advocated as a treatment for impotence, sterility, priapism, masturbation, 'wet dreams', syphilis, epilepsy, spinal paralysis, bedwetting, club foot, crossed eyes and even to prevent black men from raping white women (Dunsmuir:1999wd, http://www.icgi.org/medicalization). The sequelae from this can still be seen in the estimated 1.25million boys circumcised annually in the USA or one child every 26 s! [28]. That said there has been a reduction, in recent years, in the number of circumcisions performed annually in the western societies such as USA, UK and Australia. Circumcision rates in the USA have fallen from 65% in 1980 to 57% in 2009, continuing a downward trend from ever higher rates in the 1960s [29]. There is still marked regional variation with more circumcisions carried out in the mid-west that on the coast, with the exception of Maryland where the rate approached 83% [29, 30]. A similar downward trend though starting from a very low initial level has demonstrated in the UK. Korea where non-medically indicated 'social' circumcision is believed to be an after-effect of American occupation, is the one developed culture that is bucking this downward trend [31]. The reasons for this trend are varied. Given that the main reasons for circumcising one's child, outside of religious indications, are because his father is circumcised or because of a belief that it is cleaner or more hygienic [32]. As fewer fathers are circumcised, naturally the rate will fall and similarly position statements such as that released by the American Academy of Pediatrics suggesting that circumcision was unnecessary will have both a direct effect and an indirect one by influencing Medicaid to no longer reimburse the cost in some American states. In Australia a similar government initiative to not reimburse hospitals for carrying out non-medically indicated circumcision has had a similar effect. That said circumcision rates for phimosis in Western Australia are more than seven times the expected incidence of phimosis [33].

There is an ever growing anti-circumcision lobby driven, to be fair, by men who have been circumcised. Groups such as NOHARMM (National Organization to Halt Abuse & Routine Mutilation of Males), NORM (The National Organization of Restoring Men) and NoCirc (National Organization of Circumcision Information Resource Centers). Their objections are based on reports (from selected series of men) of dissatisfaction with penile appearance following circumcision in 1/3–1/2 men, due to scarring, or insufficient penile skin restricting erections and erectile curvature [28]. A number of women also object to routine circumcision primarily because of the pain it causes their child and some because of concerns regarding its impact on sexual function later in life for both their child and his potential female partner [34].

There is an equally strong pro-circumcision lobby promoting the public health benefits of circumcision. Ever since the first report in 1989 describing an association between circumcision status and susceptibility to HIV infection [35] there have been a number of randomized control trials in sub-Saharan Africa demonstrating a 50–60% reduction in HIV susceptibility [36–38]. Furthermore research has shown that circumcision in areas with a high prevalence of HIV is cost effective [39]. Given the high rates of circumcision required to have a significant impact, circumcision in the neonatal period has been shown to be even more effective given the potential higher take-up rates, lower procedural costs and lower complication rates [40]. Male circumcision has been shown to associated with a reduced risk of sexually transmitted diseases, penile cancer and urinary tract infections [41–43]. Despite some predictions there is no evidence that circumcision as an adult to mitigate HIV risk is associated with increased sexual risk taking behaviour. What is not clear is the protective effect on male-to-female HIV transmission of male circumcision. In the only trial to-date looking at this, what was found was an increased susceptibility of female partners of HIV-positive males who underwent circumcision and resumed sexual intercourse before complete wound healing [44]. Other advantages for female partners are a reduced susceptibility to Human Papilloma Virus infection and cervical carcinoma [45].

Extrapolating data from sub-Saharan African trials with a very high prevalence of HIV among heterosexuals to more developed westernized cultures with a higher rate of male-to-male infection is prone to error. Many of the trials had difficulty distinguishing the relative impacts of circumcision status and genital ulcer disease and hence the ongoing need to wear a condom cannot be underestimated. The high complication rates of 17–35% in adults undergoing circumcision, compared with 0.2% of neonates [46], give cause for consideration when proposing population-wide intervention [47]. Though the neonatal period is the best time to circumcise [48], the ethics and legality of performing circumcision on infants without their consent as a public health measure to minimize the risk of contracting a disease for which there are readily available and credible prevention strategies is still under discussion [49–53]. The psychological impact of circumcision both on the neonatal patient and subsequently as an adult is still being calculated [54].

Whatever the indication or justification there are a limited number of circumcision techniques. A detailed discussion of operative technique is beyond the scope of this text. Most open operative techniques are modifications of the 'sleeve resection' originally described by Treves in 1903 [23], normally carried out under general anaesthesia [55, 56]. The techniques carried out under local or regional anaesthesia generally make use of some form of clamp such as the Gomco, Winkleman or Mogen removed once the foreskin has been excised or the Plastibell designed to fall off within a week.

Whatever the technique employed circumcision, as with any procedure, is associated with some complications though the risks are largely overstated. Wiswell looking retrospectively at over 100,000 neonatal circumcisions performed at army hospitals over a 5-year period found a complication rate of 0.19% [42]. The majority of these were bleeding (43%), of which half required surgical haemostasis and only 3 (0.003% of total) required blood transfusion. Infection was a close second in 42% and only 25 boys (0.025% of overall) suffered any surgical trauma. The complication rate for circumcisions performed outside the hospital system is hard to quantify given the unknown denominator. What little is published suggests that Plastibell circumcision is associated with a higher complication rate, especially in obese children [57]. Other less frequent complications include recurrent phimosis leading to a buried penis, inclusion cysts, skin bridges and fistula. More significant but less frequent are glanular injuries. Meatal stenosis, thought to be due to contact with urine in the diaper and, historically reported to occur in 8–31% of boys is rarely seen nowadays possibly due to advances in diaper technology [24]. This is supported by the still relatively high incidence (20%) of meatal stenosis in Iran, possibly related to use of more traditional diapers [58].

Preputioplasty is an option for those boys with recurring preputial inflammation or restriction, despite topical steroids and who wish to keep an uncircumcised appearance. Not an operation to be considered in the presence of BXO, preputioplasty offers the possibility of increasing preputial girth at the expense of preputial length. There are a number of different publications advocating one, three or multiple longitudinal incisions which are closed transversely (alá Heineke-Mikulicz) [59]. A Y-V preputioplasty has been shown to be associated with higher success rates [60] and to be finding acceptibility with adult surgeons [61]. Preputioplasty as a credible alternative to circumcision is finding an expanding role in the management algorithm of phimosis [62]. It must be remembered that as with topical steroids much of the success relates to regular post intervention preputial retraction and hence patient age at selection is a crucial determinant.

Despite the absolute wealth of information, albeit largely conflicting, it would appear that providing information to parents has little impact on their decision to circumcise their newborn son or not as their decision had been made before the third trimester [32, 63].

69.1.3 Paraphimosis

Paraphimosis is an acquired condition resulting from retraction of the prepuce proximal to the coronal sulcus with consequent oedema and engorgement and entrapment of the glans. It is associated with failure to return the foreskin after male urethral catheterisation, post-coitally and post-masturbation but the majority in adolescents have no clear aetiology. The presumed association with phimosis is not born out by the fact that post reduction and resolution of swelling only 29% of patients have evidence of phimosis [10].

There are a number of differing techniques described to enable reduction, none of which have any proven superiority [9]. The most common method, initially trialled with topical anaesthesia but proceeding to penile block or general anaesthesia as necessary involves sustained manual compression of the prepuce and glans to reduce swelling (can take 15 min or more!) [64]. Then with a firm grip on the preputial ring the glans is invaginated. Others have suggested augmenting this approach with use of an 'ice' glove to help reduce the swelling. The use of topical osmotic agents such as glycerine magnesium sulphate, granulated sugar [8] or 50% dextrose. Others report the use of multiple needle punctures (the Dundee technique) to facilitate reduction of the oedema [7], enhanced by others by injection of hyalurinidase.

A failure of these methods especially under general anaesthetic may precipitate the need for a dorsal slit and either immediate or delayed circumcision. For those that did reduce without surgery it is no longer considered imperative to circumcise to prevent recurrence which is very rare [10].

69.1.4 Hypospadias

A condition that appears to be increasing in incidence, typically presenting at birth to obstetricians but occasionally detected antenatally, especially when severe [65, 66]. The term hypospadias is derived from the Greek for rent or defect "spadon" and 'hypo' meaning below. It is usually composed of three elements—a ventral opening of the urethra, ventral curvature (chordee) of the penis and an incomplete or hooded foreskin.

The development of the external male genitalia begins in the 7th week of gestation and is completed by 16–17 weeks [2]. The process begins earlier in the 4th–7th weeks with differentiation of the primitive sex streaks into testes under the influence of the SRY gene on the Y chromosome. The initial development of Sertoli cells triggers the development of germ cells and Leydig cells which in turn produce testosterone that is converted to dihydrotestosterone to exert its effect on the genital tubercle. Over the past decade a number of similarities between limb bud development and that of the genital tubercle have been discovered. The penis develops from ecto-, meso- and endodermal layers. The endodermal layer gives rise to the urethral folds on either side of the urethral groove, which fuse to form the urethra from the veru-montanum to the glans. The glanular urethra is formed by canalization and joins the tubularizing urethral plate. There is some evidence that this endodermal layer is crucial to penile development—endodermal differentiation—thus explaining the association of incomplete urethral development with incomplete preputial development [67]. These have been shown at a molecular level to interact through a number of signalling mechanisms including *Sonic hedgehog, BMP, WnT, Fgf* etc. [1]. How systemically circulating testosterone interacts with these signal transduction genes is still being elucidated.

For a long time hypospadias has been classified according to the position on the phallus of the meatal opening into Anterior (glanular and subcoronal)—50%, Middle (Distal penile, mid-shaft and proximal penile)—30% and Posterior (Peno-scrotal, scrotal and perineal)–20%. It is well recognized that this classification under-estimates the severity of hypospadias as the meatal opening tends to adopt a more proximal position once the chordee has been released. Furthermore the quality of the urethral tissue immediately proximal to the meatal opening is highly variable and tends to be hypoplastic or atretic proximally to the level of the bifurcation of the Corpus Spongiosum [68]. They describe a method of estimating the bifurcation of the spongiosum by drawing intersecting lines between the preputial skin and inner preputial mucosa. This understanding has prompted a new classification based on division of Corpus Spongiosum and pubic symphysis [69]. This changes the proportions to Middle 21% and Posterior 30%, of relevance when deciding whether the defect is best managed with a single or staged repair. This classification has the potential to enable more accurate comparisons between differing series of patients. It must be remembered though that this remains only one descriptive parameter of a complex anomaly that should also include an assessment of peno-scrotal transposition, penile size, glans size, nature of glanular groove, penile torsion and degree of chordee. Even by their own admission Orkiszewski have identified that in hypospadias with the most proximal meatal openings the division of the corpus spongiosum may be more distal on the penis than the meatal opening. Ultimately the classification of hypospadias is finalized intra-operatively. It is important that surgeons undertaking hypospadias repair be able to operate on all severities of hypospadias as pre-operative assessment will occasionally be an under-estimate.

There is marked variability in the incidence of hypospadias worldwide with 32 cases per 10,000, in 1992, reported from Southampton [70] and only 10 per 10,000 from South America [71]. In line with other male genital anomalies there are numerous reports of increasing incidence of hypospadias in recent years and this has been linked to increased environmental exposure to endocrine disrupting pollutants. Some of this variability will be due to under-reporting in less developed countries of minor degrees of hypospadias, however there is evidence of a genuine increase in the incidence of hypospadias in the developed world with a doubling of the incidence in America from 20 per 10,000 in 1970 to 39.7 per 10,000 in 1993. The majority of the increased incidence appears to be in less severe degrees of hypospadias which is consistent with some theories that the increase is not due to a real increase but rather due to increased reporting, previous under-reporting or a lowering of the threshold for reporting [72, 73]. Because of the confusion surrounding changing trends in the incidence of hypospadias there have been calls for more accurate registration of patients especially if endeavoring to link to potential emerging epidemiological data [74].

There is increasing evidence suggestive of an association between the incidence of hypospadias and environmental pollution by compounds with endocrine disrupting activity [75]. There are a large number of compounds with oestrogen-like activity (xeno-oestrogens—found in insecticides such as DDT, and industrial chemicals, phyto-oestrogens—plant derived chemicals with oestrogenic activity found in grains, nuts, Soya etc.) or with anti-androgenic activity [76]. For example the odds ratio of developing hypospadias is 2.4–3.4 if the patient's mother worked in agriculture in the month prior to conception [77, 78] and is 1.96 if the patient lives within 3 km of a landfill site [79]. A maternal professional exposure to hair spray products including phthalate is associated with a 2.4-fold increase risk of having a son with hypospadias [80]. An exclusive vegetarian diet has been demonstrated to have an almost fivefold increased risk of hypospadias [81]. The latter is felt to be due to an increased consumption of phyto-oestrogens especially found in Soy-based foods [76], hence their recommended intake in peri- and post-menopausal women. There are however a few reports that question the increased incidence and association with vegetarianism etc. [80, 82, 83]. Interestingly epidemiological data have unveiled a protective effect of folate supplementation during the first trimester [80].

There are a number of associated anomalies such as cryptorchidism (9%), persistent utriculus masculinus (10–57%), bifid scrotum and scrotal transposition all of which again suggest a common aetiology due to ineffective androgenisation. Severe forms of hypospadias can present as ambiguous genitalia. In some series up to 50% of patients with hypospadias and cryptorchidism had an underlying genetic, gonadal or phenotypic abnormality. All patients with hypospadias and cryptorchidism should be investigated to exclude congenital adrenal hyperplasia, a potentially lethal condition if undetected but eminently treatable. Apart from *in-utero* exposure [84], other risk factors for the development of hypospadias include placental insufficiency evidenced by an association with prematurity, very low birth weight, small for gestational age and multiple births [77].

A familial or genetic predisposition to hypospadias has been well described with a presumed multifactorial model of inheritance dependent on genetic-environmental interactions. The risk of a sibling developing hypospadias has been estimated to be between 6–10% [85]. It has been reported that as many as one in four boys with hypospadias will have a family member with hypospadias, and 1 in 14 will have two [86]. The more extensive the hypospadias the more likely for a family member to be affected with 3.5% of mild, 9% of moderate and 17% of severe cases having an affected relative. As our knowledge of the genetic mechanisms that underly development of the external genitalia increases so too does the ever expanding list of candidate genes associated with the development of hypospadias. These genes are not exclusively restricted to androgen development, conversion and effect such as 5 alpha-reductase type 2 gene (SRD5A2), 17 Beta-Hydroxysteroid dehydrogenase type 3 (HSD17B3) or Mastermind-like domain containing1 (MAMLD1) also known as Chromosome X open reading frame 6 mutation (CXorf6) to name but a few. They also include sonic hedgehog, fibroblast growth factors, bone morphogenic proteins (BMP), homeobox genes (HOX) and WnT/Beta catenin. For a detailed review the reader is directed to Kojima et al. and Kalfa et al. [87, 88]. There is some emerging evidence from in-vivo modelling of up-regulation of some of the candidate genes in response to exposure to oestrogen providing initial evidence to support the genetic-environmental interaction theory [89].

Hypospadias is a diagnosis that is almost always made at birth and generally investigations are not required. Exceptions include boys with associated undescended testes and those with proximal hypospadias who are known to have an increased incidence of utricular and renal abnormalities. Cryptorchidism is found in 8–10% of boys who have hypospadias [90]. The incidence of cryptorchidism increases with more severe forms of hypospadias such that almost a third of boys with a proximal hypospadias have an undescended testis. This latter group have a much greater incidence of chromosomal abnormalities (22%) than those with simple hypospadias (5–7%) or those with isolated hypospadias (3–6%). More severe degrees of hypospadias are also associated with an increased risk of disorders of sexual development, and persistent or enlarged utricular remnants. Boys with associated cryptorchidism or proximal hypospadias should at least undergo karyotyping. Endoscopic examination at the time of hypospadias repair may reveal an enlarged prostatic utricle in more than half of those with severe hypospadias. Whilst not mandating surgical immediate surgical intervention it may portend urinary tract infection, epididymo-orchitis, stone formation or urinary incontinence.

Despite the immortal words of Durham Smith "There is nothing new in surgery not previously described" [91], there have been over 250 described operations for hypospadias. All aim to produce a penis that is straight when erect, voids from the tip with a terminal meatus and looks cosmetically acceptable, whether that be with a circumcised or uncircumcised appearance. Broadly speaking the operative techniques can be subdivided in single or staged procedures, tubularised or grafted repairs and pedicled or free grafts. The majority of surgeons will only undertake half a dozen or so different types of hypospadias operation and a detailed operative description is best obtained elsewhere. For distal hypospadias the author's approach is dictated by the nature of the urethral plate, the depth of the glanular groove, the extent of any associated chordee and the parental desire for preputial reconstruction or not. The author prefers not to perform a preputial reconstruction in association with a Snodgrass repair [92, 93] and in that setting or where the urethral plate is deemed too narrow (<6 mm) prefers to use a meatal-based flap repair or Mathieu. Foreskin reconstruction as an option is being increasingly requested by parents who wish a cosmetic result more aligned with the general population.

For more proximal or severe hypospadias we perform a two-stage free graft or Bracka repair. For the Bracka repair we prefer to use inner preputial skin from the hooded prepuce as this is non-hair-bearing epithelium that is used to being in contact with urine. Other options for graft material include buccal mucosa—our next choice, bladder mucosa, as a last resort and never taken to the tip as constant exposure to a dry environment has lead in the past to unsightly mucosal overgrowth through the meatus, and finally posterior auricular skin graft. A necessary consequence of the Bracka repair is that the patients will ultimately end up looking circumcised. Again there are a wide range of alternative operations including but not limited to the single stage Koyanagi or modified Koyanagi [94], the Macedo 'three-in-one' [95] or the Duckett Onlay [96] or the two-stage Durham-Smith [97].

The ideal timing of hypospadias surgery continues to be debated with a trend towards surgery at a younger age. It is the author's preference to undertake hypospadias repair between 10 and 14 months of age for a number of reasons. Firstly there is a period after birth lasting approximately 6 months, often referred to as 'mini-puberty' where under the influence of circulating testosterone there is penile growth in excess of the remainder of the baby. Secondly, there are some emerging concerns regarding the impact of volatile anaesthetic agents on the developing brain. Thirdly, the surgery still takes place before the patient becomes 'genitally aware'. Finally, it is occasionally necessary in some patients to increase penile size prior to surgery and this can be achieved through the topical application of testosterone gel or intra-muscular depot testosterone. This can take as long as 3 months. When surgery is undertaken at around 1 year of age, the fact that the baby is still in diapers and yet to start toilet-training makes post-operative care simpler.

In part the wide variety of hypospadias operations is a response to a desire to improve functional and cosmetic outcomes but also a response to a need to reduce the complication rate associated with this surgery. The most common complication is urethrocutaneous fistula. There is marked variability in the reported incidence rate for fistula ranging from 2–30%. Fistulae account for 75% of complications [98] and have a 25–50% recurrence rate following repair [99, 100]. Other rarer complications include stricture, meatal stenosis, both of which should be excluded prior to fistula repair to minimize recurrence, meatal retraction, glans dehiscence, urethral diverticulum, residual chordee and unsatisfactory cosmesis with Bracka reporting up to 50% requesting further surgery. Most paediatric urologists believe that the repairs being currently performed have a much better cosmetic outcome than repairs performed 15–20 years ago and that Bracka's report is not applicable to current repairs. It is widely recognized however that there is poor agreement between patient and surgeon in relation to cosmetic outcome. It has also been reported that up to 33% of hypospadiacs are inhibited in seeking sexual contact compared to 12% of controls. For these reasons Bracka believes it is not appropriate to discharge these patients until they are fully grown and sexually active to allow time for both physical and psycho-sexual complications to manifest.

69.1.5 Inconspicuous or Concealed Penis

In 1986 Maizels developed a classification to describe a group of conditions resulting from or giving the appearance of a small penis. They consist of (1) poor penile suspension; (2) buried penis; (3) webbed penis; (4) trapped penis; (5) concealed penis; (6) diminutive penis and (7) micropenis.

While the majority present in infancy there is a second peak in later childhood/early adolescence (pre-pubertally) [101]. The latter group tend to be primarily buried in excess pre-pubic fat [102]. For this group time to allow penile growth, diet and exercise to encourage weight loss and only in a selected group is surgical intervention appropriate or required. When surgery is indicated it usually involves some form of lipectomy or liposuction and fixing of the penile shaft skin at the base of the penis [103]. Increasingly frequently a penis buried in excess pre-pubic fat is seen in infants, presenting prior to learning to walk, for whom surgical intervention is inappropriate and parents should be reassured that with weight loss the appearance will approve [104].

A buried penis, sometimes referred to as a Congenital Megaprepuce, tends to present between 6 and 12 months of age with a history of significant, spherical ballooning on micturition (not to be confused with the fusiform ballooning seen in physiological phimosis). Parents will usually report the need to manually express urine from within the prepuce. The exact aetiology of congenital megaprepuce is unknown. Most theories focus on abnormal attachments of fascial layers, others on penile skin deficits or crural abnormalities [105]. The overwhelming majority do not present at birth rather they become apparent over 6–12 months and hence whilst there is a congenital predisposition the act of micturition must play a contributing role in the progression of the condition. The natural history is unknown as most undergo some form of surgical intervention with generally speaking good outcomes [101]. There are a number of different surgical approaches all of which emphasize the importance of not removing external shaft skin, which tends to be deficient, and focusing instead on the inner preputial and Dartos layers [105–108].

Webbed penis is a form of peno-scrotal fusion anomaly for which surgical intervention may be necessary in severe cases. El-Gohary and El-Koutby recently proposed a classification of webbed penis into primary or secondary to circumcision and into simple or compound [109]. Simple merely describes a web that extends for variable lengths along the shaft of the penis. Compound is either a broad based web or one associated with scrotal transposition or chordee. The nature of the repair is based on the severity of the problem ranging from simple excision to the use of skin flaps [102, 110].

Trapped Penis is a post-operative complication following circumcision that if detected early may respond to topical steroid application [111]. It has been reported to occur in as many as 2.9% of boys circumcised as neonates [112]. More often surgical release is required which may be a simple scar revision or rarely a complex staged repair with skin grafting [113].

A concealed penis is one of the more poorly defined entities and could conceivably be any of those listed above. It would also include those that are masked by large herniae or hydroceles in neonates and infants.

Micropenis differs from other forms of concealed penis in that the underlying problem is the size of the penis which by definition is a stretched penile length of more than 2.5 standard deviations less than the mean for age [114]. For neonates this means less than 1.9 cm and for an adult 9.3 cm. This reference range does not take account of some ethnic differences and for that reason <7 cm is advocated for diagnosis of micropenis in adults [115]. It is essentially an endocrinological rather than a surgical problem resulting from a failure to produce gonadotrophins (hypogonadotropic hypogonadism), a failure of the testis to respond (hypergonadotropic hypogonadism) or idiopathic. For a more detailed review readers are directed to Wiygul and Palmer [114]. Treatment is essentially medical and aimed at improving appearances not restoring normality. When medical therapy fails surgical intervention may be appropriate with increases in length varying from 1 to 4 cm [115].

Peno-scrotal transposition describes the appearance when the penis is partially or completely enveloped by the scrotum. It can be an isolated presentation but more often appears in association with hypospadias and chordee. Primarily a cosmetic condition, more severe cases may have functional implications especially when associated with chordee. Most repairs involve flap rotation of the scrotum to drop it back but others move the penis [116].

69.2 Undescended Testis/Cryptorchidism

69.2.1 Introduction

Cryptorchidism is the most common congenital abnormality. The incidence is increasing and currently stands between 2.4 and 6.9%, averaging around 5% of all boys born at full term [117, 118] and being more common in pre-term and low birth weight infants. Descent of the testes has been the subject of extensive research. Despite this there are still large gaps in our knowledge of the aetiology of this condition.

69.2.2 Embryology

Currently the unifying theory describes testicular descent as occurring in two stages, the abdominal and the inguino-scrotal phase. Development of the gonads begins during the 4th intrauterine week. During the 6th week Testis Determining Factor, encoded by the SRY (sex-determining) region of the Y chromosome the developing gonad differentiates into a testis. Testicular descent begins during the 7th week. This phase, the abdominal phase, said to be under the control of Mullerian Inhibiting Substance (MIS) released from Sertoli cells, is attributed to regression of Mullerian structures and enlargement of the gubernaculum under the influence of Leydig cell produced insulin-like hormone 3 [119]. In addition testosterone causes regression of the Cranial Suspensory Ligament permitting the testis to remain near the internal inguinal ring during somatic growth and hence apparent trans-abdominal movement, complete by 15 weeks gestation.

The second or inguino-scrotal phase is largely under the control of testosterone and takes place during the 28th–35th intra-uterine weeks. During this phase testosterone is believed to act on the nucleus of the genitofemoral nerve in the spinal cord to cause the ipsilateral release of Calcitonin-gene related peptide (CGRP) from the end of the Genitofemoral nerve [120]. It is postulated that CGRP induces swelling and cavitation of the Gubernaculum into which the Processus Vaginalis protrudes. The growth and expansion of the gubernaculum has been shown to have a number of similarities with developing limb buds [121, 122]. This provides a space through which the testis can pass into the scrotum possibly driven by intra-abdominal pressure.

69.2.3 Classification

A fully descended testis is one that normally resides in the scrotum. An undescended testis is best described as one that cannot be manipulated to the bottom of the scrotum without undue tension on the cord. Undescended testes can be classified on the basis of whether they have become arrested in the line of normal descent and are described as intra-abdominal, canalicular or emergent. Testes that are not in the line of normal descent are called ectopic and can be Femoral, Perineal, Pre-penile, Transverse Testicular Ectopia. Histological examination of testicular biopsies suggests that ectopic and undescended testes have similar pathological origins [123].

The cremasteric reflex serves to elevate the testis in the scrotum either to help with the maintenance of testicular temperature in cold weather or to protect it from trauma. This reflex, weak at birth, becomes stronger in infancy and diminishes again after age 10. Retractile testes are those with a marked cremasteric reflex. They can be seen in the scrotum when the child is warm and fully relaxed, but retract into the superficial inguinal pouch with the slightest provocation. They can usually be diagnosed clinically in the out-patient department as the testes can be brought to the bottom of the scrotum, without tension on the cord. Occasionally this cannot be demonstrated in the OPD and may require examination under anaesthesia. Retractile testes per se do not require surgical intervention as the weakening of the reflex with age and the increase in testicular size make retraction in latter life unlikely. These patients should be followed up annually, until after puberty, as some will go on to develop acquired cryptorchidism, often referred to as Ascending Testes. Of boys diagnosed at 5 yo with retractile testes 1/3 will descend, 1/3 will remain retractile and 1/3 will ascend or become an acquired undescended testis [124]. With growth the distance from the bottom of the scrotum to the external inguinal ring increases and the excessive cremasteric reflex may prevent the spermatic cord from lengthening with age. It is more common in boys whose retractile testes are diagnosed before 7 yo rather than after 7 yo. Acquired cryptorchidism has been reported as occurring in almost 50% of post-pubertal boys with spastic diplegia. The other form of acquired cryptorchidism is that which occurs after inguinal surgery and can be referred to as iatrogenic testicular ascent. This has been reported to occur in 1.2% of boys following inguinal herniotomy.

What is relevant from a clinical point of view is whether the undescended testicle is palpable or impalpable. A palpable undescended testicle can usually be dealt with at open surgery. Unilateral or bilateral impalpable testes may require further investigation and laparoscopic techniques (described below).

69.2.4 Incidence

A large population-based study by the John Radcliffe Hospital Cryptorchidism Study Group reported that in the 1980s the incidence at birth was 5.4%, which fell to 1.85% by 3 months [125]. Those testes that had not descended by 3 months of age were unlikely to do so spontaneously. This represents a doubling of the incidence of undescended testes in 3-month-old boys since Scorer's report in 1964 [126]. The frequency of undescended testes is higher in premature infants. Approximately 45% of infants weighing less that 2000gms at birth will have undescended testes, many will descend spontaneously such that at 3 months of age 7.7% have persistent cryptorchidism.

There is worldwide concordance in the prevalence of cryptorchidism with no geographical sparing. There is a peculiar peak incidence in the UK amongst children born in March/April and a trough in boys born between June and October [127]. Similar Spring peaks and summer troughs have been reported in Austria, Sweden and Hungary. Additional associations include other congenital anomalies, low birth weight, twins, pre-eclampsia and previous stillbirth. These associations may be due to placental insufficiency, intrauterine infection, maternal pituitary hypogonadism and *in-utero* oestrogen or anti-androgen exposure.

69.2.5 Diagnosis

69.2.5.1 History

The history is usually straightforward when the absence of testes is noted at delivery or at the routine 6-week check-up. Children with a unilateral undescended testis can usually be seen at a routine OPD appointment at or after 3 months of age, by which stage the majority of those testes that will descend spontaneously will have done so. One must beware the newborn male with bilateral impalpable undescended testes and these must be seen more urgently. A diagnosis of bilateral cryptorchidism in association with Hypospadias must never be made on clinical grounds alone, as there is a very real possibility that these children may actually be over-androgenised females with Congenital Adrenal Hyperplasia (CAH), one form of which can be life-threatening if not treated.

69.2.5.2 Examination

When examining the scrotum a lot can be learned from inspection alone. With a relaxed patient in a warm environment both testes may be seen in the scrotum and observed to retract under the threat of palpation. Obvious scrotal asymmetry would suggest a unilateral undescended testis. The penis itself can be considered a "bio-assay" for testosterone and if a normal phallus is seen it is very suggestive that the developing penis was exposed to normal amounts of testosterone *in-utero*. Assessment of testicular size is helpful, especially in unilateral cryptorchidism, as there may be compensatory hypertrophy of a solitary testis; however this is not sufficient evidence that one would not actively look for the other testis. Testicular size can be measured by comparison to a Prader Orchidometer. In pre-pubertal boys the testes should be approximately equivalent to the size of the glans penis. When palpating for the 'impalpable' testis it is important to have a non-threatening approach and warm hands. Starting lateral to the superficial inguinal ring and 'milking' the contents of the inguinal canal towards the scrotum using the other hand to prevent retraction. Once located the testis is grasped between thumb and forefinger and under gentle traction an assessment is made of the distance into the scrotum that the testis can be drawn. If not palpable, remember to examine all potential sites (perineum, femoral, penile, other hemi-scrotum) for an ectopic testis.

69.2.5.3 Investigation

Imaging investigations and biochemical tests are usually of little benefit in the pursuit of the impalpable testis particularly in the presence of a normally descended contralateral testis. The investigation of choice for an impalpable undescended testis is laparoscopy.

69.2.5.4 Pathological Changes in UDTs

Testes that remain out of the scrotum undergo tubular dysplasia, evident on Electron Microscopy at 6–12 months of age, light microscopic changes at 3–4 years, macroscopic testicular atrophy in school-aged children and irreversible azoospermia if still not in the scrotum at puberty. There is some evidence to suggest that cryptorchid testes that are higher in the line of descent have more significant reductions in fertility index (spermatagonia per seminiferous tubule) than testes that have progressed further or fully descended testes [128]. Furthermore there is evidence that the longer a testis spends in an undescended position the more significantly the fertility index is negatively affected [129]. As well as a greater reduction in germ cells the longer a testis is undescended Cortes et al. found that reduction in germ cells starts from 28th week of gestation suggesting that there is more at play here than merely testicular location [130].

69.2.6 Management

69.2.6.1 Medical

Hormonal manipulation of undescended testes enjoyed a brief flurry of interest with the use of two differing regimens. Patients received either Human Chorionic Gonadotropin (HCG) by intramuscular injection twice weekly for 6–8 weeks or intra-nasal Leutenising Hormone Releasing Hormone (LHRH) up to 6 times a day for 3–4 weeks. Randomised trials showed no difference in incidence of testicular descent compared to untreated boys. Where hormonal studies are particularly useful are in boys with bilateral cryptorchidism [131]. In this group of patients if there are no palpable testes, a HCG stimulation test may be undertaken to detect functioning testicular tissue. A positive test suggests the presence of testicular tissue, however a negative test does not obviate the need for laparoscopy to look for the gonads, as they may be present but abnormal/dysplastic. One fifth of those testes that descend with hormonal therapy reascend at a later date [132]. There is also some evidence of testicular damage following HCG treatment and therefore hormonal treatment.

69.2.6.2 Surgical

Aims of Surgery

The purpose of orchidopexy is to locate the testis and place it in its normal environment. Testes are located in the scrotum so that they are 2–3° cooler than body temperature. This is possible because of the scrotal rugosity, which gives a large surface area relative to scrotal volume from which to lose heat, the absence of subcutaneous fat and a counter-current heat exchange mechanism—warm testicular arterial blood looses heat to the returning cooler blood of the pampiniform plexus of veins which surrounds it, with greater than 90% efficiency [133].

As well as achieving a cosmetically normal scrotum, placing the testis in the scrotum enables earlier detection of malignant transformation should it occur and may have some beneficial effect on fertility.

69.2.6.3 Palpable UDTs

The first successful orchidopexy was carried out by Thomas Annandale in Edinburgh in 1877 [134]. The surgical management of palpable undescended testes is reasonably straightforward with patients usually undergoing a single-stage, day-case open orchidopexy under general anaesthesia. Traditionally the testis is exposed via a groin crease incision but particularly for ascending testes some surgeons prefer a lateral scrotal margin incision or a trans-scrotal (Bianchi) approach with similar outcome results [135]. Whatever the approach the testis is identified, mobilized by dividing the gubernaculum, maximum length is obtained by separating and suture transfixing the associated patent processus vaginalis. The testis is delivered from within the tunica vaginalis and a Hydatid of Morgagni, if present, excised. The testis is then placed in the scrotum and secured. The most common method of securing is to place in an extra-Dartos or Sub-Dartos pouch where it is secured by co-apting the Dartos layer around the spermatic cord [136]. Whilst still commonly used I do not place sutures through the testicle to secure in the scrotum as I believe this to be unnecessary and have potential complications.

69.2.7 Impalpable Testis

Laparoscopy is the diagnostic test of choice for the impalpable testis. Open insertion of the umbilical port, CO_2 insufflation and a second port to manipulate the intestines are necessary [137]. Once visualized the vas must be followed throughout its full extent, as must the testicular vessels. There are a number of possible findings: (1) blind ending vas and vessels with no evident testis—so called 'vanishing testis'; (2) Normal or attenuated vas and vessels entering the inguinal canal through the internal ring—these patients require open surgical exploration of the inguinal canal with orchidopexy of a normal testis or more likely excision of a testicular remnant. The nubbin is excised as it provides no useful reproductive or endocrine function but retains its enhanced malignant potential. A single-stage orchidopexy, utilizing a pre-peritoneal or Jones approach is suitable for a normal sized-testis; (3) Good-sized testis within the peritoneal cavity that cannot be brought to the scrotum in a single stage—the surgical options for these patients are either a single stage microvascular transfer with the gonadal vessels being divided high near the renal vessels and anastamosed onto the inferior epigastric vessels or a two stage Fowler Stevens Orchidopexy. We favour the latter approach the basis for which is division of the gonadal vessels as a first stage; encouraging collateralisation of the remaining gonadal blood supply i.e. the cremasteric and vasal vessels. Followed 6 months later by the second stage, where the testis is mobilized on a pedicle of peritoneum that includes the vas and its now enhanced blood supply. This is brought through the abdominal wall medial to the inferior epigastric vessels (the Prentiss maneuver [138]) to reduce tension and placed in an extra-dartos scrotal pouch. Both of these stages can be performed as open operations, as originally described. However, we favor a laparoscopic approach for both. The first stage is an extension of the diagnostic laparoscopy with the addition of simple dissection of the gonadal vessels prior to their ligation. The second stage requires laparoscopic mobilization of the testis and then the introduction of a 10 mm port through the scrotal wound through which the testis is drawn into the scrotum and secured in the usual manner. A large meta-analysis by Elyas et al. has demonstrated that a 2-stage Fowler-Stephens approach is marginally better than recent attempts to undertake a single-stage orchidopexy with division of testicular vessels [139], with no difference between the open and laparoscopic approaches.

69.2.8 Complications of Surgery

Fortunately post-operative complications are rare and include the usual culprits of wound infection and bleeding. Testicular ascent occurs but the rate varies in relation to the extent of mobilization needed such that it is <1% for testes that are in the superficial inguinal pouch pre-operatively but close to 30% for those testes managed with a 2-stage Fowler-Stevens approach. Injury to the vas and vessels is very uncommon but vasal injury may be underestimated. Animal studies have demonstrated vasal injury from simple handling. Intimal vasal injury may never be detected therefore extreme care must be taken when mobilizing the vas off the sac to protect and preserve its patency.

69.2.9 Outcome Following Surgery

69.2.9.1 Testicular Size and Position

Testes that have undergone orchidopexy are usually smaller than normal testes and in general the higher the position of the testis initially, the smaller the final volume. Approximately 85% of all testes remain in the scrotum long term, 3% undergo testicular atrophy and 12% retract to a higher position requiring further surgery.

69.2.9.2 Fertility

Undescended testes have an obvious implication for fertility and it is difficult to get an accurate measure of this as the most commonly used indicator is paternity which is clearly prone to error in the absence of genetic testing. Remember that 15–20% of married couples have difficulty conceiving and of these 1/4–1/3 are identifiable as being due to an abnormality in the prospective father. When looking at couples who have attempted to conceive a child in the preceding 12 months Lee et al. [140] found that compared with controls (93.2% successful) men with a history of unilateral undescended testis were 89.7% successful and those with a history of corrected bilateral cryptorchidism were 65.3% successful [141]

69.2.9.3 Semen Analysis

Semen analysis would be a more objective way of assessing the effect of cryptorchidism on fertility. Only 25% of men with a history of bilateral UDTs have normal sperm counts and more than 50% have azoospermia. Amongst men with a history of unilateral orchidopexy, 20—70% have subnormal and about 50% have normal sperm counts. These figures are based on men who underwent surgery more than 25 years ago at which time surgery was often delayed until later in childhood. Recent studies are more optimistic of a benefit for testicular function with earlier orchidopexy such that 100% of those men whose orchidopexy was carried out at less than 4 years of age had normal semen analysis. The implications for fertility are equally optimistic with a report by McAleer who developed a fertility index based on the number of spermatagonia per cross-section of tubule in 50 tubules on histological examination of testicular biopsies [129]. When compared with normal controls patients whose orchidopexies were carried out at less than 1 year of age had a normal fertility index while those >5 years old had a decreased fertility index.

69.2.10 Malignancy

The absolute risk of developing malignancy in an undescended testis is hard to quantify. The majority does so in the third and fourth decades of life and 60% of the tumours are seminomas. The frequency for testicular malignancy in the population in general is 0.07%. The relative risk of developing cancer in an undescended testis has been calculated at between 5 and 10 times higher. There is no evidence of an association between likelihood of developing malignancy and initial location of testis. More importantly, there is no evidence of a reduction in malignant transformation with earlier surgery. Given the long lag-time of 30- to 40 years it may be some time yet before we are in a position to ascertain the impact of orchidopexy on those less than 2 years old on the subsequent development of malignancy.

69.3 Acute Scrotal Pathology

69.3.1 Introduction

A child who presents with an acute scrotum is the most urgent of urological emergencies. A torted testis may show signs of atrophy after 6 h and viability is compromised with a longer history. Surgery can be avoided if a confident diagnosis of torsion of an appendix testis, idiopathic scrotal oedema or epididymo-orchitis can be made but if in doubt—explore.

69.3.2 Torsion of Appendix Testis

Torsion of a testicular appendage almost always affects the appendix testis or Hydatid Cyst of Morgagni, a remnant of the cranial end of the Müllerian duct, present in 90% of boys. Other appendages include the appendix epididymis, the vas aberrans of Haller and the Paradidymis or Organ of Giraldes, all remnants of the Wolffian duct [142]. The peak incidence is between 10 and 12 years of age. The appendix testis is pedunculated and peri-pubertally may increase in size in response to hormonal stimulation. The pain is typically more gradual in onset, of longer duration and less severe than that of testicular torsion. If seen early in their clinical course it may be possible to distinguish between these two conditions. Torsion of the appendix testis has discrete localized tenderness, a palpable nodule and visible 'blue dot' of the infarcted appendix testis. With a history of longer duration it can be impossible to distinguish from testicular torsion and surgical exploration is imperative.

The diagnosis is clinical, substantiated with Doppler Ultrasonography if appropriate. Where doubt exists it is prudent and more rapid to explore the scrotum. Where a diagnosis of a torted appendix testis has been made the treatment options can be discussed. The choices are symptomatic management using oral analgesia and anti-inflammatory drugs. The alternative is surgical exploration under general anaesthesia with excision of the torted nodule, that is sent for histological examination. Contra-lateral scrotal exploration is not indicated [143]. Surgery is generally associated with a more rapid resolution of the patient's symptoms.

69.3.3 Testicular Torsion

The peak incidence occurs between the ages of 14 and 16 years and accounts for 90% of acutely presenting scrotal symptoms in post-pubertal boys. The annual incidence has been estimated at approximately 1 in 4000 males below 25 years of age [144]. The left side is more commonly affected than the right. Exercise, trauma, cold weather and cryptorchidism are possible predisposing factors. Testicular torsion takes two main forms, intravaginal and extravaginal.

69.3.4 Intravaginal Torsion

Intravaginal torsion is the more common, occurring at any age. It occurs because of a high attachment of the tunica vaginalis to the cord resulting in what is often referred to as a 'bell-clapper' testis. This allows the testis to rotate around the axis of the spermatic cord inside the tunica vaginalis. The testis may rotate internally or externally through one or more complete revolutions i.e. 360° or 720°. Manual detorsion is not recommended.

Numerous studies support prompt surgical exploration and detorsion. There is evidence that if torted for 6–8 h a testis will show signs of atrophy and after >8–10 h ischaemic necrosis is almost inevitable. However all acute scrotums should be explored given the often inaccurate nature of the duration of symptoms and the occasional occurrence of intermittent torsion where testes are said to have twisted and untwisted spontaneously.

Less than 50% of boys with testicular torsion present with a classic history of sudden onset of severe scrotal/testicular pain and swelling associated with a high riding, tender testis on physical examination. Because of the pathways of testicular innervation the initial pain is often referred to the groin or lower abdomen. The association of lower abdominal pain and vomiting can be misleading causing a misdiagnosis of acute appendicitis if the scrotum is not examined.

69.3.5 Extravaginal Torsion

Extravaginal torsion, also referred to as intrauterine or neonatal torsion is thought to occur pre-natally or during birth. The anatomical arrangement is normal but a lack of fixation between the tunica vaginalis and the scrotal/dartos tissues permits the testicle and tunica to rotate about the spermatic cord. Typically these patients present in the early neonatal period with an indurated and discoloured scrotum that is not tender. Published reports would suggest that testicular salvage is not possible is this setting. The anatomical arrangements are such that contra-lateral torsion is extremely unlikely. Rare cases of synchronous or metachronous extravaginal torsion have been reported. Our current policy is to not explore these testes immediately but to proceed to an elective exploration as soon as it can be arranged. This provides an opportunity to fix the contra-lateral side, remove the dead testis and exclude the rare possibility of a congenital testicular tumour.

The management of testicular torsion is based on immediate surgical exploration. The scrotum may be entered via a transverse scrotal crease incision over the affected side or through a midline sagittal incision in the raphe. Once exposed the testis and spermatic cord is untwisted and assessed for viability based on the prompt return of perfusion as evidenced by a change in colour or bleeding of oxygenated blood when the tunica albuginea is incised. In prepubertal boys there is no contraindication to detorting an apparently non-viable testis. However, in post-pubertal boys there is evidence of impaired fertility following testicular torsion. It may be that detorting and preserving a testis of dubious viability predisposes to the production of anti-sperm antibodies (there are no sperm present pre-pubertally) and may explain the reduced sperm quality, up to 50%, in later life. It is our policy to detort all testes and give the benefit of the doubt to the testis where possible. Once detorted and deemed viable the testis should be fixed, the contralateral side explored and prophylactically fixed to reduce the likelihood of torsion. There is much debate as to the method of fixation with some authors advocating placement in an extra-dartos pouch without suture fixation and others who support intra vaginal 3-point fixation with a non-absorbable suture. We employ the latter approach. All patients must be warned that testicular fixation makes recurrent testicular torsion very unlikely but not impossible and they should take the recurrence of sudden and severe testicular/scrotal pain seriously, seeking urgent medical attention.

69.3.6 Idiopathic Scrotal Oedema

Sometimes this idiopathic and enigmatic condition represents a cutaneous infection spreading forward from the anus, others that it is an allergic phenomenon and still others that it perhaps results from an insect bite. It usually presents with an asymptomatic patient whose parents have noticed a marked oedema and erythema of the scrotum. Typically the erythema involves one hemi-scrotum, but may be bilateral, extends beyond the confines of the scrotum up onto the anterior abdominal wall or back towards the anal verge. The usual age range is 5–6 years but it has been seen in up to 10 year olds. It is often confused with testicular torsion or cellulitis. The absence of testicular tenderness, pyrexia and malaise mitigate against these diagnoses. Treatment usually consists of reassurance but antibiotics and anti-histamines, of no proven benefit, have been advocated in the past. It resolves in 1–2 days and recurrence is unusual.

69.3.7 Epididymitis

Epididymitis or epididymo-orchitis, is the consequence of the retrograde passage of urine along the patent vas deferens. Because patency of the vas is critical to its aetiology it tends to occur either in early infancy (<6 months) or in adolescence as the vas is generally occluded in the intervening years becoming patent again with the onset of puberty. Though usually associated with reflux of infected urine it may occur with vasal reflux of sterile urine usually in patients with a predisposing anatomical abnormality such as ectopic ureter or persistent Müllerian remnant. All patients with epididymo-orchitis should at least undergo ultrasound examination of the urinary tract; additionally infants should have a micturating cystourethrogram.

As testicular torsion is significantly more common, a clinical diagnosis of epididymo-orchitis must be reached very carefully and ideally supported by evidence of a urinary tract infection; up to 50% of patients will have fever and pyuria, urinary tract abnormality or sonographic evidence that the testis has not torted. Management is based on administration of analgesia and antibiotics, usually intravenous Gentamicin or Ciproflaxacin, until the results of urine culture have been. If epididymo-orchitis is found at surgical exploration it is customary to take a swab or fine-needle aspirate from the epididymis for culture and sensitivity.

69.3.8 Orchitis

True orchitis is very rare but may occur in association with Mumps or septicaemia. Mumps orchitis, unilateral in 80% of patients, is extremely rare prior to puberty. In orchitis the testis tends to be larger and harder than in epididymitis. Approximately one third of patients will develop testicular atrophy and have an increased risk of infertility and malignancy.

69.3.9 Other

69.3.9.1 Hernia/Hydrocoele

Incarcerated inguino-scrotal herniae or a hydrocoeles may present as an acute scrotum but an experienced clinician can usually easily distinguish these conditions.

69.3.9.2 Malignancy

Testicular malignancy is rare but it may be primary as in adenocarcinoma, seminoma or secondary as in the malignant infiltration seen in leukemia.

69.3.9.3 Henoch-Schönlein Purpura

This vasculitic condition typically presents with a purpuric rash that extends from the buttocks and lower limbs to the remainder of the body. In addition to scrotal discolouration it occasionally affects the testis itself causing tenderness. A history of rash preceding the testicular symptoms may help with the diagnosis. Treatment is generally supportive though some paediatricians advocate steroid therapy.

69.3.10 Summary

As a general rule unless the diagnosis of testicular torsion can be confidently and completely excluded urgent surgical exploration should be undertaken in all cases. Investigations such as Doppler Ultrasonography and Isotope Scintiggraphy should not delay prompt exploration and rather are usually used to provide reassurance where testicular torsion has been clinically excluded.

69.4 Varicocele

A varicocele is an abnormal dilatation of the testicular vein and pampiniform plexus within the spermatic cord and scrotum leading to the classic description of "a bag of worms". It is rarely seen before 10 years of age but approximates 15% by late adolescence, similar to the rate seen in adults. They are typically asymptomatic, presenting as an incidental finding, although occasionally associated with vague symptoms of 'heavy scrotum' or 'dragging pain'. They are more commonly found (40%) in men with primary infertility [145] and it is the implications for fertility that cause the greatest confusion regarding treatment.

Varicoeles are graded clinically into one of three grades:

- Grade 1—small and only palpable with Valsalva
- Grade 2—easily paplable when patient examined upright
- Grade 3—visible when patient upright

Patients must be examined when both erect and supine. Varicoceles that do not resolve when the patient is recumbent and/or right-sided varicoceles are more likely to be secondary to intra-abdominal pathology and should prompt an abdominal examination and further imaging. More than 90% of varicoceles are on the left side. There are a number of possible reasons for this—the longer course of the left gonadal vein, valvular incompetence of the gonadal vein, the left vein drains into the smaller left renal vein than the right which joins the IVC, the 'nutcracker effect' where the left gonadal vein is compressed between the superior mesenteric artery and the aorta [146].

During physical examination testicular volume, using an orchidometer or an ultrasound, and testicular consistency must be assessed. The role of ultrasound is controversial. It is highly accurate, repeatable and non-invasive and more accurate than orchidometer at detecting volume differentials [146, 147]. However the cost implications of implementing Diamond et al.'s suggestion for annual surveillance ultrasonography would be somewhere between $364 and $795 million per annum [148]. For adolescent boys with equal sized testes at time of diagnosis of varicocele 25% will have demonstrable testicular growth arrest, regardless of the grade of their varicocele [149]. For those patients with right sided or non-reducing varicoceles a combined abdominal and scrotal ultrasound may yield additional benefit however for others regular self-examination and annual review with clinical examination and orchidometry makes the most sense.

Biochemical tests reported in the literature but rarely used include Gonadtrophin releasing Hormone stimulation assay, serum Inhibin levels and FSH stimulation test [146]. Semen analysis on the other hand is of immense practical use in adults and late adolescence and possible in early adolescence, however there no established norms for early adolescence [150].

The clinical significance of varicocele lies in its relation to male infertility after all 40% of men with primary infertility have a varicocele yet only 20% of men with a varicocele are infertile [150]. There are a number of theoretical pathophysiological mechanisms by which varicoceles amy impact fertility—poor venous drainage with resultant interference with counter-current heat exchange and relative hyperthermia causing oxidative stress impairing spermatogenesis [150], endocrine disruption with reduction in intra-testicular testosterone and reduced Sertoli cell response to FSH [146].

Deciding on whom to surgically intervene continues to remain controversial. The American Urological Association [151] recommends treatment for:

- Male partners in a couple attempting conception where the varicocele is palpable, they have documented infertility, the female has normal fertility or potentially correctable infertility and there are demonstrated abnormalities on semen analysis.
- Adult males with a palpable varicocele and abnormal semen analysis but are not currently attempting to conceive.
- Young men who have a varicocele and normal semen analyses should be followed with annual semen analysis.
- Adolescents who have a varicocele and objective evidence of reduced ipsilateral testicular size

should be offered repair. Those without testicular size discrepancy should be followed annually with assessment of size and semen quality.

In adults with fertility issues and poor semen analysis the decision to intervene is relatively simple however in adolescents there is still significant uncertainty of the indications for and outcome of surgery. It is the most common correctable cause of male infertility with improvement in semen qualities, especially motility, in 66% and 40% of female partners conceiving [146]. That said a Cochrane review by Evers et al. found no significant impact on fertility where the treated varicocele was the only abnormality found in either partner [152].

In adolescents a testicular discrepancy of 20% between sides is considered an indication for surgery and there are numerous studies demonstrating catch-up growth in 85% of those undergoing surgery compared with 30% when observed [150]. Given that surgery alters venous and lymphatic drainage it has been postulated that the reduction in size discrepancy may reflect testicular oedema rather than true growth [150].

Once a decision to intervene has been made next is a decision about the best approach: whether it is to be embolization by an interventional radiologist [153] or surgery. There are a number of surgical approaches—subinguinal (Marmar), inguinal (Ivanissevich) and retroperitoneal (Palomo) that may be augmented by the use of microsurgical instruments [154] in the inguinal and distal approach or laparoscopic for the retroperitoneal (Table 69.1 (A detailed discussion of the various surgical approaches is beyond the scope of this text).

Table 69.1 Comparison of surgical approaches [158]

Approach	Failure rate	Hydrocele rate
Embolization	4.3% (1.9–9.3%)	
Inguinal	15.6% (3.5–17.5%)	7.5% (4.3–17.5%)
Microscopic	2% (1.4–14.8%)	0.3% (0–0.7%)
Retroperitoneal	12.5% (7.3–15.5%)	7.6% (4.6–9%)
Laparoscopic	11% (4–26.5%)	7.5% (1.7–12.7%)

Once a decision to operate has been made and a choice of approach made all that remains is the timing and for those in whom infertility is the indication operating in those with <1 year history of infertility does not result in an increased pregnancy rate above untreated males and given the rate of spontaneous resolution of infertility in couples with a history of less than 2 years then it has been suggested to reserve surgical intervention for those with more than 2 years of fertility struggles [155].

69.5 Epididymal Cyst/ Spermatocele

Epididymal cysts are benign cystic lesions of the epididymis that contain serous fluid in pre-pubertal boys and spermatoceles which are seen post-pubertally contain sperm. These are benign lesions that for the most part (80%) are asymptomatic and incidental pick-ups [156]. The remaining 20% were either discovered on self examination or rarely presented clinically with acute torsion. The incidence of epididymal cysts increases over time from 3.3% in boys <5 yo, 4.2% in 5–10 yo, 20.1% in 10–15 yo and 35% in boys >15 yo. Surgical intervention is generally reserved for large cysts.

For a more detailed review of other intra-scrotal lesions the reader is referred to Rubenstein et al.'s review article [157].

References

1. Cohn MJ. Development of the external genitalia: conserved and divergent mechanisms of appendage patterning. Dev Dyn. 2011;240:1108–15.
2. Yiee JH, Baskin LS. Penile embryology and anatomy. ScientificWorldJournal. 2010;10:1174–9.
3. Hodges FM. Phimosis in antiquity. World J Urol. 1999;17:133–6.
4. Gairdner D. The fate of the foreskin, a study of circumcision. Br Med J 1949;2:1433–1437, illust.
5. Oster J. Further fate of the foreskin. Incidence of preputial adhesions, phimosis and smegma among Danish schoolboys. Arch Dis Child. 1968;43:200–3.
6. Babu R, Harrison SK, Hutton KAR. Ballooning of the foreskin and physiological phimosis: is there any objective evidence of obstructed voiding? BJU Int. 2004;94:384–7.

7. Reynard J, Barua J. Reduction of paraphimosis the simple way—the Dundee technique. BJU Int. 1999;83:859–60.
8. Kerwat R, Shandall A, Stephenson B. Reduction of paraphimosis with granulated sugar. Br J Urol. 1998;82:755.
9. Mackway-Jones K, Teece S. Ice, pins, or sugar to reduce paraphimosis. Emerg Med J. 2004;21:77–8.
10. Little B, White M. Treatment options for paraphimosis. Int J Clin Pract. 2005;59:591–3.
11. Clouston D, Hall A, Lawrentschuk N. Penile lichen sclerosus (balanitis xerotica obliterans). BJU Int. 2011;108(Suppl 2):14–9.
12. Gargollo PC, Kozakewich HP, Bauer SB, Borer JG, Peters CA, Retik AB, et al. Balanitis xerotica obliterans in boys. J Urol. 2005;174:1409–12.
13. Kiss A, Király L, Kutasy B, Merksz M. High incidence of balanitis xerotica obliterans in boys with phimosis: prospective 10-year study. Pediatr Dermatol. 2005;22:305–8.
14. Das S, Tunuguntla HS. Balanitis xerotica obliterans—a review. World J Urol. 2000;18:382–7.
15. Vincent MV, Mackinnon E. The response of clinical balanitis xerotica obliterans to the application of topical steroid-based creams. J Pediatr Surg. 2005;40:709–12.
16. Ashfield JE, Nickel KR, Siemens DR, MacNeily AE, Nickel JC. Treatment of Phimosis with Topical Steroids in 194 Children. J Urol. 2003;169:1106–8.
17. Lund L, Wai KH, Mui LM, Yeung CK. Effect of topical steroid on non-retractile prepubertal foreskin by a prospective, randomized, double-blind study. Scand J Urol Nephrol. 2000;34:267–9.
18. Esposito C, Centonze A, Alicchio F, Savanelli A, Settimi A. Topical steroid application versus circumcision in pediatric patients with phimosis: a prospective randomized placebo controlled clinical trial. World J Urol. 2008;26:187–90.
19. Palmer LS, Palmer JS. The efficacy of topical betamethasone for treating phimosis: a comparison of two treatment regimens. Urology. 2008;72:68–71.
20. Morley KW, Dinulos JG. Update on topical glucocorticoid use in children. Curr Opin Pediatr. 2012;24:121–8.
21. Yanagisawa N, Baba K, Yamagoe M, Iwamoto T. Conservative treatment of childhood phimosis with topical conjugated equine estrogen ointment. Int J Urol. 2000;7:1–3.
22. Pileggi FO, Martinelli CE Jr., Tazima MFGS, Daneluzzi JC, Vicente YA. Is suppression of hypothalamic-pituitary-adrenal axis significant during clinical treatment of phimosis? J Urol. 2010;183:2327–31.
23. Dunsmuir WD, Gordon E. The history of circumcision. BJU Int. 1999;83:1–12.
24. Lerman SE, Liao JC. Neonatal circumcision. Pediatr Clin North Am. 2001;48:1539.
25. Glass JM. Religious circumcision: a Jewish view. BJU Int. 2000;85:560.
26. Goodman J. Jewish circumcision: an alternative perspective. BJU Int. 1999;83(Suppl 1):22–7.
27. Rizvi SA, Naqvi SA, Hussain M, Hasan AS. Religious circumcision: a Muslim view. BJU Int. 1999;83(Suppl 1):13–6.
28. Hammond T. A preliminary poll of men circumcised in infancy or childhood. BJU Int. 1999;83(Suppl 1):85–92.
29. Cheng D, Hurt L, Horon IL. Neonatal circumcision in Maryland: a comparison of hospital discharge and maternal postpartum survey data. J Pediatr Urol. 2008;4:448–51.
30. Leibowitz AA, Desmond K, Belin T. Determinants and policy implications of male circumcision in the United States. Am J Public Health. 2009;99:138–45.
31. Kim DS, Lee JY, Pang MG. Male circumcision: a South Korean perspective. BJU Int. 1999;83(Suppl 1):28–33.
32. Binner SL, Mastrobattista JM, Day M-C, Swaim LS, Monga M. Effect of parental education on decision-making about neonatal circumcision. South Med J. 2002;95:457–61.
33. Spilsbury K, Semmens JB, Wisniewski ZS, Holman CDJ. Circumcision for phimosis and other medical indications in Western Australian boys. Med J Aust. 2003;178:155–8.
34. O'Hara K, O'Hara J. The effect of male circumcision on the sexual enjoyment of the female partner. BJU Int. 1999;83(Suppl 1):79–84.
35. Fink AJ. A possible explanation for heterosexual male infection with AIDS. N Engl J Med. 1986;315:1167.
36. Auvert B, Taljaard D, Lagarde E, Sobngwi-Tambekou J, Sitta R, Puren A. Randomized, controlled intervention trial of male circumcision for reduction of HIV infection risk: the ANRS 1265 Trial. PLoS Med. 2005;2:e298.
37. Bailey RC, Moses S, Parker CB, Agot K, Maclean I, Krieger JN, et al. Male circumcision for HIV prevention in young men in Kisumu, Kenya: a randomised controlled trial. Lancet. 2007;369:643–56.
38. Gray RH, Kigozi G, Serwadda D, Makumbi F, Watya S, Nalugoda F, et al. Male circumcision for HIV prevention in men in Rakai, Uganda: a randomised trial. Lancet. 2007;369:657–66.
39. Kahn JG, Marseille E, Auvert B. Cost-effectiveness of male circumcision for HIV prevention in a South African setting. PLoS Med. 2006;3:e517.
40. Binagwaho A, Pegurri E, Muita J, Bertozzi S. Male circumcision at different ages in Rwanda: a cost-effectiveness study. PLoS Med. 2010;7:e1000211.
41. Daling JR, Madeleine MM, Johnson LG, Schwartz SM, Shera KA, Wurscher MA, et al. Penile cancer: importance of circumcision, human papillomavirus and smoking in in situ and invasive disease. Int J Cancer. 2005;116:606–16.
42. Wiswell TE, Geschke DW. Risks from circumcision during the first month of life compared with those for uncircumcised boys. Pediatrics. 1989;83:1011–5.

43. Larke NL, Thomas SL, dos Santos Silva I, Weiss HA. Male circumcision and penile cancer: a systematic review and meta-analysis. Cancer Causes Control. 2011;22:1097–110.
44. Wawer MJ. Circumcision in HIV-infected men and its effect on HIV transmission to female partners in Rakai, Uganda: a randomised controlled trial. Lancet. 2009;374(9685):229–37.
45. Castellsagué X, Bosch FX, Muñoz N, Meijer CJLM, Shah KV, de Sanjose S, et al. Male circumcision, penile human papillomavirus infection, and cervical cancer in female partners. N Engl J Med. 2002;346:1105–12.
46. Christakis DA, Harvey E, Zerr DM, Feudtner C, Wright JA, Connell FA. A trade-off analysis of routine newborn circumcision. Pediatrics. 2000;105:246–9.
47. Kim HH, Goldstein M. High complication rates challenge the implementation of male circumcision for HIV prevention in Africa. Nat Clin Pract Urol. 2009;6:64–5.
48. Morris BJ, Waskett JH, Banerjee J, Wamai RG, Tobian AAR, Gray RH, et al. A 'snip' in time: what is the best age to circumcise? BMC Pediatr. 2012;12:1–15.
49. Freeman M. A child's right to circumcision. BJU Int. 1999;83:74–8.
50. Hodges FM, Svoboda JS, Van Howe RS. Prophylactic interventions on children: balancing human rights with public health. J Med Ethics. 2002;28:10–6.
51. Van Howe RS, Svoboda JS, Dwyer JG, Price CP. Involuntary circumcision: the legal issues. BJU Int. 1999;83(Suppl 1):63–73.
52. Gerharz EW, Haarmann C. The first cut is the deepest? Medicolegal aspects of male circumcision. BJU Int. 2000;86:332–8.
53. Payne H. UK law regarding children: essentials for the paediatrician. J Paediatr Child Health. 2008;18:207–12.
54. Goldman R. The psychological impact of circumcision. BJU Int. 1999;83(Suppl 1):93–102.
55. Tucker SC, Cerqueiro J, Sterne GD, Bracka A. Circumcision: a refined technique and 5 year review. Ann R Coll Surg Engl. 2001;83:121–5.
56. Elder JS. Surgery illustrated circumcision. BJU Int. 2007;99:1553–64.
57. Mousavi SA, Salehifar E. Circumcision complications associated with the Plastibell device and conventional dissection surgery: a trial of 586 infants of ages up to 12 months. Adv Urol. 2008;606:123.
58. Joudi M, Fathi M, Hiradfar M. Incidence of asymptomatic meatal stenosis in children following neonatal circumcision. J Pediatr Urol. 2010;7(5):526–8.
59. Barber NJ, Chappell B, Carter PG, Britton JP. Is preputioplasty effective and acceptable? J R Soc Med. 2003;96:452–3.
60. Nieuwenhuijs JL, Dik P, Klijn AJ, de Jong TPVM. Y-V plasty of the foreskin as an alternative to circumcision for surgical treatment of phimosis during childhood. J Pediatr Urol. 2007;3:45–7.
61. Munro NP, Khan H, Shaikh NA, Appleyard I, Koenig P. Y-V preputioplasty for adult phimosis: a review of 89 cases. Urology. 2008;72:918–20.
62. Huntley JS, Bourne MC, Munro FD, Wilson-Storey D. Troubles with the foreskin: one hundred consecutive referrals to paediatric surgeons. J R Soc Med. 2003;96:449–51.
63. Maisels MJ, Hayes B, Conrad S, Chez RA. Circumcision: the effect of information on parental decision making. Pediatrics. 1983;71:453–5.
64. Dubin J, Davis JE. Penile emergencies. Emerg Med Clin North Am. 2011;29:485–99.
65. Cafici D, Iglesias A. Prenatal diagnosis of severe hypospadias with two- and three-dimensional sonography. J Ultrasound Med. 2002;21:1423–6.
66. Meizner I, Mashiach R, Shalev J, Efrat Z, Feldberg D. The 'tulip sign': a sonographic clue for in-utero diagnosis of severe hypospadias. Ultrasound Obstet Gynecol. 2002;19:250–3.
67. Baskin LS, Ebbers MB. Hypospadias: anatomy, etiology, and technique. J Pediatr Surg. 2006;41:463–72.
68. Mouriquand PDE, Mure P-Y. Current concepts in hypospadiology. BJU Int. 2004;93(Suppl 3):26–34.
69. Orkiszewski M. A standardized classification of hypospadias. J Pediatr Urol. 2012;8:410–4.
70. Chambers EL, Malone PS. The incidence of hypospadias in two English cities: a case-control comparison of possible causal factors. BJU Int. 1999;84:95–8.
71. Paulozzi LJ. International trends in rates of hypospadias and cryptorchidism. Environ Health Perspect. 1999;107:297–302.
72. Toppari J, Kaleva M, Virtanen HE. Trends in the incidence of cryptorchidism and hypospadias, and methodological limitations of registry-based data. Hum Reprod Update. 2001;7:282–6.
73. Aho M, Koivisto AM, Tammela TL, Auvinen A. Is the incidence of hypospadias increasing? Analysis of Finnish hospital discharge data 1970–1994. Environ Health Perspect. 2000;108:463–5.
74. Dolk H, Vrijheid M, Scott JES, Addor MC, Botting B, De Vigan C, et al. Toward the effective surveillance of hypospadias. Environ Health Perspect. 2004;112:398.
75. Wang M-H, Baskin LS. Endocrine disruptors, genital development, and hypospadias. J Androl. 2008;29:499–505.
76. Słowikowska-Hilczer J. Xenobiotics with estrogen or antiandrogen action—disruptors of the male reproductive system. Central Eur J Med. 2006;1:205–27.
77. Sun G, Tang D, Liang J, Wu M. Increasing prevalence of hypospadias associated with various perinatal risk factors in Chinese newborns. Urology. 2009;73:1241–5.
78. Fernandez MF, Olmos B, Granada A, López-Espinosa MJ, Molina-Molina J-M, Fernandez JM, et al. Human exposure to endocrine-disrupting chemicals and prenatal risk factors for cryptorchidism and hypospadias: a nested case-control study. Environ Health Perspect. 2007;115(Suppl 1):8–14.

79. Dolk H, Vrijheid M, Armstrong B, Abramsky L, Bianchi F, Garne E, et al. Risk of congenital anomalies near hazardous-waste landfill sites in Europe: the EUROHAZCON study. Lancet. 1998;352:423–7.
80. Ormond G, Nieuwenhuijsen MJ, Nelson P, Toledano MB, Iszatt N, Geneletti S, et al. Endocrine disruptors in the workplace, hair spray, folate supplementation, and risk of hypospadias: case-control study. Environ Health Perspect. 2009;117(2):303–7.
81. North K, Golding J. A maternal vegetarian diet in pregnancy is associated with hypospadias. BJU Int. 2000;85:107–13.
82. Fisch H, Hyun G, Hensle TW. Rising hypospadias rates: disproving a myth. J Pediatr Urol. 2010;6:37–9.
83. Elliott P, Richardson S, Abellan JJ, Thomson A, de Hoogh C, Jarup L, et al. Geographic density of landfill sites and risk of congenital anomalies in England. Occup Environ Med. 2009;66:81–9.
84. Klip H, Verloop J, Van Gool JD, Koster META, Burger CW, van Leeuwen FE, et al. Hypospadias in sons of women exposed to diethylstilbestrol in utero: a cohort study. Lancet. 2002;359:1102–7.
85. Avellán L. On aetiological factors in hypospadias. Scand J Plast Reconstr Surg. 1977;11:115–23.
86. Manson JM, Carr MC. Molecular epidemiology of hypospadias: review of genetic and environmental risk factors. Birth Defects Res A Clin Mol Teratol. 2003;67:825–36.
87. Kojima Y, Kohri K, Hayashi Y. Genetic pathway of external genitalia formation and molecular etiology of hypospadias. J Pediatr Urol. 2010;6:346–54.
88. Kalfa N, Philibert P, Sultan C. Is hypospadias a genetic, endocrine or environmental disease, or still an unexplained malformation? Int J Androl. 2009;32:187–97.
89. Willingham E, Baskin LS. Candidate genes and their response to environmental agents in the etiology of hypospadias. Nat Clin Pract Urol. 2007;4:270–9.
90. Shukla AR, Patel RP, Canning DA. Hypospadias. Urol Clin North Am. 2004;31:445–60. viii
91. Durham SE. The history of hypospadias. Pediatr Surg Int. 1997;12:81–5.
92. Snodgrass WT, Nguyen MT. Current technique of tubularized incised plate hypospadias repair. Urology. 2002;60:157–62.
93. Snodgrass WT. Snodgrass technique for hypospadias repair. BJU Int. 2005;95:683–93.
94. Hayashi Y, Kojima Y, Mizuno K, Nakane A, Kurokawa S, Maruyama T, et al. Neo-modified Koyanagi technique for the single-stage repair of proximal hypospadias. J Pediatr Urol. 2007;3:239–42.
95. Macedo A, Srougi M. Onlay urethroplasty after sectioning of the urethral plate: early clinical experience with a new approach—the 'three-in-one' technique. BJU Int. 2004;93:1107–9.
96. Duckett JW. The current hype in hypospadiology. BJU Int. 1995;76:1–7.
97. Smith ED. Durham Smith repair of hypospadias. Urol Clin North Am. 1981;8:451–5.
98. Snyder CL, Evangelidis A, Hansen G, St Peter SD, Ostlie DJ, Gatti JM, et al. Management of complications after hypospadias repair. Urology. 2005;65:782–5.
99. Shankar KR, Losty PD, Hopper M, Wong L, Rickwood AMK. Outcome of hypospadias fistula repair. BJU Int. 2002;89:103–5.
100. Cimador M, Castagnetti M, De Grazia E. Urethrocutaneous fistula repair after hypospadias surgery. BJU Int. 2003;92:621–3.
101. Herndon CDA, Casale AJ, Cain MP, Rink RC. Long-term outcome of the surgical treatment of concealed penis. J Urol. 2003;170:1695–7; discussion 1697.
102. Bergeson PS, Hopkin RJ, Bailey RB, McGill LC, Piatt JP. The inconspicuous penis. Pediatrics. 1993;92:794–9.
103. Shenoy MU, Srinivasan J, Sully L, Rance CH. Buried penis: surgical correction using liposuction and realignment of skin. BJU Int. 2000;86:527–30.
104. Wan J, Rew KT. Common penile problems. Prim Care. 2010;37:627–42, x.
105. Smeulders N, Wilcox DT, Cuckow PM. The buried penis–an anatomical approach. BJU Int. 2000;86:523–6.
106. Lee T, Suh H-J, Han J-U. Correcting congenital concealed penis: new pediatric surgical technique. Urology. 2005;65:789–92.
107. Brisson P, Patel H, Chan M, Feins N. Penoplasty for buried penis in children: report of 50 cases. J Pediatr Surg. 2001;36:421–5.
108. Summerton DJ, McNally J, Denny AJ, Malone P. Congenital megaprepuce: an emerging condition–how to recognize and treat it. BJU Int. 2000;86:519–22.
109. El-Koutby M, Mohamed Amin EG. Webbed penis: a new classification. J Indian Assoc Pediatr Surg. 2010;15:50–2.
110. Chen Y-B, Ding X-F, Luo C, Yu S-C, Y-L YU, Chen B-D, et al. A new plastic surgical technique for adult congenital webbed penis. J Zhejiang Univ Sci B. 2012;13:757–60.
111. Palmer JS, Elder JS, Palmer LS. The use of betamethasone to manage the trapped penis following neonatal circumcision. J Urol. 2005;174:1577–8.
112. Blalock HJ, Vemulakonda V, Ritchey ML, Ribbeck M. Outpatient management of phimosis following newborn circumcision. J Urol. 2003;169:2332–4.
113. Zucchi A, Perovic S, Lazzeri M, Mearini L, Costantini E, Sansalone S, et al. Iatrogenic trapped penis in adults: new, simple 2-stage repair. J Urol. 2010;183:1060–3.
114. Wiygul J, Palmer LS. Micropenis. ScientificWorldJournal. 2011;11:1462–9.
115. Wylie KR, Eardley I. Penile size and the 'small penis syndrome'. BJU Int. 2007;99:1449–55.
116. Kolligian ME, Franco I, Reda EF. Correction of penoscrotal transposition: a novel approach. J. Urol. 2000;164:994–6; discussion 997.

117. Thonneau PF, Gandia P, Mieusset R, Candia P. Cryptorchidism: incidence, risk factors, review and potential role of environment; an update. J Androl. 2003;24:155–62.
118. Cortes D, Kjellberg EM, Thorup J, Breddam M. The true incidence of cryptorchidism in Denmark. J Urol. 2008;179:314–8.
119. Hutson JM, Balic A, Nation T, Southwell B. Cryptorchidism. Semin Pediatr Surg. 2010;19:215–24.
120. Hutson JM, Nation T, Balic A, Southwell BR. The role of the gubernaculum in the descent and undescent of the testis. Ther Adv Urol. 2009;1:115–21.
121. Nightingale SS, Western P, Hutson JM. The migrating gubernaculum grows like a "limb bud". J Pediatr Surg. 2008;43:387–90.
122. Nagraj S, Seah GJ, Farmer PJ, Davies B, Southwell B, Lewis AG, et al. The development and anatomy of the gubernaculum in Hoxa11 knockout mice. J Pediatr Surg. 2011;46:387–92.
123. Hutcheson JC, Snyder HM, Zuñiga ZV, Zderic SA, Schultz DJ, Canning DA, et al. Ectopic and undescended testes: 2 variants of a single congenital anomaly? J Urol. 2000;163:961–3.
124. Agarwal PK, Diaz M, Elder JS. Retractile testis—is it really a normal variant? J Urol. 2006;175:1496–9.
125. JRHCS Group. Cryptorchidism: a prospective study of 7500 consecutive male births, 1984–8. John Radcliffe Hospital Cryptorchidism Study Group. Arch Dis Child. 1992;67:892–9.
126. Scorer CG. The descent of the testis. Arch Dis Child. 1964;39:605–9.
127. Jackson MB, Swerdlow AJ. Seasonal variations in cryptorchidism. J Epidemiol Community Health. 1986;40:210–3.
128. Saito S, Kumamoto Y. The number of spermatogonia in various congenital testicular disorders. J Urol. 1989;141:1166–8.
129. McAleer IM, Packer MG, Kaplan GW, Scherz HC, Krous HF, Billman GF. Fertility index analysis in cryptorchidism. J Urol. 1995;153:1255–8.
130. Cortes D, Thorup JM, Beck BL. Quantitative histology of germ cells in the undescended testes of human fetuses, neonates and infants. J Urol. 1995;154:1188–92.
131. Esposito C, De Lucia A, Palmieri A, Centonze A, Damiano R, Savanelli A, et al. Comparison of five different hormonal treatment protocols for children with cryptorchidism. Scand J Urol Nephrol. 2003;37:246.
132. Ritzén EM. Undescended testes: a consensus on management. Eur J Endocrinol. 2008;159(Suppl 1):S87–90.
133. Sørensen H, Lambrechtsen J, Einer-Jensen N. Efficiency of the countercurrent transfer of heat and 133Xenon between the pampiniform plexus and testicular artery of the bull under in-vitro conditions. Int J Androl. 1991;14:232–40.
134. Tackett LD, Patel SR, Caldamone AA. A history of cryptorchidism: lessons from the eighteenth century. J Pediatr Urol. 2007;3:426–32.
135. Gordon M, Cervellione RM, Morabito A, Bianchi A. 20 years of transcrotal orchidopexy for undescended testis: results and outcomes. J Pediatr Urol. 2010;6:506–12.
136. Ritchey ML, Bloom DA. Modified dartos pouch orchiopexy. Urology. 1995;45:136–8.
137. Casale P, Canning DA. Laparoscopic orchiopexy. BJU Int. 2007;100:1197–206.
138. Kolon TF, Patel RP, Huff DS. Cryptorchidism: diagnosis, treatment, and long-term prognosis. Urol Clin North Am. 2004;31:469–80. viii–ix
139. Elyas R, Guerra LA, Pike J, DeCarli C, Betolli M, Bass J, et al. Is staging beneficial for Fowler-Stephens orchiopexy? A systematic review. J Urol. 2010;183:2012–9.
140. Lee PA, O'Leary LA, Songer NJ, Coughlin MT, Bellinger MF, LaPorte RE. Paternity after unilateral cryptorchidism: a controlled study. Pediatrics. 1996;98:676–9.
141. Taran I, Elder JS. Results of orchiopexy for the undescended testis. World J Urol. 2006;24:231–9.
142. Sellars MEK, Sidhu PS. Ultrasound appearances of the testicular appendages: pictorial review. Eur Radiol. 2003;13:127–35.
143. Ben-Meir D, Deshpande A, Hutson JM. Re-exploration of the acute scrotum. BJU Int. 2006;97:364–6.
144. Cuckow PM, Frank JD. Torsion of the testis. BJU Int. 2000;86:349–53.
145. Wampler SM, Llanes M. Common scrotal and testicular problems. Prim Care. 2010;37:613–26, x.
146. Paduch DA, Skoog SJ. Current management of adolescent varicocele. Rev Urol. 2001;3:120.
147. Diamond DA, Paltiel HJ, DiCanzio J, Zurakowski D, Bauer SB, Atala A, et al. Comparative assessment of pediatric testicular volume: orchidometer versus ultrasound. J Urol. 2000;164:1111–4.
148. Walker AR, Kogan BA. Cost-benefit analysis of scrotal ultrasound in treatment of adolescents with varicocele. J Urol. 2010;183:2008–11.
149. Thomas JC, Elder JS. Testicular growth arrest and adolescent varicocele: does varicocele size make a difference? J Urol 2002;168:1689–91; discussion 1691.
150. Merriman LS, Kirsch AJ. Varicocele in adolescence: where are we now? Curr Urol Rep. 2012;13:311–7.
151. Report on Varicocele and Infertility. An AUA Best Practice Policy and ASRM Practice Committee Report. April 2001. http://www.auanet.org ISBN 0-9649702-1-5 (Volume 4) ISBN 09649702-6-0 (4 Volume set)
152. Evers JHLH, Collins J, Clarke J. Surgery or embolisation for varicoceles in subfertile men. Cochrane Database Syst Rev. 2008;CD000479.
153. Tauber R, Pfeiffer D. Surgical atlas varicocele: antegrade scrotal sclerotherapy. BJU Int. 2006;98:1333–44.

154. Baazeem A, Zini A. Surgery illustrated—surgical atlas microsurgical varicocelectomy. BJU Int. 2009;104:420–7.
155. Giagulli VA, Carbone MD. Varicocele correction for infertility: which patients to treat? Int J Androl. 2011;34:236–41.
156. Posey ZQ, Ahn HJ, Junewick J, Chen JJ, Steinhardt GF. Rate and associations of epididymal cysts on pediatric scrotal ultrasound. J Urol. 2010;184:1739–42.
157. Rubenstein RA, Dogra VS, Seftel AD, Resnick MI. Benign intrascrotal lesions. J Urol. 2004;171:1765–72.
158. Diegidio P, Jhaveri JK, Ghannam S, Pinkhasov R, Shabsigh R, Fisch H. Review of current varicocelectomy techniques and their outcomes. BJU Int. 2011;108:1157–72.

Part X

Outcomes in Newborn Surgery

Long-Term Outcomes in Neonatal Surgery

70

Risto J. Rintala and Mikko P. Pakarinen

Abstract

Paediatric surgery and neonatal surgery as a part of it started to develop to an independent surgical speciality after World War II simultaneously in many Western countries. The first paediatric intensive care units and neonatal surgical units were opened in 1950s. These factors lead to rapid change in the mortality of patients with congenital malformations. Specialised paediatric surgeons and, surgical wards and operation theatres dedicated to care for children enabled survival of increasing numbers of patients with congenital defects and acquired neonatal surgical problems.

Keywords

Neonatal surgery • Paediatric surgery • Long term outcomes • Quality of life

70.1 Introduction

Paediatric surgery and neonatal surgery as a part of it started to develop to an independent surgical speciality after World War II simultaneously in many Western countries. The first paediatric intensive care units and neonatal surgical units were opened in 1950s. These factors lead to rapid change in the mortality of patients with congenital malformations. Specialised paediatric surgeons and, surgical wards and operation theatres dedicated to care for children enabled survival of increasing numbers of patients with congenital defects and acquired neonatal surgical problems. During the last 50 years the mortality of patients with congenital defects, also those with malformation complexes has continued to decrease (Figs. 70.1 and 70.2). This development is due to improved neonatology and paediatric intensive care and especially due to improved treatment possibilities of congenital cardiac defects. The downside of decreased mortality is that a significant percentage of survivors today have permanent morbidities and long-term handicaps.

Until recently there has been too little information about long-term consequences of repaired congenital defects or acquired neonatal surgical problems. For paediatric surgeons the end point and final outcome measure is the functional outcome in an adult patient. Recent research has indi-

R.J. Rintala, MD, PhD (✉)
M.P. Pakarinen, MD, PhD
Section of Paediatric Surgery, Children's Hospital, Helsinki University Central Hospital,
P O Box 281, 00029, HUS, Helsinki, Finland
e-mail: risto.rintala@hus.fi

P.D. Losty et al. (eds.), *Rickham's Neonatal Surgery*, https://doi.org/10.1007/978-1-4471-4721-3_70

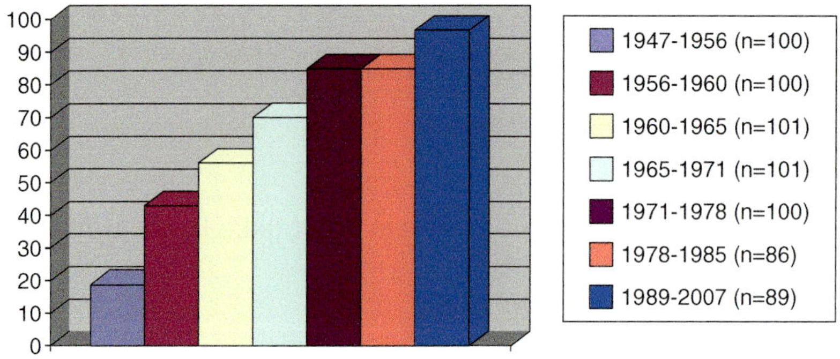

Fig. 70.1 Survival of 677 oesophageal atresia patients undergoing surgery at Children's Hospital, University of Helsinki from 1947 to 2007

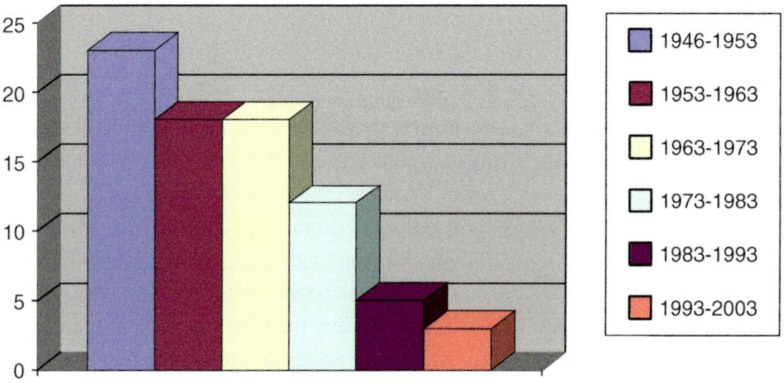

Fig. 70.2 Overall mortality of patients with anorectal malformations at Children's Hospital, University of Helsinki from 1946 to 2003

cated that a significant proportion of patients suffer from abnormal organ functions during childhood and many of these abnormalities are carried on to adulthood. These have often a significant impact on quality of life. Long-term functional results and quality of life are today as important outcome measures as early mortality and morbidity.

70.2 Rationale of Long-Term Follow-Up Programmes

There are several involved parties that are concerned on long-term outcomes of neonatal surgery. The patients' parents need to get a realistic picture on what is going to happen to their newborn child requiring surgery. The information has to be as accurate as possible without giving inappropriately positive expectations concerning functional outcomes. The parents tolerate well bad news on future problems of the patient as long as the given information is honest and consistent.

The patient himself/herself needs to get reliable information, as early as this can be given, of potential problems during later life. The information needs to include clarification of management modalities available to treat these problems. The parents may adopt to the handicaps of the patient and may not consider these as major functional problems. On the other hand, the patients may experience these handicaps as major factors that limits their social activities. For example even minor soiling in a teenager with an anorectal malformation may segregate the patient from many social activities such as sports and overnight visits to friends although the parents may consider that the patient's continence has greatly improved since earlier childhood.

The surgical team caring for newborn patients needs long-term follow-up data to guide clinical practice. In many neonatal surgical conditions the final functional outcome is not evident until the child has reached adolescence or adulthood. Longitudinal follow-up studies are required to determine the natural history of a neonatal surgical condition. Profound knowledge of possible complications that may develop during the development period of a neonatal surgical patient may guide primary treatment and definitely modifies the follow-up of the patient. For example, the recent finding of increased incidence of thyroid cancer in adult patients with Hirschsprung's disease [1] suggests that screening of thyroid cancer, especially medullary thyroid cancer, may be indicated in all patients with Hirschsprung's disease.

Health care administration need to be aware of the consequences and costs of neonatal surgery. Although the numbers are not high, the management costs of a newborn surgical patient are very high. There is a need for highly specialised intensive care facilities. In many cases the intensive care period may be lengthened significantly, e.g. patients with severe congenital diaphragmatic hernia may require weeks of intensive care. Patients with multiple malformations, especially those with combined cardiac and oesophageal anomalies may remain longer periods in the intensive care unit. On the other hand, the mortality of practically all neonatal surgical conditions has decreased significantly during the last decades. This implicates that more sick children survive with more handicaps. It is likely that these surviving children with serious primary conditions have more needs for medical care during their growth period than those with less stormy start. For planning of resource expenditure of long-term care of paediatric surgical patients, it is essential that data on long-term functional outcome and morbidities is available.

70.3 How to Analyse Long-Term Outcomes

The main problem in analysing long-term outcomes on paediatric surgical patients is the lack of standardization of surgical procedures. Although paediatric surgical conditions are usually well defined and classified, there are no standardization of procedures used to repair congenital or acquired defects in neonates. It is likely that the type of surgical procedure plays a significant role but this is very difficult to demonstrate.

The length of the follow-up period is also a crucial factor. The most valid endpoint is the outcome beyond childhood, at maturity. There is, however, paucity of long-term follow-up data in adults with congenital defects, therefore, short-term studies, often with variable age ranges of patients, have been used as measures of long-term outcome. This kind of studies have often had significant methodological problems. There has commonly been a lack of a healthy control population. Healthy controls with similar age, sex and municipality distribution as the patients are crucial for reliable outcome analysis.

Long-term outcome data, in terms of function and quality of life, is usually based on clinical history and examination. A major problem is the validity and agreement of the information attained from children and parents. Reliable data can be collected only from older children. The parents may not be able to provide truly reliable functional data for several reasons. They may not want to report unfavorable results to a surgeon who has been responsible for the treatment of their child. The parents may also ignore minor and moderate functional defects in a child who has had a congenital problem from birth or, in the case of smaller children, may consider them to be part of normal functional maturation.

The low incidence of neonatal surgical conditions poses a significant problems for outcome analysis. Institutional series are commonly too small to allow reliable comparisons between different management modalities. Pooling data from multiple centres could be a powerful tool also for long-term outcome studies but there is an increased opportunity for bias. Standardized management and follow-up protocols are very difficult to set up and long-term outcome studies commonly require many years of follow-up that is very difficult to organize in a multi-centre setting.

The study design in the evaluation of long-term outcomes is inherently problematic. Randomized controlled trials with enough power are usually unavailable for long-term outcome studies; the patients series are too small and there are to many confounding factors such as variable surgical skills and techniques, inhomogeneous patient material and problems in recruiting patients for follow-up visit/examinations. Observational studies are more commonly used for analysis of long-term outcomes. Observational studies can be performed prospectively, retrospectively or as a cross-sectional study. Prospective matched, controlled cohort studies are powerful in providing information on natural history of a congenital defect or disease. Case control studies are useful for cross-sectional studies e.g. gastrointestinal morbidity in adult oesophageal atresia patients. The critical point in case control studies is the matching of controls [2].

Recently, measures to assess the functional status and quality of life have become widely available also for children. These instruments are designed to measure health related quality of life (HRQoL) and are today validated for many languages and cultural backgrounds. Quality of life instruments can usually be divided in two categories: generic instruments that assess overall HRQoL and disease specific instruments that are validated and available for patients with for example renal diseases, gastrointestinal disease etc. A typical generic HRQoL instrument is SF-36 [3] that has 36 items and assess seven domains. SF-36 is not validated for children under 16 years of age, therefore, other instruments need to be used. Of the commonly used paediatric HRQoL generic instruments CHQ (Child Health Questionnaire) [2] includes 87 items and 11 dimensions, and PedsQL (paediatric Quality of Life Inventory) [4] that is a very flexible and easy to use tool has 23 items in four domains. Both of these come in several forms for different age groups and also for parents/caregivers. A typical disease specific instrument is GIQLI (gastrointestinal quality of life index) that has 36 items in five domains [5].

70.4 General Long-Term Consequences of Neonatal Surgery and Anaesthesia

There is very little published data concerning overall long-term effects of neonatal surgical procedures and anaesthesia. More data is available of the effects of prematurity on the incidence of disabilities later in life. Brain development is particularly vulnerable during the second and third trimesters of pregnancy. Very low birth weight (VLBW, birth weight 500–1500 g) infants have a high risk for hypoxic brain injury and intraventricular haemorrhage that are frequently associated with long-term neurodevelopmental sequelae [6]. Although the mortality of these patients has decreased during the last 20 years, the incidence of cerebral palsy has increased significantly [7]. There is an inverse correlation between the incidence of neurological damage and gestational age. Overall, 20–25% of children born with a birth weight under 800 g have at least one major disability [7].

Many studies have suggested that the prevalence of children with neurological disabilities has increased because of better survival of VLBW infants. The main problem in the assessment of neurological outcome is that the abnormalities may not become fully manifest until school age. In a follow-up study of children born at 25 weeks or earlier many, who showed no disability at the age of 30 months, demonstrated mild to moderate disabilities at the age of 6 years. The overall prevalence of neurodevelopmental disabilities in this group of extremely low birth weight children was between 90–100% depending on the gestational age [8].

Recent findings in neonatal rodents have revealed that many commonly used paediatric anaesthetic agents and sedatives are neurotoxic. Excessive neuronal apoptosis has been found to develop in rat pups immediately after exposure of standard anaesthetics [9]. The apoptosis has affected several regions of the developing brain including hippocampus and cerebral cortex. In the experimental animals the detected apoptotic effect was significant also at physiological and behavioural levels persisting into adulthood. It is controversial whether the apoptosis was caused by derangements of physiological homeostasis secondary to anaesthesia or by the direct effect of anaesthetic agents. These findings in experimental animals have raised concerns regarding safety of anaesthesia and surgical procedures in immature infants [10]. Epidemiological studies in human infants have yielded conflicting findings, some studies have suggested an association between neonatal anaesthetic exposure and later learning or behavioural problems [11], others have not shown any association [12].

The long-term neurodevelopmental effects of surgery early in life has been studied in premature infants who have developed necrotising enterocolitis. In a large meta-analysis concerning 7843 infants with necrotizing enterocolitis the median follow-up was 20 months [13]. Necrotizing enterocolitis was associated with significantly worse neurodevelopmental outcome than prematurity alone. Overall, 45% of infants with necrotizing enterocolitis were neurodevelopmentally impaired. Moreover, the need for surgery increased the risk of neurological impairment. Another study concerning surgically treated patients with necrotizing enterocolitis suggested that patients who initially underwent enterostomy formation had a worse neurodevelopmental outcome than those with primary anastomosis despite comparable severity of illness [14].

It is clear that a neonatal infant requiring surgical management is exposed to numerous adverse factors related to anaesthesia and surgical stress that can have a significant neurodevelopmental impact in future life. The effect of these factors have been demonstrated in premature infants, especially in those suffering from necrotizing enterocolitis, who are extremely ill and more vulnerable to central nervous system injuries than full-term infants. On the other hand, it is obvious that these adverse factors affect also full term surgical infants, although the long-term impact has largely not been investigated. For example, surviving infants with critical congenital diaphragmatic hernia who were treated with extracorporeal membrane oxygenation have a high incidence of developmental delay and central nervous system abnormalities [15]. Developmental delay occurs also in patients not treated with ECMO but ECMO is a very strong risk factor for adverse neurocognitive and psychomotor outcome [16].

The effect of neonatal surgery on cognitive and psychological development has been addressed only in a few studies. Most studies concern patients who have undergone neonatal correction of cardiac malformations, resulting in cyanosis, such as transposition of great arteries by arterial switch in cardiopulmonary by-pass [17, 18]. These studies have shown that these patients have lower general intelligence, more motor impairments and behavioural problems than healthy children. Risk factors for cognitive problems were the duration of operation and postoperative complications.

Ludman et al. [19, 20] studied non-cardiac neonatal surgical patients one and 3 years after surgery comparing the cognitive and developmental progress of the patients with those of healthy infants. At 1 year the surgical infants performed within normal range but less well than the controls in most areas of development. At 3 years the cognitive functioning of children whose condition resolved during first months of life was similar to the controls. Those requiring further treatment and surgery functioned at lower levels than controls. The number of operations under general anaesthesia was most strongly associated with poorer outcome.

70.5 Factors that Influence the Long-Term Outcome

70.5.1 The Type of the Malformation/Condition

The severity of the defect that is repaired in the neonatal period has a significant impact on long-term outcome. Benign conditions presenting during the neonatal period such as inguinal hernia and hypertrophic pyloric stenosis are successfully repaired with simple procedures with few complications. The long-term outcome of these conditions is usually excellent. Late complications of inguinal hernia repair include recurrence, testicular ascent and atrophy and damage to vas deferens or Fallopian tubes. These complications are uncommon but occur more frequently following neonatal repair [21] and in patients with incarcerated inguinal hernia [22]. Late surgical consequences of pyloromyotomy for hypertrophic pyloric stenosis are rare. Adhesive bowel obstructions are very uncommon as are significant dyspeptic symptoms [23, 24]. Probably the most important long term risk is inheritance; the risk of offspring of patients to inherit the disease is 20% of sons and 7% of daughters of a female proband and 5% of sons and 2.5% of daughters of s male proband [25].

The long-term outcome of defects that are life-threatening in the newborn period is influenced by severity of the anatomy, success of the anatomic reconstruction and occurrence of operative complications. Associated anomalies have a significant impact on the outcome, also. There is, however, scarcity of long-term follow-up data of many neonatal surgical conditions. In the following section examples of neonatal surgical conditions with recent consistent long-term follow-up data are considered, illustrating the factors that are involved in the outcome, especially beyond childhood.

70.5.1.1 Oesophageal Atresia

Patients with oesophageal atresia have multiple long-term consequences that are carried to adult life. One important consequence is the inherent abnormality of the oesophagus in these patients. No matter how perfect the original repair is there will always be a significant degree of oesophageal dysmotility [26]. The dysmotility is intensified in patients that have had anastomotic complications or long gap atresia. The dysmotility is associated with the incidence of epithelial metaplasia that predisposes to oesophageal malignancy [26]. Cases of oesophageal cancer in relatively young patients with repaired oesophageal atresia have been reported during the last decades [27, 28]. The dysmotility is also associated with a significant incidence of oesophageal symptoms. Symptoms of gastro-oesophageal reflux occur on average in 45% of adult patients with repaired oesophageal atresia [26, 29–31] and dysphagia in up to 85% of the patients [26, 32].

Thoracic deformities and scoliosis occur in a significant percentage of adults patients with repaired oesophageal atresia. Clinical and radiological scoliosis has been reported in more than half of patients [33]. The risk factors for developing scoliosis are thoracotomy-induced rib fusions and occurrence of associated malformations. Chest wall and shoulder asymmetries are also common occurring in 30–80% of patients [33, 34] and are associated with rib fusions and paralysis of serratus anterior and latissimus dorsi muscles.

Some of the associated defects in oesophageal atresia patients may go undetected during infancy and early childhood. In a recent report on adults with repaired oesophageal atresia 45% had vertebral anomalies that were detected at adult age [33]. Cervical spine was most commonly affected (38% of patients), many of these abnormalities were Klippel-Feil type of vertebral fusions. The radiographs obtained during the primary surgical care had revealed vertebral anomalies in only 3% of the patients. The high incidence of undetected cervical spinal anomalies is a significant and worrying finding as fused cervical vertebrae may later in life result in cervical instability and spinal stenosis. Cervical instability is associated with increased risk of spinal cord injury [35].

The overall quality of life of oesophageal atresia has been reported to be comparable with healthy peers [36, 37]. However, when disease-specific quality of life scores have been used (GIQLI: gastrointestinal quality of life; RSRQLI: respiratory quality of life), oesophageal atresia patients have obtained significantly lower scores than healthy controls [38]. Age and occurrence of associated malformations predicted poor gastrointestinal quality of life and occurrence of associated anomalies and tracheomalacia poor respiratory quality of life.

70.5.1.2 Hirschsprung's Disease

There are conflicting data regarding long-term outcome of surgery for Hirschsprung's disease. A traditional assumption has been that a great majority of patients gain more or less normal bowel function at least beyond childhood. This widely held view has been strongly challenged by several recent reports, where the follow-up has been extended to late childhood or adult age [39–43]. The reasons for this disparity remains somewhat unclear. In some older reports the data concerning patients' bowel function was retrospectively retrieved from hospital notes, that may underestimate problems in bowel function [41]. There is also an inherent bias when telephone and letter inquiries without structured questionnaires are used. Some more recent studies have used structured scoring systems that are based on questionnaires validated by healthy age- and sex-matched controls [43]. A common finding in these studies has been that the scores of Hirschsprung's disease patients are significantly lower than those of the controls.

It is commonly believed that bowel function in patients with operated Hirschsprung's disease improves with age. This is confirmed by most studies [39, 44, 45]. The critical age for final improvement is puberty [44]. Most reports describing outcome in adults or adolescents show few limitations in social functioning, occupation or sport activities despite overall reduced continence scores when compared with healthy controls [43, 44, 46]. In adults with operated Hirschsprung's disease, the gastrointestinal quality of life as measured with the GIQLI score, has been found to be marginally lower than in healthy controls [43]. The questions that gave the lowest scores were disease specific questions that were related to anorectal function. A worrying finding in this study was, however, that the only finding that correlated with poor bowel function was age. This suggests that the bowel control in patients with Hirschsprung's disease deteriorates by growing age.

A recent finding in patients with Hirschsprung's disease is that the incidence of thyroid cancer, especially medullary thyroid cancer, is significantly increased [47]. The cancer cases are often related to mutations in RET proto-ocogene in chromosome 10 and occurrence of associated MEN 2A syndrome [48]. The absence of MEN 2A does not rule out the possibility of medullary thyroid cancer, therefore, clinical and genetic screening of adults with operated Hirschsprung's disease need to be considered.

70.5.1.3 Anorectal Malformations

Anorectal malformations form an extremely diverse group of anomalies where the diversity of severity ranges between a simple and mild displacement of the anus that have little or no early or long-term consequences and extremely severe caudal regression syndromes that are often incompatible with life. Therefore, overall statements concerning long-term outcomes are not possible.

There are still very few reports on outcomes of ARM in adults. Most adult series include patients that have been operated by traditional methods, such as abdominoperineal or sacro-abdomino- and sacroperineal pull-throughs [49, 50]. There are no reports on adult outcomes following posterior sagittal anorectoplasty, the gold standard of ARM repair today.

Another problem is lack of uniformly accepted standardized methods to evaluate outcomes. Reliable comparison between reports is difficult, therefore, the outcomes can be expressed only in very general terms. Moreover, the criteria used to evaluate long-term outcome are variable and mostly designed for high anomalies [51–53]. The most recent assessment criteria are based on a consensus meeting in Krickenbeck 2005 [54]. These have, however, not gained overall acceptance. The likely reason for this is that the Krickenbeck criteria are mainly descriptive and relatively crude, and difficult to use in comparing the results.

In high anomalies a good result means usually socially acceptable continence which is not equivalent to normal anal function. A patient with a high anomaly and a good functional result rarely has normal bowel function and although socially continent may have some degree of smearing or soiling associated with physical straining or loose stools. Although many patients with low malformations have normal bowel function at long term, a method designed to assess long term outcome in high anomalies may underestimate minor defects in bowel function that are not uncommon in these patients,. These defects may become significant when the patient leads a life of an independent adult individual.

There are several prognostic factors that have impact on the long-term outcome. The level of the anomaly is an important prognostic factor in terms of bowel function. Males with a bladder neck fistula and females with a high confluence cloaca [55] have significantly poorer prognosis than patients with a lower urogenital connection

[56]. The obvious cause of worse prognosis in very high anomalies is the more marked hypoplasia of the voluntary sphincter muscles, especially the infralevator part the muscles [55].

The presence of severe sacral abnormalities is associated with hypoplastic sphincters. If more than two sacral vertebrae are missing or if the patient has other major sacral deformities, such as hemivertebrae and vertebral fusions the functional outcome is worse than in patients with normal sacrum or lesser degree of sacral maldevelopment [55, 56].

The role of the internal sphincter in anorectal malformations is a topic which has been debated for decades. The functioning internal sphincter can be demonstrated by the presence of rectoanal relaxation reflex at anorectal manometry. Most patients with a low anomaly have positive rectoanal reflex [57, 58]. In patients with high malformations rectoanal relaxation reflex has traditionally been present in only a minority of patients [58, 59]. However, when the rectourogenital fistulous connection has been preserved at the anorectal reconstruction the percentage of patients with preserved functional internal sphincter has been between 40–80% [56, 58, 60]. The presence of internal sphincter has been clearly shown to correlate with favorable functional outcome [56, 58, 59, 61].

Colonic motility disorders presenting usually as constipation have been earlier reported to be a problem in patients with low anorectal malformations and in females with a vestibular fistula [55]. Chronic constipation is also the main functional complication following repair of high anomalies by posterior sagittal anorectoplasty [55, 62, 63]. The incidence of constipation following PSARP procedure has varied between 10% [64] and 73% [63]. Constipation seems to be more common when internal sphincter preserving techniques have been used [63]. The cause of constipation is unclear; the extensive mobilization of the anorectum may cause partial sensory denervation of the rectum and impair the awareness of rectal fullness. Also, rectosigmoid hypomotility and generalized colonic motility disturbance has been suggested [55, 65].

It is likely that the surgical method of anorectal reconstruction in high malformations is a significant prognostic factor. However, this is very difficult to prove since randomized controlled studies are completely missing. Significantly better continence outcome was found in 21 patients who had posterior sagittal anorectoplasty compared with 16 patients having abdominoperineal pull-through [62]. Others [64, 66] have found no difference between patients who had undergone sacroabdominoperineal operation and those who had posterior sagittal anorectoplasty.

Associated defects may have a significant impact on life of patients with anorectal malformations. The urinary tract is the most commonly affected organ system. Urinary incontinence is today uncommon in patients that have undergone posterior sagittal anorectoplasty. Urinary incontinence occurs mainly in patients with neurogenic bladder that is caused by partial or complete sacral agenesis. In females with complex cloacal malformation continent urethral reconstruction may not be possible. Social continence, however, can be achieved by intermittent catheterizations or catheterizable continent urinary stomas. Tethering of the spinal cord is common in patients with anorectal malformations, however, neurological symptoms are uncommon. Untethering should be considered only in symptomatic patients [67]. Gynecological complications occur frequently in patients with cloacal malformations. Agenesis or duplication of Mullerian structures are found in approximately half of the cloaca patients. Uterovaginal agenesis and vaginal septum are not uncommon also in patients with vestibular fistulae [68]. Gynecological symptoms arise mostly from menstrual obstruction that occurs typically in cloaca patients. In these patients symptomatic adnexal cysts as well as endometriosis are not uncommon.

Patients with low malformations such as perineal fistulas have normal fertility [69]. The fertility of patients with more severe anomalies is a more complicated issue. Pregnancy is possible even in patients with complex cloacal malformation [68], but requires careful monitoring and delivery by caesarean section. In a long-term follow-up study concerning adults high malformations, only 39% of the patients had children, which was significantly less than healthy controls, 60% of whom had offspring [56]. Obviously, the low frequency of offspring in patients with high anomalies reflects true infertility in a significant percentage of patients. On the other hand, some patients may avoid sexual contacts because of defective fecal continence.

At adult age, defective fecal continence that is a reality in many patients with anorecatal malformations has significant social consequences. The continence related social problems are more common in patients with high lesions. The main problem is fecal soiling that restricts social activities. In a report [56] on the adult patients with high ARM 85% experienced social disability related to soiling. Other problems disturbing especially occupational life were inability to hold back flatus and fecal urgency. Hassink et al. [70] have reported that adult patients had significantly lower educational level than expected.

The literature reports on quality of life of adult patients with ARM show significant incidence of emotional problems [56, 69–74]. Up to rate of 58% of psychiatric diagnoses has been reported by Diseth et al. [74]. Psychosocial functioning also appears to be more affected in patients with severe anomalies and worse fecal continence [75].

70.5.2 Aging

The effect of aging in the outcome of neonatal surgical conditions is poorly studied. A common belief has been that most functional problems in congenital or acquired surgical conditions occur during the growth period with a general trend of global improvement in various domains of function. At adulthood the functional status stabilizes to the level that was reached at the end of the growth period. The overall health and quality of life appear to remain stable in some neonatal surgical conditions such as oesophageal atresia [37, 38]. In some conditions such as Hirschsprung's disease there is evidence that functional outcome might deteriorate by aging [43]. This is probably true also in patients with anorectal malformations.

The patients with spina bifida are vulnerable to deterioration of health at adulthood. The mortality is clearly increased in adult spina bifida patients when compared with healthy population. Those with hydrocephalus are especially at risk, the most common cause of death is unrecognized shunt malfunction. The need for repeat shunt surgery is not abolished in adulthood. The ambulatory status tends to decrease also after childhood [76, 77]. One of the greatest challenges in paediatric medicine today is to establish a network of transitional care for spina bifida patients that reach adulthood.

Biliary atresia is another condition where aging significantly affects outcome. After Kasai portoenterostomy operation the survival with native liver typically decreases to 20—40% or less until adult age. Although increasing numbers of patients with biliary atresia survive to adulthood with native liver, there remains a significant possibility of hepatic deterioration requiring liver transplantation at adult age [78]. Most surviving patients with native liver have not normal liver function. Cirrhosis and portal hypertension are typical findings and these are reflected in the laboratory parameters of hepatic synthetic capacity [79]. These patients require meticulous lifelong follow-up to detect those patients that require liver transplantation at adult age for recurrent jaundice or complications of liver cirrhosis.

70.5.3 Risk for Malignancies

Malignant degeneration occurring with advancing age is a risk that is clearly associated with congenital malformations. This is a central topic that commonly emerges when long-term outcomes are discussed. In addition to above discussed risks of malignancy that is associated with Hirschsprung's disease and possibly with oesophageal atresia, there are numerous examples of malignancy complicating congenital malformations. There is a risk of malignancy with undescended testes [80], asymptomatic cystic adenomatous malformation of the lung [81] and multicystic degeneration of the kidney [82]. Cancer may arise from a duplication cyst at any level of the gastrointestinal tract [83–86]. A unique anomaly complex is the Currarino syndrome where an anorectal anomaly and sacral defect are associated with presacral mass that is usually an anterior meningocele or presacral teratoma or a combinations of the two. The teratoma component has traditionally been considered as a benign tumor but accumulating data has confirmed that there is a significant risk of malignant degeneration both during childhood and in adults [87]. The author has encountered two malignant presacral masses in adult Currarino syndrome patients. Malignancy of the bile ducts, mainly cholangiocarcinoma; is a well established complication associated with choledochal cyst in adults. The risk is less that 1% if the cyst presents during first decade of life but increases to 14% in the third decade. Abnormal pancreaticobiliary junction probably plays a role in the pathogenesis. A possible pathogenic sequence is pancreatobiliary reflux because of pancreaticobiliary ductal malunion, inflammation, dysplasia with or without intestinal metaplasia, and invasive carcinoma. A combination of biliary stasis due to poor drainage of a stagnant pool of bile and increased mutagenicity of the bile acids may be ultimately responsible [88].

70.5.4 Undefined Factors

There are many conditions and management modalities in a newborn surgical patient of which very little is known in terms of long-term consequences. Many of these consequences may affect the neurocognitive and psychological prognosis of the patients. Little is known of long-term effects of multiple general anaesthesias that are quite commonly required in the postoperative management of neonatal surgical conditions. A typical procedures requiring multiple general anaesthesias are anastomotic dilatations of strictures following oesophageal atresia repair. Anal dilatations are usually necessary following repair of anorectal malformations. There is evidence that the duration of anal manipulation in patients with anorectal malformations is inversely related to mental and psychosocial outcome [89]. Later in childhood many of these patients undergo long-term bowel management regimens that often include invasive anal manipulations such as enemas. Psychosocial consequences of these procedures are completely unknown. It is self-evident that permanent and frequent soiling during childhood is deleterious to patients mental health, therefore, bowel management regimens are required. However, these regimens should avoid long-term anal enema administrations and use antegrade enema routes instead as they are usually well tolerated and associated with improved quality of life [90].

Intra-abdominal surgery during the neonatal period is associated with long-term complications that are related to adhesion formation. The overall risk of adhesive obstruction is less than 10% [91] but significantly higher reaching almost 20% in some conditions such as congenital diaphragmatic hernia [92]. The implications of neonatal pelvic and lower abdominal surgery in conditions like sacrococcygeal teratoma, Hirschsprung's disease and anorectal anomalies on fertility and fecundity in females is largely unknown at the moment.

Conclusions

The development of neonatal surgery after World War II and rapidly improving early outcomes has brought into light a growing group of individuals that in the past would have died or suffered from serious functional defects. The early operative and functional outcomes in these patient groups are usually well recognized, however, amazingly few reports on long-term outcomes beyond childhood are available. The medical teams and especially neonatal surgeons taking care of neonatal surgical patients have the responsibility to follow-up their patients throughout their growth period to study the true long-term outcomes. The caregivers of the patients have the right to know about possible late complications, effect of the neonatal surgical condition on growth and development, and also possible cognitive and psychosocial consequences. Proper follow-up gives also tools for development of management guidelines and surgical practice.

The follow-up of neonatal surgical patients should not end when the patients reach adulthood as congenital anomalies and neonatal surgical conditions may affect fertility and sexuality. The potential risks of malignancy and future inheritance need also be considered. The research on long-term outcomes is facilitated by development of patient registries and tracking systems. Reliable long-term outcome studies require also validated and standardized research tools and healthy control materials.

References

1. Sistonen SJ, Koivusalo A, Lindahl H, Pukkala E, Rintala RJ, Pakarinen MP. Cancer after repair of esophageal atresia: population-based long-term follow-up. J Pediatr Surg. 2008;43:602–5.
2. Killelea BK, Lazar EL, Vitale MG. Principles of outcome analysis. In: Stringer MD, Oldham KT, Mouriquand PDE, editors. Pediatric surgery and urology (Chap. 2). 2nd ed. Cambridge: Cambridge University Press; 2006. p. 17–28.
3. Ware JE Jr, Sherbourne CD. The MOS 36-item short-form health survey (SF-36). I. Conceptual framework and item selection. Med Care. 1992;30:473–83.
4. Varni JM, Limbers CA, Burwinkle TM. Impaired health-related quality of life in children and adolescents with chronic conditions: a comparative analysis of 10 disease clusters and 33 disease categories/severities utilizing the PedsQL 4.0 Generic Core Scales. Health Qual Life Outcomes. 2007;5:43–58.
5. Eypasch E, Williams JI, Wood-Dauphinee S, et al. Gastrointestinal quality of life index: development, validation, and application of a new instrument. Br J Surg. 1995;82:216–22.
6. Lemons JA, Bauer CR, Oh W, et al. Very low birth weight outcomes of the National Institute of Child health and human development neonatal research network, January 1995 through December 1996. NICHD Neonatal Research Network. Pediatrics. 2001;107:E1.
7. Vincer MJ, Allen AC, Joseph KS, Stinson DA, Scott H, Wood E. Increasing prevalence of cerebral palsy among very preterm infants: a population-based study. Pediatrics. 2006;118:e1621–6.
8. Marlow N, Wolke D, Bracewell MA, Samara M, EPICure Study Group. Neurologic and developmental disability at six years of age after extremely preterm birth. N Engl J Med. 2005;352:9–19.
9. Jevtovic-Todorovic V, Hartman RE, Izumi Y, et al. Early exposure to common anesthetic agents causes widespread neurodegeneration in the developing rat brain and persistent learning deficits. J Neurosci. 2003;23:876–82.
10. Loepke AW. Developmental neurotoxicity of sedatives and anesthetics: a concern for neonatal and pediatric critical care medicine? Pediatr Crit Care Med. 2010;11:217–26.
11. Wilder RT, Flick RP, Sprung J, et al. Early exposure to anesthesia and learning disabilities in a population-based birth cohort. Anesthesiology. 2009;110:796–804.
12. Bartels M, Althoff RR, Boomsma DI. Anesthesia and cognitive performance in children: no evidence for a causal relationship. Twin Res Hum Genet. 2009;12:246–53.
13. Rees CM, Pierro A, Eaton S. Neurodevelopmental outcomes of neonates with medically and surgically treated necrotizing enterocolitis. Arch Dis Child Fetal Neonatal Ed. 2007;92:193–8.
14. Ta BD, Roze E, van Braeckel KN, et al. Long-term neurodevelopmental impairment in neonates surgically treated for necrotizing enterocolitis: enterostomy associated with a worse outcome. Eur J Pediatr Surg. 2011;21:58–64.
15. Ahmad A, Gangitano E, Odell RM, et al. Survival, intracranial lesions, and neurodevelopmental outcome in infants with congenital diaphragmatic hernia treated with extracorporeal membrane oxygenation. J Perinatol. 1999;19(6 Pt 1):436–40.
16. Danzer E, Gerdes M, Bernbaum J, et al. Neurodevelopmental outcome of infants with congenital diaphragmatic hernia prospectively enrolled in an interdisciplinary follow-up program. J Pediatr Surg. 2010;45:1759–66.
17. Calderon J, Bonnet D, Courtin C, Concordet S, Plumet MH, Angeard N. Executive function and theory of mind in school-aged children after neonatal corrective cardiac surgery for transposition of the great arteries. Dev Med Child Neurol. 2010;52:1139–44.
18. Vahsen N, Kavsek M, Toussaint-Götz N, Schneider K, Urban AE, Schneider M. Cognitive and motor abilities and behavioural outcome in children after neonatal operation with cardiopulmonary bypass. Klin Padiatr. 2009;221:19–24.
19. Ludman L, Spitz L, Lansdown R. Developmental progress of newborns undergoing neonatal surgery. J Pediatr Surg. 1990;25:469–71.
20. Ludman L, Spitz L, Lansdown R. Intellectual development at 3 years of age of children who underwent major neonatal surgery. J Pediatr Surg. 1993;28:130–4.
21. Rescorla FJ, Grosfeld JL. Inguinal hernia repair in the perinatal period and early infancy: clinical considerations. J Pediatr Surg. 1984;19:832–7.
22. Steinau G, Treutner KH, Feeken G, et al. Recurrent inguinal hernias in infants and children. World J Surg. 1995;19:303–6.
23. Benson CD, Lloyd JR. Infantile pyloric stenosis. A review of 1,120 cases. Am J Surg. 1964;107:429–33.
24. Dietl KH, Borowski U, Menzel J, Wissing C, Senninger N, Brockmann J. Long-term investigations after pyloromyotomy for infantile pyloric stenosis. Eur J Pediatr Surg. 2000;10:365–7.
25. Carter CO, Evans KA. Inheritance of congenital pyloric stenosis. J Med Genet. 1969;6:233–54.

26. Sistonen SJ, Koivusalo A, Nieminen U, Lindahl H, Lohi J, Kero M, Kärkkäinen P, Färkkilä MA, Sarna S, Rintala RJ, Pakarinen MP. Esophageal morbidity and function in adults with repaired esophageal atresia: A population-based long-term follow-up. Ann Surg. 2010;251:1167–73.
27. Deurloo JA, van Lanschot JJ, Drillenburg P, et al. Esophageal squamous cell carcinoma 38 years after primary repair of esophageal atresia. J Pediatr Surg. 2001;36:629–30.
28. Sistonen SJ, Koivusalo A, Lindahl H, Pukkala E, Rintala RJ, Pakarinen MP. Cancer after repair of esophageal atresia: Population-based long-term follow-up. J Pediatr Surg. 2008;43:602–5.
29. Deurloo JA, Ekkelkamp S, Taminiau JA, Kneepkens CM, Ten Kate FW, Bartelsman JF, Legemate DA, Aronson DC. Esophagitis and Barrett esophagus after correction of esophageal atresia. J Pediatr Surg. 2005;40:1227–31.
30. Taylor AC, Breen KJ, Auldist A, et al. Gastroesophageal reflux and related pathology in adults who were born with esophageal atresia: A long-term follow-up study. Clin Gastroenterol Hepatol. 2007;5:702–6.
31. Krug E, Bergmeijer JH, Dees J, et al. Gastroesophageal reflux and Barrett's esophagus in adults born with esophageal atresia. Am J Gastroenterol. 1999;94:2825–8.
32. Chetcuti P, Phelan PD. Gastrointestinal morbidity and growth after repair of oesophageal atresia and tracheo-oesophageal fistula. Arch Dis Child. 1993;68:163–6.
33. Sistonen SJ, Helenius I, Peltonen J, Sarna S, Rintala RJ, Pakarinen MP. Natural history of spinal anomalies and scoliosis associated with esophageal atresia. Pediatrics. 2009;124:e1198–204. Epub 2009 Nov 9
34. Jaureguizar E, Vazquez J, Murcia J, et al. Morbid musculoskeletal sequelae of the thoracotomy for esophageal fistula. J Pediatr Surg. 1985;20:511–4.
35. Hall JE, Simmons ED, Danylchuk K, Barnes PD. Instability of the cervical spine and neurological involvement in Klippel-Feil syndrome. A case report. J Bone Joint Surg Am. 1990;72(3):460–2.
36. Koivusalo A, Pakarinen MP, Turunen P, et al. Health-related quality of life in adult patients with esophageal atresia: a questionnaire study. J Pediatr Surg. 2005;40:307–12.
37. Ure BM, Slany E, Eypasch EP, et al. Quality of life more than 20 years after repair of esophageal atresia. J Pediatr Surg. 1998;33:511–5.
38. Sistonen SJ, Pakarinen MP, Rintala RJ. Long-term results of esophageal atresia: Helsinki experience and review of literature. Pediatr Surg Int. 2011;27:1141–9.
39. Yanchar NL, Soucy P. Long-term outcome after Hirschsprung's disease: patients' perspectives. J Pediatr Surg. 1999;34:1152–60.
40. Reding R, de Ville de Goyet J, Gosseye S, et al. Hirschsprung's disease: a 20-year experience. J Pediatr Surg. 1997; 32:1221–5.
41. Catto-Smith AG, Coffey CM, Nolan TM, Hutson JM. Fecal incontinence after the surgical treatment of Hirschsprung disease. J Pediatr. 1995;127:954–7.
42. Bai Y, Chen H, Hao J, et al. Long-term outcome and quality of life after the Swenson procedure for Hirschsprung's disease. J Pediatr Surg. 2002;37:639–42.
43. Jarvi K, Laitakari EM, Koivusalo A, et al. Bowel function and gastrointestinal quality of life among adults operated for Hirschsprung disease during childhood: a population-based study. Ann Surg. 2010;252:977–81.
44. Heikkinen M, Rintala RJ, Louhimo I. Bowel function and quality of life in adult patients with operated Hirschsprung's disease. Pediatr Surg Int. 1995;10:342–4.
45. Baillie CT, Kenny SE, Rintala RJ, et al. Long-term outcome and colonic motility after the Duhamel procedure for Hirschsprung disease. J Pediatr Surg. 1999;34:325–9.
46. Diseth TH, Bjornland K, Novik TS, et al. Bowel function, mental health, and psychosocial function in adolescents with Hirschsprung's disease. Arch Dis Child. 1997;76:100–6.
47. Pakarinen MP, Rintala RJ, Koivusalo A, et al. Increased incidence of medullary thyroid carcinoma in patients treated for Hirschsprung's disease. J Pediatr Surg. 2005;40:1532–4.
48. Moore SW, Zaahl MG. Multiple endocrine neoplasia syndromes, children, Hirschsprung's disease and RET. Pediatr Surg Int. 2008;24:521–30.
49. Rintala RJ, Pakarinen MP. Imperforate anus: long- and short-term outcome. Semin Pediatr Surg. 2008;17:79–89.
50. Hassink EA, Rieu PN, Severijnen RS, et al. Are adults content or continent after repair for high anal atresia? A long-term follow-up study in patients 18 years of age and older. Ann Surg. 1993;218:196–200.
51. Stephens FD, Smith ED. Classification, identification and assessment of surgical treatment of anorectal anomalies. Pediatr Surg Int. 1986;1:200–5.
52. Stephens FD, Smith ED. Ano-rectal malformations in children. Chicago: Year Book Medical; 1971.
53. Templeton JM, Ditesheim JA. High imperforate anus—quantitative result of long-term fecal continence. J Pediatr Surg. 1985;20:645–52.
54. Holschneider A, Hutson J, Peña A, et al. Preliminary report on the International Conference for the Development of Standards for the Treatment of Anorectal Malformations. J Pediatr Surg. 2005;40:1521–6.
55. Peña A. Anorectal malformations. Semin Pediatr Surg. 1995;4:35–47.
56. Rintala R, Mildh L, Lindahl H. Fecal continence and quality of life in adult patients with an operated high or intermediate anorectal malformation. J Pediatr Surg. 1994;29:777–80.
57. Rintala R, Lindahl H, Sariola H, et al. The rectourogenital connection in anorectal malformations is an ectopic anal canal. J Pediatr Surg. 1990;25:665–8.
58. Husberg B, Lindahl H, Rintala R, et al. High and intermediate imperforate anus: Results after surgical

correction with special respect to internal sphincter function. J Pediatr Surg. 1992;27:185–9.
59. Iwai N, Hashimoto K, Goto Y, et al. Long term results after surgical correction of anorectal malformations. Z Kinderchir. 1984;39:35–9.
60. Mollard P, Meunier P, Mouriquand P, et al. High and intermediate imperforate anus: functional results and postoperative manometric assessment. Eur J Pediatr Surg. 1991;1:282–6.
61. Hedlund H, Peña A, Rodriquez G, et al. Long-term anorectal function in imperforate anus treated by a posterior sagittal anorectoplasty: manometric investigation. J Pediatr Surg. 1992;27:906–9.
62. Holschneider AM, Pfrommer W. Gerresheim B, Results in the treatment of anorectal malformations with special regard to the histology of the rectal pouch. Eur J Pediatr Surg. 1994;4:303–9.
63. Rintala R, Lindahl H, Marttinen E, et al. Constipation is a major functional complication after internal sphincter-saving posterior sagittal anorectoplasty for high and intermediate anorectal malformations. J Pediatr Surg. 1993;28:1054–8.
64. Langemeijer RATM, Molenaar JC. Continence after posterior sagittal anorectoplasty. J Pediatr Surg. 1991;26:587–90.
65. Rintala R, Marttinen E, Virkola K, et al. Segmental colonic motility in patients with anorectal malformations. J Pediatr Surg. 1997;32:453–6.
66. Mulder W, de Jong E, Wauters I, et al. Posterior sagittal anorectoplasty: functional results of primary and secondary operations in comparison to the pull-through method in anorectal malformations. Eur J Pediatr Surg. 1995;5:170–3.
67. Tuuha SE, Aziz D, Drake J, et al. Is surgery necessary for asymptomatic tethered cord in anorectal malformation patients? J Pediatr Surg. 2004;39:773–7.
68. Breech L. Gynecologic concerns in patients with anorectal malformations. Semin Pediatr Surg. 2010;19:139–45.
69. Rintala R, Mildh L, Lindahl H. Fecal continence and quality of life in adult patients with an operated low anorectal malformation. J Pediatr Surg. 1992;27:902–5.
70. Hassink EA, Rieu PN, Brugman AT, Festen C. Quality of life after operatively corrected high anorectal malformation: a long-term follow-up study of patients aged 18 years and older. J Pediatr Surg. 1994;29:773–6.
71. Hartman EE, Oort FJ, Aronson DC, et al. Critical factors affecting quality of life of adult patients with anorectal malformations or Hirschsprung's disease. Am J Gastroenterol. 2004;99:907–13.
72. Hartman EE, Oort FJ, Aronson DC, et al. Explaining change in quality of life of children and adolescents with anorectal malformations or Hirschsprung disease. Pediatrics. 2007;119:e374–83.
73. Hartman EE, Oort FJ, Sprangers MA, et al. Factors affecting quality of life of children and adolescents with anorectal malformations or Hirschsprung disease. J Pediatr Gastroenterol Nutr. 2008;47:463–71.
74. Diseth TH, Emblem R. Somatic function, mental health, and psychosocial adjustment of adolescents with anorectal anomalies. J Pediatr Surg. 1996;31:638–43.
75. Hanneman MJ, Sprangers MA, De Mik EL, et al. Quality of life in patients with anorectal malformation or Hirschsprung's disease: development of a disease-specific questionnaire. Dis Colon Rectum. 2001;44:1650–60.
76. Bowman RM, McLone DG, Grant JA, Tomita T, Ito JA. Spina bifida outcome: a 25-year prospective. Pediatr Neurosurg. 2001;34:114–20.
77. Dillon CM, Davis BE, Duguay S, et al. Longevity of patients born with myelomeningocele. Eur J Pediatr Surg. 2000;10(Suppl 1):33–4.
78. Shinkai M, Ohhama Y, Take H, et al. Long-term outcome of children with biliary atresia who were not transplanted after the Kasai operation: >20-year experience at a children's hospital. J Pediatr Gastroenterol Nutr. 2009;48:443–50.
79. Lykavieris P, Chardot C, Sokhn M, et al. Outcome in adulthood of biliary atresia: a study of 63 patients who survived for over 20 years with their native liver. Hepatology. 2005;41:366–71.
80. Hutson JM, Balic A, Nation T, Southwell B. Cryptorchidism. Semin Pediatr Surg. 2010;19:215–24.
81. Nasr A, Himidan S, Pastor AC, et al. Is congenital cystic adenomatoid malformation a premalignant lesion for pleuropulmonary blastoma? J Pediatr Surg. 2010;45:1086–9.
82. Homsy YL, Anderson JH, Oudjhane K, Russo P. Wilms tumor and multicystic dysplastic kidney disease. J Urol. 1997;158:2256–9.
83. Lee MY, Jensen E, Kwak S, Larson RA. Metastatic adenocarcinoma arising in a congenital foregut cyst of the esophagus: a case report with review of the literature. Am J Clin Oncol. 1998;21:64–6.
84. Mathieu A, Chamlou R, Le Moine F, et al. Tailgut cyst associated with a carcinoid tumor: case report and review of the literature. Histol Histopathol. 2005;20(4):1065–9.
85. Michael D, Cohen CR, Northover JM. Adenocarcinoma within a rectal duplication cyst: case report and literature review. Ann R Coll Surg Engl. 1999;81:205–6.
86. Kuraoka K, Nakayama H, Kagawa T, et al. Adenocarcinoma arising from a gastric duplication cyst with invasion to the stomach: a case report with literature review. J Clin Pathol. 2004;57:428–31.
87. Yoshida A, Maoate K, Blakelock R, et al. Long-term functional outcomes in children with Currarino syndrome. Pediatr Surg Int. 2010;26:677–81.
88. Benjamin IS. Biliary cystic disease: the risk of cancer. J Hepatobiliary Pancreat Surg. 2003;10:335–9.
89. Diseth TH, Egeland T, Emblem R. Effects of anal invasive treatment and incontinence on mental health and psychosocial functioning of adolescents with

Hirschsprung's disease and low anorectal anomalies. J Pediatr Surg. 1998;33:468–75.
90. Bau MO, Younes S, Aupy A, et al. The Malone antegrade colonic enema isolated or associated with urological incontinence procedures: evaluation from patient point of view. J Urol. 2001;165(6 Pt 2):2399–403.
91. Wilkins BM, Spitz L. Incidence of postoperative adhesion obstruction following neonatal laparotomy. Br J Surg. 1986;73:762–4.
92. Vanamo K, Rintala RJ, Lindahl H, Louhimo I. Long-term gastrointestinal morbidity in patients with congenital diaphragmatic defects. J Pediatr Surg. 1996;31:551–4.

Long Term Outcomes in Pediatric Urology

71

Joel Cazares and Atsuyuki Yamataka

Abstract

Pediatric urology has evolved in the last decades as an independent specialty from pediatric surgery covering several congenital and acquired diseases and interacts with other pediatric specialties for an early diagnosis and adequate treatment. However, in many places from all over the world, pediatric urology remains under performance by pediatric surgeons. Prenatal diagnosis has become a reality in urological pathologies and some procedures can be performed as early as fetal surgery or immediately after birth.

The long-term outcomes in the most common urological problems are presented and we look forward for new therapies and robotics in the pediatric population for the next years.

Keywords

Newborn surgery • Paediatric urology • Long term outcomes

71.1 Vesicoureteric Reflux

71.1.1 Background

Age at diagnosis has two peaks with different demographic features and distinct modes of presentation. The first group is antenatal, predominantly male and identified on ultrasonography, or if there is a family history there is no gender predominance. This vesicoureteric reflux (VUR) resolves or improves in the vast majority by 4 years of age [1]. The second group is diagnosed later, after a urinary tract infection (UTI) and is predominantly female.

71.1.2 Long-Term Outcome

Long-term follow-up studies in relation to VUR cover various scenarios; children presenting with acute UTI, VUR with renal scarring followed into adulthood, girls with asymptomatic bacteriuria and VUR and scarring, and children

J. Cazares, MD • A. Yamataka, MD, PhD FAAP(Hon) (✉)
Department of Pediatric General and Urogenital Surgery, Juntendo University School of Medicine, Tokyo, Japan
e-mail: yama@juntendo.ac.jp

P.D. Losty et al. (eds.), *Rickham's Neonatal Surgery*, https://doi.org/10.1007/978-1-4471-4721-3_71

with VUR nephropathy who had ureteric reimplantation. To summarize, there is no evidence that recognition and treatment of VUR has any impact on the development of end-stage renal disease.

The primary objective in the management of VUR is the prevention of ascending pyelonephritis secondary to bacteriuria. It has been a long held belief that antibiotic prophylaxis prevents parenchymal damage in patients with VUR, and that long-term administration is well tolerated and is the treatment of choice for all infants regardless of severity of VUR [2] and that older children with mild to moderate (I–III) reflux can be maintained infection free because spontaneous resolution is common, although recent studies [3] have shown no significant results. Approximately, up to 50% of VUR patients have renal scarring at the time of initial presentation, but relatively few new scars develop after medical or surgical treatment and no child with normal kidneys initially developed scarring. However, once deterioration in renal function commences, it progresses even when UTI are successfully prevented or treated and hypertension satisfactorily controlled. VUR repair at this stage does not affect the development of renal failure [4].

Minimally invasive endoscopic injection has been in use for more than 20 years and while highly successful for grades II–IV, its role in grade V is questionable with no effect on the subsequent incidence of UTI [5, 6].

For surgical intervention there seems to be a great discrepancy between effective and ineffective treatments, but no obvious difference between effective treatment and no treatment. There is a general trend for children over 2 years of age with persistent high-grade VUR (IV–V) to have surgery to decrease complications secondary to pyelonephritis. Cohen and Leadbetter-Politano are most commonly performed procedures with Cohen associated with lowest failure and complication rates. Again, while surgical correction can be highly successful and prevent renal damage, the overall incidence of infections is not reduced, and prophylactic antibiotics are usually required. To summarize, antireflux surgery should be reserved for patients who have high grades of reflux refractive to medical treatment, and for those with social circumstances or particular problems, which make medical treatment difficult to supervise or administer.

71.2 Pelvicuretero Junction/ Ureteropelvic Junction Stenosis

71.2.1 Background

There is no imaging or urodynamic modality that can accurately distinguish pelviureteric junction (PUJ)/ ureteropelvic junction (UPJ) obstruction from patients with inconsequential hydronephrosis, so the current approach is to observe conservatively in the short-term, reserving surgery for cases who deteriorate or become symptomatic. Symptomatic hydronephrosis in children occurs much less commonly than antenatally diagnosed hydronephrosis, but long-term follow-up studies of adults who underwent pyeloplasty many years earlier clearly identify the benefit of surgical intervention for alleviating symptoms [7, 8]. Surgery should be performed immediately regardless of age once the diagnosis of true obstruction is made [9]. Otherwise the added benefit of surgery in less severe cases is not clear since the same improvement may be observed without surgery.

71.2.2 Long-Term Outcome

The challenge for the clinician in the management of hydronephrosis is to decide who should be observed, who should be medically managed, and who requires surgery. This decision is complicated further by the challenge of cost containment. While open pyeloplasty is the gold standard for treatment, minimally invasive surgery/robotic surgery are gaining momentum but are less cost effective compared with open surgery. Earlier surgery has better results.

71.3 Megaureters

71.3.1 Background

Management of megaureter has changed markedly over the past 20 years and most patients are often entirely asymptomatic with kidneys that are functioning well [10]. Antenatal diagnosis of hydroureteronephrosis raises concern because of uncertain indications for surgical intervention. The current consensus is that megaureter represents non-obstructive dilation and therefore careful observation with antibiotic prophylaxis is all that is needed for most children [11, 12].

71.3.2 Long-Term Outcome

Should there be evidence of deteriorating renal function, worsening dilatation or breakthrough urinary tract infections, surgical intervention is mandatory and involves excision of the stenotic ureteral segment, reduction in caliber of the dilated distal ureter and ureteral reimplantation. The timing of surgery affects preservation of renal function. Ureteric reimplantation in infants below 1 year of age may be challenging due to the discrepancy between the grossly-dilated ureter and the small infantile bladder, and concern regarding possible iatrogenic bladder dysfunction [13].

71.4 Bladder Exstrophy

71.4.1 Background

Classic bladder exstrophy accounts for 60% of patients with defects in ventral coverage of several organs while cloacal exstrophy and epispadias are far less common.

Reconstruction of exstrophy-epispadias complex remains one of the greatest challenges facing the pediatric surgeon. Many modifications in surgical procedures have improved outcome, but as no formal assessment of staged repair versus total reconstruction with respect to function and cosmesis has been performed to date, the definitive approach has yet to be established. Depending on severity, surgical intervention may commence early with closure of the bladder, posterior urethra, pelvis and abdominal wall at birth, followed by genital reconstruction, and some form of continence procedure that may proceed through to adolescence. The current trend is clearly toward augmentation in patients who do not have adequate bladder capacity or in whom continence procedures involving simple closure and bladder neck reconstruction fail. Genital reconstruction that used to be common in adolescent exstrophy patients is now uncommon [14, 15].

71.4.2 Long-Term Outcome

Survival rates in bladder exstrophy patients today are normal. Long-term follow-up shows that staged repair has better outcome and less complications [16, 17], and urinary continence is achievable in at least 65% with males doing better than females [18, 19].

The psychological effects of a major congenital genitourinary malformation such as bladder exstrophy can be devastating. Although urinary continence and genital cosmesis are major issues, long-term goals for sexual function have considerably modified the surgical procedures performed in infancy over the past 20 years. Despite severe epispadias associated with exstrophy, most patients completing staged reconstruction can expect to enjoy sexual relations. Sexual response and libido of males with bladder exstrophy is normal although fertility through conventional procreation is very low because of penile shortening, dorsal chordee, poor erections and retrograde ejaculation. However, only a small proportion classify these as distressing [18]. Females tend to fare better in all aspects of sexual health with most being satisfied with the appearance of their genitalia and all being sexually active. In fact, women with bladder exstrophy have delivered children, with the commonest complication being cervical/uterine prolapse, and future urinary reconstruction should include prophylactic anterior fixation of the uterus. Cesarean section should be considered for all exstrophy patient deliveries [20].

Now that patients who have undergone modern exstrophy treatment techniques have been followed into adulthood, it is gratifying to see the successful lives these patients enjoy—a sharp contrast to lives before successful bladder closure was common.

Adenocarcinoma is approximately 400 times more common in patients with bladder exstrophy than in the normal population, accounting for up to 93% of the bladder tumors seen in these patients. Long-term monitoring with cystoscopic evaluation is recommended. Long-term follow-up of patients who have completed modern staged reconstruction with successful bladder closure is expected to reveal a diminished risk for cancer [21, 22].

71.5 Epispadias

71.5.1 Long-Term Outcome

The defect in epispadias can be closed successfully and satisfactory continence achieved without loss of renal function or normal drainage. In fact, continence can be expected in up to 90% of complete epispadias patients managed successfully. In other words, results in both complete epispadias and bladder exstrophy have improved to the point where functional closure and bladder neck reconstruction should be the aim of initial surgery, and only those patients who are proven to have special problems or who fail in achieving success at each step need to be considered for alternatives of internal or external urinary diversion or augmentation cystoplasty [21, 23].

71.6 Neuropathic Bladder

71.6.1 Background

Over the past 20 years the survival rate of these children has improved with the primary goal of treatment being preservation of renal and bladder function. Practical and functional substitutes for native bladder tissues are constantly being researched in view of the detrimental combination of intestinal tissue and urine.

71.6.2 Long-Term Outcome

Clean intermittent urethral catheterization (CIC) itself does not necessarily guarantee continence and usually requires the addition of pharmacotherapy in the form of anticholinergics and alpha adrenergics, or surgery [24, 25]. There is limited data on the long-term follow-up of children with neuropathic bladder taking medications. Oral and intravesical oxybutynin both cause side effects, more prominent in children taking oral oxybutynin. Injection of botulinum in the detrusor muscle is effective for detrusor hyperreflexia in the short term requires anesthesia for administration [26].

Prophylactic bicarbonate is mandatory, as is orthopedic follow-up to combat the impact of acidosis on growing children to prevent bone demineralization and loss of growth potential.

Symptomatic UTIs are relatively infrequent with CIC and in the absence of significant preexisting reflux, fresh renal scarring is unusual.

Surgical intervention must match the needs of the patient with those of the primary care giver. If for example, a third party is the primary care giver, then a conduit urinary diversion with collecting bag is far easier to manage than trying to assess when a bladder is full.

The most commonly performed diversions are vesicostomy, refluxing ureterostomy, and ileal conduit, usually performed temporarily for deteriorating upper tracts or failure of CIC [27, 28]. Otherwise, procedures performed with good outcome include suprapubic diversion via a suprapubic tube or button often followed by a Mitrofanoff stoma or button vesicostomy as an alternative to a Mitrofanoff channel [29].

For bladder neck surgery, revision rates are similar for all procedures performed but the incidence of complications appears highest with the Kropp procedure. Artificial urinary sphincter (AUS) should be the initial treatment of choice for the surgical management of neurogenic sphincter incontinence. However, there is limited long-term published data [30–35].

There are very few reviews of long-term outcome of augmentation cystoplasty specifically in the pediatric age group and many patients with cystoplasties performed years ago, have never been followed-up properly, and present with complications that could have been managed simply as they arose. Careful follow-up for monitoring voiding efficiency and timely use of CIC are vital to prevent decompensation. Voiding inefficiency after augmentation cystoplasty is common and can be managed by CIC especially in neuropathic bladder and is due to associated sphincter weakness that after surgical intervention can improve continence greatly [36, 37]. The competence of bladder outflow is often overlooked [38, 39].

Augmentation cystoplasty will continue to require the use of gastrointestinal tract segments until such time as an entirely urothelial bladder substitute is available. Current composite enterocystoplasties where demucosalized intestine is seeded with urothelial cells propagated in vitro could evolve to create a synthetic substitute for augmentation.

Gastrocystoplasty is an alternative and is advantageous because of decreased chloride absorption and mucus production, with lower incidence of urinary infections, stone formation, and perforation [40, 41]. However, up to 89% have decreased urinary continence postoperatively and hematuria dysuria syndrome amenable to proton pump inhibitors has been described in up to 25% of children. Suture line bleeding is the most serious surgical complication. Long-term follow-up documents improved urodynamics with increased bladder capacity and compliance [41, 42].

71.7 Mitrofanoff

71.7.1 Background

Mitrofanoff conduit is the most commonly performed continent catheterizable conduit in patients with a neuropathic bladder. Creation of a Mitrofanoff channel is usually performed concomitantly with an augmentation cystoplasty in children with neuropathic bladder and occasionally with the Malone antegrade continence enema (MACE) procedure [43].

71.7.2 Long-Term Outcome

Long-term follow-up of the Mitrofanoff channel has shown its robustness in the ability to be catheterized. High continence rates have been achieved when combined with an augmentation cystoplasty and bladder neck procedure [44].

Stomal stenosis is the most frequent complication requiring revisional surgery. Other long-term problems include UTI, bladder calculi, urine leakage, and progressive bilateral upper tract dilation [45, 46], and kinking of the channel, long stenosis of the channel, and difficulty in catheterization [47].

71.8 Posterior Urethral Valves

71.8.1 Background

Posterior urethral obstruction more than any other urinary anomaly has the capacity to affect the development and function of the whole urinary tract and can range from conditions incompatible with postnatal life when severe, to extremely mild conditions that may not manifest until later in life [48–50]. Posterior urethral valves (PUV) can be detected prenatally by ultrasonography (US) from 24 weeks' gestation when urinary tract dilation, hydronephrosis and/or a distended thick-walled bladder can be identified with a sensitivity of close to 100%. However, if prenatal US findings suggestive of PUV are noted before 24 weeks' gestation, or if there is severe bilateral hydronephrosis with oligohydramnios or renal dysplasia with oligohydramnios in the second trimester, the risk for postnatal chronic kidney disease is increased and perinatal mortality can be as high as 90–95% [51].

71.8.2 Long-Term Outcome

Although most infants with PUV are diagnosed in utero, underlying primary renal dysplasia cannot be altered by postnatal intervention, and provided bladder function can be preserved, the progressive decline in renal function associated with persistent high bladder pressures can be impeded [52, 53]. Impairment of renal function is found in around 70% of boys at presentation and over 80% of boys less than 3 months old. Although renal dysplasia is irreversible, adequate attention to urinary infections and bladder dysfunction can decrease or delay ongoing renal deterioration, and recent evidence would suggest that dysplastic kidneys do not affect infection rates or function of the remaining kidney and may be left in place. After initial management, 60% of patients recover normal biochemical renal function on short-term follow up [54]. However, renal failure can occur in up to 40% of PUV patients. In most countries transplantation is a viable treatment option and attention to bladder dysfunction and treatment of high bladder pressures associated with urge incontinence with anticholinergic therapy and frequent voiding are important to protect transplanted kidneys and prevent further deterioration. Dilated ureters attached to dysplastic kidneys may also have potential use during bladder augmentation in those rare cases of high-pressure bladder refractory to standard therapy [55, 56]. In bladders that have progressed to myogenic failure and incomplete emptying, clean intermittent catheterization (CIC) and/or overnight bladder drainage may be necessary. It must be remembered that patients with PUV do not have altered urethral sensation, and for the majority, catheterization through the penis is painful [57–59].

The presence of reflux should not change the initial overall treatment of PUV and probably does not change the long-term prognosis unless there is recurrent infection. Ureteral reimplantation is indicated only in those patients with recurrent urinary tract infection despite appropriate chemoprophylaxis and after appropriate therapy to treat bladder dysfunction.

Bladder dysfunction manifesting as incontinence, can complicate up to 38% of patients with PUV. Daytime catheterization can often be avoided in older boys if they can adhere to a strict schedule of timed voiding. Night time indwelling catheterization optimizes bladder drainage with documented improvement in hydronephrosis and bladder compliance. Compliance with catheterization can be difficult and creation of a continent catheterizable channel to the anterior abdominal wall could improve quality of life greatly and improve compliance. Patients with high-pressure voiding dynamics often benefit from the use of anticholinergic medications and conservative measures are usually effective enough for modifying bladder dynamics (i.e., keeping bladder volumes sufficiently low to maintain acceptable bladder pressure) in the medium term, but careful follow-up to assess renal dysfunction is mandatory [60–62].

Sexual function may be impaired due to higher incidence of undescended testes, the impaired function of the posterior urethra and ejaculatory mechanism and the effect of urethral surgery and renal failure. However, semen samples are fertile and fathering children is possible [63, 64].

The overall infant mortality rate has improved from about 50% to less than 3% in the past 3 decades. Early infant mortality in PUV is related to pulmonary hypoplasia and can be as high as 63% in boys less than 1 month old. With earlier, often prenatal diagnosis, possible future treatment options may include fetal cystoscopy and in utero treatment of PUV, or amnioinfusion to allow normal pulmonary development, already proven successful in bilateral renal agenesis [65, 66]. Longer follow-up has shown that chronic renal failure can cause death in up to 6.4% of boys between 3 and 12 years after presentation while end-stage renal disease can cause death between 10 and 15 years after presentation. Early management will certainly result in increasing numbers of patients surviving to be recruited into renal replacement programs. However, renal dialysis and transplantation are associated with morbidity and mortality, and prognosis may in fact prove to be closer to renal failure once follow-up extends to several decades [67].

71.9 Hypospadias

71.9.1 Background

The results of hypospadias surgery can be assessed objectively with urography or subjectively with respect to cosmesis, sexual function, psychosocial adjustment, and body image [68, 69]. Hypospadias should be repaired within the first year of life preferably around 6 months of age [70, 71]. It is an age well accepted by parents, reliable for the surgeon, and not remembered by the patient.

The most significant advance in surgical technique over the past 10 years is Snodgrass' primary tubularized urethroplasty. Reports of the success of tubularized incised plate urethroplasty are favorable and concern about strictures and meatal stenosis are unfounded [72, 73]. However, tubularized island flap urethroplasty appears to be associated with a high complication rate of up to 40% even in experienced hands and is not now commonly performed [74–76], while a vascularized preputial flap used as an onlay to preserve the urethral plate will provide a more secure result long-term. Other observations that appear to enhance outcome include: the neourethra in single-stage repairs using vascularized preputial pedicle flaps is functionally equivalent to a normal urethra in most boys using preputial island flaps; multi-stage surgery for severe hypospadias and redo surgery is acceptable if one-step surgery appears to be difficult, although additional procedures are often required to achieve an optimal outcome [77].; dorsal plication of the tunica albuginea to correct curvature has stood the test of 17 years follow-up with minimal recurvature, and is a simpler technique than ventral grafting of the corpora; buccal mucosa grafts are the best urethral replacement for redo surgery and for stricture, and the meatus will be durable [78]; an apical meatus is usually preferred, allows a good stream, and is worth the extra effort despite data to the contrary [79]; while urography is a good objective measure of caliber, observation of a good stream of urine at follow-up is more satisfying to both the patient and treating surgeon. Ideally one should have both; redundant skin after hypospadias repair in the child will often fill out and be unnoticeable after puberty [80]; utricles are not of great concern when they are small, however, they may cause inflammation or stone formation and treatment is difficult if they are large.

71.9.2 Long-Term Outcome

Long-term evaluation of surgical procedures has been largely hindered by the constant modifications made over time. What long-term results are available concern procedures that have now been abandoned. Data would suggest that most men have no lasting effects, but up to 40% of those with severe hypospadias have some degree of voiding difficulties. Although objective assessment of appearance after hypospadias surgery is also difficult, a recent study found TIP to be most cosmetically appealing [81].

Hypospadias patients appear to be inhibited when seeking sexual contact, are more likely to have a negative opinion of their genitals, and often fail to adjust sexually [82]. Size of the hypospadias penis will most often be perceived as small by the patient and parents but may not be so when compared to the range of normal. An absolutely straight erect penis is not necessary for enjoyable sex; gentle curvature is within the norm, and fixation on perfect straightness with hypospadias is unwarranted [83, 84]. The majority would appear to enjoy conventional sexual activity [85, 86]. Fertility is theoretically unaffected, but if associated with cryptorchidism, patients are unlikely to be fertile.

Complications are common and should be treated at least 6 months after the initial procedure, to allow the tissues to heal properly. Onlay urethroplasties used in severe cases would appear to be associated with a lower overall complication rate of 28.6% [87]. Unsatisfactory appearance related to irregular suture lines, scars, unevenness, or redundant skin can deflate confidence and invoke comment, but if the ventral aspect of the glans is short and there is no mucosal collar around the glans, the cosmetic result is disastrous and is related directly to the artistry of the surgeon not technical prowess [88].

Fistulas are the second most common complication of hypospadias repair, and can be seen during the first month after operation [89, 90]. Urethrocele is often related to a difference in urethral compliance between the native urethra and the reconstructed urethra.

71.10 Intersex

71.10.1 Background

Almost 90% of ambiguous genitalia patients are managed by some form of feminizing genitoplasty. While the immediate goal is to provide a feminine appearance to the external genitalia, long-term goals are to create a functional vagina sizable enough for comfortable sexual intercourse, to retain sexually sensitive tissue to allow orgasm and, if internal genitalia permit, to preserve potential for fertility.

71.10.2 Long-Term Outcome

Intersexuality does not threaten a patient's life, but rather their psychosocial status. Body image and psychosexual identification are often profoundly disturbed because despite tests that objectively define chromosomes and internal genital anatomy [91], decisions about sexual assignment and choices for treatment are made quite subjectively.

While vaginoplasty techniques have advanced to allow a responsive natural looking vagina to be fashioned, such surgery is planned in infancy to enhance social adjustment and family acceptance without any real consideration of the best interests of the patient. Unfortunately, future adjustment issues cannot be resolved in advance, and long-term follow-up data is lacking because unless patients have persistent problems, they tend to be lost to follow-up. Little is known about how adults adjust to genitoplasty, or whether the genitoplasty expresses their sexual preference. After many years of genitoplasty experience and technical revisions, gender identification mismatch tends to be consistently problematic and requires close monitoring with good counseling. Recent trends indicate that patients are not so much disturbed by unusual looking genitals but are more concerned about sensation and potential for fertility [92]. Thus, if the chromosomal and gonadal sex are compatible with fertility, gender assignment should be made to preserve fertility, if the external phenotype allows [93].

No studies of clitoral surgery address the long-term results of erotic sexual sensitivity. Sexual orgasmic response is multifactorial; however, the extent to which sexual orgasm and response is dependent on the clitoris is unknown [94].

71.11 Cloacal Malformation

71.11.1 Background

Urinary incontinence seen in patients with cloacal malformation is multifactorial. It may be secondary to structural abnormalities of the bladder, bladder neck and urethra, sacral dysplasia or agenesis, and intrinsic or iatrogenic neurovesical dysfunction (surgical denervation) [95, 96]. Despite obvious anomalies, accurate diagnosis is not always made before referral, which can potentially place the newborn at risk for sepsis, with preoperative renal scarring or dysplasia present in up to 25%.

71.11.2 Long-Term Outcome

Urinary continence after cloacal repair is often difficult to achieve and is only possible after several procedures, including bladder neck reconstruction. Associated congenital anomalies such as tethered cord and renal malformations are common, adversely affecting continence as well as general renal function [97]. Some 60% of cloacal malformation patients have an atonic type of neurogenic bladder, requiring CIC [98]. In a recent follow-up study, 66% of children had dry intervals of over 4 h; 62.5% using CIC through a Mitrofanoff channel and 12.5% through the urethra [97, 98]. Upper tract deterioration is a concern in cloacal malformation secondary to persistent hydronephrosis (in up to 60%), the need for bladder augmentation and the presence of reflux requiring reimplantation (in up to 75%), make it extremely difficult to reach an overall conclusion about renal dysfunction [99, 100]. Research data would indicate that 60% of children with common channels of at least 3 cm required bladder augmentation associated with bladder neck closure and Mitrofanoff conduit, compared with none of the patients who had common channels less than 3 cm. Thus explaining the high rate of dryness achieved after all these procedures [99, 101].

71.12 Robotics

Robotic surgery can generate extremely delicate movements in a confined working space such as are found generally in the pediatric population [102]. Initial results with robotic assistance are encouraging and have demonstrated safety comparable to open procedures and outcomes at least equivalent to standard laparoscopy, although it should be regarded as an assisted form of open surgery rather than an evolution of laparoscopy. Future development of smaller instruments, incorporating tactile feedback, will likely overcome current limitations related mainly to lack of tactile sensation or feedback to the surgeon [103, 104]. Currently, robot-assisted surgery must rely on visual clues surrounding the operative site to adjust for orientation and tactile input [105]. Ultimately, the efficacy and role of robotic surgical systems will require definition following comparison with standard procedures of choice performed open or laparoscopically.

71.13 Stem Cells

Embryonic stem cell research is generally controversial and newer semi synthetic stem cell development programs have had varying success with no real potential for active application established. Human embryonic stem (hES) cells are derived from the inner cell mass of the blastocyst stage embryo, and human embryonic germ (hEG) cells are obtained from primordial germ cells. Formation of embryoid bodies is an important intermediate step for hES and hEG cells, before differentiation into various cell types [106, 107]. With embryoid body formation, the markers of pluripotentiality decline, and ectodermal, mesodermal, and endodermal markers appear. Some research on urologic tissue engineering has been promising but has been hindered because form does not always equate with function, especially for bladder tissue.

References

1. Kenda RB, Zupancic Z, Fettich JJ, Meglic A. A follow-up study of vesico-ureteric reflux and renal scars in asymptomatic siblings of children with reflux. Nucl Med Commun. 1997;18(9):827–31.
2. Weiss SPF. Vascular changes in pyelonephritis and their relation to arterial hypertension. Trans Assoc Am Physicians. 1938;53:60.
3. Pennesi M, Travan L, Peratoner L, Bordugo A, Cattaneo A, Ronfani L, Minisini S, Ventura A, North East Italy Prophylaxis in VUR Study Group. Is antibiotic prophylaxis in children with vesicoureteral reflux effective in preventing pyelonephritis and renal scars? A randomized, controlled trial. Pediatrics. 2008;121(6):e1489–94.
4. Risdon RA. The small scarred kidney in childhood. Pediatr Nephrol. 1993;7(4):361–4.
5. Hutch J. Theory of maturation of the intravesical ureter. J Urol. 1961;86:534–8.
6. Birmingham Reflux Study Group. Prospective trial of operative versus non-operative treatment of severe vesicoureteric reflux in children: five years' observation. Br Med J (Clin Res Ed). 1987;295(6592):237–41.
7. Mikkelsen SS, Rasmussen BS, Jensen TM, Hanghoj-Petersen W, Christensen PO. Long-term follow-up of patients with hydronephrosis treated by Anderson-Hynes pyeloplasty. Br J Urol. 1992;70(2):121–4.
8. Notley RG, Beaugie JM. The long-term follow-up of Anderson-Hynes pyeloplasty for hydronephrosis. Br J Urol. 1973;45(5):464–7.
9. Freedman ER, Rickwood AM. Prenatally diagnosed pelviureteric junction obstruction: a benign condition? J Pediatr Surg. 1994;29(6):769–72.
10. Cozzi F, Madonna L, Maggi E, Piacenti S, Bonanni M, Roggini M, et al. Management of primary megaureter in infancy. J Pediatr Surg. 1993;28(8):1031–3.
11. McLellan DL, Retik AB, Bauer SB, Diamond DA, Atala A, Mandell J, et al. Rate and predictors of spontaneous

resolution of prenatally diagnosed primary nonrefluxing megaureter. J Urol. 2002;168(5):2177–80; discussion 80
12. Shenoy MU, Rance CH. Is there a place for the insertion of a JJ stent as a temporizing procedure for symptomatic partial congenital vesicoureteric junction obstruction in infancy? BJU Int. 1999;84(4):524–5.
13. de Jong TP. Treatment of the neonatal and infant megaureter in reflux, obstruction and complex congenital anomalies. Acta Urol Belg. 1997;65(2):45–7.
14. Diseth TH, Bjordal R, Schultz A, Stange M, Emblem R. Somatic function, mental health, and psychosocial functioning in 22 adolescents with bladder exstrophy and epispadias. J Urol. 1998;159(5):1684–9.
15. Feitz WF, Van Grunsven EJ, Froeling FM, de Vries JD. Outcome analysis of the psychosexual and socioeconomic development of adults born with bladder exstrophy. J Urol. 1994;152(5 Pt 1):1417–9.
16. Gearhart JP, Forschner DC, Jeffs RD, Ben-Chaim J, Sponseller PD. A combined vertical and horizontal pelvic osteotomy approach for primary and secondary repair of bladder exstrophy. J Urol. 1996;155(2):689–93.
17. Meldrum KK, Baird AD, Gearhart JP. Pelvic and extremity immobilization after bladder exstrophy closure: complications and impact on success. Urology. 2003;62(6):1109–13.
18. Stein R, Hohenfellner K, Fisch M, Stöckle M, Beetz R, Hohenfellner R. Social integration, sexual behavior and fertility in patients with bladder exstrophy--a long-term follow up. Eur J Pediatr. 1996;155(8):678–83.
19. Ben-Chaim J, Jeffs RD, Reiner WG, Gearhart JP. The outcome of patients with classic bladder exstrophy in adult life. J Urol. 1996;155(4):1251–2.
20. Gearhart JP, Sciortino C, Ben-Chaim J, Peppas DS, Jeffs RD. The Cantwell-Ransley epispadias repair in exstrophy and epispadias: lessons learned. Urology. 1995;46(1):92–5.
21. Gearhart JP. Complete repair of bladder exstrophy in the newborn: complications and management. J Urol. 2001;165(6 Pt 2):2431–3.
22. Lottmann HB, Yaqouti M, Melin Y. Male epispadias repair: surgical and functional results with the Cantwell-Ransley procedure in 40 patients. J Urol. 1999;162(3 Pt 2):1176–80.
23. Grady RW, Carr MC, Mitchell ME. Complete primary closure of bladder exstrophy. Epispadias and bladder exstrophy repair. Urol Clin North Am. 1999;26(1):95–109, viii
24. Wolraich ML, Hawtrey C, Mapel J, Henderson M. Results of clean intermittent catheterization for children with neurogenic bladders. Urology. 1983;22(5):479–82.
25. Cass AS, Luxenberg M, Gleich P, Johnson CF, Hagen S. Clean intermittent catheterization in the management of the neurogenic bladder in children. J Urol. 1984;132(3):526–8.
26. Schlager TA, Clark M, Anderson S. Effect of a single-use sterile catheter for each void on the frequency of bacteriuria in children with neurogenic bladder on intermittent catheterization for bladder emptying. Pediatrics. 2001;108(4):E71.
27. Jayanthi VR, Churchill BM, McLorie GA, Khoury AE. Concomitant bladder neck closure and Mitrofanoff diversion for the management of intractable urinary incontinence. J Urol. 1995;154(2 Pt 2):886–8.
28. Nguyen HT, Baskin LS. The outcome of bladder neck closure in children with severe urinary incontinence. J Urol. 2003;169(3):1114–6; discussion 6
29. Kass EJ, Koff SA, Diokno AC, Lapides J. The significance of bacilluria in children on long-term intermittent catheterization. J Urol. 1981;126(2):223–5.
30. Kropp KA, Angwafo FF. Urethral lengthening and reimplantation for neurogenic incontinence in children. J Urol. 1986;135(3):533–6.
31. Salle JL, de Fraga JC, Amarante A, Silveira ML, Lambertz M, Schmidt M, et al. Urethral lengthening with anterior bladder wall flap for urinary incontinence: a new approach. J Urol. 1994;152(2 Pt 2):803–6.
32. Young HH. Exstrophy of the bladder: the first case in which a normal bladder and urinary control have been obtained by plastic operation. Surg Gynecol Obstet. 1942;74:729–37.
33. Dees JE. Congenital epispadias with incontinence. J Urol. 1949;62(4):513–22.
34. Leadbetter GW Jr. Surgical Correction of Total Urinary Incontinence. J Urol. 1964;91:261–6.
35. Hoebeke P, De Kuyper P, Goeminne H, Van Laecke E, Everaert K. Bladder neck closure for treating pediatric incontinence. Eur Urol. 2000;38(4):453–6.
36. Palmer LS, Franco I, Kogan SJ, Reda E, Gill B, Levitt SB. Urolithiasis in children following augmentation cystoplasty. J Urol. 1993;150(2 Pt 2):726–9.
37. Mathoera RB, Kok DJ, Nijman RJ. Bladder calculi in augmentation cystoplasty in children. Urology. 2000;56(3):482–7.
38. Krishna A, Gough DC. Evaluation of augmentation cystoplasty in childhood with reference to vesicoureteric reflux and urinary infection. Br J Urol. 1994;74(4):465–8.
39. Quek ML, Ginsberg DA. Long-term urodynamics followup of bladder augmentation for neurogenic bladder. J Urol. 2003;169(1):195–8.
40. DeFoor W, Minevich E, Reeves D, Tackett L, Wacksman J, Sheldon C. Gastrocystoplasty: long-term followup. J Urol. 2003;170(4 Pt 2):1647–9; discussion 9–50
41. Chadwick Plaire J, Snodgrass WT, Grady RW, Mitchell ME. Long-term followup of the hematuria-dysuria syndrome. J Urol. 2000;164(3 Pt 2):921–3.
42. Abdel-Azim MS, Abdel-Hakim AM. Gastrocystoplasty in patients with an areflexic low compliant bladder. Eur Urol. 2003;44(2):260–5.
43. Liard A, Séguier-Lipszyc E, Mathiot A, Mitrofanoff P. The Mitrofanoff procedure: 20 years later. J Urol. 2001;165(6 Pt 2):2394–8.
44. McAndrew HF, Malone PS. Continent catheterizable conduits: which stoma, which conduit and which reservoir? BJU Int. 2002;89(1):86–9.

45. De Ganck J, Everaert K, Van Laecke E, Oosterlinck W, Hoebeke P. A high easy-to-treat complication rate is the price for a continent stoma. BJU Int. 2002;90(3):240–3.
46. Narayanaswamy B, Wilcox DT, Cuckow PM, Duffy PG, Ransley PG. The Yang-Monti ileovesicostomy: a problematic channel? BJU Int. 2001;87(9):861–5.
47. Cain MP, Rink RC, Yerkes EB, Kaefer M, Casale AJ. Long-term followup and outcome of continent catheterizable vesicocstomy using the Rink modification. J Urol. 2002;168(6):2583–5.
48. Thomas DF, Gordon AC. Management of prenatally diagnosed uropathies. Arch Dis Child. 1989;64(1 Spec No):58–63.
49. Parkhouse HF, Barratt TM, Dillon MJ, Duffy PG, Fay J, Ransley PG, Woodhouse CR, Williams DI. Long-term outcome of boys with posterior urethral valves. Br J Urol. 1988;62(1):59–62.
50. Parkhouse HF, Woodhouse CR. Long-term status of patients with posterior urethral valves. Urol Clin North Am. 1990;17(2):373–8.
51. Jee LD, Rickwood AM, Turnock RR. Posterior urethral valves. Does prenatal diagnosis influence prognosis? Br J Urol. 1993;72(5 Pt 2):830–3.
52. Reinberg Y, de Castano I, Gonzalez R. Influence of initial therapy on progression of renal failure and body growth in children with posterior urethral valves. J Urol. 1992;148(2 Pt 2):532–3.
53. Ellis EN, Pearson D, Champion B, Wood EG. Outcome of infants on chronic peritoneal dialysis. Adv Perit Dial. 1995;11:266–9.
54. Sedman A, Friedman A, Boineau F, Strife CF, Fine R. Nutritional management of the child with mild to moderate chronic renal failure. J Pediatr. 1996;129(2):s13–8.
55. Connolly JA, Miller B, Bretan PN. Renal transplantation in patients with posterior urethral valves: favorable long-term outcome. J Urol. 1995;154(3):1153–5.
56. Dinneen MD, Fitzpatrick MM, Godley ML, Dicks-Mireaux CM, Ransley PG, Fernando ON, Trompeter RS, Duffy PG. Renal transplantation in young boys with posterior urethral valves: preliminary report. Br J Urol. 1993;72(3):359–63.
57. Cass AS, Stephens FD. Posterior urethral valves: diagnosis and management. J Urol. 1974;112(4):519–25.
58. Whitaker RH, Keeton JE, Williams DI. Posterior urethral valves: a study of urinary control after operation. J Urol. 1972;108(1):167–71.
59. Churchill BM, Krueger RP, Fleisher MH, Hardy BE. Complications of posterior urethral valve surgery and their prevention. Urol Clin North Am. 1983;10(3):519–30.
60. Silver RK, MacGregor SN, Cook WA, Sholl JS. Fetal posterior urethral valve syndrome: a prospective application of antenatal prognostic criteria. Obstet Gynecol. 1990;76(5 Pt 2):951–5.
61. Muller F, Dommergues M, Mandelbrot L, Aubry MC, Nihoul-Fekete C, Dumez Y. Fetal urinary biochemistry predicts postnatal renal function in children with bilateral obstructive uropathies. Obstet Gynecol. 1993;82(5):813–20.
62. Lipitz S, Ryan G, Samuell C, Haeusler MC, Robson SC, Dhillon HK, Nicolini U, Rodeck CH. Fetal urine analysis for the assessment of renal function in obstructive uropathy. Am J Obstet Gynecol. 1993;168(1 Pt 1):174–9.
63. Krueger RP, Hardy BE, Churchill BM. Cryptorchidism in boys with posterior urethral valves. J Urol. 1980;124(1):101–2.
64. Woodhouse CR, Reilly JM, Bahadur G. Sexual function and fertility in patients treated for posterior urethral valves. J Urol. 1989;142(2 Pt 2):586–8; discussion 603–5
65. Freedman AL, Bukowski TP, Smith CA, Evans MI, Johnson MP, Gonzalez R. Fetal therapy for obstructive uropathy: diagnosis specific outcomes [corrected]. J Urol. 1996;156(2 Pt 2):720–3; discussion 723–4
66. Ansari MS, Singh P, Mandhani A, Dubey D, Srivastava A, Kapoor R, Kumar A. Delayed presentation in posterior urethral valve: long-term implications and outcome. Urology. 2008;71(2):230–4.
67. Reinberg Y, Gonzalez R, Fryd D, Mauer SM, Najarian JS. The outcome of renal transplantation in children with posterior urethral valves. J Urol. 1988;140(6):1491–3.
68. Baskin LS, Himes K, Colborn T. Hypospadias and endocrine disruption: is there a connection? Environ Health Perspect. 2001;109(11):1175–83.
69. North K, Golding J. A maternal vegetarian diet in pregnancy is associated with hypospadias. The ALSPAC Study Team. Avon Longitudinal Study of Pregnancy and Childhood. BJU Int. 2000;85(1):107–13.
70. Baskin LS, Duckett JW, Ueoka K, Seibold J, Snyder HM 3rd. Changing concepts of hypospadias curvature lead to more onlay island flap procedures. J Urol. 1994;151(1):191–6.
71. Snodgrass W. Tubularized, incised plate urethroplasty for distal hypospadias. J Urol. 1994;151(2):464–5.
72. Bracka A. Hypospadias repair: the two-stage alternative. Br J Urol. 1995;76(Suppl 3):31–41.
73. Beck C. Hypospadias and its treatment. Surg Gynecol Obstet. 1917;24:511–32.
74. Elbakry A. Complications of the preputial island flap-tube urethroplasty. BJU Int. 1999;84(1):89–94.
75. Browne D. An operation for hypospadias. Lancet. 1936;1:141–3.
76. Byars LT. A technique for consistently satisfactory repair of hypospadias. Surg Gynecol Obstet. 1955;100(2):184–90.
77. Retik AB, Bauer SB, Mandell J, Peters CA, Colodny A, Atala A. Management of severe hypospadias with a 2-stage repair. J Urol. 1994;152(2 Pt 2):749–51.
78. Duckett JW, Coplen D, Ewalt D, Baskin LS. Buccal mucosal urethral replacement. J Urol. 1995;153(5):1660–3.
79. Devine CJ Jr, Horton CE. A one stage hypospadias repair. J Urol. 1961;85:166–72.

80. van der Werff JF, Boeve E, Brussé CA, van der Meulen JC. Urodynamic evaluation of hypospadias repair. J Urol. 1997;157(4):1344–6.
81. Snodgrass W, Koyle M, Manzoni G, Hurwitz R, Caldamone A, Ehrlich R. Tubularized incised plate hypospadias repair for proximal hypospadias. J Urol. 1998;159(6):2129–31.
82. Mureau MA, Slijper FM, Nijman RJ, van der Meulen JC, Verhulst FC, Slob AK. Psychosexual adjustment of children and adolescents after different types of hypospadias surgery: a norm-related study. J Urol. 1995;154(5):1902–7.
83. van der Werff JF, Ultee J. Long-term follow-up of hypospadias repair. Br J Plast Surg. 2000;53(7):588–92.
84. Park JM, Faerber GJ, Bloom DA. Long-term outcome evaluation of patients undergoing the meatal advancement and glanuloplasty procedure. J Urol. 1995;153(5):1655–6.
85. Mureau MA, Slijper FM, van der Meulen JC, Verhulst FC, Slob AK. Psychosexual adjustment of men who underwent hypospadias repair: a norm-related study. J Urol. 1995;154(4):1351–5.
86. Mondaini N, Ponchietti R, Bonafè M, Biscioni S, Di Loro F, Agostini P, Salvestrini F, Rizzo M. Hypospadias: incidence and effects on psychosexual development as evaluated with the Minnesota Multiphasic Personality Inventory test in a sample of 11,649 young Italian men. Urol Int. 2002;68(2):81–5.
87. Hayashi Y, Mogami M, Kojima Y, Mogami T, Sasaki S, Azemoto M, Maruyama T, Tatsura H, Tsugaya M, Kohri K. Results of closure of urethrocutaneous fistulas after hypospadias repair. Int J Urol. 1998;5(2):167–9.
88. Emir L, Erol D. Mathieu urethroplasty as a salvage procedure: 20-year experience. J Urol. 2003;169(6):2325–6; author reply 2326–7
89. Secrest CL, Jordan GH, Winslow BH, Horton CE, McCraw JB, Gilbert DA, Devine CJ Jr. Repair of the complications of hypospadias surgery. J Urol. 1993;150(5 Pt 1):1415–8.
90. Mingin G, Baskin LS. Management of chordee in children and young adults. Urol Clin North Am. 2002;29(2):277–84.
91. Kuhnle U, Krahl W. The impact of culture on sex assignment and gender development in intersex patients. Perspect Biol Med. 2002;45(1):85–103.
92. O'Connell HE, Hutson JM, Anderson CR, Plenter RJ. Anatomical relationship between urethra and clitoris. J Urol. 1998;159(6):1892–7.
93. Rink RC, Adams MC. Feminizing genitoplasty: state of the art. World J Urol. 1998;16(3):212–8.
94. Passerini-Glazel G. Feminizing genitoplasty. J Urol. 1999;161(5):1592–3.
95. Hendren WH. Urological aspects of cloacal malformations. J Urol. 1988;140(5 Pt 2):1207–13.
96. Brock WA, Pena A. Cloacal abnormalities and imperforate anus (Chap. 19). In: Kelais PP, King LR, Belman AB, editors. Clinical pediatric urology, vol. 2. 3rd ed. Philadelphia: WB Saunders; 1992. p. 920–42.
97. Warne SA, Wilcox DT, Ransley PG. Long-term urological outcome of patients presenting with persistent cloaca. J Urol. 2002;168(4 Pt 2):1859–62; discussion 1862
98. Warne S, Chitty LS, Wilcox DT. Prenatal diagnosis of cloacal anomalies. BJU Int. 2002;89(1):78–81.
99. Peña A, Levitt MA, Hong A, Midulla P. Surgical management of cloacal malformations: a review of 339 patients. J Pediatr Surg. 2004;39(3):470–9; discussion 470–9
100. Levitt MA, Peña A. Cloacal malformations: lessons learned from 490 cases. Semin Pediatr Surg. 2010;19(2):128–38.
101. Peña A, Hong A. Advances in the management of anorectal malformations. Am J Surg. 2000;180(5):370–6.
102. Casale P. Robotic pediatric urology. Curr Urol Rep. 2009;10(2):115–8.
103. Behan JW, Kim SS, Dorey F, De Filippo RE, Chang AY, Hardy BE, Koh CJ. Human capital gains associated with robotic assisted laparoscopic pyeloplasty in children compared to open pyeloplasty. J Urol. 2011;186(4 Suppl):1663–7.
104. Yamzon J, Kokorowski P, De Filippo RE, Chang AY, Hardy BE, Koh CJ. Pediatric robot-assisted laparoscopic excision of urachal cyst and bladder cuff. J Endourol. 2008;22(10):2385–8; discussion 8
105. Peters CA. Laparoscopic and robotic approach to genitourinary anomalies in children. Urol Clin North Am. 2004;31(3):595–605, xi
106. Jones DR, Bui TH, Anderson EM, Ek S, Liu D, Ringdén O, et al. In utero haematopoietic stem cell transplantation: current perspectives and future potential. Bone Marrow Transplant. 1996;18(5):831–7.
107. Albanese CT, Barcena A. Ontogeny of the fetal immune system: implications for fetal tolerance induction and postnatal transplantation. In: Harrison MR, editor. The unborn patient: the art and science of fetal therapy. Philadelphia: W.B. Saunders; 2001. p. 605–15.

Evidence Based Neonatal Surgery

72

Nigel J. Hall, Simon Eaton, and Agostino Pierro

Abstract

Surgical intervention has, quite rightly, a well-established role in the management of a number of congenital and acquired neonatal conditions. Surgical approaches have been developed over a period of time, from the initial endeavours of pioneering neonatal surgeons, to the procedures commonly in everyday use today. Such development has been predominantly a result of necessity, learning from past experience and translation of techniques in use in other surgical fields into neonatal surgery. As neonatal surgical experience has grown, surgeons have begun to develop alternatives to what were once thought to be traditional techniques such that for a number of conditions we now have the luxury of choice in the treatment of these often fragile infants. With choice, there comes a dilemma. Which approach should be used? How should we make the decision?

Keywords

Evidence based neonatal surgery • Evidence based paediatric surgery Systematic review and meta-analysis • RCTs

72.1 Introduction

Surgical intervention has, quite rightly, a well-established role in the management of a number of congenital and acquired neonatal conditions. Surgical approaches have been developed over a period of time, from the initial endeavours of pioneering neonatal surgeons, to the procedures commonly in everyday use today. Such development has been predominantly a result of necessity, learning from past experience and translation of techniques in use in other surgical fields into neonatal surgery. As neonatal surgical experience has grown, surgeons have begun

N.J. Hall, PhD, MRCPCH, FRCS(Paed) (✉)
Faculty of Medicine, University Surgery Unit, University of Southampton, Southampton, UK
e-mail: n.j.hall@soton.ac.uk

S. Eaton, PhD
Developmental Biology and Cancer Programme, UCL Great Ormond Street Institute of Child Health, London, UK

A. Pierro, MD, FRCS(Eng), OBE
Division of General and Thoracic Surgery, The Hospital for Sick Children, Toronto, ON, Canada

P.D. Losty et al. (eds.), *Rickham's Neonatal Surgery*, https://doi.org/10.1007/978-1-4471-4721-3_72

to develop alternatives to what were once thought to be traditional techniques such that for a number of conditions we now have the luxury of choice in the treatment of these often fragile infants. With choice, there comes a dilemma. Which approach should be used? How should we make the decision?

The practice of evidence based medicine means integrating clinical expertise with the best available external clinical evidence from systematic research. Given that evidence based medicine is now an integral part of routine practice, we are required to draw on the available evidence to guide us in our decisions and justify them. The application of such evidence to surgical specialties, termed *evidence based surgery (EBS)*, has lagged behind our non-surgical counterparts. In the field of paediatric and neonatal surgery we are hindered further in our ability to perform evidence based surgery by a paucity of patient numbers from which we are able to draw high quality evidence. Compared with adult general surgeons, who may perform many hundreds of similar operations, general paediatric surgeons perform a great variety of different operations, but each of them may be in relatively small numbers. One consequence of this is that the evidence base for many paediatric and neonatal surgical procedures is limited compared with comparable procedures in adults. However, this problem is not just related to number of operations, as some very frequently performed paediatric operations such as hydrocele repair are also performed with very little evidence base.

This lack of evidence has been highlighted previously by Baraldini et al., who performed a study to determine the type of research evidence supporting operations in a tertiary referral paediatric surgical unit [1]. All patients admitted over a 4-week period to two surgical teams were enrolled in the study and all major operations carried out on each patient since birth were evaluated. Twenty-six percent of the operations were supported by a randomised controlled trial (RCT, level 1 evidence), but the vast majority of these trials had been conducted on adult patients. At that time, the only operation supported by an RCT *in children* was repair of congenital diaphragmatic hernia. The majority of the operations (68%) were based on evidence from non-randomised, prospective or retrospective studies.

More recently, Ostlie and St Peter scrutinised the Paediatric Surgical literature searching for RCTs in the field of Paediatric Surgery [2]. They identified only 56 RCTs relating to paediatric surgical conditions over a 10 year period and only four relating to neonatal conditions. A Paediatric Surgical RCT comprised just 0.04% of the manuscripts published in the 26 journals containing at least one RCT during the study period. An updated study of the Baraldini paper has recently been published, in which the evidence base for paediatric surgical operations, including specifically neonatal operations, was reviewed, in which it was concluded that although there had been an improvement in evidence base, more than one third of the procedures still lacked evidence-based literature support [3].

Whilst these three studies highlight the lack of EBS within the field of paediatric surgery as a whole and within the field of neonatal surgery in particular, a number of groups are striving to improve the evidence base on which Paediatric Surgeons base their daily practice.

This review examines the current available evidence for neonatal surgical procedures. We focus on those conditions of the term and preterm neonate which would be managed by the general paediatric and neonatal surgeon, excluding conditions affecting the cardiovascular, genitourinary and nervous systems. The evidence that we present will be primarily of level 1. There are many retrospective reviews and case series amongst the literature which may give some guidance as to which approach to a given condition may be superior. By their very nature, these have internal flaws and are subject to bias. We are firmly of the view that the correct way to determine the best approach to a condition where a choice exists is by means of a RCT. We have therefore reviewed primarily RCTs as they relate to neonatal surgery and we include non-randomised studies only where no RCTs exist and the alternative evidence is of sufficient quality or interest to make it noteworthy. We present the published evidence up relating to the more common surgical conditions of the neonatal period is presented. It is hoped that in future editions of this book further evidence will be available in neonatal surgery.

72.2 Oesophageal Atresia

Following the first classic description of oesophageal atresia with tracheo-oesophageal fistula by Gibson in 1697, it was not until the early twentieth century that the first attempts at repair of this congenital anomaly were made. Initially mortality remained high but during the course of the twentieth century oesophageal atresia was changed from a condition incompatible with life to a condition having a survival rate in excess of 90% [4]. With high survival rates now commonplace, surgeons have looked for interventions to refine both operative technique and outcome. The introduction of minimally invasive surgery has presented one such opportunity and thoracoscopic repair of oesophageal atresia has been performed, reportedly with good results [5, 6]. However, concern has been raised regarding acidosis during thoracoscopic repair of oesophageal atresia and congenital diaphragmatic hernia in infants, although a pilot randomised controlled trial suggested that this acidosis was not as severe in oesophageal atresia as in congenital diaphragmatic hernia [7]. In this pilot randomised controlled trial, there was no significant difference in outcomes between those operated thoracoscopically and those operated via a thoracotomy, although it should be noted that only ten oesophageal atresia patients were included and that clinical outcomes were not the primary aim of the study [7].

A proportion of infants with oesophageal atresia are born such that the interruption of the oesophagus between upper and lower pouches is too great to permit a primary anastomosis ("long-gap"). This may be managed in a staged manner using techniques including delayed primary repair with gastrostomy, cervical oesophagostomy, oesophageal replacement, and continuous extracorporeal tension of the oesophageal ends to encourage longitudinal growth (Foker technique [8]). Despite the lack of quality evidence, it is interesting that the United Kingdom National Institute of Clinical Excellence (NICE) has reviewed the evidence relating to the Foker technique and approved its use despite the unclear evidence considered relating to a limited number of infants who underwent this procedure [9]. Although experience with the technique is increasing it remains predominantly limited to a few centres [10]. Whilst the Foker technique may have a role in the management of selected infants with oesophageal atresia, we feel that this technique should be used cautiously and due consideration given to alternative approaches. It has not been subjected to the true scientific interrogation required to unanimously support its use.

Post-operatively the main challenges faced are anastomotic leakage, the development of anastomotic strictures requiring dilatation, gastro-oesophageal reflux, oesophageal dysmotility and tracheomalacia. Various techniques have been proposed to minimise the incidence of these post-operative complications. Elective paralysis and ventilation [11, 12] has been proposed as effective method of minimising anastomotic leakage following 'tight' oesophageal anastomosis. Both elective oesophageal dilatation and the routine use of anti-reflux medications [13] have been proposed to reduce the incidence of anastomotic strictures. None of these methods of treatment have been subjected to the rigorous scientific interrogation of a RCT.

72.3 Congenital Diaphragmatic Hernia

Congenital diaphragmatic hernia (CDH) remains one of the most interesting and challenging congenital anomalies of the newborn. Once a condition that carried an extremely poor prognosis, overall survival rates are now in the range of 40–70% with some centres reporting mortality of less than 20%. Central to our understanding of this condition has been the recognition that early surgical repair is not crucial for survival but that delayed surgical approach following improvement in cardiorespiratory function is preferable. However, even though most centres now delay repair until stabilisation, the evidence base for delayed repair is limited. Only two small RCTs of emergency early repair vs. delayed repair have been performed, neither of which showed a significant advantage of delayed repair [14, 15], and a systematic review concluded that a large multicentre RCT should be performed [16]. Such a trial would be very difficult to perform, however, because of the widespread perceived benefit of delaying surgery until haemodynamic stability is established. Survival rates are still far from desirable. This has prompted the pursuit of alternative strategies including extracorporeal membrane oxygenation (ECMO) and fetal intervention. A number of groups worldwide have led these pursuits and several RCTs performed. This is the neonatal condition that boasts the highest number of RCTs investigating various aspects of its treatment.

Prenatal diagnosis of CDH has permitted the identification of those fetuses with characteristics suggestive of poor prognosis and high postnatal mortality. A number of prenatal interventions have been suggested in attempts to improve outcome. Whilst technically feasible, prenatal repair of CDH by means of open fetal surgery failed to improve outcome and resulted an increased incidence of premature birth with no survival benefit [17]. Fetal endoluminal tracheal occlusion (FETO) has been investigated as a means of promoting prenatal lung growth in the anticipation that this would improve survival. Following *in-utero* FETO in experimental models of CDH, investigators found an increase in lung growth, improvement in lung compliance and improved postnatal oxygenation and ventilation. Initial reports [18–21] in the human suggested great promise using this technique but a recent RCT investigating FETO in what were considered to be high risk infants with CDH (lung to head ratio <1.4) was stopped before completion due to a higher than anticipated survival in the control (untreated) group [22]. This resulted in the study being underpowered to demonstrate any benefit in the treatment group. Another RCT investigating the effect of a modified FETO technique, in infants deemed to be at particularly poor prognosis (liver herniation and significantly reduced lung to head ratio), is currently ongoing [23].

Post-natally, it has been suggested that alternative ventilator strategies may improve outcome from CDH. Studies (some of them RCTs) have been performed investigating the effect of inhaled nitric oxide (NO) [24], routine ECMO [25], surfactant usage [26], partial liquid ventilation [27] and high-frequency oscillatory ventilation [28] in CDH infants. At present there is no evidence of improved outcome in infants with CDH following any of these interventions.

The technique of surgical repair of the diaphragmatic defect is of far lesser importance than management of the infant's cardio-respiratory compromise secondary to pulmonary hypoplasia and associated pulmonary hypertension. Surgical repair of the defect can proceed once the infant's cardio-respiratory status has stabilised. Following the return of the abdominal contents from the thorax to the abdomen, the defect is repaired primarily when possible but using a patch when the defect is too large for primary repair. Retrospective evidence suggests that a biological patch may confer a lower recurrence rate when compared with a synthetic alternative [29]. Surgical repair is possible through a traditional laparotomy incision or via minimal access techniques through both the abdomen and thorax. There is no evidence of improved outcome following minimal access repair when compared with conventional open surgical approach; and a recent meta-analysis of retrospective data suggests that the recurrence rate may be higher following minimally invasive repair [30], and the pilot randomised controlled trial of thoracoscopic vs. open repair of oesophageal atresia and congenital diaphragmatic hernia described above under oesophageal atresia showed that acidosis was significant during thoracoscopic repair of congenital diaphragmatic hernia [7].

72.4 Atresia of the Mid and Hind Gut

The surgical principle behind operative repair of duodenal, jejuno-ileal and colonic atresias is restoration of continuity from mouth to anus whilst maintaining as much intestinal length as possible. In the majority of cases, primary repair of the defect is possible. A laparoscopic approach to repair of duodenal atresia has been reported [31] but there is no evidence to support the preferential use of either open surgery or laparoscopy. The most significant long term adverse outcome following intestinal atresia is that of short bowel syndrome in a small group of infants. The underlying aetiology of this is usually the anatomical nature of the underlying anomaly rather than the technique of surgical repair. The high (>90%) survival rates and acceptable long term gastrointestinal function in the majority of infants provide evidence in support of current techniques [32]. Controversy does exist, however, in post-operative feeding strategies; some surgeons advocate parenteral feeding for some types of atresia whereas others do not [33]. There is no good quality evidence base either for or against parenteral nutrition.

72.5 Anorectal Malformations

The management of anorectal malformations remains a challenge for paediatric surgeons mainly due to the high incidence of functional long-term impairment including faecal incontinence, urinary incontinence, sexual dysfunction and fertility problems. The introduction and widespread use of the posterior sagittal anorectoplasty (PSARP; [34]) is generally perceived to have improved functional outcome from this complex group of anomalies. However, gathering reliable evidence to support this statement is difficult due to the diversity of anomalies, the functional (and therefore often subjective) nature of the outcomes of interest and indeed the widespread usage of the PSARP procedure thereby precluding meaningful comparison with alternative surgical approaches. A laparoscopically-assisted anorectoplasty has also been advocated, with the rationale of minimising perineal dissection [35]. However, whether there is advantage of the laparoscopically-assisted anorectoplasty over the PSARP remains a matter of debate.

72.6 Anterior Abdominal Wall Defects

The anterior abdominal wall defects (gastroschisis and exomphalos) are often considered together due to their anatomical similarities and similarities in their management strategy. The principles of surgery relating to these conditions are to protect the bowel and other eviscerated organs and to achieve their return to the abdominal cavity as soon as possible so that the defect in the abdominal wall can be closed. Reduction and closure may be undertaken as single stage primary procedure or as a staged approach with the use of a silo.

Infants in whom primary closure is possible have traditionally had the procedure performed under general anaesthetic. However, the need for this in selected infants with gastroschisis (but not exomphalos) has been questioned and the concept of primary reduction without anaesthesia at the bedside has been reported [36]. There is a lack of quality evidence in support this approach. A Cochrane review failed to identify any RCT addressing this issue and recommended that they be undertaken [37]. None has been.

When a staged approach is required this involves the use of a protective bag known as a 'silo' into which the eviscerated abdominal contents are placed. The silo serves to protect the bowel from the outside environment particularly preventing the bowel from dehydration. It also facilitates reduction of its contents into the abdominal cavity by containing it in such a way that gravity and external pressure can be applied to enhance reduction. Traditionally silos were attached to the abdominal wall musculature surgically but recently the 'preformed silo' product has become available that can be tucked under the musculature and held in place without the need for general anaesthesia or surgical attachment. Following return of the abdominal contents to the abdomen, the abdominal wall defect is closed. This has usually been a surgical closure under general anaesthetic but a number of centres are now performing this at the bedside without the need for anaesthesia and achieving excellent cosmetic results.

The advent of the preformed silo has led clinicians to consider whether such a technique should be used for all cases of gastroschisis and that attempted primary closure should be avoided altogether. The potential complications of primary closure include a sudden rise in intra-abdominal pressure which may result in respiratory compromise, organ failure and significant complications. Pastor and colleagues [38] have performed a RCT comparing routine placement of a preformed silo without anaesthetic at the bedside with attempted primary closure either under general anaesthetic or at the bedside. In the group randomised to undergo attempted primary closure, a preformed silo was placed if primary closure was not possible either due to a large discrepancy between volume of eviscerated contents and abdominal capacity or due to an unacceptable increase in intra-abdominal pressure. Unfortunately their study was stopped early due to poor recruitment and analyses demonstrated no difference between the groups in outcome measures of number of days on a ventilator, duration of PN dependency, length of hospital stay, incidence of sepsis and NEC and intra-abdominal pressure at the time of closure. However due to the smaller than anticipated numbers in this study, the trial was significantly underpowered to detect any difference in this outcome measures between the groups. Previous retrospective studies have demonstrated improved outcomes following routine use of preformed silos although there are significant biases in patient allocation attributable to the retrospective nature of these reports [39, 40]. More recently however, a national non-randomised cohort study from the UK [41] has not shown any proven benefit of one approach over the other and has raised some concerns about the safety of pre-formed silos based on a higher incidence of intestinal ischaemia in cases treated with a pre-formed silo. A systematic review and meta-analysis on this topic suggested although that routine use of a pre-formed silo is associated with fewer days on a ventilator, strong evidence to support either strategy was not available [42].

One of the most challenging aspects of the treatment of the infant with gastroschisis is the management of intestinal dysfunction following return of the bowel to the abdomen and abdominal wall closure. The precise aetiology of this dysfunction is unclear but it is proposed that there is a degree of intestinal damage sustained *in utero*. A number of interventions have been proposed to improve the intestinal dysfunction including prenatal amniotic fluid exchange, elective pre-term delivery [43, 44], elective Caesarian section delivery [45], early onset of enteral feeds [46] and administration of pro-kinetic agents [47]. The efficacy of early delivery and of pro-kinetic agents has been investigated in RCTs. Logghe et al. performed a RCT comparing elective delivery at 36 weeks gestation with spontaneous onset of labour [43]. They found no clear benefit in terms of time to full enteral feeding or hospital stay in infants who were electively delivered at 36 weeks although the sample size was small. Curry et al. investigated the effect of enteral erythromycin as a prokinetic agent on time taken to achieve full enteral feeds compared with placebo in a prospective randomised study comprising 62 infants with gastroschisis [47]. No benefit was observed in time taken to achieve full enteral feeds nor episodes of sepsis, duration of PN requirement or total hospital stay in infants receiving erythromycin.

72.7 Congenital Lung Lesions

Congenital cystic adenomatous malformation (CCAM) and bronchopulmonary sequestration are congenital lung lesions often detected on routine antenatal scanning. Whilst there is general consensus that symptomatic CCAMs should be surgically excised to allow symptomatic relief, controversy exists surrounding the optimal management of asymptomatic lesions. Justification for surgical excision of asymptomatic lesions is the avoidance of symptoms or other complications (e.g. malignant transformation) in the future. However such an approach is not without risk and involves exposing the child to potentially significant surgical complications [48]. Whilst there are no randomised studies comparing surgical excision with non-operative observation,

Stanton et al. have performed a meta-analysis of the postnatal management of antenatally diagnosed lung lesions [49]. They concluded that the risk of an asymptomatic lesion becoming symptomatic is extremely low and that a non-operative approach may be appropriate for small lesions. A more recent study confirmed that non-operative observation does appear to be an acceptable management strategy [50]. Further prospective studies are required to provide reliable data to guide clinicians and parents on the optimum management of asymptomatic lesions.

72.8 Hirschsprung Disease

Hirschsprung disease, characterised by an absence of ganglion cells in the nerve plexi of the large bowel, most commonly presents in the neonatal period with failure of passage of meconium within the first 48 h of birth and is often associated with abdominal distension, with or without vomiting. Diagnosis is based on rectal biopsy and following diagnosis, definitive surgery is planned to excise the affected colonic segment. There are a number of operative techniques, the main differences between them being the nature of the anastomosis between the 'pulled through' section of normal bowel, proximal to the excised aganglionic segment and the rectum. Evaluating and comparing these procedures is problematic for many reasons. Firstly, the main outcome measures of interest are long term and primarily relate to bowel function. As is the case following surgical correction of anorectal malformations, there are difficulties in quantifying bowel function in such a way that meaningful results can be achieved. In additional there is inter-patient variability in the severity of disease, length of affected intestine and susceptibility to enterocolitis, a well-established complication of Hirschsprung disease. Thus strong evidence in support of one operative technique over the others is lacking.

Despite this, significant advances in the management of neonates with Hirschsprung disease have been made in recent times. With the advent of laparoscopic surgery, many surgeons are performing a pull through procedure either with the assistance of the laparoscope [51] or in a completely minimally invasive fashion [52]. Early experience suggests that the traditional benefits of minimally invasive surgery can be achieved with functional outcome similar to that reported following open surgery. However, long term follow-up of these children is, at present, lacking.

The other recent advance is the use of the primary pull-through procedure in selected infants. The traditional approach to the infant with Hirschsprung disease has been to achieve intestinal decompression with a stoma, to perform a pull-through procedure with this covering stoma and then to close the stoma following successful healing of the pull-through. However it is now clear that selected infants can be successfully managed with a primary pull-through procedure with intestinal decompression achieved preoperatively with rectal washouts and avoiding the need for a stoma altogether. One potential disadvantage of this is a higher incidence of postoperative enterocolitis [53] but this is not a consistent finding across series [54] and it is evident that the primary pull-through is here to stay.

72.9 Inguinal Hernia

Inguinal herniotomy is the procedure of choice for neonates with an inguinal hernia (IH). Gross et al.'s report in 1953 of 3874 children who underwent inguinal herniotomy reported a recurrence rate of just 0.15% [55]. The standard approach to inguinal herniotomy was by an open groin incision but laparoscopic repair is now routinely practised with comparable outcomes [56]. In the neonatal population there are a number of issues which remain largely unanswered. These are: how the contralateral groin should be managed, whether laparoscopic repair confers any benefit over open repair in this age group and whether repair should be undertaken on an urgent or even emergent basis due to the perceived higher risk of incarceration in the neonatal population.

Despite being debated for over 50 years, management of the contralateral groin in infants with unilateral IH remains controversial. It is recognised that a proportion of infants with IH will develop a metachronous contralateral hernia but identification of such infants has proved difficult. Some surgeons advocate routine contralateral open groin exploration at the time of repair of IH but this places the contralateral vas deferens and testicular vessels at potentially unnecessary risk. A systematic review estimated that the incidence of metachronous contralateral hernia in infants <6 months of age was 11% and that 9 contralateral groins would need to be routinely explored to prevent one metachronous contralateral hernia [57].

The introduction of laparoscopic IH repair has serendipitously provided a unique insight into this problem. Laparoscopy enables the surgeon to visualise both deep inguinal rings at the time of inguinal hernia repair and perform bilateral closure should the contralateral deep ring be open. Fundamental to the role of laparoscopic repair of IH repair in neonates must remain the efficacy of the procedure. Initial reports of laparoscopic repair of IH in children suggested a higher recurrence rate than could be achieved with open surgery [58, 59]. Recent RCTs comparing open and laparoscopic IH repair in children have reported similar recurrence rates with both techniques although none have focussed specifically on neonates [60–62]. The role of laparoscopy in the treatment of IH and prevention of metachronous IH in infants (<1 year) is currently being investigated in a prospective randomised study (www.marchtrial.org).

The optimal timing of IH repair in neonates is also unclear. The risk of incarceration of IH is believed to be higher in infants, in particular infants born pre-term, when compared with older children [63]. This has led to some surgeons repairing inguinal hernias on an urgent basis in infants, and for pre-term infants with an IH to have a hernia repair prior to discharge home. The precise risk of incarceration, however, is unknown as there are no observational studies where children known to have a hernia have been observed without planned elective surgery.

One important consideration in hernia repair in boys is future fertility, because of the possibility of damage to the vas or vessels, either during repair, or if a hernia becomes incarcerated. Very little is known about testicular size and fertility following herniotomy, but hopefully infants who have been recruited to RCTs will provide cohorts who will be followed up into puberty to answer this important question. This further demonstrates a significant problem for top-level evidence in neonatal surgery, that important outcomes may not be apparent for many years. This provides problems, particularly where populations are relatively mobile, as in the UK.

72.10 Necrotising Enterocolitis

The general principles of surgery for the infant with advanced necrotising enterocolitis (NEC) are to control intra-abdominal sepsis and remove ischaemic or irreversibly diseased intestine whilst preserving as much intestinal length as possible. A number of techniques have been proposed to achieve these aims, including resection of bowel with primary anastomosis, resection with stoma formation and the ‘clip and drop’ technique with subsequent ‘second look’ laparotomy [64–66]. None of these techniques has been subjected to a RCT to determine superiority over the others and they are all in common usage today with justification for their use coming from a number of series all reporting, in general terms, similar outcomes. However the landscape is beginning to change with an on-going trial of stoma versus primary anastomosis in infants with NEC requiring intestinal resection.

In addition to laparotomy, peritoneal drainage has been proposed as a useful intervention in the infant with perforated NEC. Initially described by Ein et al. [67] as a procedure for infants thought too unwell to tolerate laparotomy, it has subsequently been described as a stabilising manoeuvre [68, 69] in the smallest and sickest infants and even proposed as primary definitive treatment [70–72]. Recently, two RCTs have addressed the issue of whether primary peritoneal drainage or laparotomy is superior in the smallest infants with NEC. These are summarised in Table 72.1 [73, 74].

Post-operative treatment of infants who have had surgery for NEC is also open to debate. The

Table 72.1 RCTs comparing laparotomy with primary peritoneal drainage in infants with perforated necrotising enterocolitis

Study	Included infants (g)	Number	Main outcomes	Authors conclusion
Moss 2006 [73]	<1500	PPD 55 Lap 62	No difference in mortality or dependence on PN at 90 days or length of hospital admission	No effect of procedure on outcome
Rees 2008 [74]	<1000	PPD 35 Lap 34	No difference in survival, ventilator or PN dependence at 1 or 6 months or length of hospital admission. 74% of infants undergoing PPD required delayed laparotomy	Recommend early laparotomy

PPD primary peritoneal drain, *Lap* laparotomy, *PN* parenteral nutrition

Table 72.2 RCTs comparing open and laparoscopic pyloromyotomy in infants with pyloric stenosis

Study	Detail	Number	Recovery time	Complications	Other significant findings	Authors conclusion
Greason 1997 [79]	LP vs. UMB	LP 10 OP 10	LP < OP	Similar	-	Recommend LP
St Peter 2006 [77]	LP vs. Open[a]	LP 100 OP 100	Similar	Similar	Less pain and vomiting with LP	Recommend LP
Leclair 2007 [78]	LP vs. UMB	LP 50 OP 52	Similar	Similar	Less pain with LP	Recommend OP
Hall 2009 [76]	LP vs. UMB	LP 87 OP 93	LP < OP	Similar	Less analgesia with LP	Recommend LP

[a]Open in this study was either by supra-umbilical or transverse upper abdominal incision
Umb supraumbilical, *LP* laparoscopic pyloromyotomy, *OP* open pyloromyotomy, <, denotes shorter than

period of antibiotic usage, time to introduction of enteral feeds, and type of enteral feed are all areas where practise is based on weak evidence. Although there have been no RCTs, a retrospective cohort study suggested that an early re-introduction of enteral feeds is associated with benefit in terms of hospital stay and decreased incidence of central venous catheter-related sepsis, but apparently without increased risk of recurrent NEC [75].

72.11 Pyloric Stenosis

The standard surgical approach to the infant with pyloric stenosis is the pyloromyotomy based on the technique originally described by Ramstedt. A number of modifications to this procedure have been introduced over time. Whilst the underlying surgical procedure has remained constant, the approach to the pylorus has been modified in attempts to improve cosmetic outcome, shorten post-operative recovery and reduce post-operative pain. The pyloromyotomy may be performed via an open incision in the right upper quadrant (RUQ), an open supra-umbilical incision or via a laparoscopic approach.

Four RCTs have studied the effect of surgical approach to the pyloromyotomy on post-operative recovery all comparing laparoscopic pyloromyotomy (LP) with open pyloromyotomy (OP) [76–79]. These are summarised in Table 72.2. Whilst three of these studies recommend LP over OP on the basis of shorter post-operative recovery and/or less post-operative pain or vomiting, one study is notable in its recommendation of OP over LP [78]. Although the incidence of complications was similar in both groups in this study, the authors felt that although there was not a statistically significant difference, the trend towards a higher incidence of incomplete pyloromyotomy following LP (LP 3/50 *vs.* OP 0/52; p = 0.11) precluded the use of this approach.

A meta-analysis [80] including the three large scale RCTs concluded that post-operative recovery was shorter following LP with a similar incidence in overall complications between the groups. However, there was a trend (p = 0.06) towards a higher incidence of incomplete pyloromyotomy following LP when compared with OP. A further meta-analysis, which included prospective cohort studies as well as the RCTs reached similar conclusions. The findings of a trend towards an increased rate of incomplete pyloromyotomy in both these meta-analyses highlight another problem in conducting RCTs and meta-analyses of RCTs in neonatal surgery. Major complications, such as incomplete pyloromyotomy, are rare such that individual RCTs are frequently not powered to detect them. Even when several RCTs are meta-analysed, rare complications are problematic as RCTs without any complications (e.g. the zero rate of incomplete pyloromyotomy in each arm one of the trials [77]) do not contribute to the overall effect sizes in the meta-analysis when odds ratios or relative risks are used. Thus the strong trend towards a higher rate of incomplete pyloromyotomy following LP is critically dependent on precisely how the meta-analysis is performed. A large multicentre retrospective study of incomplete pyloromyotomy following open and laparoscopic pyloromyotomy showed that although there was a significantly increased risk following laparoscopy, the risk difference was <1%. One could argue that although important, such complications are so rare that they do not pose a *clinically significant risk* on an individual patient basis.

In summary, it appears that duration of post-operative recovery and post-operative pain are shorter following a laparoscopic approach to the pyloromyotomy and that LP is a valid technique so long as due care and attention is paid to avoiding incomplete pyloromyotomy.

72.12 Commentary

Despite the well-established and accepted role for surgical intervention in the management of many conditions affecting the term and pre-term neonate, a quality evidence base supporting many of these interventions is lacking. Surgical approaches and techniques have largely evolved over time with outcomes being compared to history rather than being formally compared prospectively. There is a clear need for well designed, prospective, randomised studies in improving the outcomes of infants with surgical conditions as well as advancing our knowledge. Neonatal surgery is a difficult area in which to conduct randomised controlled trials because of the relatively small number of patients, and the perceived difficulty in getting surgeons to participate and parents to consent to randomisation. In addition, some outcomes are difficult to assess or compare.

There is now clear evidence that successful surgical randomised controlled trials can be achieved even in this patient population. Of note, however, only a few trials have randomised and studied the number of patients required by their power calculation. Due to the relative small number of surgical neonates in each hospital it is necessary to: (1) develop a collaboration among paediatric surgical units to foster multicentre RCTs; (2) change the attitude of clinicians, nurses and parents similarly to encompass the concept of widespread routine recruitment into RCTs; (3) appreciate the importance of protocol, equipoise and clinical relevance in the management of surgical neonates. Evidence based neonatal surgery is, quite rightly, here to stay; we must encompass it, develop it and excel in it for the future benefit of those in our care.

References

1. Baraldini V, Spitz L, Pierro A. Evidence-based operations in paediatric surgery. Pediatr Surg Int. 1998;13:331–5.
2. Ostlie DJ, St Peter SD. The current state of evidence-based pediatric surgery. J Pediatr Surg. 2010;45:1940–6.

3. Zani-Ruttenstock E, Zani A, Bullman E, Lapidus-Krol E, Pierro A. Are paediatric operations evidence based? A prospective analysis of general surgery practice in a teaching paediatric hospital. Pediatr Surg Int. 2015;31:53–9.
4. Houben CH, Curry JI. Current status of prenatal diagnosis, operative management and outcome of esophageal atresia/tracheo-esophageal fistula. Prenat Diagn. 2008;28:667–75.
5. Bax KM, Van DZ. Feasibility of thoracoscopic repair of esophageal atresia with distal fistula. J Pediatr Surg. 2002;37:192–6.
6. Rothenberg SS. Thoracoscopic repair of tracheo-esophageal fistula in newborns. J Pediatr Surg. 2002;37:869–72.
7. Bishay M, Giacomello L, Retrosi G, Thyoka M, Garriboli M, Brierley J, et al. Hypercapnia and acidosis during open and thoracoscopic repair of congenital diaphragmatic hernia and esophageal atresia: results of a pilot randomized controlled trial. Ann Surg. 2013;258:895–900.
8. Foker JE, Linden BC, Boyle EM Jr, Marquardt C. Development of a true primary repair for the full spectrum of esophageal atresia. Ann Surg. 1997;226:533–41.
9. National Institute for Health and Clinical Excellence. Foker technique for long-gap oesophageal atresia IPG153.London: National Institute for Health and Clinical Excellence; 2006.
10. Foker JE, Kendall Krosch TC, Catton K, Munro F, Khan KM. Long-gap esophageal atresia treated by growth induction: the biological potential and early follow-up results. Semin Pediatr Surg. 2009;18:23–9.
11. Uchida K, Inoue M, Otake K, Okita Y, Morimoto Y, Araki T, et al. Efficacy of postoperative elective ventilatory support for leakage protection in primary anastomosis of congenital esophageal atresia. Pediatr Surg Int. 2006;22:496–9.
12. Beasley SW. Does postoperative ventilation have an effect on the integrity of the anastomosis in repaired oesophageal atresia? J Paediatr Child Health. 1999;35:120–2.
13. Losty PD, Jawaid WB, Khalil BA. Esophageal atresia and tracheo-esophageal fistula. In: Puri P, editor. Newborn surgery. London: Hodder Arnold; 2011. p. 388–400.
14. de la Hunt MN, Madden N, Scott JES, Matthews JNS, Beck J, Sadler C, et al. Is delayed surgery really better for congenital diaphragmatic hernia? A prospective randomized clinical trial. J Pediatr Surg. 1996;31:1554–6.
15. Nio M, Haase G, Kennaugh J, Bui K, Atkinson JB. A prospective randomized trial of delayed versus immediate repair of congenital diaphragmatic-hernia. J Pediatr Surg. 1994;29:618–21.
16. Moyer VA, Moya FR, Tibboel D, Losty PD, Nagaya M, Lally KP. Late versus early surgical correction for congenital diaphragmatic hernia in newborn infants. Cochrane Database Syst Rev. 2002;(3):CD001695.
17. Harrison MR, Adzick NS, Bullard KM, Farrell JA, Howell LJ, Rosen MA, et al. Correction of congenital diaphragmatic hernia in utero VII: a prospective trial. J Pediatr Surg. 1997;32:1637–42.
18. Harrison MR, Albanese CT, Hawgood SB, Farmer DL, Farrell JA, Sandberg PL, et al. Fetoscopic temporary tracheal occlusion by means of detachable balloon for congenital diaphragmatic hernia. Am J Obstet Gynecol. 2001;185:730–3.
19. Harrison MR, Sydorak RM, Farrell JA, Kitterman JA, Filly RA, Albanese CT. Fetoscopic temporary tracheal occlusion for congenital diaphragmatic hernia: prelude to a randomized, controlled trial. J Pediatr Surg. 2003;38:1012–20.
20. Harrison MR, Langer JC, Adzick NS, Golbus MS, Filly RA, Anderson RL, et al. Correction of congenital diaphragmatic hernia in utero, V. Initial clinical experience. J Pediatr Surg. 1990;25:47–55.
21. Harrison MR, Adzick NS, Flake AW, Jennings RW, Estes JM, MacGillivray TE, et al. Correction of congenital diaphragmatic hernia in utero: VI. Hard-earned lessons. J Pediatr Surg. 1993;28: 1411–7.
22. Harrison MR, Keller RL, Hawgood SB, Kitterman JA, Sandberg PL, Farmer DL, et al. A randomized trial of fetal endoscopic tracheal occlusion for severe fetal congenital diaphragmatic hernia. N Engl J Med. 2003;349:1916–24.
23. Randomized control trial of fetoscopic endoluminal tracheal occlusion with a balloon versus expectant management during pregnancy in fetuses with left sided congenital diaphragmatic hernia and moderate pulmonary hypoplasia (TOTAL). gov/ct2/show/NCT00763737 2009. http://clinicaltrials.gov/ct2/show/NCT00763737|FCC|
24. The Neonatal Inhaled Nitric Oxide Study Group (NINOS). Inhaled nitric oxide and hypoxic respiratory failure in infants with congenital diaphragmatic hernia. Pediatrics. 1997;99:838–45.
25. The Congenital Diaphragmatic Hernia Study Group. Does extracorporeal membrane oxygenation improve survival in neonates with congenital diaphragmatic hernia? J Pediatr Surg 1999;34:720–4.
26. Lally KP, Lally PA, Langham MR, Hirschl R, Moya FR, Tibboel D, et al. Surfactant does not improve survival rate in preterm infants with congenital diaphragmatic hernia. J Pediatr Surg. 2004;39:829–33.
27. Hirschl RB, Philip WF, Glick L, Greenspan J, Smith K, Thompson A, et al. A prospective, randomized pilot trial of perfluorocarbon-induced lung growth in newborns with congenital diaphragmatic hernia. J Pediatr Surg. 2003;38:283–9.
28. Snoek KG1, Capolupo I, van Rosmalen J, Hout Lde J, Vijfhuize S, Greenough A, et al. Conventional mechanical ventilation versus high-frequency oscillatory ventilation for congenital diaphragmatic hernia: a randomized clinical trial (The VICI-trial). Ann Surg. 2016;263:867–74
29. Mitchell IC, Garcia NM, Barber R, Ahmad N, Hicks BA, Fischer AC. Permacol: a potential biologic patch

alternative in congenital diaphragmatic hernia repair. J Pediatr Surg. 2008;43:2161–4.
30. Lansdale N, Alam S, Losty PD, Jesudason EC. Neonatal endosurgical congenital diaphragmatic hernia repair: a systematic review and meta-analysis. Ann Surg. 2010;252:20–6.
31. Spilde TL, St Peter SD, Keckler SJ, Holcomb GW III, Snyder CL, Ostlie DJ. Open vs laparoscopic repair of congenital duodenal obstructions: a concurrent series. J Pediatr Surg. 2008;43:1002–5.
32. Kumaran N, Shankar KR, Lloyd DA, Losty PD. Trends in the management and outcome of jejuno-ileal atresia. Eur J Pediatr Surg. 2002;12:163–7.
33. Bishay M, Lakshminarayanan B, Arnaud A, Garriboli M, Cross KM, Curry JI, et al. The role of parenteral nutrition following surgery for duodenal atresia or stenosis. Pediatr Surg Int. 2013;29:191–5.
34. deVries PA, Peña A. Posterior sagittal anorectoplasty. J Pediatr Surg. 1982;17:638–43.
35. Georgeson KE, Inge TH, Albanese CT. Laparoscopically assisted anorectal pull-through for high imperforate anus—A new technique. J Pediatr Surg. 2000;35:927–30.
36. Bianchi A, Dickson AP. Elective delayed reduction and no anesthesia: 'minimal intervention management' for gastrochisis. J Pediatr Surg. 1998;33:1338–40.
37. Davies MW, Kimble RM, Woodgate PG. Ward reduction without general anaesthesia versus reduction and repair under general anaesthesia for gastroschisis in newborn infants. Cochrane Database Syst Rev 2002;CD003671
38. Pastor AC, Phillips JD, Fenton SJ, Meyers RL, Lamm AW, Raval MV, et al. Routine use of a SILASTIC spring-loaded silo for infants with gastroschisis: a multicenter randomized controlled trial. J Pediatr Surg. 2008;43:1807–12.
39. Minkes RK, Langer JC, Mazziotti MV, Skinner MA, Foglia RP. Routine insertion of a silastic spring-loaded silo for infants with gastroschisis. J Pediatr Surg. 2000;35:843–6.
40. Owen A, Marven S, Jackson L, Antao B, Roberts J, Walker J, et al. Experience of bedside preformed silo staged reduction and closure for gastroschisis. J Pediatr Surg. 2006;41:1830–5.
41. Bradnock TJ, Marven S, Owen A, Johnson P, Kurinczuk JJ, Spark P, et al. Gastroschisis: one year outcomes from national cohort study. BMJ. 2011;343:d6749.
42. Ross AR, Eaton S, Zani A, Ade-Ajayi N, Pierro A, Hall NJ. The role of preformed silos in the management of infants with gastroschisis: a systematic review and meta-analysis. Pediatr Surg Int. 2015;31:473–83.
43. Logghe HL, Mason GC, Thornton JG, Stringer MD. A randomized controlled trial of elective preterm delivery of fetuses with gastroschisis. J Pediatr Surg. 2005;40:1726–31.
44. Moir CR, Ramsey PS, Ogburn PL, Johnson RV, Ramin KD. A prospective trial of elective preterm delivery for fetal gastroschisis. Am J Perinatol. 2004;21:289–94.
45. Reigstad I, Reigstad H, Kiserud T, Berstad T. Preterm elective caesarean section and early enteral feeding in gastroschisis. Acta Paediatr. 2011;100:71–4.
46. Walter-Nicolet E, Rousseau V, Kieffer F, Fusaro F, Bourdaud N, Oucherif S, et al. Neonatal outcome of gastroschisis is mainly influenced by nutritional management. J Pediatr Gastroenterol Nutr. 2009;48:612–7.
47. Curry JI, Lander AD, Stringer MD. A multicenter, randomized, double-blind, placebo-controlled trial of the prokinetic agent erythromycin in the postoperative recovery of infants with gastroschisis. J Pediatr Surg. 2004;39:565–9.
48. Hall NJ, Chiu PP, Langer JC. Morbidity after elective resection of prenatally diagnosed asymptomatic congenital pulmonary airway malformations. Pediatr Pulmonol. 2016;51:525–30.
49. Stanton M, Njere I, de-Ajayi N, Patel S, Davenport M. Systematic review and meta-analysis of the postnatal management of congenital cystic lung lesions. J Pediatr Surg. 2009;44:1027–33.
50. Ng C, Stanwell J, Burge DM, Stanton MP. Conservative management of antenatally diagnosed cystic lung malformations. Arch Dis Child. 2014;99:432–7.
51. Georgeson KE, Robertson DJ. Laparoscopic-assisted approaches for the definitive surgery for Hirschsprung's disease. Semin Pediatr Surg. 2004;13:256–62.
52. Dasgupta R, Langer JC. Transanal pull-through for Hirschsprung disease. Semin Pediatr Surg. 2005;14:64–71.
53. Teitelbaum DH, Cilley RE, Sherman NJ, Bliss D, Uitvlugt ND, Renaud EJ, et al. A decade of experience with the primary pull-through for Hirschsprung disease in the newborn period: a multicenter analysis of outcomes. Ann Surg. 2000;232:372–80.
54. Wulkan ML, Georgeson KE. Primary laparoscopic endorectal pull-through for Hirschsprung's disease in infants and children. Semin Laparosc Surg. 1998;5:9–13.
55. Gross RE. Inguinal hernia. The surgery of infancy and childhood. Philadelphia: WB Saunders; 1953. p. 449–62.
56. Dutta S, Albanese C. Transcutaneous laparoscopic hernia repair in children: a prospective review of 275 hernia repairs with minimum 2-year follow-up. Surg Endosc. 2009;23:103–7.
57. Ron O, Eaton S, Pierro A. Systematic review of the risk of developing a metachronous contralateral inguinal hernia in children. Br J Surg. 2007;94:804–11.
58. Hassan ME, Mustafawi AR. Laparoscopic flip-flap technique versus conventional inguinal hernia repair in children. JSLS. 2007;11:90–3.
59. Yang C, Zhang H, Pu J, Mei H, Zheng L, Tong Q. Laparoscopic vs open herniorrhaphy in the management of pediatric inguinal hernia: a systemic review and meta-analysis. J Pediatr Surg. 2011;46:1824–34.
60. Saranga BR, Arora M, Baskaran V. Pediatric inguinal hernia: laparoscopic versus open surgery. JSLS. 2008;12:277–81.
61. Koivusalo AI, Korpela R, Wirtavuori K, Piiparinen S, Rintala RJ, Pakarinen MP. A single-blinded, randomized comparison of laparoscopic versus open hernia repair in children. Pediatrics. 2009;123:332–7.

62. Chan KL, Hui WC, Tam PK. Prospective randomized single-center, single-blind comparison of laparoscopic vs open repair of pediatric inguinal hernia. Surg Endosc. 2005;19:927–32
63. Zamakhshary M, To T, Guan J, Langer JC. Risk of incarceration of inguinal hernia among infants and young children awaiting elective surgery. CMAJ. 2008;179:1001–5.
64. Fasoli L, Turi RA, Spitz L, Kiely EM, Drake D, Pierro A. Necrotizing enterocolitis: extent of disease and surgical treatment. J Pediatr Surg. 1999;34:1096–9.
65. Hall NJ, Curry J, Drake DP, Spitz L, Kiely EM, Pierro A. Resection and primary anastomosis is a valid surgical option for infants with necrotizing enterocolitis who weigh less than 1000 g. Arch Surg. 2005;140:1149–51.
66. Ron O, Davenport M, Patel S, Kiely E, Pierro A, Hall NJ, et al. Outcomes of the "clip and drop" technique for multifocal necrotizing enterocolitis. J Pediatr Surg. 2009;44:749–54.
67. Ein SH, Marshall DG, Girvan D. Peritoneal drainage under local anesthesia for perforations from necrotizing enterocolitis. J Pediatr Surg. 1977;12:963–7.
68. Cass DL, Brandt ML, Patel DL, Nuchtern JG, Minifee PK, Wesson DE. Peritoneal drainage as definitive treatment for neonates with isolated intestinal perforation. J Pediatr Surg. 2000;35:1531–6.
69. Rovin JD, Rodgers BM, Burns RC, McGahren ED. The role of peritoneal drainage for intestinal perforation in infants with and without necrotizing enterocolitis. J Pediatr Surg. 1999;34:143–7.
70. Ein SH, Shandling B, Wesson D, Filler RM. A 13-year experience with peritoneal drainage under local anesthesia for necrotizing enterocolitis perforation. J Pediatr Surg. 1990;25:1034–6.
71. Lessin MS, Luks FI, Wesselhoeft CW Jr, Gilchrist BF, Iannitti D, DeLuca FG. Peritoneal drainage as definitive treatment for intestinal perforation in infants with extremely low birth weight (<750 g). J Pediatr Surg. 1998;33:370–2.
72. Morgan LJ, Shochat SJ, Hartman GE. Peritoneal drainage as primary management of perforated NEC in the very low birth weight infant. J Pediatr Surg. 1994;29:310–4.
73. Moss RL, Dimmitt RA, Barnhart DC, Sylvester KG, Brown RL, Powell DM, et al. Laparotomy versus peritoneal drainage for necrotizing enterocolitis and perforation. N Engl J Med. 2006;354:2225–34.
74. Rees CM, Eaton S, Kiely EM, Wade AM, McHugh K, Pierro A. Peritoneal drainage or laparotomy for neonatal bowel perforation? A randomized controlled trial. Ann Surg. 2008;248:44–51.
75. Bohnhorst B, Muller S, Dordelmann M, Peter CS, Petersen C, Poets CF. Early feeding after necrotizing enterocolitis in preterm infants. J Pediatr. 2003;143:484–7.
76. Hall NJ, Pacilli M, Eaton S, Reblock K, Gaines BA, Pastor A, et al. Recovery after open versus laparoscopic pyloromyotomy for pyloric stenosis: a double-blind multicentre randomised controlled trial. Lancet. 2009;373:390–8.
77. St Peter SD, Holcomb GW III, Calkins CM, Murphy JP, Andrews WS, Sharp RJ, et al. Open versus laparoscopic pyloromyotomy for pyloric stenosis: a prospective, randomized trial. Ann Surg. 2006;244:363–70.
78. Leclair MD, Plattner V, Mirallie E, Lejus C, Nguyen JM, Podevin G, et al. Laparoscopic pyloromyotomy for hypertrophic pyloric stenosis: a prospective, randomized controlled trial. J Pediatr Surg. 2007;42:692–8.
79. Greason KL, Allshouse MJ, Thompson WR, Rappold JF, Downey EC. A prospective, randomized evaluation of laparoscopic versus open pyloromyotomy in the treatment of infantile hypertrophic pyloric stenosis. Pediatr Endosurg Innov Tech. 1997;1:175–9.
80. Jia WQ, Tian J-H, Yang K-H, Ma B, Liu Y-L, Zhang P, Li R-J, Jia R-H. Open versus laparoscopic pyloromyotomy for pyloric stenosis: a meta-analysis of randomized controlled trials. Eur J Pediatr Surg. 2011;21:77–81.

Index

P.D. Losty et al. (eds.), *Rickham's Neonatal Surgery*, https://doi.org/10.1007/978-1-4471-4721-3

B

C

E

J

K

O

W

X

Y

Z

Printed by Printforce, the Netherlands